De
Yale Medical School

W9-CFF-708

Given to
Audrey Annabel Moore
1976

Principles of INTERNAL MEDICINE

Principles of INTERNAL MEDICINE

Principles of
INTERNAL MEDICINE

EDITORS

T. R. HARRISON, A.B., M.D., M.S. (Hon.), D.SC. (Hon.)
Professor of Medicine, The Medical College of the University of Alabama, Distinguished
Professor, University of Alabama, Birmingham

RAYMOND D. ADAMS, B.A., M.A., M.D., M.A. (Hon.)
Bullard Professor of Neuropathology, Harvard Medical School, Boston

IVAN L. BENNETT, Jr., A.B., M.D.
Baxley Professor of Pathology and Director of the Department of Pathology, Johns Hopkins
University School of Medicine, Baltimore

WILLIAM H. RESNIK, PH.B., M.D.
Clinical Professor of Medicine, Yale University School of Medicine, New Haven

GEORGE W. THORN, M.D., M.A. (Hon.), LL.D. (Hon.), SC.D. (Hon.)
Hersey Professor of the Theory and Practice of Physic, Harvard Medical School, Physician-in-
Chief, Peter Bent Brigham Hospital, Boston

M. M. WINTROBE, B.A., M.D., B.SC. (Med.), PH.D., D.SC. (Hon.)
Professor and Head, Department of Medicine, and Director, Laboratory for Study of Hereditary and Metabolic Disorders, University of Utah College of Medicine, Salt Lake City

FIFTH EDITION

Volume 1, Pages 1 to 587

The Blakiston Division
McGRAW-HILL BOOK COMPANY
New York Toronto Sydney London

PRINCIPLES OF INTERNAL MEDICINE

Copyright © 1966, 1962, and 1958 by McGraw-Hill, Inc. Copyright 1954 and 1950 by McGraw-Hill, Inc. All Rights Reserved. Printed in the United States of America. This book, or parts thereof, may not be reproduced in any form without permission of the publishers.

Library of Congress Catalog Card Number: 65–20973

26843

34567–CO–10987

To all those who have taught us,
and especially to our younger colleagues
who continue to teach and inspire us

Contributors

RAYMOND D. ADAMS, B.A., M.A., M.D., M.A. (HON.)
Bullard Professor of Neuropathology, Harvard Medical School; Chief of Neurology Service and Neuropathologist, Massachusetts General Hospital, Boston.

JAMES C. ALLEN, M.D.
Assistant Professor of Medicine, Johns Hopkins University School of Medicine, Baltimore.

ARTHUR K. ASBURY, M.D.
Instructor in Neurology, Harvard Medical School, Boston.

KARL-ERIK ÅSTRÖM, M.D.
Associate Professor in Pathology, Karolinska Institutet, Stockholm, Sweden.

HENRY T. BAHNSON, M.D.
George V. Foster Professor and Chairman, Department of Surgery, University of Pittsburgh, Pittsburgh.

ALBERT R. BEHNKE, B.A., M.D., M.S. (HON.)
Formerly Radiological Medical Director, U.S. Naval Radiological Defense Laboratory, San Francisco.

IVAN L. BENNETT, JR., A.B., M.D.
Baxley Professor of Pathology and Director of the Department of Pathology, Johns Hopkins University School of Medicine, and Pathologist-in-Chief, Johns Hopkins Hospital, Baltimore.

DANIEL S. BERNSTEIN, M.D.
Associate in Medicine, Harvard Medical School, Boston.

ALFRED BLALOCK, M.D.
Formerly Professor of Surgery and Chairman, Department of Surgery, Johns Hopkins Medical School, and Surgeon-in-Chief, Johns Hopkins Hospital, Baltimore.

STUART BONDURANT, M.D.
Associate Professor of Medicine, Indiana University Medical Center, Indianapolis.

PHILIP K. BONDY, B.A., M.D.
Ensign Professor of Medicine, Yale University School of Medicine, New Haven, Connecticut.

BEN V. BRANSCOMB, M.D.
Associate Professor of Medicine, The Medical College of the University of Alabama, Birmingham.

ABRAHAM I. BRAUDE, M.D.
Professor of Medicine, University of Pittsburgh; Director of Microbiology, Presbyterian-University Hospital, Pittsburgh.

RALPH W. BRAUER, A.B., M.SC., PH.D.
Professor of Physiology, Duke University; Director of the Marine Biomedical Research Laboratory, Wrightsville Beach, North Carolina.

CHARLES H. BURNETT, M.D.
Professor of Medicine, University of North Carolina School of Medicine; Attending Physician, North Carolina Memorial Hospital, Chapel Hill.

GEORGE F. CAHILL, JR., B.S., M.D., M.A. (HON.)
Associate Professor of Medicine and Director, Elliott P. Joslin Research Laboratories, Harvard Medical School; Senior Associate in Medicine, Peter Bent Brigham Hospital, Boston.

EVAN CALKINS, M.D., A.B.
Professor and Chairman, Department of Medicine, State University of New York at Buffalo; Head, Department of Medicine, The Buffalo General Hospital, Buffalo.

CHARLES C. J. CARPENTER, M.D.
Assistant Professor of Medicine, Johns Hopkins University School of Medicine, Baltimore.

GEORGE E. CARTWRIGHT, B.A., M.D.
Professor of Medicine, University of Utah College of Medicine, Salt Lake City.

LEIGHTON E. CLUFF, M.D.
Professor and Chairman, Department of Medicine, University of Florida College of Medicine, Gainesville.

ROBERT E. COOKE, B.S., M.D.
Given Foundation Professor of Pediatrics and Chairman of the Department, Johns Hopkins University School of Medicine; Pediatrician-in-Chief, Johns Hopkins Hospital, Baltimore.

LEWIS L. CORIELL, M.A., PH.D., M.D., F.A.A.P.
Professor of Pediatrics, University of Pennsylvania School of Medicine, Philadelphia; Senior Physician, The Children's Hospital, Philadelphia; Director, South Jersey Medical Research Foundation, Camden, New Jersey.

JOHN F. CRIGLER, JR., M.D.
Assistant Professor of Pediatrics, Department of Pediatrics, Harvard Medical School, Boston; Senior Associate in Medicine, Department of Medicine, The Children's Hospital Medical Center, Boston.

EUGENE P. CRONKITE, M.D.
Head, Division of Experimental Pathology, Medical Research Center Brookhaven National Laboratory, Upton, New York.

PRAFUL M. DALAL, M.D.
Professor of Medicine and Neurologist, Departments of Medicine and Neurology, T.N. Medical College and B.Y.L. Nair Hospital, Bombay, India.

JOSEPH F. DINGMAN, M.D.
Director of Medical Research, Lahey Clinic Foundation; Lecturer on Medicine, Harvard Medical School, Boston.

WILLIAM DOCK, B.S., M.D.
Professor of Medicine, State University of New York Downstate Medical Center; Chief, Medical Service, Veterans Administration Hospital, Brooklyn.

PHILIP R. DODGE, M.D.
Assistant Professor of Neurology, Harvard Medical School (at the Massachusetts General Hospital); Pediatrician, Massachusetts General Hospital; Neurologist, Massachusetts General Hospital, Boston.

E. E. EDDLEMAN, JR., B.S., M.D.
Professor of Medicine, University of Alabama Medical College; Associate Chief of Staff for Research and Education, Veterans Administration Hospital, Birmingham.

HENRI VANDER EECKEN, HM., M.D.
Professor of Neuro-Psychology and Agrégé in Neurology, Faculty of Medicine, University of Ghent, Ghent, Belgium.

KENDALL EMERSON, JR., B.S., M.D.
Associate Clinical Professor of Medicine, Harvard Medical School; Physician, Peter Bent Brigham Hospital; Visiting Physician, Boston Lying-in Hospital, Boston.

EDWIN ENGLERT, JR., A.B., M.D.
Associate Professor of Medicine and Chairman, Subdivision of Gastroenterology, Department of Medicine, University of Utah College of Medicine; Associate Physician, University of Utah Medical Center; Chief, Medical Service, Veterans Administration Hospital, Salt Lake City.

FRANKLIN H. EPSTEIN, M.D.
Professor of Medicine, Yale University School of Medicine, New Haven, Connecticut.

E. HARVEY ESTES, JR., M.D.
Professor of Medicine, Duke University School of Medicine, Durham, North Carolina.

STEFAN S. FAJANS, M.D., B.S.
Professor of Internal Medicine, University of Michigan Medical School, Ann Arbor.

F. ROBERT FEKETY, JR., M.D.
Assistant Professor of Medicine, Johns Hopkins University School of Medicine, Baltimore.

HARRY A. FELDMAN, A.B., M.D.
Professor and Chairman, Department of Preventive Medicine, State University of New York Upstate Medical Center at Syracuse, New York.

RICHARD A. FIELD, M.D.
Assistant Professor of Medicine, Harvard Medical School; Assistant Physician and Chief of the Diabetes Unit, Massachusetts General Hospital, Boston.

C. MILLER FISHER, M.D.
Associate Clinical Professor of Neurology, Harvard Medical School; Neurologist, Massachusetts General Hospital, Boston.

RUSSELL S. FISHER, M.D., B.S.
Chief Medical Examiner, State of Maryland; Professor of Forensic Pathology, University of Maryland Medical School; Lecturer in Forensic Pathology, Johns Hopkins Medical School; Associate in Public Health Administration, Johns Hopkins School of Hygiene and Public Health, Baltimore.

THOMAS B. FITZPATRICK, M.D., PH.D.
Edward Wigglesworth Professor of Dermatology and Head of the Department of Dermatology, Harvard Medical School, Boston.

RICHARD H. FOLLIS, JR.
Formerly Armed Forces Institutes of Pathology and the Veterans Administration Central Laboratory for Anatomic Pathology and Research, AFIP, Washington, D.C.

PETER H. FORSHAM, M.A., M.D.
Professor of Medicine and Pediatrics, Chief of Endocrinology, Department of Medicine, and Director, Metabolic Research Unit, University of California School of Medicine, San Francisco.

HENRY M. FOX, M.D.
Associate Clinical Professor of Psychiatry, Harvard Medical School; Physician, Peter Bent Brigham Hospital, Boston.

DONALD S. FREDRICKSON, M.D.
Clinical Director and Head, Section of Molecular Diseases, Laboratory of Metabolism, National Heart Institute, National Institutes of Health, Bethesda.

LAWRENCE R. FREEDMAN, M.D.
Associate Professor of Medicine, Yale University School of Medicine, New Haven, Connecticut.

DALE G. FRIEND, M.D.
Assistant Professor of Medicine, Harvard Medical School, Harvard University, Boston.

FRANK H. GARDNER, M.D.
Associate Clinical Professor of Medicine, Harvard Medical School; Physician, Peter Bent Brigham Hospital, Boston.

SEYMOUR J. GRAY, B.A., M.D., PH.D.
Associate Clinical Professor of Medicine, Harvard Medical School; Physician, Peter Bent Brigham Hospital, Boston; Visiting Professor of Nutrition, Massachusetts Institute of Technology, Cambridge.

SHELDON EDWARD GREISMAN, M.D.
Associate Professor of Medicine, University of Maryland School of Medicine, Baltimore.

T. R. HARRISON, A.B., M.D.
Professor of Medicine, The Medical College of the University of Alabama, Birmingham, and Distinguished Professor of the University of Alabama.

LLOYD L. HEFNER, B.S., M.D.
Professor of Medicine, The Medical College of the University of Alabama, Birmingham.

ALBERT HEYMAN, B.S., M.D.
Professor of Neurology, Duke University School of Medicine, Durham, North Carolina.

ROGER B. HICKLER, M.D.
Assistant Professor of Medicine, Harvard Medical School, Harvard University, Boston.

FREDERIC L. HOCH, M.D.
Assistant Professor of Medicine, Harvard Medical School; Senior Associate in Medicine, Peter Brent Brigham Hospital, Boston.

PAUL D. HOEPRICH, M.D.
Associate Professor of Internal Medicine and Associate Research Professor of Pathology, University of Utah College of Medicine, Salt Lake City.

EDWARD W. HOOK, M.D.
Professor of Medicine, Cornell University Medical College, New York.

JUSTIN H. HOPE, B.S., M.D.
Professor of Neurology and Psychiatry, Howard University, Washington, D.C.

RICHARD B. HORNICK, M.D.
Assistant Professor of Medicine, Division of Infectious Disease, University of Maryland School of Medicine, Baltimore.

FRANK LYNN IBER, M.D.
Associate Professor of Medicine, Johns Hopkins University School of Medicine, Baltimore.

SIDNEY H. INGBAR, M.D.
Associate Professor of Medicine, Harvard Medical School, Harvard University; Associate Director (Clinical Research Center) Thorndike Memorial Laboratory, Boston City Hospital, Boston.

FRANZ J. INGELFINGER, B.A., M.D.
Professor of Medicine, Boston University School of Medicine, Boston.

KURT J. ISSELBACHER, M.D.
Associate Professor of Medicine, Harvard Medical School, Harvard University, Boston.

ELIZABETH B. JACKSON, M.S.
Assistant Professor in Medicine, University of Maryland School of Medicine, Baltimore.

LEONARD W. JARCHO, A.B., M.A., M.D.
Professor and Head, Department of Neurology; Associate Professor of Medicine, University of Utah College of Medicine, Salt Lake City.

MICHEL JEQUIER, M.D.
Professor de Neurologie, Faculté de Médecine, Université de Lausanne, Lausanne, Switzerland.

CAROL J. JOHNS, M.D.
Instructor in Medicine, Johns Hopkins University School of Medicine, Baltimore.

RICHARD J. JOHNS, M.D.
Associate Professor of Medicine, Johns Hopkins University School of Medicine, Baltimore.

BYRON A. KAKULAS, M.D., M.R.A.C.P., M.C. Path.
Department of Pathology, School of Medicine, Victoria Square, Perth, Western Australia.

JULIAN I. KITAY, A.B., M.D.
Associate Professor of Medicine and Assistant Professor of Physiology, School of Medicine, University of Virginia, Charlottesville.

VERNON KNIGHT, M.D.
Professor of Medicine, Baylor University School of Medicine, Houston, Texas.

JOHN H. KNOWLES, M.D.
General Director and Physician, Massachusetts General Hospital; Lecturer on Medicine, Harvard Medical School, Boston.

W. EUGENE KNOX, M.D.
Associate Professor of Biological Chemistry, Harvard Medical School; The New England Deaconess Hospital, Boston.

M. GLENN KOENIG, M.D.
Assistant Professor of Medicine, Vanderbilt University School of Medicine, Nashville, Tennessee.

JOHN C. LAIDLAW, M.A., PH.D., M.D., F.R.C.P. (c).
Associate Professor of Medicine, University of Toronto; Senior Physician, Toronto General Hospital, Toronto, Canada.

DAVID P. LAULER, M.D.
Associate in Medicine, Harvard Medical School; Associate in Medicine, Peter Bent Brigham Hospital, Boston.

GUSTAF E. LINDSKOG, B.S., M.D., M.A. (HON.)
William H. Carmalt Professor of Surgery, Yale University School of Medicine, New Haven, Connecticut.

BERNARD LOWN, M.D.
Assistant Professor of Medicine, Department of Nutrition, Harvard School of Public Health; Senior Associate in Medicine and Director, S. A. Levine Cardiac Center, Peter Bent Brigham Hospital, Boston.

CHAMP LYONS, A.B., M.D.
Formerly Professor and Chairman, Department of Surgery, The Medical College of the University of Alabama, Birmingham.

BERNARD LYTTON., M.B.B.S., F.R.C.S. (Eng.)
Assistant Professor of Urology, Yale University School of Medicine, New Haven, Connecticut.

ALEXANDER MARBLE, M.D.
Associate Clinical Professor of Medicine, Harvard Medical School; Physician, Joslin Clinic and New England Deaconess Hospital; Boston.

FRED McCRUMB, M.D.
Associate Professor of Medicine, University of Maryland School of Medicine, Baltimore.

VICTOR A. McKUSICK, M.D.
Professor of Medicine and Chief, Division of Medical Genetics, Department of Medicine, Johns Hopkins University School of Medicine, Baltimore.

ALBERT I. MENDELOFF, M.D.
Associate Professor of Medicine, Johns Hopkins University School of Medicine; Physician-in-Chief, Sinai Hospital of Baltimore, Baltimore.

JOHN P. MERRILL, A.B., M.D.
Associate Professor of Medicine, Harvard Medical School; Physician, Peter Bent Brigham Hospital; In-

vestigator of the Howard Hughes Medical Institute, Boston.

JOST J. MICHELSEN, M.D.
Instructor in Surgery, Harvard Medical School, and Clinical Associate in Neurosurgery, Massachusetts General Hospital, Boston.

EDWARD S. MILLER, M.D.
Associate Clinical Professor in Medicine, University of Colorado School of Medicine, Denver.

WILLIAM R. MILNOR, A.B., M.D.
Associate Professor of Physiology and Medicine, Johns Hopkins University School of Medicine; Physician, Johns Hopkins Hospital, Baltimore.

CARL A. MOYER, B.A., M.S., M.D.
Director of Research, Michigan Technological University, Houghton.

DON H. NELSON, M.D.
Professor of Medicine, University of Southern California School of Medicine, Los Angeles.

GEORGE NICHOLS, JR., M.D.
Clinical Professor of Medicine, Harvard Medical School; Chief of Medicine, Cambridge City Hospital; Senior Associate, Peter Bent Brigham Hospital, Boston.

PHILIP SIDNEY NORMAN, M.D.
Associate Professor of Medicine, Department of Medicine, Johns Hopkins University School of Medicine, Baltimore.

VINCENT PERLO, M.D.
Instructor in Neurology, Harvard Medical School, and Neurologist, Massachusetts General Hospital, Boston.

ROBERT G. PETERSDORF, M.D.
Professor and Chairman, Department of Medicine, University of Washington School of Medicine, Seattle.

SIR GEORGE PICKERING, M.A., M.D., F.R.C.P., F.R.S.
Regius Professor of Medicine, University of Oxford, Oxford, England.

DONALD M. PILLSBURY, M.D., D.SC.
Professor and Former Chairman, Department of Dermatology, University of Pennsylvania School of Medicine, Philadelphia.

CHARLES H. RAMMELKAMP, JR., B.A., M.D., D.SC. (HON.)
Professor of Medicine and Associate Professor of Preventive Medicine, Western Reserve University School of Medicine; Director, Department of Medicine and Research Laboratories, Cleveland Metropolitan General Hospital, Cleveland.

T. J. REEVES, M.D.
Professor of Medicine, Director of Cardiovascular Division, University of Alabama School of Medicine, Birmingham.

EDWARD C. REIFENSTEIN, JR., B.A., M.D.
Senior Associate Medical Director, Clinical Research Division, The Squibb Institute for Medical Research,

E. R. Squibb & Sons Division, Olin Mathieson Chemical Corporation; Assistant Clinical Professor of Medicine, New York Medical College, Flower and Fifth Avenue Hospitals, New York.

WILLIAM H. RESNIK, M.D.
Clinical Professor of Medicine, Yale University; Consultant Physician, Yale-New Haven Hospital; Consultant Physician, Stamford Hospital, Stamford, Connecticut.

JOHN CHARLES RIBBLE, M.D.
Assistant Professor of Medicine, Cornell University School of Medicine, New York.

CLAYTON RICH, M.D.
Associate Professor of Medicine, University of Washington School of Medicine, Seattle; Associate Chief of Staff and Chief, Radioisotope Service, Veterans Administration Hospital, Seattle.

EDWARD P. RICHARDSON, JR., M.D.
Assistant Professor of Neuropathology, Harvard Medical School; Neurologist and Neuropathologist, Massachusetts General Hospital, Boston.

EUGENE ROBIN, M.D.
Professor of Medicine, University of Pittsburgh Medical School, Pittsburgh.

DAVID E. ROGERS, M.D.
Professor of Medicine, Department of Medicine, Vanderbilt University School of Medicine; Physician-in-Chief, Vanderbilt University Hospital, Nashville, Tennessee.

JEAN RUBEIZ, M.D.
Rockefeller Fellow in Neuropathology from the American University of Beirut; Research Fellow in Neuropathology, Harvard Medical School, and Research and Clinical Fellow in Neuropathology, Massachusetts General Hospital, Boston.

FUAD SABRA, M.D.
Professor of Medicine (Neurology) and Acting Chairman of Department of Medicine, American University of Beirut.

MARIA Z. SALAM, M.D.
Assistant Professor of Pediatrics, in Charge of Children's Neurology, American University of Beirut; Research Associate in Neuropathology, Harvard Medical School, and Research Associate in Neurology (Pediatric), Massachusetts General Hospital, Boston.

ROBERT S. SCHWAB, A.B., B.A., M.A., M.D.
Associate Clinical Professor of Neurology, Harvard Medical School; Neurologist and Director of the Brain Wave Laboratory, Massachusetts General Hospital, Boston.

HERBERT A. SELENKOW, M.D.
Assistant Professor of Medicine, Harvard Medical School; Senior Associate in Medicine and Director, Thyroid Laboratory, Peter Bent Brigham Hospital, Boston.

ARNOLD M. SELIGMAN, M.D.
Associate Professor of Surgery, Johns Hopkins University School of Medicine; Surgeon-in-Chief, Sinai Hospital, Baltimore.

WALTER B. SHELLEY, PH.D., M.SC.
Professor and Chairman, Department of Dermatology, University of Pennsylvania School of Medicine, Philadelphia.

LAWRENCE E. SHULMAN, M.D., PH.D.
Associate Professor of Medicine and Director, Connective Tissue Division, Department of Medicine, The Johns Hopkins University School of Medicine, Baltimore.

J. LAWTON SMITH, M.D.
Associate Professor of Ophthalmology and Neurosurgery, University of Miami School of Medicine, Miami, Florida.

PHILIP SNODGRASS, M.D.
Associate in Medicine, Harvard Medical School; Associate in Medicine, Peter Bent Brigham Hospital, Boston.

WESLEY W. SPINK, B.A., M.D., D.SC. (HON.)
Professor of Medicine, University of Minnesota Hospitals and Medical School, Minneapolis.

EUGENE A. STEAD, JR., B.S., M.D.
Professor and Chairman, Department of Medicine, Duke University School of Medicine; Physician-in-Chief, Duke Hospital, Durham, North Carolina.

WILLIAM W. STEAD, M.D.
Professor of Medicine, Marquette University School of Medicine, Milwaukee Medical Director, Muirdale Sanatorium, Milwaukee; Chief of Medical Chest Service, Milwaukee County General Hospital, Milwaukee.

JURGEN STEINKE, M.D.
Instructor in Medicine, Harvard Medical School, Harvard University, Boston; Junior Associate in Medicine, Peter Bent Brigham Hospital, Boston.

JOHN H. TALBOTT, M.D.
Editor, Journal of the American Medical Association, Chicago.

MELVIN L. TAYMOR, M.D.
Assistant Clinical Professor of Gynecology, Harvard Medical School, Boston.

GEORGE W. THORN, M.D., M.A. (HON.), LL.D. (HON.), SC.D. (HON.), M.D. (HON.), F.R.C.P.
Hersey Professor of the Theory and Practice of Physic, Harvard Medical School; Physician-in-Chief, Peter Bent Brigham Hospital, Boston.

ANSGAR TORVIK, M.D.
Assistant Professor of Pathology, Department of Pathology, Ullevaal Hospital, Oslo, Norway.

PHILIP A. TUMULTY, M.D.
Professor of Medicine, Johns Hopkins University School of Medicine, Baltimore.

FRANK H. TYLER, B.A., M.D.
Professor of Medicine, University of Utah College of Medicine, Salt Lake City.

MAURICE VICTOR, M.D.
Professor of Neurology, Western Reserve University School of Medicine; Chief, Neurology Service, Cleveland Metropolitan General Hospital, Cleveland.

WARREN E. WACKER, M.D.
Assistant Professor of Medicine, Harvard Medical School, Boston.

ROBERT R. WAGNER, M.D.
Professor of Microbiology, Johns Hopkins University School of Medicine, Baltimore.

FRANK B. WALSH, M.D.
Professor Emeritus of Ophthalmology, Johns Hopkins University School of Medicine, Baltimore.

JOHN N. WALTON, T.D., M.D., F.R.C.P.
Neurologist, Newcastle-upon-Tyne General Hospital and Newcastle Regional Hospital Board; Physician in Neurology, Royal Victoria Infirmary, Newcastle-upon-Tyne, England.

HENRY deF. WEBSTER, M.D.
Associate in Neurology, Harvard Medical School; Associate Neurologist and Assistant Neuropathologist, Massachusetts General Hospital, Boston.

LOUIS WEINSTEIN, M.S., PH.D., M.D.
Professor of Medicine, Tufts University School of Medicine; Lecturer on Infectious Disease, Harvard Medical School; Lecturer in Medicine, Boston University School of Medicine; Chief, Infectious Disease Service, New England Medical Center Hospitals, Boston.

LOUIS G. WELT, A.B., M.D.
Professor and Chairman, Department of Medicine, University of North Carolina, Chapel Hill.

M. M. WINTROBE, B.A., M.D., B.SC. (MED.), PH.D., D.SC. (HON.)
Professor and Head, Department of Medicine, and Director, Laboratory for Study of Hereditary and Metabolic Disorders, University of Utah College of Medicine, Salt Lake City.

SUMNER WOOD, JR., M.D.
Associate Professor of Pathology, Johns Hopkins University School of Medicine, Baltimore.

T. E. WOODWARD, M.D.
Professor of Medicine and Head, Department of Medicine, University of Maryland School of Medicine, Baltimore.

GEORGE W. WRIGHT, B.S., M.D.
Head of Medical Research, Department of Medicine, St. Luke's Hospital; Associate Clinical Professor of Medicine, Western Reserve University School of Medicine, Cleveland.

Preface

It has been said that prefaces are written for the benefit of the writers and not the readers of a book. Though the latter will ultimately judge the book by the style and substance of its contents, it is relevant that the editors present their point of view. As pointed out by Victor Hugo in his famous preface to *Cromwell*, one seldom inspects the cellar of a house after visiting its salons nor examines the root of a tree after eating its fruit.

But prefaces still seem to have a place, as evidenced by the fact that most books have one. They are always put at the beginning of books, as if the authors wished to prepare the reader for what lies within or perhaps distract the prospective critic from too careful an analysis of its contents. To pursue our analogy a bit further, the reader may not be interested in the cellar, but nevertheless he would like to examine the foundations of the book in which he is about to invest.

This book represents the Editors' basic approach to medicine. In fact, the plan of it conforms to the *clinical method* which they have found most useful both as students and as teachers. This method is described on the next pages. We do not presume that senior physicians reading this book should adopt our method, for in a sense this would imply that we, the writers, are more able than the readers. Instead, we suggest only that the clinical method here discussed has served us well and others may find it helpful.

When the Editors first met nineteen years ago, they resolved to write a book embodying the principles of general medicine and presenting clinical and laboratory data in a fashion which would be logical and hence appealing to the intellect. It was thought then, and we have since been confirmed in this belief, that a textbook of medicine should recapitulate the steps in the process of thinking by which a physician reaches a diagnosis: the interpretation of the patient's symptoms, the recognition of a constellation of symptoms—the syndrome, and finally a consideration of the various disorders that could give rise to the clinical picture.

The Editors have found this process of observation and reasoning, the stepwise interpretation of symptoms and syndromes proceeding usually from the general to the particular, to be the most effective approach in attempting to reach a correct diagnosis. This method also corresponds to the teaching methods which we have found to be most successful for undergraduate students and residents. These are the reasons for the arrangement of the contents of the book with consideration first of the cardinal manifestations of disease (Part II), and only later the presentation of various diseases (Parts IV to VIII), following a section containing material of fundamental biological importance (Part III). The syndromic approach is emphasized insofar as possible, and the reader will find at the beginning of most of the sections, either in the Introduction and/or in the first chapter of each section, a discussion of the approach to the patient having the type of disease considered in that section.

With each edition the Editors have striven to achieve logical coherence by extending this plan to every section of the book. In the present edition, by further rearrangement and rewriting, this goal has been approached more completely than before. New clinical manifestations, such as those of the integument, have been included among the cardinal manifestations of disease, and others which might more properly be considered syndromes have been transferred to later parts of the book.

The method of approaching a diagnosis which is based on an analysis of the symptoms, recognition of the syndromes, and the ultimate listing of the possible diseases affecting the patient is one which ensures consideration of the many possible interpretations of the clinical picture which the patient presents. Thus it is less likely that a disorder which should be considered will be overlooked.

Those who are accustomed to the classical medical textbook will find it helpful to peruse the chapters on cardinal manifestations of disease and the introductory chapters on common syndromes. For the beginning medical student familiarity with this introductory material is essential. The interne, resident, or practicing physician confronted with a diagnostic problem or an unfamiliar manifestation or disorder will find these discussions helpful, especially the sections on syndromes. The experienced physician will find it more useful to turn directly to the disease with which he is concerned, though a more leisurely review of cardinal manifestations may also serve to update his knowledge of the recent advances in medical science which are pertinent to this field of interest. By the use of many cross references and the more complete index which the Editors have personally prepared, it is hoped that the fragmentation and duplication that are inevitable in a work of this kind have been held to a minimum and that a book of greater usefulness has been produced.

Since past editions have met with favor in foreign countries, the Editors have found it necessary to include diseases which are not common in the USA. People are now mingling throughout the world, because of ease of transport, and this has turned our attention to the medical problems of the underdeveloped countries. A major one is undernutrition, and for this reason the section on nutrition has been entirely rewritten and expanded in the fifth edition.

A deliberate attempt has been made to avoid long bibliographies. The references at the end of the chapters are limited, for the most part, to reviews and monographs which contain comprehensive bibliographies, together with older works of historical significance.

Once again we wish to express appreciation to our many colleagues who have so generously responded to editorial suggestions. We continue to be indebted to numerous friends and colleagues for valuable criticisms. Among them are:

Drs. Walter Frommeyer and Basil I. Hirschowitz of Birmingham, Attilio D. Renzetti, John R. Ward, Charles A. Nugent, and C. Donald West of Salt Lake City, and Dr. Ben Friedman of Dallas.

The preparation of the new edition would have presented insuperable problems without the loyal and effective aid of our several secretarial coworkers. We are especially indebted to Mrs. Ann Zurek of Baltimore, Miss Minnie Mae Tims and Mrs. Geraldine Haynes of Birmingham, Alabama, Miss Eulalia Grzebieniowska, Mrs. Ruth Simonds, Mrs. Dorothy Starrett, Mrs. Shirley Howe, and Miss Mara Eglitis of Boston, Miss Ruth Compton of New York, Mrs. Shirley Broadhurst, Mrs. Joan Lyman, and Mrs. Barbara Sessions of Salt Lake City, and Mrs. Dolores Ready of Stamford, Connecticut.

Our relations with the McGraw-Hill Company, particularly with its Blakiston Division, have been cordial and friendly rather than merely agreeable and satisfactory.

RDA
ILB
TRH
WHR
GWT
MMW

Contents

PART SIX

Disorders Due to Chemical and Physical Agents

PART SEVEN

Disorders Caused by Antigens and Other Foreign Substances

PART EIGHT

Disorders Caused by Biologic Agents

Color Plates

Principles of Internal Medicine

Principles of Internal Medicine

Part One

The Physician and the Patient

Section 1

The Physician and the Patient

█ APPROACH TO THE PATIENT

The Editors

No greater opportunity, responsibility, or obligation can fall to the lot of a human being than to become a physician. In the care of the suffering he needs technical skill, scientific knowledge, and human understanding. He who uses these with courage, with humility, and with wisdom will provide a unique service for his fellowman, and will build an enduring edifice of character within himself. The physician should ask of his destiny no more than this; he should be content with no less.

In the practice of medicine the physician employs a discipline which seeks to utilize scientific methods and principles in the solution of its problems, but it is one which, in the end, remains an art. It is an art in the sense that rarely, if ever, can the individual patient be considered the equivalent of an experiment so completely controlled that it is possible to exclude judgment and experience from the interpretation of the patient's reactions. It is an art, too, in the sense that the practicing physician can never be content with the sole aim of endeavoring to clarify the laws of nature; he cannot proceed in his labors with the cool detachment of the scientist whose aim is the winning of the truth, and who, theoretically, is uninterested in the practical outcome of his work. The practicing physician must never forget that his primary and traditional objectives are utilitarian—the prevention and cure of disease and the relief of suffering, whether of body or mind.

THE PATIENT AS A PERSON

The student receives much expert coaching in the methods of physical and laboratory diagnosis, and it is in these areas that he will most easily develop the skills which permit him to be comfortable with the patient. Mastery of the more intangible psychologic aspects of medicine is not so easily learned, however. The skills essential here depend not simply on instruction but on emotional maturity, manifested by sensitive self-cultivation of the capacity to see deeply and

accurately the problems of another human being. The challenge is further magnified by the fact that the examining physician is himself a human instrument, subject to error due to the events in his own biography. The irritability and exasperation of even the kindest and most conscientious physician may sometimes represent not the legitimate protest at the patient's lack of cooperativeness but a basic and not wholly conscious sense of his own insecurity. The successful management of the patient properly begins with the development of emotional maturity on the part of the physician.

Just as the physical growth of each person depends on an adequate and balanced supply of appropriate foodstuffs, so does emotional growth depend on the receipt of proper psychologic nutrients. Although each individual is born with manifold potentialities determined by his genes, the emotional climate in which he grows and develops will shape his eventual character and abilities just as surely as foodstuffs will modify his physique. Just as invading bacteria influence multitudinous bodily reactions, so do emotions possess the capacity to exert force and thereby alter behavior, including certain of the biochemical processes of the body.

Any departure from good health carries a potential threat of physical disintegration or crippling disability, and even the most intelligent and best-informed patient should not be considered immune to forebodings just because he refrains from mentioning them. It is especially important that these fears be borne in mind when dealing with the elderly patient, who is rarely unmindful that "the trap is laid" and death is always near.

The attitude of the patient approaching the doctor must always be tinged—for the most part unconsciously—with distaste and dread; its deepest desire will tend to be comfort and relief rather than cure, and its faith and expectation will be directed towards some magical exhibition of these boons. Do not let yourselves believe that however smoothly concealed by education, by reason, and by confidential frankness these strong elements may be, they are ever in any circumstances altogether absent. (Wilfred Trotter)

In the long development of growth from infancy to adult life, there is a progressive change in social relationships, from one of complete dependence on parent, family, and teacher to one of relative independence. At the same time, the process of maturation requires the partial suppression of egocentric drives to the point that the affairs of other members of one's family and social group assume increasing importance. These trends and their modification during the life experience are part of the elaborate theory of personality development to be found in the writings of psychologists, particularly those of the psychoanalytically related schools. Deviations in these natural developments have been shown to prevent satisfactory social adjustment and to result in neuroticism.

Illness constitutes a threat not only to the physical integrity of the individual but also to his status in his social group, a fact that is soon learned by every thoughtful physician. Prolonged invalidism during childhood tends invariably to leave behind an excessive egocentricity, which may become the basis of a lifelong neurosis. In the adult, illness often enforces a return to a posture of dependency, a change usually accompanied by feelings of apprehension and discouragement, sometimes leading to frank anxiety and depression. It is for these reasons that many adults in positions of responsibility express greater concern about the economic and social implications of their illness than about the illness itself. This explains a number of common psychologic defenses which the patient exercises against illness. He may refuse medical aid or if he summons the courage to consult a physician, he may minimize or even fail to mention the very symptom about which he is most deeply concerned. On the other hand, there are individuals whose attainment of maturity has been tenuous and uncertain, so that the position of dependency imposed by illness comes as a welcome relief from adult responsibility. They appear to enjoy illness and to resent anything that menaces their state of invalidism. Lesser degrees of this tendency are to be noted among those who consult the physician at the appearance of every new symptom and who are continuously preoccupied with their past illnesses and operations.

It is not easy to keep these basic facts in mind when examining a draped patient in the relatively neutral domain of the hospital ward or even in the private examining room. There are potent obstacles that stand in the way of the physician's making an adequate study of the patient's emotional life. Organic lesions have a way of compelling attention to themselves, and it is less exhausting to limit one's focus to the sphere of physical disease. More time, energy, and experience are necessary to view the patient as an active participant in an enormous moving pageant which includes the personal eccentricities of his forebears, his own fears and patterns of reaction, as well as the hopes for his children's future. It is not enough to know that poverty, insecurity, and perhaps poor vocational and domestic relations are now keeping the patient unhappily depressed, for all too often it is apparent that present socioeconomic (external) factors are not crucial determinants in the contemporary scene. To explain many of the manifestations of illness, it is necessary to view the patient more deeply as an organism with a vast repository of past experiences dating from the earliest days of life, many of which are vaguely remembered, yet have become the foundation of its current system of meeting daily problems. Under the threat of disease, defensive attitudes, which were useful in infancy and childhood but inappropriate in adult life, have a way of reasserting themselves; one of the oldest, the state of readiness for fight or flight (Cannon), may be a precipitating cause of illnesses such as peptic ulcer or hypertension when called upon too frequently.

The young physician usually finds himself inadequate in his dealings with the patient, for not only does he experience an inevitable sense of insecurity with respect to the patient's problems, but he feels equally uneasy about his newly acquired role of authority and responsibility. Moreover, both he and his older colleague often find it difficult to control their own reactions: disinterest because the patient presents no fascinating problem of organic disease, irritation at his verbosity and lack of clarity and consistency in the recital of the history, annoyance because the patient's illness fails to respond to treatment in the expected manner. The physician can hardly expect to achieve a deep appreciation of the patient's psychologic problems unless he learns to recognize and control his own.

More broadly stated, the physician has a special function in society because he should be a trained biologist in human behavior as well as in human diseases. He brings highly technical knowledge and skills to bear upon the problems of his patient as a person as well as upon the patient's physiologic functioning. He should bring to the suffering patient a quiet humanity, a confidence and security based upon the conviction that all will be done that can be done. The patient must feel that his unique individuality is recognized and appreciated and that his life's problems are meaningful. This is important in patients with well-defined organic disease as well as in the "stress" syndromes largely due to emotional pressures expressed through the body. If we can accept the principle of causality in human behavior, we can, with patience and diligence, learn to fathom the large outlines of a person's motivations even though many of the details very often remain obscure.

"Let me see in the sufferer the man alone. . . . Let me be intent upon one thing, O Father of Mercy, to be always merciful to Thy suffering children." (Maimonides)

THE ART OF MEDICINE

Despite the constantly increasing application of scientific methods to the problems of medicine, there remain large areas that are as yet insusceptible of solution by the use of precise methods. To extract the telltale clue from a maze of confusing symptoms, to determine from a mass of conflicting physical signs and laboratory data the ones that are of crucial significance, to know in a borderline case when to initiate and when to refrain from a line of treatment—these decisions are not usually the outcome of laboratory study alone. In the end, these decisions are expressions of judgment acquired through "assimilated experience."

Concerning the more personal relations with the patient and the understanding and capacity to peer beyond surface motivations and behavior, no instruction or training can entirely replace an intuitive talent and maturing wisdom. The astute physician will recognize when the casual mention of an apparently trivial complaint is the device for seeking reassurance regarding a feared disorder such as cancer or heart disease. He will know or suspect how profitable it will be to continue probing the more intimate aspects of the patient's life, when to overcome a reluctance to discuss them, and when to permit them to remain undiscussed. Knowing when to express a bright and reassuring prognosis and when and how to utter doubt and caution requires more than a knowledge of disease.

No problem can be more distressing than that presented by the patient with incurable disease, particularly when death is imminent and inevitable. There should be no ironclad, inflexible rule that the patient must be told "everything." All patients do not have the courage or faith or stoicism that the advocates of this conviction think they may or should have. "One thing is certain: it is not for you to don the black cap and, assuming the judicial function, take hope away from any patient . . . hope that comes to us all." (William Osler) The proponents of this principle do not really adhere to their philosophy when they tell the "truth" in such a manner that the kernel of the truth is not conveyed to the patient. How much, for example, is communicated to the patient when the physician says to the patient who has leukemia: "You have more white corpuscles in your blood than is normal, but we have found no evidence that any damage has been done." Nor can one conscientiously follow the opposite rule of never telling the patient the truth. How much the patient is to be told will depend on his religious convictions, the wishes of his family, the state of his affairs, and his own desires and character. But even this platitude solves nothing, since it is not merely the recognition of these factors but the physician's wisdom in assessing the relative importance of each that determines how complete a discussion of the facts will best serve the interests of the patient. The younger physician may extract some small measure of consolation from the knowledge that his older and more experienced colleague has no simple and easy formula for meeting the question.

The physician must also be prepared to deal with sentiments commonly experienced at a time of death in the family.

I do not know that I have anything to reproach in my conduct, and certainly nothing in my feelings and inten-

tions towards the dead. But it is a moment when we are apt to think that, if this or that had been done, such event might have been prevented. (Letter to Shelley from Lord Byron on the death of his daughter.)

These words express the feelings of guilt that almost invariably afflict the members of a family when parent or child or spouse has died. The doctor must be prepared to tender what assurance is possible that no fault need be attached to the living.

Somewhat related to this problem is the expiatory attitude of the family when a member becomes gravely or hopelessly ill. The meager resources that may represent the savings of a lifetime of toil may be dissipated in weeks or months in payment for needlessly expensive rooms, private nursing services, and consultations. It is difficult for the physician to oppose these futile gestures too strenuously for they serve more to bring consolation to the family than to assuage the distress of the patient.

Tact, sympathy, and understanding are expected of the physician, for the patient is no mere collection of symptoms, signs, disordered functions, damaged organs, and disturbed emotions. He is human, fearful, and hopeful, seeking relief, help, and reassurance. To the physician, as to the anthropologist, nothing human is strange or repulsive. The misanthrope may become a smart diagnostician of organic disease, but he can scarcely hope to succeed as a physician. The true physician has a Shakespearean breadth of interest in the wise and the foolish, the proud and the humble, the stoic hero and the whining rogue. He cares for people.

2 APPROACH TO DISEASE
The Editors

HISTORY

The history of an illness should embody all the facts of medical significance in the life of the patient up to the time he consults the physician; but, of course, the most recent ones attract the most attention, for these, obviously, are the reason the patient seeks medical advice. Ideally the narration of symptoms should be in the patient's own words, the principal events being presented in the temporal order in which they occurred. Few patients possess the necessary powers of observation and talent for lucid, coherent description. Usually the help of the physician is needed. He must guide them by questions but at the same time avoid influencing them by inserting his own ideas, especially if the patient is suggestible.

Often it happens that a symptom which has greatly concerned a patient possesses little significance as a medical datum, whereas a seemingly minor complaint may be of importance. Therefore the mind of the physician must be constantly alert to the possibility that any event related by the patient, any symptom however trivial or apparently remote, may be the key to the solution of the medical problem.

An informative history is more than an orderly listing of symptoms. Something always is gained by listening to the patient and noting the way in which he talks about his symptoms. Inflection of voice, facial expression, and attitude may betray important clues to the meaning the symptoms have to the patient. Thus, listening to this recitation, one learns not only something about the disease but also something about the patient behind the disease.

With experience one learns the pitfalls of history taking. What patients relate for the most part are subjective phenomena elusively filtered through minds that vary in their background of past experience. Patients obviously differ widely in their responses to the same stimuli. Their remarks are variably colored by fear of disease, disability, and death and by concern over the consequences of illness to their families. And as if these difficulties were not enough, there are the additional ones created by language barriers, by failing intellectual powers which deprive the subject of accurate recall, or by a disorder of consciousness that makes him oblivious of his illness. It is not surprising, then, that even the most careful physician may at times despair of collecting factual data; and often he is forced to proceed with evidence that represents little more than an approximation of the truth.

Viewed in another way, the symptom marks, in the patient's mind, a departure from normal health; in the physician's mind, it initiates a process of inductive and deductive reasoning that culminates in diagnosis. In pondering the various possible explanations of a given symptom or clinical state the physician begins a search for other data, elicited by further questioning of the patient and his family, by physical examination, or by special laboratory tests. The symptoms alone sometimes will provide the most certain clue, as in angina pectoris or epilepsy, where physical findings and laboratory data collected between attacks may fail to corroborate the existence of heart or brain disease even when it is manifestly present. In most illnesses, however, the history will not be so decisive, though it may still narrow the number of diagnostic possibilities and guide the subsequent investigation.

It is in the taking of the history that the physician's skill, knowledge, and experience are most clearly in evidence. He has learned from experience how to weigh each given symptom, depending on its nature and the context in which it occurs. He knows when to be incredulous and turn to more reliable sources of information, and he never lets his skepticism blind him to an unusual symptom, a manifestation of some new condition that has previously lain beyond the reach of medical knowledge. Moreover, he knows when to press an interrogation more deeply in a search for further details and when to cast about more broadly, realizing that "disease often tells its secrets in a casual

parenthesis." And, finally, he knows how to take advantage of the interview in which the history is gathered to obtain the confidence of his patient and to allay apprehension and fear, the first steps in therapy.

PHYSICAL EXAMINATION

Little need be said about the importance of the physical examination, for early in his training the physician learns that physical signs are the objective and verifiable marks of pathology. But although the physical sign represents a solid, indisputable fact, its significance is enhanced when it confirms a functional or structural change already evidenced by the patient's history. The physical sign may stand as the only evidence of disease, especially in those cases where the history has been inconsistent and confused or is completely lacking.

If full advantage is to be gotten from the physical examination, it must be performed methodically and thoroughly. Although attention has usually been directed by the history to the offending organ or part of the body, nevertheless the examination must extend to all parts of the body. The patient must be literally scrutinized from top to bottom in an objective search for abnormalities that may yield information concerning present and also future illnesses. Unless the examination procedure is systematic, important parts of it may be forgotten, an error against which even the most skilled clinician must guard. The results of the examination, like the details of the history, should be recorded at the time they are elicited and not hours later when they are subject to the distortions of memory. Many inaccuracies in case study stem from the careless practice of writing or dictating notes long after the examination has terminated.

Skill in physical diagnosis is acquired with experience, but it is not merely technique that determines success in eliciting signs. The detection of a few scattered petechiae or a faint diastolic murmur or a small mass in the abdomen is not a question of keener eyes and ears or more sensitive fingers, but of a mind directed by long experience to be alert to these findings because of the nature of the illness. Skill in physical diagnosis reflects a way of thinking more than a way of doing.

All investigations of the body should be regarded as part of the physical examination. The use of various instruments, such as the ophthalmoscope, sphygmomanometer, galvanometer, or roentgen tube, are mere extensions of the examination to less accessible structures. All these special methods are in common use, and their proficient use is part of internal medicine. Tests made on fluids or tissues removed from the patient are laboratory examinations. They must be selected carefully; even though the physician may not do the tests, he is responsible for the proper collection of the material and for the interpretation of the results.

INSTRUMENTAL AND LABORATORY EXAMINATIONS

The last century has witnessed the introduction of newer methods of instrumental and laboratory investigation of ever-increasing precision and refinement, and inevitably there has been a drift toward reliance on knowledge gained from these special means of study in the solution of clinical problems. It is essential that one always bear in mind the limitations of these newer methods of examination and their proper use in the practice of medicine. By virtue of their impersonal quality and the complexity of the techniques involved in obtaining them, data secured by instrumental and laboratory methods are frequently surrounded by an aura of authority, without heed to the fact that the data are collected by fallible human beings who are capable of committing errors of technique, or who may misinterpret the most precise evidence. Too great emphasis may be placed on minor deviations that may yet lie well within the range of normality. These and other possible errors serve to indicate that even these data cannot release the physician from the necessity of careful observation and study of the patient. The wise physician is he who understands the merits and limitations of each source of information, whether it be the history, or the physical examination, or the laboratory investigations. Barring those exigencies that make careful study impracticable or impossible, the history and physical examination should be thorough and painstaking, and the special examinations and laboratory tests should be adequate to furnish what additional information may be necessary. In some cases, it will suffice to use merely the simple tests that should be at the disposal of every practicing physician; in the more obscure cases the full resources of the most advanced teaching hospital may be essential for the successful unraveling of the clinical problem. The physician should weigh carefully not only the hazards but also the expense involved in every test that he demands. Every procedure that does not have a specific purpose toward contributing to the management of the patient's illness is a pretentious economic waste resulting from ignorance or callousness or plain charlatanism. Scientific study of a clinical problem does not consist merely of filling a patient's record with endless data. Discrimination in the ordering of laboratory procedures and judgment in appraising the risk and expense of a procedure as against the value of the information to be derived from it are among the criteria by which one estimates the manner in which the art and science of medicine have been fused by the physician.

THE CLINICAL METHOD AND THE SYNDROMIC APPROACH TO DISEASE

The steps described above have as their object the collection of accurate data concerning all the diseases to which human beings are subject, namely, all conditions that "limit life in its powers, enjoyment and duration." But much more is required in making a diagnosis. Each datum must be interpreted in the light of the known facts of anatomy, physiology, and chemistry. The synthesis of these interpretations yields information concerning the affected organ or body system. Further, from the vantage point afforded by an anatomic diagnosis the physician may then turn to other data, such as the mode of onset and clinical course of the illness, and finally to the results of laboratory tests, in order to ascertain the cause of the disease.

All these steps comprise the clinical method, which always proceeds in a series of logical steps. The perceptive student will note certain similarities between the clinical method and the scientific method. Each begins with observational data which suggest a series of hypotheses. These latter are tested in the light of further observations, some clinical, others contrived laboratory procedures. Finally, a conclusion is reached, which in science is called a *theory* and in medicine a *working diagnosis*. The modus operandi of the clinical method, like that of the scientific method, cannot be reduced to a single principle or a type of inductive or deductive reasoning. It involves both analysis and synthesis, the essential parts of cartesian logic. The physician does not start with an open mind any more than does the scientist, but with one prejudiced from knowledge of recent cases; and the patient's first statement directs his thinking in certain channels. He must struggle constantly to avoid the bias occasioned by his own attitude, mood, irritability, and interest.

It is particularly in the study of more difficult patients that one observes most clearly the logical order of the clinical method. Anatomic diagnosis regularly precedes etiologic diagnosis. One seldom succeeds in determining the cause and mechanism of a disease before ascertaining which organ has been involved. An intermediate step is syndromic diagnosis. Most physicians attempt consciously or unconsciously to fit a given problem into one of a series of syndromes. The syndrome, in essence, is a group of symptoms and signs of disordered somatic function, related to one another by means of some anatomic, physiologic, or biochemical peculiarity of the organism. It embodies a hypothesis concerning the deranged function of an organ, organ system, or tissue. Congestive heart failure, Cushing's disease, and dementia are examples. In congestive heart failure dyspnea, orthopnea, cyanosis, dependent edema, engorged neck veins, pleural fluid, pulmonary râles, and enlargement of the liver are known to be connected by a single pathophysiologic mechanism—failure of the heart, leading to salt and water retention and high venous pressure. In Cushing's disease the moon facies, hypertension, diabetes, and osteoporosis, are the recognized effects of excess corticosteroids acting on many target organs. In dementia deterioration of memory, incoherence in thinking, faulty judgment, etc., are related through a neuroanatomic and a neurophysiologic principle, i.e., all these disordered intellectual functions are related to slow impairment of the function and destruction of the association areas of the cerebrum.

A syndromic diagnosis usually does not indicate the precise cause of an illness, but it greatly narrows the number of possibilities and, thus, suggests whatever further clinical and laboratory studies are required. The derangements of each organ system in human beings are reducible to a relatively small number of syndromes. Diagnosis is greatly simplified if a given clinical problem conforms neatly to a well-defined syndrome. Then one need only turn to a book for a list of the various diseases that may cause it. The search for the cause of an illness that does not conform to a syndrome is much more difficult, for a seemingly infinite number of diseases may then have to be considered. Nevertheless, the principle remains: the clinical method is an orderly intellectual activity which proceeds almost invariably from symptom to sign, to syndrome, and to disease.

3 CARE OF THE PATIENT
The Editors

Enormous strides have taken place during the past few decades in our knowledge of the mechanisms of disease and in the development of powerful and effective treatment agents. The responsibilities of the physician in his management of the patient have correspondingly magnified. When little was known about the pathogenesis of a disorder and when, with rare exceptions, practically all the drugs in the huge pharmacopoeias were virtually placebos when given in the recommended doses, the therapeutic decisions of the physician were seldom of crucial importance. The scientific physician of the time practiced in a golden era of therapeutic nihilism. He was aware of the worthlessness of most of the drugs that were available to him, and he displayed his skill as a scientific physician by not tampering mischievously with the natural recuperative powers of the body.

Throw out opium, which the Creator himself seems to prescribe, for we often see the scarlet poppy growing in the cornfields as if it were foreseen that where ever there is hunger to be fed there must also be pain to be soothed; throw out a few specifics which our art did not discover and is hardly needed to apply; throw out wine which is a food and the vapors of which produce the miracle of anesthesia, and I firmly believe that if the whole materia medica, as now used, could be sunk to the bottom of the sea it would be all the better for mankind,—and all the worse for the fishes. (O. W. Holmes, 1860)

The discovery during the past several decades of therapeutic agents capable of exerting decisive influence on the course of disease has made it essential that the physician have some understanding of the disturbed functions induced by disease, of the manner of treatment most likely to exert a beneficial effect, and of the risks involved in the proposed therapeutic plan.

Ideally, treatment should strive for the complete restoration of the patient's health, physical and mental.

But medicine contemplates other subjects besides cure. It aims still to postpone the progress of incurable disease and to put off its evil consequences; and, when, they can no longer be postponed, it seeks to render them more tolerable. (Latham)

These goals, which were hardly attainable at the time of Latham, seldom fail to be achieved with at least some degree of success at the present time. Remedies are available. It is the responsibility of the doctor to use them wisely, with due regard for their action, cost, and potential dangers. For every medical procedure, whether diagnostic or therapeutic, contains within it the potentiality of harm, and it would be impossible to afford the patient all the benefits of modern scientific medicine if every reasonable step in diagnosis and therapy were withheld because of the possible risks. "Reasonable" here implies that the physician has weighed the pros and cons of a procedure and has concluded on rational grounds that it is advisable or essential for the relief of discomfort or the cure or amelioration of disease. When the deleterious effects of the physician's action exceed any advantages that could logically have been anticipated, we are justified in designating these effects as *iatrogenic*. It is necessary only to recall the occasionally dangerous or fatal reactions that followed the use of antibiotics given for a trivial respiratory infection, or the gastric hemorrhage or perforation caused by cortisone administered for a mild arthritis, or the fatal homologous serum jaundice that followed needless transfusions of blood or plasma.

It is equally important to consider the harm physicians may do to patients through ill-considered or unjustified remarks. No matter how placid the patient may seem, he approaches the physician with at least some degree of fear and concern. His anxiety can be enhanced by a too serious demeanor, a flippant remark, or an impressive conference. Many persons have been crippled by a cardiac neurosis because the physician expressed a grave prognosis on the basis of a misinterpreted electrocardiogram.

The good physician appreciates the fact that he is always in a position to cause injury by his treatment, by his words, and by his behavior. Skill in handling patients cannot be taught; all that one can do is emphasize the importance of tact, caution, judgment, and wisdom—ideals to be striven for but never fully attained. Better than words are the examples of thoughtfulness and understanding exhibited by the medical teacher or senior staff physician in his ward or clinic conferences with students and younger colleagues. But even if it were possible finally to achieve the goal—a generation of flawless physicians with infallible judgment and infinite wisdom—there would still be the patients who have uncanny capacity to misinterpret the most innocent remarks and the most cautiously expressed opinions. In the end, iatrogenic illness is largely a matter of incomplete knowledge and fallacious judgment on the part of the physician conjoined with the fears and anxieties of the patient. So long as medicine remains an art, iatrogenic illness will remain. The best hope for diminishing its incidence is ceaseless consideration by the physician of the wisdom of each of his decisions and acts and greater appreciation of the mood and attitude of the patient.

It is trite to emphasize that the physician must never become so absorbed in the disease that he forgets the patient who harbors it. Nevertheless, this exhortation cannot be repeated too often. As the science of medicine advances, it is all too easy to become so fascinated by the various manifestations of a malady that one disregards the ailing person: his fears, his concerns about his job and the future of his family, the cost of medical care, the specter of economic insecurity, and similar related problems. Treatment of a patient consists in more than the dispassionate confrontation of a disease. It embodies also the exercise of warmth, compassion, and understanding. In the now famous words of Peabody, "one of the essential qualities of the clinician is interest in humanity, for the secret of the care of the patient is in caring for the patient."

Part Two
Cardinal Manifestations of Disease

Section 1

Pain

4 GENERAL CONSIDERATIONS
Raymond D. Adams and William H. Resnik

Pain, it has been said, is one of "Nature's earliest signs of morbidity." Few will deny that it stands preeminent among all the sensory experiences by which man judges the existence of disease within himself. There are relatively few maladies that do not have their painful phases, and in many of them pain is a characteristic without which diagnosis must always be in doubt. It seems appropriate, therefore, to begin a section on the cardinal manifestations of disease with a discussion of the more general aspects of pain.

The painful experiences of the sick pose manifold problems for the practitioner of medicine, and the student should know something of these problems in order to prepare himself properly for the task ahead. He must be ready to diagnose disease in patients who have felt only the first rumblings of discomfort, before other symptoms and signs of disease have appeared. To cope effectively with problems of this type requires a sound knowledge of the sensory supply of the viscera and a familiarity with the typical symptoms of many diseases. He will be consulted by some patients who seek treatment for pains that appear to have no obvious structural basis, and further inquiry will disclose that worry, fear, and other troubled emotional states may have aggrandized relatively minor aches and pains. To understand problems of this type requires insight into the psychologic factors which influence behavior and a knowledge of psychiatric disease. Next, he must manage the "difficult pain cases," in which no amount of investigation will bring to light either medical disease or psychiatric illness, and it is here that he will sense the need of a sound and assured clinical approach to the pain problem. Finally, he must care for the patients with intractable pain, often from an established and incurable disease, who demand relief either by drug or the "less moderate means of surgery." The possibilities of the latter require a comprehension of the anatomic pathways of pain.

END ORGANS, AFFERENT TRACTS, AND NUCLEI OF TERMINATION OF PAIN PATHWAYS

Pain is now regarded by most physiologists and psychologists as a sensation which depends on its own specific sensory apparatus. The receptors in the skin and deep structures are fine, freely branching nerve endings, which form an intricate network. A single primary pain neurone, with its cell body in the posterior root ganglion, subdivides into many small peripheral branches to supply an area of skin of at least several square millimeters. The cutaneous area of each neurone overlaps with those of other neurones, so that every spot of skin is within the domain of from two to four sensory neurones. These free nerve endings are also found in many of the other specialized sensory receptors in the skin, such as the Krause endbulbs, the Ruffinian plumes, and Pacinian corpuscles, which may account for the extremes of hot, cold, and pressure sensation becoming painful. However, the whole subject of specific nerve endings for each modality of sensation is being reinvestigated, and a final statement cannot be made at this time. It appears now that free nerve endings themselves may serve as receptors for other types of sensation. They are the only end organ in the cornea where touch, temperature, and pain are felt.

The sensory nerve fibers for pain course through somatic and visceral nerves, where they are mixed with motor fibers, and they enter the spinal cord and brain stem through the posterior roots and the cranial nerves, respectively. The fibers are of two sizes, one very small, 2 to 4 μ in diameter, with a slow conducting velocity, the other somewhat larger, 6 to 8 μ, with more rapid transmission rates. As the posterior root fibers enter the spinal cord they terminate in the posterior horn of gray matter, where they synapse with the secondary sensory neurone, the axone of which ascends and crosses the anterior commissure of the spinal cord within three or four segments to find its place in the anterolateral spinothalamic tract. Some of the nerve cells in the posterior horns send their axones to the central gray matter and to anterior horn cells of the same segment and adjacent segments and subserve such reflex functions as the flexor reflex, of which Babinski's sign is but a part. The anterolateral spinothalamic tract continues upward to the posterolateral nucleus of the thalamus. This tract lies in the anterior part of the lateral and the anterior funiculi of the spinal cord and passes through the retroolivary part of the medulla and the dorsolateral parts of the pons and midbrain (Fig. 4-1, see also Fig. 4-2). The most superficial fibers are those from the opposite foot and leg and the successively deeper ones from the trunk, arm, neck, and face. Before reaching the thalamus, collateral branches are given off to other segmental structures, such as the reticular formation of the brain stem and the hypothalamus. In addition there appears to be a great diminution in the number of fibers as one pursues the tract upward, which means that many of the ascending fibers are terminating in structures located in the brain stem. The thalamic termination of the spinothalamic tracts along with the secondary trigeminothalamic tracts synapse with the third sensory neurones, which project to the cortex in the parietal lobes. Physiologists are not agreed, however, as to the cortical terminus, for electrical stimulation of the cortex in the conscious human being does not produce a painful sensation but only a tingling as a rule, nor do parietal lobe lesions cause central pain. Nearly all pain fibers from the periphery cross to the contralateral half of spinal cord, brain stem, and thalamus, but a few are believed to ascend ipsilaterally, at least for a considerable distance. This point is still being studied.

The pain-sensitive structures in the viscera and integuments of the body, the mechanisms of their excitation, and the peripheral nervous pathways are now fairly well established. The skin and mucous membranes are sensitive to pain, as are also many of the mesodermal tissues. As a means of quick orientation it should be remembered that the facial structures and anterior cranium are the field of the trigeminal nerves; the back of head, second cervical; the neck, third cervical; epaulet area, fourth cervical; deltoid area, fifth cervical; the thumb, sixth cervical; the index finger, seventh cervical; middle finger, eighth cervical; the little finger, first thoracic; the nipple segment, fifth thoracic; the umbilicus, tenth thoracic; the groin, first lumbar; the medial side of knee, third lumbar; the great toe, fifth lumbar; the little toe, first sacral; the back of thigh, second sacral; and genitosacral areas, third, fourth, and fifth sacrals (Figs. 49-1 and 49-2). The first to fourth thoracic nerves are the important dermatomes for the intrathoracic viscera, and the sixth, seventh, and eighth thoracic segments for the upper abdominal organs (see Figs. 49-1 and 49-2). The student should memorize these facts just as he has the multiplication table.

The stimuli that are effective in arousing the sensation of pain vary to some degree for each tissue. The very existence of pain impulses arising from

viscera was debated until it was demonstrated that the adequate stimuli for pain originating in the heart or digestive tract, for example, are different from those which cause pain in the skin. The latter is sensitive to pricking, cutting, and burning, whereas these same forms of stimulation give rise to no distress when applied to the stomach or intestine. Pain in the gastrointestinal tract is produced by local trauma of an engorged or inflamed mucosa, distension or spasm of smooth muscle, and traction upon the mesenteric attachment. Severe pain may be induced in voluntary muscles by ischemia, the basis for the condition known as *intermittent claudication*, and also by the injection of water or irritating solutions. Also, prolonged contraction of muscles is a source of pain.

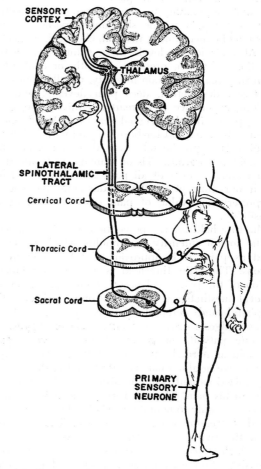

Fig. 4-1. Diagram of pain pathways. Stimuli acting on free nerve endings in the skin, muscles, blood vessels, and viscera give rise to sensory impulses, which are transmitted along the primary sensory neurones into the posterior horn of the spinal cord. The secondary sensory neurones cross to the opposite side of the spinal cord almost immediately, within one or two segments, and combine to form the lateral spinothalamic tract, which terminates in the posterolateral nucleus of the thalamus. The third sensory neurone conveys the impulse from the thalamus to the cortex of the postcentral convolution. Visceral pain fibers, although they pass through the sympathetic ganglions en route to the spinal cord, do not differ from other somatic pain fibers.

Joints are insensitive to pricking, cutting, or cautery, but the synovial membrane responds to hypertonic saline solution and inflammation. Ischemia, the only proved cause of pain in the heart muscle, is responsible for the pain of angina pectoris and myocardial infarction. Arteries give rise to pain when punctured with a needle, when induced to pulsate excessively, as in migraine, and in certain diseases affecting their walls, such as temporal arteritis. Distortion of cranial vessels by traction, displacement, or distension is a common cause of headache.

PHYSIOLOGY AND PSYCHOLOGY OF PAIN

SUPERFICIAL PAIN. There are distinct differences in the characteristics of pain arising in the skin and that originating in the viscera. The effective stimulus for pain in the skin and superficial structures may be mechanical, thermal, chemical, or electrical. At their lowest levels these stimuli may evoke sensations of touch, pressure, warmth, or cold. Only when they reach a certain intensity, usually approaching tissue destruction, does pain develop, and the resulting experience is thereafter a mixed one, combining pain with the original sensation. Wolff points out that the threshold for burning pain with a thermal stimulus is approximately two thousand times the threshold for warmth. Tissue damage is believed to be a common effect of all pain stimuli, a fact from which our concept of the fundamental biologic or self-preservation value of pain derives much of its plausibility.

The threshold for the perception of pain is defined as the lowest intensity of stimulus which is recognized as pain. It is approximately the same in all persons. The pain threshold is lowered by inflammation of the peripheral nerve endings and is raised by local anesthetics (such as procaine), lesions of the peripheral and cerebral nervous system, centrally acting analgesic drugs, and distraction or suggestion. Neurotic patients in general have the same pain threshold as normal subjects, but their reaction may be excessive or abnormal. The threshold in the frontal-lobotomized patient is undiminished, but he no longer reacts to his pain. The intensity of the pain stimulus bears a roughly quanitative relationship to the reported degree of sensory experience. The ratio between the two is expressed by the Weber-Fechner law, which states that when a series of progressively increasing stimuli is applied, in order for minimal sensory differences to be perceived, the new stimulus must be increased by a constant fraction of the previously effective one.

Pain arising in the skin has a pricking or burning quality and is localized with a high degree of precision. Pricking pain has a more rapid rate of conductivity than burning pain, being transmitted by the larger pain fibers. Together they constitute the "double response" of Lewis. A painful stimulus to the toe produces first a pricking pain and about 2 sec later a burning pain. Ischemia of the nerve subserving an area of skin produced by application of a tourniquet abolishes pricking pain before burning pain.

In the skin, localization of the pain stimulus is achieved by the simultaneous stimulation of multiple overlapping sensory neurones. Analgesia results from the interruption of all sensory neurones, and hypalgesia from the interruption of a few leaving others intact.

DEEP (INCLUDING VISCERAL) PAIN. The existence of visceral pain was long disputed, but it is now generally accepted that pain arising in the viscera does occur, provided that the stimuli are adequate. There is sound evidence that pain from viscera and deep skeletal structures is mediated through a common sensory apparatus and that the character and behavior of both are essentially the same. Hence, when we discuss visceral pain, the same principles will apply to deep skeletal pain. The pain is recognized by the patient as being "deep," i.e., deep to the skin; it is dull and aching in quality (although occasionally burning, as in the heartburn of esophageal disorders and rarely in anginal pain); the double response is absent; the pain is poorly localized and its borders are only vaguely delineated. It is probable that the high threshold and poor localization of deep pain are related, in part at least, to the relatively sparsely occurring sensory endings in the deep structures, in contrast to the closely distributed and overlapping terminals in the skin where pain threshold is low and accurately localized. Probably the most important characteristics are its relatively crude segmental localization beneath the surface of the body and its frequent reference to certain areas of the body. The simplest explanation for these latter phenomena is that suggested by Lewis:

If we suppose that certain tissues are represented in great detail in the sensorium, we can also understand that pain arising in these tissues may be localized with accuracy. But in other tissues having only a massive cerebral representation, localization may be expected to be less accurate. Segmental reference of deep pain may mean no more than that, centrally, the deep tissues supplied by a given cord segment have a general but little detailed representation. Thus, the impulses received whether these are derived from a viscus or from a deep somatic tissue, would tend to awaken very similar sensory impressions, and to be localized over a general sphere having no precise margins. And it may be regarded as natural enough that the general reference should be to regions that are relatively superficial, regions from which we are habitually receiving sensory impressions, and which are endowed with some positional sense.

The above concept implies that when pain originates in a viscus or deep skeletal tissue, the sensorium recognizes and localizes the pain as arising not in the exact region wherein it occurs but roughly in any or all structures innervated by cord segments subserving the affected viscus or deep somatic tissue. The pain appears to be projected toward the body surfaces supplied by these segments. For **example**, the sensory fibers from the heart terminate in the first through the fourth thoracic cord segments (possibly in some cases the fifth thoracic); and pain arising in the heart as the result of ischemia is not localized specifically in the region of the heart or in the precise region of the injured myocardium but in those superficial and deep structures whose sensory nerves also end in the first through the fourth thoracic spinal segments (see Fig. 4-2, showing theoretic distribution of heart pain in the first through fourth thoracic segments). Unfortunately, from the standpoint of diagnosis, the same cord segments receive fibers from the aorta, pulmonary artery, esophagus, and skeletal structures, which explains why pain arising in them may resemble that of myocardial infarction.

Referred Pain. All that has been said about segmental localization of deep pain applies also to referred pain, a term used in clinical medicine to indicate the appearance of pain in a location of the body some distance from the viscus in which the pain originates. According to the hypothesis of Lewis and Kellgren, presented above, the referred pain is an integral part of the phenomenon of visceral pain. Thus, with cardiac pain in which sensory impulses enter mainly the left half of the first through fourth thoracic cord segments, the reference of pain to the arms is explained by the anatomic fact that the first thoracic segment supplies the inner surface of the arm as well as the thorax and heart. Thus it is just as natural for heart pain to appear in the characteristic location in the left arm as it is in the anterior midchest.

This view of visceral and referred pain is obviously incomplete. It does not explain why, in the total area bounded by the first through fourth thoracic myotomes, heart pain should so commonly appear only in the anterior midline. Possibly this is related to the fact that the anterior surfaces of the body are more profusely supplied with sensory fibers. It does not explain, also, why in exceptional cases the pain may be experienced only in some unusual part of the "normal" area, for example, an anginal pain occurring only in the interscapular region of the chest. Nor do we know why visceral pain may sometimes overflow into territories completely unrelated to the known innervation of the involved viscus, for example, the appearance of anginal pain in the jaws. Clinical experience teaches us that spread of pain beyond the limits that are "normal" is due in some cases to an unusual intensity of pain; thus an anginal pain that is ordinarily confined to the midsternal region (second through fourth thoracic nerves) may spread to the neck and shoulders (third through seventh cervical nerves). In other cases, extension of pain outside the normal boundaries may be due to coexistent lesions in structures with innervation not too distant from the cord segments primarily involved in the cardiac pain. Thus an anginal pain may be localized high in the epigastrium (seventh and eighth thoracic nerves) when peptic ulcer or gallbladder disease is also present. This may be because of summation of stimuli reaching the affected cord segments. We do not know

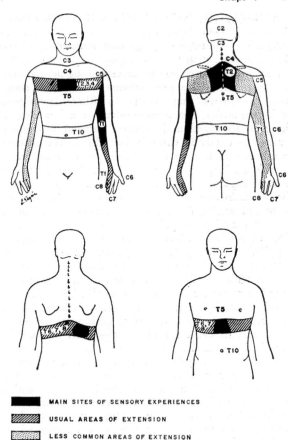

MAIN SITES OF SENSORY EXPERIENCES

USUAL AREAS OF EXTENSION

LESS COMMON AREAS OF EXTENSION

Fig. 4-2. Radiation and sites of reference of cardiac pain (*upper*); gallbladder pain (*lower*)

why visceral pains overflowing into neighboring cord segments beyond the limits that are normal for the viscus tend preferentially to wander into higher rather than lower segments, except that cephalad structures have a more abundant representation in consciousness than do caudad ones.

Deep Skeletal Pain. Since there is sound experimental evidence for the view that visceral pain and deep skeletal pain are mediated through a common deep sensory system, it is not surprising that their characteristics should be similar and that on occasion differentiation between the two may be extremely difficult. Thus a small tear or injury in a lumbar muscle or ligament innervated by the twelfth thoracic or first lumbar nerve may give rise to a pain whose quality and localization, including radiation into the groin and scrotum, are indistinguishable from those of pain caused by renal colic. A similar injury in the right upper rectus muscle may cause a pain that mimics closely the pain of gallbladder colic; and a lesion in a muscle or ligament deep in the chest wall may cause pain with radiation to the left arm, identical in localization with that of angina. Under these circumstances, differentiation of somatic from visceral pain must be made on grounds other than the location and reference of pain.

HYPERALGESIA, HYPERPATHIA, AND INVOLUNTARY MUSCLE SPASM. Superficial pain is often accompanied by hyperalgesia (increased sensitivity) of the skin, and deep pain by hyperalgesia of the subcutaneous tissue and muscle in the corresponding dermatomes and myotomes. This phenomenon of excessive sensitivity or soreness may be due to either hyperalgesia or hyperpathia. The former refers to a lowering of the pain threshold and is often induced by inflammations not only in the skin but also in the mucous membrane of the nose, stomach, colon, bladder, or esophagus. Hyperpathia refers to an alteration in the sensory experience without reduction in the sensory threshold, in which instance stimuli evoke a more intense and persistent sensation than usual. Unlike other sensory experiences, pain from deep structures may also cause involuntary spasm in skeletal muscles supplied by the same or adjacent segments of the spinal cord, e.g., spasm of the right upper rectus muscle with a gallstone impacted in the cystic duct or of the pectoral muscles in myocardial infarction.

Pain sensation may be induced by stimulation of the receptors or by irritation of peripheral nerves or roots, and in certain areas of the body it may be abolished by diseases which affect the peripheral or cerebral nervous system or by a surgical procedure which may accomplish the same result. Pain in a circumscribed region may be terminated by section of the nerve which supplies that region (neurotomy) or the spinal roots (posterior rhizotomy); pain in a limb or one side of the trunk may be interrupted by section of the anterolateral spinothalamic tract (lateral spinal tractotomy in the spinal cord or lateral medullary tractotomy in the medulla).

PERCEPTION OF PAIN. The arrival of pain impulses at the thalamocortical level of the nervous system is attended by conscious awareness of the pain stimulus. Clinical study has not informed us of the exact localization of the nervous apparatus for this mental process. It is not entirely abolished by a total hemispherectomy including the thalamus on one side. It is often said that impulses reaching the thalamus create awareness of the attributes of sensation and that the parietal cortex is necessary for the appreciation of the intensity and localization of the sensation. This seems an oversimplification. Probably a close and harmonious relationship between thalamus and cortex must exist in order for a sensory experience to be complete. The traditional separation of sensation (in this instance awareness of pain) and perception (awareness of the painful stimulus) has been abandoned in favor of the view that sensation, perception, and the various conscious and unconscious responses to a pain stimulus comprise an indivisible process.

Although similar to other sensory or perceptive phenomena in certain respects, such as predictable response to given intensity of stimulus, pain differs in other ways. One of its most remarkable characteristics is the strong feeling tone, or affect, with which it is endowed, nearly always one of unpleasantness.

Furthermore, pain does not appear to be subject to negative adaptation. Most stimuli, if applied continuously, soon cease to be effective, whereas pain may persist as long as the stimulus is operative and, by establishing a central excitatory state, may even outlast the stimulus.

PSYCHOLOGIC ASPECTS OF PAIN. A discussion of this problem could hardly be complete without some reference to the influence of emotional states or to the importance of racial, cultural, and religious factors on the pain response, especially the overt expressions. It is common knowledge that some individuals, by virtue of training, habit, or phlegmatic character, are relatively stoical and that others are excessively responsive to pain. Rarely one encounters individuals who are totally incapable of experiencing pain throughout their lifetime, not from any lack of sensory endings or peripheral sensory apparatus but from some peculiarity of central reception.

Lastly, it is important to keep in mind the devastating effects of chronic pain. As Ambroise Paré is alleged to have said, "There is nothing that abateth so much the strength as paine." Continuous pain can be observed to have an adverse effect on the entire nervous system. There is increased irritability, fatigue, troubled sleep, poor appetite, and loss of emotional stability. Courageous men are reduced to a whimpering, pitiable state that may arouse only the scorn of a healthy person. They are irrational about illness and may make unreasonable demands of family and physician. Of course the effect of narcotic drugs often complicates the picture. This state, which may be termed *pain shock*, once established, requires delicate but firm management.

CLINICAL APPROACH TO THE PATIENT WITH PAIN AS THE PREDOMINANT SYMPTOM

One of the most frequent errors is to think of pains always in terms of the severe intractable pains of disease, overlooking the fact that there are thousands of other pains which are part of the daily sensory experience of otherwise healthy individuals. To mention but a few, there is the momentary, hard pain over an eye, in the temporal region, or in the ear or jaw, which strikes with alarming suddenness; the more persistent ache which arises in some fleshy part such as the shoulder, neck, thigh, or calf; the darting pain in an arm or leg; the fleeting precordial discomfort that arouses momentarily the thought of heart disease; the breath-taking catch in the side; the cluster of abdominal pains with their associated intestinal rumblings; and the brief discomfort upon movement of a joint. These *normal pains*, as they should be called, occur at all ages, tending to be brief and to depart as obscurely as they came. They acquire medical significance only when elicited by the inquiring physician or when presented as a complaint by the worried patient;

and of course they must always be distinguished from the *abnormal pains* of disease.

When pain by its intensity, duration, and the circumstance of its occurrence appears to be abnormal or constitutes one of the principal symptoms of disease, an attempt should be made by careful analysis of it to reach a tentative decision as to its cause and the mechanism of its production. This can usually be accomplished by a very thorough interrogation of the patient in which he is encouraged to relate as accurately as possible the main characteristics of the pain. This is followed by a physical examination and not infrequently by special laboratory tests, of which there has been much refinement in recent years.

LOCATION OF PAIN. When the pain is caused by a superficial lesion, the cause and effect are usually so obvious that no problem is posed. It is the deep lesion, whether involving somatic or visceral structures, that causes trouble, and here exact localization becomes especially important. We have already seen that pain originating from such tissues no longer is sensed as coming from them but is instead roughly segmental, i.e., within the territory of the cord segments innervating the structure. The identification of the segments involved is of value, for it sets the limit on the diagnostic possibilities that must be considered, i.e., to those structures having a corresponding innervation. Thus an epigastric or subxiphoid pain or one in the opposite region in the back obliges one to search for its cause in all those structures innervated by the sixth through eighth thoracic cord segments, i.e., the esophagus, stomach, duodenum, pancreas, biliary tract, the upper retroperitoneal structures, as well as the deep somatic tissues in this region. Also one must consider the possibility that a lesion in a viscus innervated by spinal segments above or below the sixth through eighth thoracic cord segments may at times be the source of pain that has spread outside its normal boundaries and involved the epigastrium (Fig. 4-2).

PROVOKING AND RELIEVING FACTORS. These factors are of greater value than quality of pain in providing important data concerning its mechanism. Pain related to breathing, swallowing, and defecation focuses attention on the respiratory apparatus, the esophagus, and the lower bowel, respectively. A pain coming on a few minutes after the beginning of general bodily movement and relieved within a few minutes by rest indicates ischemia as the probable cause. Pain occurring several hours after meals and relieved by food or alkali suggests the irritative effect of acid on the raw lining of the stomach or duodenum. Pain that is brought on or relieved by certain movements or postures of parts of the body is usually due to the activity of diseased skeletal structures (bones, muscles, ligaments). Pain that is enhanced by cough, sneeze, and strain is usually radicular in origin or arises in ligamentous structures. Pain that is increased or altered by cutaneous stimuli is due to disease in sensory tracts in the peripheral or central nervous system. These are a few examples illustrating the paramount importance of determining with the greatest possible accuracy the factors that influence the appearance or relief of pain.

QUALITY AND TIME-INTENSITY CHARACTERISTICS OF THE PAIN. These features are of importance. However, too much stress should not be laid on the adjectives that the patient uses to describe his pain. His choice of words will depend, in part at least, on his vocabulary and on what he imagines is taking place. "Crushing" or "squeezing" are commonly employed to describe an anginal pain, and this implication of pressure does have some significance, since the pain may depend on an associated involuntary contraction of the pectoral muscles. Another patient with the same disease, however, may describe the pain as "exploding" or "burning." Far more important than the adjective used is the information that the pain is steady and does not fluctuate. Similarly, the ulcer pain is frequently designated as "gnawing"; but again, the deep, steady quality is more important than the word used to denote it. Gallbladder colic and renal colic are misnomers, if by colic is meant a "paroxysmal abdominal pain due to spasm, obstruction or distension of any of the hollow viscera." *In both these disorders, the pain is steady.* The aching quality of all deep pains is usually characteristic, but there are in addition several other informative attributes. A true colicky pain, one that is rhythmic and cramping, suggests an obstructive lesion in a hollow viscus. If the patient is a woman and has had children, it is a good idea to ask whether her "cramp" resembles the pains she had during childbirth. A pain that is steady and varies little or not at all from moment to moment means that the stimulus to pain is steady and unwavering, as in angina pectoris and peptic ulcer. Thus a pain in the anterior midsternal region whose intensity fluctuates appreciably within the space of a minute or two is not due to angina, even though the history may appear to suggest a relation to exertion. Similarly, a high epigastric pain appearing several hours after a meal and even apparently relieved by food is not caused by an ulcer if the pain fluctuates perceptibly within seconds or a few minutes. The stimulus to ulcer pain does not quickly vary in intensity. A throbbing pain indicates that an arterial pulsation is giving rise to painful stimuli. Sharp, transitory pain is caused by disease of nerve roots or ganglions, as exemplified by tic douloureux or tabes, or by some disorder in a somatic tissue such as a tear of a muscle or ligament; and often there is a background of dull, aching pain. Particularly noteworthy here is the abrupt intensification of the dull ache of root pain by cough, sneeze, or strain which momentarily increases the intraspinal pressure and stretches or alters the position of the root.

MODE OF ONSET OF THE PAIN. This factor is also important. A pain reaching its full intensity almost immediately after its appearance suggests a rupture of tissue. The pain of a dissecting aortic aneurysm often develops in this manner. In fact, the suddenness and the severity of the pain, reaching a peak of intensity within seconds or minutes, sometimes provides the first clue differentiating this type of chest pain from that caused by myocardial infarction. A similarly rapid accession of pain may occur with the rupture of a peptic ulcer.

DURATION OF THE PAIN. This is another important attribute. Anginal pain rarely lasts less than 2 or 3 min or more than 10 or 15 min. Ulcer pain may continue for an hour or more, unless terminated by the ingestion of food or alkali or a tumbler of water.

SEVERITY OF PAIN. In any given disease, the severity of pain is subject to wide variation, and also patients differ in their tolerance to it. Therefore one cannot judge the gravity of an illness by the intensity of the pain. As a rule, pains that completely interrupt work and pleasurable activity, require opiates for relief, enforce bed rest, and awaken the patient from sound sleep are to be taken more seriously than those which have the opposite characteristics.

TIME OF OCCURRENCE. An accurate determination must be made of the time of occurrence. The relationship of ulcer pain to the preceding meal has already been described. Postural aches come after prolonged activity and disappear with rest, whereas arthritic pains are usually most severe during the first movements after prolonged inactivity. The mechanism for this latter phenomenon is not known; nor do we understand why painful lesions of the bone, such as those caused by metastatic cancer, are likely to be most disturbing during the night. It is possible that the occurrence or aggravation of such pains is due to enhanced awareness of painful stimuli at a time when the mind is not distracted by other stimuli; or it may be that the pains are now more easily evoked by unconscious movements made during sleep when protective reflexes are in abeyance.

It should be obvious from these remarks that the full significance of a pain is usually not revealed by any one single characteristic. It is only by combining all these data that one can determine its anatomic site and its mechanism. In general, *the most important and revealing clues are obtained from the answers to the questions: What brings on the pain? What relieves it?* Pain is a subjective manifestation, not a state to be observed or measured. The accuracy of our data depends on the skill with which we frame our questions and on the powers of observation and memory of the person answering them.

Finally the diagnostic value of measures which *reproduce* and *relieve the pain* should be stressed. Not only are they important for diagnosis, but they convince the patient that the physician understands and can control the mechanism of his pain and the illness behind it. Climbing several flights of stairs under the physician's supervision may settle the question of the presence or absence of angina pectoris. An injection of procaine into a tender area in the chest wall or some other skeletal structure with complete disappearance of the pain may establish a skeletal origin and exclude the possibility of visceral disease. Reproducing the distress sometimes caused by aerophagia merely by distending the esophagus or stomach with air, or re-

producing the vague but sometimes alarming sensation of pressure in the chest caused by unconscious hyperventilation by having the patient hyperventilate are other examples of how the principle of the reproduction of pain may be usefully employed.

A systematic interrogation of the patient will not lead to accurate diagnosis in every instance, but the habit of searching for the identifying characteristics of pain will enable the physician to increase his skill in this difficult field. Furthermore, after becoming familiar with the customary responses to these questions, he becomes more alert to the anxious, the hysterical, or the depressed patient who while complaining of pain seems incapable of describing any of its details, or unwilling to do so. Instead, there is preoccupation with theories of what is wrong or with the treatments or mistreatments already given. Finally, there will always be cases that defy solution, when the physician can proceed only by repeatedly reexamining the patient, explaining the need for continued observation, and enlisting his aid and forbearance during this trying period. Asking the patient to tolerate a certain amount of pain without the use of powerful analgesics is usually effective, particularly when the possibility of drug addiction is explained to him.

INTRACTABLE PAINS

In the relatively rare circumstances when all manner of investigation has failed to throw light on the cause and mechanism of the pain, demands for pain-relieving surgery may become increasingly insistent. The physician may in desperation turn to measures which are more dangerous than the disease. Here the commonest source of error is to operate unnecessarily on the hysterical patient (see Chap. 214), only to discover too late that each operative procedure leaves a new pain, often at a higher level than the first. Depressive psychosis may masquerade as a painful state, and electric shock therapy may dramatically terminate the illness. Sometimes a half dozen or more operations are unsuccessfully performed on a single patient. The safest rule to follow in these cases is not to use opiates continuously or to recommend operation for the relief of pain unless a reasonable diagnosis has been made. For the pains of metastatic cancer, the thalamic pain of vascular disease of the brain, and other incurable diseases, the relative advantages of the controlled use of opiates versus lateral spinothalamic tractotomy or frontal lobotomy must be carefully weighed in each patient. The age of the patient, life expectancy, and mental state are all of importance in selecting the treatment procedure. Too often today an operation on the spinal cord or brain is chosen in preference to narcotics and the controlled use of drugs. Forgotten is the fact that many patients with cancer were formerly kept relatively comfortable and active by the judicious use of morphine and its analogues and were never subjected to costly operations or deprived of any of those qualities of mind and character which are so treasured by their families.

Superficial pain arising in integumentary structures rarely presents a problem in therapy. Acetylsalicylic acid, 0.30 to 0.60 Gm orally every 4 hr, usually suffices. Acetophenetidin may be added. These two drugs are a particularly effective combination when one element of pain is integumentary. Commercial proprietary preparations of these drugs containing caffeine or amphetamine such as A.S.A., Empirin compound, or Edrisal are available in most pharmacies. The caffeine or amphetamine is particularly useful if there is central nervous system depression. When this type of pain is not effectively controlled by nonnarcotic analgesics, codeine should be given. Usually the addition of small amounts (8 to 30 mg) of codeine phosphate to the standard dose of acetylsalicylic acid and acetophenetidin is effective. A preparation containing codeine phosphate 8 to 30 mg, acetylsalicylic acid 0.23 Gm, acetophenetidin 0.16 Gm, and caffeine 0.032 Gm is commercially available (Empirin compound with codeine phosphate). Codeine, 30 to 45 mg every 3 hr, gives maximal analgesia with minimal side effects. Adequate rest and relief of muscle tension should also be encouraged. The application of heat, especially moist heat, is usually beneficial. Occasionally, cold applications are preferred; but with the exception of cooling packs applied to an inflamed, burning skin or to a causalgia, cold is more likely to aggravate than to soothe the painful condition.

Occasionally integumental and deep pains of skeletal structures are of such severity as to require more powerful narcotic analgesics, such as meperidine hydrochloride (Demerol) in doses of 50 to 100 mg orally or intramuscularly, methadone hydrochloride 5 to 10 mg orally or subcutaneously, or dihydromorphine hydrochloride (Dilaudid) 1.0 to 2.0 mg orally or subcutaneously. These drugs are most useful in conditions when sedation is not required. When pain is unusually severe and some degree of euphoria is desired, morphine is the ideal drug. It should be given in doses of 8.0 to 15.0 mg orally or subcutaneously. Frequently a dose as small as 4.0 to 6.0 mg will relieve pain without causing undesirable nausea and vomiting. If the original dose is too small, a second dose of the same or slightly larger size can be given in 2 hr. This divided dose is less likely to induce nausea and vomiting than the larger single dose, because the stimulating effect of the first dose is insufficient to produce these symptoms and the depressant effect which follows reduces the sensitivity of the vomiting mechanism or renders it refractory to the second dose. Since all these narcotic analgesics are, for the most part, detoxified by the liver, they either should not be used or should be given in only half the usual dosage in cases of liver disease, myxedema, adrenal insufficiency, and other states in which the metabolic rate is reduced. Morphine and related narcotic analgesics tend to cause pruritus and therefore should be used with care in patients with skin irritability. The possibility of initiating addiction in susceptible individuals must be carefully evaluated in every instance.

If the patient exhibits mental tension, insomnia, and restlessness, a sedative drug such as phenobarbital or sodium barbital may be given with the analgesic agents. Sedative medication, especially the quick-acting barbiturates, should not be used alone for the control of pain, because they sometimes cause excitement and confusion under these circumstances.

Visceral pain originating in the stomach, gall-bladder, intestines, or heart is usually very poorly controlled by the nonnarcotic analgesics. Various combinations of acetylsalicylic acid and acetophenetidin usually prove to be ineffective unless given with sedatives. The narcotic analgesics are the agents of choice, but of course they should never be given until the physician is certain that the relief of the pain will not mask the state of his patient. If sedation is not desirable, and if constipation is a troublesome problem, the newer synthetic analgesics, meperidine in doses of 50 to 100 mg orally or intramuscularly or methadone 5 to 10 mg by mouth or subcutaneously every 4 to 6 hr, are recommended. Like morphine, these drugs are habit-forming, but they do not share with morphine the properties of strong analgesia, sedation, and euphoria. Patients with severe visceral pain who are also anxious or fearful and unable to relax or sleep should be given morphine sulfate in doses of 8 to 15 mg subcutaneously. The well-known spasmogenic effects of morphine are partially counteracted by atropine sulfate, 0.3 to 0.4 mg. Aminophylline, 0.5 Gm intravenously, overcomes much of this undesirable spastic action; a rectal suppository of 0.5 Gm, although less effective, may be substituted.

Intractable pain due to incurable diseases such as metastatic carcinoma is one of the most difficult of therapeutic problems. As a rule, one resorts to narcotic drugs because of their strong analgesic action, and habituation is accepted as the lesser of two evils. An alternative is "pain-relieving surgery." Section of peripheral nerves, the lateral spinothalamic tracts in the spinal cord (cordotomy), or the lateral part of the medulla and lobotomy are relatively safe procedures which have advantages in certain cases over the continuous use of opiates.

REFERENCES

Cohen, H.: The Mechanism of Visceral Pain, Trans. Med. Soc. London, 64:35, 1944.

Feindel, W. H., G. Weddell, and D. C. Sinclair: Pain Sensibility in Deep Somatic Structures, J. Neurol., Neurosurg. Psychiat., 11:113, 1948.

Hardy, J. D., H. G. Wolff, and H. Goodell: "Pain Sensations and Reactions," Baltimore, The Williams & Wilkins Company, 1952.

Lewis, T.: "Pain," New York, The Macmillan Company, 1942.

Ryle, J. A.: "The Natural History of Disease," London, Oxford University Press, 1936.

White, J. C., and W. H. Sweet: "Pain, Its Mechanisms and Neurosurgical Control," Springfield, Ill., Charles C Thomas, Publisher, 1955.

5 HEADACHE
George Pickering

Interpreted literally, headache signifies ache or pain located anywhere in the head; but its meaning has been narrowed by long usage to signify ache or pain experienced in the region of the cranial vault.

Headache is thus an experience or sensation which can be described. As in other forms of pain, its description can be analyzed into certain components—namely, quality, location, intensity, time relations, and the manner in which it is influenced by other events in the immediate environment of the patient. These characteristics, the associated sensations, and the presence of certain physical signs are the means whereby it is possible to decide which disorder is responsible for headache in a given instance. The characteristics of headache may now be discussed briefly in general terms.

QUALITY. The quality of pain is often described in terms of past experience, actual or imagined. Such descriptions are of limited value in deciding the origin of pain. There is strong evidence for the belief that if associated sensations are excluded, the subject can recognize only two types of pain by its quality: superficial pain arising from the skin, which is sharp and burning in character; and deep pain arising from all structures deep to the skin, which is dull or aching. With very few exceptions, headache is a dull, aching pain, and thus of the type that arises from structures deep to the skin.

LOCATION. Pain arising from the skin is localized fairly precisely to its point of origin. Pain arising from structures deep to the skin is less accurately localized the farther the point of origin is beneath the surface, and both pain arising from really deep somatic structures and pain from visceral tissues are referred in a segmental pattern. These same principles apply to headache. Thus pain arising from a localized lesion not far beneath the surface, such as temporal arteritis, may be fairly well localized over the lesion itself. But with deep extracranial lesions, such as those affecting the accessory sinuses of the nose and the upper cervical vertebras and their joints and ligaments, pain may be more widely referred in an area that is not directly over the lesion; still more is this true of intracranial lesions. Although headache is not necessarily located directly over the lesion, the reference of pain arising from the various structures from which it may arise is fairly constant from one subject to another, and is thus of some diagnostic value.

INTENSITY. The intensity of pain is notoriously hard to assess. Patients' statements on intensity are not of themselves of much value, for it is not unusual to find that the most extravagant epithets are applied to pains for which there is little organic basis, and where the physician is forced to conclude that the major disturbance is not of the body but of the mind. The sensitivity to pain varies with different individuals, and with the same individual under different circumstances. Intensity may be judged by other criteria.

Thus headache which wakens the patient at night and, to a lesser extent, headache which prevents sleep are nearly always of organic origin. Severe headaches again are often accompanied by vomiting, but this is more common in those of intracranial than of extracranial origin. The severest headaches are probably those associated with meningitis, and here the patient may frequently sweat with the pain and be obliged to cry out.

TIME-INTENSITY CURVE. Very rarely is headache a momentary flash of severe pain, and then usually it is due to trigeminal neuralgia affecting the supraorbital division of the nerve. More usually the pain lasts minutes or hours, and the duration of pain may be of assistance, diagnostically. Thus in cerebral tumor the pain occurs at first in paroxysms lasting several minutes. In many forms of headache of extracranial origin and of little pathologic import, the pain may at the outset last for some days. Some pains, though continuous, wax and wane with the pulse beat, and it is clear that in such instances of throbbing pain the pain arises from a structure which is moved by the arterial pulse.

RELATIONSHIP OF HEADACHE TO OTHER EVENTS IN THE ENVIRONMENT. In many instances of organic headache, the tissue disturbance which leads to the excitation of the pain nerves is influenced by events in the environment. Thus exposure to cold may act as a trigger to that ill-defined process that will be considered under nodular or fibrositic headache. In cerebral tumor, circumstances influencing the inflow or outflow of blood from the cranial cavity may precipitate headache. The headache of hypertensive disease is most frequent on waking in the morning, as is that of cerebral tumor, and that of infection of the nasal accessory sinuses may recur at certain hours of the day with almost astronomic regularity. Other examples will be found later, but these instances serve to show that an analysis of this feature of headache is of considerable value from the diagnostic aspect, and the facts so elicited must, of course, be accounted for in any hypothesis that seeks to explain the mechanism of pain.

PAIN-SENSITIVE STRUCTURES. The structures which may give rise to headache are, in general, those of the cranial cavity, the cranium itself, the covering of the skull, and other adjacent structures such as the orbital contents, the accessory nasal sinuses, and the deep structures of the neck close to the occipital region of the skull. Of intracranial structures, the brain itself is insensitive. Its pial covering is likewise insensitive except over the great vessels of the circle of Willis, and their chief branches such as the anterior, posterior, and middle cerebral, for a variable distance from their origin. Pain from these structures is referred to the same side of the head, if far from the midline, or bilaterally, if near the midline. From the anterior and middle cerebral arteries the pain is referred to the forehead and temple, from basilar to the occiput. The parietal dura mater is sensitive only along the course of the main arteries such as the middle meningeal, from which pain is referred to the temple on the same side, and along the course of the large venous sinuses such as the superior longitudinal sinus, where the cerebral veins enter. Deflection of the falx, or of the tentorium, also produces pain. Pain from the superior longitudinal sinus and straight sinus is referred to behind or above the eye, from the lateral part of the lateral sinus to the ear. Deflection of the tentorium produces supraorbital pain. The periosteum of the skull is sensitive but the bone not so. Of superficial structures, the galea, muscles, ligaments, arteries, and skin are all sensitive to pain. Pain arising from the more superficial of these deep structures—that is, the coverings of the cranial vault over most of its extent—is referred fairly well to the point stimulated. But with the deeper ligaments, muscles, and tendons of the occipital region, reference over the upper cervical segments is found. The nerves conveying sensory impulses are the trigeminal, particularly the ophthalmic division from structures above the tentorium; from structures below the tentorium the glossopharyngeal and the upper cervical spinal nerves.

FATIGUE AND PSYCHOLOGIC DISTURBANCE. It is not infrequent for headache to develop in otherwise healthy individuals during times of great mental or emotional stress or when their tolerance is lowered by infection or other debilitating agents. Such a tendency may be enhanced by such common disturbances of the mind as anxiety, fear, conflict, and fatigue. In such cases headache tends to occur toward the end of the day and to be experienced as a dull ache in the forehead which may spread to the temples or occiput; it is not usually throbbing and usually is relieved by sound sleep. There has been a tendency to assume that this headache is feigned or imagined or determined by psychologic factors, but this seems an unlikely explanation. It is accepted that fear and worry may accentuate pain by focusing attention on it, but it is held that the pain itself nearly always has as its basis the stimulation of pain nerves. It is suggested that many such cases result from excessive and maintained contraction of the muscles of facial expression, particularly the frontalis and the muscles of the scalp and neck. It may often be observed in such persons that the forehead is unusually deeply furrowed, and this type of headache can sometimes be abolished by conscious relaxation of the muscles of the forehead and scalp.

A sensation of pressure on the head, particularly on the vertex—as of a tightly fitting hat—is also met with in psychologic disorders, but while this is often described as headache, it is not true pain. It seems that in those with a disorder limited to the mind, the symptoms referred to the head are not so much simple sensations as expressions of the disordered personality.

Aside from the importance of fatigue and psychologic disorders as primary causes of headache, these factors are of great secondary importance in precipitating and aggravating headache due to almost any other primary cause. It is important that the physician should bear this consideration in mind, for if he does not, he will be unable to assess the relative parts played in the production of the symptom by local disturbances of the body, and by the mind. On such assessment must depend his whole therapeutic approach.

VARIETIES OF HEADACHE

In perusing the following account, the reader should realize that our knowledge is by no means complete and that both the classification presented and the explanations offered may require modification as knowledge advances. The classification to follow is presented from the standpoint of logical arrangement rather than clinical importance, and hence such frequent causes of headache as migraine and fever are not discussed first. The main classification used here is (1) headache arising from cranial and extracranial structures, (2) headache arising from intracranial structures, and (3) headache which cannot as yet be classified in this way.

FROM CRANIAL AND EXTRACRANIAL STRUCTURES

By their peculiar structure and function the viscera naturally interest the student and practitioner much more than the body wall, and in the case of headache the idea of an intracranial cause occurs most readily. But it is very probable that the cause of headache lies outside the skull at least as frequently as inside.

FROM ARTERIES OR THEIR NEIGHBORHOOD. As will be discussed later, there is evidence that dilatation of the temporal arteries, with stretching of surrounding sensitive structures, is responsible for most of the pain in migraine and some of the pain in febrile headache. In addition, the temporal or occipital arteries may rarely be the seat of a subacute inflammation involving the periarterial tissues and the arterial wall, often leading to occlusion of the vessel ("temporal arteritis"). Pain begins in the region of the affected vessel and, as it becomes more severe, spreads more widely over that side of the head; sometimes pain is more or less bilateral throughout, though it is not yet certain whether in such cases arteries are affected bilaterally. The pain is dull, with or without a throbbing or shooting element. It is often severe, sometimes interfering with sleep, and commonly lasts for weeks or months. The disease affects individuals over the age of fifty-five, and other arteries—retinal, cerebral, and the major branches of the aorta—may be affected. Disturbances of vision, particularly blindness, which is usually permanent, and transient diplopia, are common, and periods of disorientation are not infrequent. Blindness is due to obstruction of the ophthalmic artery or of the central retinal artery or one of its branches, and lesions of these may be seen on ophthalmoscopic examination. Other evidences of a constitutional upset are found, such as fever, malaise, anorexia, night sweats, a raised sedimentation rate, and anemia. The affected arteries of the scalp are always tender, and the overlying skin may be reddened; the arterial pulse distal to the lesion is usually lost for a while.

ASSOCIATED WITH MYOFIBROSITIS. In certain cases of headache, tender nodules may be felt near the cranial insertion of the sternomastoids; in muscles near their insertions to the superior and inferior nuchal lines; in the occipitalis, frontalis, and trapezius muscles; or in the temporalis and the galea aponeurotica. The pathologic basis of these nodules, as of those in myofibrositis of the trunk, is obscure, and it is also uncertain whether the tenderness of these nodules signifies that pain arises from them or is a secondary consequence of pain. It is thus possible that the tenderness of these nodules and the pain itself are referred from a distant and deep-seated focus, for nodules may be felt in the absence of pain or tenderness, and pain of deep origin is widespread and accompanied by deep tenderness in the area of the pain. The pain, which is of the deep aching type, often begins in a localized area in the forehead, temple, or nape of neck, and spreads to involve one or both sides of the head. It is often precipitated by exposure to cold or draft, and intense paroxysms may be added to an ache which may continue for weeks or months at a lower level of intensity. The pain may be severe but rarely keeps the patient awake at night. It can be abolished in many cases by massage applied to the nodules, but massage may make the pain worse at first. The frequency of this type of headache is disputed; by some it is said to be the commonest of all, but the general opinion seems to be that it is rather uncommon.

FROM LIGAMENTS AND DEEP STRUCTURES ATTACHED TO THE OCCIPUT AND UPPER CERVICAL VERTEBRAS. If hypertonic saline solution is injected into ligament, muscle, tendon, fascia, periosteum, or periarticular tissue situated deep in the neck near the occiput, pain is referred to the back of the head and the nape of the neck on the same side. One of the commonest causes of pain in these areas is cervical osteoarthritis. A similar pain may be seen in spondylitis ankylopoietica and in rheumatoid arthritis affecting the cervical spine. This pain is often produced or increased by movement of the head, and it may disappear when ankylosis becomes virtually complete. These structures are also subject to trauma, and occasionally headache initially occipital in distribution is found to follow a sudden flexion, extension, or torsion of the head on the neck. The pain may last days or weeks. Headache arising from these deep cervical structures is not uncommon, but it is often difficult to elucidate the causal lesion.

THE NASAL ACCESSORY SINUSES. Acute or subacute suppuration in the maxillary antrum gives pain over the antrum or in the forehead. In suppuration of the frontal ethmoid and sphenoid sinuses, the pain is around the eyes on one or both sides, but it may be in the vertex or other part of the cranium, especially in disease of the sphenoid sinuses. In all cases, pain may be associated with tenderness of the skin in the same distribution. Other signs are usually present, such as nasal or postnasal discharge of pus, fever, and opacity of the sinuses to transillumination or

x-ray. Unless such clinical evidence of infection is present, headache is unlikely to be due to sinusitis. The pain may have two remarkable properties: (1) when throbbing, it may be abolished by compressing the carotid artery on the same side; (2) it tends to recur and get better at the same hours on successive days, most frequently occurring when the patient wakes, and disappearing after the patient gets out of bed. These time relations are generally ascribed to the sinuses filling up during the night and discharging after the erect posture has been assumed. The pain can usually be abolished by inhaling vasoconstrictors such as amphetamine (Benzedrine) or by anesthetizing the orifices of the sinuses. Although some believe that sinus pain arises chiefly at nasal orifices of the sinuses, it is generally assumed that the headache arises from the mucous membrane lining the sinus, and that the pain nerves are stimulated by tension. If so, it seems probable that sinus headache, like earache, is usually due to suction on the mucous membrane when aeration is impeded by block; it is then relieved when aeration is effected. During airplane flight both earache and sinus headache tend to occur on descent, when the relative pressure in the blocked viscus falls, rather than on ascent, when such pressure tends to rise.

EYESTRAIN. Errors of refraction of the eyes are a well-recognized cause of headache. In such cases pain tends to be referred to the orbit, forehead, and temple, does not throb with the pulse, and tends to occur during intensive use of the eyes as in reading or close work, and to persist for some time afterward. It is particularly obtrusive toward evening and if the subject is fatigued. There is evidence to show that, in the presence of refractive error, use of the eyes produces sustained contraction of the extraoccular muscles of the orbit and of the frontal, temporal, and even occipital muscles, and it is suggested that the pain results from this contraction. A similar mechanism is postulated for the headache of glaucoma. The relief of such refractive errors by use of the correct spectacles abolishes the headache. Headache from eyestrain is probably not so frequent as would be indicated by the number of spectacles prescribed for its relief. Hyperopic astigmatism is a more frequent cause than myopia.

OSTEITIS. Syphilitic osteitis of the skull, now rare, Paget's disease, and metastases from primary tumors elsewhere may all produce headache, which is sometimes severe.

FROM INTRACRANIAL STRUCTURES

HISTAMINE HEADACHE. Although opinions vary concerning the existence and frequency of spontaneous headache due to histamine, the relation of the drug to the symptom is, nevertheless, of some interest, since it was the first kind of headache in which the mechanism of the pain was demonstrated. The headache can be produced easily in a normal subject by quick intravenous injection of 0.1 mg histamine acid phosphate. Headache begins about a minute after the injection, as the facial flush is beginning to fade, is maximal at about the second minute when the flush is nearly gone, and disappears about the eighth minute (Fig. 5-1). At first, it throbs conspicuously with each beat of the pulse but is felt in both sides of the forehead, and at its height it extends to the vertex and occiput. It can be established that:

1. Headache does not arise from an extracranial structure, because arrest of the circulation to the scalp before injection of histamine does not prevent the pain.

2. Headache arises from a structure innervated by the trigeminal nerve, since it does not occur on that side of the head when the sensory root has been severed or the ganglion injected with alcohol.

3. It probably arises from structures in the meninges, as it is greatly increased by shaking the head gently, and the meninges are the structures which will be chiefly strained in this movement.

4. It arises from the territory supplied by the internal carotid artery, since injection of histamine into the internal carotid produces headache, but injection into the external carotid does not.

The most striking events following the intravenous injection of histamine are consequences of vasodilatation; thus the face flushes, the blood pressure falls, and the cerebrospinal fluid pressure rises. Curiously enough, headache begins only when these signs of vasodilatation are subsiding and, in fact, is prevented from appearing by the phenomena occurring during the phase of obvious vasodilatation. Thus, when histamine is slowly infused into a vein, headache does not usually appear until after the infusion is stopped; and an established headache is temporarily relieved at the moment the face flushes after a second injection of histamine. It can further be shown that any event which leads to a fall in arterial pressure tends to relieve the histamine headache, as does any event which tends to increase the cerebrospinal fluid pressure. Thus the headache throbs with the pulse and is abolished on the same side of the head by digital obliteration of the common carotid artery. The headache is relieved by compression of the jugular veins, or by injecting saline solution into the subarachnoid space, both of which raise cerebrospinal fluid pressure. These facts are most easily explained by supposing that headache results from stretching of pain-sensitive tissue around the large intracranial arteries derived from the internal carotid, such as the anterior and middle cerebral. It is supposed that these arteries are relaxed by histamine but that the headache does not occur when they are prevented from expanding by low blood pressure and high intracranial pressure.

It is probable that a similar mechanism is concerned in producing the headache of fever.

The injection of histamine is being increasingly used as a diagnostic method, but caution should be used in interpreting the results. The reproduction of a patient's headache by histamine probably points to an abnormality in the structures concerned but does not necessarily mean that histamine is the cause. Thus the

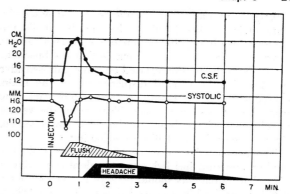

Fig. 5-1. Chart showing the course of the cerebrospinal fluid (CSF) pressure, the systolic blood pressure, the facial flush, and the headache following intravenous injection of 0.1 mg histamine. (*Pickering: Clin. Sci.*, 1:82, 1933.)

localized headache of cerebral tumor can be reproduced, and the localized headaches of trauma and the generalized headache of fever increased, by histamine.

A rather peculiar syndrome reproduced in this way has been termed *histamine cephalagia* or *paroxysmal nocturnal orbital cephalagia*. The patients are usually adult males and are awakened from sleep by an intense pain in and around the orbit, which reaches a peak of severity within a few minutes and after 15 to 45 min subsides. The pain is accompanied by lacrimation, blockage of the nostril, sweating, and sometimes by swelling over the temporal vessels on the same side of the head. The attacks may occur every day or night for weeks or months and then subside completely, only to recur in exactly the same locality at some later time. The attacks may also occur by day, but this is less frequent. The attacks themselves may be cut short by inhalation of oxygen or by intravenous injection of ergot alkaloids as described for migraine (p. 1295).

LUMBAR PUNCTURE HEADACHE. A very characteristic headache occasionally occurs a few hours to a few days following lumbar puncture, particularly if the patient has been allowed up or if several attempts have been made to enter the spinal theca. The headache is usually, but not always, throbbing and is felt chiefly in the occiput but also widely over the cranial vault; the pain may spread into the neck and back. It may be accompanied by vomiting and neck rigidity and other signs of meningeal irritation. The most characteristic feature of the headache is its very conspicuous increase when the patient sits up and its relief on lying down. The headache is caused by a leakage of cerebrospinal fluid along the tract left at lumbar puncture. For if, when the headache is present, a second lumbar puncture is performed with the patient horizontal, the pressure of cerebrospinal fluid is found to be zero, and if the pressure is restored by the injection of normal saline solution into the theca, the headache is abolished, though it usually returns after some hours, presumably because the leakage continues. The headache is increased by compression of the jugular veins and is usually unaffected by digital obliteration of one carotid artery. From these facts it seems probable that the headache results from the tension exerted on some pain-sensitive structure by the caudad displacement of the brain, consequent on the emptying of cerebrospinal fluid from the subarachnoid space. Tension on the venous attachments of the brain to the great dural venous sinuses seems the most likely mechanism.

The occasional occurrence of headaches following lumbar puncture has led some to adopt the point of view that all patients should be kept in the recumbent position, preferably prone, following the procedure. Headache following cisternal puncture is rare.

A similar headache syndrome sometimes occurs after straining or a fall on the buttocks. Presumably, there is a tear in the arachnoid membrane, with a leakage of cerebrospinal fluid. The pressure of the cerebrospinal fluid is low and there may be a slight pleocytosis. The condition subsides spontaneously within a few days to weeks.

RAISED INTRACRANIAL PRESSURE. Headache is an outstanding symptom in a number of diseases in which intracranial pressure becomes elevated, and the suggestion has been widely accepted that such headache results from stretching the pain-sensitive parietal dura mater. This hypothesis must now be rejected for the following reasons:

1. It is difficult to see how the parietal dura mater, supported as it is by the bony skull, can be stretched by a rise in intracranial pressure, except at the various foramens of the skull.

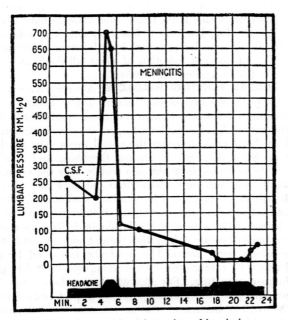

Fig. 5-2. Chart showing the relationship of headache to cerebrospinal fluid pressure in a case of meningococcal meningitis in which the pressure was altered by withdrawal of cerebrospinal fluid and injection of saline solution through the lumbar puncture needle. (*Pickering. Brit. Med. J.,* 1:907, 1939.)

2. The cerebrospinal fluid pressure may be raised to very high levels (500 or 600 mm H_2O) by injecting saline solution into the subarachnoid space at lumbar puncture or by jugular compression, without headache resulting.

3. A critical examination of the behavior of headache in several diseases reveals facts which cannot be reconciled with the hypothesis. These facts will be described separately, under the several diseases.

MENINGITIS. One of the most severe headaches is that associated with meningitis—particularly the acute inflammations produced by the pyogenic microbes, the meningococcus, streptococcus, pneumococcus, and staphylococcus; in the less acute tuberculous meningitis, headache is often less intense. The headache is more or less generalized over the calvarium and may be throbbing or not; it is associated with rigidity of the neck muscles, so that when the head is flexed the neck muscles contract strongly and pain is felt in the occiput and neck; Kernig's and Brudzinski's signs may also be present but are less reliable. The patient commonly lies on his side with the head extended and the hips and knees flexed, and he shuns the light. This headache is very greatly increased by shaking the head, and the patient may resent any movement of his bed.

In all forms of meningitis the cerebrospinal fluid pressure is commonly raised, sometimes to very high levels of over 600 mm H_2O, and it is not infrequent to find that removal of cerebrospinal fluid by lumbar puncture relieves the pain (Fig. 5-2). Nevertheless, it is found that if the pressure is reduced still further—below the normal level—pain is increased, to be relieved by reinjection of fluid and restoration of pressure to normal. It seems probable that in this instance pain is due to a chemical irritation of the pain nerve endings of the meninges, consequent on the tissue damage of bacterial action, and that mechanical distortion of these inflamed tissues, as by distension or depletion of the subarachnoid space, may further increase pain. The mechanism of pain thus is probably identical with that occurring in acute inflammatory conditions elsewhere, such as those affecting the pulp of the finger and the peritoneum.

CEREBRAL TUMOR. Headache is the outstanding symptom of cerebral tumor. Its features are very variable, and while there are certain features of headache which strongly suggest tumor, these features will not be found in all cases. Headache in cerebral tumor at first occurs in attacks lasting only a few seconds to 3 hr, and typically about 1 hr. The paroxysms may be precipitated by any activity, especially such as involves abrupt changes in position of the head, and they diminish in frequency when the patient is kept in bed. With the patient at rest the attacks often occur when the patient wakes in the morning. Usually no simple event is found to abolish the pain, and relief is sought from anodynes and bed rest. Frequently, as the tumor grows, headache may increase in frequency, duration, and intensity. In the later stages the pain may become continuous. The pain may be slight but can be intolerably severe. In fact, the most severe headaches occurring in disease are those of meningitis, subarachnoid hemorrhage, and tumor, rivaled only by that of intrathecal air insufflation. Brief paroxysms of most intense headache, during which the subject writhes in agony and is oblivious to events around him, are highly suggestive of tumor. Headache is essentially a deep, aching pain, though the epithets used vary with the patient's experience, imagination, and command of language. The pain may throb with the pulse, or it may be continuous or "smooth." Not infrequently the headache is accompanied by nausea or vomiting. In some cases the two are related, vomiting occurring with the worst but not with the least pain; but vomiting also occurs in tumor without headache, and it occurs without preceding nausea. (See Chap. 206.)

Most frequently in tumor, headache is bilateral and frontal, but there is some relation between sites of pain and tumor, in the absence, but not in the presence, of papilledema. Thus occipital headache is more frequent with tumors below than with those above the tentorium, and when headache is unilateral, the tumor is on the same side in about 90 per cent of cases. Sometimes headache is localized to an area roughly 5 cm in diameter, which may correspond fairly closely to the site of the tumor. Headache is more frequent in quickly growing tumors, such as gliomas, than in the slower-growing varieties, such as meningiomas. It is also more frequent and begins earlier when the mass is smaller in tumors involving the ventricles, or below the tentorium, than when the frontal or parietal lobes are involved; tumors of the temporal and occipital lobes occupy an intermediate position with respect to time of onset and severity of headache.

It may be accepted that the afferent impulses responsible for tumor headache arise within the cranial cavity for, as will be mentioned, pain can be induced and relieved by procedures which affect only the cranial content; also that the stimulus is mechanical, for the common effect of such procedure is to alter the stresses and strains inside the skull. The stimulus is probably not stretching of the parietal dura mater by raised intracranial pressure, because:

1. The parietal dura mater is firmly suffixed by the skull.

2. In a given case, cerebrospinal fluid pressure measured in the presence of headache is not significantly higher than in its absence.

3. Lumbar puncture may relieve, but it may also increase or induce, headache.

4. Raising intracranial pressure by jugular compression, or by intrathecal injection of saline solution, may relieve as well as increase headache in cerebral tumor.

5. It has been shown at operation under local anesthesia that headache may sometimes be reproduced by emptying or distending the ventricles on the same or opposite side.

From these experimental findings, as well as from the clinical features of headache, it seems that sudden changes of intracranial pressure, either up or down, may precipitate pain. Two ideas of the origin are widely entertained: that it arises from the arteries at the base of the brain and that it arises from tension on the dural attachments of, and supports for, the brain. The first explanation finds support in the observation that histamine may, in a given patient, reproduce precisely the headache of tumor, even when this has a highly individual localization. The second explanation is not easily compatible with certain details of observations made on individual cases, though it agrees with much of the evidence; for it is well known that tumor gives rise to distortions of the intracranial septums and that such distortions can give rise to pain, presumably, by tension on the pain-sensitive tissues around the dural sinuses. That headache is due to such distortion would be in harmony with many of the facts about tumor headache, namely, that it may be either relieved or increased by lowering cerebrospinal fluid pressure, that the headache may frequently be relieved by intravenous or rectal injections of hypertonic solutions, and that the headache may disappear following operations for decompression. Moreover, this hypothesis would be compatible with its high incidence in posterior fossa and rapidly growing tumors.

SUBARACHNOID HEMORRHAGE. Headache is a constant feature of spontaneous subarachnoid hemorrhage resulting from rupture of a miliary aneurysm of the circle of Willis or its main branches, and the stories given by such patients indicate that headache must begin at about the time when the aneurysm ruptures. Thus, a patient who up to that time has been perfectly well is seized abruptly with the most severe generalized headache, and a few moments later he sinks to the ground unconscious. The headache is invariably severe when the patient recovers consciousness and lasts for some days or weeks afterward. It has been supposed that the headache arises, as does that of meningitis, from inflammation of the meninges evoked by the presence of blood, and it is true that neck rigidity is a constant feature of subarachnoid hemorrhage, as it is in meningitis. Pain may also arise from the pain-sensitive tissue in the region of the aneurysmal sacs; and it is possible that sudden stretching of the perivascular tissue, with consequent headache, may precede the actual rupture into the subarachnoid space. However, it is to be noted that accounts of pain produced at operation by stimulating the great vessels at the base of the brain describe pain as unilateral, while in subarachnoid hemorrhage it is nearly always bilateral. Moreover, there is evidence from intracranial aneurysm that headache from the region of the artery is more localized, for in unruptured aneurysms headache occurring in paroxysms restricted to the same side of the head is common. (See Chap. 204.)

VASCULAR LESIONS. Headache is relatively uncommon in cerebral embolism and cerebral thrombosis. Intracerebral rupture of an artery, as in atheroma or hypertension, usually produces loss of consciousness and often results in death. If the patient recovers consciousness, he often complains of severe headache and may show neck rigidity, as in subarachnoid hemorrhage. Blood may be present in the cerebrospinal fluid. But it is now becoming clear that smaller amounts of bleeding are more frequent than had been thought. Headache as a presenting feature of a cerebral vascular accident should always arouse suspicion that hemorrhage is the cause; when the headache assumes the characteristics of meningeal headache and is accompanied by neck rigidity, suspicion becomes near certainty. The idea that the imminence of cerebral hemorrhage can be foretold by headache is, in general, entirely without foundation, but it has obvious commercial value and appeals to the intellectually feeble or the morally unscrupulous.

SUBDURAL HEMATOMA. An effusion of blood into the subdural space may follow severe head injury, when it constitutes from the beginning a surgical problem, but it may also occur from minor trauma, particularly in elderly subjects. Its clinical picture is that of an expanding intracranial lesion, and its differentiation from other such lesions may be difficult. Usually after a latent period of days to weeks or months, headache develops and increases in frequency and severity. The patient has periods of drowsiness, amnesia, and confusion, and he may lapse into coma. In the earlier stages there may be no physical signs; later spastic hemiparesis, sensory loss, papillary inequality, abnormal ocular movement, and papilledema may occur, probably owing to compression of the brain stem at the temporal opening. Dysphasia and hemianopia are rare. The physician should always inquire for minor trauma in an elderly subject presenting with otherwise unexplained headache and confusion. The diagnosis is suspected by finding lightly bloodstained or xanthochromic CSF, often with raised protein content. Pineal shift may be seen on plain x-rays. The diagnosis is confirmed by angiography. The treatment is surgical.

MIGRAINE. This common, sometimes disabling, but otherwise benign malady will be described fully in Chap. 218.

OTHER FORMS OF HEADACHE

FROM HYPERTENSION. Hypertension is now a diagnosis so commonly made, and carrying with it in the public mind such fear of its consequences, that many of its symptoms are to be attributed not so much to the disease as to the state of mind that its diagnosis endangers. Headache is not a common complaint of patients with mild hypertension before diagnosis; occurring in such patients after diagnosis, the headache has no peculiar features. But in severe hypertension a characteristic headache is common and is frequently the symptom bringing the patient to the doctor. It may be troublesome and may be severe. Characteristically, the pain is occipital and is noticed on waking in the morning, to improve as the day advances; it may last an hour or longer. The headache may be associated with nausea and vomiting. Over a large series of cases there is some relationship between intensity of headache and intensity of hypertension, and the severest headaches are thus commonly found in hypertension of the malignant type. As papilledema also occurs in malignant hypertension (and cerebral hemorrhage is by no means rare in that condition), a mistaken diagnosis of cerebral tumor may be made unless the level of the blood pressure and the total clinical picture are taken into consideration.

The precise mechanism of headache in hypertension remains obscure. The cerebrospinal fluid pressure is raised in rough proportion to the diastolic arterial pressure but it is the same in the presence and absence of headache. That the headache may have an intracranial source is indicated by its often being increased by withdrawal of cerebrospinal fluid at lumbar puncture. Evidence has been produced to show that headache of hypertension is often due to stretching of the walls of extracranial arteries. Thus the headache is said to be relieved by compression of the superficial arteries supplying the scalp and abolished by tying these arteries. Pain is often uninfluenced by carotid artery compression, nor is its morning incidence dependent on whether the patient sleeps with one or several pillows.

FROM FEVER. Headache occurs in many diseases in which the temperature rises—for example, acute tonsillitis, typhoid fever, malaria, and sandfly fever. The pain may be throbbing with the pulse, or steady; it may be frontal, occipital, or generalized. The headache is very much like the histamine headache in being relieved on the same side by carotid artery compression, on both sides by compression of the jugular veins, or by the injection of saline solution into the subarachnoid space; it is increased by shaking the head. Like histamine headache, pain is temporarily relieved by injection of histamine or amyl nitrite during the time the arterial pressure is lowered and the cerebrospinal pressure raised by these drugs. It seems probable, therefore, that the headache arises in the same way as that following histamine—namely, from stretching of pain-sensitive tissue around the large arteries at the base of the brain. In certain cases, however, pain may be lessened by compression of temporal or angular arteries, and in these a component of the headache seems to be derived from the walls of extracranial arteries, as in migraine.

FROM ANEMIA. Some patients suffering from severe anemia experience headache which is abolished when the hemoglobin content of the blood is restored by treatment. The headache is usually frontal or generalized and may or may not be throbbing. It tends to occur toward evening. This headache has been insufficiently investigated to reveal its mechanism. Headache is, however, a common experience after exposure to high altitudes and thus to oxygen lack, and it is tempting to suppose that the two may be related.

Curiously enough, if exposure to a high altitude (over 14,000 ft) is brief—say, 4 hr—headache is experienced not during the exposure but afterward. The explanation of this curious fact is unknown. Likewise, the explanation for the headache which may occur in patients with polycythemia is uncertain.

POSTTRAUMATIC. After head injury, especially one that has caused loss of consciousness, over 50 per cent of patients suffer from headache. Other associated symptoms are dizziness, amounting to a sense of instability rather than to true vertigo, and mental change, of which loss of memory and inability to concentrate are the chief signs. (See Chap. 205.)

Considerable divergence of opinion exists as to the mechanism of headache in such cases. In a small series with dull pain more or less localized to the area of injury and persisting up to 8 years afterward, Penfield recorded localized changes in the subarachnoid and subdural spaces revealed by air insufflation into the spinal theca. He also described the relief of headache after such insufflation. In cases not so relieved, he reported success from dividing adhesions formed near the site of injury between the dura and piarachnoid. Consequently, he ascribed the headache in these cases to tension set up in these adhesions between the brain and its coverings, the adhesions being formed when the brain was out of place due to the local tissue reaction to injury. The fuller experience of the Second World War suggests that headache of this type and origin is uncommon. More usually, the headache is bilateral, frontal, or generalized, often throbbing, and usually occurring in paroxysms or liable to paroxysmal exacerbations. The paroxysms may be induced by stooping, physical exertion, noise, and excitement. The pain may be increased by lying down and relieved by raising the head on pillows, or relieved by recumbency, and is worst in the erect posture. These observations suggest an organic cause for the headache, but the nature of this has not been worked out. The headaches usually pass off with the improvement of the patient, consequent on modern rehabilitation management, and are relieved by the ordinary anodynes.

The evolution of posttraumatic headache is often complicated by the presence of economic problems in relation to compensation.

APPROACH TO THE PATIENT WITH HEADACHE

From the foregoing account it will be appreciated that certain forms of headache may be diagnosed and others suspected, when a lucid description of the pain has been obtained from the patient. Headache occurring toward the end of the day and relieved by sound sleep may be due to fatigue or eyestrain; that due to a disturbed mind is less often relieved by sleep. Paroxysmal headache, often unilateral, preceded by an aura and accompanied by vomiting is recognizable as migraine. Occipital headache occurring on waking, and declining as the day wears on, usually is due to hypertension but may be due to cerebral tumor. Headache persisting without remission for weeks or months, and unaccompanied by other manifestations of disease, is commonly due to an affection of the deep structures of the neck and head, such as myofibrositis; occasionally, its abrupt onset following sudden movement indicates a traumatic lesion. Following head injury, headache is common and often associated with dizziness, inability to concentrate, and impaired memory. Headache recurring over short periods, at a definite hour of the day, suggests a sinus infection. Headache that is accompanied by symptoms of fever and acute infection probably is due to a febrile illness; when meningitis is present, the headache is very severe and neck rigidity is almost invariable. Headache occurring in brief and severe paroxysms, becoming recently longer and more frequent, is suggestive of cerebral tumor; the headache has localizing value. Sudden severe headache, followed by loss of consciousness, suggests a subarachnoid hemorrhage. After lumbar puncture, headache may develop when the patient sits up and may be relieved when the patient lies down.

These points in the history which have been noted are very important; but they are often no more than pointers as to which investigations should be carried out in a specific case. Many of the conditions named have physical signs that should be sought.

The central nervous system, the eyes, the ears, nose, and throat, the skull, the scalp, the neck, the blood pressure, and the urine should be examined in all cases, particular attention being paid to the fundus oculi. Anemia and syphilis may have to be excluded, and an x-ray examination of the head and neck may be needed. Other special examinations particularly relevant to the cranial content should be done if there are clear indications for them. It is equally important that the physician should try to assess the contribution made by disturbances of the mind. While mental disturbance per se produces a feeling of pressure or confinement of the head rather than ache or pain, pain may arise from secondary effects on the muscles of the head and neck, and any pains, however trivial, may appear severe to a mind that is tormented with fear or doubt.

REFERENCES

GENERAL

Kellgren, J. H.: On the Distribution of Pain Arising from Deep Somatic Structures with Charts of Segmental Pain Areas, Clin. Sci., 4:35, 1939.

Lewis, T.: "Pain," New York, The Macmillan Company, 1942.

—— and W. Hess: Pain Derived from the Skin and the Mechanism of Its Production, Clin. Sci., 1:39, 1933.

HEADACHE

Graham, J. R., and H. G. Wolff: The Mechanism of Migraine Headache and Action of Ergotamine Tartrate, Arch. Neurol. Psychiat., 39:737, 1938.

Horton, B. T.: Use of Histamine in Treatment of Specific Types of Headache, J.A.M.A., 116:377, 1941.

Northfield, D. W. C.: Some Observations on Headache (Especially That of Cerebral Tumor), Brain, 61:133, 1938.

Penfield, W.: Chronic Meningeal (Post-traumatic) Headache and Its Specific Treatment by Lumbar Air Insufflation, Surg. Gynecol. Obstet., 45:747, 1927.

Pickering, G. W.: Experimental Observations on Headache, Brit. Med. J., 1939, I:907.

——: Observations on the Mechanism of Headache Produced by Histamine, Clin. Sci., 1:77, 1933.

Wolff, H. G., et al.: "Pain," Baltimore, The Williams & Wilkins Company, 1943.

6 PAIN IN THE CHEST

T. R. Harrison, William H. Resnik, and T. J. Reeves

The common problem in patients who complain of chest pain involves the distinction of trivial disorders from coronary disease, which is attended by the threat of sudden death. *There is little parallelism between the severity of the pain and the gravity of its cause. An incorrect positive diagnosis of a hazardous condition such as angina pectoris is likely to have harmful psychologic and economic consequences.* In no field of medicine is accurate diagnosis more important or, at times, more difficult.

The apparently bizarre radiation of pain arising in the thoracic viscera can usually be explained in terms of the known facts concerning nerve supply. These have been considered in the fourth chapter. One occasionally sees a patient with extension of pain to a location which cannot be logically explained. In most instances, such an individual will be found to have more than one disorder capable of causing pain in the chest. The presence of the second and often silent condition may affect the radiation of the pain produced by the primary disorder. Thus when the pain of angina pectoris extends to the back, the patient will usually be found to have also a significant degree of spinal arthritis. Similarly, the radiation of anginal pain to the abdomen commonly occurs only in individuals who have some upper abdominal disorder, such as hiatal hernia, disease of the gallbladder, pancreatitis, or peptic ulcer. When such instances are excluded, there is only an occasional patient who presents a distribution of pain which cannot be logically explained in terms of the known facts about nerve supply.

The common tendency to assume that the presence of an objective abnormality, such as a hiatal hernia or right bundle branch block, necessarily means that an atypical chest pain is arising in the stomach or the heart is to be strongly condemned. Such an assumption is justified only provided that the careful history indicates that the behavior of the pain is entirely compatible with the site of origin which is suggested by the objective finding.

THE LEFT-ARM MYTH. There is a long tradition, widely accepted by physicians and laymen, that pain in the left arm, especially when appearing in conjunction with chest pain, has a unique and ominous significance as being almost certain evidence of the presence of ischemic heart disease. This is a myth that has neither theoretic nor clinical foundation. From a theoretic standpoint, *any* disorder involving the deep afferent fibers of the upper thoracic region should be capable of causing pain in either area, both areas, or neither area (p. 13). Hence a pain of trivial significance arising in skeletal tissues innervated by upper (first to fourth) thoracic nerves would be expected to produce left-arm-area pain. These expectations are exactly in accord with clinical observation. Almost any condition which is capable of causing pain in the chest may induce radiation to the left arm. Such localization is common not only in patients with coronary disease but also in those with numerous other types of chest pain. Neither the location, radiation, nor quality of pain is of crucial diagnostic significance. Rather, it is the careful history of the behavior of the pain, in terms of the conditions which induce it and relieve it.

Table 6-1. CLASSIFICATION OF CHEST PAIN

I. Heart
  A. Myocardium: oxygen deficiency
    1. Infarction (permanent anoxia)
    2. Angina pectoris (temporary hypoxia)
    3. Preinfarctional angina (usually combining some features of both 1 and 2, above)
  B. Pericardium: inflammation
  C. Periapical pain and precordial ache (these are really varieties of chest wall pain and are not of cardiac origin)

II. Aorta: dissecting aneurysm (the pain of saccular aneurysm is usually due to pressure on surrounding structures)

III. Other thoracic organs
  A. Pleura (including pleuritis, pneumothorax, and pleurodynia)
  B. Mediastinum (emphysema, inflammation, masses)
  C. Esophagus (esophagitis, spasm, carcinoma, diverticulum)

IV. Chest wall (musculoskeletal pain—the commonest cause of pain in the chest)
  A. Primary, with no associated cardiovascular disease
    1. "Rheumatic"
    2. Psychogenic
  B. Secondary (indirectly induced by underlying visceral disease, usually cardiac; the shoulder-hand syndrome is the classic example)
    1. Shoulder-hand syndrome
    2. Pectoral syndrome
  C. Associated (not initially caused by cardiovascular disease but conditioned and aggravated by it)

V. Abdominal disorders causing chest pain:
  A. Stomach: aerophagia and pouches (especially hiatal hernia, rarely diverticulum)
  B. Splenic flexure
  C. Gallbladder, duodenum, and pancreas (rare causes of anterior chest pain, except when radiation is conditioned by coexisting coronary disease)

VI. Rare and miscellaneous

Only the more important or more common conditions listed in Table 6-1 will be considered in the text. No attempt has been made to enumerate all the causes of chest pain.

PAIN DUE TO OXYGEN DEFICIENCY OF THE MYOCARDIUM

PHYSIOLOGIC CONSIDERATIONS OF THE CORONARY CIRCULATION. Pain due to myocardial ischemia occurs when the oxygen supply to the heart is deficient in relation to the oxygen need. The oxygen consumption of this organ is closely related to the physiologic effort made during contraction. Thus the oxygen consumption depends not only on the energy involved in expelling blood but also on the "wasted" isometric energy required to raise the ventricular pressure sufficiently to open the semilunar valves. When other factors remain constant, an elevation of stroke volume produces an efficient type of response because it leads to increase in ejection work only, the isometric factor per minute remaining relatively constant. Thus a rise in flow load causes less increment in myocardial oxygen consumption than does a comparable increase in cardiac work per minute, brought about by elevation either of pressure or of heart rate. However, the net effects of these hemodynamic variables depend not on oxygen need alone but rather on the balance between the demand and the supply of oxygen. Since the heart is always active, the coronary venous blood is normally much more desaturated than that from other areas of the body. Thus the removal of more oxygen from a unit of blood, which is one of the two adjustments commonly utilized by exercising skeletal muscle, is already employed in the "resting" heart. Therefore, this organ has only one effective means of obtaining the additional oxygen required for greater work, and this is by increase in the coronary blood flow.

It follows, from Poiseuille's equation, that the flow of blood through the coronary arteries is proportional to the gradient between the aortic and intramural (during systole) or intraventricular (during diastole) pressures, but is proportional to the *fourth power of the radius* of the coronary arteries. Thus a relatively slight alteration in coronary diameter will produce a large change in coronary flow, provided that other factors remain constant.

The coronary dilatation associated with increased stroke volume, which normally compensates for the tachycardia of exercise, is impaired when there is fixed coronary narrowing. Thus physical exertion, or any other condition which increases heart rate, tends to precipitate anginal attacks. Bradycardia usually has the opposite effects, and this apparently explains the rarity of angina in persons with complete heart block, even when this disorder is caused by coronary disease. However, extreme bradycardia is associated with pronounced decline in diastolic pressure, which may reduce the coronary flow.

CAUSES OF MYOCARDIAL HYPOXIA. By far the most frequent underlying cause is disease of the coronary arteries. This is usually the result of atheroma, which is often complicated by blood clots. Much less frequently, narrowing of the coronary orifices due to syphilitic aortitis or to distortion by a dissecting aneurysm may be responsible. A drug, such as ergot, which causes constriction of the coronary arteries, may occasionally induce anginal attacks in the absence of organic disease. There is no evidence that vasoconstriction or increased cardiac work (rise in rate or blood pressure, or liberation of catecholamines) due to emotion can precipitate angina unless there is also structural narrowing of the vessels. However, when this is present, it is likely that reflex vasoconstriction from abdominal or other disorders, as well as emotional vasoconstriction, may precipitate episodes.

Aside from conditions which narrow the lumen of the coronary arteries, the only other frequent causes of myocardial hypoxia are disorders, such as aortic stenosis, which cause a marked disproportion between the perfusion pressure and the ventricular work. Under such conditions the systolic rise in left ventricular pressure is not, as in hypertensive states, balanced by corresponding elevation of aortic pressure, and most of the coronary flow occurs in diastole. Therefore, increase in heart rate is especially harmful because it shortens diastole more than systole and thereby decreases the total available perfusion time per minute.

Patients with marked right ventricular hypertension may have exertional pain which is, in most respects, identical with that of the common type of angina. It is likely that this discomfort results from relative ischemia of the right ventricle brought about by the increased oxygen need and by the elevated intramural resistance, with sharp reduction of the normally large systolic perfusion of this chamber.

In persons with syphilitic aortitis, angina is not uncommon and the relative roles of aortic insufficiency and of coronary ostial narrowing are difficult to assess. However, the latter factor is absent in patients with rheumatic aortic insufficiency, and unless there is coexistent stenosis, angina is exceptional. Apparently, the reduction in diastolic perfusion pressure is usually balanced by the greater systolic perfusion due to coronary dilatation. Angina may be severe when marked regurgitation is associated with a relatively slight degree of stenosis.

The importance of tachycardia, decline in blood pressure, or diminution in arterial oxygen content will be apparent from the above discussion. However, these are precipitating and aggravating rather than underlying causes of angina.

THE EFFECTS OF MYOCARDIAL HYPOXIA. The most common of these is *anginal pain,* which is considered in some detail in Chap. 148. The exact mechanism of the pain stimulus is still unknown. The evidence that oxygen deficiency is in some way responsible appears to be overwhelming, but the precise mechanism of its action has not been established.

As a rule, myocardial infarction is associated with a pain similar in quality and distribution to that of angina but of greater intensity and much longer duration. It is not relieved by coronary dilator drugs. Occasionally, the pain is minimal or even completely absent. In such instances, it is probable that pre-existing long-standing myocardial ischemia has caused damage to the nerve fibers which would otherwise conduct the pain impulses.

A second effect of myocardial ischemia is often seen in the *electrocardiogram*. Most persons with angina have normal tracings between attacks, and the record may even remain normal during the seizures. However, in many instances, depression of the S-T segments appears in leads I, II, AVL, or in those from the left precordium. There is strong experimental evidence that such depressions, as well as the elevations which are usually seen in patients with infarction and are observed in a few patients during anginal attacks, are related to alterations in ionic balance. These changes affect the diastolic base-line (T-P) potential and thus produce relative depression (low plasma potassium or high plasma sodium) or elevation (low sodium or high potassium) of the S-T segment. It would appear that the net effect of very severe ischemia is to produce S-T elevation, while less marked ischemia has the reverse effect. The value and limitation of electrocardiographic changes occurring after exercise in the diagnosis of angina pectoris is discussed in Chap. 148.

A third effect of myocardial hypoxia is alteration in contraction. It has been shown that the pulmonary capillary (wedge) pressure may rise during anginal attacks. This indicates *temporary left ventricular failure*, which is presumably induced by the decreased contractility of the ischemic areas.

The beneficial effect of nitrites was originally ascribed by Lauder Brunton to reduction in tension in the arteries and thus, presumably, in the heart. Subsequent studies in animals pointed toward absolute increase in coronary flow. However, direct measurements in man suggest that the increase is relative and dependent on a greater decrease in the work and in the oxygen consumption of the heart than in coronary flow, because of a reduction in the resistance in the myocardial vessels.

Another characteristic effect of myocardial hypoxia is *liability to sudden death*. This may never occur, despite hundreds of anginal episodes. However, it may supervene early in the disease and even in the first attack. When the conducting system is involved, the patient may die from atrioventricular block, with standstill of the ventricle. However, the usual mechanism is probably ventricular fibrillation, which can often be seen to occur in animals following ligation of a coronary artery.

PAIN DUE TO IRRITATION OF SEROUS MEMBRANES OR JOINTS

PERICARDITIS. Experimental studies made on man indicate that the visceral and the internal surface of the parietal pericardium are ordinarily insensitive to pain, although when the latter is sufficiently inflamed, painful stimuli may originate from it. The most highly sensitive region is the lower part of the external surface of the parietal layer, and the pain associated with inflammation of the remaining part usually arises in the adjacent pleura. These observations explain why noninfectious pericarditis (that associated with uremia and with myocardial infarction) with relatively mild inflammation is usually painless or accompanied rarely with very mild pain, whereas infectious pericarditis, being nearly always more intense and spreading to the neighboring pleura, is usually associated with typical pleuritic pain (i.e., aggravated by breathing, coughing, etc.). Since the central part of the diaphragm receives its sensory supply from the phrenic nerve, which arises from the third to fifth cervical segments of the spinal cord, pain arising from the lower parietal pericardium and central tendon of the diaphragm is felt characteristically at the tip of the shoulder, the adjoining trapezius ridge, and the neck. Involvement of the more lateral part of the diaphragmatic pleura, supplied by branches from the intercostal nerves (sixth to ninth thoracic), causes pain not only in the anterior chest but also in the upper abdomen and corresponding region of the back, thus sometimes simulating the pain of acute cholecystitis or pancreatitis.

Pericarditis causes three distinct types of pain. By far the commonest is the pleuritic pain, related to respiratory movements and always aggravated by cough or deep inspiration, sometimes brought on by swallowing, because the esophagus lies just beyond the posterior portion of the heart, sometimes by change of bodily position. This type of pain is due to the pleuritic component of the pleuropericarditis so commonly present in the infectious forms. The next commonest pericardial pain is the steady, crushing substernal pain identical with that of acute myocardial infarction; if the pleuritic component is absent, differentiation on the basis of the pain alone is impossible. The mechanism of this steady substernal pain is not certain, but it is probable that it arises from the highly inflamed inner parietal surface of the pericardium or from the irritated afferent cardiac nerve fibers lying in the periadventitial layers of the superficial coronaries. The third type of pain, one that *a priori* should appear to be the most common and characteristic, is actually quite uncommon. This pain is synchronous with the heartbeat and is felt at the left border of the heart and left shoulder. Rarely, all three types may be present simultaneously.

The painful syndromes which may follow operations on the heart ("post commissurotomy syndrome"), myocardial infarction, or trauma to the heart are discussed in later chapters (pp. 826 and 850). Such pains often but not always arise in the pericardium.

Pleural pain is very common and may be identical with that of pericarditis. However, its sharp superficial quality (p. 12) and its aggravation by each breath readily distinguishes it from the deep dull steady unwavering pain of myocardial ischemia. The pain of mediastinitis or of mediastinal emphysema (p. 950) usually resembles that of pleuritis but is more likely to be maximal in the substernal region, and the associated feeling of constriction may cause confusion with myocardial infarction.

The *costochondral and chondrosternal articulations* are the commonest sites of anterior chest pain. Objective signs of arthritis, in the form of swelling (Tietze's syndrome), redness, and heat are very rare, but sharply localized tenderness is common. The pain may be "neuritic," i.e., darting and lasting for only a few seconds, or a dull ache enduring for hours or days. An associated feeling of tightness due to muscle spasm (see below) is frequent. When the discomfort endures for a few days only, a story of minor trauma or of some unaccustomed physical effort can be obtained. The chronic variety of this discomfort is common in persons with arthritis of the spine and also in patients with ischemic heart disease, but in many instances no associated disorder is found. It should be emphasized that *pressure on the chondrosternal and costochondral junctions is an essential part of the examination of every patient with chest pain.* A large percentage of patients with this disorder, and especially those who also have minor and innocent T-wave alterations (p. 83), are erroneously labeled as having coronary disease. The dire consequences of such a mistake have already been emphasized.

PAIN DUE TO TISSUE DISRUPTION

Rupture or tear of a structure may give rise to pain that sets in abruptly and reaches its peak of intensity almost instantly. Such a story would, therefore, arouse the suspicion of dissecting aneurysm, pneumothorax, mediastinal emphysema, a cervical disk syndrome (p. 44), or rupture of the esophagus. However, the patient may be too ill to recall the precise circumstances, or the pain may be atypical and increase gradually in severity. Likewise, other and more benign conditions, such as a slipped costal cartilage or an intercostal muscle cramp, may produce pain with an abrupt onset.

PAIN DUE TO INCREASED MUSCLE TENSION

This is of two varieties, depending on whether the discomfort arises in skeletal or smooth muscle. The former is very frequent, and the usual causes are discussed later in some detail. A very rare type is *intercostal cramp*, which, except for the location, is identical with the common night cramp in the valves. Here, again, the coexistence of insignificant variations in the electrocardiogram *often* leads to the tragedy of a false positive diagnosis of ischemic heart disease.

It is likely that increased tension in visceral musculature is responsible for the chest pain associated with some esophageal disorders, the splenic flexure syndrome, aerophagia, and diverticulum of the stomach. There is uncertainty whether the same mechanism or pinching of nerve fibers causes the discomfort of hiatal hernia, a disorder that can mimic the pain of

myocardial ischemia exactly as regards location, quality, and intensity but not as regards precipitating and alleviating factors.

CLINICAL ASPECTS OF SOME OF THE COMMONER CAUSES OF CHEST PAIN

Some of the features of pericarditis have already been described, and those of the more serious causes of chest pain such as myocardial ischemia (angina pectoris and infarction), dissecting aneurysm, and disorders of the pleura, esophagus, stomach, duodenum, and pancreas are considered in the appropriate chapters dealing with these problems. Here, we are concerned with the discussion of those causes which are not considered in more detail elsewhere.

PAIN ARISING IN THE CHEST WALL OR UPPER EXTREMITY. This may develop as a result of muscle or ligament strains brought on by unaccustomed exercise and felt in the costochondral or chondrosternal junctions or in the chest wall muscles. We mention the upper extremities and especially the left because of the deeply ingrained legend that pain in the left arm has a specific significance in indicting the heart. Another cause is spinal arthritis. Finally, pains in the upper extremity (shoulder-hand syndrome) and in the pectoral muscles may, through unknown mechanisms, occur in patients with ischemic heart disease.

Skeletal pains in the chest wall or shoulder girdles or arms are usually recognized quite easily. Localized tenderness of the affected area is usually present, and the pain is sometimes clearly related to movements involving the painful locus. Thus deep breathing, turning or twisting of the chest, and movements of the shoulder girdle and arm will elicit and duplicate the pain of which the patient complains. The pain may be very brief, lasting only a few seconds, or dull and aching and enduring for hours. The duration is, therefore, likely to be either longer or shorter than untreated anginal pain, which usually lasts for only a few minutes.

These skeletal pains often have a sharp or sticking quality. In addition, there is frequently a feeling of tightness which is probably due to associated spasm of intercostal or pectoral muscles. This may produce the "morning stiffness" seen in so many skeletal disorders. The discomfort is unaffected by nitroglycerin but often abolished by infiltration of the painful areas with procaine (Novocain).

When chest wall pain is of recent origin and follows some unusual activity involving the pectoral muscles, it presents no problem in diagnosis. However, *longstanding skeletal pain is frequent in persons who also have angina pectoris.* This association is sometimes coincidental, because both disorders are very common. In other instances, it seems that the coronary disease is responsible for the chest wall pain, the exact mechanism being uncertain but similar to that responsible for the well-known shoulder-hand syndrome. This coexistence of the two different types of chest pain in the same patient is a frequent cause of a confusing history because in the patient's mind the anginal needle may be hidden in the skeletal haystack. Thus every middle-aged or elderly patient who has long-standing anterior chest wall pain merits careful study.

Detailed questioning will sometimes reveal that what was originally thought by the patient to be a single type of discomfort actually comprises two different pains which, though similar in quality and area, differ as regards duration and initiating factors. When the history is inconclusive, the postexertional electrocardiogram may furnish decisive information. However, both false positive and false negative tracings may be obtained, according to whether they are interpreted loosely or critically (p. 831). It may thus be necessary to study the pain itself and to learn by direct observations whether exercise alone or postprandial exertion, or even postprandial effort undertaken holding an ice cube, is capable of producing it. Repeated tests may be required, the effects of preceding placebos, as compared to nitroglycerin, on the amount of exertion required to induce the pain being compared. *The confusion created by the presence of innocent skeletal pain impairs the reliability of the history and is probably the commonest cause of errors—both positive and negative—in the diagnosis of angina pectoris.*

Emotional disorders are also common causes of chest wall pain. Usually, the discomfort is experienced as a sense of "tightness," sometimes called "aching," and occasionally it may be sufficiently severe as to be designated a pain of considerable magnitude. Since the discomfort has almost always the additional quality of tightness or constriction and, furthermore, since it is often localized across the sternum, although it may be felt in other areas of the anterior chest, it is not surprising that this type of pain is frequently confused with that of myocardial ischemia. Ordinarily, it lasts for a half hour or more and may persist for a day or less with slow fluctuation of intensity. The association with fatigue or emotional strain is usually clear, although it may not be recognized by the patient until called to his attention. The pain probably develops through unconscious and prolonged increase of muscle tone (as in frowning in the face, or as can be quickly produced in the hand by tightly clinching the fist), often enhanced by an accompanying hyperventilation (by causing a contraction of the chest wall muscles similar to the painful tetany of the extremities). When the hyperventilation and/or the associated adrenergic effect due to anxiety also causes innocent changes in the T waves and S-T segments, the confusion with coronary disease is strengthened. However, the long duration of the pain, the lack of any relation to exertion but association rather with fatigue or tension, and the usual periodic occurrence on successive days without any limitation of capacity for exercise usually make the differentiation from ischemic pain quite clear.

As compared to these two causes (the chest wall muscle and ligament strains and the contraction of the pectoral muscles due to reflex influences, fatigue, or tension) the various other conditions that may cause skeletal discomfort are uncommon and readily recognized after appropriate observation: spinal arthritis, herpes zoster, anterior scalene and hyperabduction syndromes, malignant disease of the ribs, etc.

The several *abdominal disorders* which may at times mimic anginal pain may usually be suspected from the history, which ordinarily will indicate some relationship to swallowing, eating, belching, the expulsion of flatus, etc. Occasionally, as in some patients with hiatal hernia, the gastrointestinal x-ray will be of crucial significance. Rarely, it may be necessary to inflate the stomach or the splenic flexure with air, in order to satisfy both the doctor and the patient that one of these organs is responsible for a tight pain in the lower chest. It should be emphasized again that the demonstration of the presence of a coexistent abdominal disorder such as hiatal hernia does not constitute proof that the chest pain of which the patient complains is due to this. Such disorders are frequently asymptomatic and are not at all uncommon in patients who also have angina pectoris.

APPROACH TO THE PATIENT WITH PAIN IN THE CHEST

Most individuals with this complaint will fall into one of two general groups. The first consists of persons with prolonged and often severe pain without obvious initiating factors. Such persons will frequently be gravely ill. The problem is that of differentiating such serious conditions as myocardial infarction, dissecting aneurysm, and pulmonary embolism from each other and from less grave causes. In some such instances, the careful history will provide significant clues, while objective evidence of crucial importance will appear within the subsequent 2 or 3 days. Thus, when the initial examinations are not decisive, a watch and wait policy, with repeated electrocardiograms coupled with measurements of the transaminase, sedimentation rate, etc., will commonly provide the correct answer.

The second group of patients comprises those who have brief episodes of pain, with otherwise apparently excellent health. Here, the resting electrocardiogram will rarely supply decisive information, but records taken after exercise will often reveal characteristic changes (p. 831). However, in many instances it is the study of the subjective phenomenon, i.e., of the pain itself, that will lead to the diagnosis. Of the several methods of investigation which are available for such patients, three are of cardinal importance.

A detailed and *meticulous history* of the behavior of the pain is the most important method. The location, radiation, quality, intensity, and, especially, duration of the episodes are important. Even more so is the story of the aggravating and alleviating factors. Thus a history of sharp aggravation by breathing, coughing, or other respiratory movements will usually point toward the pleura, pericardium (because of the associated pleuropericarditis), or mediastinum as the site, although chest wall pain is likewise affected by respiratory motions. Similarly, a pain which regularly appears on rapid walking and vanishes within a few minutes upon standing still will usually mean angina pectoris, although here, once again, a similar story will rarely be obtained from patients with skeletal disorders.

When the history is inconclusive, the *study of the patient at the time of the spontaneous episode* will often supply crucial information. Thus the electrocardiogram, which may be normal both at rest and after exercise in the absence of pain, will occasionally demonstrate striking changes when recorded during an anginal episode. Similarly, x-ray of the esophagus or of the stomach may show no evidence of cardiospasm or of hiatal hernia except when the observation is made during the pain.

The third method of study represents the *attempt to produce and alleviate the pain at will*. This procedure is necessary only when doubt exists following the history or when needed for psychotherapeutic purposes. Thus the demonstration that a localized pain, which can be reproduced by pressure on the chest, is completely relieved by local infiltration with procaine will often be of conclusive importance in convincing the patient that the heart is not the site. The discomfort due to distension of the stomach or of the splenic flexure with air is frequently mistaken by the patient, and occasionally by the physician, for pain of cardiac origin. The simple demonstration, by passing a tube to the appropriate area and inflating with air, that the pain can be exactly reproduced may be not only of diagnostic but also of psychotherapeutic value. However, the demonstration that such procedures will reproduce the patient's pain may be misleading in persons who have angina in addition to another disorder. It may, therefore, be necessary to study also the effect of exercise on the pain and on the electrocardiogram.

When, as is not rarely the case, the history is atypical, the correct diagnosis of angina pectoris will often depend in large measure on the response to nitroglycerin. Here, a number of pitfalls should be avoided. If the patient has previously had the drug, careful questioning may be necessary to avoid errors. Thus disappearance after its sublingual administration does not necessarily prove that there is a cause and effect relationship. It is necessary to be certain that the pain vanishes more rapidly (usually within 5 min) and more completely when the drug is used than when it is not employed. A false negative impression concerning the effect of nitroglycerin may be the result of the use of a deteriorated preparation which has been exposed to light. It is thus necessary to be sure that the dosage used is sufficient to induce a pharmacologic effect in the form of a slight flush or a mild pounding headache. In doubtful instances, repeated exercise tests, with and without preceding administration of nitroglycerin, are necessary. The demonstration that the time required for a given exercise to produce pain is consistently and considerably longer when it is under-

taken within a few minutes after a sublingual nitroglycerin pill than after a placebo may, in some instances, represent the sole method for accurate recognition of angina pectoris. A completely negative response to such repeated tests constitutes almost conclusive evidence against angina.

SUMMARY

The location of a pain in the chest has little diagnostic import. The concept that radiation from the anterior chest to the left arm necessarily indicates coronary disease as a cause is an old wives' tale. The several thoracic viscera and the chest wall have nerve fibers which pass by a final common pathway to the pain-receptive areas of the brain. One can no more identify the cause of the pain by its location alone than one can hear the ring of a telephone and know the city from which the call originated. Differences in the quality and duration of pain may be of diagnostic value. However, the most important aspect of the history in the diagnosis of *brief and recurrent chest pain is the relationship to various precipitating and alleviating factors*. The observation of the effect of exercise on the electrocardiogram and on the pain is often conclusive. In many instances the study of the effect of nitroglycerin on the amount of exercise required to produce pain is crucial.

In the spontaneously arising pains of long duration, as in myocardial infarction, dissecting aneurysm, pulmonary embolism, acute pericarditis, gallbladder colic, incarcerated hiatal hernia, acute pancreatitis, in all of which the pain may be identical in location, severity, character, and sites of reference, it is often the corollary data, clinical and laboratory, that finally determine the diagnosis.

Reproducing and alleviating the discomfort is not only sometimes of value in establishing the diagnosis but of immense psychologic benefit to the patient when he learns that an apparently mysterious and disturbing disorder can be mimicked and relieved at will.

When, as will occasionally occur, the thorough examination leaves one in doubt, observation over a period of time will often clarify the question, at least to the extent of establishing or excluding the more serious causes of the pain. Under such circumstances the patient should be advised to follow the same exertional and dietary regime which one would advise in any healthy middle-aged person, because this is essentially the same as that advised for a person with minimal myocardial ischemia (p. 832). At the same time, fear can be alleviated by the reassurance that this regime is aimed not at treatment of an existing condition but at preventing future vascular disease.

REFERENCES

Capps, J. A.: Pain from the Pleura and Pericardium, Assoc. Research Nervous and Mental Disease, Proc. (1942) 23:263, 1943.

Edwards, W. L. Jack: Musculoskeletal Pain Following Myocardial Infarction, Am. Heart J., 49:713, 1955.

Keefer, C. S., and W. H. Resnik: Angina Pectoris: A Syndrome Caused by Anoxemia of the Myocardium, Arch. Internal Med., 41: 769, 1928.

Müller, O., and K. Rørvik: Haemodynamic Consequences of Coronary Heart Disease with Observations during Anginal Pain and on the Effect of Nitroglycerine, Brit. Heart J., 20:302, 1958.

Prinzmetal, M., and R. A. Massumi: Anterior Chest Wall Syndrome: Chest Pain Resembling Pain of Cardiac Origin, J.A.M.A., 159:177, 1955.

Wehrmacher, William H.: "Pain in the Chest," Springfield, Ill., Charles C Thomas, Publisher, 1964.

7 ABDOMINAL PAIN

Carl A. Moyer

Abdominal pain may be defined as a consciousness of distress in the abdomen. Under certain conditions this manifests itself as indigestion, which will be considered later. It may have a parenchymatous, metabolic, or neurogenic origin. The etiologic classification in Table 7-1, while not complete, includes the important causes of this symptom.

Table 7-1. ETIOLOGIC CLASSIFICATION
OF ABDOMINAL PAIN

I. Pain associated with parenchymatous disease
   A. Pain referred to the abdomen from extraabdominal disorders (i.e., from thorax, spine, or genitalia)
   B. Pain having its origin within the abdomen
      1. Incident to disturbances of function or obstruction of hollow organs { Bowel / Bile ducts / Ureter / Bladder / Pancreatic duct
      2. Incident to peritoneal inflammation
         a. Chemical { Gastric juice / Pancreatic juice / Urine / Bile / Blood extravasation from a parenchymatous organ* (liver, spleen, kidney, ovary)
         b. Bacterial { Gastrointestinal contents / Bacterial invasion of uterus and oviducts / Rupture of abscesses into the remaining free peritoneal cavity / Invasion of peritoneal cavity from the blood stream—primary peritonitis
      3. Incident to disturbances in blood supply
         a. Pressure or torsional occlusion { Volvulus / Strangulated hernias / Twisted pedunculated cysts / Uterine fibroids

         b. Embolism and thrombosis { Arterial / Venous
         c. "Inflammatory" (e.g., visceral angiitis)
      4. Incident to disruption of a viscus (e.g., rupture of a viscus or tearing apart of arterial walls)
      5. Incident to an increase in tension upon supporting elements
         a. Traction on mesenteries
         b. Rapid swelling of capsules (e.g., congested liver, carcinomatous lymph nodes)
         c. Rapid separations of leaves of mesenteries { New growths / Rupture of vessels
      6. Incident to disease of muscle
         a. Traumatic myopathy
         b. Infectious myositis { Viral / Bacterial / Parasitic
II. Pain associated with metabolic disease
   A. Endogenous
      1. Toxic (uremia, diabetic coma, porphyria)
      2. Allergic
   B. Exogenous
      1. Toxic (e.g., lead poisoning)
      2. Biologic (e.g., bite of the black widow spider)
III. Central or neurogenic pain
   A. Organic
      1. Lesions of the central nervous system (post-apoplectic pain)
      2. Root pain (including the "lightning" pain of tabes dorsalis)
      3. Causalgia
   B. Ideogenous ("mind pain," "psychogenic pain")

* Blood introduced into the peritoneal cavity through a needle or from torn mesenteric vessels usually produces no pain.

The differentiation of abdominal pain is difficult. The location of the pain, its type (colicky, steady, boring), its mode of onset, its rate of change in intensity, its relationship to eating and to evacuation of bowel and bladder are historically important in the determination of cause. The degree and location of muscle spasm, changes in the pattern of breathing, the location of tenderness to percussion and to steady increase in pressure, the threshold of counter pain necessary to remove abdominal pain from consciousness, and the determination of changes in cutaneous sensitivity are signs of importance in the differentiation of abdominal pain.

PAIN OF PARENCHYMATOUS ORIGIN

REFERRED ABDOMINAL PAIN. This type of pain is the enigma of the surgeon, for he recognizes that the lower thoracic cavity and the upper abdomen are neurologically and lymphatically one unit. For example, early acute lobar pneumonia, with basilar pleurisy, may be attended by severe abdominal pain and a degree of "spasm" of the abdominal muscles so intense as to lead one to think that a duodenal ulcer has perforated or that the gallbladder has ruptured and peritonitis is present. To make matters more confusing, the abdominal pain of pneumonia may be present before any physical or roentgenologic signs of pneumonia are detectable. Conversely, acute cholangitis and acute subphrenic abscesses are often associated with pleuritic pain in the lower right chest and signs of fluid in or atelectasis of the lower lobe of the lung. Coronary occlusive disease and acute cholecystitis, with cystic duct obstruction, may also be mistaken one for the other.

The differentiation of referred abdominal pain from that arising within the abdominal cavity may depend solely upon the course that the illness takes during a brief period of careful observation. However, a tentative opinion of the probable anatomic location of the primary difficulty can often be made from the elucidation of a few clinical signs.

Abdominal pain referred from within the chest is usually associated with alterations in breathing, lag and restriction of motion of the lower thoracic segment that are much more apparent than those associated with pain of intraabdominal origin. In addition, pain that accompanies intraabdominal flammatory processes (exclusive of those limited to the lesser omental cavity) is generally associated with spasm of the abdominal muscles that *does not* perceptibly relax during the inspiratory phase of the respiratory cycle; whereas the spasm occasioned by the referred type does relax during inspiration. Evidently the reciprocal inhibition of the abdominal muscles, which are expiratory muscles, that normally takes place during inspiration still occurs with referred abdominal pain but does not occur with that of peritonitis. Another point of difference that may be of help is that steady, gentle pressure over the painful area does not materially increase, and may actually relieve, the pain if it is referred, but generally increases it if it is of intraabdominal inflammatory origin.

It is especially important that referred and intraabdominal inflammatory pain be differentiated, because the latter often indicates immediate surgical intervention. Intrathoracic diseases more commonly associated with abdominal pain are lobar pneumonia, coronary occlusive disease, infectious pericarditis, and "cardiospasm." The routine careful search for specific clinical signs of their existence will often lead to the correct inference as to the origin of pain that appears superficially to be of abdominal origin. However, it is well to remember that diseases may be coexistent, and the existence of intrathoracic or intraabdominal disease before the acute disease develops, even though it may be "asymptomatic," may result in unusual areas of reference of the acute pain. For example, a painless healed abdominal incision, especially if it is recent, often becomes the point of reference for pain arising from widely separated organs within the abdomen. Though it has not as yet been proved, it is thought that the same principle may explain the peculiar references of pain with acute gallbladder disease to the left shoulder, if coronary occlusive disease exists; and the radiation of the pain of myocardial infarction to the epigastrium or right upper quadrant of the abdomen, if preexisting, though asymptomatic, gallbladder or duodenal disease is present.

Referred pain arising from the testis is acutely intensified by light testicular pressure, and that arising from the seminal vesicle is usually relieved by expression of its contents. That arising from vertebral disease often has the characteristics of root pain.

The commonest causes of abdominal pain having their origins within that cavity are disturbances in the function of hollow organs, intraabdominal inflammation, and increase in tension of supporting elements.

PAIN ASSOCIATED WITH DISTURBANCES IN FUNCTION OF HOLLOW ORGANS. This pain is, at least initially, intermittent or colicky. It is generally associated with definite organic disease but may occasionally accompany variations in physiologic function without visible organic disease. Anyone who has observed the terrific colic of acute coccal food poisoning or who, having made a diagnosis of acute intestinal obstruction, has had the misfortune of performing a celiotomy upon an individual who is actually suffering from porphyria, and has seen the unbelievable contortions performed by the intestine, is convinced that severe colic can be associated solely with changes in physiologic function.

Pain which is incident to disturbances in the function of various hollow organs has certain relatively specific areas of reference. That associated with obstruction of the cystic duct or distension of the gallbladder is referred most commonly to the epigastrium, then to the right posterior chest about the scapula, and occasionally to the left lower quadrant of the abdomen. Sudden common bile duct or pancreatic duct obstruction by stone produces pain that is felt in the epigastrium and in the upper lumbar region of the back. The colicky pain of midgut obstructive origin, or in other words, terminal duodenal, small intestinal, appendiceal, ascending and proximal transverse colonic obstructive origin, is generally supraumbilical or circaumbilical. That associated with lesions in the flexures of the colon is felt in the region of these structures. Obstructive lesions of the lower descending and sigmoid colon produce pain that is felt most often in the left iliac region and over the sacrum.

Obstruction of the ureter from below the ureteropelvic junction to its intravesical portion is productive of pain that is initially felt directly over the point of obstruction, but after spasm of lumbar and flank muscles develops, the pain becomes diffuse and tends to cover the flanks. Acute occlusion of the intravesicular portion of the ureter, and of the proximal urethra, tends to produce pain which is referred to the shaft of the penis, the scrotum, and the inner surface of the thigh in the male, to the inner surface of the thigh in the female, and to the suprapubic regions of both sexes.

Rapid distension of the bladder is productive of suprapubic pain. Obstruction of the ureteropelvic junction is associated with pain in the costovertebral angle.

PAIN INCIDENT TO AN INFLAMMATORY PROCESS INVOLVING A PARIETAL PERITONEAL SURFACE. Pain of this sort is located over the area involved and is steady and aching in character. The rate of its development and intensity are dependent upon the amount and character of the chemical substances which impinge upon a given surface per unit of time. For example, a milliliter of highly acid sterile gastric juice or a milliliter of sterile alkaline pancreatic juice (which, in addition to their acidity and alkalinity, are enzymatically potent) in the peritoneum is immediately productive of much more intense inflammation and pain than is a milliliter of bacteria-laden, neutral, enzymatically impotent liquid feces from the ascending colon.

Ultimately, as the bacteria multiply and elaborate irritants, the peritoneal surface over which the organisms spread becomes severely inflamed and painful. The differentiation between inflammatory processes of bacterial chemical and body chemical origin is primarily dependent upon the analysis of progression of the inflammation or pain (Fig. 7-1).

Another factor that must be considered in the analysis of the severity of the pain that accompanies an inflammatory process is the rate of change in the intensity of the stimulus. If the rate of change in the intensity of a stimulus is sufficiently slow, no sensation of pain will be felt, even if a very intense, widespread inflammatory reaction is present (e.g., tuberculous peritonitis); if the rate of change is very rapid, the pain is intense (e.g., ruptured duodenal ulcers). In general, the intensity of pain is more intimately related to the rate of change in strength of stimulus than it is to the area to which the stimulus is applied.

The location and extent of tonic muscle spasm, which usually occurs with peritonitis, is fundamentally dependent upon the surface area involved in the process. The intensity of the spasm is usually related directly to the rate of development of the inflammation and is related inversely to the functional integrity of the central nervous system. The latter relationship is especially important. A severely ill or a dying man will not show spasm of the abdominal muscles, even if his stomach or gallbladder ruptures. Degenerated psychotic (schizophrenic) patients and those suffering from advanced Parkinson's disease and from extensive multiple sclerosis have been observed in whom the acute rupture of a viscus (gallbladder or duodenum) with widespread generalized peritonitis has been unattended by any significant degree of muscle spasm.

The pain incident to inflammation is aggravated by pressure on the abdomen.

Abdominal pain that attends vascular occlusive disease is characteristically rapid in onset, and agonizing, if the process is at all extensive. It tends to be constant and diffuse. If it is not complicated by coexistent inflammatory pain, the tonic spasm of muscles is much less in relation to the severity of the pain than is the muscle spasm associated with an acute peritoneal inflammation.

The pain attending the rupture of a viscus (except those containing potent chemicals) is a sudden, sharp, terrifying pain that is quickly over. The pains of rupture of the gravid uterus, of the spleen, or of the distended, obstructed appendix are of this type.

PAIN FREQUENTLY ASSOCIATED WITH INCREASE IN TENSION UPON SUPPORTING ELEMENTS OF ORGANS (CAPSULES, LIGAMENTS, AND MESENTERY). This pain tends to be steady and aching in character, increased by muscular activity and relieved by rest, and may vary considerably with change of posture. It may be absent in the morning, following a well-slept night, but increase gradually during the activities of the day. It is not well localized; it tends to be circaumbilical and supraumbilical if the organ involved lies in the abdominal cavity and infraumbilical, suprapubic, and in the low-back region if the organ involved is located in the pelvis. Gentle percussion with the closed fist or pressure over the organ involved aggravates this type of pain. The area of tenderness to percussion shifts with position if the organ involved is mobile (e.g., lymph nodes in the mesentery). Abdominal muscle spasm is usually minimal if present at all.

Abdominal pain associated with generalized myositis of infectious origin mimics pain of intraabdominal inflammatory origin. It is constant, aching, aggravated by movement and pressure, and associated with tonic muscle spasm. The main differential point between the pain of myositis and the pain of peritoneal inflammation is the presence, in the former, of tenderness and spasm of muscle masses not innervated by the nerves supplying the peritoneum and, in the latter, limitation of muscle spasm and tenderness to their areas of distribution.

Abdominal pain of "metabolic" origin may mimic all other types, and its recognition depends upon the constant awareness on the part of the doctor that it may simulate early small intestinal obstruction, appendicitis, cholecystitis, ruptured ulcer, etc.

The abdominal pain with sickle-cell anemia tends

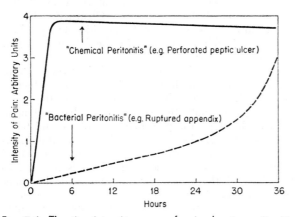

Fig. 7-1. The time-intensity curve of pain due to peritonitis depends on the underlying cause. When enzymatic digestion of the peritoneum is responsible, the pain rapidly reaches a maximal degree of intensity. When bacterial inflammation is responsible, the progression is much slower and is apparently related to the rate of bacterial growth.

to migrate, and the areas of tenderness likewise tend to shift within brief periods of time (1 to 3 hr).

That associated with diabetes and uremia has no specific characteristics.

The bite of the black widow spider produces severe pain and rigidity, not only in the abdominal muscles but also in the long muscles of the back (sacrospinalis), a region rarely affected by pain of intra-abdominal origin.

The abdominal crisis of chronic porphyria mimics acute intestinal obstruction and is characteristically attended by unusually prominent signs of increased peristaltic activity.

The pain of lead colic has no specific characteristics.

Ileus, or obstruction of the intestine, may accompany all types of abdominal pain. (See Chap. 183.)

PAIN OF NEUROGENIC OR CENTRAL ORIGIN

Pain associated with abnormalities of the spinal nerves and roots such as tumors and degenerative diseases (diabetic and syphilitic) or incident to impingement of bone (arthritis and fractures of the spine) or soft tissue (ruptured nucleus pulposis) upon nerve roots or elements of the cauda equina is usually localized. Cord and root pains tend to have a sudden onset (lightning pains) and a lancinating character and are often limited to a few neural segments. They have no consistent relationship to eating. The abdominal pain arising from the impingement of bone or a ruptured nucleus upon nerve roots is aggravated by movements of the spine. Muscle spasm is often intense, but it is not particularly increased by gentle pressure on the abdomen. Changes in nerve thresholds are common (hyperesthesia, hypesthesia). Distension of the abdomen is uncommon, and persistent changes in breathing are not seen often.

CAUSALGIA (PERIPHERAL TYPE). This quality of pain is usually limited to areas of distribution of peripheral nerves that have been partially severed or have partially regenerated after complete severance or pressure block. Its quality is variable; usually the person cannot describe it with clarity and precision; it is most troublesome during periods of rest.

In persons with causalgic pain the respiration and muscle tonus are normal; the threshold of counter pain necessary to remove abdominal causalgic pain from consciousness is low; the light touch of a pinpoint to the forehead is frequently enough. The geographic distribution of cutaneous pain spots is grossly altered in the painful area. These spots are very irregularly spaced, with frequent gaps of a centimeter between them. In fact, disturbance in pain-spot distribution may be the only significant clue that a pain is causalgic. In general, peripheral causalgia seems to be fundamentally related to a change in the relationships of the various cutaneous sensory stimuli that simultaneously impinge upon the skin and deep structures.

For example, feeling a rough surface is not a painful experience, but it may be if the ulnar or median nerves are partially severed. The recognition that a surface is rough is dependent upon a pattern of stimuli arising in touch, pressure, and pain endings. Unequal interference with the receptive capacity of various sensory endings or fibers so changes the central appreciation of feeling a rough surface as to make it distressful to the individual. The painful sensations that accompany the stepping on a "sleeping" foot are similar to causalgia, and the differential disturbances of various peripheral sensory components are relatively easily demonstrable.

PSYCHOGENIC PAIN. This pain is characterized by indefiniteness of onset, diffuseness of location, and casual definition of type, with little or no relationship to meals or evacuation. Generally, irregularly cyclic muscle spasms may be felt, and many bizarre types of change in the character of breathing may be seen. The commonest type of change in breathing is a restriction of the depth of inspiration without accentuation of the speed of expiration. The expiratory accessory muscles of respiration may be tonically (not rhythmically) active. If generalized abdominal muscle spasm is present, the abdomen will be protuberant in the lateral view and normal or narrow in the anterior view. Generally speaking, no persistent localized point of tenderness will be present excepting when the abdomen is scarred. The physical signs of central psychogenic pain can be obliterated by the suppression of consciousness [drowsiness or sleep or with thiopental (Pentothal) N_2O "analgesia"], or by inducing a powerful stimulation of breathing with 10 per cent carbon dioxide.

The foregoing chapter has been concerned, in the main, with the more severe types of abdominal pain. The milder types of abdominal discomfort will be considered in Chap. 25, in the section dealing with Indigestion.

REFERENCES

Association for Research in Nervous and Mental Disease: "Pain: Proceedings of the Association, December 18 and 19, 1942," Baltimore, The Williams & Wilkins Company, 1943 (Research Publications, vol. 23, 1942).

Bishop, G. H.: Response to Electrical Stimulation of Single Sensory Units of Skin, J. Neurophysiol., 6:361, 1943; The Peripheral Unit of Pain, ibid., 7:71, 1944; The Structural Identity of the Pain Spot in Human Skin, ibid., 7:185, 1944.

Fine, J., B. M. Banks, and L. Hermanson: The Treatment of Gaseous Distention of the Intestine by the Inhalation of 95 Per Cent Oxygen, Ann. Surg., 103:375, 1936.

Lewis, T.: "Pain," New York, The Macmillan Company, 1942.

Olivecrona, H.: Inhibition Ileus (Paralytic), chap. 23, pp. 425–422, in "Intestinal Obstruction," 2d ed., O. H. Wangensteen (Ed.), Springfield, Ill., Charles C Thomas, Publisher, 1942.

Wangensteen, O. H.: "Therapeutic Problem in Bowel Obstructions," Springfield, Ill., Charles C Thomas, Publisher, 1937.

8 PAIN IN THE BACK AND NECK

Raymond D. Adams, Michel Jequier,
and Jost Michelson

The following remarks concern mainly the lower back since it is most frequently the site of disabling pain. The lower spine and pelvis, with their many muscular and tendinous attachments, are relatively inaccessible to palpation and also to inspection, even through the medium of x-ray. For want of reliable physical signs and laboratory tests, it is often necessary to depend on the patient's description of his pain, which may not be altogether accurate, and his behavior during the execution of certain maneuvers. Seasoned clinicians, for these reasons, come to appreciate the need of a systematic clinical approach, the description of which will be one of the main purposes of this chapter.

ANATOMY AND PHYSIOLOGY OF THE LOWER BACK

The spine is roughly divisible into two parts: an anterior column of articulated vertebral bodies and intervertebral disks held together by the anterior and posterior longitudinal ligaments, which together constitute the supporting pillar of the body; and a posterior segment consisting of pedicles and laminas, fused to form the walls of the spinal canal, which provides protection of paravertebral muscles.

The stability of the spine depends on two types of supporting structures, the ligamentous (passive) and muscular (active). Active muscular support and movement are contributed by the erectores spinae, abdominal, glutei maximus, psoas, and hamstring muscles.

The vertebral and paravertebral structures derive their innervation from the recurrent branches of the spinal nerves. Pain endings and fibers have been demonstrated in the ligaments, muscles, periosteum of bone, annulus fibrosus, and synovia of the articular facets. The sensory fibers from these structures and the sacroiliac and lumbosacral joints join to form the sinovertebral nerves which pass via the recurrent branches of the spinal nerves of the first sacral and the fifth to first lumbar vertebras into the gray matter of the corresponding segments of the spinal cord. Efferent fibers emerge from these segments and extend to the muscles through the same nerves. The sympathetic nerves contribute only to the innervation of blood vessels and appear to play no part in voluntary and reflex movement, though they do contain sensory fibers.

The parts of the back that possess the greatest freedom of movement, hence are most frequently subject to injury, are the lumbar and cervical. The majority of these movements are reflex and are the basis of posture.

GENERAL CLINICAL CONSIDERATIONS

TYPES OF LOW BACK PAIN. Of the several symptoms of disease of the spine (pain, stiffness or limitation of movement, and deformity), pain is of foremost importance by virtue of its frequency and disabling effects. Four types of pain may be differentiated: local, referred, radicular, and that arising from secondary (protective) muscular spasm. One must identify these several types of pain by the patient's description, and here reliance is placed mainly on the character, location, and the conditions which modify them. The mechanism of the several types of pain has already been described in Chap. 4.

Local pain is caused by any pathologic process which impinges upon or irritates sensory endings. Involvement of structures which contain no sensory endings is painless. The substance of the vertebral body may be destroyed by tumor, for example, without evocation of pain, whereas lesions of periosteum, synovial membranes, muscles, annulus fibrosus, and ligaments are often exquisitely painful. Although painful states are often accompanied by swelling of the affected tissues, this is not apparent if a deep structure of the back is the site of disease. Local pain is steady, of the aching type, and rather diffuse but is always felt in or near the affected part of the spine. Often there is involuntary splinting of the spine segments by paravertebral muscles, and certain movements or postures which alter the position of the injured tissues aggravate or relieve the pain. Firm pressure upon superficial structures in the region of the involved structure usually evokes tenderness which is of aid in identifying the site of the abnormality.

Referred pain is of two types, that projected from the spine into regions lying within the area of the lumbar and upper sacral dermatones and that projected from the pelvic and abdominal viscera to the spine. Pain due to diseases of the upper lumbar spine is usually referred to the anterior aspects of the thighs and legs; and that from the lower lumbar spine is referred to the gluteal regions, posterior thighs, and calves. Pain of this type tends also to be deep, of aching quality, and rather diffuse. In general the referred pain parallels in intensity the local pain in the back. In other words, maneuvers which alter local pain have a similar effect on referred pain, though not with such precision and immediacy as in "root pain." Pain from visceral disease usually is felt within the abdomen or flanks and may be modified by the state of activity of the viscera. Its character and temporal relationships are those of the particular visceral structure involved, and posture and movement of the back have relatively little effect, either on the local pain or that referred to the back.

Radicular, or "root," *pain* has some of the characteristics of referred pain but differs in its greater intensity, distal radiation, circumscription to the territory of a root, and the factors which excite it. The mechanism is distortion, stretching, irritation, or compression of a spinal root, most often at the intervertebral foramen but sometimes central to this point. The pain is sharp, often quite intense, and nearly always radiates from a central position near the spine to some part of the lower extremity. It is usually superimposed on the dull ache of referred pain. Cough, sneeze, and strain characteristically evoke this sharp radiating pain, though these maneuvers may also jar or move the spine and enhance local pain. Any motion which stretches the nerve, i.e., forward bending with the knees extended or "straight-leg raising," excites radicular pain; and jugular vein compression, which raises intraspinal pressure and may cause a shift in the position of the root, has a similar effect. The fourth and fifth lumbar and first sacral roots, which form the sciatic nerve, if involved in disease, cause pain which extends mainly down the posterior aspect of thigh, the postero- and anterolateral aspects of the leg, and into the foot, in the distribution of this nerve—so-called "sciatica." Tingling, paresthesias, and numbness or sensory impairment of the skin, soreness of the skin, and tenderness along the nerve usually accompany radicular pain. Also reflex loss, weakness, atrophy, fascicular twitching, and often stasis edema may occur if motor fibers are involved in the anterior roots.

Pain resulting from muscular spasm is usually mentioned in relation to local pain, but it deserves separate consideration. As stated above, muscle spasm is associated with most conditions which result in local pain. Muscles in a state of persistent tension pull on their periosteal attachments and give rise to a dull ache, which Smith-Petersen has called "secondary pain." One can feel the tautness of the erector spinae and gluteal muscles and demonstrate by palpation that the pain is localized to them.

Other pains often of undetermined origin are sometimes described by patients with chronic disease of the lower back. In the legs drawing, pulling, cramping sensations (without involuntary muscle spasm), tearing, throbbing, or jabbing pains, feelings of burning or coldness are difficult to interpret and, like paresthesias and numbness, should always suggest the possibility of nerve or root disease.

Since it is often difficult to obtain physical or laboratory confirmation of painful disease of the lower spine, the importance of an accurate history and description of symptoms cannot be overemphasized. Frequently the most important lead comes from knowledge of the mode of onset and circumstances which initiated the pain. Inasmuch as many painful affections of the back are the result of injury incurred during work or in an accident, the possibility of exaggeration or prolongation of pain for personal reasons, or even hysteria or malingering, must always be kept in mind.

THE EXAMINATION OF THE LOWER BACK. *Inspection* of the spine, buttocks, and legs when standing erect, walking, stooping, and squatting is of value. The patient's resting posture should be noted because faulty posture, whether from congenital abnormalities or other diseases, predisposes to strain of the lumbosacral and sacroiliac regions. With sciatica the lumbar spine is often scoliotic, with the convexity toward the normal side, though the converse may occur. Also, flattening or even a slight flexion of the lumbar lordosis is common with acute painful states. The presence of

a definite kyphosis usually signifies deformity of one of the vertebral bodies, e.g., fracture. Spasm of paravertebral muscles on one or both sides is often obvious during inspection. One may also notice a hypotonia of the glutei on the affected side, with drooping of the gluteal fold.

The next step in the examination is observation of the spine, hips, and legs during certain motions. During the procedure it is well to remember that no advantage accrues from trying to find out how much the patient can be hurt. Instead, it is much more important to determine when and under what conditions the pain commences. The natural motions of the patient should be observed as he disrobes and while he is standing, sitting, and reclining, except when certain positions cannot be tolerated because of pain. When standing, the motion of forward bending normally produces flattening and reversal of the lumbar lordotic curve and exaggeration of the dorsal curve. With lesions of the lumbosacral region which involve the posterior ligaments, articular facets, or erector spinae, the patient attempts to avoid stretching these structures. As a consequence, the erectores spinae remain taut and prevent motion in the lumbar spine. Forward bending then occurs at the hips and at the lumbar-thoracic junction. With disease of the lumbosacral joints and spinal roots, the patient bends in such a way as to avoid tensing the hamstring muscles and putting leverage upon the pelvis. In unilateral "sciatica," with its increased curvature toward the side of the lesion, lumbar and lumbosacral motions are splinted and bending is mainly at the hips; at a certain point the knee on the affected side is flexed to relieve hamstring spasm and tilting of the pelvis, which stretch the roots and sciatic nerve.

Lateral bending is usually less instructive than forward bending. However, in unilateral ligamentous or muscular sprain, bending to the opposite side aggravates the pain by stretching the damaged tissues. Moreover, in lateral disk lesions, bending of the spine may be fuller toward the opposite side.

In diseases of the lower spine, flexion while sitting can normally be performed easily, even to the point of bringing the knees in contact with the chest. The reason for this is that knee flexion relaxes the hamstring muscles and the principal motion is then at the hips. The lumbar and lumbosacral joints and the normal curve of the spine need not be altered under these conditions. On the other hand, if the knees are extended, the same impedance of movement noted during forward bending, while standing with the legs straight, is observed.

The study of motions in the reclining position yields the same information as those in the standing and sitting positions, with the difference that they may also be performed passively by the examiner. Passive lumbar flexion is like active forward bending in the standing position. With lumbosacral lesions and sciatica, it causes little pain and is not limited as long as the hamstrings are relaxed (knee flexed). With lumbosacral and lumbar spine disease (e.g., arthritis), passive flexion of the hips is free, whereas flexion of the lumbar spine is impeded and painful. Passive straight-leg raising (possibly up to 90° except in those who are congenitally stiff), like forward bending in the standing posture with the leg straight, places the sciatic nerve and its roots, also the hamstrings, under tension, thereby producing pain. Consequently, in diseases of the lumbosacral joints and of the lumbosacral roots, this movement is limited on the affected side and, to a lesser extent, the opposite side. Lasègue's sign (pain and limitation of movement during elevation of the leg when the knee is extended) is but a variation of this test, as are Golthwaite's sign (limited extension at the knee after the thigh has been flexed on the trunk) and Lewin's sign (snapping back of the knee into flexion when released). The evoked pain is always referred to the diseased side, no matter which leg is flexed. In disease of the lumbosacral joints there may also be slight limitation of straight-leg raising, though rarely to the degree seen in disease of the lumbosacral roots.

The motion of hyperextension is best performed with the patient standing or lying prone. If the condition causing back pain is acute, it may be difficult to extend the spine in the standing position. A patient with lumbosacral sprain can usually extend or hyperextend the spine without aggravation of pain, since this motion tenses the iliopsoas and thereby rotates the ilium forward, relieving the pull on the lumbosacral and to some extent the sacroiliac joints. If involved in an active inflammatory or other acute process, however, tightening of the iliopsoas muscles lateral to the sacroiliac joints will exert pressure upon these joints. Also, if there is ligamentous sprain, no enhancement of pain occurs because the posterior segments of the spine are relaxed during extension. The converse is true if there is sprain of extensor muscles, for hyperextension places the muscular attachments to the periosteum under tension. Although disease of articular facets may limit extension, little or no pain is produced. In lumbar disk disease, extension of the spine is usually tolerated well, though in some patients with a displaced disk fragment situated posterolaterally pain is evoked by extension rather than flexion. A reversed Lasègue's sign (limitation in the hyperextension of straight leg while in prone position) suggests spinal nerve involvement at the midlumbar level or a lesion of the lumbosacral joint.

Palpation and percussion of the spine are the last steps in the examination. The approach must always be gentle since rough percussion of the designated area of pain only confuses the physician and antagonizes the patient. It is preferable to palpate first those regions which are the least likely to evoke pain. At all times the examiner should know what structures are being palpated (see Fig. 8-1). Localized tenderness, if pronounced, means a lesion of that region, but it is more apt to be significant in disease of the spine because the involved structures are so deep that they less often give rise to surface tenderness. Mild superficial and poorly localized tenderness signifies only a disease process within the affected segment of the body.

Tenderness over the costovertebral angle often indicates genitourinary disease, adrenal disease (Rogoff's sign), or an injury to the transverse process of the first lumbar vertebra [Fig. 8-1(1)]. Hypersensitivity on palpation of the transverse processes of the other lumbar vertebras as well as the overlying erector spinae muscles may signify fracture of the transverse process or a sprain of muscle attachments.

Upon palpation of the spinous processes and interspinous ligaments any deviation in the anteroposterior or lateral plane must be particularly noted. Such a deviation usually indicates a fracture of the spinous processes or of the vertebral bodies or other disease of these structures. Tenderness of the interspinous ligaments is indicative of acute sprain or strain [Fig. 8-1 (2)].

Tenderness in the region of the articular facets between the fifth lumbar and first sacral vertebras is consistent with a lumbosacral sprain from a hyperflexion or hyperextension injury or from strain due to faulty posture [Fig. 8-1(3)]. It is also not infrequent

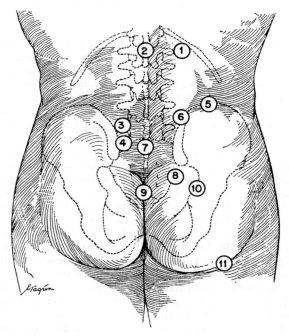

Fig. 8-1. (1) Costovertebral angle. (2) Spinous process and interspinous ligament. (3) Region of articular fifth lumbar to first sacral facet. (4) Dorsum of sacrum. (5) Region of iliac crest. (6) Iliolumbar angle. (7) Spinous processes of fifth lumbar to first sacral vertebras (tenderness = faulty posture or occasionally spina bifida occulta). (8) Region between posterior superior and posterior inferior spines. Sacroiliac ligaments (tenderness = sacroiliac sprain; often tender with fifth lumbar to first sacral disk). (9) Sacrococcygeal junction (tenderness = sacrococcygeal injury, i.e., sprain or fracture). (10) Region of sacrosciatic notch (tenderness = fourth to fifth lumbar disk rupture and sacroiliac sprain) (11) Sciatic nerve trunk (tenderness = ruptured lumbar disk or sciatic nerve lesion).

in disease of the lumbar disks with nerve root involvement.

Pain or tenderness referable to the dorsum of the sacrum is usually due to an exaggerated congenital lordosis with a postural and muscular strain and protective muscle spasm [Fig. 8-1(4)].

Tenderness in the region of the iliac crests may signify muscle sprain at the origin of the iliocostalis muscle [Fig. 8-1(5)]. Most commonly this point is used as a landmark in locating the spinous process of the third lumbar interspace. A useful sign of radicular involvement is radiation of pain in a nerve root distribution upon pressure lateral to the affected vertebra, over the point of exit of the spinal nerve.

In palpation of the iliolumbar angles, the transverse process of the fifth lumbar vertebra, the iliolumbar ligaments, and the erector spinae are the structures under the probing finger [Fig. 8-1(6)]. Tenderness at this point suggests possible fracture of the transverse process, strain of the iliolumbar ligaments due to faulty posture, as well as an acute sprain of the same structure of the erector spinae. A unilateral sacralized transverse process of the fifth lumbar vertebra sometimes gives rise to tenderness and pain referable to the iliolumbar angle.

Rectal and pelvic examination constitute an essential part of the diagnostic study of all cases of low back pain and sciatica.

Upon completion of the examination of the back a search for motor, reflex, and sensory changes (see Syndrome of Ruptured Disk, p. 40), particularly in the lower extremities, should be made.

SPECIAL LABORATORY PROCEDURES. Laboratory tests often aid in diagnosis. Depending on the circumstances, these may include measurement of the serum proteins, phosphatases (alkaline and acid), calcium, phosphorus, or uric acid. X-rays should be taken in every case of low back pain and sciatica in the anterior-posterior, lateral, and oblique planes of the lumbar spine and, at times, the thoracic spine. Stereoscopic or laminographic films may provide further information, if the regular x-rays show abnormalities. In many cases of low back pain with neurologic manifestations, examination of the spinal canal with a contrast medium (myelogram) is necessary. This study can be combined with tests of dynamics of the cerebrospinal fluid, and a sample of the fluid should always be removed for cytologic and chemical examination prior to the installation of the contrast medium (Pantopaque, Myodil, or air). Injection and removal of Pantopaque require special skill and should not be attempted without previous experience with the procedure. If done properly, the procedure is harmless. Injection of contrast medium directly into the intervertebral disk (diskograms) has recently become popular. The technique of this procedure is more complicated than that of myelographic examination, and the risk of damage to nerve roots or the introduction of infection is not inconsiderable. In the authors' opinion, the results do not warrant the risk involved.

PRINCIPAL CONDITIONS WHICH GIVE RISE TO DISABLING PAIN IN THE LOWER BACK

CONGENITAL ANOMALIES OF THE LUMBAR SPINE

Anatomic variations of the spine are not at all infrequent, and although not of themselves the source of pain and functional derangement, they may be of importance because they dispose to strain by permitting excessive mobility or the adoption of abnormal postures.

There may be a lack of fusion of the laminas of the neural arch—a spina bifida—of one or several of the lumbar vertebras, or of the sacrum. Hypertrichosis or hyperpigmentation in the sacral area may betray the condition, but it may remain entirely occult until disclosed by x-ray. The anomaly induces pain only when accompanied by malformation of vertebral joints or stretching and distortion of nerve roots. The anomaly may also condition the spine in such fashion as to encourage postural low back pain.

Spondylolysis, another important anomaly, consists of a bony defect in the pars interarticularis, which is replaced by cartilage, permitting a forward displacement of the vertebral body (spondylolisthesis), usually the fifth lumbar. Although of congenital origin, the first symptoms of disordered function (low back pain radiating to the thighs, tightness of back muscles, and signs of involvement of spinal roots—paresthesias and sensory loss, muscle weakness, and reflex impairment) may not appear until later in life and are often precipitated by an injury.

Articular facets of the vertebras may be set in an unusual plane, either oblique or frontal, rather than the sagittal one as in the normal lumbar spine; they are then unusually susceptible to injury. There may also be an abnormality of the number of mobile lumbar vertebras (either six or four). The lowest vertebra, if asymmetric in its relation to the sacrum, may give rise to chronic back pain.

TRAUMATIC AFFLICTIONS OF THE LOWER BACK

Trauma constitutes the most frequent cause of low back pain.

In severe acute injuries, the examining physician must be careful to avoid further damage. In tests of motility, all movements must be kept to a minimum until an approximate diagnosis has been made and adequate measures have been instituted for the proper care of the patient. If the patient complains of pain in his back and cannot move his legs, his spine may have been fractured. The prone position is then most advantageous, and his neck should not be flexed nor should he be allowed to sit up. (See Chap. 203 for further discussion of spinal cord injury.)

SPRAINS AND STRAINS. The terms *strain* and *sprain* are used loosely by most physicians. Strain should designate a minor injury which does not produce gross structural damage. The abnormal mechanical force may be acute, as in heavy lifting, or mild and persistent, due to maintenance of an abnormal posture. The latter is often occupational. Rest and relaxation promptly alleviate the discomfort, attesting to the lack of major structural change. Sprain, properly speaking, refers to an injury of joints, muscles, tendons, and ligaments (i.e., annulus fibrosus). In other words, definite structural damage has occurred. Both strains and sprains of the back are caused by lifting heavy objects, with the spine in a position of imperfect mechanical balance, as when lifting and turning at the same time. Sudden unexpected motion is particularly dangerous.

The diagnosis of strains and sprains of the various structures of the lower back depends upon the description of the injury, the localization of the pain by the patient, the finding of localized tenderness, and the augmentation of pain when tension is exerted on the involved muscles, ligaments, and joints by the appropriate maneuvers. The prompt alleviation of the pain by rest and relaxation indicates the existence of a strain. Sprain of the back responds less rapidly to such simple measures. It may, however, be relieved by local infiltration of an anesthetic agent, a finding which is also helpful in diagnosis.

Sacroiliac sprain, one so popular as an explanation of unilateral back pain, is now highly controversial. Because of their irregular surfaces the sacroiliac bones are interlocked, and joint movement is minimal and is further restricted by strong sacroiliac ligaments. Only violent injury could derange this well-protected and stable joint. When the joint is injured, the principal symptom is a localized ache which is made worse by rotatory movements of the pelvis, local percussion, and reverse Lasègue sign. It must be remembered that involvement of a spinal nerve root (fifth lumbar or first sacral) associated with injury to the disk is the more common cause of pain and local tenderness in the area of the sacroiliac joint.

VERTEBRAL FRACTURES. Fractures of the lumbar vertebral body are usually the result of flexion injuries. Spasm of the lower lumbar muscles, limitation of movements of the lumbar spine, and the x-ray appearance of the damaged portion of the lumbar spine (with or without neurologic abnormalities) are the basis of clinical diagnosis. The pain is usually immediate, though occasionally it may be delayed for days, and some patients are found to have had crushed fractures of the vertebral body without being able to recall any traumatic episode.

Fractured transverse processes, which are almost always associated with tearing of the psoas muscle, are diagnosed by the finding of deep tenderness at the site of the injury, local muscle spasm on one side, and limitation of all movements which stretch the lumbar muscles. Radiologic evidence provides the final confirmation.

PROTRUSION OF LUMBAR INTERVERTEBRAL DISKS. This is now recognized as the major cause of severe and chronic or recurrent low back and leg pain. This condition is most likely to occur between the fifth lumbar and first sacral vertebras and with lessening frequency between the fourth to fifth lumbar, the third to fourth lumbar, the second to third lumbar, and the first to second lumbar vertebras. Almost nonexistent in the thoracic spine, it is next most frequent at the sixth to seventh and fifth to sixth cervical vertebras. The cause is usually a flexion injury, but in a considerable proportion of cases no trauma is recalled. Degeneration and minor trauma of posterior longitudinal ligaments and the annulus fibrosus, which occurs in many adults of middle and advanced years, may have taken place silently or have been manifested by mild, recurrent lumbar ache. A sneeze, lurch, or other trivial injury may then cause the nucleus pulposus to extrude through the frayed ligament.

The fully developed syndrome of ruptured intervertebral disk consists of a combination of orthopedic and neurologic abnormalities. The orthopedic symptoms and signs comprise backache, abnormal posture, and limitation of motion of the spine (particularly flexion). The neurologic manifestations are those of nerve root involvement and include radicular pain, sensory disturbances (paresthesias, hyper- and hyposensitivity in dermatome pattern), motor abnormalities (weakness and atrophy, coarse twitching and fasciculation, and muscle spasms), and impairment of tendon reflexes. Since herniation of the intervertebral lumbar disks most often occurs between the fourth and fifth lumbar vertebras and the fifth lumbar and first sacral vertebras with irritation and compression of the fifth lumbar and first sacral roots, respectively, it is important to recognize the clinical characteristics of lesions of these two roots. *Lesions of the fifth lumbar* root produce pain in the region of the hip, groin, posterolateral thigh, lateral calf to the external malleolus, dorsal surface of the foot, and the first or second and third toes. Paresthesias may be in the entire territory or only the distal parts of these territories. The tenderness is in the lateral gluteal region and near the head of the fibula. Weakness, if present, involves the extensor of the big toe and of the foot. Either the knee or ankle reflex may be diminished, but these reflexes are usually unchanged. Walking on the heels may be more uncomfortable than walking on the toes. In *lesions of the first sacral* root the pain is felt in the midgluteal region, posterior thigh, posterior calf to the heel, and the plantar surface of the foot and fourth and fifth toes. Tenderness is most pronounced over the midgluteal region (sacroiliac joint), posterior thigh, and calf. Paresthesias and sensory loss are mainly in the lower leg and outer toes, and weakness, if present, involves the flexor muscles of the foot and toes, abductors of the toes, and hamstring muscles. The angle reflex is diminished to absent in the majority of cases. Walking on the toes is more uncomfortable than on the heels. Straight-leg raising during the acute, painful stages is present with lesions of either root.

The rarer *lesions of the fourth and third lumbar roots* give rise to pain in the anterior part of the thigh and knee, with corresponding sensory loss. The kneejerk is diminished or abolished. An inverted Lasègue sign is positive when the third lumbar root is affected.

The syndrome is usually unilateral. Only with massive derangements of the disks do bilateral symptoms and signs occur, and these may then be associated with paralysis of the sphincters. The pain may be mild or severe. All or part of the above syndrome may be present. There may be back pain with little or no leg pain; rarely leg pain may be experienced without pain in the back. The rupture of multiple lumbar or lumbar and cervical disks is not infrequent, attesting to a basic disorder of the annulus fibrosus.

When all parts of the syndrome are present, both the skeletal as well as the neurologic components, the diagnosis is easy; when only one part is present, particularly backache, it may be difficult, especially if there has been no accident. Since similar symptoms may occur without demonstrable disk rupture, other diagnostic procedures are required. Plain x-rays usually show no abnormality or at most a narrowing of the intervertebral space; hence one must resort to Pantopaque myelography. This will reveal in most cases an indentation of the lumbar subarachnoid space or deformity of the root sleeve. Unfortunately, a small ruptured disk may not show. The electromyogram is helpful in showing denervation of leg muscles (see p. 1363). The protein of the cerebrospinal fluid is elevated in some instances.

Tumor of the spinal canal, epidural or intradural, may produce a syndrome similar to that of ruptured disk (see Chap. 206).

ARTHRITIS

Arthritis will be discussed more fully elsewhere. It need only be mentioned that hypertrophic arthritis is much more frequent than rheumatoid and that the latter may take two forms, one in which the spine involvement is but a part of a generalized arthritis, often with other signs of "connective tissue disease," and the other limited almost exclusively to the spine, sacroiliac joints, and hips (rheumatoid spondylitis or Marie-Strümpell arthritis) (p. 1363). An extreme form of hypertrophic arthritis in the cervical region, sometimes leading to spinal cord or nerve compression, is called *spondylosis* (see Chap. 237).

Rheumatoid spondylitis, which often begins with involvement of the sacroiliac joints, induces continuous aching pain and stiffness in the back or in the buttocks and thighs. Rarely, however, the disease reaches an advanced degree without pain. Acute painful exacerbations are probably due to involvement of the apophyseal joints. The pain is centered in the spine and is worse on movement, especially after the patient has been inactive. Pain during the night or in the early morning hours is another common feature. It may be partially relieved by activity and is often aggravated by seasonal and barometric changes. The effect of salicylates, which usually alleviate the pain to some degree, may be taken as another diagnostic feature. Signs of root involvement are incompatible with the diagnosis of rheumatoid arthritis.

In *hypertrophic arthritis,* by contrast, pain in the spine may or may not be accompanied by the motor, reflex, or sensory changes of root involvement. The pain in the spine is of the same type as in rheumatoid spondylitis and is also accompanied by a sense of stiffness and limitation of movement. It differs slightly in being more clearly aggravated by motion, more readily relieved by rest, and less pronounced at night. The severity of the pain is not clearly related to the degree of the process as seen in the x-ray. X-ray evidence of the disease in the spine is found in a majority of individuals beyond the age of fifty as is also clicking in the neck on head movement. The presence of such changes should not be accepted as establishing an arthritic source of a severe and progressive pain, since it may be due to a more serious unrelated condition, such as a neoplasm.

Injury may exacerbate the pain of both rheumatoid and hypertrophic arthritis. (See Chap. 237 for further discussion of spondylitis.)

DESTRUCTIVE DISEASES

These may be neoplastic, infectious, or metabolic. Metastatic carcinoma (breast, bronchus, prostate, thyroid, hypernephroma, stomach, uterus), multiple myeloma, and lymphoma are the common tumors which involve the spine; tuberculosis and pyogenic osteomyelitis are the most frequent infections, though brucellosis, typhoid fever, actinomycosis, and blastomycosis are known to occur.

Special mention should be made of the spinal *epidural abscess* (usually staphylococcal), which necessitates urgent surgical treatment. The symptoms are a localized pain, spontaneous as well as on percussion and palpation, often with radicular radiation, and a rapidly developing flaccid paraplegia appearing in a febrile patient.

Destructive lesions of any type may develop silently, i.e., without any pain, as long as they are limited to the osseous tissue. Upon spreading to the periosteum or to the adjacent spinous structures, however, they become the source of much pain of both local and referred type, and often one or more spinal roots are implicated as well, with the typical radicular type being added to the clinical picture. Pain caused by neoplasms of the spine is of aching character and more or less steady, though occasionally waxing and waning. It is especially severe at night, seeming to be only slightly benefited by rest; yet activity during the day also worsens the pain. As the disease progresses, the pain increases in duration and severity. It may then be of a throbbing character. The most important physical finding, which should lead one to suspect a destructive lesion, is an intensification of the pain by jarring the spine, by percussing the spinous processes gently with the fist or a reflex hammer, or by exerting a steady pressure upon these parts. Axial compression (downward pressure exerted on the head or falling on the heels) may also serve to intensify the pain. Nocturnal pain, spinal ache, and percussion sensitivity are also characteristic of Pott's disease and osteomyelitis. The establishment of the cause of the pain is often delayed because the first x-rays may not disclose the lesion. If these are negative, they should be repeated after an interval of a few weeks. Other laboratory data such as white blood count and smear, sedimentation rate, and levels of globulin, acid and alkaline phosphatase in the serum are helpful.

In so-called "metabolic bone diseases" (osteoporosis of either the postmenopausal or senile type or osteomalacia) a considerable degree of demineralization may occur without any symptoms whatsoever. Many such patients do, however, complain of aching in the lumbar or thoracic area. This is most likely to occur following an injury, sometimes of trivial degree, which leads to collapse or wedging of a vertebra. Certain movements greatly enhance the pain, and certain positions relieve it. One or more spinal roots may then be involved. Paget's disease of the spine is nearly always painless. The recognition of these bone disorders is discussed in some detail elsewhere (Chaps. 226 to 231).

REFERRED PAIN FROM VISCERAL DISEASE

The pain of disease of the pelvic, abdominal, or thoracic viscera is often felt in the region of the spine; i.e., it is referred to the more posterior parts of the spinal segment which innervates the diseased organ. Occasionally back pain may be the first and only sign. The general rule is that pelvic diseases are referred to the sacral region, lower abdominal disease to the lumbar region (centering around the second to fourth lumbar vertebras), and upper abdominal diseases to the lower thoracic spine (eighth thoracic to the first and second lumbar vertebras). Characteristically there are no local signs, no stiffness of the back, and motion is of full range without augmentation of the pain. However, some positions, e.g., flexion of the lumbar spine in the lateral recumbent position, may be more comfortable than others.

LOW THORACIC AND UPPER LUMBAR PAIN IN ABDOMINAL DISEASE. Peptic ulceration or tumor of the wall of the stomach and of the duodenum most typically induces pain in the epigastrium (see Chaps. 24 to 26 and 180); but if the posterior wall is involved and particularly if there is retroperitoneal extension, the pain may be felt in the region of the spine. Usually the pain is central in location or is more intense on one side. If very intense it may seem to encircle the body. It tends to retain the characteristics of pain from the affected organ; e.g., if due to peptic ulceration, it is relieved by food and soda and appears about 2 hr after a meal.

Diseases of the pancreas (peptic ulceration with extension to the pancreas, cholecystitis with pancreatitis, tumor) are apt to cause pain in the back, being more to the right of the spine if the head of the pancreas is involved and to the left if the body and tail are implicated.

Diseases of retroperitoneal structures, e.g., lymphomas, sarcomas, and carcinomas, may evoke pain in this part of the spine with some tendency toward radiation to the lower abdomen, groins, and anterior thighs. A secondary tumor of the ileopsoas region on one side often produces a unilateral lumbar ache with radiation toward the groin and labia or testicle; there may also be signs of involvement of the upper lumbar spinal roots. An aneurysm of the abdominal aorta may induce a pain which is localized to this region of the spine but may be felt higher or lower, depending on the location of the lesion.

The sudden appearance of obscure lumbar pain in a patient receiving anticoagulants should arouse the suspicion of retroperitoneal bleeding.

LUMBAR PAIN WITH LOWER ABDOMINAL DISEASES. Inflammatory diseases of segments of the colon (colitis, diverticulitis) or tumor of the colon cause pain which may be felt in the lower abdomen between the umbilicus and pubis, or in the midlumbar region, or in both places; and if very intense, it may have a beltlike distribution around the body. A lesion in the transverse colon or first part of the descending colon may be central or left-sided, and its level of reference to the back is to the second to third lumbar vertebras. If the sigmoid colon is implicated, the pain is lower, in the upper sacral region and anteriorly in the midline suprapubic region or left lower quadrant of the abdomen.

SACRAL PAIN IN PELVIC (UROLOGIC AND GYNECOLOGIC) DISEASES. Although gynecologic disorders may manifest themselves by back pain, the pelvis is seldom the site of a disease which causes obscure low back pain. For the most part the diagnosis of painful pelvic lesions is not difficult, for a thorough palpation of structures by abdominal, vaginal, and rectal examination may be supplemented by methods (sigmoidoscopy, barium enema, pyelography) which adequately visualize all these parts.

Menstrual pain itself may be felt in the sacral region. It is rather poorly localized, tends to radiate down the legs, and is of a crampy nature. The most important source of chronic back pain from the pelvic organs, however, is the uterosacral ligaments. Endometriosis or carcinoma of the uterus (body or cervix) may invade these structures, while malposition of the uterus may pull on them. The pain is localized centrally in the sacrum below the lumbosacral joint but may be more on one side. In endometriosis the pain begins during the premenstrual phase and often continues, merging with menstrual pain. Malposition of the uterus (retroversion, descensus, and prolapse) characteristically leads to sacral pain, especially after the patient has been standing for several hours. Posture may also evoke pain here when a fibroma of the uterus pulls on the uterosacral ligaments. Carcinomatous pain due to implication of nerve plexuses is continuous and becomes progressively more severe; it tends to be more intense at night. The primary lesion may be inconspicuous, being overlooked upon pelvic examination. Papanicolaou smears and a pyelogram are the most useful diagnostic procedures. X-ray therapy of these tumors may produce sacral pain consequent to swelling and necrosis of tissue, the so-called "radiation phlegmon of the pelvis." Low back pain with radiation into one or both thighs is a common phenomenon during the last weeks of pregnancy.

Chronic prostatitis, evidenced by prostatic discharge, frequency of urination, and slight reduction in sexual potency, may be attended by a nagging sacral ache; it may be mainly on one side, with radiation into one leg if the seminal vesicle is involved on that side. Carcinoma of the prostate with metastases to the lower spine is another cause of sacral or lumbar pain. It may be present without urinary frequency or burning. Spinal nerves may be infiltrated by tumor cells, or the spinal cord itself may be compressed if the epidural space is invaded. The diagnosis is established by rectal examination, x-rays of the spine, and measurement of acid phosphatase (particularly the prostatic phosphatase fraction). Lesions of the bladder and testes are usually not accompanied by back pain. When the kidney is the site of disease, the pain is ipsilateral, being felt in the flank or lumbar region.

Visceral derangements of whatever type may intensify the pain of arthritis, and the presence of arthritis may alter the distribution of visceral pain. With disease of the spine in the lumbosacral region, for example, distension of the ampulla of the sigmoid by feces or a bout of colitis may aggravate the arthritic pain. In patients with arthritis of the cervical or thoracic spine, the pain of myocardial ischemia may radiate to the back.

OBSCURE TYPES OF LOW BACK PAIN AND THE QUESTION OF PSYCHIATRIC DISEASE

The practicing physician is consulted by many individuals who complain of low back pain of obscure origin. A safe rule is to assume that all of them have some type of primary or secondary disease of the spine and its supporting structures or of the abdominal or pelvic viscera. If the pain is of acute onset and short duration, it may be due to only a minor trauma, a "fibrositis," or some form of articular disease. If it is recurrent, the possibility of a ruptured disk, an instability of the spine due to a congenital malformity, or the effects of bad posture must be considered. If it is severe and progressive, neoplasia, a tuberculous infection, and rheumatoid spondylitis should be kept in mind. Adolescent girls are subject to an obscure form of epiphyseal disease of the spine (Scheuermann's disease) which may cause low back pain with exercise over a period of 2 to 3 years.

POSTURAL BACK PAIN

Many slender asthenic individuals, some with a disposition to anxiety or neurocirculatory asthenia, have discomfort in the back. Their backs ache much of the time, and the pain interferes with effective work. The physical examination is negative except for slack musculature and poor posture. The pain is diffuse in the mid or low back and characteristically is relieved by bed rest and induced by the maintenance of a particular posture over a period of time. Pain in the neck and between the shoulder blades is a common complaint among thin, tense, active women and seems to be related to taut trapezius muscles.

PSYCHIATRIC ILLNESS

Low back pain may be encountered in compensation hysteria and malingering, in anxiety or neurocirculatory asthenia (formerly called neurasthenia), in depression and hypochondriasis, and in many nervous individuals whose symptoms and complaints do not fall within any category of psychiatric illness.

Again it is probably correct to assume that pain in the back in such patients usually signifies disease of the spine and adjacent structures, and this should always be carefully looked for. However, the pain may be exaggerated, prolonged, or woven into a pattern of invalidism or disability because of coexistent or secondary psychologic factors. This is especially true when there is the possibility of personal gain (notably compensation). The patients seeking compensation from protracted low back pain without obvious structural disease tend, after a time, to become suspicious, hostile toward the medical profession or anyone who might question the authenticity of their illness, and they are uncooperative. One notes in them a tendency to describe their pain poorly and to prefer, instead, to discuss the degree of their disability and their mistreatment in the hands of the medical profession. These features and a negative examination of the back should lead one to suspect a psychologic factor. A few patients, usually frank malingerers, adopt the most bizarre attitudes, being unable to straighten up, walking with trunk flexed at almost a right angle (camptocormia) (see Chap. 214).

The depressed and hypochondriac patient represents a troublesome problem, and a common error is to minimize the importance of anxiety and depression or to ascribe them to worry over the illness and its social effects. The more common and minor back ailments, e.g., those due to osteoarthritis and postural ache, are enhanced and rendered intolerable by the irritable moodiness and self-concern. The disability seems excessive for the degree of spinal malfunction, and misery and despair are the prevailing features of the syndrome. One of the most reliable diagnostic measures is the response to drugs which alleviate the depression (see Chap. 215).

PAIN IN THE NECK AND SHOULDER

This topic has been discussed to some extent in the chapter on thoracic pain, and further references will be found under Pain in the Extremities.

It is useful to distinguish here three major categories of painful disease—those of the spine, cervical plexus, and shoulder. Although the pains in these three regions of the body may overlap, the patient himself usually can indicate the site of the origin. Pain arising from the cervical spine is nearly always felt in the spine (though it may be projected to the shoulder and arm), is evoked or enhanced by certain movements or positions of the neck, and is accompanied by tenderness and limitations of motions of the neck. Similarly, pain of brachial plexus origin is experienced in and around the shoulder, is induced by the performance of certain tasks with the arm and by certain positions, and is associated with tenderness of structures above the clavicle. There may be a palpable abnormality above the clavicle (aneurysms of subclavian artery, tumor, cervical rib). The combination of circulatory symptoms and signs referable to the lower part of the brachial plexus, manifested in the hand by obliteration of pulse when the patient takes and holds a full breath with the head tilted back or turned (Adson's test), unilateral Raynaud's phenomenon, trophic changes in the fingers, sensory loss over the ulnar side of the hand with or without interosseous atrophy, completes the clinical picture. X-rays showing a cervical rib or deformed thoracic outlet or superior sulcus tumor of the lung (Pancoast syndrome) offer confirmation of the diagnosis. Shoulder pain is localized to the shoulder region, is influenced by motion, and is associated with tenderness and limitation of motions (extension, abduction, external and internal rotation). Here, the most common diseases are bursitis and tear of the rotator cuff. Spine, plexus, and shoulder pain all may radiate into the arm or hand, but sensory, motor, and reflex changes always indicate involvement of nerve roots (in disease of the spine), plexus, or nerves.

Hypertrophic arthritis of the cervical spine may cause pains which radiate into the back of the head, shoulders, and arms on one or both sides of the thorax. Coincident involvement of nerve roots is manifested by paresthesias, sensory loss, weakness, or tendon reflex change. Should bony ridges form in the spinal canal (spondylosis), the spinal cord may be compressed, with resulting weakness and atrophy and sometimes sensory disturbances in the arms and spastic weakness and ataxia with loss of vibratory and position sense in the legs. A Pantopaque cervical myelogram reveals the degree of encroachment on the spinal canal and the level at which the spinal cord is affected. The authors have experienced the greatest difficulty in distinguishing spondylosis with spinal cord compression from primary neurologic diseases (syringomyelia, amyotrophic lateral sclerosis, ruptured disk, or tumor) with an unrelated hypertrophic arthritis of the cervical spine, particularly at the fifth to sixth and sixth to seventh cervical vertebras, where the disk spaces are often narrowed in the adult. A combination of nervous tension with hypertrophic arthritis of the cervical spine or a painful injury to ligaments and muscles after an accident in which the neck is forcibly extended and flexed (e.g., whiplash injury to spine) are extremely vexatious clinical syndromes. If the pain is persistent and limited to the neck, the problem will usually prove to have been complicated by psychologic factors.

One of the commonest causes of neck, shoulder, and arm pain is disk herniation in the lower cervical region. As with rupture of the lumbar disks, the syndrome includes the aforementioned disorder of spinal function and evidence of neural involvement. It develops after a trauma which may be major or minor (sudden hyperextension of the neck, diving, forceful manipulations, chiropractic treatment, etc.). Virtually every patient exhibits an abnormality in full motion of the neck (limitation and pain). Hyperextension is the movement that most consistently aggravates the pain. With laterally situated disk lesions between the fifth to sixth cervical vertebras, the symptoms and signs are referred to the sixth cervical roots, i.e., pain felt at the trapezius ridge, tip of the shoulder, anterior upper arm, radial forearm, and often in the thumb; paresthesias and sensory impairment or hypersensitivity in the same regions; tenderness in the area above the spine of the scapula and in the supraclavicular and biceps regions; weakness in flexion of the forearm; diminished to absent biceps and supinator reflexes (triceps retained or exaggerated). With sixth to seventh cervical disk disease and involvement of the seventh cervical root, the pain is in the region of the shoulder blade, pectoral region and medial axilla, posterolateral upper arm, dorsal forearm and elbow, index and middle fingers, or all the fingers; tenderness is most pronounced over the medial aspect of the shoulder blade opposite the third to fourth thoracic spinous processes, in the supraclavicular area and triceps region; paresthesias and sensory loss are most pronounced in the second and third fingers or tips of all the fingers; weakness is in extension of the forearm (occasionally wrist drop is present) and in the hand grip; the triceps reflex is diminished to absent, and the biceps and supinator reflexes are preserved. Cough, sneeze, and downward pressure on the head in the hyperextension position exacerbate pain, and traction (even manual) tends to relieve it.

Unlike lumbar disks, the cervical ones, if large and centrally situated, may result in compression of the spinal cord (central disk, all of the cord; paracentral disk, part of the cord, i.e., Brown-Séquard syndrome). The central disk is often nearly painless, and the cord syndrome may simulate a degenerative disease (amyotrophic lateral sclerosis, combined system disease). A common error is to fail to think of a ruptured disk in the cervical region in patients with obscure symptoms in the legs. The diagnosis of ruptured cervical disk should be confirmed by the same laboratory procedures that were mentioned under lumbar disk.

Metastases in the cervical spine may be very painful, but the problem is not different from that of secondary deposits of tumor in other parts of the spine.

Shoulder injuries (rotator cuff), subacromial or subdeltoid bursitis, the frozen shoulder (periarthritis or capsulitis), tendinitis, and arthritis may develop in patients who are otherwise well, but these conditions are more frequent in hemiplegics or in individuals suffering from coronary heart disease. The pain is often severe and extends toward the neck and down the arm into the hand. The dorsum of the latter may tingle without other signs of nerve involvement. Vasomotor changes also may occur in the hand (shoulder-hand syndrome), and after a time osteoporosis and atrophy of cutaneous and subcutaneous structures occur (Sudeck's atrophy or Sudeck-Leriche syndrome). These conditions fall more within the province of orthopedics than of medicine and will not be discussed in detail.

The carpal tunnel syndrome with paresthesias and numbness in palmar distribution of the median nerve and aching pain which extends up into the forearm may be mistaken for disease of the shoulder or neck.

MANAGEMENT OF BACK PAIN

A muscular sprain is always benign in character, and one may expect full recovery in 2 to 4 weeks. Ligamentous sprains, if severe, may last longer, from 6 to 12 weeks. The underlying principle of therapy in both is immobilization or protection in a position that relaxes and removes pressure from the injured structure. If the erector spinae are sprained, the optimal position is hyperextension; the same is true of sprains of the posterior and sacroiliac ligaments. This position is best maintained by having the patient lie with a small pillow or blanket under the lumbar spine or lie face down. During the acute phase of any injury of this type, the application of cold, in the form of an ice bag or cold water bottle (ethyl chloride spray of the skin is said to give dramatic relief at times), is indicated. It reduces the circulation and consequently the swelling. After the third or fourth day, heat is desirable to improve the circulation and to relax protective muscle spasm. Analgesic medication should be given liberally during the first few days [codeine 30 mg and aspirin 0.6 Gm, meperidine (Demerol) 50 mg, or morphine 10 to 15 mg]. When ready for ambulation, after some days in bed, the patient may need protection of the injured part, preferably adhesive strapping in case of muscle sprain or a belt or brace. Plaster casts should be avoided. Ambulatory treatment is supplemented by corrective exercises designed to overcome faulty position and to increase the mobility of the spinal joints. Only if these measures prove inadequate and the patient is partially disabled over long periods of time by an unstable, painful lower back (recurrent lumbosacral backache) should operative intervention, usually some form of fusion operation, be considered.

In the treatment of an acute rupture of a lumbar or cervical disk, complete bed rest is essential and strong analgesic medication is required. Traction is of little value in lumbar disk disease, and it is best to permit the patient to find the most comfortable position. Later, traction, if of any value, keeps the patient confined to bed. In contrast, traction is of great help in rupture of cervical disks. Often the pain subsides after 2 to 3 weeks in bed, and the patient may remain free of pain upon resuming normal activities. Or he may suffer some minor recurrence but be able to carry on his usual activities, and eventually he will recover. There is always danger of relapse. To prevent this, mild muscle-strengthening exercises of the spine

after the pain has subsided (see Fig. 8-2) and avoidance of activities which favor spine injury (see Fig. 8-3) are recommended. If the pain does not subside after a trial of prolonged bed rest (several weeks) and the myelogram demonstrates a large disk, an operative removal, preferably without spine fusion, should be undertaken. The final decision as to the time and necessity of surgery depends on the duration and gravity of the pain and the neurologic disorder.

For the many patients with back pain who do not fall into any one of the above categories, simple measures are beneficial. For the adolescent with a suspicion of epiphyseal disease, restricted activity (avoidance of vigorous sports) for a few months or years and a supporting garment help. Muscle-strengthening exercises and a physical conditioning program are indicated for postural backache (see Fig. 8-2). Spine fusion should be reserved only for the exceptional patient with disabling and persistent pains.

Spondylosis of the cervical spine, if painful, is helped by bed rest and traction; if signs of spinal cord involvement are present, a collar to limit movement may halt the progression and even lead to improve-

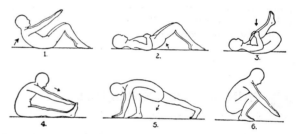

Fig. 8-2. Front of postural instruction sheet. Patient is instructed as follows:

Exercises should be taken on a padded floor. Exercise 4 should be omitted unless otherwise instructed. Start exercises by doing each one ——— times morning and evening, increasing the series one a day until you are doing each one ——— times morning and evening. Exercises are essential in obtaining a proper muscular balance, but a correct posture is acquired only through conscious effort.

Remember—
1. When standing or walking, toe straight ahead and take most of your weight on heels.
2. Try to form a crease across the upper abdomen by holding the chest up and forward and elevating the front of the pelvis.
3. Avoid high heels as much as possible.
4. Sit with the buttocks "tucked under" so that the hollow in the low back is eradicated.
5. When possible, elevate the knees higher than the hips while sitting. This is especially important when driving (driver's seat forward) or riding as a passenger in an automobile.
6. Sleep on your back with knees propped up or on your side with one or both knees drawn up. Bed should be firm.
7. Do not lift loads in front of you above the waist line.
8. Never bend backward.
9. Do not bend forward with knees straight. Always "squat."
10. Avoid standing as much as possible.
Learn to Live 24 Hours a Day without a Hollow in the Lower Part of Your Back

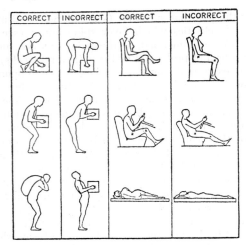

| CORRECT | INCORRECT | CORRECT | INCORRECT |

Fig. 8-3. Reverse side of postural instruction sheet showing correct and incorrect methods of lifting, sitting, and sleeping.

ment. Decompressive laminectomy with sectioning of denticulate ligaments is reserved for severe instances of the disease with advancing neurologic symptoms. The shoulder-hand syndrome may benefit from stellate ganglion blocks or ganglionectomy, but the basic treatment is physiotherapy, with surgical procedures being used only as measures of last resort.

9 PAIN IN THE EXTREMITIES

Eugene A. Stead, Jr.

Pain in the extremities comes from disturbances within the tissues of the extremities or from irritation at any level of the sensory nerve paths serving the extremity, or it is referred from deep somatic or visceral structures.

DISTURBANCES WITHIN THE TISSUES

Any lesion causing inflammation, swelling, ischemia, or destruction of pain-sensitive tissues of the extremity may cause pain. Burns, frostbite, and chemical injuries are painful. Arthritis, cellulitis, abscesses, osteomyelitis and hematomas, tumors, Paget's disease, and bone changes with hyperparathyroidism cause varying degrees of pain. Degeneration of nerves and trauma to nerve trunks are painful. Damage to nerves or to muscles from ischemia is painful.

IRRITATION OF SENSORY NERVES

Involvement of the nerves at any point in their course from the extremity to the spinal cord may cause pain in the extremity. The pain of cervical rib, ruptured intervertebral disk, spinal cord tumor, and tabes dorsalis falls into this group. Central pain from involvement of the spinothalamic tract and thalamus is occasionally seen.

PAIN REFERRED FROM DEEP STRUCTURES

The pain of angina pectoris and myocardial infarction frequently radiates to the inner surfaces of the arms. Pain from the hip may be referred to the knee. Pain from the deep muscles of the back or from the vertebras may be the source of pain referred to the extremity.

CAUSES OF PAIN IN THE EXTREMITIES

PAIN FROM TRAUMA, INFLAMMATION, AND SWELLING. The immediate response to trauma is due to mechanical stimulation of nerve endings. Pain persisting after the injury may result from chemical stimuli produced by the injured tissues. Lewis has described the reactions in skin made hyperalgesic by injury. Needle pricks too light to awaken pain in uninjured skin will arouse a response in a traumatized area. Pain is easily induced by friction or warming, and often by cooling. Distension of the skin by direct stretching or by venous congestion causes pain. If injured skin is rubbed, pain is felt immediately; this subsides and is followed in about 15 sec by a second pain which lasts a minute or more. If the circulation to the part is obstructed, the initial pain is unaltered, but the second pain rises to a greater intensity and persists until approximately 1 min after the circulation is restored. The first pain comes from direct stimulation of sensory nerves, the second from a relatively stable pain-giving substance released into, and held within, the tissue space. The chemical nature of this substance is not known. Skin made hyperalgesic by injury, regardless of the mechanism of the injury, will respond to heat and congestion with burning pain. If this reaction occurs diffusely in the skin of the extremities without obvious cause, the burning pain from warmth and congestion is called *erythromelalgia*.

The injury to the skin caused by heat is well recognized. That prolonged cold will cause tissue damage in many ways comparable to burns is less commonly realized. Prolonged immersion of the feet or prolonged exposure to cold with the feet in wet boots will cause severe tissue damage to the point of gangrene, even though actual freezing does not occur. Freezing, of course, causes tissue damage and may produce gangrene. Fibrosis and ischemic neuritis are common after any form of injury from cold and may cause persistent tenderness and pain.

In bacterial infections, the mechanical factor of rapidly forming edema increases local tissue pressure and causes pain in skin already made hyperalgesic by chemical factors associated with injury. Congestion aggravates the pain, and elevation of the part alleviates it. Less rapid edema formation usually does not cause pain, because the tissues stretch gradually. Patients with cardiac edema complain of heaviness of the legs and occasionally of diffuse tenderness. Edema associated with varicose veins may cause a sense of fullness and dull ache. In acute thrombophlebitis, pain may arise from the involved veins. It may be aggra-

vated by ischemia secondary to sympathetic vasoconstriction resulting from the sensory stimuli from the
inflamed veins. Tumor masses may cause pressure on
bone or peripheral nerves.

Arthritis is a common cause of pain in the extremities. When the process is *acute,* as in pyogenic arthritis, gout, and many cases of rheumatic fever, pain
is likely to be severe at rest and intensified by the
slightest movement. The other signs of inflammation
—swelling, redness, and warmth—are pronounced.

In chronic arthritis of the degenerative type, which
is especially common in the knees (p. 1358), pain is
usually present only on motion, although there may
be minimal discomfort at rest because of local spasm
of muscles. Heat and redness are lacking, and swelling
may be present or absent. In elderly women with
arthritis of the distal interphalangeal joints (Heber-
den's nodes), pain may be lacking despite striking
deformity.

Rheumatoid arthritis (p. 1352), which is often most
pronounced in the hands, is characterized by marked
fluctuations in the intensity of the inflammation, and
hence of the pain. Prolonged periods of freedom from
symptoms other than slight stiffness in the morning
and minimal swelling alternate with exacerbations of
mild to severe aching, associated with swelling and
heat and lasting a few hours to many weeks.

Pain arising in the bones of the extremities is likely
to be severe, throbbing, worse at night, and associated
with pronounced localized tenderness. Trauma, osteomyelitis, neoplasms, metabolic diseases of bone (p.
1335), and pulmonary osteoarthropathy are the most
important causes.

The syndrome of sore, painful shoulder with superficial and deep areas of exquisite tenderness is common. It frequently begins as wryneck and at times occurs in a number of persons closely associated with
one another. Marked spasm prevents abduction of
the arm at the shoulder. The entire upper extremity
may feel numb and queer. There is no fever. Biopsy
of the skin and muscles shows apparently normal tissues. Light freezing of the skin with ethyl chloride or
procainization of the superficial and deep tender areas
frequently gives dramatic relief of pain, relief which
may be permanent. The mechanism of pain production in this syndrome is not known.

**PAIN FROM ISCHEMIA, THROMBOSIS, EMBOLISM,
AND ARTERITIS.** Interference with blood supply may
result from obliterative arterial disease or embolus or
from arteriolar spasm secondary to stimulation of
sensory receptors or nerves. It may be aggravated in
polycythemia by the adverse effect of increased viscosity of the blood. The pain may be produced by the
action on sensory nerve endings of metabolites accumulating in the muscles or by changes in the nerves
themselves.

The sensations produced by ischemia to the extremity are familiar to all. When the blood supply is
occluded, the part gradually becomes numb and
paralyzed and we say the part has "gone to sleep." If
the part is not moved, pain does not develop. The

sensation at the end of the fingers becomes dulled in
about 12 to 15 min. At that time, light pressure on
the fingers may hurt, and stroking the finger tips
causes an unpleasant sensation. Later, pain is dulled,
and much later, analgesia develops. On release of the
arterial occlusion, unpleasant tingling occurs, particularly in the fingers. This tingling is not the result
of the inrush of blood into the fingers, because it
occurs if blood is released only into the proximal part
of the extremity. It results from changes in the main
nerves of the arm during recovery. Stroking the fingers
accentuates it. The paresthesias produced by the
injury and recovery of the nerve from ischemia are
similar to those produced by chronic disease processes
involving the peripheral nerves or nerve roots.

If the extremity is exercised while the circulation
is completely occluded, a continuous diffuse aching
pain develops in the muscles because the sensory
nerves are stimulated by the formation of stable
metabolites. The pain is present during and between
contractions. It is frequently described as a cramp,
but the muscles are flaccid. If the contractions are
continued, the muscles become tender. On release of
the tourniquet, the pain disappears in a few seconds,
probably as the result of the carrying away of readily
diffusible metabolites.

If the brachial artery at the elbow or the femoral
artery at the inguinal ligament is occluded by digital
pressure for ½ hr, instead of by application of a cuff,
much less change in the circulation occurs, because
collateral circulation is not stopped. Loss of sensation
does not occur, and on release of the occlusion, the
reactive hyperemia is much less intense than with the
cuff.

In occlusive vascular disease of the vessels of the
legs, a common symptom is pain with tenderness of
the muscles which is relieved by rest. It is called
intermittent claudication, and it represents in the
muscles of the extremities the same changes which
occur in the heart with angina pectoris. The resting
muscle is receiving an adequate supply of blood for
normal metabolism. When muscle metabolism is increased by exercise and occlusive vascular disease
prevents increase of the blood supply, metabolites
accumulate in the muscles and stimulate the sensory
nerve endings. The nature of the chemical substances
has not been determined. The more severe the circulatory impairment, the less exercise is required to produce the pain and the more slowly the pain disappears
on rest.

In occlusive vascular disease, the nerves themselves
may become ischemic and cause severe and persistent
pain. This pain, in certain instances, is aggravated by
dependency because of stimuli resulting from congestion. In addition to Buerger's disease and arteriosclerosis, ischemic neuritis is a prominent symptom in
small-vessel involvement of the type seen in periarteritis nodosa.

Embolus or thrombus in the brachial or femoral
vessels frequently produces sufficient circulatory impairment to cause pain. The pain in thrombosis is

indistinguishable from the pain of embolism. The pains do not occur at the site of occlusion but in the muscles and tissues distal to it. The time of onset of the pain will depend on the temperature of the part, the amount of activity, and the amount of associated vasospasm. If the part is warm and still, the limb may become numb before the muscle pain is produced. Heat applied to a limb with poor circulation may cause gangrene from (1) increased metabolism of tissue without corresponding increase in blood supply or (2) lack of cooling effect of the blood. When heat above body temperature is applied to the skin, the blood normally acts as a cooling system; in the presence of arterial occlusion, local heating causes an immediate rise in temperature of the part. If the part is exercised, the muscle pain occurs early. Twenty-four hours after an embolus has lodged, the vessel wall may be tender because of periarterial inflammation. Occlusion of small blood vessels does not cause pain unless ischemia of muscle or nerve is produced.

Normal skin hurts when warmed after severe exposure to cold. This is a response to direct injury from the cold. The white, cold fingers in Raynaud's phenomenon may be painful. In scleroderma the thickening of the connective tissue combined with spasm of the digital arteries may result in painful ulceration of the fingers and eventual loss of the terminal phalanges.

The pain from ischemia or infection is frequently altered or absent in patients with diabetes because of associated peripheral neuropathy. Whenever a painful-looking lesion of the extremity is treated casually by the patient, neuropathy should be suspected. Tabes dorsalis, leprosy, senile cortical atrophy, and syringomyelia should be considered.

The circulation to the extremities can be greatly modified by overactivity of the sympathetic nervous system. In many instances of injury, inflammation, or thrombophlebitis, sensory stimuli arising in the extremity may produce intense reflex vasoconstriction, and the resulting ischemia may cause diffuse pain. Relief of the vasoconstriction by paravertebral procaine block of the appropriate sympathetic ganglions may cause striking relief of pain. Similarly, sensory impulses arising from ischemic areas after arterial occlusion by an embolus or thrombus may stimulate sympathetic nervous system activity and reflex spasm. Paravertebral block will relieve the spasm of collateral vessels, and if circulation improves sufficiently, pain will disappear.

PAIN FROM NEUROPATHY, NEURITIS, GANGLIONITIS, AND PRESSURE ON NERVES OR NERVE ROOTS. Involvement of the peripheral nerves frequently causes unpleasant sensations in the extremities. In diabetic neuropathy, numbness may be accompanied by diffuse pains through both lower extremities. Any combination of sensory loss and pain may occur in peripheral nerve damage from infection, poisons, or mechanical factors such as trauma or pressure. Spinal cord tumors and slipped intervertebral disks are common causes of nerve root pain. Inflammation of the dorsal root ganglions results in the syndrome of herpes zoster. The redness and blistering is attributed to antidromic vasodilatation from stimulation of the sensory nerves. Impulses arising in sensory nerves or ganglions and passing peripherally to the sensory end organs are called *antidromic*. Involvement of the dorsal root ganglions, dorsal roots, and adjacent spinal cord produces the lightning pains in the extremities typical of tabes dorsalis. Paralysis from pressure in the axilla may be caused by crutches or by sleeping with the arm thrown over the back of a chair. The latter usually occurs in alcoholic stupor and is called "Saturday night paralysis."

PAIN FROM IMMOBILIZATION, SPASM, AND CRAMPS. Prolonged immobilization of a part results in stiffness of muscles and joints. The muscles tighten and splint the joint, and motion is prevented. An attempt to move the part produces pain. Local infiltration with procaine will frequently allow a great improvement in motility, which may be permanent. Similar spasm occurs after trauma. A painful sprain of the ankle which prevents walking may be relieved in a few minutes by procainization. Even in acute arthritis part of the pain may be secondary to spasm and may respond to curare or procaine, which relax the muscle. In acute poliomyelitis, nonparalyzed muscles may be sore and contracted. Application of hot packs gives relief.

Muscles placed in unusual positions may go into intense contraction and cause severe pain. Cramps in the foot or leg occurring at night are common. They are relieved by forcefully extending the joint so as to stretch the cramped muscles. In nocturnal cramps, pain occurs so quickly that simple ischemia would seem unlikely. They differ from the cramps of arterial disease in that the pain is not brought on by exercise. Painful muscle cramps occur in tetany and in chloride deficiency. Whether the pain of tetany is caused by ischemia from the prolonged contraction or related to damage because of the intensity of the contraction is not known.

Unaccustomed, strenuous exercise causes aching, tender muscles, tendons, and joints. The pain results from low-grade injury to the muscles from repetitive maximal contractions.

GLOMUS TUMOR. Tumor of the glomus, the specialized arteriovenous anastomosis of the skin, produces unusual vasomotor phenomena and radiating pain. It is characteristically a small (a few millimeters in diameter), extremely painful, purplish nodule either in the skin of the extremity or under the nail. Pain is caused by contact or change of temperature and may spread to involve the entire extremity. Why these tumors are so painful is not clear. While most observers have noted an unusually rich nerve supply, others have not found it.

PAIN FROM CAUSALGIA. Pain in the extremity associated with signs of local circulatory dysfunction is seen in nerve injuries after amputations and in persons with coronary arterial disease with or without myocardial infarction. It occurs in the hand-shoulder syndrome. The above conditions have one thing in common: local injury sets up a reaction which at first appears to be the result of sensory stimuli from the injured part. Later changes occur in the peripheral nerves, spinal cord, or central nervous system so that the process continues after the injury has apparently healed.

Classic Causalgia. Injury to any nerve, more commonly the medial or sciatic nerve, may give rise after a few days or weeks to a burning pain. The gross injury to the nerve may have been severe or trivial. The pain will be caused by light friction; deep pressure is less painful. Heat usually provokes the pain. The skin becomes smooth and glossy and is frequently wet with sweat. It has a red or purplish tint. The temperature of the involved part is usually said to be increased. The pain is frequently relieved by sympathectomy. Causalgic pain may result from the activation of sensory fibers by sympathetic impulses. If injury links the two systems so that leakage of efferent sympathetic impulses into the sensory nerves can occur, most of the clinical phenomena of causalgia, including the relief by sympathetic block, can be explained.

The initiating mechanisms of causalgia are unknown. Several theories have been advanced: (1) The sensitivity of the skin may result from vasodilator substances released by repeated centrifugal impulses arising in the injured area. It is known that stimulation of the paralyzed end of a cut cutaneous nerve results in vasodilatation which may be accompanied by itching and burning pain. (2) The sensitivity of the skin may result from a summation of impulses from normal skin with those from the injured nerve.

Regardless of the local mechanism, it appears that other mechanisms central to the extremity are capable of continuing the process once the causalgia has been present for some time. At this stage, dorsal root section or sections of the spinothalamic tract may not modify the pain. Chain reactions within the short interconnecting nerves in the spinal cord have been postulated. Paravertebral block or sympathectomy should be done early before these central changes occur and before the patient becomes a drug addict. Because the patient's complaints are so bizarre and because the original injury may be mild, causalgia is frequently mistaken for a compensation neurosis.

Phantom Limb Pain. After amputation of a limb, the patient may complain of pain which he localizes in the removed part. At times this may be caused by a neuroma of the cut nerves or by the faulty construction of the stump. The stump may show vasomotor changes. In most instances, therapy directed toward the stump does not relieve the pain; at times, paravertebral block of the sympathetic ganglions does. The clinical observations suggest that, as in causalgia, pain may begin locally but that changes may take place in the central nervous system which are responsible for its continuation.

Hand-Shoulder Syndrome. Myocardial infarction is frequently complicated by persistent shoulder pain with marked limitation of motion. At times, swelling of the hand and wrist and contraction of the palmar fascia are present. The elbow is not involved. Atrophy of skin and osteoporosis may follow. Similar disturbances in shoulder and hand function have occurred in association with trauma, hemiplegia, herpes zoster, and cervical osteoarthritis. This syndrome may occur without recognized associated diseases. The exact mechanism of this fairly common syndrome is unknown.

APPROACH TO THE PATIENT

A careful history will usually yield important clues. The pain may be felt in the region of the knee when the disease is in the hip or in the foot when the knee is the seat of the disorder. Pain on first arising in the morning, particularly when associated with stiffness, suggests a disturbance of joints or muscles. When the bone is affected, there is commonly nocturnal aggravation. Pain of throbbing character usually arises in tense tissues with free blood supply, and hence suggests bone as the source. Sharp shooting pain of brief duration, brought on by coughing or sneezing, is common with disorders of the vertebral column or of the posterior nerve roots. Relief of discomfort by elevation suggests venous obstruction; relief by dependency suggests an arterial lesion. Pain ascribed to walking may actually be due to standing and may have its source in the feet. Pain due to ischemia of muscles is characteristically induced by walking, with latency of onset and of offset. Disorders of joints are likely to be accompanied by pain on local movement, the duration of the discomfort paralleling that of the movement.

The history having suggested the responsible structure, the suspicion is confirmed or disproved by the physical findings and the appropriate special procedures. Since these are mentioned in the later chapters dealing with the disorders of the various systems of the body, they need not be cited here. However, it should be emphasized that x-ray examination, while often invaluable in the case of long-standing disease of the bones, may be entirely negative in the presence of serious skeletal disorders of recent origin. This is especially important in regard to acute osteomyelitis and to the earlier stages of metastatic neoplasms of bone.

REFERENCES

Allen, E. V., N. W. Barker, and E. A. Hines, Jr.: "Peripheral Vascular Diseases," Philadelphia, W. B. Saunders Company, 1946.

Doupe, J. C., C. H. Cullen, and G. Q. Chance: Post-traumatic Pain and the Causalgic Syndrome, J. Neurol., Neurosurg. Psychiat., 7:33, 1944.

Lewis, Thomas: "Pain," New York, The Macmillan Company, 1942.

——: "Vascular Disorders of the Limbs," New York, The Macmillan Company, 1946.

Steinbrocker, O.: Shoulder-Hand Syndrome: Associated Painful Homolateral Disability of Shoulder and Hand with Swelling and Atrophy of Hand, Am. J. Med., 3:402, 1947.

Sweet, W. H.: Pain, chap. 19, p. 459, in "Handbook of Physiology," vol. 1, Sec. 1, Neurophysiology, The American Physiological Society, Washington, D.C., 1959.

Section 2

Alterations in Body Temperature

10 DISTURBANCES OF HEAT REGULATION

Ivan L. Bennett, Jr.

In health, the body temperature of man is maintained within a narrow range despite extremes in environmental conditions and physical activity. To a lesser but nonetheless remarkable extent, this is true of other mammals as well. An almost invariable accompaniment of systemic illness is a disturbance in temperature regulation, very often an abnormal elevation, or *fever*. In fact, fever is such a sensitive and reliable indicator of the presence of disease that thermometry is probably the commonest clinical procedure now in use.

Even in the absence of a frank febrile response, interference with heat regulation by disease is evident. This may take the form of flushing, pallor, sweating, and abnormal sensations of cold or warmth (an example is the sensitivity of persons with coryza to drafts), or it may consist of erratic fluctuations of body temperature within normal limits when a patient is at bed rest.

CONTROL OF BODY TEMPERATURE

The principal source of body heat is the combustion of foods. The greatest amount of heat is generated in the liver and the voluntary muscles. Heat production by muscle is of particular importance because the quantity can be varied according to the need. In most circumstances this variation consists of small increases and decreases in the number of nerve impulses to the muscles, causing unapparent tensing or relaxing. When, however, there is a strong stimulus for heat production, muscle activity may increase to the point of shivering, or even to a generalized rigor.

Heat is lost from the body in several ways. Small amounts are used in warming food or drink and in the evaporation of moisture from the respiratory tract. Most heat is lost from the surface of the body, by radiation, convection, and evaporation. The relative importance of these processes depends upon environmental factors. When the outside temperature is equal to or above that of the body, the only means of heat loss is evaporation.

The principal method of regulating heat loss is by varying the volume of blood flowing to the surface of the body. A rich circulation in the skin and subcutaneous tissues carries heat to the surface, where it can escape. In addition, sweating increases heat loss by providing water to be vaporized; this is under control of cholinergic elements of the autonomic nervous system. When the need is for conservation of warmth, adrenergic autonomic stimuli cause a sharp reduction in the blood flow to the surface. This transforms the skin and subcutaneous tissue into layers of insulation.

The control of body temperature, integrating the various physical and chemical processes for heat production or loss, is a function of cerebral centers located in the hypothalamus and brain stem. An animal whose brain stem has been sectioned loses ability to control body temperature, which consequently tends to vary with the environment, a condition referred to as *poikilothermia*. Working with monkeys and cats, Ranson and his associates found that stimulation of areas in the cephalic portion of the hypothalamus caused activation of mechanisms for heat loss, such as sweating and panting. Stimulation of the caudal part of the hypothalamus activated mechanisms for warming the body and conservation of heat, such as shivering and erection of hair. Clinical experience indicates that the thermoregulatory centers have similar locations in human beings. Lesions which damage the anterior portion of the hypothalamus may be associated with high levels of body temperature, whereas lesions in the posterior part may cause marked hypothermia.

It is probable that the cerebral temperature-regulating centers are affected by more than one kind of stimulus. Experiments on animals show that variation in the temperature of the blood flowing through the brain can cause activation of the appropriate counteracting mechanisms, either for heat loss or for heat production. There is evidence that these centers may be stimulated by sensory impulses, e.g., the flushing and sweating which may occur after ingestion of highly seasoned food. That physiologic variations in endocrine function may affect the body temperature is shown by the fact that the mean body temperature of women is higher during the second half of the menstrual cycle than it is between the onset of menstruation and the time of ovulation. The sensations of intense heat followed by diaphoresis that characterize the vasomotor instability experienced by some women at the menopause are undoubtedly a result of endocrine imbalance (see Chap. 90).

A basic problem on which information is needed is why the normal body temperature of warm-blooded animals is in the neighborhood of 98 to 103°F. Animals or human beings whose cervical cords have been severed maintain about the same body temperature, although fluctuations tend to be greater because of lack of neural control. There may be some intrinsic chemical regulating mechanism in the tissues.

Sweating, so important in man, is supplanted by panting and radiation from the body surface in many animals. In the rabbit, for example, the surface of the large ears is of great importance in dissipating heat.

As has been previously mentioned, diseases of many types derange temperature regulation and fever is the result in many animals, but notable exceptions exist. The laboratory mouse responds to most "pyrogenic" stimuli with a profound drop in body temperature, and the rat gives variable responses, sometimes showing an elevation of temperature and sometimes showing a hypothermic response to disease. It has been found by Atwood and Kass that when mice or rats are maintained at high ambient temperatures, their response to materials known to be pyrogenic in man is no longer irregular but is constantly febrile. This is a striking demonstration of the influence of environment and other factors upon the outward expression of the derangement in body temperature control which occurs in disease.

NORMAL BODY TEMPERATURE

It is not practical to designate an exact upper level of normal body temperature, since there are small differences among normal persons. There are rare individuals whose temperatures are always elevated slightly above accepted "normal" levels. The physician must use some judgment in deciding what constitutes an abnormal temperature in a given case. In general, however, it is safest to regard an oral temperature above 98.6°F in a person who has been lying in bed as an indication of disease. A temperature above 99.0°F in a person who has been engaged in moderate activity has the same significance. The temperature may be as low as 96.5°F in healthy individuals. Rectal temperature is usually 0.5 to 1.0°F higher than oral temperature. In very hot weather the body temperature may be elevated by 0.5° or perhaps even 1.0°F.

There is a distinct diurnal variation in body temperature in the healthy human being. Oral readings of 97°F are relatively common on arising in the morning. Body temperature rises steadily through the day, reaches a peak of 99°F or greater between 6 P.M. and 10 P.M., and then drops slowly to reach a minimum at 2 A.M. to 4 A.M. Although it might be postulated immediately that this diurnal variation is dependent upon increasing activity during the day and rest at night, it was shown conclusively by Kleitman that the pattern is not reversed in individuals who work at night and sleep during the day for long periods of time.

Diurnal variations in the body temperature of animals undoubtedly exist but have been studied to no great extent.

It is important to note that the febrile patterns of most human diseases tend to follow this normal diurnal pattern. Fevers tend to be higher, to "spike," in the evening, and many patients with febrile disease will be found to have relatively normal temperatures in the early morning hours.

Severe or prolonged exercise or very hot baths can produce a transient elevation in body temperature, which is quickly compensated for by increased dissipation from the skin and lungs. Such elevations are not properly classified as fevers.

Body temperature is somewhat labile in young children, and transient elevations after relatively slight exertion in warm weather are frequently observed in this group.

DISORDERED THERMOREGULATION

All fevers are accompanied by an *increase in heat production*. Abrupt rises after shaking chills may involve as much as a 600 per cent increase for a short time, according to DuBois. Elevation of body temperature itself increases metabolic activity about 7 per cent for each degree Fahrenheit. There is no question, however, about the major importance of *decrease in heat loss* in fevers of any duration. Abrupt rises after severe exertion in healthy individuals are compensated for within a few minutes, but in illness the compensatory mechanism fails and the elevation is sustained. When it is considered that a decrease of 10 per cent in heat loss will result in a body temperature of 106°F within a few hours, the cardinal role of defective heat loss in fever is more easily appreciated. DuBois has pointed out the existence of a "safety valve" in human adults. When hyperthermia reaches dangerous levels, the mechanisms for heat loss are suddenly activated; consequently, oral temperatures of 106°F are rare in man. While the operation of this cutoff can be spoken of as analogous to the action of a thermostat, there is no evidence to support the existence of any physiologic equivalent of a "thermostat" in the regulation of body temperature; the analogy should not be substituted for a frank admission of ignorance of the basic mechanisms involved.

DISEASES OF THE NERVOUS SYSTEM. Disease of the regulatory centers in the hypothalamus may affect body temperature. Cases have been observed in which there was destruction of the centers controlling heat-conserving mechanisms, with resulting hypothermia. More commonly, cerebral lesions are manifested by hyperthermia; this may occur with tumors, infections, degenerative diseases, or vascular accidents. It is not uncommon in cerebral apoplexy for the temperature to rise to 105 to 107°F during the last few hours before death.

Heat stroke ("sunstroke") is an interesting example of fever due to interference with the controlling mechanism. Here the central mechanisms for cooling seem suddenly to fail and the patient ceases to sweat, despite the fact that his temperature is rising. Some of the highest temperatures ever observed in human beings (112 to 113°F) have been in cases of heat stroke. A temperature higher than 114°F is not compatible with life (Chap. 253).

INCREASED HEAT PRODUCTION. Patients with thyrotoxicosis frequently have an elevation in temperature 1 to 2°F above the normal range. This is ascribable to the increased amount of heat produced by an increase in the activity and rate of the metabolic processes. Dinitrophenol, a drug which was formerly used for weight reduction in obese persons, causes elevation of temperature; this too seems to be caused by an increased metabolic activity, produced by some mechanism outside the thyroid.

IMPAIRMENT OF HEAT LOSS. Patients with congestive heart failure nearly always have an elevation of body temperature. Usually this is only a matter of 0.5 to 1.5°F. It has been thought by many that the elevation is caused by impairment of heat dissipation as a result of diminished cardiac output, decline in cutaneous blood flow, the insulating effect of edema, and the increased heat production incident to the muscular activity of dyspnea. Others have objected to this explanation because patients with congestive heart failure are likely to have other causes of fever, such as venous thrombosis, embolism, myocardial infarction, rheumatic fever, and urinary tract infection. However, since slight fever is so regularly present even in the absence of such complications, it would appear that the circulatory disturbance may be responsible.

Patients with skin disorders such as ichthyosis or congenital absence of sweat glands may have fever in a warm environment because of inability to lose heat from the surface of the body. Similarly, individuals taking drugs which impair sweating [atropine, propantheline (Pro-Banthine)] may have fever in warm weather.

HYPOTHERMIA. From the clinical standpoint, reduction of body temperature is of far less frequency and importance than is elevation. Daily variation of temperature within the "subnormal" range, i.e., 97 to 98.6°F, is observed in all healthy individuals. The temperature range may be somewhat lower than normal, i.e., 96 to 97.5°F, in patients with myxedema and during the first day or so after critical fall in temperature associated with infectious disease. Oral temperatures below 96°F are rarely encountered, as there is apparently a potent countering mechanism which

opposes fall below that level. This barrier may, of course, be broken through by exposure to extreme cold (Chap. 254). Furthermore, when cerebral function has been impaired, as by alcohol or large doses of sedative drugs, less severe chilling can result in fall in body temperature. The lowered body temperature in shock may be due to impaired cerebral regulation or to inability to produce adequate heat.

One condition in which profound hypothermia may develop is myxedema with coma (Chap. 82). Body temperature in such a patient may gradually sink to 80 to 85°F. Attending personnel may fail to recognize this because the clinical thermometer registers only as low as it has been shaken; hence a series of readings in the range of 95 to 97°F may be erroneously recorded.

REFERENCES

DuBois, E. F.: "Fever and the Regulation of Body Temperature," Springfield, Ill., Charles C Thomas, Publisher, 1948.

Pickering, G. W.: Regulation of Body Temperature in Health and Disease, Lancet, 1:1 and 59, 1958.

11 CHILLS AND FEVER
Ivan L. Bennett, Jr.

In view of the extensive knowledge of physiologic mechanisms controlling body temperature mentioned in the previous chapter, it is surprising that so little is known about the ways in which diseases upset thermoregulation.

Some bacteria, particularly gram-negative species, produce endotoxins which are pyrogenic (see Chap. 276), and a few viruses cause immediate fever when injected into man or animals. Many microorganisms, however, possess no demonstrable pyrogenic toxin and, of course, fever accompanies diseases which do not involve invasion of the body by any known parasite. Omitting disorders which involve cerebral thermoregulatory centers directly, febrile diseases may be grouped as follows: (1) It is safe to generalize that all *infections*, whether caused by bacteria, rickettsias, viruses, or more complex parasites, may cause fever. (2) *Mechanical trauma,* as in crushing injuries, frequently gives rise to fever lasting 1 or 2 days. (3) Most *neoplastic diseases* can cause fever. Carcinoma of the stomach or pancreas, with metastasis to the liver, is nearly always associated with temperature elevation. Hypernephroma can produce hectic fever with daily chills. In lymphosarcoma or Hodgkin's disease, fever may be one of the prominent early manifestations. (4) Many *hematopoietic disorders* are characterized by pyrexia, examples being acute hemolytic episodes and the leukemias. (5) *Vascular accidents* of any magnitude nearly always cause fever, examples being myocardial and pulmonary infarctions. (6) *Diseases due to immune mechanisms* are almost always febrile. These include the so-called collagen diseases, drug fevers, and serum sickness. (7) Certain *acute metabolic disorders* such as gout, porphyria, and thyroid crisis are associated with fever.

PATHOGENESIS OF FEVER

Several hypotheses have been offered to explain disturbed temperature regulation in noninfectious disease. Some investigators have attributed fever to shifts in body water which interfere with heat production and heat loss. It is true that newborn infants may become febrile when fluid intake is inadequate and that the temperature elevation subsides promptly when fluid is administered. In adults, there are occasional instances of fever associated with extracellular fluid deficit when the ambient temperature is above 90°F. On the other hand, "dehydration" is not ordinarily associated with fever in adults, and the clinical practice of attributing fever to this cause is to be deprecated.

Some have attempted to account for fever on the basis of alterations in endocrine function, with particular reference to the thyroid and adrenals. There is little clinical or experimental evidence to support this idea. Temperature regulation is normal in Addison's disease and in Cushing's syndrome. Body temperature is slightly above normal in thyrotoxicosis and a little below in myxedema, but these differences are entirely in keeping with the metabolic rate and there is no real evidence of impaired thermoregulation in either disease.

There was a renewal of interest in a role of the endocrines in the pathogenesis of fever with the finding that abnormalities of etiocholanolone metabolism exist in some patients with "periodic" fever (see Chap. 387). The finding by Kappas that many steroids are pyrogenic for man cannot yet be translated into clinical terms.

The common factor in febrile diseases is *tissue injury*. The hypothesis which best fits clinical and experimental observations is that fever results from disturbance of cerebral thermoregulation brought about by a product or products of tissue injury. It has been shown experimentally that inflammatory exudates cause fever when injected intravenously into normal animals and similar results have been obtained in human subjects. Further work indicates that one source of pyrogenic material is the polymorphonuclear leukocyte, although other cells may also release fever-producing substances.

While considering the pathogenesis of fever, it is worth noting the sequence of events which follows intravenous injection of killed bacteria or of purified bacterial endotoxin. Figure 11-1 shows a typical human response to injection of typhoid vaccine. It is to be noted that body temperature does not begin to rise until about an hour after injection of the pyrogen. During this interval, the patient notes no discomfort and his appearance is unchanged. Then, rather sud-

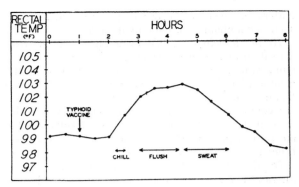

Fig. 11-1. Typical temperature response of a human being to intravenous injection of a comparatively large dose of typhoid vaccine—100,000,000 organisms.

denly, there is malaise, he complains of cold, and within minutes he is burrowing down into the bedclothes, asking for more blankets. He begins to shiver and is soon having a shaking chill which lasts 10 to 20 min. During this time, the skin is pale and cold but rectal temperature rises steeply. After subsidence of the rigor, the patient gradually feels warmer, skin circulation increases, and within 2 hr he is flushed and complains of feeling feverish. After another hour, profuse sweating begins and body temperature begins to return toward normal.

Much remains to be learned about the nature of the events which follow intravenous injection of a pyrogenic substance. It has been established that endotoxin is removed from the circulation within a few minutes by the fixed phagocytes of the reticuloendothelial system. It may be assumed that the febrile reaction involves an effect on the cerebral thermoregulatory centers. Experimental evidence suggests that two mechanisms may be involved: a direct effect on the brain by the bacterial toxin and an indirect effect by an endogenous substance such as the pyrogen contained in polymorphonuclear leukocytes.

ACCOMPANIMENTS OF FEVER

The perception of fever by patients varies enormously. Some individuals can tell with considerable accuracy whether their body temperatures are elevated, apparently by sensations of warmth in the skin. Other persons, notably patients with tuberculosis, may be wholly unaware of body temperatures as high as 103°F. Often, also, patients may pay no attention to fever because of other unpleasant symptoms such as headache and pleuritic pain.

The *headache* of fever is discussed in Chap. 5. The pain often experienced in the back and muscles during acute infectious diseases seems to be an effect of the causative organisms, not a direct manifestation of fever.

Abrupt onset of fever with a *chill* or *rigor* is characteristic of some diseases and, in the absence of antipyretic drugs, rare in others. Although repeated rigors suggest pyogenic infection with bacteremia, a similar pattern of fever may occur in noninfectious diseases such as lymphoma and hypernephroma.

Herpes labialis, so-called fever blister, results from activation of the herpes simplex virus by elevation of temperature, as evidenced by the frequency of this complication in patients undergoing artificial fever therapy. For reasons which are obscure, fever blisters are common in pneumococcal infections, streptococcosis, malaria, meningococcemia, and rickettsioses but are rare in primary atypical pneumonia, tuberculosis, brucellosis, smallpox, and typhoid.

Delirium can result from elevation of body temperature and is particularly common in patients with alcoholism or cerebral arteriosclerosis.

Convulsions are not infrequent in febrile children, especially those with a family history of epilepsy, although febrile convulsions do not signal the onset of serious cerebral disease.

CLINICAL IMPORTANCE OF FEVER

The clinical thermometer was one of the first instruments of precision to be introduced into the practice of medicine. Its objectivity and simplicity make it an immensely valuable aid to physical diagnosis. Nowadays we are so accustomed to graphic temperature charts in hospitals and the ready availability of the clinical thermometer for use in the home that we scarcely realize our great dependence upon them. Determination of the body temperature assists in estimating the severity of an illness, its course and duration, and the effect of therapy, or even in deciding whether a person has an organic illness.

A question frequently asked is whether fever is beneficial. There are a few infections of man in which pyrexia appears definitely to be beneficial to the host, examples being neurosyphilis, some gonococcal infections, and chronic brucellosis. Certain other diseases, such as uveitis and rheumatoid arthritis, sometimes improve after fever therapy. In experimental animals some pneumococcal and cryptococcal infections have been influenced in favor of the host animal by raising the body temperature. Aged and debilitated patients with infection may exhibit little or no fever, and this is generally interpreted as a bad prognostic sign. In the great majority of infectious diseases, however, there is no reason to believe that pyrexia accelerates phagocytosis, antibody formation, or other defense mechanisms.

Fever has its detrimental aspects. The greater velocity of all metabolic processes accentuates weight loss and nitrogen wastage. The work and the rate of the heart are increased. Sweating aggravates loss of fluid and salt. There may be discomfort due to headache, photophobia, general malaise, or unpleasant sensation of warmth. The rigors and profuse sweats of hectic fevers are particularly unpleasant for the patient.

MANAGEMENT OF FEVER. Since fever ordinarily does little harm and imposes no great discomfort, antipyretic drugs are rarely necessary and may obscure the effect of a specific therapeutic agent and of the natural course of the disease. There are situations, however, in which lowering of the body temperature is of vital importance: heat stroke, postoperative hyperthermia, delirium due to high pyrexia, shock associated with fever. Under these circumstances, sponging the body surface with alcohol or the application of cool compresses to the skin and forehead may be employed. When high internal temperature is combined with cutaneous vasoconstriction, as in heat stroke or postoperative hyperthermia, the cooling measures should be combined with massage of the skin in order to bring blood to the surface, where it may be cooled. Immediate immersion in a tub of ice water should be considered a lifesaving emergency procedure in patients with heat stroke if the internal body temperature is in excess of 108°F.

If antipyretic drugs, such as aspirin (0.3 to 0.6 Gm), are employed to bring about a fall in temperature, the ill effects of the unpleasant diaphoresis, sometimes associated with an alarming fall in blood pressure and the subsequent return of fever, occasionally accompanied by a chill, can be mitigated by enforcing a liberal fluid intake and by administering the drug regularly at 3- or 4-hr intervals.

The discomfort of a rigor can be alleviated in many patients by the intravenous injection of calcium gluconate. This procedure will stop the shivering and chilliness but has no influence on the ultimate height of the fever.

DIAGNOSTIC SIGNIFICANCE OF FEVER

Physicians frequently have the problem of dealing with illnesses of unknown etiology in which fever is a prominent or the only manifestation. Fever is not an indication of any particular type of disease; it is merely a reaction to injury comparable to alterations in leukocyte count, increased erythrocyte sedimentation rate, etc. The more important probabilities to be considered in dealing with a patient with "F.U.O.," or fever of unknown origin, are discussed below.

FEBRILE ILLNESSES OF SHORT DURATION

Acute febrile illnesses of less than 2 weeks' duration are a common occurrence in medical practice. In many instances they run their courses, progressing to complete recovery; yet the physician in attendance is never able to arrive at a precise diagnosis. In most instances, however, it is safe to assume that the illness is of infectious origin; for although short febrile illnesses can be of noninfectious origin, e.g., allergic fevers due to drugs or serums, thromboembolic disease, hemolytic crises, gout, etc., such are decidedly in the minority.

Most of these acute febrile infectious diseases are probably viral infections, since diagnostic methods for bacterial infection are better, and since most bacterial infections are rapidly brought under control by the chemotherapeutic agents now in common use. It is not practicable to carry out tests needed to identify all the viruses at present known, and furthermore there must be a considerable number of as yet unidentified viruses pathogenic for man.

The following attributes, while not restricted solely to acute infections, are highly suggestive:

1. Abrupt onset
2. High fever, i.e., 102 to 105°F, with or without chills
3. Respiratory symptoms—sore throat, coryza, cough
4. Severe malaise, with muscle or joint pain, photophobia, pain on movement of the eyes, headache
5. Nausea, vomiting, or diarrhea
6. Acute enlargement of lymph nodes or spleen
7. Meningeal signs, with or without spinal fluid pleocytosis
8. Leukocyte count above 12,000 or below 5,000 per cu mm

To repeat, none of the symptoms or signs listed is encountered only in infection. Many of these features could be seen in acute myeloblastic leukemia or disseminated lupus erythematosus. Nevertheless, in a given instance of acute febrile illness with some or all of the manifestations listed, the probabilities strongly favor infection, and the physician is able to give reasonable assurance that the patient will probably recover in a week or two, regardless of a precise diagnosis.

It is desirable of course to establish an accurate diagnosis, and the physician should take whatever steps are practicable in the circumstances to establish the cause. Cultures of the throat, blood, urine, or feces should be obtained *before* institution of antibacterial chemotherapy. Diagnosis by means of skin tests or serologic test should be carried out.

PROLONGED FEBRILE ILLNESSES

Some of the knottiest problems in the field of internal medicine are found in cases of prolonged fever in which the diagnosis remains obscure for weeks or even months. Eventually, however, the true nature of the illness usually reveals itself, since a disease which causes injury sufficient to evoke temperature elevations of 101°F or higher for several weeks does not often subside without leaving some clue as to its nature.

The elucidation of problems of this sort calls for skillful application of all diagnostic methods—careful history, thorough physical examination, and the considered application of good laboratory examinations.

It is obviously not possible or practical in this section to mention all the known entities which may cause prolonged febrile disease, or even to give an adequate discussion of the differential diagnosis of the more frequent ones. Additional details about the manifestations and differential diagnosis of the entities mentioned will be found elsewhere.

INFECTIOUS DISEASES

The infections occupy a less prominent position among the causes of prolonged fever now than formerly, because of the common practice of administer-

ing antibiotic drugs to any patient in whom fever persists for more than a few days. Consequently, many infections are at present being eradicated by more or less "blind" therapy, without their nature or location ever accurately being determined.

Certain infections do not respond to the usual antibiotic therapy and must be thought of in differential diagnosis at the present time. In general, this does not apply to virus diseases, for although chemotherapy rarely affects them, they tend to run their courses more or less acutely and do not often cause continued illness lasting many weeks or months. The following infections must be mentioned.

TUBERCULOSIS. This disease proves to be responsible for puzzling febrile disease with surprising frequency, despite the facts that there is a fairly effective therapy and that the simple procedure of chest x-ray is usually sufficient for diagnosis of the commonest clinical form. The drugs given as therapeutic trials may not include those with tuberculostatic activity such as streptomycin or isoniazid. Extrapulmonary forms of tuberculosis may not be easily located, e.g., disease of the bones, deep lymph nodes, genital or urinary organs. Furthermore the pulmonary lesions of miliary tuberculosis may not be detectable by x-ray until very late in the course of the disease. In considering the possibility of tuberculous infection, the skin test may be of great assistance, since negative reaction to a properly executed skin test rules out the possibility of tuberculosis except in rare instances of overwhelming disease. A positive skin reaction, on the other hand, does not prove that tuberculosis is causing the patient's illness, but in its presence the experienced physician will continue to keep tuberculosis in mind as a possibility until another cause for the fever and other symptoms are found.

BACTERIAL ENDOCARDITIS. In the classical subacute form of the disease, a heart murmur is nearly always present; therefore absence of murmur largely eliminates this disease from consideration. The correct diagnosis is likely to be missed in middle-aged or elderly patients, in whom the presence of a heart murmur may not be given much weight. For example, an elderly patient with subacute bacterial endocarditis may first present himself following the occurrence of a cerebral embolus and may be regarded as having had a hemorrhage or thrombosis because of arteriosclerosis. The best clinical practice is to culture the blood of *every* patient who has fever and a heart murmur. One cannot take the risk of overlooking this curable disease.

BRUCELLOSIS. The point to be emphasized is that this infection is a most unlikely possibility in an American city dweller. It has to be considered in the case of farmers, veterinarians, or slaughterhouse workers. There is a common misconception that brucellosis frequently causes arthritis. Although arthralgia and myalgia are common, actual redness and swelling of joints are rare in this disease. Peripheral leukocytosis is seldom seen in brucellosis. In active febrile disease the blood culture and bone marrow culture frequently are positive, and specific agglutinins are *nearly always* present in the serum. Precise diagnosis is therefore a relatively easy matter.

SALMONELLA INFECTION. Although typhoid fever is subject to great variability and may cause fever for several weeks, it should not often be a cause of prolonged fever of obscure origin, since cultures of feces or blood will be positive, and the specific antibodies are detected in the agglutination reaction. Other salmonella organisms may, however, cause prolonged febrile illness, and these may present greater diagnostic difficulty. Routine serologic tests are not helpful, and few laboratories can or will carry out serologic tests to detect antibody responses to all possible infecting strains. Antibiotics, including chloramphenicol (Chloromycetin), may not be effective. Repeated culture of the blood or of bone marrow may yield the causative organism. There may eventually be localization of infection in a joint or the pleural cavity from which the etiologic agent can be obtained.

PYOGENIC INFECTION. Chemotherapy does not succeed in eradicating all localized pyogenic infection, and in certain locations inflammation may be relatively asymptomatic. These infections include osteomyelitis of the vertebras or pelvic bones, abscess (subdiaphragmatic, hepatic, perinephric, renal cortical, retropharyngeal, mediastinal), cholangitis, and bronchiectasis. If these possibilities are thought of, appropriate questioning, examination, and x-ray studies will usually reveal their presence.

AMEBIASIS. Amebic colitis usually evokes symptoms pointing to disease of the colon. Hepatic involvement, on the other hand, may not give a distinctive clinical picture, and prolonged fever may be the principal manifestation. Some assistance may be obtained from a history of dysentery, or from the elicitation of tenderness or enlargement of the liver, and elevation of the right leaf of the diaphragm. The complement fixation test has little diagnostic value, either when positive or when negative. Therapeutic trial of an antiamebic drug, such as chloroquine or emetine, which acts on the hepatic form of amebiasis, may be justified.

HISTOPLASMOSIS. This infection is prevalent in the region of the Mississippi Valley of the United States, although in most individuals it is not clinically recognizable. The disease may, however, be manifested as a chronic febrile illness, with localizing manifestations pointing to many organ systems. Fever, leukopenia, anemia, hepatomegaly, and splenomegaly in a person who has resided in a geographic area where histoplasmosis occurs should suggest the possibility. The skin reaction to histoplasmin should be positive. The organisms may be demonstrated in biopsy or by culture of involved tissue or in bone marrow, occasionally even in the peripheral blood.

COCCIDIOIDOMYCOSIS. This disease need be considered only in persons who have traveled through, or resided in, the Southwest part of the United States. Clinical manifestations are like those of the various forms of tuberculosis. The coccidioidin skin test and serologic reaction to this antigen are positive.

SCHISTOSOMIASIS. Persons who have lived in the Caribbean islands, in Africa, or in the Far East may have prolonged febrile illness associated with this infestation. Diarrhea, bladder symptoms, cough, hepatosplenomegaly, and anemia are suggestive. Diagnosis is made by finding the ova in feces or urine or in rectal or hepatic biopsy.

COLLAGEN DISEASES

Under this term is included a broad spectrum of diseases in which there are histologic evidences of disorders of the collagen and the blood vessels. Some of these diseases are particularly important causes of prolonged febrile illness.

DISSEMINATED LUPUS ERYTHEMATOSUS. This disease is by no means rare, being encountered with greater frequency in American hospitals than typhoid fever. The possibility should receive special consideration in a young woman with fever, polyarthritis, low or low-normal leukocyte count, anemia, pulmonary infiltrations or pleural involvement, and hematuria and other evidence of acute nephritis. Behavioral abnormalities, orbital edema, and salivary gland swelling are less common features. The diagnosis can be made with confidence in patients who develop the full clinical picture, or by demonstration of the LE cell or LE phenomenon. The diseases likely to be confused with disseminated lupus erythematosus are rheumatic fever and rheumatoid arthritis.

PERIARTERITIS NODOSA. Features which particularly point to this syndrome are febrile illness in a male of any age, with leukocytosis, eosinophilia, anemia, asthma, peripheral neuritis, arthritis or muscle pain, hypertension, and evidence of renal involvement. Lesions in medium-sized arteries can give rise to the clinical pictures of myocardial infarction, mesenteric embolism, and peripheral vascular disease. There may be a variety of cutaneous eruptions. The only conclusive method of diagnosis is biopsy of a muscle or a skin lesion or of other tissue excised at operation.

RHEUMATOID ARTHRITIS. In its earlier stages there may not be characteristic swelling and deformity of joints but only vague pains in muscles and joints, together with fever, slight anemia, and malaise. Differentiation from rheumatic fever and from disseminated lupus erythematosus may be difficult. Sometimes diagnosis cannot be made until the more characteristic picture of the disease develops.

RHEUMATIC FEVER. Fever, with or without muscle and joint pains, may persist for weeks and months at a time. A history of preceding attacks or of an upper respiratory infection before onset of the systemic illness, the presence of a heart murmur, relative tachycardia, and prolonged P-R interval in the electrocardiogram are suggestive findings. Significant elevation of the antistreptolysin O titer is present in 80 per cent of cases.

HENOCH-SCHÖNLEIN, OR ALLERGIC, PURPURA. There may be fever, joint pains, and evidences of renal and pulmonary involvement. The results of the capillary fragility test and platelet count are normal. Differentiation from lupus erythematosus, rheumatic fever, and acute glomerulonephritis may be difficult. Diagnosis will depend on the finding of hemorrhagic occurrences, usually in the intestinal lumen or in joints.

NEOPLASTIC DISEASES

Fever is a common manifestation of malignant growth but a very rare accompaniment of benign tumors. In patients in the age range where cancer is common, unexplained fever should always suggest the possibility of neoplasm.

CARCINOMAS AND SARCOMAS. Certain malignant processes seem especially likely to cause fever. Notable are sarcomas involving bone or lymphoid tissue, hypernephroma, carcinoma of the pancreas or stomach, and metastatic cancer of the liver. Occasionally the clinical picture is strongly suggestive of pyogenic infection, with hectic fever, chills, sweats, and marked leukocytosis; and patients have been subjected to laparotomy with preoperative diagnoses such as empyema of the gallbladder, localized peritonitis, or liver abscess.

HODGKIN'S DISEASE. Fever may be the principal symptom and only objective finding early in the course of Hodgkin's disease, especially when the principal involvement is in the abdominal viscera. Cases with splenomegaly and vague abdominal distress have been confused with typhoid fever. The Pel-Ebstein fever seen in a minority of cases of Hodgkin's disease will be mentioned later. Diagnosis of this disorder is made by biopsy.

HEMATOPOIETIC DISEASES

Disorders of blood formation or blood destruction are frequently associated with fever.

LEUKEMIAS. It is not uncommon for acute leukemia to be mistaken for acute infection at the onset. The acute leukemias are nearly always accompanied by fever, sometimes as high as 105°F. The correct diagnosis will be suggested by rapid development of anemia and characteristic changes in peripheral blood and bone marrow. Chronic leukemia, particularly lymphatic, may be characterized by low-grade fever, but because of the typical changes in circulating leukocytes, it is not often a diagnostic problem.

HEMOLYTIC EPISODES. Most of the hemolytic diseases are characterized by bouts of fever. Acute crises of hemolysis may give rise to shaking chills and marked elevations of temperature. The difficulty sometimes encountered in differentiating sickle-cell disease from acute rheumatic fever is now well known. The presence of these hemolytic disorders is suggested by the more rapid development of anemia than occurs in other febrile illnesses and by the usual accompaniment of icterus. Diagnosis is confirmed by appropriate laboratory tests.

Fever is not characteristic of severe anemia due to external blood loss or of the anemia of uremia.

VASCULAR DISEASE

Reference has already been made to the fever of collagen diseases, all of which are accompanied by vascular lesions. In addition, certain other diseases of the blood vessels, not always regarded as being in the same category as the collagen diseases, may cause chronic febrile illness.

TEMPORAL, OR CRANIAL, ARTERITIS. This is a disease of old people, featured by severe aching pain in the temporal area, with fever and leukocytosis. There may be accompanying visual defect or blindness due to involvement of the retinal artery. The temporal or occipital arteries may be inflamed and tender. Diagnosis is not difficult if the condition is thought of and the superficial arteries are carefully palpated.

THROMBOEMBOLIC DISEASE. In migratory thrombophlebitis, segments of large veins become inflamed and thrombosed. There is usually local pain and swelling, but sometimes the lesions have to be searched for. Symptomless thrombosis of deep calf or pelvic veins may cause prolonged febrile illness as a result of repeated small emboli. These emboli may not be manifested by pleuritic pain or hemoptysis, but cough, dyspnea, or vague thoracic discomfort is likely to be present. Careful examination of the legs and repeated examination of the lungs should reveal the diagnosis.

MISCELLANEOUS

LIVER DISEASE. Most patients with cirrhosis exhibit low-grade fever at times. Rarely there are chills and high fever, owing either to salmonella infection or to bacteremia due to coliform bacteria.

SARCOIDOSIS. Ordinarily fever is not characteristic of sarcoidosis, but it is prominent in a minority of cases, especially those characterized by arthralgia and cutaneous lesions resembling erythema nodosum, or in those with extensive hepatic lesions. Diagnosis is suggested by lymphoid enlargement, ocular lesions, and hyperglobulinemia and is clinched by biopsy of skin, lymph nodes, or liver.

DRUG FEVER. Great emphasis should be placed on this category of febrile disease. One of the first things the consultant should inquire into is the matter of drug ingestion. Fever due to allergy to one of the antibiotics may become superimposed on the fever of the infection for which the drug was given, resulting in a very confusing picture. Other drugs capable of causing fever are the sulfonamides, arsenicals, iodides, thiouracils, and barbiturates. One should not forget laxative drugs in this connection, especially those containing phenolphthalein. Any question of drug fever can be resolved rapidly by discontinuing all medication. The diagnosis can be further substantiated by giving a test dose of the drug after fever has subsided, but this may result in a very unpleasant or even dangerous reaction.

MALINGERING. Rarely, a patient will wish to seem to be having fever. Many methods have been employed to cause the thermometer to register higher than the true temperature. If malingering is suspected, all that is necessary to prove it is to repeat the temperature determination immediately after a high reading has been obtained, with someone remaining at the bedside while the thermometer is in place.

PROLONGED LOW–GRADE TEMPERATURE ELEVATIONS

Not infrequently the physician is consulted because it has been observed that a patient, while not appearing acutely ill, has been subject to elevation of body temperature above the "normal" level, i.e., his temperature has been in the range of 99.0 to 100.5°F. Prolonged low-grade fever may be a manifestation of serious illness, or it may be a matter of no real consequence. Possibly there are some individuals whose "normal" temperatures are in this range. However, there is no certain way of identifying such individuals. The possibilities which the physician has to consider in such cases vary considerably according to the age groups concerned.

In children it should not be forgotten that temperature regulation may be somewhat erratic even up to the age of twelve years. Children may therefore have slight temperature elevations when excited or after exercise. A mother may note that her child's skin feels hot when he has been playing and find his temperature slightly above the normal line. Reexamination on subsequent days may reveal the same elevation from time to time. The physician consulted about this has to decide whether the "fever" is an indication of disease or of imperfect thermoregulation. If the physical examination reveals no abnormality, if the appetite is good and the child is gaining weight, and if there is no anemia or urinary abnormality, it is fairly safe to advise the parent to cease taking temperatures and forget about "fever." Real harm can be done by restricting the activity of an otherwise healthy child, owing to misinterpretation of the significance of low-grade fever.

In young adults chronic low-grade temperature elevation cannot easily be imputed to imperfect thermoregulation. Here one has to consider tuberculosis, brucellosis, and rheumatic fever or other collagen disease, as well as many of the conditions mentioned in the preceding section. A special problem encountered in females of this age group is that which has been called *habitual hyperthermia*. Every experienced physician has encountered examples of the syndrome. The patient may have temperatures of 99.0 to 100.5°F regularly or intermittently for years. The patient usually has a variety of complaints characteristic of psychoneurosis, such as fatigability, insomnia, bowel distress, vague aches, and headache. Prolonged careful study and observation fail to reveal evidence of organic disease. Unfortunately, many of these people go from doctor to doctor and are subjected to a variety of unpleasant, expensive, and even harmful tests, treatments, and operations. The diagnosis of this syndrome can be made with reasonable certainty after a suitable period of observation and study, and if the patient can be convinced of it, a real service will have been rendered.

In a patient past middle age, fever, even low-grade, should always be regarded as a probable indication of organic disease. The possibilities to be considered in this age group are the same as those discussed above in the section Prolonged Febrile Illnesses.

RELAPSING AND RECURRENT FEVERS

Occasionally patients are encountered who have recurrent bouts of high fever at more or less regular intervals. The following are among the diseases which have to be considered:

MALARIA. The disease has almost completely vanished from the United States and Canada, but cases are encountered occasionally in persons recently arrived from foreign countries. It is most unusual, however, for malaria to recur after a symptom-free interval of 1 year or more. Seizures recur at 2- or 3-day intervals, depending on the maturation cycle of the parasite. Diagnosis depends on demonstration of the parasites in the blood.

RELAPSING FEVER. This disease occurs in the Southwest part of the United States, extending as far east as Texas. Again the recurrences are doubtless related to some cycle in the development of the parasites. Diagnosis is by demonstration of the spirochetal organisms in stained films of the blood.

RAT-BITE FEVER. Two etiologic agents—*Spirillum minus* and *Streptobacillus moniliformis*—can be transmitted by the bite of a rat. Both may cause an illness characterized by periodic exacerbations of fever. The clue as to the diagnosis depends on obtaining a history of rat bite 1 to 10 weeks previous to the onset of symptoms. The causative organism can be established by appropriate laboratory procedures.

PYOGENIC INFECTION. In rare instances, localized pyogenic infections give rise to periodic bouts of fever separated by afebrile and relatively symptom-free intervals. The so-called "Charcot's intermittent biliary fever," i.e., cholangitis with biliary obstruction due to stones, is an example. The febrile attacks are sometimes associated with slight jaundice. There should be a history suggestive of cholelithiasis, and during the attacks tenderness can be elicited in the right upper quadrant. *Urinary tract infection*, with episodes of ureteral obstruction due to small stones or inspissated pus, can also cause recurrent fever.

HODGKIN'S DISEASE. In perhaps 5 to 10 per cent of cases, there is seen at some time during the course of the disease the so-called "Pel-Ebstein fever"— bouts of fever lasting 3 to 10 days, separated by afebrile and asymptomatic periods of 3 to 10 days. These cycles may be repeated regularly over a period of several months. In rare instances this periodicity of the fever has been sufficiently striking to suggest the correct diagnosis before lymph node swelling or splenomegaly had become evident.

DIAGNOSTIC PROCEDURE

When faced with so large a number of possibilities, it is obvious that no single plan can be outlined for the systematic study of every problem in unexplained fever. One must develop the course of study according to the probabilities in a given case, depending upon leads provided by the history and the physical examination. Obviously if the features suggest the presence of infectious disease, the main dependence will be upon bacteriologic and immunologic methods of diagnosis, whereas in an obscure febrile disorder in a person in the "cancer age group" the best chance of early diagnosis may lie in x-ray studies.

Careful elicitation of the patient's past *history* and the chronologic development of his symptoms may give the important leads. In respect to infection we are interested in places of recent residence, contact with domestic or wild animals and birds, preceding acute infectious diseases such as diarrheal illness or boils, contact with persons with tuberculosis, etc. Knowledge as to drugs ingested may be important. Localizing symptoms may give a clue to an organ system affected by neoplasm or infection.

In the *physical examination,* careful search is made for skin lesions and for petechial hemorrhages in the ocular fundi, conjunctivas, nail beds, and skin. The lymph nodes are carefully palpated, with special attention to the retroclavicular and axillary areas. The finding of a heart murmur or of change in the character of a preexisting one may be important. Detection of an abdominal mass may be the first lead to diagnosis of neoplastic disease. Palpable enlargement of the spleen suggests infection, leukemia, or lymphoma and points away from a diagnosis of cancer. Enlargement of the liver and spleen suggests lymphoma, leukemia, chronic infection, or cirrhosis. A large liver without palpable spleen would point to liver abscess or metastatic cancer. Nowadays the rectum and the female pelvic organs are sure to be examined, but the male patient's testicles may not be examined, with resulting failure to discover a teratoma or tuberculosis.

References have already been made to a variety of laboratory examinations which may be needed: cultures of blood, bone marrow, urine, or other body fluids; examination of blood smears for parasites or for evidence of hematologic disorder; tests for hemolysins, LE phenomenon; serologic studies; etc. X-ray studies are of course of the greatest assistance also. In all patients the chest should be examined early in the study, and the examination should perhaps be repeated occasionally. It may be expedient to proceed with studies of the gastrointestinal and urinary tracts even in the absence of symptoms referable to these areas, especially in the case of patients in the older age groups.

It will have been noted how often biopsy has been mentioned as the best means of definitive diagnosis. Bone marrow aspiration may be helpful, not only for the histology of the marrow but also for occasional demonstration of other disease processes such as metastatic carcinoma or granulomas and for culture. Aspiration biopsy of the liver is a very useful procedure and can be done with reasonable safety. It may be helpful not only with primary or metastatic disease of the liver, but also because the liver may reveal existence of other diseases such as histoplasmosis, schistosomiasis, brucellosis, tuberculosis, sarcoidosis, or lymphoma. Lymph node biopsy is, of course, helpful in diagnosis of many diseases, including the lymphomas, metastatic cancer, tuberculosis, and mycotic infections. Careful examination and consideration should precede excision of a node. The inguinal nodes are notoriously unsatisfactory for biopsy, yet are too frequently chosen because of their easy accessibility. Axillary, cervical, and supraclavicular nodes are much more likely to yield helpful information, and the node excised need not necessarily be large. Muscle biopsy may be of assistance in the recognition of dermatomyositis, periarteritis nodosa, sarcoidosis, and trichinosis.

Exploratory laparotomy is to be recommended occasionally, since it may be the only means of finding a cryptic abscess or other remediable lesion.

THERAPEUTIC TRIALS

It is common practice to give a trial of antibiotic therapy to patients with unidentified febrile disorders. While this kind of marksmanship has had its good effects, one cannot applaud "blind" therapy. Undesirable features include drug toxicity, superinfection due to resistant pathogenic bacteria, and interference with accurate diagnosis by cultural methods. Furthermore, a coincidental fall in temperature not due to the therapy is likely to be interpreted as response to treatment, with the conclusion that one is dealing with an infectious disease. If, in spite of these disadvantages, decision is made to proceed with therapeutic trial of antibiotics, streptomycin or isoniazid should not be omitted, since they are the only ones which affect tuberculosis.

Other drugs may be given on a trial basis where there is a question of such infections as amebiasis, schistosomiasis, malaria, etc.

One does not obtain much information from a trial of cortisone or ACTH therapy. These have an antipyretic effect, and also produce a euphoric state in many individuals, so that apparent improvement while receiving these agents tells little about the nature of the underlying disease.

REFERENCES

Atkins, E.: Pathogenesis of Fever, Physiol. Rev., 40:580, 1960.

Geraci, J. E., L. A. Weed, and D. R. Nichols: Fever of Obscure Origin—The Value of Abnormal Exploration in Diagnosis, J.A.M.A., 169:1306, 1959.

Petersdorf, R. G., and P. B. Beeson: Fever of Unexplained Origin: Report of 100 Cases, Medicine, 40:1, 1961.

Section 3

Alterations in Respiratory and Circulatory Function

12 COUGH AND HEMOPTYSIS
George W. Wright

COUGH

There is great variability in the concentration and character of air contaminants presented at the "breathing level" of human beings. The "self-cleansing" mechanisms of the lung (Chap. 170) can be augmented to meet intensified challenges. In general, this leads to an increase of secretions and activity of the mucociliary apparatus. When the macrophage and leukocyte responses increase, the secretions become purulent. The augmented secretions of the supralaryngeal area are removed by voluntary mechanical means. Those from the tracheobronchial system are removed by cough.

Like sneezing, cough may be a reflex mechanism, and to some degree it can be inhibited voluntarily. It arises by stimulation of the mucosa or deeper structures in the major bronchi or trachea, or of the vagus nerve itself, which supplies this area. Cough also can be initiated voluntarily with various degrees of violence. Accumulation of mucus on the surface or inflammation, drying, cooling, or chemical stimulation of the mucosa will initiate this reflex, or desire to cough. The mechanical details of the expulsive action of cough are complex. Cinefluorographic plus pressure studies indicate the following train of events. The intrathoracic pressure is raised against the closed glottis. When the trachea is subsequently abruptly opened, the pressure in the lumen of the tracheobronchial system falls far more rapidly than in the surrounding structures. This imbalance of pressure leads to a bronchial transmural pressure gradient that momentarily causes marked narrowing, if not complete closure, of the trachea and bronchial lumens. At the time this narrowing occurs, air is forced from the distal parts toward the larynx at an ever-increasing velocity. These two events, namely, lumen narrowing and augmented velocity of air flow, push mucus toward the oral pharynx in the same manner that a pea is expelled far better from a close-fitting tube than from a loose-fitting one. Preliminary closure of the glottis is helpful but not absolutely essential because laryngectomized persons cough effectively through a patent tracheostomy. Studies of this sort have not confirmed the concept of a "peristaltic milking" of the tracheobronchial tree during cough.

As a symptom of disease, cough has little intrinsic value in differential diagnosis. It is, however, an important warning that disease is present and, when persistent, *always demands* a full exploration of possible causes, since at times it is the earliest symptom of curable disease. No person with a chronic cough should ever be dismissed lightly as having a "cigarette cough," even though this is commonly enough found to be the case.

Anything causing inflammation or necrosis of the bronchial mucosa will lead to the symptom of coughing. In most forms of *acute bronchitis* the cough is nonproductive at the onset, but may become productive of purulent sputum in a day or so. Substernal burning almost always occurs, and some degree of wheezing is common. If the cough occurs as a complication of the common cold, the diagnosis is usually apparent. As a rule, the symptoms associated with acute bronchitis are not severe and the cough subsides in a few days. Cough of an acute onset may, of course, be associated with more profound evidences of infection or lung damage, and in such instances the physical examination and the chest roentgenogram will usually reveal the underlying cause. Occasionally, a *pulmonary infarction* will be associated with no other symptom than cough.

If a changed pattern of coughing persists for more than a few days, other causes must be sought. Sputum examination and x-ray are indicated. Films taken in the posteroanterior and lateral projections will usually reveal evidence of inflammatory disease such as *tuberculosis, fungous infection,* or other granulomas by the time any one of these has progressed to the stage of causing a cough. At times, however, the roentgenogram fails to reveal the cause. Bronchoscopic examination may then be necessary because localized diseases of the bronchi such as *tumors* or inflammatory disease may first be disclosed only by this procedure. Sometimes even this method of examination fails to reveal disease in the distal and nonvisualized bronchi. Cytologic studies of bronchial washings and sputum and bronchography must then be used to explore the possibility of disease of the distal bronchi. Occasionally, fluoroscopy of the lungs will demonstrate "trapping" of air in a segment whose supplying bronchus is obstructed by intrabronchial disease. Emphasis must be placed upon the fact that cough may precede any other evidence of lung disease. Hence, if cough persists and no cause is found, the entire gamut of studies must be repeated after a brief lapse of time.

There are other causes of cough which do not manifest their presence readily in the roentgenogram. *Chronic bronchitis,* a disease characterized by a productive cough of several years' duration, cough occurring *throughout* the day and especially in the morning on arising and also at night, usually associated with one or more attacks of purulent bronchitis each winter and often ultimately associated with respiratory insufficiency is diagnosed primarily by history and exclusion of other causes of the symptoms such as bronchiectasis (see Chap. 171).

Another common but often unrecognized cause of chronic cough is *diffuse obstructive disease of the lung* (diffuse obstructive emphysema). The cough associated with this disease is not always productive, but it may be paroxysmal and severe.

At times, cough of a chronic nature may be caused by *congestion of the lungs.* Mitral stenosis and left ventricular failure, especially of a slight degree, may cause a rather characteristic cough. The episodes under these circumstances are characterized by a frequently recurring single cough, at times little more than a "clearing of the throat." The cough has a particularly annoying feature in the frequency with which it is repeated, although no single episode is as a rule very prolonged or violent. In frank *pulmonary edema* the cough may, of course, be much more severe.

Cough has a protective purpose as a rule, but it can also be harmful. Distal bronchial secretions tend to be spread peripherally during cough and thus may spread disease within the lung. The exact mechanism of this is not known. Trauma to the tracheobronchial wall or larynx may occur during cough and lead to bleeding or to implantation of infection. The muscular effort involved in coughing is relatively great and may aggravate heart failure in patients who have passive congestion of the lungs.

Ribs may be fractured as a result of cough. Muscle soreness also develops from chronic prolonged cough. The pain thus induced often is a difficult problem. In a prolonged paroxysm of cough, the persistent high intrathoracic pressure may so impede venous return that cardiac output falls and cerebral ischemia occurs. Fainting or convulsions (laryngeal syncope) may occur. Such attacks developing in a person operating a mechanical device may lead to disastrous results.

HEMOPTYSIS

Bleeding from the lungs is an important and fairly common medical problem. It is, of course, necessary to ascertain that the blood is actually coming from the pulmonary tree, not from the gastrointestinal tract or the nasopharynx. Blood which comes from the lungs is often bright red and frothy in appearance, whereas that from the stomach may be dark red, brown, or black and may be mixed with particles of food. Vomiting of blood is usually preceded by a feeling of nausea and commonly accompanied by retching, whereas hemorrhage from the lung may begin without antecedent symptoms and usually is accompanied either by coughing or by clearing of the throat.

HEMOPTYSIS ASSOCIATED WITH HARD COUGHING. Very commonly, persons who have a hard, forceful cough will produce sputum which is blood streaked. This is a result of trauma to the air passages from the force of the coughing and is of little clinical significance. This type of hemoptysis usually can be identified by the history and by inspection of the sputum, noting that the blood is streaked on the surface, not intimately mixed with it.

Allied to this is the blood spitting which occurs rarely in patients with calcified lymph nodes adjacent to large bronchi. There may be erosion of the bronchial wall by the calcified mass, with bleeding and eventual ingress of the foreign body to the bronchial lumen (broncholith). Or conceivably bleeding may be caused by tearing the mucosa during the act of coughing, owing to acute angulation of a bronchus over the unyielding node.

PNEUMONIA. The sputum in bacterial pneumonia nearly always contains blood; only rarely is this the case with the viral pneumonias. In pneumococcal pneumonia the sputum may be pink or red, but more commonly, because of bacterial growth, it is the color of rust or prune juice. In staphylococcal pneumonia the sputum may be "rusty" or it may be a bright cherry red. In Friedländer bacillus pneumonia the sputum is characteristically bloody and tenacious, varying in color from dark brown to bright red. In pneumonia of any etiology the sputum seldom resembles pure blood; nearly always it is a mixture of mucopurulent material with blood.

PULMONARY INFARCTION. This is the commonest cause of hemoptysis in patients hospitalized for reasons other than lung infection. The excellent studies of Hampton and Castleman have shown that the incidence of pulmonary infarction following embolism is approximately 90 per cent in patients with heart disease, contrasted with an incidence of about 60 per cent in patients with other diseases. The higher incidence in cardiac patients probably reflects the influence of preexisting chronic pulmonary abnormalities resulting from chronic congestion of the pulmonary vascular circuit. Pulmonary infarction is discussed in more detail on p. 926. The condition should be suspected as the cause of hemoptysis (1) when there is associated pleural pain without clear evidence of pneumonia, (2) in all patients with congestive heart failure, (3) in the postoperative and post-traumatic states, (4) in all bedridden patients, (5) whenever there are signs of phlebothrombosis, and

(6) in patients exhibiting transient elevations of serum bilirubin and lactic dehydrogenase with normal values for serum transaminase.

BRONCHIECTASIS. It is estimated that hemoptysis occurs in 50 per cent of patients with bronchiectasis, and in young persons this is one of the most frequent causes of the symptom. Erosion of the inflamed bronchial mucous membrane, by infection or the trauma of coughing, causes bleeding. Diagnosis in this type of hemoptysis is usually not difficult, in view of the history of chronic productive cough and positive findings on the bronchogram.

PULMONARY TUBERCULOSIS. Small hemorrhages may occur early in the exudative phase of tuberculosis, as a result of direct erosion of vessels. In chronic ulcerative tuberculosis, bleeding occurs from incompletely obliterated pulmonary vessels which run through or along the walls of cavities. In some cases the source of bleeding is an aneurysmal dilatation, and this may bleed profusely.

Although hemorrhage in pulmonary tuberculosis is seldom immediately fatal, it may have serious effects. The plugging of a large bronchus with blood may cause atelectasis. Of even greater seriousness is the widespread dissemination of the tuberculous infection which may occur. Blood from a tuberculous cavity may be heavily contaminated with tubercle bacilli, and, as discussed previously, because of its fluidity it may be widely distributed throughout the lungs by coughing.

Because bleeding may occur at a relatively early stage of the disease, bronchial carcinoma should be suspected as the cause of the hemoptysis in any man aged forty-five or more, especially a heavy smoker.

PULMONARY NEOPLASMS. Adenomas of the bronchi nearly always cause hemoptysis, which is likely to be profuse. In bronchogenic carcinoma, the symptom is present in 25 to 50 per cent of cases. The source of bleeding is erosion of the surface of the tumor, within the lumen of the bronchus.

MITRAL STENOSIS. This is secondary only to tuberculosis as a cause of hemoptysis in young women. With mitral stenosis of long duration and in patients with advanced congestive failure, hemoptysis is more unusual. Recurrent, profuse hemoptysis is likely to be relieved by mitral valvulotomy (p. 825). The bleeding is assumed to result from rupture of small vessels of the pulmonary circulation consequent to an increase in the pulmonary venous pressure. It may also be the result of rupture of collateral varices, which have been shown to develop between the bronchial and pulmonary veins. The relative infrequency of the hemoptysis in long-standing mitral stenosis may reflect a general thickening in the supporting structures and walls of these vessels as a result of prolonged pulmonary venous hypertension.

OTHER CAUSES. The diseases mentioned previously are the principal causes of pulmonary hemorrhage, although various others occasionally may be responsible. In aneurysm of the aorta there may be bleeding through an eroded bronchus. Rarely, hemoptysis occurs in patients with arterial hypertension, presumably because of rupture of a submucous artery. Abscess in the lung may cause bleeding, as may the various purpuric states. Patients with hereditary hemorrhagic telangiectasia may bleed from the lungs repeatedly.

Episodes of hemoptysis occasionally are encountered in persons without other symptoms in whom careful study fails to reveal the cause. Possibly some of these episodes are associated with small areas of bronchiectasis of such limited extent that diagnosis by present methods is impossible.

REFERENCES

Berguson, F. C., R. E. Kobilak, and J. E. Deitrick: Varices of the Bronchial Veins as a Source of Hemoptysis in Mitral Stenosis, Am. Heart J., 28:445, 1944.

Hampton, A. O. and B. Castleman: Correlation of Postmortem Chest Teleroentgenograms with Autopsy Findings, with Special Reference to Pulmonary Embolism and Infarction, Am. J. Roentgenol., 43:305, 1940.

Johnston, R. N., W. Lockhart, R. T. Richie, and D. H. Smith: Hemoptysis, Brit. Med. J., 1:592, 1960.

13 HICCUP (SINGULTUS)
William H. Resnik and Raymond D. Adams

Hiccup is defined as a "spasmodic contraction of the diaphragm causing inspiration, followed by a sudden closure of the glottis." A classification of the causes of hiccup follows:

1. Disorders of the diaphragm and adjacent abdominal and thoracic organs
2. Phrenic nerve stimulation originating in the brain
3. Irritation of the phrenic nerve along course in neck and thorax

DISORDERS OF THE DIAPHRAGM AND ADJACENT ABDOMINAL AND THORACIC ORGANS. These constitute the most frequent cause of hiccup, which appears to be especially prone to occur in acute peritonitis, acute intestinal obstruction, acute pancreatitis (especially the severer hemorrhagic type), all post-abdominal-operative states (particularly after operations involving the upper abdominal organs), and, indeed, any disorder associated with ileus. Thus, the symptom may be encountered after a severe myocardial infarction, and in the preantibiotic era hiccup was common in severely ill patients with acute lobar pneumonia. Hiccup in conjunction with dysphagia is occasionally seen in disorders involving the terminal esophagus, such as carcinoma, achalasia, and hiatus hernia. Transitory and inconsequential bouts of hiccup may occur with any digestive disorder. Rarely, it may be associated with carcinoma of the pancreas.

The hiccup in the above group is usually attributed to reflex stimulation of the phrenic nerve. However, the common factor in all the above conditions is either significant distension of the stomach or intestines, possible trauma of diaphragm (upper abdominal operations), or actual peritonitis, possibly involving the diaphragm. These suggest the alternative mechanisms of direct irritative lesions of the diaphragm or mechanical impingement of the distended stomach or loops of intestines on the diaphragm as possible causes of the symptom.

PHRENIC NERVE STIMULATION ORIGINATING IN THE BRAIN. Any lesion, such as trauma or any of the various types of meningitis, encephalitis, or vertebral-basilar ischemia, involving the base of the brain, and hence the region of the respiratory center, may cause persistent hiccup. The symptom occurs in uremia and is usually of grave prognostic significance. The mechanism in uremia is unknown, but the symptom is probably of central origin and caused by chemical irritation of the respiratory center. The hiccup of acute and chronic alcoholism is well-known. Whether this, too, is of central origin or caused by an associated gastritis is uncertain. There is a form of hiccup, thought to be of hysterical origin, persisting for days but disappearing during sleep.

DIRECT IRRITATION OF THE PHRENIC NERVE. Any lesion causing direct irritation of the phrenic nerve can cause intractable hiccup, such as mediastinal lymphoma, mediastinitis of any etiology, or injury of phrenic nerve after thoracic surgery.

The mechanism of the distressing and persistent crises of hiccup in tabes dorsalis is unknown.

TREATMENT. Assuming that appropriate measures have been instituted toward control of the specific cause of the hiccup and toward relief of abdominal distension by gastric suction through a Levin tube, symptomatic relief can usually be obtained with chloral hydrate, 0.6 Gm, or chlorpromazine, 25 to 50 mg (or any of the other phenothiazine drugs) every 3 or 4 hr. It has been reported that a skeletal-muscle relaxant, such as orphenadrine citrate (Norflex), 60 mg, given intravenously, followed by 100 mg orally every 12 hr has been effective. In other cases, inhalation of 5 to 10 per cent carbon dioxide for 10 min every hour may be effective; in the most resistant cases, blocking of a phrenic nerve may be required.

14 DYSPNEA
George W. Wright

Patients with pulmonary or heart disease, anemia, or neuroses often consult a physician for the first time because they are "out of breath" or "can't get their breath." Some complain that breathing "does not satisfy them," or they "feel the air goes in only a little distance," or they feel that they are "smothering." These complaints characterize dyspnea. For our purposes, it is defined as "the awareness of respiratory distress or of unusual breathlessness." It is a subjective phenomenon and liable to all the influences of emotion, ignorance, fatigue, and other factors that make human beings such variable creatures from day to day. Dyspnea is a form of breathlessness that is distressing or unusual because of the circumstances under which it develops, or because the sensation itself is unusual. It may or may not be associated with the labored breathing or other signs of respiratory embarrassment.

Physiologic dyspnea occurs during vigorous exercise in young healthy persons. Moderate exertion may cause the same sensation in normal elderly sedentary persons, and especially in those who are obese. Dyspnea at rest or during such minimal exertion as slow horizontal walking may occur during the last few weeks of pregnancy, but it is otherwise to be considered as a manifestation of some disease process.

Pathologic dyspnea is usually due to disorders of the heart, lungs or emotions. Less common causes are anemia and disturbances of the respiratory neuromuscular apparatus (e.g., poliomyelitis) or of the chest wall (e.g., advanced scleroderma). However, these latter conditions are likely to be accompanied by other and more pressing symptoms. Thus when dyspnea is the prime complaint, one thinks first of cardiac, pulmonary, and emotional disorders.

In normal persons the sensation of a need for augmented breathing during heavy exercise is not a distressing one. This may be because we are accustomed to the sensations associated with the increase of respiratory drive. It may also be because of an inhibition or neutralization of respiratory drive by each act of inspiration, so that a steady state of respiratory drive exists in which each act of inspiration satisfies the demand for more air. Stretch receptors resident within the lung and chest wall may be activated by inspiration in such a manner as to inhibit the sensation of respiratory need. When, however, the act of inspiration does not sufficiently neutralize the respiratory drive, a persistent activity of the inspiratory center may accumulate and finally reach a level that in some ways sends impulses to the cortex which are recognized as "unsatisfied need for breathing." There is some experimental evidence to support this concept of the genesis of the abnormal sensation of dyspnea. Fatigue of the respiratory muscles, which cannot be measured, probably contributes to the sensation.

One can examine the individual who complains of dyspnea from the viewpoint of three variables: load, capacity, and sensitivity of the cerebral cortex. The estimated load during effort would be best expressed in units of work performed by the muscles of respiration. Measurements of the relationship between volume of air flow and transthoracic or transpulmonary pressure gradient are, however, not readily available. A usable, though not perfect, substitute for the work of breathing is the "effect" of that work, namely, the liters of air breathed per minute. The load at the time when dyspnea is experienced during exercise can, therefore, be expressed in terms of minute ventilation.

The capacity of the breathing apparatus can be measured in the same terms, namely, the maximal breathing capacity expressed in liters per minute. The ratio of the breathing load at the time that dyspnea develops to maximal breathing capacity, expressed in liters per minute, is referred to by some as the *dyspnea index*. The strain or sensation associated with respiratory effort will be related to this quotient, and the normal person is unaware of any strain until the "index" exceeds 0.30 to 0.35. It is apparent that the dyspnea index can exceed 0.35 at lower than normal intensities of exercise *if the maximal breathing capacity is reduced or if the minute ventilation is abnormally augmented*. If the sensations of respiration intrude upon consciousness at lower values, one may infer that the cortex has been made more aware of or is more sensitive than normal to these sensations. Thus some persons, usually classed as neurotic, are exquisitely sensitive to the breathing sensation, while others, because of powerful or engrossing distractions, completely ignore them.

Dyspnea usually appears first during exercise and is present at rest only when impairment of function is severe. Those diseases which weaken the neuromuscular system, or reduce the mobility of the thorax or the flexibility of the lung, or increase obstruction to air flow induce dyspnea chiefly, but not entirely, by causing a loss of breathing power. Those diseases which pose an abnormal barrier to the transit of oxygen across the alveolocapillary membrane or which are associated with increased lung rigidity induce dyspnea chiefly by causing an abnormally high load of breathing. Often both loss of breathing power and

abnormally high load of breathing coexist. In some patients, undoubted dyspnea occurs when there is no significant demonstrable abnormality of the respiratory or circulatory system. The cerebral cortex in these patients is perhaps more sensitive than usual to the sensations associated with respiration.

The simple methods of testing pulmonary function will be considered first. Although these do not pinpoint a precise locus of the abnormality of function, they do provide a useful estimate of the capacity of the respiratory apparatus to carry out its ventilatory activity. The history and physical examination are relatively insensitive methods for this purpose. Auscultation of wheezes throughout the lungs, inability to augment the normal respiratory murmur by rapid inspiration and expiration, plus the observation of limited thoracic cage motion virtually assures a diminished ability to move air into and out of the lungs. Regional wheezing suggests localized bronchial narrowing and should arouse the suspicion of carcinoma.

A very useful maneuver for a rough estimate of the capacity for air movement into and out of the lungs is careful fluoroscopic examination of the chest with observation of motion of the thoracic cage and diaphragm and the changes in lung density that accompany emptying and filling of the lung during quiet breathing and during explosive forced full inspiration and expiration. Unfortunately, this method lacks quantitation.

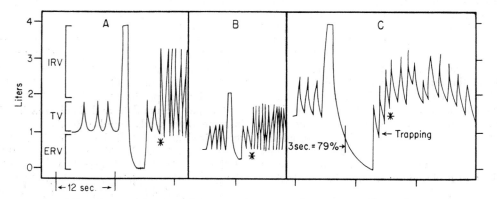

Fig. 14-1. *IRV* = Inspiratory reserve volume. *ERV* = Expiratory reserve volume. The inspiratory capacity is the sum of the inspiratory reserve and the tidal volume (*TV*). The vital capacity is the inspiratory capacity plus the expiratory reserve, or the largest expiration possible from the position of full inspiration. Each of the three spirograms begins with a few tidal breaths, followed by a vital capacity breath blown at maximal velocity. At the asterisk, each subject began to breathe as rapidly and deeply as possible (the maximal breathing capacity).

   A. The spirogram of a normal person. The vital capacity is rapid and smooth and completed in less than 3 sec. The maximal breathing is not only rapid but deep.

   B. The spirogram of a patient with severe diffuse interstitial fibrosis without emphysema. It is a typical record illustrating restrictive ventilatory insufficiency. Because of increased retractive force within the lungs, tidal breathing is shallow and near the position of complete expiration. Consequently, the expiratory reserve volume is small. The respiratory rate is rapid to compensate for the greater percentage of dead-space breathing. The vital capacity is small but rapidly exhaled. The maximal breathing capacity is reduced but not so severely as the vital capacity, since an increased rate partially offsets the loss of depth.

   C. Spirogram characteristic of obstructive ventilatory insufficiency obtained from a patient with emphysema. Although the vital capacity is large, expiration is severely obstructed, so only 79 per cent is exhaled in 3 sec. Trapping of air in the lungs is indicated by the shifting level of the end-expiratory position of the breath following the vital capacity effort. The maximal breathing effort is carried out near full inspiration and is irregular and severely reduced below normal.

MEASUREMENTS OF PULMONARY VOLUMES

These are simple and valuable in assessing the integrity of the respiratory apparatus. A study of Fig. 14-1 indicates the useful information that may be gleaned from spirometry. The pulmonary volumes are static measurements and lack the element of time. The respiratory pump is capable of augmenting its action manyfold, and dynamic measurements of this function are important. A single explosive full expiratory effort started from a position of full inspiration adds the element of velocity to volume of air flow. Various segments of this expiratory act can be measured, as, for example, the peak flow rate, the maximal midexpiratory flow rate, the maximal flow rate during the last liter of the vital capacity, and the absolute volume and proportion of total vital capacity expelled in the first second of such an effort. These single expiratory efforts fail to take into consideration the fact that respiration is a repetitive phenomenon; for this reason, plus others, a measurement of the maximal voluntary breathing capacity has some advantages. These measurements are quite sensitive to any change occurring in an individual, provided the measurement is made before and after the alteration of function occurs. Unfortunately, there is a wide range of variation in the maximal capacity for air flow among normal persons. Hence, although the test faithfully reveals the ability of the person, it will not indicate with certainty that an abnormal state exists, until a reduction of capacity to approximately 75 per cent, or less, of the predicted normal is observed. Even so, these methods are superior to purely clinical observations.

At the end of a maximal forced expiration, a volume of gas known as the residual volume still remains in the lung. Incomplete emptying of the lung, such as occurs in diffuse obstructive disease, will be revealed by an enlargement of the residual volume. This can be measured either by physical or by gas-rinsing procedures.

MECHANICS OF RESPIRATION AND ALVEOLAR VENTILATION

Movement of air into and out of the lungs is a consequence of enlargement and reduction in the size of the thorax. The force developed by contraction of the muscles of respiration is used for the following purposes:

1. Movement of the thoracic cage
2. Movement of the underlying lung structures
3. Movement of air through the tracheobronchial tree

Thus it is seen that the respiratory muscles are used to overcome resistive forces, which can be considered under three categories:

1. Elastic resistances, such as the "spring" of the ribs and stretch of the elastic tissues of the lung

2. Nonelastic resistances, such as those tissues of the chest wall and lung which have no property of recoil

3. Resistance to air flow in the tracheobronchial tree

Two of these forces, namely, those caused by resistance to air flow and motion of nonelastic tissue, can be measured only during respiratory movement, whereas elastic resistance is a static force measured in the absence of movement. The minor forces involved in overcoming inertia can be neglected. The ratio of volume of air inspired to the drop in intrapleural pressure is spoken of as "mechanical compliance" of the lung and is customarily expressed in liters of air per centimeter of water pressure.

Diseases which increase the rigidity of the lung parenchyma or which reduce the number of available lung units will decrease the compliance of the lung and thereby increase the work of breathing. Also, diseases which alter the elastic character of the lung in such a manner as to reduce the recoil will increase the compliance of the lung and, by the same token, diminish the force of the elastic recoil which is used during passive or slow expiration. While, on the one hand, this reduces the work of breathing during inspiration, it increases the work of breathing during expiration.

Resistance to air flow is related to three primary factors, namely, the diameter and length of the lumen of the tubes and the presence or absence of turbulent and eddy flow as contrasted with laminar flow. Disease processes leading to a reduction in the size of the lumen will increase the resistance to flow in those areas. Moreover, anything that produces irregularities in the lumen or changes the branching angle may set up turbulent or eddy flow and, consequently, increase the resistance to transbronchial air flow. This is especially likely to occur during augmented rates of flow. During rates of flow that accompany the resting-state, expiration, in contrast to inspiration, is for the most part a passive phenomenon, the forces that accomplish this act arising by virtue of recoil of elastic tissue within the lung and chest wall. During greater rates of flow, however, active expiratory effort utilizing muscular contraction is required. Under these circumstances, a decrease in thoracic or lung compliance or an increase in airway resistance will require unusually augmented work of breathing.

Relatively little is known concerning the magnitude of the work of breathing because of the difficulty with which such measurements are made. Studies currently available indicate that during the resting state approximately 2 per cent of the total body oxygen uptake is utilized by the muscles of respiration. In normal persons, at the rate of ventilation developed during maximal intensity of exercise, approximately 10 to 15 per cent of the total body oxygen uptake is utilized by the respiratory muscles. This may amount to as much as 400 to 500 ml per min. In diseased states that lead to a marked augmentation of the work of breathing, it seems obvious that much larger portions of the total body oxygen uptake, especially in the resting state, would be used for metabolic purpose by the respiratory muscles. It is apparent that therapeutic efforts aimed at reducing the work of breathing in pathologic situations may be very important, not only by reducing stress on the respiratory muscles, with consequent reduction in their oxygen need, but also by reducing their carbon dioxide production, which may be a large contributing factor in the maintenance of high CO_2 levels in the blood, where ventilation is impaired and the work of breathing is augmented.

DISTURBANCES OF ALVEOLAR VENTILATION

The mere fact that large volumes of air can be respired does not assure optimal alveolar ventilation. If the volume respired per minute is too small to satisfy the metabolic demand, alveolar hypoventilation exists. Normally, the volume of respired air is increased in direct proportion to augmented demand for oxygen and carbon dioxide exchange during exercise, so that the partial pressure of these gases in the alveoli stays within narrow limits over a wide range of physical effort. When the respiratory apparatus cannot augment ventilation sufficiently to keep pace with the demand for gas exchange, the alveolar P_{O_2} drops and P_{CO_2} rises. A second situation leading to alveolar hypoventilation has to do with the relationship of the tidal volume to the anatomic dead space. During shallow breathing, the majority of each tidal breath moves into and out of the anatomic dead space and relatively little alveolar ventilation occurs, with the consequence that the turnover of alveolar gas is reduced and the P_{O_2} drops and P_{CO_2} rises. A third type of alveolar hypoventilation occurs when the distribution of each breath is uneven, so that some clusters of alveoli are over- and others underventilated. This causes regional variations in alveolar P_{O_2} and P_{CO_2}. If the hypoventilated alveoli, either regional or generalized, are perfused with pulmonary artery blood, the natural consequence is apt to be arterial hypoxia and hypercapnia. On the other hand, the consequences of alveolar hypoventilation will vary, dependent upon whether or not the alveoli are perfused. The auscultation of wheezes or evidence of impaired respiratory mechanics of various sorts strongly suggests that alveolar hypoventilation either exists or can be made to exist under the stress of physical exercise.

DISTURBANCES OF TRANSMEMBRANE DIFFUSION OF O_2 AND CO_2

Oxygen and carbon dioxide move between the blood and gas phases of the lung across the alveolocapillary structure because of the pressure gradient for the gases between these two media. The highly complex chemical and physical forces governing this transit will not be discussed here. In the presence of pulmonary disease, this process can become one of the chief limiting factors in physical performance. The integrity of this process can be examined, but instrumentation is needed for such studies. Two approaches can be used.

In normal persons the blood leaving the alveolar capillaries has its hemoglobin fully oxygenated, but when a sample of peripheral systemic arterial blood is examined, a measurable amount of hemoglobin will be found to be in the reduced form. It is believed that approximately 5 per cent of the blood leaving the left ventricle represents venous admixture from various sources within the lung, and this accounts for the fact that the arterial hemoglobin at sea level is only 95 per cent oxygenated.

Methods of acceptable accuracy are available for the direct measurement of P_{O_2} in the blood by calculation of the P_{O_2} in the alveolar gas. As might be expected, because of the venous admixture factor, there is a higher P_{O_2} in the alveolar gas than in the arterial blood. This difference of approximately 10 ml Hg is referred to as the *alveolar-arterial (A-a) gradient*. The A-a gradient may be increased by disease if the alveolocapillary membrane is thickened or otherwise altered in character, or if a portion of the pulmonary artery blood flow bypasses the alveoli entirely, as, for example, in arteriovenous fistula. Arterial hypoxia may occur, therefore, as a result of three entirely different conditions: alveolar hypoventilation, altered alveolocapillary membrane, and direct arteriovenous communications that bypass the alveoli. When alveolar hypoventilation is the cause, the A-a gradient will be normal or only slightly increased but other abnormalities, discussed under Mechanics of Respiration, will be disclosed. Alveolar bypass and alteration of the alveolocapillary membrane (alveolocapillary block) are associated with an increased A-a gradient, and evidences of alveolar hypoventilation are usually absent.

One can distinguish between alveolocapillary block and arteriovenous fistula in most instances in the following way: If one respires a mixture containing 30 to 40 per cent oxygen, the alveolar P_{O_2} is raised sufficiently to drive the necessary molecules of oxygen across the alveolocapillary membrane and restore a normal degree of arterial hemoglobin saturation. Blood passing through an arteriovenous communication within the lung does not perfuse alveoli, and hence will not be influenced by the elevated alveolar P_{O_2}. Raising the alveolar P_{O_2} will alter the arterial saturation only slightly, if at all, in the arterial hypoxia caused by arteriovenous fistulas.

A second approach to the integrity of the alveolocapillary membrane is a more direct one. The capacity of the lung to permit the transit of oxygen from the gas to the blood phase can be expressed in terms of milliliters of gas per millimeter of pressure gradient per unit of time. This is commonly referred to as the D_L for O_2, and it has been found to be larger during exercise than in the resting state. This property of the lung is dependent primarily upon the following factors: the effective surface area of the pulmonary capillary bed, the thickness and character (tissue components) of the membranes separating the gas from the blood phase, and the volume of blood in the capillaries to which the gas is exposed.

The D_L for other gases differs from that of O_2. Carbon dioxide, because it passes across animal membranes approximately twenty times as easily as does oxygen, has a much larger D_L. For this reason, disease involving the alveolocapillary membrane rarely interferes with carbon dioxide removal from the blood (at least to a clinically significant degree), whereas serious impediment to oxygen does occur. Because of much greater technical convenience, it is customary today to use carbon monoxide as the gas for studying these characteristics of the lung. Using this gas, it is possible to distinguish between the membrane component and the capillary blood volume component, but it is still not possible to discriminate between the effective surface area and the nature of the membrane itself. Current experience indicates that abnormalities of the diffusion characteristics of the lung are more common than heretofore believed, and they may play an important role in the symptoms and physical limitations of diseased organs.

VENTILATION-PERFUSION RELATIONSHIPS

Alveolar hypoventilation and alveolocapillary block may occur as generalized lung phenomena in which all, or the vast majority, of the units are involved, or they may occur in isolated clusters of units scattered throughout the lung, or they may involve chiefly one lung. The effects of scattered areas of hypoventilation are not the same as those of generalized hypoventilation because, commonly, the alveoli not involved by hypoventilation actually undergo hyperventilation. Since the dissociation curves of oxygen and of carbon dioxide have different shapes, clusters of hyperventilated alveoli cannot effectively augment amounts of oxygen put into the blood but they can remove significant quantities of carbon dioxide. As a consequence, the arterial blood-gas findings differ in these two situations. In generalized hypoventilation, hypoxia and hypercapnia coexist, whereas in the patchy varieties of alveolar hypoventilation, hypoxia may exist without any attending hypercapnia.

The final effect of hypo- or hyperventilation of alveoli upon arterial blood gases will depend also upon the degree to which these alveoli are perfused with mixed venous blood. In the resting state, for reasons poorly understood, alveolar hypoventilation of the patchy type is often not associated with arterial hypoxia or hypercapnia because a reduction in capillary perfusion occurs to a degree commensurate with the hypoventilation, so that the ventilation and perfusion ratios actually are normal, although the oxygen uptake and CO_2 output per lung unit are reduced. This relationship may be grossly disturbed during exercise, however. The need to use the stress of physical exercise to unmask abnormal conditions in the lung cannot be emphasized too greatly. Not only must one increase the metabolic demand and thus unbalance the ventilation/perfusion ratio, but also it would appear that some of the arterial-venous shunt mechanisms are responsive to intravascular pressure changes and operate only during the periods of increased blood flow or of pulmonary hypertension that may accompany physical exercise.

Regional areas of hypoperfusion may also occur in the presence of normally ventilated alveoli. If, for example, one suddenly ligated the main pulmonary artery on one side, the tremendous increase in blood flow through the other lung would greatly augment the rate of removal of oxygen and delivery of carbon dioxide to that perfused lung. Hypoxia and hypercapnia would ensue unless these perfused alveoli were physically hyperventilated. The alveoli of the ligated lung, of course, continue to be ventilated but perform no useful function and, therefore, constitute a physiologic dead space. Although this precise circumstance rarely occurs, a similar situation involving scattered clusters of alveoli is common. This leads to a persistent hyperventilation state with abnormally large physiologic dead space.

The mechanism whereby variations in perfusion can occur is not entirely clear. Arteriolar or capillary thrombosis or actual destruction of the tissues are obvious mechanisms. On the other hand, a reduction in perfusion paralleling that of ventilation, even to the point that perfusion virtually ceases in nonventilated portions of lung, has been observed without attending anatomic obstruction to blood flow. Studies during recent years have shown that some mechanism is available whereby alveolocapillary perfusion is diminished (presumably by narrowing or closure of these vessels) whenever the alveolar P_{O_2} is diminished by hypoventilation. The important thing is to realize that the respiratory system exhibits a great ability to tailor its perfusion to whatever ventilation exists in various regions of the lung.

It is apparent from these comments that the pulmonary vascular bed may undergo a considerable reduction in size as a result of intrinsic pulmonary disease, some of which is on an organic basis and some on a functional basis. This restriction of the vascular bed may lead to serious circulatory consequences that will be discussed in detail in Chap. 169.

INTEGRATION AND CONTROL OF RESPIRATION

The rate and depth of respiration are controlled directly by impulses arising within the brain stem from cells designated as the *respiratory centers*. The discharge of these cells is modified as to rate and intensity by a host of impulses coming to them from many parts of the body. The cerebral cortex, chemo- and pressoreceptors, thermoreceptors, muscle-tension receptors, sensory bodies in the lung, pain receptors, and other less certainly established sensory bodies elsewhere in our anatomy send out such regulatory impulses. The cells of the respiratory center also vary their discharge in response to their own tissue environment. Hence, the rate of flow of blood to these cells and its chemical character, in terms of pH, P_{O_2} and P_{CO_2} will modify the discharge of the respiratory center. With so many influences, one marvels that the respiratory discharge is other than chaotic. Normally, the stimuli are well integrated so that there is reciprocal stimulation and inhibition of the various parts of the center, and the final discharge pattern has an orderly character. During the "resting state" the volume of air respired per minute depends to a large measure on environmental stimuli and conscious, or perhaps even subconscious, activity of the cortex. Excitement, interest in surrounding events, etc., have a large influence on the pattern and rate of ventilation at rest. Because of this, our ability to recognize abnormal respiratory drive at rest is limited. If, at rest, the minute volume consistently exceeds 10 liters for men and 7 liters for women, unusual respiratory drive probably exists. In contrast, sustained physical work by a normal person under normal physiologic conditions will cause the respired minute volume to increase directly in a straight-line fashion with the measured increment of oxygen uptake. The ratio of these two measurements over a wide range of physical activity is 25 ± 5 liters of air respired for each liter of oxygen uptake in the steady state. This ratio may be termed the *oxygen ventilation equivalent* (O_2V). At the extremes of hard physical exercise, this ratio becomes increased because oxygen uptake reaches a plateau, whereas the respiratory minute volume continues to rise.

APPROACH TO THE PATIENT WITH DYSPNEA

When muscular disorders, anemia, thyrotoxicosis, or metabolic acidosis are responsible for dyspnea, this symptom is a relatively minor phenomenon and the clinical picture is dominated by other and more specific manifestations of the underlying diseases. The problems arise in differentiating the psychogenic, pulmonary, and cardiac varieties of dyspnea from each other and, more especially, in evaluating the relative significance of each of these types when two of them coexist, as they frequently do.

Emotional dyspnea is characterized by a sensation of smothering often described as "a need for more oxygen," or "my breathing does not get in enough air." Associated complaints such as numbness of the face or the extremities, tightness of the chest muscles with slight pain, "drawing" of the hands, faintness, lightheadedness, "floating away," palpitation, or aerophagia with belching are usually present. In most instances the symptoms are episodic, and there is little relation of dyspnea to exertion. The manifestation of panic or of the acute anxiety state (p. 1267) may be pronounced.

Unless there is coexistent cardiac or pulmonary disease, the various tests of respiratory function yield normal findings, although during an attack there is hypocapnia and increased ventilation in relation to oxygen uptake.

As a general rule, dyspnea of pulmonary or cardiac origin appears initially during exertion. However, bronchial asthma and acute left ventricular failure (p. 792) may first occur at rest. Cough of long duration is a frequent concomitant of pulmonary dyspnea, but acute episodic coughing may accompany either type. Clinical, radiologic, or electrocardiographic evidence of primary pulmonary or cardiac disease is of obvious importance.

Seizures of dyspnea which awaken the patient speak for a cardiac origin, but early morning episodes associated with cough and expectoration point toward pulmonary disease.

The arm-to-tongue circulation time is usually prolonged in patients with cardiac dyspnea but normal when the distress is of pulmonary origin. A decrease in the rate of air flow (i.e., in the "timed vital capacity" or "forced expiratory volume") is more likely to signify pulmonary dyspnea. Both types of dyspnea are associated with decrease in total vital capacity, which is usually reduced less in relation to the decline in maximal breathing capacity in the pulmonary than in the cardiac disorders. This relative disproportion, which is due to airway obstruction, may, however, be present in those patients with cardiac failure who have pronounced wheezes (cardiac asthma, p. 792).

Arterial hypoxia, which is common in patients with pulmonary disease, is absent or minimal in those with acquired cardiac disorders, except when edema of the lungs is pronounced or some complication such as pulmonary infarction supervenes. Hypercapnia is the rule in the advanced stages of those disorders of the lungs associated with alveolar hypoventilation; it is absent in patients with cardiac failure except for those instances due to primary pulmonary disorders (cor pulmonale).

As dyspnea and limitation for physical exercise become progressively more severe, orthopnea begins to be experienced by the patient who has heart failure. In contrast, orthopnea rarely occurs in primary pulmonary disease, even though the dyspnea associated with exercise may be severe. When the pulmonary cripple begins to experience orthopnea, he is apt to be developing cor pulmonale and heart failure.

For further discussion of the differentiation between pulmonary and cardiac dyspnea, the reader is referred to p. 794.

HYPERCAPNIA AND HYPOCAPNIA

Although hypercapnia, an abnormally elevated P_{CO_2} in tissues and blood, is a relatively common clinical state as a result of pulmonary disease, it occurs only in those situations leading to alveolar hypoventilation. Alveolocapillary block does not lead to clinically significant hypercapnia because of the greater ability for carbon dioxide to traverse the membrane and the common occurrence of alveolar hyperventilation. All the conditions discussed earlier that lead to alveolar hypoventilation will, if severe enough, lead to hypercapnia, provided, of course, that the hypoventilated alveoli are also perfused with pulmonary artery blood.

Hypocapnia, the development of a subnormal P_{CO_2} in the tissues and blood, is unusual. It may occur in those pulmonary diseases which lead to hyperventilation of alveoli that are relatively well perfused with pulmonary artery blood. More often it is the result of emotional disturbances.

For further discussion of hypercapnia and hypocapnia, the reader is referred to Chap. 61. Hypoxia is considered in Chap. 15.

REFERENCES

Arnott, W. M.: The Syndrome of Alveolar-Capillary Block and Its Functional Pathology, Progr. in Cardiovascular Diseases, 1:435, 1959.

Brisco, W. A., and A. B. DuBois: The Relationship between Airway Resistance, Airway Conductance and Lung Volume in Subjects of Different Age and Body Size, J. Clin. Invest., 37:1279, 1958.

Comroe, J. H., Jr., et al.: "The Lung," Chicago, Year Book Publishers, Inc., 1955.

Forster, R. E.: Exchange of Gases between Alveolar Air and Pulmonary Capillary Blood: Pulmonary Diffusing Capacity, Physiol. Rev., 37:391, 1957.

Fry, D. L., R. B. Ebert, W. W. Stead, and C. C. Brown: The Mechanics of Pulmonary Ventilation in Normal Subjects and in Patients with Emphysema, Am. J. Med., 16:80, 1954.

Harvey, R. M., M. I. Ferrer, D. W. Richards, Jr., and A. Cournand: Influence of Chronic Pulmonary Disease on the Heart and Circulation, Am. J. Med., 10:719, 1951.

West, J. R., E. de F. Baldwin, A. Cournand, and D. W. Richards, Jr.: Physiopathologic Aspects of Chronic Pulmonary Emphysema, Am. J. Med., 10:481, 1951.

Wright, G. W., and G. F. Filley: Pulmonary Fibrosis and Respiratory Function, Am. J. Med., 10:642, 1951.

—— and B. V. Branscomb: The Origin of the Sensations of Dyspnea, Trans. Am. Clin. & Climatol. A.. 66:116, 1954.

15 CYANOSIS, HYPOXIA, AND POLYCYTHEMIA

T. R. Harrison and M. M. Wintrobe

CYANOSIS

The term *cyanosis*, in its strictest sense, means blueness, but it is ordinarily restricted to a special type of blueness—namely, that which is due to an increased amount of reduced hemoglobin, or derivatives of hemoglobin, in the small blood vessels of the skin and mucous membranes. Hence it is to be distinguished from argyria, a condition in which there is a bluish discoloration of the skin as the result of the deposi-

tion of silver salts. In the latter condition there is a metallic tint and the blue color persists despite pressure, whereas the truly cyanotic skin becomes pale when sufficient pressure is exerted to express the blood from the vessels.

Cyanosis is usually most marked in the lips, the nail beds, the ears, and the malar eminences. In the last region the line of distinction between true cyanosis and the ruddy color which is commonly seen in robust elderly subjects cannot always be clearly drawn. Furthermore, the "red cyanosis" of polycythemia vera (Chap. 113) must be distinguished from the true cyanosis discussed here. A cherry-colored flush, rather than cyanosis, is caused by carboxyhemoglobin (Chap. 241).

Certain modifying factors influence the degree of cyanosis. These include the thickness of the epidermis, the quantity of cutaneous pigment, and the color of the blood plasma, as well as the state of the capillaries of the skin. The accurate clinical detection of the presence and degree of cyanosis is difficult, as proved by oxymetric studies.

The *fundamental mechanism of cyanosis* was shown, by Lundsgaard and Van Slyke, to consist of an increase in the amount of reduced hemoglobin in the vessels of the skin. This may be brought about either by increase in the amount of venous blood in the skin as the result of dilatation of the venules and venous ends of the capillaries, or by a decrease in the oxygen saturation in the capillary blood.

As a general rule, cyanosis becomes apparent when the mean capillary concentration of reduced hemoglobin exceeds 5 Gm per 100 ml. It is the absolute rather than the relative amount of reduced hemoglobin which is important in producing cyanosis. Thus, in a patient with severe anemia the relative amount of reduced hemoglobin in the venous blood may be very large when considered in relation to the total hemoglobin. However, since the latter is markedly reduced, the absolute amount of reduced hemoglobin may still be small. It is for this reason that patients with severe anemia do not display cyanosis. Conversely, the higher the total hemoglobin content, the greater the tendency toward cyanosis; thus, patients with marked polycythemia may be cyanotic in the absence of any other demonstrable abnormality. Likewise, local passive congestion, which causes an increase in the total amount of hemoglobin in the vessels in a given area, may cause cyanosis even though the average percentage unsaturation is not altered.

Cyanosis also is observed when nonfunctional hemoglobin is present in the blood, as little as 1.5 Gm per 100 ml or 0.5 Gm sulfhemoglobin being sufficient to produce cyanosis (Chap. 114).

It follows from this discussion that cyanosis is intimately related to hypoxia, i.e., to reduction in the oxygen concentration or tension in the body. We may, therefore, now consider certain causes and effects of hypoxia. This term is preferable to the less exact expression *anoxia*, which means the complete absence of oxygen and thus a state incompatible with life.

MECHANISM OF HYPOXIA

The following classification is adapted from those of Barcroft and of Van Slyke:

I. *Arterial hypoxia*, i.e., hypoxia consequent to failure of the arterial blood to become normally saturated with oxygen
   A. Diminished oxygenation in the lungs
   B. Admixture of venous blood via shunts
II. *Anemic hypoxia*, i.e., hypoxia due to a decline in the quantity of hemoglobin capable of transporting oxygen per unit volume of blood
   A. Diminished concentration of hemoglobin
   B. Chemical alteration of hemoglobin to derivatives which do not carry oxygen
III. *Circulatory hypoxia*, arising from
   A. Ischemia
   B. Stagnation
IV. *Metabolic hypoxia*, arising from
   A. Need for oxygen beyond the capacity of normal respiratory mechanisms to supply it
   B. Failure of tissues to employ available oxygen

ARTERIAL HYPOXIA. This term refers to a condition in which the oxygen tension is diminished in the ar-

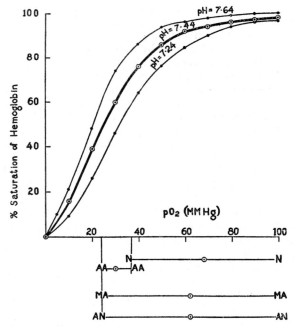

Fig. 15-1. Relationship between oxygen tension and oxygen saturation of the hemoglobin of the blood. The heavy line is for blood at pH 7.44. The curves to the right and left are for bloods of pH 7.24 and 7.64, respectively, and indicate quantitatively the magnitude of the Bohr effect for hydrogen ion concentration changes of these magnitudes.

During vigorous muscular effort the increase in acidity of the blood causes the dissociation curve to shift to the right, raises the tissue oxygen tension for any given degree of saturation of the hemoglobin, and thus makes oxygen more available to the muscles. On the other hand, any condition such as high altitude, which causes respiratory alkalosis (p. 329), moves the dissociation curve to the left. This facilitates oxygen uptake in the lungs by increasing the oxygen saturation at a given level of alveolar oxygen tension.

terial blood, with consequent diminution in the percentage saturation of the hemoglobin (Fig. 15-1). Such a diminution in the arterial tension may be brought about when there is a corresponding decline in the tension of oxygen in the inspired air (e.g., at high altitude), the respiratory mechanism remaining otherwise unimpaired, by interference with the free passage of air through the respiratory pathways or by increase in the barriers to diffusion through which the gas must pass to reach hemoglobin. In the case of many types of chronic pulmonary disease attended by fibrosis and obliteration of the capillary vascular bed, arterial hypoxia does not occur because there is no significant volume of circulation through the unaerated portions. The occurrence of arterial hypoxia is favored by disorders such as pulmonary edema and emphysema, in which there is considerable circulation through areas of the lungs in which ventilation is impaired.

Another, but less common, cause of arterial hypoxia is a congenital malformation of the heart that allows unaerated blood to pass into the arterial system. Congenital heart disease of several types is attended by abnormal communications between the right and left sides of the heart. Under ordinary conditions the transfer of blood tends to be from the left side, with its higher pressure, to the right side. However, under certain conditions, such as exist in patients with the combination of pulmonary stenosis and an interventricular septal defect, or in patients with a three-chambered heart, a significant proportion of the blood returning to the right side of the heart passes directly into the left side without passing through the lungs, the quantity sometimes varying with posture. Under such conditions arterial hypoxia tends to occur (Chap. 137).

When hypoxia occurs as the result of decline in oxygen tension in the inspired air, the respiration is stimulated, the alveolar ventilation increases, and the carbon dioxide tension in the alveoli and in the arterial blood declines. This causes a shift to the left in the oxygen dissociation curve (Fig. 15-1) and enables a given tension of alveolar oxygen to cause a greater degree of oxygen uptake by the hemoglobin (the Bohr effect).

When, on the other hand, hypoxia results from interference with the passage of air into the lungs, or from impairment of oxygen diffusion in the lungs, the resulting respiratory stimulation is less effective in causing carbon dioxide elimination. The carbon dioxide tension, therefore, remains normal or rises; and the oxygen dissociation curve tends to remain unchanged or to move to the right (Fig. 15-1). Under such conditions the percentage saturation of the hemoglobin in the arterial blood at a given level of alveolar oxygen tension does not rise and may even decline. Thus arterial hypoxia and cyanosis are likely to be more marked in proportion to the degree of depression of alveolar oxygen tension when such depression results from pulmonary disease than when the depression occurs as the result of a decline in the partial pressure of oxygen in the inspired air.

Figure 15-1 illustrates why the respiratory mechanisms may be considerably impaired without a significant degree of arterial hypoxia developing. This is because the properties of the hemoglobin are such that its dissociation curve is practically flat above 100 mm of oxygen tension, and almost flat down to about 80 mm. When the tension of oxygen in the alveoli falls below the point at which the slope of the dissociation curve tends to become more nearly vertical, a rapid decline in the amount of oxygen in the arterial blood occurs. A clear understanding of the physiologic significance of this S shape of the oxygen dissociation curve enables one to see why hypoxia and cyanosis do not occur in significant degree in a person ascending in an airplane to about 8,000 ft, and why a further ascent to 16,000 ft is associated with development of well-marked cyanosis and hypoxia. At 8,000 ft the tension of oxygen in the inspired air is about 120 mm Hg and the alveolar tension approximately 80 mm Hg. At such pressures of oxygen the blood is well-nigh completely saturated. On the other hand, at 16,000 ft the oxygen tensions in atmospheric air and alveolar air are about 85 and 50 mm Hg, respectively, and the oxygen dissociation curve shows that under such conditions the arterial blood is only about 75 per cent saturated. This leaves an excess of 25 per cent of the hemoglobin in the reduced form, an amount which, as explained already, is likely to be associated with cyanosis.

The moderate hyperventilation associated with arterial hypoxia causes a shift in the oxygen dissociation curve. The hemoglobin will, under these circumstances, take up more oxygen at a given oxygen tension (Bohr effect). Thus, at an alveolar oxygen pressure of 55 mm Hg, a rise in pH from 7.44 to 7.64 will cause the arterial saturation to increase from 80 to nearly 90 per cent (Fig. 15-1).

If the flow of blood through the tissues and the oxygen consumption of the tissues remain constant, then the amount of oxygen extracted in the tissues as the blood passes through the capillaries will remain constant. Therefore, if the oxygen content of arterial blood is reduced, the venous blood emerging from the capillary will have less oxygen by an amount corresponding to the initial abnormal reduction in the arterial blood.

The clinical features of arterial hypoxia depend upon the acuteness with which it sets in. Barcroft pointed out that when hypoxia develops rapidly, the picture resembles drunkenness; when it develops slowly, it simulates fatigue. In either case cyanosis is likely to be striking. When the arterial hypoxia is of long duration, clubbing of the fingers usually appears.

ANEMIC HYPOXIA. This includes different states, one of which is associated with anemia and others in which there is a partial conversion to non-oxygen-carrying derivative pigments (Chap. 114). Any decrease in hemoglobin concentration is attended by a corresponding decline in the oxygen-carrying power. Under such conditions the tension of oxygen in the arterial blood remains normal, but the absolute amount of oxygen transported per unit volume of blood is diminished. As the anemic blood passes through the capillaries, and the usual amount of oxygen is removed from it, the tension of oxygen in the venous blood declines to a greater degree than would normally be the case.

Carbon monoxide intoxication is accompanied by the equivalent of anemic hypoxia in that the hemoglobin which is combined with the carbon monoxide (carboxyhemoglobin) is unavailable for oxygen transport. But, in addition to this, the presence of carboxyhemoglobin increases the affinity of normal hemoglobin for oxygen at low oxygen tensions (i.e., shifts the lower portion of the dissociation curve of hemoglobin to the left), so the oxygen can be unloaded only at lower tensions. By such formation of carboxyhemoglobin a given degree of reduction in oxygen-carrying power produces a far greater degree of tissue hypoxia than the equivalent reduction in hemoglobin due to simple anemia.

The tension of oxygen in the venous blood is decreased in both conditions—anemic hypoxia and arterial hypoxia. But the tension of oxygen in the arterial blood is not reduced in anemic hypoxia, and the decrease in mean capillary oxygen tension and in tissue oxygen tension is less than in arterial hypoxia. Patients with anemia of moderate severity do not exhibit any manifestations of oxygen deficiency while at rest but are likely to display such symptoms on exertion. With severe anemia, symptoms of hypoxia may be present even at rest.

CIRCULATORY HYPOXIA. Even though the blood is normal as regards quantity and kind of pigment and is normally saturated with oxygen, and even though the oxygen consumption of the tissues remains normal, reduced oxygen tension at the venous end of the capillary will necessarily occur if the volume flow of blood through the tissues is reduced. Such a decrease in circulation to the tissues may be purely local, as in the case of obstruction to arteries and veins, or more general, as in the case of circulatory failure. When the obstruction is local and is primarily on the arterial side of the circulation, the affected members are likely to be pale, often with a slight bluish tint, and cold. When the obstruction affects the veins primarily, the tissues may be swollen and blue. The circulatory type of hypoxia may, therefore, be subdivided into two varieties, the ischemic type, in which the arterial flow is primarily affected, and the congestive or stagnant type, in which the venous flow is primarily at fault.

In *ischemic hypoxia*, the blood flow through the tissues is reduced and the actual volume of blood in the tissues is less than normal, but the rate of movement of the blood may remain relatively normal. When venous pressure rises, the volume of blood in the tissues increases, the velocity of movement diminishes, and the volume of blood flow per unit of time may or may not decrease. Because the velocity of flow is diminished under such circumstances, the term *stagnant hypoxia* is applicable.

The clinical pictures which occur when circulatory

hypoxia is general, as the result of circulatory failure, are discussed in some detail in Chaps. 128 and 135.

METABOLIC HYPOXIA. Increased Oxygen Need of Tissues. Even if oxygen diffusion into arterial blood is unhampered, with hemoglobin qualitatively and quantitatively normal, the tension of oxygen in venous blood (hence, mean capillary tension) may be reduced if the oxygen consumption of the tissues is elevated without a corresponding increase in volume flow per unit of time. Such a situation may be encountered in febrile states and in thyrotoxicosis. Under such conditions the circulation may be considered deficient relative to the metabolic requirements. Thus, this type of metabolic hypoxia is comparable to circulatory hypoxia in that in both conditions the volume flow of blood is decreased relative to the needs of the tissues, the difference being that in one case the primary defect is in the volume flow of blood and in the other the primary defect is an increased oxygen need by the tissues.

Ordinarily, the clinical picture of patients with hypoxia due to an elevated basal metabolic rate is quite different from that of other types of hypoxia; the skin is warm and flushed, owing to increased cutaneous blood flow which dissipates the excessive heat produced, and cyanosis is absent in these patients.

Failure of Tissues to Employ Available Oxygen. The administration of cyanide (and several other similarly acting poisons) leads to a paradoxic state in which the tissues are unable to utilize oxygen and the venous blood, in consequence, tends to have a high oxygen tension. This is a type of metabolic disturbance in which the defect is not in oxygen supply to the tissues but in the capacity of the tissues to utilize oxygen. The number of mechanisms transferring electrons to oxygen is limited. It is only by a defect in one or more of these mechanisms, or by failure of preceding oxidations to provide electrons for them, that diminution in oxygen utilization can occur. Thus, cyanide paralyzes the electron-transfer function of cytochrome oxidase so that it cannot pass electrons to oxygen, whereas reduction of tissue temperature slows the rates of metabolic reactions that produce such electrons. Diphtheria toxin is believed to inhibit the synthesis of one of the cytochromes and thus interfere with oxygen consumption and energy production by the cells involved.

EFFECTS OF HYPOXIA

The symptoms of local oxygen deficiency depend on the tissues affected and are, therefore, protean in nature; they will not be discussed here. When hypoxia is general, all parts of the body may suffer some impairment of function, but those parts which are most sensitive to the effects of hypoxia give rise to symptoms which dominate the clinical picture. The *changes in the central nervous system* are especially important, and here the higher centers are most sensitive. Acute hypoxia, therefore, produces impaired judgment, motor incoordination, and a clinical picture closely resembling acute alcoholism. When hypoxia is long-standing, the symptoms consist of fatigue, drowsiness, apathy, inattentiveness, and delayed reaction time, simulating manifestations of severe fatigue. As hypoxia becomes more severe, the centers of the brain stem are affected and death usually results from respiratory failure. The gasping reflex, being a primitive mechanism, persists to the last. Measurements of cerebral blood flow indicate that with reduction of arterial oxygen tension, cerebral vascular resistance decreases and cerebral blood flow increases. This finding tends to minimize the cerebral hypoxia. On the other hand, reduction of arterial oxygen tension, when accompanied by diminution of carbon dioxide tension, increases cerebral vascular resistance, and volume flow per unit of time is decreased. It would appear, therefore, that when hypoxia is associated with increased ventilation and hypocapnia, it is enhanced, at least in the higher levels of the central nervous system, by a reduction in volume flow of blood per unit of time. Compared with the brain, the phylogenetically older spinal cord and peripheral nerves are relatively insensitive to hypoxia, and symptoms due to disturbance of these structures usually do not appear. There is evidence that hypoxia causes constriction of pulmonary arteries. This has the advantage of shunting blood away from poorly ventilated areas toward better ventilated portions of the lung. However, it has the disadvantage of causing increased pulmonary resistance and increased burden on the right ventricle.

Some of the *metabolic effects of severe acute hypoxia* are well known in regard to the liver and muscles. In these structures the breakdown of the primary foodstuff, carbohydrate, normally proceeds anaerobically (i.e., without oxidation) to the stage of formation of pyruvic acid. The further oxidation of pyruvate requires the availability of oxygen. When this is deficient, the breakdown is impaired and increasing proportions of pyruvate become reduced to lactic acid, which cannot be further broken down anaerobically (Chap. 62). Hence, there is an increase in the blood lactate, with decrease in bicarbonate and a corresponding acidosis. As, under these circumstances, the total energy obtained from foodstuff breakdown is greatly reduced, the amount of energy available for continuing resynthesis of energy-rich phosphate compounds becomes inadequate. As the breakdown of the latter substances is the immediate source of energy driving the myriad of anabolic reactions which take place in tissues, such deficiency of energy-rich phosphate compounds produces a complex disturbance of cellular function which at present is only poorly understood. Whether or not the more subtle effects of mild hypoxia upon, for example, the central nervous system are mediated through lesser degrees of such disordered metabolism remains to be demonstrated.

Hypoxia has a double effect upon the respiratory center. The structure is rendered less sensitive, but acid accumulation at the same time tends to stimulate it. This latter effect is augmented by discharge from the chemoreceptors of the carotid and aortic bodies. Within certain limits, the degree of respiratory stimulation is the result of these influences; however, profound hypoxia is likely to cause degeneration of the center to dominate. Then death results from respiratory failure.

The acute effects of hypoxia on the *reaction of the blood* are likewise complicated, because two different antagonistic influences are at work. If breathing is stimulated by hypoxia, the resulting increase in ventilation, with loss of carbon dioxide, tends to make the blood more alkaline. On the other hand, the diffusion of unoxidized lactic acid from the tissues into the blood tends to make the blood more acid. In either case the total bicarbonate, and hence the carbon dioxide–combining power, tends to be diminished. With mild hypoxia there is likely to be respiratory alkalosis; severe hypoxia is attended by metabolic acidosis (see Chap. 61).

One of the important mechanisms of compensation for prolonged hypoxia is an increase in the amount of hemoglobin in the blood. This is not due to direct stimulation of the bone marrow but may be the effect of a hormonelike substance called *erythropoietin*. This is a glycoprotein, produced in some manner through the mediation of the kidney and possibly other tissues, which acts upon the stem cells. Assayable levels of erythropoietin are increased by hypoxia. The production of this hormone has been found to be regulated by the balance between tissue oxygen supply and demand. The titer of erythropoietin in plasma increases when oxygen supply is reduced. On the other hand, when the oxygen requirement is lowered, as in starved or in hypophysectomized animals, the erythropoietin response to hypoxia is also reduced.

The *heart*, although relatively sensitive to hypoxia as compared to most of the structures of the body, is less sensitive than the nervous system. Consequently, serious manifestations of cardiac impairment do not commonly occur when there is generalized hypoxia, and the manifestations arising in the nervous system dominate the picture. It is known that diminished oxygen tension in the tissues favors increase in local blood flow, with increased venous return, and an elevation of the cardiac output. This increase in cardiac work, which is one of the means of compensation for hypoxia, may precipitate congestive failure in patients with preexisting heart disease.

Other effects of hypoxia include stimulation of erythrocyte production, which is discussed later, and cyanosis, which can now be considered in more detail.

DIFFERENTIAL DIAGNOSIS OF CYANOSIS

Causes of Cyanosis

I. Circulatory disorders
  A. Cardiac disease
    1. Congenital (intense cyanosis, clubbed fingers, polycythemia)
    2. Acquired (slight cyanosis, no clubbed fingers, no polycythemia)
  B. Peripheral circulatory failure or local obstruction (pallid or ashen cyanosis, cold extremities)

II. Pulmonary disorders
  A. Acute (pneumonia, edema, infarction) (no clubbing and no polycythemia)
  B. Chronic (emphysema, extensive fibrosis) (clubbing and polycythemia often present)
III. Hematogenous disorders
  A. Polycythemia; erythrocytosis of high altitudes (cyanosis, more or less clubbing, and other varieties of erythrocytosis); erythremia (plum-red cyanosis, no clubbing)
  B. Abnormality in hemoglobin (methemoglobinemia, sulfhemoglobinemia) (no clubbing, minimal polycythemia)
    1. Exogenous (various drugs and chemicals)
    2. "Enterogenous cyanosis"
    3. Hereditary methemoglobinemias

From a practical standpoint it is useful to divide cyanosis into the *circulatory, pulmonary* and *hematogenous* groups. The circulatory group includes cardiac and peripheral types. When cyanosis is due to acquired disease of the heart, it is usually slight in degree and is accompanied by evidence of mitral stenosis, congestive failure, or both these conditions. Cyanosis due to congenital lesions is likely to be intense and to be associated with enlargement of the heart and clubbing of the fingers. Cyanosis dependent on disorders of the peripheral circulation is either local and accompanied by evidence of arterial or venous obstruction, or general and associated with the manifestations of peripheral circulatory failure or shock (Chap. 128). Pulmonary cyanosis, whether acute or chronic, is accompanied by the clinical and radiographic evidences of the responsible process, while hematogenous cyanosis is associated with polycythemia or with abnormal pigments in the blood (see Chap. 114).

In a given patient with cyanosis the following points are likely to be especially important in arriving at a correct interpretation of the cause:

1. The history, particularly the duration (cyanosis present since birth usually is due to congenital heart disease) and the possible exposure to various drugs or other agents which may produce abnormal types of hemoglobin.

2. Objective evidence by radiographic or physical examination of disorders of the respiratory or circulatory systems.

3. The presence or absence of clubbing of the fingers. (Clubbing without cyanosis is frequent in patients with subacute bacterial endocarditis and in association with nonspecific ulcerative colitis, and it may occasionally occur in healthy persons or as an occupational effect.) Slight cyanosis of the lips and cheeks, without clubbing of the fingers, is common in well-compensated patients with mitral stenosis and is probably due to minimal arterial hypoxia resulting from fibrotic changes in the lungs secondary to long-standing congestion. The combination of cyanosis and clubbing is frequent in many patients with certain types of congenital cardiac disease and is seen occasionally in persons with advanced pulmonary disease

or pulmonary arteriovenous shunts. Cyanosis due to acquired cardiac disease, to acute disorders of the lungs, or to acute intoxications is not associated with clubbed fingers.

4. Spectroscopic and other examinations of the blood for abnormal types of hemoglobin in instances where there is a story of suitable exposure, or where examination of the circulatory and respiratory systems affords no adequate explanation for the presence of cyanosis (Chap. 114).

POLYCYTHEMIA

The term *polycythemia* signifies an increase above the normal in the number of red corpuscles in the circulating blood. This increase is usually, though not always, accompanied by a corresponding increase in the quantity of hemoglobin and in the volume of packed red corpuscles. The increase may or may not be associated with an increase in the total quantity of red cells in the body. It is important to distinguish between *absolute* polycythemia (an increase in the total red corpuscle mass) and *relative* polycythemia, which occurs when, through loss of blood plasma, the concentration of the red corpuscles becomes greater than normal in the circulating blood. This may be the consequence of abnormally lowered fluid intake or of marked loss of body fluids, such as occurs in persistent vomiting, severe diarrhea, copious sweating, or acidosis (Chaps. 61, 128). Loss of electrolytes from the extracellular compartment, when not accompanied by corresponding loss of water, leads to a decline of osmolar concentration in the extracellular fluid. The resulting shift of water into the tissue cells may produce relative polycythemia, sometimes of high grade. In certain types of peripheral circulatory failure there is a loss of plasma into the interstitial fluid. Such a shift takes place largely in the periphery, with the result that the polycythemia may be more marked in capillary blood than in that from central blood vessels.

Because the term *polycythemia* is loosely used to refer to all varieties of increase in the number of red corpuscles, the terms *erythrocytosis* and *erythremia* are preferred in referring to two forms of absolute polycythemia. *Erythrocytosis* denotes absolute polycythemia which occurs in response to some known stimulus; *erythremia* refers to the disease of unknown etiology, which is discussed elsewhere (Chap. 113).

Erythrocytosis develops as a consequence of a variety of factors and represents a physiologic response to conditions of hypoxia. As noted above, sojourn at high altitudes leads to defective saturation of arterial blood with oxygen and stimulates the production of more red corpuscles. Immediately on ascent to a high altitude, symptoms such as fatigue, dizziness, headache, nausea, vomiting, ringing in the ears, and prostration may appear. In most persons adaptation soon occurs, with the development of polycythemia and other compensatory adjustments. However, a disorder may set in insidiously a few years later, or even as long as 20 years after continued residence at high altitudes,

leading to the development of a condition known as *chronic mountain sickness* or *seroche* (*Monge's disease*). Two forms have been described, an emphysematous type in which dyspnea is prominent and bronchitis is common; and an erythremic type in which prominent manifestations are a florid color which turns to cyanosis on the least exertion, mental torpor, fatigue, and headache. Those affected are usually in the fourth to sixth decade. Return to sea level promptly relieves the symptoms. Brisket disease of cattle, a disorder of young calves grazing at high altitudes in Utah and Colorado, which is characterized by pulmonary hypertension and subsequent right heart failure, is not a true counterpart of Monge's disease since it is not associated with sustained oxygen unsaturation or polycythemia.

Emphysema is the commonest of the chronic pulmonary conditions which may lead to erythrocytosis. Silicosis, with extensive pulmonary fibrosis, is another. Pulmonary arteriovenous fistula may lead to impaired saturation of arterial blood with oxygen, with the consequent development of erythrocytosis and of a clinical picture resembling closely that of certain types of congenital heart disease. Cavernous hemangioma of the lung may be associated with polycythemia. Hypertension of the lesser circulation, with pulmonary arterial and arteriolar sclerosis, may be accompanied by a train of symptoms such as asthma, bronchitis, dyspnea, and cyanosis, as well as erythrocytosis.

Under the mechanical conditions existing in obese patients, periods of shallow breathing may develop and result in alveolar hypoventilation and erythrocytosis. The fat, somnolent, red-faced boy of Dickens' *The Pickwick Papers* may well have been an example of this disorder. The claim that abnormal function of the respiratory center may be the cause of hypoxemia and absolute polycythemia requires substantiation.

The partial shunting of blood from the pulmonary circuit, such as occurs in congenital heart disease, causes the most striking erythrocytosis from abnormality in the circulation. Erythrocyte counts as high as 13 million, which are possible only when the red corpuscles are smaller than normal, have been observed in such cases, with volumes of packed red cells even as high as 86 ml per 100 ml of blood. The commonest defect producing such polycythemia is pulmonary stenosis associated with a right-to-left shunt that allows venous blood to enter the systemic arterial tree without transversing the lungs. Although erythrocytosis does not usually occur in patients with acquired heart disease, it may occasionally be seen in persons with mitral stenosis.

The excessive use of coal-tar derivatives and other forms of chronic poisoning, by producing abnormal hemoglobin pigments such as methemoglobin and sulfhemoglobin (Chap. 114), may cause erythrocytosis. Another chemical agent, cobalt, has produced erythrocytosis in experimental animals, but the mechanism is obscure.

Erythrocytosis is found in Cushing's syndrome and can be produced by the administration   large amounts of adrenocorticosteroids. Especially intriguing are the instances of polycythemia observed in association with various tumors. These have been chiefly of two varieties, infratentorial and renal. The tumors in the posterior fossa of the skull have usually been vascular (hemangioblastomas). The renal tumors have included renal carcinoma, adenoma, sarcoma, and hypernephroma. Other tumors which have been associated with polycythemia include uterine myomas and hepatic carcinoma. Polycythemia has also been reported in association with polycystic disease of the kidneys and hydronephrosis. However, only a small proportion (0.3 to 2.6 per cent) of the various renal disorders mentioned above have been associated with polycythemia. What is of special interest is the fact that plasma erythropoietin levels have been found elevated in a number, though not all, of the cases so studied, erythropoiesis-stimulating activity has been demonstrated in tumor extracts and in renal cyst fluid, and polycythemia has disappeared after the associated tumor was removed.

The term *stress erythrocytosis* has been applied to the polycythemia seen occasionally in very active, hard-working persons in a state of anxiety, who appear florid but who have none of the characteristic signs of erythremia—no splenomegaly nor leukocytosis with immature cells in the blood. In such individuals the total red cell mass is normal and the plasma volume below normal.

In essence, then, erythrocytosis is known to develop when there is:

1. Defective saturation of arterial blood with oxygen, resulting from (*a*) decreased atmospheric pressure and (*b*) impaired pulmonary ventilation.

2. Congenital disorders that permit right-to-left shunts.

3. Defect in circulating blood pigment.

It is clear, however, that some instances of erythrocytosis cannot be explained by these long-recognized mechanisms.

4. The adrenocortical secretions may produce polycythemia.

5. Humoral mechanisms of less well-defined nature may play a role, as suggested by the cases of polycythemia associated with a variety of tumors, malignant and benign, and with certain renal disorders mentioned above.

The differential diagnosis of polycythemia will be discussed in the chapter on Hemolytic Anemias (Chap. 113).

REFERENCES

Barcroft, J.: "The Respiratory Functions of the Blood," London, Cambridge University Press, 1925.

Burwell, C. S., E. D. Robin, R. D. Whaley, and A. G. Bickelmann: Extreme Obesity Associated with Alveolar Hypoventilation: A Pickwickian Syndrome, Am. J. Med., 21:811, 1956.

Donati, R. M., R. D. Lange, and N. I. Gallagher: Nephrogenic Erythrocytosis, A.M.A. Arch. Internal Med., 112:960, 1963.

Donati, R. M., J. M. McCarthy, R. D. Lange, and N. I. Gallagher: Erythrocythemia and Neoplastic Tumors, Ann. Internal Med., 58:47, 1963.

Gordon, A. S.: Hemopoietine, Physiol. Rev., 39:1, 1959.

Heymans, C.: Chemoreceptors and Regulation of Respiration, Acta Physiol. Scand., 22:4, 1951.

Hurtado, A.: Some Clinical Aspects of Life at High Altitudes, Ann. Internal Med., 53:247, 1960.

Jacobson, L. O., C. W. Gurney, and E. Goldwasser: The Control of Erythropoiesis, pp. 297–327, in Advances in Internal Medicine, W. Dock and I. Snapper (Eds.), vol. 10, Chicago, Year Book Publishers, Inc., 1960.

Lundsgaard, C., and D. D. Van Slyke: Cyanosis, Medicine, 2:1, 1923.

Stickney, J. C., and E. J. van Liere: Acclimatization to Low Oxygen Tensions, Physiol. Rev., 33:13, 1953.

Wintrobe, M. M.: "Clinical Hematology," 5th ed., Philadelphia, Lea & Febiger, 1961.

16   EDEMA
Louis G. Welt and Charles H. Burnett

Edema is defined as an increase in the extravascular component of the extracellular fluid volume. It may be localized or have a generalized distribution depending on the primary lesion. It is recognized by the clinician in its gross generalized form by puffiness of the face (which is most readily apparent in the periorbital areas) and by the persistence of an indentation of the skin following pressure. This is known as *"pitting" edema*. In its more subtle form it may be detected by the fact that the rim of the bell of the stethoscope leaves an indentation on the skin of the chest that lasts a few minutes. One of the first symptoms a patient may note is the ring on a finger fitting more snugly than in the past. Lastly, it should be cautioned that the volume of the interstitial space may increase by several liters before edema is recognized by the patients from the symptoms or by the physician through physical examination. *Ascites* and *hydrothorax* refer to accumulation of excess fluid in the peritoneal and pleural cavities, respectively. *Anasarca*, or *"dropsy,"* refers to gross generalized edema.

PATHOGENESIS

A more detailed discussion of the volume and distribution of body fluids is presented in Chap. 60. About one-third of the total body water is confined to the extracellular space. This compartment, in turn, is composed of the plasma volume and the interstitial space. Under ordinary circumstances the plasma volume represents about 25 per cent of the extracellular space, and the remainder is in the interstitium. The forces that regulate the disposition of fluid between these two components of the extracellular compartment are frequently referred to as the *Starling forces*, owing to the masterful description presented by that noted physiologist.

In general terms, two forces tend to promote a movement of fluid from the vascular to the extravascular space, and these forces are the *hydrostatic pressure within the vascular system* and the *colloid osmotic pressure* in the interstitial fluid. In contrast, the factors which promote a movement of fluid into the vascular compartment are the *colloid oncotic pressure,* contributed by the plasma proteins, and the *hydrostatic pressure within the interstitial fluid,* referred to as the *tissue tension.* These forces are balanced so that there is a large movement of water and diffusible solutes from the vascular space at the arteriolar end of the microcirculation and back into the vascular compartment at the venous end.[1] In addition, fluid is returned from the interstitial space into the vascular system by way of the lymphatics, and unless these channels are obstructed, lymph flow tends to increase if there is a tendency toward a net movement of fluid from the vascular compartment to the interstitium. In this fashion, all these forces are usually balanced so that a given steady state exists with respect to the size of the two compartments, and yet a large exchange between them is permitted. However, should any one of these factors be altered significantly, one can see how there may be a net movement of fluid from one component of the extracellular space to the other.

An increase in pressure in the vessels of the microcirculation may readily result from an increase in venous pressure due to local obstructive phenomena in the venous drainage, or to congestive heart failure, or to the simple expansion of the vascular volume by the administration of large volumes of fluid at a rate in excess of the ability of the kidneys to excrete these excesses. The colloid oncotic pressure of the plasma may be reduced owing to any of the factors that may induce hypoalbuminemia, such as malnutrition, liver disease, and loss of protein into the urine or into the gastrointestinal tract, or to a severe catabolic state.

Damage to the capillary endothelium increases the permeability of these vessels, which permits the transfer to the interstitial compartment of a fluid containing more protein than usual. Injury to the capillary walls may be the result of chemical, bacterial, thermal, or mechanical agents. Increased capillary permeability may also be a consequence of a hypersensitivity reaction. Lastly, damage to the capillary endothelium is presumably responsible for inflammatory edema, which is easily recognized by the presence of other signs of inflammation—redness, heat, and tenderness.

In any attempts to formulate a hypothesis concerning the pathophysiology involved in edematous states, it is exceedingly important to discriminate between the primary events, which account for the maldistribution of fluid between the two components of the extracellular space, and the predictable secondary consequences, which include the retention of salt and water.

[1] At this time there is no final resolution of the argument whether the exchange of fluid and solutes occurs between capillary endothelial cells or through the cells themselves.

There are instances in which an abnormal retention of salt and water may, in fact, be the *primary* disturbance. In these circumstances the edema is a secondary manifestation of the generalized increase in volume of the extracellular fluid. These special instances are usually related to those conditions characterized by an acute reduction in renal function (such as acute tubular necrosis or acute glomerulonephritis) and other disorders characterized by the primary production of excess mineralocorticoid or inappropriate secretion of the antidiuretic hormone.

These latter circumstances aside, one can create a hypothesis which is admittedly at least incomplete but within which one can begin to understand the concatenation of events in a variety of edematous states and perceive many of the features common in the pathophysiology of each. The basic premise is that the primary disorder concerns one or more alterations in the Starling forces such that there is a net movement of fluid from the vascular system into the interstitium or from the arterial compartment of the vascular space into the chambers of the heart or into the venous circulation itself. In either event, a diminished arterial volume may be anticipated to have certain consequences that lead to retention of salt and water. If retention of an increment of salt and water repairs the volume deficit, the stimuli to retain salt and water should be dissipated and a new steady state achieved. If, on the other hand, retention of salt and water does not repair the volume deficit because the increased volume of fluid cannot be sustained in the appropriate component of the vascular bed, the stimuli are not dissipated and the retention of salt and water continues. The sequence of events can be explored in a variety of circumstances.

Obstruction of Venous and Lymphatic Drainage to a Limb

The simplest condition to examine may be the consequences of lymphatic and venous obstruction to a limb. This must increase the hydrostatic pressure in the microcirculation so that more fluid is transferred from the circulation than can be reabsorbed at the venous end; furthermore, the alternate route, the lymphatic channels, are stipulated to be obstructed as well. This event must of necessity cause an increased volume of interstitial fluid in the limb at the expense of the plasma volume. The diminished plasma volume has a variety of consequences:

RENAL HEMODYNAMIC CHANGES. The diminished volume of plasma can be expected to reduce the perfusion of the kidney and decrease the glomerular filtration rate. Since one of the most important influences regulating the excretion of salt (and water) may be the filtered load itself, this would promote the excretion of lesser quantities of salt and smaller volumes of water. Other consequences of a hemodynamic nature are presumably conditioned by alterations in plasma volume. For reasons that are as yet unclear, it seems quite well established that an influence of "volume" on the rate of excretion of salt functions independently of its filtered load and independently of mineralocorticoid secretion. The nature of this regulatory mechanism is unknown, but a direct correlation occurs between alterations in volume and alterations in the excretion of salt. The phenomenon may be related to the character and distribution of blood flow to the kidney, but there are other alternatives. In any event, a diminished plasma volume can readily diminish the excretion of salt owing to alterations in renal hemodynamic parameters.

HUMORAL FACTORS. Ample evidence reveals that a diminished volume of plasma in some fashion promotes an increased secretion of aldosterone. This is due to an increase in an aldosterone-stimulating agent, which is dependent on the presence of intact kidneys and may well be angiotensin. This, in turn, may be increased in the plasma owing to some influence on the renal circulation related to alterations in flow or pressure, or to the chemical composition of intraluminal fluid that may stimulate the release of renin from the juxtaglomerular apparatus. In turn, the renin reacts with renin substrate to form angiotensin I, and the latter is converted enzymatically to angiotensin II, which stimulates the secretion of aldosterone. Whatever the precise sequence of events, a diminished plasma volume promotes increased secretion of this mineralocorticoid which implements the renal tubular reabsorption of sodium.

The retention of sodium owing to the hemodynamic and humoral factors alluded to above may, in turn, be accompanied directly by an increased reabsorption of water. If not, then the primary retention of sodium thus dictates some increase in the effective osmolality of body fluids, promotes thirst and the acquisition of water, and promotes the secretion of antidiuretic hormone, which then implements the retention of water.

In the context of the disorder under discussion, the volume of the extracellular fluid (about 140 mM sodium per liter of water) is increased. This increment tends to accumulate in the interstitium of the limb in which venous and lymphatic drainage are obstructed until the tissue tension is great enough to counterbalance the primary alteration in the Starling forces, at which time no further fluid will accumulate in that limb. At this point the additional accumulation of fluid will repair the deficit in plasma volume, and the stimuli to retain more salt and water are dissipated. The net effect is an increase in the volume of interstitial fluid in a local area, and the secondary responses repair the plasma volume deficit incurred by the primary event.

This same sequence may be translated easily to many other edematous states.

Nephrotic Syndrome

The primary alteration in this disorder is a diminished colloid oncotic pressure due to exorbitant loss of protein into the urine. This should promote a net movement of fluid into the interstitium and initiate the sequence of events described above. However, so long as the hypoalbuminemia is severe, the increment of fluid cannot be restrained within the vascular compartment, and hence the stimuli to retain salt and water are not abated.

Cirrhosis with Ascites

Measurements of blood volume in cirrhosis of the liver are commonly increased when the disorder is accompanied by a fairly large system of dilated venous radicles. Nevertheless, the arterial volume is quite likely diminished in size. If the primary event in the formation of ascites is due to obstruction of the lymphatic drainage of the liver as well as obstruction of the portal venous system, it is likely that the enlarged venous system has promoted a deficit in the arterial component. Once again, the sequence of events already described will come into play, and salt and water will be retained. So long as the venous bed continues to enlarge and the collection of fluid in the peritoneal cavity increases, the deficit in volume of the arterial side of the circulation is not repaired and the stimuli persist to retain salt and water. In addition, considerable data suggest that there are arteriovenous shunts in this disorder. One consequence of these shunts is a reduced renal blood flow despite an increase in cardiac output. In this fashion the alterations due to renal hemodynamic factors are fortified.

Although the diseased liver admittedly may not inactivate aldosterone and antidiuretic hormone in a competent fashion, it is unlikely that this plays a significant role in salt and water retention. Some suggest that this difficulty in inactivation permits the development of higher levels of these humoral agents, which may amplify the responses in terms of salt and water retention. This seems unlikely since, in the first place, a tendency to diminished inactivation of these hormones might be expected to retard their rates of secretion; furthermore, it is apparent that if one provides a mechanism for the loculated ascitic fluid to reach the interstitium of the abdominal wall by the use of a prosthetic device, there is an immediate diuresis of salt and water. This is presumably because if the ascitic fluid reaches the interstitial space elsewhere, it can be reabsorbed into the circulation and this, in turn, will repair the volume deficit and dissipate the stimuli responsible for the retention of salt and water. Unfortunately, these devices are soon obstructed by scar tissue and hence have not been a practical form of therapy. Nevertheless, this experience emphasizes that deficient inactivation of these hormones by the diseased liver plays no important role in implementing the edematous state.

Congestive Heart Failure

In this disorder it is postulated that the defective systolic emptying of the chambers of the heart promotes an accumulation of blood in the heart and venous circulation at the expense of the arterial volume, and the oft-repeated sequence of events is initiated. In many instances of mild heart failure a small increment of volume may be achieved, which may repair the volume deficit and establish a new steady state. This may result because up to a point an increase in the volume of blood within the chambers of the heart appears to promote a more forceful contraction and may thereby increase the volume ejected in systole. However, if the cardiac disorder is more severe, retention of fluid cannot repair the arterial volume deficit. The increment accumulates in the venous circulation, and the increase in hydrostatic pressure therein promotes the formation of edema in the lungs as well as elsewhere. The pulmonary edema impairs gas exchange and may induce hypoxia, which embarasses cardiac function still further. The volume of blood within the chambers of the heart becomes ever larger and reaches a point where this increase affects systolic emptying adversely, thus worsening the heart failure.

Cyclic Edema

There is a syndrome characterized by periodic episodes of edema without obvious cause. It has been observed most commonly (but not exclusively) in women, and there appears to be some relationship to the menstrual cycle. The fact that most cases are seen in women may be due, in part at least, to the unfortunate cosmetic consequences of facial edema which is more likely to disturb women than men. Another feature of this disorder is fairly constant, large, diurnal alterations in weight so that the patient

may weigh several pounds more in the evening than in the morning after having been in the upright posture most of the day.

No one knows whether all these patients represent a single type of disorder with varying degrees of intensity. A large diurnal weight change suggests the possibility that patients may well have increased capillary permeability in general, which is emphasized daily by the upright posture and the consequent increased hydrostatic pressure in the vessels. The episodes of more frankly sustained edema may be the result of a further increase in capillary permeability due to some other influence. If, in fact, it truly occurs more commonly in women and is correlated with the menstrual cycle, there may be some hormonal influence on the permeability of vessels which permits the loss of plasma volume into the interstitial space and the sequence of events secondary to a contraction in plasma volume. An occasional patient has been reported in whom the loss of plasma volume was so striking as to induce peripheral vascular collapse; and in one instance, at least, this was so severe as to cause death.

This general formulation is represented graphically in Fig. 16-1. As mentioned earlier, this is certainly incomplete, and the amplification presented in this discussion may well have serious defects of omission and error. Allusion has been made to some of the unknown areas. One more which deserves further comment concerns the precise role of the mineralocorticoid hormone in these problems. Although increased quantities of aldosterone have been demonstrated to be secreted in these various edematous states, it must be emphasized

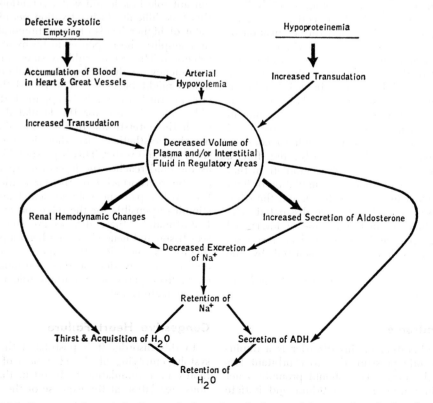

Fig. 16-1. Sequence of events leading to the formation of edema and the retention of salt and water.

that augmented levels of aldosterone (or other mineralocorticoids) do not always promote the accumulation of edema, as witnessed by the lack of striking fluid retention in most instances of primary aldosteronism. Furthermore, although normal subjects will retain some salt and water under the influence of a potent mineralocorticoid such as deoxycorticosterone acetate or 9-alpha-fluorohydrocortisone, this accumulation appears to be self-terminative despite continued exposure to the steroid and to salt and water. It is probable that the failure of normal subjects to accumulate fluid indefinitely reflects an increase in glomerular filtration rate or other hemodynamic influences, alluded to earlier, that result from some increase in the volume of the extracellular fluid compartment. The role of such a hormone in the accumulation of fluid in these edematous states discussed above may be more effective because these patients are unable to repair the crucial deficit in volume.

Throughout this discussion it has been assumed that the retention of sodium salts is primary to water retention. This is attested to by (1) the usual failure to accumulate edema if sodium is not available in the diet and (2) the successful use of pharmacologic agents and other measures that promote the excretion of sodium in the urine. In most circumstances the mechanisms responsible for maintaining a normal effective osmolality in the body fluids continue to operate efficiently so that sodium retention promotes thirst and secretion of the antidiuretic hormone, which, in turn, lead to the ingestion and retention of approximately 1 liter of water for each 140 mM sodium retained. Similarly, measures which promote the loss of sodium into the urine are accompanied by antithetical responses leading to the net loss of an equivalent volume of water from the body.

DIFFERENTIAL DIAGNOSIS

Despite numerous inconsistencies encountered in the explanation for the various factors and mechanisms concerned in edema formation, the primary cause can usually be determined. As a rule, localized edema can be readily differentiated from generalized edema. The great majority of patients with noninflammatory generalized edema of significant degree suffer from cardiac, renal, hepatic, or nutritional disorders. Consequently, the differential diagnosis of generalized edema should be directed toward implicating or excluding these several conditions. The considerations listed below should suffice to differentiate the common causes of edema.

Localized Edema

Edema originating from inflammation or hypersensitivity is usually readily identified; allusion has been made to characteristics of this type of edema. Localized edema due to venous or lymphatic obstruction (thrombophlebitis, chronic lymphangitis, resection of regional lymph nodes, filariasis, etc.) may demonstrate in a local area all the characteristics of edema occurring from generalized retention of salt and water. It should be reemphasized that lymph edema is peculiarly intractable because restriction of lymphatic flow results in increased protein concentration in interstitial fluid, a circumstance which severely impedes removal of retained fluid.

Edema of Heart Failure

Evidence of heart disease as manifested by cardiac enlargement, diastolic murmurs, and gallop rhythm plus evidences of cardiac failure, such as dyspnea, basilar rales, diminished vital capacity, prolonged circulation time, venous distension, increased venous pressure, and hepatomegaly, usually provides abundant evidence of the pathogenesis of edema resulting from heart failure.

Edema of the Nephrotic Syndrome

The classic triad—massive proteinuria, hypoproteinemia, and hypercholesterolemia is usually present. This syndrome may occur during the course of a variety of kidney diseases, which include glomerulonephritis, diabetic glomerulosclerosis, amyloid infiltration, renal vein thrombosis, diffuse connective tissue diseases, and hypersensitivity reactions. A history of previous renal disease may or may not be elicited; more commonly, it is not.

Edema of Acute Glomerulonephritis

The edema occurring during the acute phases of glomerulonephritis is characteristically associated with hematuria, proteinuria, and hypertension. Some evidence supports the view that the fluid retention is due to increased capillary permeability; but probably in most instances the edema in this disease results from primary retention of sodium and water by the kidneys owing to acute renal insufficiency and the consequent development of a congested state. However, discrimination between congestive heart failure and a congested state in acute renal insufficiency is often difficult. The congested state differs from congestive heart failure since it is characterized by a normal or increased cardiac output, a normal or diminished circulation time, a reduction in the packed cell volume, a normal arteriovenous oxygen difference, and failure to respond to a digitalis preparation. Patients commonly have severe evidence of pulmonary congestion on chest x-ray before cardiac enlargement is significant, and these patients frequently lie supine in bed with no tachypnea. If one cannot discriminate between the congested state and congestive heart failure, use of a cardiac glycoside is more prudent but especial care should be taken to avoid digitalis intoxication.

Edema of Cirrhosis

Ascites plus evidence of hepatic disease (collateral venous channels, hepatomegaly, spider angiomas, and jaundice) characterize edema of hepatic origin. The ascites is frequently extremely refractory to treatment; the lack of therapeutic response can be ascribed to the fact that intraabdominal fluid collects as a result of a combination of obstruction of hepatic lymphatic drainage, portal hypertension, hypoalbuminemia, and relatively high protein content of the ascitic fluid. The latter may be due to escape of a protein-containing fluid through the lymphatic vessels of the liver capsule or through the portal vessels, the lymphatic drainage of which is impeded. Edema may also occur in other parts of the body in patients with cirrhosis as a result of hypoalbuminemia. Furthermore, the sizable accumulation of ascitic fluid may be expected to increase intraabdominal pressure and impede venous return from the lower extremities; hence, it tends to promote accumulation of edema in these limbs as well.

Edema of Nutritional Origin

An inadequate diet over a prolonged period may produce hypoproteinemia and edema. In some instances of extreme malnutrition the degree of transudation appears to be disproportionately great for the degree of serum protein deficit observed. Coexisting beriberi heart disease may augment edema of this origin. In the latter condition, increased cardiac output and blood flow, in addition to those factors usually present in heart failure and capillary dilatation, may further favor edema formation. More striking edema is commonly observed when these famished subjects are provided with an adequate diet. The mechanism is not clear, but the ingestion of more food may increase the quantity of salt taken, which is retained along with water. The edema may be more apparent than under other circumstances, because the subcutaneous tissue is so depleted of fat that modest collections of edema may be more obvious than they would be in an obese subject.

GENERAL DIFFERENTIAL CRITERIA

Aside from the criteria already mentioned, certain other points may help elicit the cause of edema.

The distribution of edema is an important guide to the cause. Thus, edema of one leg or of one or both arms is usually the result of vascular or lymphatic obstruction. Edema resulting from hypoproteinemia characteristically is generalized, but it is especially evident in the eyelids and face and tends to be most pronounced in the morning because of the recumbent posture assumed during the night. Edema associated with heart failure, on the other hand, tends to be more extensive in the legs and to be accentuated in the evening, a feature also determined largely by posture. In the rare types of cardiac disease, such as tricuspid stenosis and constrictive pericarditis, in which orthopnea may be absent and the patient may prefer the recumbent posture, the factor of gravity may be equalized and facial edema observed. Less common

causes of facial edema include trichinosis, allergic reactions, and myxedema. Unilateral edema occasionally results from cerebral lesions affecting the vasomotor fibers on one side of the body; paralysis also reduces lymphatic and venous drainage on the affected side.

The color, thickness, and sensitivity of the skin are important. Local tenderness and increase in temperature suggest inflammation. Local cyanosis may signify a venous obstruction. Generalized but usually slight cyanosis commonly indicates congestive heart failure. In individuals who have had repeated episodes of prolonged edema, the skin over the involved area may be thickened, hard, and often red.

The venous pressure is of great importance in evaluating edema. Elevation of this measurement in an isolated part of the body usually reflects venous obstruction. Generalized elevation of venous pressure is almost pathognomonic of congestive heart failure, although it may be present in the congestive state that accompanies acute renal insufficiency. Ordinarily significant increase in venous pressure can be recognized by the level at which cervical veins collapse; in doubtful cases and for accurate recording, the venous pressure should be measured.

Determination of the concentration of serum proteins, and especially of serum albumin, clearly differentiates those patients in whom edema is due entirely or in part to diminished intravascular colloid osmotic pressure. The presence of proteinuria affords useful clues. The complete absence of protein in the urine is evidence against (but does not exclude) either cardiac or renal disease as a cause of edema. In a patient with edema without proteinuria, the presence of a palpable liver constitutes strong evidence that hepatic disease may be the cause of the edema. Slight to moderate proteinuria is the rule in patients with heart failure, whereas persistent massive proteinuria usually reflects the presence of the nephrotic syndrome. Since the liver may be palpable in subjects with heart failure or hepatic disease, the presence of proteinuria in a patient who does not have a palpable liver suggests the possibility of the nephrotic syndrome. Aside from the points mentioned, which bear directly on the question of the type of edema, much valuable information can be obtained from other features of the examination. Some of these are the presence or absence of heart disease, the character of the urinary sediment, the dietary history, and a history of alcoholism.

It should be emphasized that edema may originate from a variety of abnormal states; it is not, therefore, necessarily a consequence of only one of the disorders enumerated above. For example, in a diabetic patient, edema may be the result of hypoalbuminemia associated with the nephrotic syndrome with intercapillary glomerulosclerosis, increased venous pressure associated with congestive heart failure due to atherosclerotic and hypertensive heart disease, and the anemia consequent to uremia.

SUMMARY

Edema limited to a local area suggests either obstruction or local capillary damage. The obstruction may be lymphatic, venous, or both, and the local capillary damage may be due either to inflammation or to allergy. Significant generalized edema may occur before it can be appreciated clinically. It appears first in tissues that are expansible and may be demonstrable only by pressure against a bony eminence such as the tibia. The presence of generalized edema requires investigation especially for evidence of cardiac, renal, or hepatic disease and occasionally for manifestations of nutritional deficiency.

The primary factors promoting transfer of fluid from the intravascular to the extravascular compartment of the extracellular fluid space are reasonably clear. The secondary factors that induce salt and water retention include a variety of hemodynamic humoral mechanisms, the nature of which, although clarified by recent investigations, can still not be formulated by any single hypothesis with confidence.

REFERENCES

Bricker, N. S., P. A. F. Morrin, and S. W. Kime: The Pathologic Physiology of Chronic Bright's Disease, Am. J. Med., 28:77, 1960.

Gottschalk, C. W.: Osmotic Concentration and Dilution of the Urine, Am. J. Med., 36:670, 1964.

Kleeman, C. R., H. W. L. Hew, and L. B. Guzé: Pyelonephritis, Medicine, 39:3, 1960.

Pitts, R. F.: "Physiology of the Kidney and Body Fluids," Chicago, Year Book Publishers, Inc., 1963.

Strauss, M. B., and L. G. Welt, "Diseases of the Kidney," Boston, Little, Brown & Company, 1964.

17   PALPITATION

William H. Resnik

Palpitation is a subjective phenomenon and may be defined as consciousness of the beating of the heart. From the standpoint of diagnosis, it is not usually a very important symptom. Palpitation, except for certain cardiac arrhythmias, is not pathognomonic of any particular group of disorders; even when it occurs as a more or less prominent complaint, the diagnosis of the underlying malady is made largely on the basis of other associated symptoms and data, rather than by an analysis of the palpitation alone. Nevertheless, palpitation frequently constitutes a symptom of considerable importance in the minds of patients. The clear association of this symptom with the function of the heart and the fear engendered by the suspicion that heart disease may be present account for the apprehension frequently inspired by consciousness of the heartbeat. This anxiety is all the more pronounced in patients who know or who have been told that they may have heart disease; to them palpitation may seem to be an omen of impending disaster.

In the following paragraphs a number of conditions will be discussed primarily from the standpoint of palpitation. It must not be inferred, however, that in all these disorders palpitation is always a symptom of great magnitude, even from the patient's standpoint. Palpitation may be absent without affecting the ultimate diagnosis; but in the various conditions discussed below, palpitation *may* be the chief source of the patient's discomfort and the outstanding complaint.

Palpitation may be expressed by the patient in various terms, such as "pounding," "fluttering," "flopping," and "skipping," and in most cases it will be obvious that the complaint is of a sensation of disturbance of the heartbeat. Not infrequently, the patient complains of throbbing in the neck or upper abdomen, when under similar circumstances most persons would refer the palpitation to the precordium.

PATHOGENESIS OF PALPITATION

Under ordinary circumstances the rhythmic heartbeat is imperceptible to the healthy individual of average or placid temperament. Palpitation may be experienced by normal persons who have engaged in strenuous physical effort or have been strongly aroused emotionally. This type of palpitation is physiologic and represents the normal awareness of an overactive heart—that is to say, a heart that is beating at a rapid rate and at the same time expelling more than the usual amount of blood with each beat. Since palpitation accompanies physiologic overactivity of the heart as well as certain pathologic forms of overactivity, such as are seen in severe anemia or thyrotoxicosis, it is commonly assumed that it is the overactivity per se or the associated increased stroke output that is responsible for the symptom. However, overactivity of the heart is associated with several alterations in cardiac function: increased stroke output, acceleration of heart rate, steeper gradient of development of intraventricular pressure during the period of isometric contraction, increased intensity of the heart sounds, especially of the first sound. Of these various factors, the last two are probably the ones chiefly concerned with the appearance of palpitation, whereas increased stroke output, both on clinical and experimental grounds, appears to play no immediate role in the causation of this symptom. For example, complete heart block is characterized by a considerably increased output per beat; in this condition palpitation is inconspicuous and occurs only when the atrial contraction precedes the ventricular by a very brief interval, thus giving rise to a loud first sound (*bruit de canon*).

On the basis of clinical experience, there seems to be a closer correlation between palpitation and intensity of the first heart sound than between this symptom and any other single phenomenon related to cardiac function. Intensity of the first heart sound depends mainly on the vigor with which the atrioventricular valve leaflets are brought into apposition by ventricular systole. In turn, the force with which the valves are snapped together depends on (1) the position of the AV valves at the onset of ventricular contraction and (2) the rapidity with which intraventricular tension increases after the beginning of ventricular systole.

The influence of the position of the AV valves may be explained as follows. In general, when diastole is abbreviated, as after a short P-R interval or in the case of a premature beat occurring during the early filling phase of diastole, the AV valves are widely separated and pressed against the ventricular walls. When contraction starts, the valves are forced to make a maximal excursion in order to come into closure; hence the loud sound. On the other hand, after a long P-R interval or at the onset of a premature beat occurring during the phase of diastasis, the AV valves in late diastole have already floated back into a position of semiclosure. The final movement of the AV valves to closure after the onset of ventricular systole is through a reduced arc, and the first sound is correspondingly diminished in intensity.

The rate at which intraventricular pressure rises during systole also has an important effect on the abruptness and force with which the AV valves are closed, and hence on the intensity of the first sound. Thus, following the administration of epinephrine, the speed of contraction of the left ventricle increases, the duration of the isometric contraction phase is diminished (both phenomena are the result of an increased gradient of intraventricular pressure), and the intensity of the first sound is increased. It has also been suggested that this mechanism as well as the wide separation of the valve leaflets is responsible for the loud first sound after a brief P-R interval. When the AV leaflets are widely separated, more time is required to close the valves, and in the additional increment of time, more ventricular fibers are excited and contracting at the moment of closure than is normally the case. Hence, the ventricular systole is more vigorous, the ventricular pressure rises more rapidly, and vibrations of greater intensity are induced by closure of the AV valves. Experimentally, it has been demonstrated that the vibrations chiefly responsible for the intensity of the first sound occur during isometric contraction, and these vibrations increase as isometric pressure increases.

Thus, palpitation is probably a sensation accompanying an unusually rapid and forceful closure of the atrioventricular valves which gives rise to a first sound of greater than normal intensity. These circumstances prevail in any clinical condition characterized by an increased stroke volume in conjunction with a rapid rate.

These various considerations indicate that whether or not palpitation appears will often depend on the summation of numerous conflicting forces. To illustrate: In paroxysmal tachycardia the intensity of the first sound will tend to be increased by the shortening of the diastole and the quickening of the P-R interval which keep the AV valves wide open at the onset of ventricular systole. On the other hand, the diminished cardiac output tends to cause a fall in the gradient of intraventricular pressure, and this in turn diminishes the intensity of the first sound. Moreover, as myocardial fatigue supervenes and incomplete emptying of the ventricle increases the residual blood in the ventricles, the AV valves are floated back from a position of wide patency to one of semiclosure and the intensity of the first sound is thereby diminished further, an effect enhanced by the reduced velocity of ventricular contraction. In mitral stenosis the first sound is characteristically sharp and loud; yet palpitation is usually absent. The probable explanation is that the quality of the first sound in this condition is due chiefly to the altered physical characteristics (scarring) of the leaflets rather than to the force of the mitral valve closure.

Actually, there are available no carefully controlled studies undertaken to investigate the problem of palpitation, and further speculation regarding the importance of the various factors involved in the causation of the symptoms would be fruitless at present.

IMPORTANT CAUSES OF PALPITATION

It is impracticable to enumerate all the circumstances under which palpitation may occur. Hence, only those disorders will be mentioned in which palpitation *may* be a prominent symptom.

PALPITATION DUE TO DISORDERS OF THE MECHANISM OF THE HEARTBEAT. Extrasystoles. The symptoms are fairly consistent, and in most cases the diagnosis will be suggested by the patient's story. The actual premature contraction is often described as a "flopping" or as if "the heart turns over." The pause following the premature contraction may be felt as an actual cessation of the heartbeat, in contrast to the complete unconsciousness of the pause when the heart beats normally or at a slow rate, and the patient will often magnify the duration of the interval and sometimes express apprehension as to whether the heart will actually resume its beat. The first ventricular contraction succeeding the pause may be felt as an unusually vigorous beat and will be described as "pounding" or "thudding." Any one or all three of these different symptoms initiated by the premature contraction may be experienced by the patient. It should be strongly emphasized that, *in the absence of clinical or other evidence of organic heart disease, premature beats have no significance whatever.* Usually the identification of the extrasystole as the cause of palpitation is a simple matter. When numerous extrasystoles are present, differentiation from atrial fibrillation can be made by any procedure that will bring about a definite increase in the ventricular rate; at increasingly rapid heart rates, the extrasystoles usually diminish in frequency and then disappear, whereas the irregularity of atrial fibrillation increases. Heart block, with dropped beats, is the only other common arrhythmia with which the premature contraction is likely to be confused; here, simple auscultation will reveal the absence of the premature beat prior to the pause.

The Ectopic Tachycardias. These conditions, which are considered in some detail in Chap. 140, are common and important causes of palpitation. Ventricular tachycardia is an exception, and this may be related to the abnormal sequence, and hence impaired coordination and vigor, of ventricular contraction. If the patient is seen between attacks, the diagnosis of ectopic tachycardia will depend upon the history of abrupt onset and offset.

The specific type of ectopic tachycardia can often be surmised from a consideration of all the data obtained from the history, but a precise diagnosis can be made only when an electrocardiogram and observations on the effect of carotid sinus pressure are made during a seizure.

The diagnosis of paroxysmal tachycardia from the history alone, regardless of the type, depends on securing a story of abrupt onset and offset. In many cases of rapid heart action, it is difficult or impossible to determine with certainty whether there was an actual sudden onset or whether there was a preceding period of anxiety followed by the rapid, but not abrupt, development of sinus tachycardia. It is usually even more difficult to ascertain the exact characteristics of the offset of the tachycardia.

PALPITATION DEPENDENT ON THE PRESENCE OF SOME ORGANIC OR FUNCTIONAL DISTURBANCE ORIGINATING OUTSIDE THE CIRCULATORY SYSTEM. Once again, only the more important and common conditions, particularly those which may not be readily recognized, will be mentioned.

Thyrotoxicosis. In its fully developed form, thyrotoxicosis will usually be evident and offers little difficulty in the way of diagnosis. It is the lesser grades, particularly those which are complicated by the presence of myocardial failure, that are likely to be overlooked. The suspicion that thyrotoxicosis is present may be aroused by the detection of any one of its characteristic features, and confirmation of the diagnosis will be obtained by the procedures mentioned in Chap. 82.

Anemia. When mild, anemia may cause palpitation during exertion; when severe, it causes palpitation at rest. In some patients the coloring of the skin may not reveal the cause of the symptom, but appropriate studies of the blood will clarify the situation.

Fever. Palpitation may be present in acute infections, particularly in the early stages; but here the symptom is merely an insignificant phenomenon in the midst of other obviously more important ones. Palpitation may be one of the more prominent symptoms in an individual suffering from one of the chronic and sometimes more obscure febrile illnesses, such as incipient tuberculosis, chronic brucellosis, subacute bacterial endocarditis, or acute rheumatic fever with carditis and relatively few or no joint manifestations.

Carditis in acute rheumatic fever and subacute bacterial endocarditis cannot of course be considered causes of palpitation originating outside the heart. They are considered in this group because the presenting symptoms, including palpitation, are often only those of an infection without localizing symptoms that direct suspicion to the heart. The problem is to determine that the cause of the palpitation is an infectious illness and to carry out the usual procedures to reveal the type of infection.

Hypoglycemia. Palpitation is often a prominent feature of this condition and appears to be related to release of epinephrine. Confirmation of the diagnosis is obtained by appropriate blood sugar estimations and by prompt relief of all symptoms on the administration of glucose in one form or another (Chap. 88).

Aerophagia. Many patients who complain of "gas" and belching also complain of palpitation, possibly due in some cases to an associated anxiety state. This type of palpitation is readily recognized by the history of relief through eructation.

Tumors of Adrenal Medulla (Pheochromocytomas). Such tumors may give rise to recurrent attacks whose symptoms, including paroxysms of hypertension and palpitation, are identical with those seen following the injection of epinephrine or norepinephrine. This type of tumor is rather uncommon and is mentioned chiefly because cure may be effected by surgical removal. An identical syndrome may be produced when monoamine oxidase (MAO)–inhibitor drugs are taken concurrently with sympathomimetic drugs, such as ephedrine or amphetamine, or with foods, such as ripened cheese, that contain amines.

Drugs. The relationship between the development of palpitation and the use of tobacco, coffee, tea, alcohol, epinephrine, ephedrine, aminophylline, atropine, or thyroid extract will usually be obvious, and further elaboration is unnecessary.

PALPITATION AS A MANIFESTATION OF THE ANXIETY STATE. Persons who are healthy physically and well-adjusted emotionally may have palpitation under certain circumstances. Thus, during or immediately after vigorous physical exertion or during sudden emotional tension, palpitation is common and is usually associated with outspoken tachycardia. Occasionally such a person may be conscious of the heartbeat when lying on the left side, but this type of palpitation is clearly due to the better transmission of the heart sounds to the ear. Lifting the head from the pillow will bring about a striking diminution or immediate disappearance of the symptom.

In some patients, palpitation may be one of the outstanding manifestations of a transitory episode of acute anxiety which may never recur. That is, after this one episode or between infrequent bouts of increased nervous tension, he may experience no palpitation which is not normal for the otherwise healthy, well-adjusted individual. In other persons the palpitation may, with other symptoms, represent a lifelong disorder indicative of disturbed autonomic function.

Whether this illness is simply an expression of a chronic, deep-seated anxiety state superimposed on a normal autonomic nervous system or depends on a constitutional or inherited autonomic instability, as some believe, is not yet entirely clear. At any rate, the clinical significance of this differentiation between the transitory and the enduring forms is that the former is often dissipated by emphatic reassurance from the physician, whereas the latter is usually resistant even to the most thorough and expert psychiatric care. In the latter case, the patient must be given constant psychologic support and should be taught to live within the limits of his physical capabilities.

This chronic form of palpitation is known by various names such as *Da Costa's syndrome, soldier's heart, effort syndrome, irritable heart, neurocirculatory asthenia,* and *functional cardiovascular disease.* Aside from palpitation, the chief symptoms are one or more of those of an anxiety state (p. 1267).

Physical examination usually reveals the typical findings of the hyperkinetic syndrome (p. 787). Electrocardiograms may display minor depressions of the S-T junction and inversion of T waves and so occasionally lead to a mistaken diagnosis of coronary disease; this is particularly likely to occur when these findings are associated with complaints by the patient of an aching feeling of substernal tightness, commonly present in emotional stress (p. 30). Minimal elevation of body temperature is sometimes present and may be responsible for an erroneous diagnosis of subacute rheumatic carditis (Chap. 272). A normal sedimentation rate and a tendency for the tachycardia to decrease sharply during sleep constitute strong evidence against rheumatic carditis. The two conditions may coexist. In fact, the presence of any kind of organic disease is one of the commonest causes of the underlying anxiety which frequently produces this functional syndrome.

The diagnosis of this type of anxiety state depends on the positive phenomena mentioned above. Even when a patient presents undoubted objective evidence of structural cardiac disease, a superimposed anxiety state should be considered responsible for the symptoms when the clinical picture is that which has been described. Normal values for vital capacity and for circulation time make it extremely improbable that dyspnea is due to organic cardiac disease which does not cause a sighing type of dyspnea. Pain localized to the region of the apex, lasting for hours or days, and accompanied by hyperesthesia is rarely due to structural cardiac disease but is common in the functional syndrome. Palpitation associated with organic cardiac disease is nearly always accompanied by arrhythmia or by marked tachycardia, but the symptom may exist with regular rhythm and with a heart rate of 80 or less in patients with the anxiety state. Giddiness due to this syndrome can usually be reproduced by hyperventilation (Chap. 44) or by change from the recumbent to the erect posture.

The treatment of the anxiety cardiac syndrome depends on removal of the cause. *In many instances the examination itself and the physician's attitude are the treatment.* A very thorough history followed by a detailed explanation, emphatic assurance, and instructions to take more rather than less physical exercise will produce dramatic relief in many instances. Frequently, the demonstration that the physician can reproduce not only the palpitation but many other symptoms of the anxiety state merely by the hypodermic injection of 0.5 to 1.0 ml epinephrine serves to convince the patient that his symptoms are not the result of some mysterious disorder but rather the effect of a well-understood physiologic mechanism. This is especially true when the initial anxiety has been mainly the result of fear of heart disease. When the cause is more deep-seated, or when the physician has not been able to gain the complete confidence of the patient, little or no benefit is the usual outcome. Even so, the psychiatrist may be able to do much toward emotional and economic rehabilitation.

Management of these patients is facilitated by a clear understanding on the physician's part of the mechanisms of the symptoms. The palpitation is probably related to release of epinephrine and to the lowered perception threshold. The pain probably arises in the intercostal tissues as the result of the pounding of the heart. The hyperventilation with its ensuing train of symptoms (Chap. 44) is analogous

Table 17-1

Does the palpitation occur:	If so, suspect:
As isolated "jumps" or "skips"?	Extrasystoles
In attacks, known to be of abrupt beginning, with a heart rate of 120 or over, of regular or irregular rhythm?	Paroxysmal rapid heart action
Independent of exercise or excitement adequate to account for the symptom?	Atrial fibrillation, auricular flutter, thyrotoxicosis, anemia, febrile states, hypoglycemia, anxiety state
In attacks developing rapidly though not absolutely abruptly, unrelated to exertion or excitement?	Hemorrhage, hypoglycemia, tumor of the adrenal medulla
In conjunction with the taking of drugs?	Tobacco, coffee, tea, alcohol, epinephrine, ephedrine, aminophylline, atropine, thyroid extract, MAO inhibitors
On standing?	Postural hypotension
In middle-aged women, in conjunction with flushes and sweats?	Menopausal syndrome
When the rate is known to be normal and the rhythm regular?	Anxiety state

to emotional sighing. There is evidence that the entire syndrome is related to decline of the normal inhibitory effect of the cerebral cortex on those hypothalamic centers which normally control the sympathetic system ("cortical-hypothalamic imbalance"). Explanation of these physiologic mechanisms to the patient is one of the most important features of therapeutic reassurance.

The commonest causes for palpitation have been enumerated and briefly discussed. Since this symptom occurs in such a wide variety of disorders which have no common or closely related underlying disturbance of structure or function, aside from the alterations in the intensity of the heart sounds, it is impossible to follow closely any predetermined plan of study in elucidating the significance of the symptom. The exact procedure will vary, of course, with the circumstances under which the patient is seen. Table 17-1 summarizes the main points of information that will be ascertained in the history. These questions, and others formulated according to circumstances of the individual case, will serve to suggest the additional lines of inquiry that may be necessary for analysis and appraisal of palpitation.

Two points merit special emphasis. The first is that in a person with a regular rhythm the presence of palpitation is usually good evidence against the simultaneous presence of myocardial failure. The second

point is that as a rule palpitation produces anxiety and fear out of all proportion to its seriousness. When the cause has been accurately determined and its significance explained to the patient, the symptom is often ameliorated and may disappear entirely.

REFERENCES

Cohen, M. E., and P. D. White: "Life Stress and Bodily Disease," chap. 56, vol. 29, 1949, in Research Publications of the Association for Research Nervous Mental Disease, Baltimore, The Williams & Wilkins Company, 1950.

Kjellberg, S. R., V. Rudhe, and T. Sjöstrand: The Effect of Adrenaline on the Contraction of the Human Heart under Normal Circulatory Conditions, Acta Physiol. Scand., 24:333, 1952.

Lewis, J. K., and W. Dock: Origin of Heart Sounds and Their Variation in Myocardial Disease, J.A.M.A., 110: 271, 1938.

Siecke, H., and H. E. Essex: Relation of the Difference in Pressure across the Mitral Valve to the Amplitude of the First Heart Sound in Dogs with Atrioventricular Block, Am. J. Physiol., 192:135, 1958.

Yu, P. N., B. J. B. Yim, and C. A. Stanfield: Hyperventilation Syndrome. Changes in the Electrocardiogram, Blood Gases, and Electrolytes during Voluntary Hyperventilation; Possible Mechanisms and Clinical Implications, A.M.A. Arch. Internal Med., 103:902, 1959.

Section 4

Alterations in Genitourinary Function

18 DYSURIA, INCONTINENCE, AND ENURESIS

Bernard Lytton and Franklin H. Epstein

NORMAL MICTURITION

An appreciation of the anatomic and physiologic mechanisms involved in micturition is necessary for a rational approach to the difficult problems of urinary incontinence, enuresis, and other disorders of bladder function.

The bladder muscle or detrusor consists of interlacing bundles of muscle that form an arc around the internal vesical orifice and continue down into the urethra, where they are interspersed with elastic fibers. The normal tone of these fibers constitutes the internal vesical sphincter. The bladder receives a dual nerve supply from the autonomic system and the sacral parasympathetic, via the pelvic nerves (second, third, and fourth sacral segments), from which the ganglions of the pelvic plexus and bladder wall receive pre-

ganglionic fibers and give off postganglionic fibers to the detrusor muscle and bladder neck. The sympathetic preganglionic fibers (last two dorsal and first two lumbar segments) pass via the lumbar splanchnic nerves to synapse in the paraaortic and pelvic plexuses. The postganglionic fibers supply mainly the blood vessels in the bladder wall and the muscles around the bladder neck. The sympathetic innervation has little influence on bladder function but is probably concerned with closure of the bladder neck at the time of ejaculation; removal of the first lumbar sympathetic ganglion bilaterally is usually followed by infertility due to retrograde ejaculation.

Afferent fibers subserving the sensations of distension and pain pass mainly via the pelvic nerves to the sacral segments of the spinal cord. Some of these fibers are said to pass via the sympathetic nerves, but it is probable that any residual sensation of bladder filling after section of the sacral nerves is due to stretching of the peritoneum overlying the bladder. The internal pudendal nerve supplies motor and sensory fibers, from the second, third, and fourth sacral segments, to the external sphincter muscle, urethra, and perineal muscles. The action of the detrusor and sphincter muscles is, therefore, both reflex and voluntary.

Micturition is normally a voluntary act. As the bladder fills, a fairly constant low pressure is maintained by the detrusor muscle as it accommodates itself to the increasing volume. When it reaches its capacity, 400 to 500 ml in the normal adult, the stretch receptors transmit impulses via the pelvic afferent nerves, the sacral reflex center, and the fasciculus gracilis to the brain. This initiates the desire to void. Impulses from the brain, which arise in the paracentral lobules, are transmitted via descending fibers just anterior to the corticospinal tracts, the micturition center in the sacral part of the cord, and the pelvic and pudendal nerves to initiate the act of micturition. An initial relaxation of the perineal muscles is followed by detrusor contraction. At this point there is usually tensing of the abdominal muscles and diaphragm, although the resultant rise in abdominal pressure alone cannot initiate voiding normally and is not essential for evacuation. The intravesical pressure rises rapidly to 18 to 43 cm water, the external sphincter relaxes, the bladder neck opens, and voiding occurs with a pressure of 50 to 150 cm. The opening of the bladder neck is the result of active detrusor contraction which widens the bladder neck and shortens the urethra, thus lowering the resistance of the bladder outlet. Closure of the bladder neck occurs with relaxation of the detrusor, which allows a return of the musculature to its normal position assisted by recoil of the elastic fibers. It is apparent that any interference with detrusor activity or the anatomy of the bladder neck will interfere with the opening mechanism and lead to incomplete emptying or some loss of continence.

DYSURIA

Dysuria denotes difficulty or pain associated with voiding. It may result from a wide variety of pathologic conditions. Frequency, hesitancy, burning, urgency, and strangury (slow, painful emission of urine) are often referred to under the more general term dysuria.

Urgency occurs as a result of trigonal or posterior urethral irritation by inflammation, stones, or tumor. The urge may be so great and so sudden that a patient voids involuntarily.

Frequency of urination in bladder lesions occurs when there is a decreased capacity or when there is pain on distension. In acute inflammatory lesions, edema and loss of elasticity of the bladder wall cause pain or an urge to void when only a small quantity of urine is present in the bladder. Chronic inflammatory lesions such as tuberculosis produce a similar effect and may proceed to permanently diminished capacity from scarring.

The majority of conditions producing these symptoms arise in the bladder and urethra. Diseases of other organs and systems may, by invading, compressing, or distorting the lower urinary tract, produce dysuria. Diseases of the nervous system, which involve the nerve supply of the bladder either centrally, as in tabes and multiple sclerosis, or peripherally, as in diabetic neuropathy, produce difficulty in voiding and sometimes pain when secondary infection occurs as a result of residual urine.

The evaluation of a patient with dysuria must include a complete history and physical examination as well as a complete urologic examination, together with relevant radiologic or laboratory investigations suggested by abnormalities detected during the clinical examination.

Inflammatory lesions in the bladder, prostate, or urethra are the commonest causes of dysuria. These include acute bacterial infections, chronic prostatitis in men, and chronic posterior urethrotrigonitis in women. A great deal may be learned from examination of the external urinary meatus. About 20 per cent of children with urinary complaints have a degree of *meatal stenosis*, which may interfere sufficiently with bladder function to result in recurrent infection. Meatal stenosis is often an important etiologic factor in the development and persistence of chronic prostatitis in men and chronic posterior urethritis and trigonitis in women. Adult men with unsuspected meatal stenosis of long standing have to strain to produce a thin stream and may take 5 min to empty their bladder. They may develop trabeculation of the bladder and elevation of blood urea. Meatotomy results in relief or considerable improvement.

A *urethral caruncle* may present with symptoms of severe discomfort on voiding. This tumor appears as a small cherry-red polyp protruding from the posterior lip of the external meatus and is generally exquisitely tender on palpation. The latter feature helps to distinguish it from the commoner condition of urethral prolapse. Simple excision is the treatment of choice.

Benign overgrowth of the prostate commonly causes frequency, hesitancy, straining, slowing of the stream, and dribbling in older men. Pain is uncommon unless the condition is complicated by infection or vesical calculi.

Frequency and urgency may follow *radiation injury* to the bladder. In the acute phase this may be amenable to treatment with bladder sedatives containing antispasmodics and with small doses of steroids to combat the inflammatory reaction. The persistence of symptoms or bleeding may necessitate surgical intervention. *Malignant tumors of the bowel, diverticulitis*, or *regional ileitis* may involve the bladder and cause frequency. Fistula formation results in severe dysuria and pneumaturia.

Chronic interstitial cystitis, a nonspecific chronic inflammatory disease of the bladder wall manifested by small, shallow, stellate hemorrhagic ulcers (Hunner's ulcers), gives rise to a fairly characteristic pattern of dysuria. The patients, generally middle-aged women, complain of persistent frequency and often have severe suprapubic pain, relieved by voiding. There may be an associated terminal hematuria. The urine contains a few white cells and red cells but no bacteria. It may ultimately lead to fibrosis with permanent contraction of the bladder.

Frequency without discomfort on voiding may be associated with a normal bladder capacity and be due to the *polyuria* of diabetes, to conditions causing hypercalcemia or hypokalemia, to the *nocturia* of early congestive heart failure, or to loss of renal parenchyma resulting in the passage of a large volume of poorly concentrated urine. The absence of nocturia in a patient with frequency suggests that it may be of psychogenic origin or due to a polyp or irritative lesion in the posterior urethra that is relieved by recumbency. A patient who complains of recent onset of nocturia should be carefully questioned about diuretic medication.

It should always be remembered that frequency may be due to *paradoxic incontinence* (see below).

Expanding lesions in the pelvis that reduce bladder capacity by external compression are exemplified by pregnancy. Large ovarian cysts and uterine fibroids will have a similar effect. A retroverted gravid uterus or pelvic tumor which becomes impacted may result in stretching and elongation of the urethra and produce difficulty in voiding and finally complete retention.

INCONTINENCE

Paradoxic Incontinence

True incontinence must be distinguished from *paradoxic incontinence*, which accompanies bladder distension caused by mechanical or functional obstruction and is characterized by small, frequent "overflow" voidings. In obstruction the increased power of the detrusor suffices to overcome the block, but as soon as a small quantity of urine is voided, the intravesical pressure drops and a large residual remains. Ultimately, the detrusor becomes paralyzed by overdistension, and complete retention ensues. With neurogenic bladders, small voidings occur, sometimes involuntarily, as the pressure of accumulating urine overcomes the resistance at the bladder outlet. With loss of a small amount of urine, pressure falls and a large residual is left. Often both neurologic and obstructive elements contribute, as in elderly arteriosclerotic patients with prostatic enlargement or in cases of diabetic neuropathy with secondary bladder neck obstruction. The bladder in these patients is flaccid and painless, which may make it difficult to palpate, and the residual urine predisposes to infection. This response of the bladder muscle to obstruction might be compared to that seen in striated and heart muscle under an increased work load.

Congenital Incontinence

Congenital incontinence may be due to a congenital malformation such as vesical extrophy, epispadias, ectopic urethral openings in the female, patent urachus, and defects in the spinal cord which occur in association with spina bifida and meningomyelocele. The results of primary reconstructive surgery in cases of extrophy are cosmetically satisfactorily, but sphincter control is rarely achieved. Furthermore, most of these children have persistent vesicoureteral reflux, which can lead to progressive renal damage. The majority therefore are still best treated by some form of urinary diversion with excision of the bladder. The results of urethral and bladder neck reconstruction in simple epispadias are better. The management of neurogenic bladder disturbance is principally directed toward the establishment of timed reflex voiding, diminution of residual urine, and control of infection. When there is progressive renal impairment, due to persistent infection and vesicoureteral reflux, urinary diversion is necessary.

Acquired Incontinence

This occurs either in diseases involving the spinal tracts, such as tabes, multiple sclerosis, and tumor, or as a result of trauma. The disruption of the neural mechanism results in complete relaxation of the detrusor and bladder outlet or in ineffective contractions of the detrusor, so there may be paradoxic incontinence with a flaccid bladder or uncontrollable frequent voidings with a spastic bladder. Cerebral vascular accidents or senility can produce loss of voluntary control of bladder and bowel function.

Parturition can stretch and disrupt the structures of the pelvic floor and perineum to the point that urethral resistance, while sufficient to maintain continence at rest, gives way under stress of straining or coughing and incontinence ensues. This is probably the result of loss of the urethrovesical angle and urethral shortening. This type of incontinence usually occurs when the patient is up and about.

Stress incontinence may be aggravated by urgency due to an associated urethrotrigonitis. Relief of the trigonitis will sometimes result in satisfactory control. Treatment is directed toward repair of the pelvic floor, restoration of urethral length, and correction of the urethrovesical angle.

Surgical or radiation injuries can produce vesicovaginal and ureterovaginal fistulas. Incontinence in ureterovaginal fistula occurs with normal voiding, but in vesicovaginal fistula there is generally no normal evacuation of the bladder. The treatment of these fistulas is always surgical. Temporary urinary diversion will enable spontaneous closure to occur in some instances. Excision and reconstruction of a damaged ureter is the treatment of choice, but implantation of the ureter into the bowel or substitution with an ileal segment may be necessary. Nephrectomy is the simplest procedure in the elderly or debilitated patient or when there are serious technical difficulties, provided there is adequate function in the other kidney.

Injury to the sphincter mechanism can occur with pelvic fractures or after prostatic or bladder neck surgery in elderly patients. Gradual improvement may occur for up to a year after injury. Postsurgical incontinence may be controlled with a penile clamp, but this has the disadvantage of producing edema and occasionally ulceration of the penis. A condom catheter may lead to maceration of the penile skin and is often difficult to apply. An indwelling catheter invariably leads to problems of chronic infection. A variety of surgical operations are used with indifferent success.

ENURESIS

Enuresis is generally understood to mean the unintentional voiding of urine, usually at night, when it is synonymously referred to as bedwetting. The term should be restricted to those children in whom there is an absence of any gross urologic abnormality.

Micturition in infancy is governed by a simple spinal reflex. Maturation of the nervous system and development of control over the simple reflexes by the higher centers occurs during the second year of life. By the age of thirty months, most children have voluntary control over rectal and urinary sphincters. The child who persistently wets the bed after the age of three or who, after a period of control, begins to wet the bed again presents a clinical problem. Enuresis may result from a delay in development or from loss of bladder control. It may be affected by physical and psychologic factors. There appears to be no constant single cause.

It is estimated that 15 per cent of boys and 10 per cent of girls at the age of five are enuretic, but by the age of nine only 5 per cent of all children remain bedwetters. The majority of children with simple enuresis are dry by the time they reach puberty. It is commoner among children with similarly affected siblings and in children of parents in the lower-income groups. This latter finding could be due to the later institution of toilet training.

It is important to distinguish incontinence due to organic urologic disease from enuresis early in the management of these patients. A careful evaluation at the outset should exclude chronic retention with dribbling incontinence due to either bladder neck obstruction or neurologic disease. Patients with organic disease of the bladder are usually incontinent during the day as well as at night, and there is often constant dribbling. Occasionally, however, serious degrees of bladder neck obstruction present with nocturnal enuresis as the only symptom. Occasionally a patient with petit mal epilepsy may present with wetting. Urinalysis will reveal any unsuspected infection. Enuresis occurring in retarded children or those with serious psychiatric disturbances requires treatment directed to management of their primary problem.

Contributory factors such as the child's general health, physical environment, and emotional state should be evaluated, and the parents should be encouraged to adopt an understanding rather than a punitive attitude. Correction of minor urologic abnormalities such as meatal stenosis, balanitis, vulvovaginitis, and posterior urethritis will sometimes give relief, but this is perhaps attributable only to the dysuria that follows instrumentation or to the understanding interest shown by the physician. The administration of antiparasympathetic agents to reduce bladder activity, or amphetamines to lighten sleep, have been advocated with doubtful results. The results of formal psychotherapy are uncertain. Considerable success has been claimed for alarm systems that waken the child when an electrical circuit is completed by wetting, and this method seems to be worth a trial in older children who prove resistant to simpler therapy.

19 OLIGURIA, POLYURIA, AND NOCTURIA

Louis G. Welt and Charles H. Burnett

INTRODUCTION

The kidneys provide the main channel for the excretion of water and solutes, and the urine flow and composition is adjusted so as to maintain the internal environment in a remarkably constant steady state away from equilibrium. The volume and solute content of the urine in health may vary widely. It is largely dependent on the magnitude and characteristics of the fluid and food ingested and on the quantity of water lost from other routes such as perspiration and insensible water loss. There are many ways in which urine flow can be varied in both health and disease, and it appears essential to review briefly, and in a general fashion, the manner in which urine is formed so that the vicissitudes of life and the impact of disease on urine volume and osmolality may be better understood.

PHYSIOLOGIC CONSIDERATIONS

The final bladder urine represents the net effect of a host of reactions that begin with the formation of an almost protein-free ultrafiltrate of plasma in the glomeruli. The quantity of fluid filtered at the glomeruli per unit of time is the net effect of the difference in the chemical potential of the water of plasma and that of the ultrafiltrate as well as the surface area available for filtration. These factors apply to the filterable solutes as well. The volume of water excreted per unit of time is, then, the difference between the volume filtered and the volume reabsorbed. The quantity of solutes excreted per unit of time is the difference between that which is filtered and that which is reabsorbed or secreted by the renal tubules. Many things remain obscure about these mechanisms, but there is now a general concept around which a description may be presented and from which implications may be drawn with respect to the influence of a variety of circumstances and disease processes. We are indeed indebted to the brilliant micropuncture studies started by Richards and his group in Philadelphia, and continued more recently by Wirz, by Gottschalk and his colleagues, and now by many others.

The water filtered by the glomeruli is reabsorbed at several areas along the nephron by passive diffusion along osmotic gradients, which, in turn, are established by the active transport of solutes. The osmotic gradient is maximized in the medulla and papilla owing to the anatomic arrangement of the loops of Henle and their accompanying blood vessels, which permit the establishment of an ever-increasing osmolality as the papilla is approached. This latter mechanism is referred to as the *countercurrent multiplication system*.

The *initial* step in the reabsorption of water, and the step that represents the largest volume, occurs in the proximal convolution of the nephron. The active transport of solutes, which are primarily sodium, chloride, bicarbonate, and glucose, creates an osmotic gradient so that water follows immediately. In this fashion, approximately two-thirds to three-fourths of the filtered solutes and water are reabsorbed by the end of the proximal tubule. The characteristics of this fluid are altered considerably, not only in volume but in composition. However, it is still iso-osmotic with the parent filtrate.

Another phase in the reabsorption of water occurs in the more distal portions of the nephron, which include the loop of Henle, the distal convolution, and, lastly, the collecting ducts. Although the reabsorption at these levels is smaller in volume than that which occurs in the more proximal segment of the nephron, these latter mechanisms are responsible in one circumstance for the formation of a maximally concentrated urine, and in other circumstances for the formation of a dilute urine. There are, obviously, circumstances wherein the urine osmolality occupies positions intermediate between these polar extremes.

The formation of a *maximally concentrated* urine depends on the presence of antidiuretic hormone, which permits the distal convolution and collecting duct membranes to be completely permeable to water. The micropuncture data reveal that the fluid in the early part of the distal convolution is always hypotonic (whether or not there is maximal antidiuretic hormone activity) to plasma. Furthermore, water is lost between the end of the proximal convolution and the early distal convolution. This clearly implies that solutes have been transported in excess of water, and hence some part of the ascending limb is presumably impermeable to water in the presence or absence of the antidiuretic hormone.

In the presence of antidiuretic hormone activity, the fluid within the distal convolution becomes more concentrated. Where one distal convolution meets with another to form a collecting tubule, the fluid is invariably iso-osmotic (in the rodent) with the parent filtrate. As the fluid courses through the collecting duct (in the presence of antidiuretic hormone activity) and is exposed to a fluid with an ever-increasing osmolality, a passive movement of water causes the fluid within the collecting ducts to remain in osmotic equilibrium with the fluid in the interstitium; thus, it increases in concentration until it exits into the pelvis of the kidney and moves down into the bladder for excretion.

Allusion has been made to the mechanism whereby the fluid in the interstitium is rendered continuously more hyperosmotic from outer medulla to papillary tip. It is dependent upon the anatomic arrangement of the loops of Henle and their blood vessels and is achieved by the transport of sodium salts (in excess of water) from the ascending limb of the loop. This renders the fluid in the interstitium hyperosmotic to the fluid entering the descending limb of the loop of Henle. This difference in osmolality promotes a movement of water from the descending limb fluid; and, in addition, there is entry of solutes into this portion of the limb. The net result is an increase in the osmolality of the fluid in the descending limb. This same process is repeated over and over again, and the fluid in the limb and interstitium becomes more concentrated along its course. When the fluid reaches the ascending portion of the limb and solutes are transported out of the luminal fluid, this fluid and the interstitium become ever less concentrated and are, finally, made hypotonic by the time it reaches the early distal convolution.[1]

In this setting the fluid coursing through the collecting ducts is made more hyperosmotic. Since urea can presumably permeate the collecting ducts largely by passive diffusion, urea moves from the collecting system into the interstitium as water moves along the osmotic gradient. In this fashion, urea contributes significantly to the total solute concentration in the medullary and papillary interstitium and serves to counterbalance the concentration of urea within the collecting ducts.

In man, the maximal concentration of the final urine may be as high as 1,200 to 1,400 mOsm per kg water. This may be considerably higher in rodents, the experimental animals from which the data that permit this formulation have been obtained.

In contrast, in the "complete" absence of antidiuretic hormone, the fluid in the distal convolution is not only hypotonic to plasma in the earliest portions but remains so and is excreted as bladder urine with the same or even lower osmolality. Data reveal that salt is transported from the distal convolutions and from the collecting ducts themselves. In the absence of antidiuretic hormone, this aids and abets formation of minimally concentrated urine.

In this fashion, one can visualize the manner in which a highly concentrated or a minimally concen-

[1] The antidiuretic hormone possibly serves to increase the rate of transport of solutes from the ascending limb in addition to its influence on the permeability of the distal tubular and collecting duct permeability.

trated urine can be formed. Varying amounts of anti-diuretic hormone between none and maximal provide a graded response.

Furthermore, it must be pointed out that even in the two polar situations of maximal antidiuretic hormone activity, or none, the rate of excretion of solutes determines the volume and osmolality of urine. This is to state that a urine may have an osmolality approaching that of the plasma with no antidiuretic hormone activity in the face of a solute diuresis; in contrast, the urine volume may be large and the osmolality may approach that of plasma despite maximal antidiuretic hormone activity in the presence of a solute diuresis. The manner in which a solute diuresis influences the concentration and the volume of urine is not completely clear.

However, within the context of the discussion presented above, it is apparent that a good deal of the water removed from the initial volume of filtrate depends on the active transport of salt and other solutes from the luminal fluid. Even if a constant *percentage* of filtered salt were reabsorbed in the proximal tubule, an increased filtration *rate* would provide a larger volume of fluid to the descending limb of the loop of Henle. Furthermore, to the extent that limitations are placed on the transport of salt from the proximal tubule (owing to the presence in filtrate of a larger concentration of a poorly reabsorbable solute), less water will be reabsorbed. If less salt is transported out of the loop of Henle, or if the flow of fluid through the loop is hastened, the countercurrent multiplier system will operate less efficiently; hence, the maximal osmolality will not be achieved in the interstitium of the medulla and papilla. By the same token, if the reabsorption of solutes is diminished in the distal convolution (e.g., glucose is not reabsorbable at this site), less water will be reabsorbed and a greater volume will reach the collecting duct system. Hence, a large solute excretion will increase the volume and diminish the osmolality of the final urine despite maximal antidiuretic hormone activity.

In contrast, it will be recalled that the efficient transport of solutes prior to, in, and beyond the distal convoluted tubule, coupled with the relative impermeability to water of these latter structures in the absence of antidiuretic hormone, are responsible for the formation of minimally dilute urine. If reabsorption of solutes is less efficient, owing to the filtered load or to the presence of less readily reabsorbable solutes, it is clear that urine osmolality cannot reach minimally dilute levels. As the solute diuresis becomes more intense, urine osmolality will approach that of the plasma.

In summary, a small solute excretion in the absence of antidiuretic hormone would be anticipated to be accompanied by the most dilute urine, and in the presence of antidiuretic hormone, with the most maximally concentrated urine. Varying quantities of antidiuretic hormone will have obvious influences; and the character of the urine anticipated in the presence of maximal antidiuretic hormone activity or none will be modified by the quantity and character of the solute load destined for excretion.

PATHOLOGIC CONSIDERATIONS

Oliguria

DEHYDRATION. There are many causes for oliguria, and the commonest may well be simple dehydration. In the face of a diminished volume of body fluids (especially if the loss has been water in excess of salt to provide an osmotic as well as a volumetric stimulus for the secretion of antidiuretic hormone), one anticipates a diminished filtration rate and a reduced excretion of solutes owing to the influence of a plasma volume deficit on renal hemodynamics. The diminished rate of excretion of solutes accompanied by antidiuretic hormone activity should ensure a small volume of highly concentrated urine.

CONGESTIVE HEART FAILURE. Since the volume of the filtrate plays an important role in the rate of excretion of urine, any circumstance which causes a reduced glomerular filtration rate is likely to be associated with some diminution in the rate of flow of urine. The defective systolic emptying of the heart, which is a characteristic of congestive heart failure, is commonly associated with a reduced flow of blood to the kidney and with a reduced filtration rate. This becomes more and more intense as the failure becomes more profound. Furthermore, in congestive heart failure (see Chap. 16 for more details) the renal excretion of salt is diminished, and the combination is obviously likely to result in a small volume of urine. This may be a striking feature of heart failure.

CIRRHOSIS OF THE LIVER. Cirrhosis is frequently accompanied by diminished renal blood flow and filtration rate (despite a coexistent increase in cardiac output) and by a strikingly low urine flow. In cirrhosis of the liver, as in congestive heart failure, the renal tubular reabsorption of salt is presumably more efficient, and this contributes to a diminished urine volume.

ACUTE RENAL INSUFFICIENCY. A low urine volume is one of the cardinal manifestations of this condition. In acute glomerulonephritis (or disorders with the same basic pathology) this low volume is presumably almost entirely a consequence of the drastic reduction in filtration rate. In acute tubular necrosis there is almost certainly a reduced filtration rate, but other factors as well may contribute to the striking oliguria. It is quite possible that in this latter disorder, the necrotic epithelium represents a nonfunctioning and simply passive membrane. Under these circumstances the intraluminal fluid would be under the same influences with respect to the Starling forces as is the interstitial fluid of the kidney. It could be anticipated, therefore, that the bulk of the diminished filtrate might be reabsorbed directly into the peritubular vessels, since the tubular walls no longer function as more than a passive diffusion barrier.

In the much more rare instances of renal cortical

necrosis, where all elements of the nephron are destroyed, total anuria is common. This may obtain because there is virtually no filtration whatsoever; what little does occur is likely to be subject to the influences suggested above in the context of acute tubular necrosis.

CHRONIC RENAL INSUFFICIENCY. The ability to form a maximally concentrated urine is disturbed reasonably early in chronic renal insufficiency. This is accredited to at least two factors. One suggestion is that with a reduced population of nephrons the filtration rate per nephron may well be increased, and in this circumstance there is an osmotic diuresis in terms of those nephrons which are still functioning. In the context of the discussion in the section on physiologic considerations, a framework was provided in an attempt to clarify the influence of the rate of excretion of solutes on the urine concentrating mechanism. Furthermore, if the destruction of renal mass occurs primarily in the medulla (as is so common in pyelonephritis) the nephrons with the longest loops of Henle are more likely to be destroyed. Since these longest loops of Henle set up the highest interstitial osmolality, it is apparent why urine concentrating defects are seen early. Hence, although chronic renal insufficiency may be associated with some polyuria, this is usually not striking. In the patient with end-stage kidney disease, striking reductions in urine flow are frequently observed. This is primarily a consequence of the magnitude of the destruction of renal mass.

OBSTRUCTION OF THE URINARY TRACT. Obstruction of the lower urinary tract, that is, from the bladder to the urethral meatus, is common and is due most frequently to stricture, to compression of the prostatic urethra by an enlarged gland, and, less commonly, to congenital malformations with valve formations that make emptying the bladder difficult. These patients may develop fairly striking acute reductions in urine flow, and this should always be a consideration when a patient is seen with oliguria.

Although it is less common to see oliguria as a consequence of obstruction of the upper urinary tract, it does occur. The reason for its rarity is that there are two kidneys and two ureters, and in order to achieve oliguria from obstruction above the bladder, both ureters must be compromised. However, this does occur in a variety of circumstances which include neoplastic infiltration of the ureters, and bilateral constriction consequent to a retroperitoneal sclerosing inflammatory process. On occasion constrictions may occur at the ureterovesical junctions bilaterally. Hence, although uncommon, bilateral obstruction of the upper urinary tracts may cause oliguria. Unilateral ureteral calculus with ureteral spasm on the opposite side is also possible.

Polyuria

DIABETES INSIPIDUS. This condition results from inability to synthesize and secrete antidiuretic hormone and is the achetype of a disorder accompanied by the excretion of large volumes of dilute urine. In a compilation of several reports, intracranial tumors accounted for 40 per cent of the variety of causes for diabetes inspidus, 33 per cent were so-called *idiopathic,* and the remainder were scattered among a variety of disorders including trauma. Although not a rare disorder, diabetes insipidus is certainly uncommon. The primary condition from which it must be discriminated is primary polydipsia, which may be due to an intracranial organic lesion but perhaps more often accompanies a basic emotional disorder. These two disorders can be distinguished one from the other in a relatively simple fashion (see Chap. 81).

NEPHROGENIC DIABETES INSIPIDUS. Inability of the renal tubules to respond to antidiuretic hormone of endogenous or exogenous origin characterizes nephrogenic diabetes insipidus. It is a heritable disorder with full expression in males and partial expression in females, which manifests itself quite early in life; these patients are frequently referred to as "water babies." Their management had been difficult since they do not respond to any of the available posterior pituitary preparations. However, they do respond to chlorothiazide drugs. The probable manner in which this agent influences the water turnover is by promoting a salt deficit. This, in turn, causes a smaller urine volume. This may be a consequence of a diminished filtration rate but is more likely to be associated with a larger fractional reabsorption of salt, and hence water, in the more proximal portions of the nephron. In this fashion less fluid is delivered to sites where it may escape into the bladder urine.

ACQUIRED RENAL LESIONS. There are acquired renal lesions associated with inability to concentrate the urine maximally.

Potassium depletion is commonly, if not invariably, associated with inability to concentrate the urine appropriately. The nature of the defect is not clear. Although it is at some risk that one translates data from rodents to human beings, information from rats and hamsters does exclude certain possibilities. Micropuncture data obtained by Gottschalk and his colleagues show that the osmolality of fluid in the distal convolution is the same in potassium-depleted rats as in control animals. Hence, there appears to be no lack of osmotic equilibration at this site. Furthermore, more recent data from the same laboratory utilizing normal and potassium-depleted hamsters reveal that there is no osmotic disequilibrium across the collecting duct epithelium. Other data indicate that the interstitial fluid deep in the papilla is not as hyperosmotic in potassium-depleted as in normal animals. The reasons for this are still unclear. Some published data on rats tend to deny the possibility that this is a consequence of a greater flow of fluid through the loop of Henle, since, if anything, the fractional reabsorption of water in the proximal convolution appears to be greater in a state of potassium depletion. Two obvious influences have not yet been evaluated, namely, the rate of medullary blood flow and the rate of active transport of salt in the ascending limb. An increase in medullary blood flow would tend to diminish the hypertonicity of the medullary and papillary interstitium; and a diminished rate of transport of salt across the ascending limb of the loops of Henle would diminish the efficiency of the countercurrent multiplier mechanism. The defect is reversible with potassium repletion.

Hypercalcemia has been known for some time to be accompanied by diminished ability to concentrate the urine maximally. In this instance as well, the precise mechanism is unknown. At this time the available data are somewhat similar to those discussed with respect to potassium depletion. There is no evidence of an osmotic disequilibrium across the collecting ducts and no evidence of an increased flow of fluid through the loop of Henle. The facets that have not been examined in the state of potassium depletion also raise questions about the hypercalcemic state.

Other examples of acquired renal lesions characterized by inability to concentrate the urine are seen frequently in patients with *chronic renal insufficiency,* as alluded to earlier. In addition, some rather striking examples of extreme polyuria have been seen in patients with multiple myeloma, amyloidosis, and, more commonly, after relief of an obstructive uropathy. Marked diuresis is commonly observed in the recovery phase of acute tubular necrosis from a variety of insults. This is frequently referred to as the "diuretic phase" of acute tubular necrosis and may be due in part to the delivery of accumulated fluid but very likely also due in part to renal tubular abnormalities with reference to the reabsorption of solutes and water.

SOLUTE DIURESIS. Large solute diureses, such as are noted in patients with uncontrolled diabetes mellitus and constant glycosuria, are almost always accompanied by large urine flows and complaint of polyuria. Solute diuresis may also occur in patients suffering a "reaction to injury" who are unable to utilize protein but are given large quantities of this foodstuff. In such instances protein is converted to a very large extent to urea and excreted. This increase in solute excretion promotes a large urine flow as described earlier.

Nocturia

The diurnal rhythm that applies to urine flow is such that a larger volume is excreted in the waking 12 hr than during the 12-hr period spent mostly asleep. The precise mechanisms underlying this particular rhythm are not clear, although the evidence suggests a correlation with filtration rate and solute excretion. This rhythm is lost in several circumstances, and in other instances it may appear to have been lost owing to mechanical problems.

The rhythm characterized by a relatively diminished volume of urine at night is frequently disturbed in patients with edema. This may very well be because edema accumulates more during the day owing to activity and the influence of gravity through posture. At night, when the patient is supine, some of the edema may be resorbed into the plasma volume,

thereby promoting an alteration in renal hemodynamics that leads to increased excretion of urine.

Nocturia is common in patients with chronic renal insufficiency primarily because they excrete urine at a fairly constant rate, and hence the benefits to sleep of the normal diurnal rhythm are lost. The reasons for this may be similar to those relating to a concentrated urine. In this instance it may be due to a constant osmotic diuresis per nephron.

Partial obstruction of the bladder is often accompanied by nocturia simply because the stimulus to void is so frequently present.

For reasons that are certainly unclear, the patient with untreated adrenal cortical insufficiency loses the normal diurnal rhythm and hence may complain of nocturia.

Lastly, anything that causes dysuria is almost certain to promote nocturia. In this instance, as is the case with obstruction of the bladder, nocturia is characterized by frequent but *small* volumes in contrast to the other cases noted above.

APPROACH TO THE PATIENT

Carefully taken histories usually reveal evidence of disturbances characterized by excretion of small or large volumes of urine, or the presence or absence of nocturia. The associations with disease processes of this type of disturbance have been alluded to, and the questions suggested by these clues are, in a sense, implicit.

The point that bears some emphasis, perhaps, is that wide variations in urine flow exist in health as well as in disease, and a reasonable interpretation can be made only by careful evaluation of the characteristics of the symptom equated with other problems displayed by the patient. The specific evaluation of these disorders is discussed in other sections of this text.

REFERENCES

Starling, E. H.: The Fluids of the Body, in "The Herter Lectures," New York, W. T. Keener & Co., 1909.

Welt, L. G.: Volume Receptors, Circulation, 21:1002, 1960.

Welt, Louis G.: Water Balance in Health and Disease, chap. 6, in "Diseases of Metabolism," 5th ed., G. G. Duncan (Ed.), Philadelphia, W. B. Saunders Company, 1964.

20   HEMATURIA

Bernard Lytton and Franklin H. Epstein

Bleeding from the urinary tract, whether microscopic or gross, is a serious sign. It should be regarded with the same gravity as abnormal bleeding occurring from any other body tract. Hematuria is usually classified as initial, terminal, or total. Total hematuria indicates that the bleeding occurs throughout the urinary stream and suggests that the bleeding originates from either the kidney or the ureter. Initial bleeding is generally associated with lesions in the urethra distal to the bladder neck; terminal bleeding, with lesions in the bladder, usually in the area of the trigone. Severe hemorrhage from the bladder, however, will present as total hematuria. These distinctions as to the type of bleeding are, therefore, only rough indications as to the origin of the bleeding; too much reliance should not be placed on them. About 20 per cent of the patients who come to the physician with hematuria have it as the only symptom of their urinary tract disease; it is often difficult to persuade these patients to undergo a complete urologic investigation to establish the origin of the bleeding. Ureteral colic is often associated with renal bleeding and is due to the passage of clots.

The finding of an occasional red blood cell in a centrifuged specimen of urine is probably of no significance, since Addis showed that up to 500,000 red cells may normally be excreted in the urine in 12 hr. Vigorous exercise or even intense excitement may increase the numbers of red cells, epithelial cells, and casts in the urinary sediment of normal subjects. Microscopic hematuria may also be increased during certain febrile diseases without implying serious disease of the kidneys. The presence of red blood cell casts is pathologic and further indicates that the source of the bleeding is in the kidneys rather than the lower part of the urinary tract.

Certain dyes and pigments, such as phenolsulfonphthalein, azo dyes, and the indole alkaloids found in beet roots, may produce red discoloration of the urine which must be distinguished from bleeding. The appearance of the red dye from beet roots occurs only in certain individuals; it is thought to be related to the degree of absorption of the dye from the gastrointestinal tract.

Diseases of the renal parenchyma, such as glomerulonephritis, malignant hypertension, polycystic kidneys, renal infarction, periarteritis, or poisoning with a nephrotoxic agent, will in most instances be detected by a careful history, physical examination, and the usual laboratory tests. Hematuria may result from a *disorder of blood clotting,* produced by blood dyscrasias, scurvy, or anticoagulant drugs. The increased tendency to bleed in patients on long-term anticoagulant therapy may bring to light another, previously unsuspected, pathologic condition in the urinary tract. Sickle-cell anemia or sickle-cell trait may cause bleeding into the urine from disrupted capillaries and microinfarcts in the renal medulla. The afore-mentioned conditions account for only a small proportion of all patients with hematuria.

Tumors, urinary tract obstructions, calculi, and infections account for the bleeding in about 75 per cent of patients with hematuria. Tumors alone account for some 20 per cent of all cases. It is therefore mandatory

in those patients in whom no other cause is found for the bleeding, to visualize the upper part of the urinary tract by intravenous pyelography supplemented by retrograde pyelography as indicated, and to visualize the bladder and urethra by instrumental examination. Retrograde pyelography may be supplemented by injections of air rather than opaque dye when one is trying to delineate suspected nonopaque calculi or small tumors in the renal collecting system. Doubtful lesions in the kidney may be further investigated by nephrotomography or aortography. The latter is probably best performed by the transfemoral route which allows selective injections into individual renal vessels to be made if required. Renal tumors generally have greater opacification than the surrounding kidney tissue on tomography, and the aortogram shows the characteristic pooling of the dye in the venous sinusoids which occurs in these tumors and which is a result of the small arteriovenous communications which develop.

On cystoscopy, acute and chronic cystitis, interstitial cystitis, bladder tumors, and vesical calculi may be readily diagnosed. Bleeding from engorged veins in the prostatic urethra due to benign prostatic hypertrophy is a common source of hematuria. Like prostatitis in men and chronic nonspecific posterior urethritis in women, it should be accepted as the origin of the bleeding only if more serious conditions have been excluded.

Acute cystitis may produce gross hematuria, initially overshadowing all other symptoms. *Chronic infections* such as *tuberculosis* of the urinary tract or infection with *Schistosoma hematobium* may also have hematuria as their only presenting symptom. Schistosomiasis causes ulceration of the bladder mucosa at the site of deposition of the ova by the adult flukes which inhabit the venules of the bladder and pelvis. It is probably the commonest cause of hematuria in those areas in the Middle East and Africa where it is endemic.

Bleeding associated with the menses should suggest the possibility of *endometriosis* of the urinary tract, provided contamination from the vagina has been excluded.

Trauma to the kidney nearly always manifests itself as hematuria which is often painless and may persist for several days. The incidence of renal injury is increasing because of the increased number of serious automobile accidents. The majority of these cases may be treated conservatively with bed rest and careful observation. Follow-up intravenous pyelography should be carried out, as occasionally the renal injury may produce an anatomic deformity leading to either stone formation or hypertension. A blow on the lower part of the abdomen when the bladder is distended, particularly in children where the bladder is an abdominal organ, may produce a contusion of the bladder, giving rise to painless hematuria.

A small group of patients, about 5 to 8 per cent of all cases seen, have a condition known as *essential or idiopathic hematuria.* In these patients a complete investigation reveals no abnormality to account for the bleeding. Further management consists of another complete urologic and hematologic investigation 3 to 4 months after the first episode of bleeding. It has been found that the cause of the bleeding is subsequently discovered in just under half of these patients.

The cause in the remainder, however, is not found. Such patients occasionally have severe, persistent, recurrent hematuria over several years and sometimes undergo surgical exploration of the kidney without the source of the bleeding being discovered.

21 DISTURBANCES OF MENSTRUATION

George W. Thorn

Since normal menstrual cycles depend upon the integrated action of the endocrine and nervous systems, it is to be expected that abnormalities in the menstrual cycle may occur in association with a wide variety of systemic disorders as well as with specific pathologic changes in the reproductive organs. (See Chap. 90 for a discussion of disease of the ovaries and uterus.)

MENARCHE. In temperate climates the menstrual cycle usually begins between the ages of twelve to fifteen, whereas in tropical climates it may appear as early as nine or ten. During the first year or two, the menstrual cycles are likely to be irregular, since many are anovulatory.

Uterine bleeding in the newborn may be noted for 3 to 4 days following delivery and is thought to be due to the sudden decrease in circulating estrogen level which had previously induced endometrial growth in the fetus.

Vaginal bleeding in very young girls should suggest injury from a foreign body introduced into the vagina. Very rarely vaginal bleeding will occur in association with precocious development of breasts due to an ovarian or adrenal tumor.

The delayed onset of menses, beyond the age of sixteen years, suggests *abnormalities* in the development *of the reproductive system,* such as imperforate hymen, uterine hypoplasia, and ovarian agenesis; *endocrine dysfunction,* such as anterior pituitary or thyroid deficiency; or *psychologic disturbances,* which mediate their effect through neurohumoral pathways.

MENSES. Normally periods occur at intervals of 27 to 32 days, and flow lasts an average of 5 days. Approximately 60 to 250 ml blood is lost, with the greatest quantity lost during the first or second day. The volume of menstrual flow can be estimated by the fact that each well-soaked pad will contain approximately 30 to 50 ml blood.

MENOPAUSE. Naturally occurring menopause may be expected by age fifty. Menopause represents the period of change between the years of reproduction and the regression of ovarian function. A gradual re-

duction in the duration of the menstrual cycle is to be expected at this time. *Irregular bleeding* or *hypermenorrhea* is most often caused by anovulatory cycles, but *neoplasms* should always be suspected. Induced or artificial menopause follows extirpation or irradiation of the ovaries. *Premature menopause* may occur as early as thirty-five without definitive cause; occasionally a familial tendency for this will be noted. However, other causes of amenorrhea such as endocrine abnormalities and emotional factors must be excluded.

ABNORMAL UTERINE BLEEDING. During the reproductive cycle abnormal uterine bleeding should always suggest pregnancy and one of its complications, such as threatened abortion, ectopic pregnancy, or hydatid mole. Having excluded the complications of pregnancy by history, physical examination, and a rapid serologic test, one should consider uterine pathology such as polyps, leiomyomas, and carcinoma of the cervix or body of the uterus. For these a pelvic examination and diagnostic curettage will be required. Ovarian disease, pelvic inflammation, and hormonal abnormalities such as *hypothyroidism* also can induce abnormal uterine bleeding. Systemic disturbances, particularly those associated with anemia, leukemia, abnormalities in blood clotting, and circulatory disturbances such as hypertension should be excluded. The anemia that follows prolonged menstrual bleeding may predispose a patient to further excessive menstruation. In view of the widespread use of hormones, particularly estrogens, progesterone, and androgens, for such varied conditions as osteoporosis, coronary artery disease, deficient erythropoiesis, and metastatic neoplasm, one should consider the *administration* or *withdrawal* of sex hormonal preparations as potential causes of abnormal uterine bleeding. Finally, disturbed emotional states or serious psychologic difficulties may predispose to abnormal uterine bleeding.

Hypermenorrhea, characterized by excessively long or too profuse menstrual bleeding, may result from delay in the repair of the endometrium and, of course, frequently accompanies anovulatory cyclic bleeding.

Polymenorrhea refers to regular menstrual cycles that occur more frequently than every 23 to 24 days. It is the least common of the menstrual irregularities and tends to occur very early or late in menstrual life. It is due to a shortening of the follicular or luteal phase of the menstrual cycle.

Intermenstrual bleeding refers to the occurrence of irregular bleeding between normally spaced periods. Spontaneous bleeding of this type is more likely to be endometrial in origin in contrast to bleeding of the cervix or vagina.

AMENORRHEA AND OLIGOMENORRHEA. Physiologic amenorrhea precedes the menarche, follows the menopause, and characterizes pregnancy and lactation. *Primary amenorrhea* indicates that menstruation has never occurred, whereas *secondary amenorrhea* refers to cessation of menstruation.

Uterine abnormalities such as agenesis or hypoplasia, give rise to primary amenorrhea, whereas destruction of endometrium by irradiation or excessive curettage or removal of the uterus can induce secondary amenorrhea. *Vaginal abnormalities* include such conditions as imperforate hymen. The continued retention of blood may lead to hematometra, hematosalpinx, and eventually hematoperitoneum.

Ovarian agenesis or dysgenesis (Turner's syndrome) is a cause of primary amenorrhea, whereas polycystic disease of the ovary (Stein-Leventhal syndrome), masculinizing tumors of the ovary or adrenal, destruction of ovarian function by irradiation, and hormonal imbalance give rise in most instances to secondary amenorrhea or oligomenorrhea. Hypopituitarism with Simmond's cachexia, Sheehan's syndrome, or the Chiavi-Frommel syndrome will, of course, result in reduced ovarian function and predispose to oligomenorrhea or amenorrhea. With pituitary deficiency, one would expect associated evidence of reduced adrenal and thyroid function (Chap. 80). Diabetes mellitus and hyperthyroidism may induce menstrual abnormalities characterized by oligomenorrhea or hypermenorrhea. Malnutrition, obesity, debilitating disease, intoxication, and severe anemia may be associated with oligomenorrhea or amenorrhea as well as with abnormal uterine bleeding. Fear, anxiety, and grief are frequent causes of temporary amenorrhea, and indeed psychologic factors acting on hypothalamic centers constitute one of the most frequent causes of secondary amenorrhea. Amenorrhea is almost an invariable accompaniment of anorexia nervosa.

DYSMENORRHEA. Some form of discomfort normally accompanies ovulatory menstruation in contrast to anovulation bleeding, which is almost never associated with pain. Dysmenorrhea may reflect itself as lower abdominal cramps, backache, headache, and occasionally nausea and vomiting. Of these symptoms, the commonest is abdominal cramps. Many women suffer some discomfort for a few hours on the first day of menstruation, but in the majority of cases this is not incapacitating. Obviously, the degree of pain and discomfort experienced by any individual will depend upon concurrent involvement of the pelvic organs in disease or anatomic abnormalities. The pain threshold of the patient and the effect of emotional and psychologic problems, particularly those related to ignorance or misconception about the significance of the menstrual cycle, are important factors in evaluating the pathogenesis of dysmenorrhea. In *primary spastic* or *intrinsic dysmenorrhea*, there is no evidence of pelvic pathology. It may gradually disappear later in reproductive life, and relief is usually afforded by the birth of a full-term fetus. *Characteristic of secondary dysmenorrhea is the onset of pain after several years of relatively painless periods.* Pain may begin several days before menstrual flow and radiate throughout the entire lower abdomen, into the lower back, and down the legs. It is more constant in nature and not as sharp or cramplike as that noted in the primary type. Secondary dysmenorrhea is usually associated with pelvic pathology such as endometriosis, retroversion of the uterus, pelvic neoplasm, or inflammatory disease such as salpingitis or parametritis. In rare instances intense pain at the time of menstruation may accompany the expulsion of a large mass of shaggy, uterine membrane, i.e., membranous dysmenorrhea. Such events are infrequent and isolated and do not occur with successive periods.

PREMENSTRUAL TENSION. This term is applied to a constellation of symptoms which increase in intensity for 5 to 10 days before menstruation. The most frequent complaints are a sense of abdominal bloating, breast tenderness, headache, irritability, mental depression, and an increase in weight which may be associated with edema of the legs. The abdominal distension and tight feeling may be present without any great increase in weight and ofttimes without gaseous distension of the intestines. It is thought to be due to a relaxation of the abdominal musculature and to some degree mimics "pseudocyesis."

Patients with serious organic disease such as cardiovascular disease, chronic nephritis, hepatic disease, and hypoproteinemia may exhibit a marked gain in weight with fluid retention during the premenstrual period. In the majority of patients, however, serious organic disease is not found, whereas symptoms of emotional disturbance are prominent. Although therapy designed to minimize salt and water retention will prevent excessive gain in weight, it is rare to observe significant improvement in the symptomatology until the important role of deep-seated conflicts is better appreciated by the patients. There is no doubt that the wide fluctuation in female sex hormone levels which occurs during the reproductive period, with their important effect on electrolyte and water metabolism as well as upon mood and drive, provide critical "triggering" mechanisms for pathophysiologic changes in peripheral tissues as well as in the central nervous system.

REFERENCES

Behrman, S. J., and J. R. G. Gosling: Fundamentals of Gynecology, chaps. 6–11, New York, Oxford University Press, 1959.

Rogers, J.: Menstrual Disorders, New England J. Med., 270:194, Jan. 23, 1964.

Thorn, G. W.: Cyclical Edema: Editorial, Am. J. Med., 23:507, 1957.

22 DISTURBANCES OF SEXUAL FUNCTION

George W. Thorn

GENERAL CONSIDERATIONS

In men disturbances in sexual function may result from alterations in one or all of three distinct entities.

1. Libido, or the sexual impulse
2. Potentia, or penile erection
3. Ejaculation of semen

In women aberrations of sexual function are more difficult to analyze. Lack or diminution of sexual drive or failure to attain orgasm (frigidity) is much more frequent than in men.

ALTERATIONS IN LIBIDO. Loss of Libido. Loss of libido may occur as a result of either psychologic or somatic factors. It may be complete in the presence of serious organic disease or with advanced age. On the other hand, lost or diminished libido may occur only under particular circumstances or in relation to a particular person, indicating the predominance of psychologic factors. In instances such as these, it is not unusual for a patient to experience nocturnal penile erection and emission of semen. Although loss of libido may accompany serious endocrine disorders such as anterior pituitary deficiency, Addison's disease, or diabetic acidosis or ketosis, it is not likely to be a *primary complaint* of the patient under these circumstances since the impairment in general health and activity is so overwhelming. Under these circumstances, it is more likely that the patient's spouse will have noted or called attention to the difficulty. For practical purposes it is important to bear in mind that the primary complaint of lost or decreased libido in male patients, in the absence of *severe* organic disease or *advanced* age, is almost certainly dependent *upon emotional or psychologic disturbances.*

Frigidity. Inability on the part of women to consummate the sexual act is a distressing complaint of relatively frequent occurrence. The sexual drive of the normal woman is primarily conditioned by psychologic factors, with endocrine functions in a supporting role. The changes in sexual drive produced by alterations in hormonal level are of relatively little importance in contrast to the role of emotional and psychologic factors. Conditioning from birth or early childhood most often results in a woman's belief that she is frigid. Many experiences in childhood can, later in life, result in incapacity to consummate the sexual act. Such experiences develop a climate of fear, insecurity, and dread concerning the whole subject of sex. Because of these deep-seated emotional conflicts, most patients will require intensive psychotherapy. With an understanding of the real basis of the problem and in conjunction with medical and psychiatric assistance, a small dose of androgenic hormone such as methyl testosterone, 10 mg twice daily, may be given. This may increase sexual drive and more specifically increase the sensitivity of the clitoris. Its continued use, however, may result in menstrual irregularities as well as in hirsutism and acne.

Excessive Libido. Excessive libido may occur in conjunction with serious neurologic disease such as encephalitis or brain tumor as well as with psychologic and emotional disturbances. *Nymphomania* refers to women who exhibit abnormal behavior that reflects greatly heightened libido.

ALTERATIONS IN POTENTIA. Impotence. Impotence implies the presence of sexual desire in a patient who cannot attain or sustain penile erection. Impotence is rarely of endocrine origin. More frequently it accompanies a neurologic or emotional disorder. In neurologic disorders absence or impairment of parasympathetic nerve activity prevents the development of tumescence of the corpora cavernosa. Impotence is common among patients who suffer disease of the sacral cord segments and their afferent and efferent connections, e.g., cord tumor, tabes, and multiple sclerosis. Approximately one-fourth of male diabetics in the younger age group and about one-half in the fifth decade develop impotence as a consequence of diabetic polyneuritis. Loss of both sexual desire and erection may occur in hypopituitarism, hypothyroidism, and severe eunuchoidism as well as in association with many general debilitating diseases. Patients with trauma to the prostatic urethra and those subjected to perineal operations frequently have reduced potentia. Malformation of the genitals such as extreme degrees of epispadias, pseudohermaphroditism, growths and edema of the penis, as well as large hernias, hydroceles, and elephantiasis may interfere with sexual function. In the majority of patients, however, impotence is of psychologic origin and fortunately temporary. Fears and phobias which arise about the sexual act, as well as feelings of guilt, may be responsible.

Priapism. True priapism is a state of sustained erection of the penis not accompanied by sexual desire. It is most frequent in the third or fourth decades and is usually accompanied by pain. Two types are recognized: the sustained and the recurrent nocturnal type. Priapism may result from urethral inflammation, from new growth involving the corpora, or from systemic disease such as leukemia or sickle-cell anemia. Diseases of the spinal cord may be accompanied by penile erections, reflexly induced and sustained for long periods of time. The neural apparatus for the control of sexual function is organized through the lower spinal segments, and hence may function effectively even when completely removed from voluntary control by spinal cord lesions. Recurrent, nonsustained, painful priapism is of unknown etiology, although it is often associated with prostatitis. It frequently subsides spontaneously and should be left untreated except for sedation.

EJACULATION. Another type of disturbance consists of *premature ejaculation* of semen, a common complaint in neurotic individuals, though by no means peculiar to them. After lumbar sympathectomy the semen may be ejected into the bladder because of paralysis of the periurethral muscle at the verumontanum.

DYSPAREUNIA. Dyspareunia, or *pain on intercourse*, may be present for a short time at the onset of marriage or sexual intercourse. Pain that continues long after marriage or develops later in life suggests local disease or emotional disturbance. Vaginal and pelvic examination should be made to exclude pelvic inflammatory disease, endometriosis, or tumor. In the absence of demonstrable organic disease, psychologic or emotional factors must be considered. Fear of pregnancy, fear of cancer if contraceptives are used, and tension between husband and wife can prevent enjoyment of intercourse with consequent spasm of vaginal musculature. Explanation of these facts with reassurance by an understanding physician may be followed by appreciable improvement.

STERILITY. In the male sterility may result from lack of or impairment of spermatogenesis due to testicular agenesis, hypogenesis, or cryptorchidism; to castration or exposure to roentgen rays or toxic substances; to injury or inflammation; or to endocrine or nutritional disorders. Obstruction of the seminal vesicles and epididymis and pronounced deformity of the penis interfere with the normal passage of the spermatozoa. Infection of the prostate or seminal vesicles may be injurious to the spermatozoa (Chap. 91).

In the female sterility may result from impaired oogenesis as a consequence of deficient ovarian tissue, e.g., ovarian agenesis or hypoplasia, polycystic disease of the ovary with thickened capsule; or as a consequence of the inability of the ovum to become impregnated due to disease of the fallopian tubes, such as infection and endometriosis; or to uterine, cervical, or vaginal abnormalities in structure and function. In addition, debilitating diseases, endocrine abnormalities, and nutritional deficiencies may impair ovulation as well as fertilization and implantation of the ovum.

INFERTILITY. Infertility represents one of the most important and serious disturbances of sexual function. It is estimated that 10 per cent of couples in the United States are involuntarily infertile. Of this number it is thought that approximately one-third of cases are due to infertility of the women, one-third to infertility of the man, and one-third to *decreased fertility* of both partners. Absolute infertility is said to exist when there is complete aspermia or absent or sedimentary ovarian tissue. *Relative infertility* applies to men who have oligospermia, when conception has not taken place. In contrast to other disturbances of sexual function such as impotence, frigidity, and dyspareunia, which are so frequently dependent upon psychologic and emotional factors, sterility and infertility are due primarily to functional and organic disease of the urogenital tract. In most instances the problem of infertility or sterility will be presented by the woman.

The approach to the problem of infertility in both men and women as well as suggestions for corrective therapy are discussed in detail in Chap. 91.

The genesis of *sexual perversions* remains obscure. Endocrine, biochemical, and psychologic studies have failed thus far to clarify either their cause or their mechanism.

REFERENCES

Hamm, F. C., and S. R. Weinberg: "Urology in Medical Practice," 2d ed., Philadelphia, J. B. Lippincott Company, 1962.

Calderone, M. S.: "Release from Sexual Tension," New York, Random House, 1960.

Schöffling, K., K. Federlin, H. Ditschuneit, and E. F. Pfeiffer: Disorders of Sexual Function in Male Diabetics, Diabetes, 12:519, 1963.

Section 5

Alterations in Gastrointestinal Function

23 ORAL MANIFESTATIONS OF DISEASE

William H. Resnik

In this brief discussion will be described some of the commoner or more important manifestations of systemic or local disease affecting the mouth, emphasis being placed on those that tend to be diagnostic or suggestive of a specific disorder; little or no mention will be made of oral manifestations of conditions otherwise readily recognizable.

BURNING OF THE TONGUE AND MOUTH. This symptom may occur in any of the numerous forms of *ulceration* and *stomatitis*. It is important to bear in mind that when the cause of the stomatitis is not obvious, hematologic study is mandatory, particularly when drugs capable of causing neutropenia are being administered. *Aphthous stomatitis* (canker sores) is a common cause of such ulceration, the lesion consisting of a shallow ulcer about 2 to 3 mm in diameter, surrounded by a bright red areola. The ulcers are caused by the rupture of vesicles suspected of being of viral origin, although some are unquestionably related to specific food allergens. A far more severe and extensive glossitis and stomatitis may follow the use of antibiotics, especially of the broad-spectrum type. Burning of the tongue may be an early manifestation of *nutritional deficiencies*, as discussed below. Burning of the tongue in the absence of a visible lesion is sometimes related to smoking or to a psychoneurotic state, and vitamins are ineffectual in abolishing the symptom. In many instances no satisfactory explanation for the symptom can be discovered.

MALODOROUS BREATH (HALITOSIS). A distinctly unpleasant odor to the breath may emanate from any patient suffering an *infection in the respiratory tract*, a notable example being the stench issuing from the unfortunate victim of chronic atrophic rhinitis (ozena); other examples are bronchiectasis and lung abscess. Halitosis is also likely to occur in patients with *oral sepsis* and putrefaction, such as those with *pyorrhea alveolaris*, or badly *carious teeth*, or any of the various types of *ulcerative stomatitis*, particularly those occurring in neutropenic states and acute leukemia. Some persons who smoke excessively may display halitosis, and a similar price is paid by lovers and users of garlic and onion. Occasionally, otherwise normal persons will exhibit halitosis without obvious cause, and the symptom has been attributed to the exhalation of volatile substances thought to result from the improper digestion of fats, particularly when large quantities of milk and milk products have been consumed. Some physicians with a keen sense of smell are able to suspect quickly in obtunded or comatose patients *hepatic failure* by the fishy odor of the breath, *uremia* by the ammoniac, urinary odor, and *diabetic acidosis* by the sweetish, overripe fruity odor.

PIGMENTATION OF GUMS AND BUCCAL MEMBRANES. Absorption of lead in persons with poor oral hygiene but whose teeth still remain leads to the deposition of lead sulfide at the gingival margin and the formation of the bluish-black *lead "line."* Similar "lines," practically identical in appearance, may be caused by the deposition of bismuth and of silver. *Addison's disease* is usually associated with a patchy dark-brown pigmentation of the gums, inner surfaces of the lips, and buccal mucosa. The pigmentation is similar to that normally seen in Negroes and many persons of Mediterranean ancestry and altogether different from the discrete macules of the mouth and lips of the *Peutz-Jeghers syndrome. Acanthosis nigricans* frequently involves the mouth, the importance of this rare disorder arising from the fact that in adults a high percentage of cases is associated with visceral cancer.

WHITE OR GRAYISH PATCHES. Rarely a whitish *plaque of lichen planus* may be seen in the absence of the characteristic skin lesions. White or grayish patches of *leukoplakia,* a precancerous lesion, sometimes covering large surfaces of the buccal membrane and tongue, are common in persons who smoke excessively. Even more important is the grayish patch of varying size, the highly contagious *mucous patch of secondary syphilis,* which frequently escapes recognition because early syphilis is rarely seen now and this disease is easily forgotten. The diagnosis should be suspected when the grayish surface can be scraped off easily, leaving a raw bleeding membrane.

The grayish-white membranes of *diphtheria, Vincent's angina,* and *streptococcal infections,* or the patches sometimes seen in *infectious mononucleosis* should be recognized promptly as manifestations of an acute infection and appropriate diagnostic procedures initiated at once.

SIZE AND APPEARANCE OF TONGUE. *Macroglossia* is occasionally congenital and is also seen in myxedema, acromegaly, mongolism, primary amyloidosis, tumor, or glycogen-storage disease. An abrupt nontender and painless swelling may be caused by

angioneurotic edema. *Injury to the hypoglossal nerve or nucleus,* as in progressive bulbar palsy or the bulbar form of poliomyelitis, leads to atrophy of the tongue on the affected side. The scarlet-red tongue of *pellagra,* the magenta-colored tongue of *ariboflavinosis,* and the smooth, slick tongue of *pernicious anemia* and occasionally of *iron deficiency* are rarely encountered now that vitamins and reasonably adequate diets are available for all and vitamin B_{12} and iron are given so freely. The *geographic tongue* is given its name because of its resemblance to a contour map by the transitory and often migrating loss of papillae in large areas of the tongue. This lesion has no known significance, nor has the *coated, furred tongue* frequently present in normal persons or with many harmless digestive disorders. The tongue in some elderly persons in excellent health has the appearance and color of raw beef, unaffected by vitamins or any other therapy. A black hairy appearance of the tongue is sometimes, but not necessarily, preceded by the use of antibiotic troches; it is caused by the overgrowth of fungi.

MISCELLANEOUS FINDINGS. Bleeding from the gums is usually caused by local lesions, but it may be an early manifestation of *scurvy* or *thrombocytopenic states.* The pathognomonic *Koplik spots* may be the first clue to the presence of *measles,* just as a reddening and slight swelling of the orifice of Stenson's duct may indicate the probable diagnosis of *mumps.* Bullous lesions in the mouth, caused by *pemphigus* or by *erythema multiforme* (Stevens-Johnson) may occasionally occur long before the characteristic skin lesions develop. Biopsy may be required for diagnosis. It is sometimes very difficult to differentiate between *chancre* and *epithelioma.* Serologic tests and biopsy may be required. Dilantin therapy may be revealed by a conspicuously hyperplastic gingivitis. The famous Hutchinsonian teeth, the pegged and notched central incisors, are indicative of *congenital syphilis. Xerostomia* (persistent abnormal dryness of the mouth) is, with other manifestations, one of the features of Sjögren's syndrome; at other times, it may be an isolated phenomenon, and in both instances this distressing symptom is unresponsive to any form of therapy.

24 DYSPHAGIA
William H. Resnik

Dysphagia implies a difficulty in the passage of food or water from the mouth into the stomach. Dysphagia may be classified according to the three chief mechanisms that cause it.

1. Mechanical obstruction in the esophagus
2. Disturbance in the neuromuscular mechanisms of swallowing
3. Lesions of the mouth, pharynx, or larynx causing pain or mechanical hindrance to passage of food into the esophagus

The most characteristic manifestation of dysphagia is the sensation of food "sticking" some place in its passage to the stomach, usually at the level of the obstructive lesion, sometimes referred to the *suprasternal notch,* even though the structural lesion may be at the lower end of the esophagus. *Pain,* usually behind the sternum, but sometimes radiating into the arms or back, associated with or aggravated by the act of swallowing is another common symptom of esophageal disorder. This may occur in conjunction with the "sticking" sensation or with an ulcerative or inflammatory lesion of the mucosa. The pain is usually steady and sometimes severe, and these qualities, in addition to the location and radiation of the pain, may occasionally make differentiation from the pain of myocardial ischemia difficult. The sensory innervation of the esophagus is derived from both the vagus and the sympathetic system (probably the inferior cervical ganglion and upper line thoracic sympathetic ganglia). This extensive innervation explains the wide reference of pain sometimes encountered in disorders of the esophagus. *Heartburn* is a third manifestation of esophageal disorder, a burning sensation behind the sternum, usually extending to the suprasternal notch or into the pharynx and often associated with regurgitation of gastric juice into the mouth. The mechanism of this symptom is uncertain and has been attributed to tension in the esophageal wall or reflux of gastric contents or both. For further details regarding these symptoms, see Chap. 179.

DYSPHAGIA DUE TO MECHANICAL OBSTRUCTION IN THE ESOPHAGUS. This group is by far the most important and comprises 90 per cent or more of all cases of dysphagia. The causes of the obstruction are *carcinoma, esophagitis* and *benign stricture, diaphragmatic hernia, pharyngoesophageal diverticulum (Zenker's pouch), esophageal spasm, foreign bodies, extraesophageal lesions,* and, rarely, *hypertrophic spurring of the cervical vertebras* protruding into the pharynx or esophagus. In addition, certain disorders affect esophageal motility in such a manner as to mimic mechanical obstruction: *scleroderma* and *other connective tissue disorders, achalasia* (cardiospasm), and *amyloidosis.* These disorders are discussed more fully in Chap. 179.

DYSPHAGIA DUE TO DISTURBANCES IN THE NEUROMUSCULAR MECHANISMS OF SWALLOWING. In the act of swallowing, food is transferred from the oral cavity by contraction of the tongue against the hard palate, by the action of the pharyngeal constrictors, and by the relaxation of the pharyngoesophageal sphincter. Food is thereby prevented from being forced into the nasopharynx, and it fails to enter the larynx by virtue of the elevation of this structure beneath the protective cover of the base of the tongue. Dysphagia results when any part of this coordinated and complex series of movements is disturbed. The features witnessed in varying degree in these disorders are difficulty in maneuvering food into the esophagus in the absence of pain or mechanical hindrance, regurgitation

of fluids through the nasopharynx, aspiration of food into the larynx, nasal character of the voice, and weakness of the palate. Examples of this type of dysphagia are *myasthenia gravis, oculopharyngeal muscular dystrophy, bulbar palsy, diphtheritic polyneuritis, acute bulbar poliomyelitis, cerebral vascular accidents, hepatolenticular degeneration (Wilson's disease),* and *botulism.* The *Plummer-Vinson syndrome* may also be listed here, since the difficulty of swallowing in this condition resembles that due to a neuromuscular disorder, although pain may be an additional disturbing feature. The actual mechanism of the dysphagia is not entirely clear but is due sometimes to esophageal webs, membranous structures stretching across the esophagus and partially occluding it. At other times, no web can be demonstrated, and the dysphagia may then be caused by atrophic changes in the pharynx, possibly associated with disturbances of the intrinsic nervous apparatus in the pharyngeal wall. *Dermatomyositis* is another muscular disorder that causes dysphagia by involvement of the pharyngeal and hypopharyngeal musculature.

DYSPHAGIA DUE TO LESIONS OF THE MOUTH, PHARYNX, OR LARYNX, CAUSING PAIN OR MECHANICAL HINDRANCE TO PASSAGE OF FOOD INTO THE ESOPHAGUS. In most cases the cause of trouble in this group is obvious, and detailed consideration of the various lesions is unnecessary; examples are acute tonsillitis, peritonsillar abscess, infiltrating carcinoma of the tongue, and angioneurotic edema of the tongue or pharynx.

DIFFERENTIAL DIAGNOSIS. A common complaint, not to be confused with dysphagia, is *globus hystericus.* This symptom consists of a sense of constriction in the throat; the patient usually believes there is a lump in the throat that is not visible. He is likely to be fearful that the imagined tumor may interfere with swallowing, although careful questioning reveals that there is actually no dysphagia. This fear is naturally enhanced if any enlargement of the thyroid coexists. Globus hystericus is always a manifestation of emotional stress or fatigue. The symptom is usually considered to be due to increased tonus of the hypopharyngeal musculature, although this is rarely demonstrable by x-ray. It is, of course, important to reassure the patient of the benign nature of the symptom, but it is equally mandatory not to overlook an organic disturbance of which the vague sense of dysphagia may be the early manifestation.

Determination of the basic mechanism responsible for the dysphagia is usually a simple matter, but identification of the exact disorder is not infrequently quite difficult. For example, cancer of the esophagus sometimes presents a sudden rather than a gradual onset, and the roentgenogram may have the smooth, symmetric appearance more commonly seen with benign stricture or cardiospasm; even esophagoscopy may be inconclusive, and biopsy may yield deceptive results if the bit of tissue happens to contain no neoplastic cells. Similarly, *mediastinal disorders* causing mechanical obstruction may be difficult to classify, and the same is true of the neurologic disturbances interfering with swallowing.

Certain symptoms associated with dysphagia have diagnostic value. Hiccups, together with difficult swallowing, indicate a lesion at the terminal portion of the esophagus, such as carcinoma, achalasia, or hiatal hernia. Dysphagia, followed after an interval or some duration by hoarseness, usually means extension of a malignant growth beyond the walls of the esophagus and the involvement of a recurrent laryngeal nerve. When the hoarseness comes first and the dysphagia later, the primary lesion is almost always in the larynx. Dysphagia and unilateral wheezing practically always indicate a mediastinal mass involving the esophagus and a main or large bronchus. Coughing with each swallow of food or drink means a fistulous communication between the esophagus and the trachea. Coughing occurring some time after swallowing may be due to regurgitation of food, commonest in achalasia and pharyngeal pouch.

PROCEDURE. Examination of the mouth and pharynx should disclose those lesions the effect of which is to impede the transfer of food from the mouth to the esophagus, either because of pain or mechanical interference. When lesions of the hypopharynx (e.g., *chronic abscess secondary to tuberculosis of the spine*) or of the larynx (e.g., *tuberculosis or carcinoma*) are suspected, examination with a mirror is necessary.

The investigation of mechanical obstructions in the esophagus is accomplished mainly by x-ray examination and, in doubtful cases, by esophagoscopy and biopsy of the suspected tissue. Barium mixtures should not be used in cases of suspected foreign body, since the latter may be obscured; nor should a thick barium mixture be employed when the history indicates the presence of an almost complete obstruction, since complete occlusion may be precipitated. In cases of obstruction at the cardiac orifice, a large thick-walled stomach tube should be introduced. If the tube enters the stomach without difficulty, cardiospasm or some other neuromuscular disorder such as scleroderma may be assumed to be present; otherwise, a benign or malignant stricture is responsible for the obstruction.

Studies of esophageal motility with the aid of tiny electromagnetic transducers have been found to contribute information of great value in problems of disturbed esophageal function when the usual methods of examination are indecisive. Cytologic studies are important when malignancy is suspected.

When a neuromuscular disturbance of the pharynx is thought to be the cause of dysphagia, this can be demonstrated most readily by fluoroscopic examination. When barium mixture is swallowed, some of the opaque material will be seen to cling to the pharyngeal walls and in the pyriform sinuses, and almost invariably a small amount of the barium will trickle into the trachea. If there is a question of myasthenia gravis being present, a mixture of 1.5 mg neostigmine and 0.6 mg atropine is given intramuscularly, which should bring about very striking relief of dysphagia within 30 min in cases of myasthenia gravis, and little or no improvement in other forms of neuromuscular dysphagia. Similar dissipation of the dysphagia of myasthenia gravis can be effected within 2 min by intravenous administration of 10 mg edrophonium chloride (Tensilon).

REFERENCES

Benedict, E. B., and G. L. Nardi: "The Esophagus," Boston, Little, Brown & Company, 1958.

Heitzman, E. J., G. C. Heitzman, and C. F. Elliott: Primary Esophageal Amyloidosis, A.M.A. Arch. Int. Med., 109:595, 1962.

Hilding, D. A., and M. O. Tachdjian: Dysphagia and Hypertrophic Spurring of the Cervical Spine, New England J. Med., 263:11, 1961.

Stevens, M. B., et al.: Aperistalsis of the Esophagus in Patients with Connective-Tissue Disorders and Raynaud's Phenomenon, New England J. Med., 270:1218, 1964.

Victor, M., R. Hayes, and R. D. Adams: Oculopharyngeal Muscular Dystrophy. A Familial Disease of Late Life Characterized by Dysphagia and Progressive Ptosis of the Eyelids, New England J. Med., 267:1267, 1962.

Wynder, E. L., and J. H. Fryer: Etiologic Considerations of Plummer-Vinson (Patterson-Kelly) Syndrome, Ann. Internal Med., 49:1106, 1958.

25 INDIGESTION
William H. Resnik

DEFINITION. Indigestion, or dyspepsia, has no sharply defined meaning. Some authors restrict the term to a multitude of symptoms aside from outspoken pain: heartburn and acid regurgitation, nausea and vomiting, gaseous distension and belching, and the various forms of distress such as a feeling of fullness or pressure that cannot be catalogued strictly as pain. Here we shall consider indigestion as constituting any of the above symptoms which the patient attributes to a deranged digestion, including the chronic recurrent types of pain the severity and character of which fall short of placing them among the acute abdominal emergencies—a distinction not always easy to make.

VISCERAL PAIN. The characteristics of visceral pain have been described in previous chapters (Chaps. 4 and 7). The researches of Kellgren and Lewis have demonstrated that there are two main categories of pain: *superficial,* which tends to be sharp, stinging, or burning in quality and is susceptible of accurate localization; and *deep,* which tends to be more aching, diffuse, and segmentally distributed. Abdominal pain or distress may be *somatic,* when it arises in the parietal peritoneum or dome of the diaphragm, the impulses being conveyed by the intercostal or phrenic nerves. This type of pain is of the superficial variety. Or abdominal discomfort may be of the *visceral* or *splanchnic* type, originating in certain of the viscera or closely contiguous structures such as the mesentery, the afferent impulses being carried in the sensory nerves that run in the sympathetic system. The various forms of distress associated with indigestion are almost always of the deep visceral type.

CHARACTERISTICS OF VISCERAL PAIN. The importance of localization and reference of pain, of the factors that provoke and relieve it, and of its quality and severity have been discussed in Chap. 4.

There are very few types of abdominal or digestive tract pain that are so definitely characteristic as to have diagnostic significance. One exception is *heartburn* (a sensation of warmth behind the lower sternum). This has been shown to arise predominantly, if not exclusively, from irritation of the lower esophagus. *Rebound tenderness,* associated with involuntary muscular rigidity, cutaneous hyperesthesia, and localized tenderness, usually indicates irritation of the parietal peritoneum. However, occasionally no peritonitis may be present, and it is probable that the rebound tenderness is then due to intense muscle spasm, so severe that the slight distortion incidental to the sudden release of pressure is sufficient to cause a pain identical with that characteristic of peritonitis.

Table 25-1. DISTRIBUTION OF PAIN ON THE BASIS OF CLINICAL AND EXPERIMENTAL DATA

Origin of pain	*Location of referred pain*
Esophagus...........	Behind sternum, predominantly at level of xiphoid or suprasternal notch
Stomach and first part of duodenum	High epigastrium
Gallbladder and extrahepatic bilary ducts	High epigastrium, right side of back
Pancreas............	High epigastrium, left side of back
Liver...............	Epigastrium
Small intestine.......	Region of umbilicus
Colon...............	Below umbilicus
Rectosigmoid........	Low in abdomen, just above symphysis

Obviously, the presence of other associated manifestations that have localizing value is also important: localized rigidity and tenderness of the abdominal musculature, hematemesis, melena, and jaundice. An elevated sedimentation rate should serve as a warning signal in any condition presumed to be due to a functional disorder. The appraisal of abdominal pain or indigestion requires a careful consideration of the location of the discomfort, its character and intensity, the circumstances provoking and relieving it, and the associated findings, as well as the data pertaining to the age, sex, and environmental factors surrounding the individual.

COMMON SYMPTOMS AND SYNDROMES EXPRESSED AS INDIGESTION. The digestive tract responds to abnormal stimuli by alterations in secretory and motor activity. It is abnormal motor activity which is, in large part, the cause of most of the symptoms that fall into the category of indigestion: heartburn (which is due to primary or reflex disturbances in the lower esophagus), regurgitation, and the various other symptoms mentioned below under Early Postprandial Indigestion.

Belching. This is the eructation of gas from the stomach or esophagus. It may result from ingestion of carbonated drinks or bicarbonate of soda. Usually, however, the gas is due to swallowed air or air that is sucked into the esophagus by negative intrathoracic pressure in individuals who consciously or unconsciously relax the superior esophageal spincter. Once having gained entrance into the esophagus, part of the air is passed on into the stomach; part is eructated from the esophagus without ever entering the stomach. The gas is not due to fermentation in the stomach. Entrance of excessive quantities of air into the esophagus or stomach may occur in patients suffering from practically any form of indigestion, but the most spectacular belching occurs in neurotics who may continue the sequence of gulping and eructating for hours, in the vain effort to rid themselves of gas that they assume is being formed in the stomach in prodigious amounts. The simple device of persuading them to place a cigarette holder or pencil between the teeth often serves to convince them that the symptom is self-induced.

Flatulence. Flatulence, or meteorism, is due to excessive quantities of gas in the small or large intestine. To some degree it may be due to unusual bacterial action on foods or to impaired absorption of gases into the blood stream. Possibly, diffusion of gas from the blood stream into the intestinal lumen may play a role in same cases. However, it is generally agreed that most of the gas is air that has gained entrance into the stomach by the mechanisms described above and then passed on into the intestines. Gastric distension due to air swallowing is often associated with palpitation and precordial distress and not infrequently leads to fear of heart disease.

Early Postprandial Indigestion. When food is ingested by a normal individual, a prompt diminution in the tone and peristaltic activity of the gastric musculature ensues. The subsequent motor activity incidental to the process of digestion goes on below the level of consciousness. When the normal motor responses are disturbed and gastric tone is enhanced rather than relaxed by the entrance of food into the stomach, the resultant effects of the abnormal tension in the gastric wall are felt as indigestion coming on immediately or shortly after the taking of food. The symptoms appear in different forms and combinations: a feeling of pressure or fullness or actual pain, nausea and vomiting, belching of gas, heartburn (presumably due to reflex alterations in the lower esophageal wall or irritation of the esophagus by regurgitation of gastric contents), etc. These symptoms persist for a variable period of time, sometimes curtained by vomiting, spontaneous or induced, and the subject then experiences relative or complete relief until the next meal is taken. Such early postprandial discomfort may be due to a wide variety of causes and hence has little diagnostic significance.

Late Postprandial Indigestion. In other individuals, indigestion is experienced only after a period of time has elapsed after the ingestion of food—usually 1 hr or more. As in early postprandial indigestion, the symptoms may consist of heartburn, nausea, epigastric fullness, or fluctuating symptoms in various combinations. The location of these symptoms indicates their origin to be in the esophagus, stomach, or duodenum, and they are probably due to disturbances in the muscular tension of these organs. At times the discomfort is in the distribution of colon pain, either below the umbilicus or in the region of the flexures, presumably because of an overactive gastrocolic reflex. The classic example of late postprandial indigestion is encountered in uncomplicated peptic ulcer, typically described as a deep gnawing, *steady* pain of long duration, felt high in the epigastrium.

Several hypotheses have been advanced as explanations of the mechanism of ulcer pain. The three most widely held and vigorously defended by their proponents attribute the pain to (1) increased tension in the muscular walls of the stomach or duodenal cap, (2) irritation by the acid of the gastric juice, (3) increased sensitivity of the inflammatory tissue in and around the ulcer influenced by alterations in blood flow. In all probability, all three factors play important roles in the causation of ulcer pain, and it may be a question of semantics to declare that one factor alone is the essential one. Ulcer pain has been observed in the absence of free acid; nevertheless, in the vast majority of cases, the behavior of ulcer pain *appears* to be in accord with the concentration of acid bathing it, and from a practical standpoint this is important because (1) deep, steady pain occurring an hour or more after eating and relieved by food, alkali, or vomiting (in each instance diminishing the concentration of acid) implies the irritating effect of acid on a defective membrane of the stomach or duodenum; (2) such pain occurring during the course of ulcer treatment implies inadequate neutralization of acid.

The types of indigestion do not always divide themselves neatly into these patterns of early and late postprandial discomfort. In some instances both the early and the late forms may be seen in the same subject, as well as indeterminate types that are so irregular that they defy classification. Late postprandial indigestion of the kind described above as characteristic of ulcer pain immediately suggests benign peptic ulcer, but essentially the same pain may be witnessed in other disorders such as carcinoma of the stomach with hyperacidity, ulcerative gastritis, or duodenitis. Late postprandial indigestion that does not conform to the characteristics of ulcer pain may be due to a wide variety of other primary or reflex disturbances of the stomach.

Pyloric Obstruction. Obstruction of the pylorus due either to organic stenosis or to spasm and edema usually is associated with the early appearance of indigestion, sometimes continuous, culminating hours later in colicky epigastric pains and the retention type of vomiting.

Postgastrectomy Syndromes. Following resection of a large part of the stomach, the patient may experience early satiety and nausea following the ingestion of even small amounts of food, owing to the loss of the reservoir function of the stomach. In addition, many patients experience the "dumping" syndrome characterized by nausea, palpitation, sweating, epigastric distress, weakness—a clinical picture very much like that caused by hypoglycemia. When this group of symptoms occurs soon after eating, it has been demonstrated that alterations in blood sugar are not responsible for the syndrome, the exact pathogenesis of which is still uncertain. It is generally agreed that the basic difficulty stems from the rapid entrance of food, containing osmotically active substances, into the gut. This results in a transfer of fluid into the jejunum and distension of this segment of the bowel, following which a highly complex series of functional derangements occurs. The precise mechanism whereby these numerous dysfunctions contribute to the development of the syndrome is controversial (Chap. 80). Somewhat similar symptoms occurring 1½ to 3 hr after eating have been found to be associated with hypoglycemia, the latter being due to a reactive hyperinsulinism in response to a preceding rapid rise in blood sugar. Finally, these patients may suffer from malnutrition and inability to maintain weight, owing to the "small-stomach" symptoms and fat and nitrogen loss in stools.

Partial Intestinal Obstruction. Acute obstruction of the bowel, if complete, is an emergency of such magnitude that it cannot be considered to fall into the province of the disorders now under discussion. However, incomplete obstruction may give rise to periodic bouts of cramplike pain, nausea, and vomiting, sometimes accompanied by distension. These symptoms, when mild, may be considered "indigestion" by the patient. The characteristic picture is less likely to be evidenced in partially obstructive lesions of the large bowel, particularly in the cecum, where extensive lesions may be present without giving rise to any obstructive phenomena.

DIFFERENTIAL DIAGNOSIS. A detailed outline of all the causes of recurrent indigestion is obviously impossible. However, certain principles that may be used as a guide in the analysis of chronic indigestion may be discussed. In every case the following questions must be answered: (1) Are the symptoms due to organic disease outside the digestive tract, or to organic disease within the digestive tract (including the gallbladder and extrahepatic biliary passages), or to a functional disturbance? (2) If organic disease of the digestive tract is present, is the lesion malignant or benign? (3) If the disorder is functional, is its origin psychogenic or nonpsychogenic (allergy, hypoglycemia, drugs, reflex effects)? The classification of indigestion on the basis of whether the fundamental lesion is primarily in the alimentary canal or outside it must in some instances be an arbitrary one. For example, indigestion may be a prominent feature of pernicious anemia, a condition which is associated with structural alterations in the stomach that may be the actual root of the disease. Nevertheless, tradition has placed this disorder among the diseases of the hematopoietic system.

Indigestion Due to Organic Disease outside the Digestive Tract. A complete catalog of all the conditions outside the digestive tract capable of causing indigestion would serve to do little more than call attention to the fact that diseases of practically all systems of the body may at times be accompanied by indigestion in one form or another. The presenting complaint of the patient with pernicious anemia, pulmonary tuberculosis, myocardial failure, chronic infection of the urinary tract, or disease of the pelvic organs may be dyspepsia. Migraine, epilepsy, or other disturbances of the central nervous system may manifest themselves in chronic abdominal complaints. The digestive symptoms vary in detail and severity and have no characteristics that betray the fact that they are secondary to some more remote malady.

Gastritis. In recent years the concept of gastritis has been resurrected after being long held in disfavor. A good deal of ambiguity continues to surround the subject, at least from the clinical standpoint. Various causes are responsible, the most important being the lack of a constant relationship between clinical, gastroscopic, and histologic findings and also the fact that in the same individual gastroscopic pictures of hypertrophic or atrophic gastritis may depend solely on the emotional status of the patient. Many poorly defined syndromes indicative of gastric dysfunction, now ascribed to functional disorders of the stomach, may have as their basis an actual gastritis. The clinician may surmise that such is the case when there is a previous history of exposure to excessive use of alcohol or tobacco or to drugs; or when "indiscreet" eating is followed by indigestion; or when there is a history somewhat suggestive of ulcer or cancer, neither of which can be demonstrated by objective methods.

Confirmation by gastroscopy lends weight to the diagnosis, but even this method is not conclusive, since mucosal alterations deviating from the normal may be transitory and caused by emotional factors. There can be no doubt that massive hematemesis may be due to gastritis, and occasionally a hypertrophic gastritis localized in the antral and prepyloric region may simulate cancer so closely that differentiation can be made only by histologic study. Conversely, patients with clear-cut gastroscopic evidence of gastritis may be free of suggestive symptoms.

Peptic Ulcer. The characteristic qualities of the pain of uncomplicated ulcer of the stomach or duodenum are its rhythmicity and periodicity. "Rhythmicity" refers to the pain-food-ease sequence, the classic prototype of the late-postprandial form of indigestion. "Pe-

riodicity" expresses the tendency for the indigestion to appear for weeks at a time and later to disappear for months, over the course of a number of years. As complications develop, the clinical picture tends to become distorted and to lose its usually sharply drawn lines. In cases of penetration with extension into the surrounding tissue, the characteristic pain-food-ease pattern tends to be less clearly delineated; the pain becomes more continuous and radiates more widely as the nerves of the involved tissues become affected. Obstruction at the pylorus is also heralded by alteration of the classic ulcer syndrome; there is earlier onset of pain, relief of which often is no longer afforded by food and alkali, and vomiting of the retention type makes its appearance. (See Chap. 180.)

Carcinoma of the Stomach. The traditional history of anemia, loss of weight, strength, and appetite, and discomfort of variable intensity and form after eating usually represents an advanced carcinoma of the stomach. It is now appreciated that the early stage of carcinoma of the stomach presents a picture of considerable diversity, dependent on the location and extent of the lesion. If the growth exists at the cardia or pylorus, early obstructive phenomena may be witnessed. If the lesion is small and ulcerated and if the gastric juice contains free hydrochloric acid, the clinical picture of a benign peptic ulcer may be simulated, and there may even be a temporary response to treatment. Nevertheless, with integration of roentgenologic, gastroscopic, and cytologic studies and careful observation of completeness of healing, differentiation between benign and malignant ulcer is practically always possible. In some cases the digestive symptoms, though present, may be so mild and vague as to be hardly suggestive of the disorder. Finally, in a considerable number of instances, especially those with achylia, no gastric symptoms occur until anemia, wasting, or other changes are fully displayed. In short, not only is the indigestion of early carcinoma of the stomach lacking in any definitive features that indicate the causative lesion, but the entire clinical picture may be equally uninformative. *The inevitable consequence of these observations is that any indigestion in the upper abdomen not otherwise clearly accounted for, particularly when it occurs in a male over the age of forty, should be suspected of having its origin in a malignant lesion of the stomach and should be carefully studied by every available method with this possibility in mind.*

Chronic Gallbladder Disease. The symptoms of chronic gallbladder disease are of two kinds, indigestion and colic. The indigestion may occur early or late after a meal and is lacking in any distinctive qualities that permit a diagnosis of the basic disorder. Intolerance of fats is sometimes described as a characteristic feature. Carefully taken histories disclose that, when the patient does have an intolerance of certain foods, nonfatty foods are frequently incriminated as well as the fatty ones, that some fats are acceptable when others are not, and that the particular fats that bring on symptoms vary with different individuals. Fat intolerance is, therefore, not a symptom that is an expression of an inability to handle fats alone but is rather one feature of a much broader food intolerance that applies to nonfatty foods as well and differs in its details from patient to patient. *It is more accurate to speak of food intolerance rather than fat intolerance as a common symptom in chronic gallbladder disease.* However, this kind of food intolerance is not peculiar to gallbladder disease alone. Exactly the same intolerance of foods, fatty as well as nonfatty, is encountered in patients who suffer from functional disorders or from a variety of other organic ailments in the absence of any demonstrable disease of the biliary tract. In other words, *neither the indigestion nor the so-called fat intolerance that is sometimes ascribed to gallbladder disease is distinctive.* It may be added that, since there is no evidence that in the absence of obstructive jaundice all fats are poorly digested and tolerated, there is no justification for the common practice of severely restricting the use of all fats in the diets of patients with chronic gallbladder disease. As in patients suffering from allergic disorders, dietary restrictions should be made according to the individual problems of the patient. There is no rational basis for any diet that is applicable to all patients with chronic gallbladder disease. The relationship of an indigestion to a coexistent disorder of the gallbladder, even when proved roentgenographically, is difficult to define. In one patient, surgical removal of the diseased gallbladder may bring about complete relief of the indigestion. In other individuals, removal of the gallbladder may afford no amelioration of the indigestion, and this is especially likely to be the case when the gallbladder is merely thickened but contains no stones and when there has been no previous history of acute cholecystitis.

Apart from the indigestion, the patient with chronic gallbladder disease is often subject to more or less severe attacks of biliary colic. It is these acute attacks of pain, localized high in the epigastrium or in the right (rarely in the left) hypochondrium, radiating to the right subscapular or to the interscapular regions, or sometimes to the tip of the right shoulder, which are really suggestive of gallbladder disease; when they are associated with jaundice, the diagnosis becomes clear. The frequency of this condition renders suspect every woman over the age of twenty-five, particularly if she has borne children, and all individuals over the age of forty, complaining of indigestion. Fortunately, the diagnosis is capable of confirmation in a high percentage of cases by cholecystography and cholangiography. Biliary drainage is useful only if the gallbladder has been previously removed or if it is believed that a nonfilling gallbladder is secondary to parenchymal liver disease.

Disorders of the Pancreas. Clinically, the symptoms of pancreatitis are so similar to those of gallbladder disease as to be practically indistinguishable. Probably the most important factor in making the diagnosis of pancreatitis is to keep in mind that such a condition may be present when one would ordinarily consider gallbladder disease to be the cause of the patient's complaints. In the acute exacerbations of chronic relapsing pancreatitis, the differentiation hinges primarily on finding an increased serum amylase or serum lipase at the onset of the attack. In the chronic phases of the disorder, the recognition of its presence will depend chiefly on the discovery of steatorrhea or diabetes mellitus or x-ray demonstration of calcification or enlargement of the pancreas. Numerous studies have revealed that the classic picture of painless, progressive jaundice is not the commonest form in which carcinoma of the pancreas presents itself. Jaundice occurs in about half the cases, upper abdominal pain with no definite pattern or constant form of radiation in a much higher percentage. In the absence of jaundice, diagnosis is sometimes suggested by the roentgenologic demonstration of deformity of neighboring structures by extrinsic pressure.

Diaphragmatic (Hiatal) Hernia. There has been a growing appreciation of the fact that diaphragmatic (hiatal) hernia may be responsible for a variety of clinical pictures, one of which is chronic indigestion. In the typical case, an overweight individual of middle age or over tends to have symptoms on assuming the recumbent position or on leaning forward after a full meal. The herniation may be associated with a nondescript form of indigestion or may cause a more severe attack of pain, sometimes strongly suggestive of biliary colic. At other times the pain is identical in type and distribution with that due to angina pectoris or myocardial infarction, although the characteristic relation to effort in respect to the former, or the diagnostic electrocardiographic findings in respect to the latter, are absent (Chap. 6). The diagnosis is established with certainty when an awareness of the possible existence of diaphragmatic hernia leads to confirmation by roentgenologic examination made with this condition in mind.

Disorders of the Small Intestine. When organic disease of the bowel arouses recurrent attacks of abdominal pain of the type that may be considered to fall in the category of chronic indigestion, the clue to the site of the trouble will come from the recognition of the significance of the localization of the pain in the region of the umbilicus. More exact definition of the lesion will depend primarily on x-ray examination, which should be carried out with more careful attention to the small intestine than is ordinarily given in a routine gastrointestinal series.

Chronic Disease of the Appendix (Recurrent Obstructive Disease of the Appendix). In a small number of cases, chronic disease of the appendix may be the basis for a persistent indigestion of either the early or the late postprandial type. Experimental observations have demonstrated that irritation in the colon or over the appendix may produce pain in the epigastrium, owing to reflex peristaltic activity in the prepyloric region. The mere presence of continued pain and tenderness in the right lower quadrant does not signify chronic disease of the appendix; the commonest cause of this type of pain is an irritable colon. The diagnosis of chronic disease of the appendix cannot be made with reasonable certainty until evidence of appendiceal inflammation (localization of pain in the right lower quadrant, tenderness and rigidity in McBurney's region, fever, and leukocytosis) has occurred in the midst of one or more attacks of appendiceal colic. It is worth bearing in mind that bouts masquerading as attacks of appendiceal colic may be caused by terminal ileitis (see Chap. 182).

Organic Disease of the Colon. In most cases organic disease of the colon is characterized by the appearance of one or a combination of the following symptoms: (1) diarrhea or constipation, or both; (2) bleeding from the bowel; (3) abdominal pain. The following statements regarding disease of the colon are made primarily with respect to pain and the possibility that such pain may be interpreted by the patient to be "indigestion." The character of the pain is determined by the site of the lesion, the presence or absence of obstruction, and the extent to which neighboring structures are involved. In general, pain due to disorders of the colon is referred to the lower half of the abdomen, although lesions in the hepatic or splenic flexure may give rise to pain in the upper right or left quadrants of the abdomen, respectively, while lesions in the cecum may cause periumbilical pain not infrequently mistaken for appendicitis. Obstructive phenomena, which are relatively rare in disorders of the proximal part of the colon, occur much more frequently on the left side of the colon, owing to the more solid contents of the colon in this region and also to the frequency of fibrous annular lesions due to cancer or diverticulitis, the latter two lesions often being clinically indistinguishable. Indigestion, frequently associated with nausea, is common, usually because of reflex disturbances in the stomach. The symptoms of the different organic diseases of the colon have so many features in common that exact diagnosis usually must rest on the results of the more precise methods of examination, the most important of which are x-ray and proctoscopic examination. It hardly needs to be emphasized that in every such case a careful digital examination of the rectum should be performed. Any symptom referable to the colon warrants a thorough investigation with the special aim of searching for a carcinoma. Particularly in the colon, but also in the stomach, a normal x-ray study does not rule out cancer. If symptoms fail to clear under therapy, the x-ray examination, like any other physical examination, should be repeated.

Indigestion Due to Functional Disorders of the Digestive Tract. Several circumstances afford presumptive evidence of the functional origin of chronic indigestion: clear association of symptoms with states of fatigue or emotional stress, youth of the patient, duration of the illness over a long period of time, variability of symptoms, absence of serious deterioration of health. The diagnosis may be considered established, however, only when history and physical examination, laboratory data, x-ray examination, and, in appropriate cases, endoscopic examination fail to reveal organic disease, in or out of the digestive tract, that can logically explain the digestive symptoms. Even when the investigation has been carried out in the most thorough and expert manner, unavoidable error will occur in a small percentage of cases, and the passage of time will disclose organic disease not previously demonstrable.

Psychogenic factors, excessive use of tobacco, coffee, or alcohol, improper habits of eating, cathartic habituation—each alone or in combination with the others may be responsible for the faulty functioning of the digestive tract. The symptoms vary widely, sometimes mimicking organic diseases involving the stomach or colon so closely that only after the most intensive survey and prolonged observation will it be possible to conclude that no structural disease of the digestive tract is present. One needs hardly to be reminded that almost any drug taken by mouth may cause indigestion. When this indigestion is precipitated by highly alkaline drugs such as diphenylhydantoin sodium (Dilantin), the customary treatment with alkali will tend to aggravate rather than ameliorate the trouble.

Even when demonstrable structural disease exists, the symptoms may be markedly influenced by coexistent, although less apparent, emotional disturbances. When no structural disease is found, one is not justified in assuming that psychologic factors are responsible for the symptoms unless the patient presents clear evidence of emotional disturbance. Mistakes will be minimized if one bears in mind that, though psychogenic disorders are a very common cause of indigestion, it is unsafe to make such a diagnosis in an individual case unless the evidence, both positive and negative, points unequivocally toward such a conclusion (Chap. 42).

Indigestion Due to Food Intolerance. Hypersensitiveness to specific foods is a frequent cause of digestive symptoms. In some cases, the constant association of symptoms with the ingestion of certain foods, even when the recipient is unaware that the offending foods are incorporated in the diet, the personal and familial history of an allergic background, the demonstration of positive skin tests and of antibodies that are capable of being transferred passively, the prompt cessation of symptoms on elimination of the offending foods from the diet—all these afford a chain of incontestable evidence. However, in a much higher percentage of cases, the proof that indigestion is caused or aggravated by a suspected food allergy rests on much more uncertain ground. This uncertainty is common to most disorders ascribed to an allergic reaction to foods. The immunologic tests may be negative, the provocation of symptoms by the offending foods may not be immediate and clear-cut, and the harmful influence of the suspected foods may have no better support than the statement of the patient himself. In the absence of objective proof, it is frequently difficult or impossible to know how much a supposed food sensitivity is attributable to a genuine food intolerance and how much to the fears and suspicions of an apprehensive patient. When the intolerance to specific foods seems real, it is again a problem to decide whether the symptoms are due to the relative indigestibility of the foods or their content of chemical irritants that may be more potent in some individuals than others, or whether an allergic reaction in the digestive tract is the basis of the disturbed function. One such non-allergic form of milk intolerance has been found to be caused by a deficiency of intestinal lactase. The fact remains that, however obscure may be the mechanism by which these various food intolerances operate, there are frequent instances in which indigestion seems to be related to the specific effect of certain foods, varying for each individual case. In some persons food intolerance appears to be the sole cause of symptoms; in others it may exert its effects in conjunction with obvious psychogenic influences, while in still others the food intolerance may be expressed only when demonstrable organic disease is present.

Suspicion with regard to the allergic basis of the indigestion is aroused by a family history of allergy or a personal history, in the past or present, of some unquestionably allergic disorder such as hay fever or asthma. Frequently the patient recognizes that certain foods, such as eggs or milk, may be responsible for his symptoms but may be unmindful of the fact that these same foods are commonly used in the preparation of other articles of his diet.

For the detection of the offending foods, skin tests are so unreliable as to be usually valueless. More helpful information can be obtained from elimination diets or from a careful, time-consuming history in which the patient is questioned regarding his experience with all the common articles of a dietary. Only by testing and retesting the effects of suspected foods is it possible to arrive at a reasonably clear conclusion as to the role that specific food idiosyncrasies are playing in the particular case. It should be emphasized again that the discovery of a food intolerance and the temporary relief of symptoms by elimination of the offending substance do not prove the absence of concomitant organic disease. It is not uncommon, for example, for the indigestion of chronic gallbladder disease to be considerably relieved or completely abolished for long periods of time merely by eliminating the known food offenders.

GENERAL DIAGNOSTIC CONSIDERATIONS. The introduction of more exact methods of diagnosis has brought about a steady diminution in the importance of the clinical picture alone for arriving at a conclusion as to the nature of the specific disorder responsible for a malady. However varied may be the types of injury or stress, the responses of the digestive tract and the resulting symptoms are relatively limited. Accurate information regarding the localization and projection of the pain and, hence, the cord segments affected by the sensory stimuli affords an invaluable starting point from which one may consider the various structures that could be responsible for the symptoms. Additional data pertaining to the age and sex of the patient, duration of the illness, factors precipitating or relieving the symptoms, and accessory details narrow still further the diagnostic possibilities. In the main, however, a definite diagnosis will rest chiefly on the results

of x-ray or direct inspection of the affected organ by endoscope or at the time of operation. The similarity of symptoms produced by a variety of lesions in the same structure or in other structures innervated from the same cord segments makes diagnosis on clinical grounds alone a hazardous undertaking, particularly in the detection of disease in its early and most remediable stages. Reliance on x-ray or endoscopic examination must be tempered with a recognition of the shortcomings of even these methods of investigation; in some cases only microscopic examination of the suspected tissues can define the character of the morbid process.

Difficulties in ascertaining the primary site of a gastrointestinal disorder are frequently aroused by the reciprocal relationships between the upper and lower digestive tract. Lesions in the upper tract, such as gallbladder disease or peptic ulcer, commonly give rise to reflex disturbance in the colon, and in some cases the symptoms referable to the irritable colon may preponderate to such an extent that they actually occupy the forefront of the patient's attention. Similarly, primary disorders in the colon may be associated with reflex alterations in the functions of the stomach, and indigestion, characterized by high epigastric distress, may be the predominant symptom, distracting the attention from the original site of the trouble.

PROCEDURE IN INVESTIGATION OF CHRONIC INDIGESTION. The first step in the elucidation of chronic indigestion must cover the ground encompassed in every thorough initial examination: a painstaking and complete history and physical examination and the routine blood and urine tests. The results of this first survey and the additional special procedures that may be suggested by it will serve to indicate whether any organic disease can explain the symptoms of which the patient complains. In some cases, as in angina pectoris or myocardial failure, where the diagnosis is clearly ascertained, further investigation of the digestive tract is unnecessary.

X-ray examination of the alimentary tract and gallbladder is the cornerstone on which the diagnosis of gastrointestinal disease is built; elaboration on the importance of this procedure is unnecessary. Lesions of the stomach and colon ordinarily are readily disclosed. The standard gastrointestinal series frequently fails to reveal the small intestine in adequate detail; special studies of the small intestine should be made when involvement of this structure is suspected.

As far as indigestion is concerned, the chief value of stool examinations is in the detection of occult blood and, occasionally, microscopic detection of ova and parasites. The persistence of bleeding in a case of gastric ulcer that is being properly treated arouses the strong presumption that the lesion is malignant.

Gastric analysis no longer occupies a position of importance in the diagnosis of disorders of the stomach and duodenum. Normal individuals exhibit variations in the acidity of gastric juice that may range from complete absence of hydrochloric acid to high figures that tend to overlap those seen in disease. Moreover, aside from the measurement of the volume and acidity of the gastric juice, the information afforded by the various special test meals is ascertained more easily and accurately by x-ray examination. Nevertheless, with appreciation of its limitations, gastric analysis continues to be employed as a procedure that provides helpful data in cases where the x-ray evidence is equivocal.

Fasting gastric juice of large volume and high concentration of acid is an almost constant finding in the presence of duodenal ulcer. In benign gastric ulcer, the volume and the level of acid concentration tend to be lower, but acid is rarely completely and persistently absent. Nevertheless, even after histamine stimulation, anacidity has been present, at least for periods of time, in authenticated cases of benign peptic ulcer. On the other hand, while histamine anacidity bespeaks strongly of the malignant character of a gastric ulcer, free acid does not rule out malignant disease of the stomach. In cases of pernicious anemia, in which indigestion may be the presenting symptom, anacidity refractory to histamine is invariably present.

Proctoscopic examination and digital examination of the rectum are indicated in most conditions suggestive of organic disease of the colon and are obligatory when there is any suspicion that cancer of the rectum exists.

Gastroscopy is useful determining the completeness of healing of a gastric ulcer and in disclosing lesions unseen by x-ray, notably hemorrhagic and ulcerative gastritis. Moreover, the accuracy of gastroscopic diagnosis has been enhanced by the introduction of an operating gastroscope which makes biopsy possible. However, gastroscopy is not to be considered a substitute for x-ray. A better conjecture about the status of the stomach can be made after both gastroscopic and x-ray studies than after either alone.

Cytologic examination of the gastric contents has been found, in experienced hands, to be extremely accurate in differentiating between benign and malignant disorders. Further experience with the tetracycline fluorescence test for the detection of cancer is required before its value can be assessed.

Finally, when organic disease of the digestive tract has been excluded and the possibility of an allergic disorder is entertained, elimination diets should be employed.

The question of procedure in the investigation of chronic indigestion in a patient on the wards of a large teaching hospital or at a diagnostic clinic poses no difficult problems. All the methods mentioned above may be employed; under these circumstances the patient expects and usually submits to any examination that will throw light on his illness. The problem is different in private practice, away from such institutions, and it is essentially an economic one. There would be no serious problem if the necessary examinations were as inexpensive as a blood count or a simple blood chemical analysis. A high percentage of gastrointestinal disorders seen in patients who make up the practice of the average physician are of func-

tional origin. To subject all persons complaining of indigestion to an immediate routine survey involving all the indicated procedures would be difficult, if not impossible, from the standpoint of expediency and expense. On the other hand, the alert physician must be constantly aware of the fact that any compromise with thoroughness inevitably exposes the patient to the risk of losing the opportunity, possibly an irretrievable one, of discovering an early and curable malignant disease. For the average conscientious physician in private practice, this dilemma is well-nigh insoluble.

REFERENCES

Bloomfield, A. L.: Mechanism of Pain with Peptic Ulcer, Am. J. Med., 17:165, 1954.

Cummins, A. J., M. L. Gompertz, and J. H. Kier: An Evaluation of the Tetracycline-Fluorescence Test in the Diagnosis of Gastric Cancer Comparison with Cytology, Am. Int. Med., 61:56, 1964.

Haemmerli, U. P., et al.: Acquired Milk Intolerance in the Adult Caused by Lactase Malabsorption Due to a Selective Deficiency of Intestinal Lactase Activity, Am. J. Med., 38:7, 1965.

Kinsella, V. J.: Pain in Chronic Gastric Ulcer: Basic Anatomy and Mechanism, Lancet, 2:353, 1953.

Maddock, W. G.: The Importance of Air in Gastro-Intestinal Distention, Surg. Clin. North Am., 32:71, 1952.

Miller, L. D., and G. W. Peskin: The Postgastrectomy "Dumping Syndrome," Am. J. Med. Sc., 245:218, 1963.

Palmer, W. L.: Mechanism of Pain with Peptic Ulcer: A Reply, Am. J. Med., 18:513, 1955.

Smith, A. W. M.: The Pain of Peptic Ulceration, Quart. J. Med., 24:293, 1955.

Wolf, S., and H. G. Wolff: "Human Gastric Function," 2d ed., New York, Oxford University Press, 1947.

The above papers of Bloomfield, Palmer, Kinsella, and Smith present concise expositions of the leading theories regarding the mechanism of peptic ulcer pain: disturbed motility, acid irritation, and local inflammatory reaction, respectively.

26 ANOREXIA, NAUSEA, AND VOMITING

William H. Resnik

ANOREXIA

Anorexia is a symptom which should be distinguished from satiety. There seems to be no single physiologic basis for loss of appetite. In some (probably most) cases in which correlation of gastric function with anorexia has been made, inhibition of gastric activity has been found. However, it has been shown that under certain conditions the converse may be true; loss of appetite may occur when gastric functions (secretory and motor activity) are enhanced. These contradictory findings emphasize the more complex nature of appetite as compared with hunger and indicate the large role that various psychic influences play in determining the presence or absence of appetite. In many illnesses, return of appetite after a period of anorexia is a favorable prognostic sign.

Clinically, anorexia occurs in so many conditions of ill health, both psychogenic and organic, that its diagnostic significance is small in the light of other more positive manifestations that signify the nature of the underlying disorder. In some cases loss of appetite may be the only symptom in a person in whom the history, physical examination, and routine laboratory examinations reveal no adequate cause. Under these circumstances, it is important to remember that anorexia may be the sole clue to the presence of a malignant growth in the digestive tract, particularly in the stomach or colon. Anorexia is often also the only symptom suggesting the existence of a subacute hepatitis.

NAUSEA AND VOMITING

Nausea and vomiting may each occur independently, but they are so closely allied that they may be conveniently treated as one symptom. Commonly, nausea precedes vomiting. This symptom is usually associated with a diminution of the functional activity of the stomach, alterations of the motility of the duodenum, and other evidences of autonomic acitvity: pallor of the skin, increased perspiration, salivation, and the occasional association of hypotension and bradycardia (vagal stimulation). Anorexia is also present, and it is assumed that the loss of appetite and nausea are devices developed in the course of evolution to protect the organism against the ingestion and absorption of harmful materials.

Vomiting is a more complicated symptom, depending on the coordinated activity of a number of structures: closure of the glottis, contraction and then fixation of the diaphragm in the inspiratory position, closure of the pylorus and relaxation of the rest of the stomach including the cardiac orifice, and contraction of the abdominal muscles. It is the latter act that is primarily responsible for the expulsion of the gastric contents, the stomach playing a relatively passive role. When vomiting is prolonged and forceful, reverse peristalsis in the small intestine may force bile-stained duodenal contents, or even material from lower levels of the small bowel, into the stomach.

These various activities involved in the act of vomiting are controlled and coordinated in the proper sequence by the vomiting center, which lies in the dorsal portion of the lateral reticular formation of the medulla. This center receives afferent stimuli from emetic receptor sites in the periphery of the body as well as from the brain, and then, if adequately stimulated, sends out efferent impulses to the appropriate structures: larynx, diaphragm, stomach, abdominal muscles.

It was long held that vomiting stimuli fell into two main groups: those that acted primarily by enhancing the activity of the vomiting center ("central" vomiting) and those that arose in the peripheral parts of the body and were then conveyed to the vomiting center ("reflex" vomiting). Newer evidence has modified this concept of the vomiting mechanism. It has been demonstrated that in addition to the vomiting center there exists an accessory medullary center that is responsive to chemical stimuli such as apomorphine and digitalis, but which mediates also the vestibular impulses responsible for motion sickness. In other words, the "central" vomiting due to apomorphine and digitalis is not due to direct stimulation of the vomiting center, but rather to stimulation of the medullary chemoreceptor trigger zone, which then forwards impulses to the vomiting center. Indeed, it is now believed that no drug, or other circulating emetic agent such as occurs in infections and uremia, causes "central" vomiting in the old sense, through direct stimulation of the vomiting center. All emetic stimuli originate at peripheral or central receptor sites. These latter are not autonomous since, when they are stimulated, vomiting can occur only if an intact vomiting center is present.

Probably all sensory nerves, cranial and peripheral as well as autonomic, are capable of transmitting emetic impulses. Any stimulus, if sufficiently painful, may be associated with nausea and vomiting: the "sickening" pain of a blow to the testis is an example. However, pain associated with abdominal disorders is far more likely to be associated with nausea and vomiting than is pain due to extraabdominal disturbances. In the abdomen, afferent stimuli are carried by the vagus and sympathetic nerves. Experimental work on structures subserved by both sets of nerves shows that the vagi are usually the more important in this respect. Cortical stimuli as a result of psychic disturbances, disagreeable sights, odors, or tastes, stimuli from the labyrinth and pharynx, as well as impulses from the digestive and biliary tracts, peritoneum, and urinary and pelvic organs, are common causes of nausea and vomiting. In addition, vomiting may result from the action of drugs and poisons introduced into the body, as well as from toxic substances generated in the organism. In the latter category are the "toxins" of acute infectious diseases and, presumably, the retention products responsible for the vomiting of uremia.

Although the general principles concerned with the mechanism of vomiting appear to be clear, the precise application of these principles in the elucidation of vomiting as it appears in specific clinical conditions is not always possible. In many instances multiple factors may be operative, and it is difficult to estimate the part played by each. In others, the stimuli to vomiting are unknown, and we are uncertain whether their effect is peripheral or central. For example, the cause of vomiting in uremia is still a matter of conjecture. It has been variously attributed to the irritating effect on the gut of ammonium salts converted by bacterial action from urea; to the retention of guanidine, phenol, and other as yet unknown "toxic" substances; to ulceration of the intestinal mucosa; and to dehydration and electrolyte disturbances. Further enumeration of the uncertainties of our knowledge is unnecessary to stress the point that in many clinical conditions the mechanism of vomiting is complex and imperfectly understood.

There is one form of vomiting that occurs in conditions associated with increased intracranial pressure and is quite distinctive—the so-called "projectile" vomiting. This is characterized by a sudden unexpected and sometimes violent ejection of gastric contents. The reason for its chief peculiarity, absence of nausea, is unknown.

EFFECTS OF VOMITING. As is true in any condition accompanied by profuse loss of water and salts, excessive vomiting may lead to a state of deficiency of sodium, potassium, and chloride, and hence to a loss of extracellular fluid volume (Chap. 60) and plasma volume, and finally to acute peripheral circulatory failure (Chap. 135). However, vomiting is distinctive in that the loss of chloride is greater than the loss of base. Normally, hydrochloric acid is formed in the stomach by removing the chloride ion from the blood. When, as the result of vomiting, there is excessive loss of hydrochloric acid from the body, a characteristic chemical pattern develops in the blood. This is characterized by deficiency of chloride and excess of bicarbonate (formed from the base no longer balanced by chloride), and elevation of nonprotein nitrogen as the result of prerenal deviation (Chap. 29). This chemical pattern is most typically seen in persons with pyloric or intestinal obstruction but may be observed whenever there is excessive vomiting (Chap. 60).

CLASSIFICATION. Vomiting is so common a manifestation of bodily dysfunction, and its mode of origin so uncertain in many disorders, that a simple, logical classification, according to either mechanism or etiology, is impossible. The one given below has no special merit and serves only as a basis for brief comments on certain specific conditions.

Acute Infectious Diseases. In children nausea and vomiting may be encountered at the onset or during practically any acute infection of a severity sufficient to cause the usual constitutional symptoms. In adults, nausea and vomiting are likely to occur when the infectious process is one primarily involving the gastrointestinal tract, the liver (e.g., acute infectious hepatitis, probably due to an associated duodenitis), or the meninges (in the latter case, the vomiting may be of the projectile type).

Acute Abdominal Emergencies ("Surgical Abdomen"). All the various disorders that fall into this category, and that need not be enumerated, are associated with nausea and vomiting. When the biliary tract is involved, these symptoms are far more intense in obstructions of the common duct than when the gallbladder alone is affected. In general, the most severe and persistent vomiting is seen in acute peritonitis and in acute obstructions of the small bowel (including paralytic ileus).

In certain cases of acute appendicitis, pain may be minimal and vomiting outspoken, although the reverse relationship is commoner.

Chronic Indigestion. Spontaneous and frequent nausea and vomiting are uncommon in uncomplicated peptic ulcer; more often, vomiting is induced by the patient to relieve pain. The regular appearance of nausea and the vomiting of copious quantities of material a number of hours after eating indicate the presence of pyloric obstruction due to either a benign or a malignant lesion. Unexplained nausea and loss of appetite may be the earliest symptoms of a carcinoma of the stomach or of almost any type of diffuse disease of the liver.

Diseases of the Heart. Congestive heart failure is frequently associated with nausea and vomiting, which may be the chief complaints of the patient. Under such circumstances these symptoms may result from drugs (more especially from digitalis, opiates, and xanthines), from congestion of the abdominal viscera, or from the frequently associated uremia, sometimes due to salt depletion.

Metabolic Disorders. During the crises of hyperthyroidism, in hypoparathyroidism as well as acute hyperparathyroidism, in the course of Addison's disease (especially during the acute phases), and at the onset of diabetic acidosis, nausea and vomiting may be prominent symptoms. Anorexia and, less commonly, vomiting may result from disorders of the pituitary gland (Simmonds' disease). The familiar morning sickness of the early weeks of pregnancy is listed here because there is some evidence that this phenomenon, so frequent as to be considered physiologic by some, is due to endocrine metabolic alteration initiated by the implantation of the fertilized ovum—possibly to the increased production of estrogens. Psychogenic factors undoubtedly play a role in some cases, and in the more severe form (pernicious vomiting of pregnancy) there are superimposed additional causes of vomiting due to the effects of the prolonged vomiting itself: starvation, dehydration, etc. Reference has already been made to the sometimes severe and persistent nausea and vomiting of uremia, which are to be differentiated from the somewhat similar manifestations that may occur in acute nephritis or hypertensive disease, without nitrogen retention (pseudouremia). In this latter condition the symptoms have long been considered to be due to cerebral edema or spasm of the cerebral vessels; in some cases the symptoms are actually due to thrombosis in the cerebral vessels.

Disorders of the Nervous System. Meningitis, migraine, and tabetic crises are associated with nausea and vomiting, sometimes severe and prolonged. Occasionally, nausea and vomiting may be the predominant or only symptoms in migraine. The projectile vomiting caused by lesions associated with increased intracranial pressure has already been mentioned. The coexistence of nausea, vomiting, and well-marked vertigo is suggestive of a labyrinthine disturbance such as occurs in motion sickness and in the characteristic seizures of Ménière's syndrome. It is extremely unlikely that nausea and vomiting alone are ever a manifestation of basilar artery insufficiency; practically invariably these symptoms are associated with others, such as dysphopia, diplopia, and vertigo.

Drugs and Poisons. Since the majority of these substances are capable of inducing vomiting which subsides after withdrawal of the offending substance, detailed comment is unnecessary.

Pharyngeal Irritation. A prosaic but common and sometimes disturbing cause of morning vomiting is the irritating effect of a postnasal discharge, frequently due to excessive smoking.

Psychogenic Vomiting. This term is applied to the nausea and vomiting that may occur as transitory phenomena, the result of some emotional upset, or persistent as a consequence of a more profound psychic disturbance. The condition known as *anorexia nervosa*, in which, as the result of an emotional disturbance, the patient may suffer from a profound loss of appetite and may vomit after every meal, with consequent rapid weight loss, constitutes one example of this type of vomiting. More commonly, patients with emotional disorders and vomiting maintain a relatively normal state of nutrition, because only a relatively small fraction of the ingested food is vomited.

DIFFERENTIAL DIAGNOSIS. Vomiting is to be differentiated from regurgitation, which implies the expulsion from the esophagus of undigested food retained because of some obstruction such as occurs with cardiospasm or esophageal diverticulum, or the expulsion of gastric contents without preceding nausea. Regurgitation is caused by the intrinsic activity of the esophagus or stomach and is not accompanied by the forceful contraction of the abdominal muscles (retching) that characterizes vomiting.

The character of the vomitus and the circumstances under which vomiting occurs are sometimes of importance in estimating the significance of this symptom. When several hundred milliliters of material are vomited regularly a number of hours after the preceding meal, and particularly when particles of undigested food can be recognized, pyloric obstruction is a practical certainty. If this vomitus contains free hydrochloric acid, the obstruction may be due either to ulcer or to carcinoma; absence of free hydrochloric acid suggests a malignant growth. Fecal odor after protracted vomiting indicates the presence of low obstruction of the small bowel or of peritonitis. Streaks of blood have no significance. Large quantities of blood, either bright red or dark brown (when it has been chemically altered by the acid of gastric juice), usually denote an intragastric lesion or a ruptured esophageal varix. Bile is commonly present in the gastric contents whenever vomiting is prolonged. It has no significance unless constantly present in large quantities, when it may signify an obstructive lesion below the ampulla of Vater.

In general, nausea and vomiting due to lesions or functional derangement of the stomach bear some definite relationship to eating. Unfortunately, this state-

ment is less helpful than would appear at first glance. Indigestion associated with nausea and vomiting, especially occurring shortly after eating, may be caused by a functional disturbance of the stomach dependent on an obscure lesion such as a chronic infection in the urinary tract or pelvic organs. Vomiting, practically always self-induced, which relieves an epigastric pain of the postprandial type and often occurring during the night, is highly suggestive of a peptic ulcer.

Vomiting which is entirely unrelated to eating is often due to exogenous (drugs) or endogenous (uremia, hepatic and diabetic coma) intoxication, to disorders of the nervous system, or to the various metabolic disturbances which have been mentioned. Vomiting occurring before breakfast in a young woman is commonly due to pregnancy.

Nausea and vomiting are symptoms too widespread to be investigated by any definite program of study. In most cases the associated symptoms are of more value in defining the cause of the underlying disorder. It may be well, however, to mention some of the conditions in which the cause of the nausea and vomiting may not be readily apparent: carcinoma of the stomach in an early stage, chronic indigestion due to lesions remote from the stomach, diabetic acidosis, uremia, Addison's disease, pregnancy, tabetic crises, migraine when the headache is brief and overshadowed by the nausea and vomiting, acute hepatitis at the onset and before jaundice appears, or the acute epidemic infectious disease whose only manifestation is nausea and vomiting (epidemic nausea and vomiting).

REFERENCES

Borison, H. L., and S. C. Wang: Physiology and Pharmacology of Vomiting, Pharmacol. Rev., 5:193, 1953.

Cummins, A. J.: Nausea and Vomiting, Am. J. Digest. Diseases, 3:710, 1958.

Wolf, S., and H. G. Wolff: "Human Gastric Function," 2d ed., New York, Oxford University Press, 1947.

27 CONSTIPATION, DIARRHEA, AND DISTURBANCES OF ANORECTAL FUNCTION

Albert I. Mendeloff

NORMAL COLONIC FUNCTION

MOTOR AND ABSORPTIVE FUNCTIONS. When one considers that a north-woods lumberjack may consume several kilograms of foodstuffs per day, furnishing him nearly 6,000 cal, and yet produce a stool which weighs only 100 to 200 Gm, of which nearly three-quarters is water, the efficiency of the gut becomes clearly evident. Just as slight changes in renal function may result in abnormal amounts of urine being excreted, so relatively minor deviations in the absorption of water, in intestinal tone, in propulsive motility, or in rectal sensitivity may result in dramatic changes in the caliber and consistency of the stools.

On a normal mixed diet the stomach is nearly empty several hours after food is ingested. By the time the head of the food column reaches the ileocecal valve, 99 per cent of the carbohydrate, 99 per cent of the protein, and 97 per cent of the fats have been broken down into absorbable form and entered the portal venules and the lacteals.

When the intestinal bolus reaches the terminal ileum, it tends to proceed very sluggishly unless the stomach empties; the so-called "gastroileal reflex" causes the ileum to empty into the cecum by a rapid series of small squirts. The ileocecal valve is a puzzling structure which offers no resistance to the incoming ileal bolus but is supposed to prevent regurgitation, at least of gas, from the cecum into the ileum. The ileal contents reaching the cecum daily comprise a volume of less than 500 ml, a slurry thoroughly churned in the right colon by segmental contractions of the haustra. Every now and then a coordinated wave involving a short length of colon pushes the soggy mass along into the next area; reflexes brought on by eating sweep from duodenum or stomach to the colon, and an occasional movement occurs by means of which a fairly large section of colon is emptied of its contents, and the left colon fills with a more desiccated mass. Defacatory reflexes originate from the rectal walls, which normally are approximated around a small lumen empty of feces; when sigmoid contraction distends the rectal musculature, the defecatory reflex center in the sacral cord causes the levatores ani to pull the lower rectum and both sphincters up and almost around or over the descending fecal mass; forced expiration and contraction of abdominal muscles supply the additional pressure required to force the stool past the external sphincter. However, if the sphincter is voluntarily contracted, the sigmoid colon relaxes, and the fecal mass slips back up into the rectosigmoid.

INNERVATION. The colon and rectum are supplied with both sympathetic and parasympathetic nerves carrying both sensory and motor fibers. Sympathetic elements from the lower six thoracic segments travel to the right colon via the superior mesenteric plexus; the left colon receives sympathetic fibers originating in the lumbar segments of the cord gathered into the inferior mesenteric plexus, branches of which follow the inferior mesenteric artery. The rectum receives sympathetic innervation from the hypogastric or presacral nerve. Parasympathetic cholinergic fibers to the right colon are assumed to be part of the vagus, passing through the celiac plexus. The left colon and rectum receive all their parasympathetic innervation via the nervi erigentes, originating in the sacral nerves and joining the sympathetic fibers in the pelvic plexuses, from which some accompany the inferior mesenteric artery. The anus and external anal sphincter are supplied by the inferior hemorrhoidal branch of the internal pudendal nerve and by the perineal branches of the fourth sacral nerves, which nerves also innervate the levatores ani muscles. Sensory nerves from the skin and mucous membrane of the anal canal are plentiful and go to the sacral cord.

The functional significance of the sympathetic supply to the lower bowel is unclear. Careful studies in man following dorsolumbar sympathectomy have failed to reveal any consistent dysfunction of colon or rectum. Attempts to relieve colon pain syndromes by presacral neurectomy have been unavailing. The parasympathetic cholinergic innervation of the colon seems to be of sole importance in the motor and secretory functions of that organ; cholinergic drugs correspondingly activate such functions and result, when large enough dosages are employed, in watery diarrhea, cramps, and pain.

The mechanism of defecation has been previously described, and the important contribution of the abdominal musculature, the levatores ani, and the external anal sphincter noted. The internal anal sphincter, a smooth muscle, relaxes when the rectum is distended, and seems to help allow gas to escape without full defecatory movements. Sensory innervation of the anal canal permits the brain to discriminate as to whether rectal contents are liquid, gaseous, or solid.

CONTINENCE AND INCONTINENCE

The integrity of the defecation reflex depends upon the presence of a neuroreceptor system beginning in the smooth muscle of the upper rectum. When its tension reaches a threshold, this musculature contracts, joining and augmenting an entire complex of abdominal wall contraction, internal anal sphincter relaxation, and opening of the external anal sphincter. The reflex is believed to be further augmented by the anal sensation of feces passing through the anal canal, and perhaps also by associated reflexes like that of micturition. The central representation of defecation lies, in experimental animals, in the medulla near the vomiting center, and it may be transiently disturbed in many vascular insults to the brain. Voluntary inhibition of defecation, described earlier, is mediated through rapid relaxation of the abdominal musculature and the contraction of the external anal sphincter.

This sequence of events can take place in persons whose sacral cord has been destroyed—i.e., all its elements can function in the absence of an intact peripheral nerve supply—but the strength of such a denervated contraction is weak, and evacuation is generally incomplete unless laxation, usually by enema, reenforces the reflex. Cord transection abolishes the cerebral appreciation of the urge to defecate. Thus disease or trauma to the higher spinal cord and the brain can produce in the function of colon and rectum the same range of disturbances of function as occur in the bladder (see Chap. 18). The colon may become hypotonic, the external sphincter ineffective, and the defecatory reflexes dulled; the levatores ani muscles are often weak and the abdominal musculature unable to produce and sustain effective pressure increases.

The inability to appreciate anal sensation, whether due to central disease, peripheral neuritis of sacral nerves, or surgical interruption of anal innervation, as in treatment of hemorrhoids and perirectal abscess, may also weaken the responses and is often particularly troublesome when the stool is semisolid or liquid. The "sensing" of the consistency of rectal contents by anal receptors has been demonstrated only recently; it provides some explanation for the unpleasant fact that many surgical repairs of the anorectal area look anatomically excellent, but the patient is incontinent of any fecal material other than a hard dry stool.

Sudden interruption of function of the central nervous system, as by cerebral vascular accident, interferes with this whole defecatory complex at many levels, and usually results in fecal incontinence of some degree. The dysfunction is maximal at the onset of the process and generally returns toward normal over a period of weeks. In most forms of neurologic disease resulting in incontinence, the reflex may be satisfactorily activated by rectal distension, most practically produced by a combination of aperients and enemas, which results in a mass movement in the more proximal bowel, augmenting the reflex evacuation from the rectum. As sensation from the anal area returns, the passage of stool through the anus reenforces the reflex. Since the bowel is filled infrequently, and irrigation techniques are generally effective and not dangerous, fecal incontinence in such patients is usually much less troublesome than is urinary incontinence. Fecal impactions may be prevented by regularly administered enemas, control of diet, use of drugs, and regular exercises for strengthening the voluntary anal muscles.

DISORDERED BOWEL FUNCTION

SYMPTOMS. Exaggerations of the motor components of normal gastrointestinal activity constitute the most important early symptoms of gastrointestinal diseases. In the small intestine rapid propulsive motility may be associated with dyssynergy, the combination giving rise to cramping contractions. Because of the rather imprecise character of man's system for the detection and recognition of the sources of visceral pain, these cramps are usually projected to the midline—if they originate in the duodenum, to the epigastrium; if from the jejunum, to the umbilicus; if from the lower ileum, to the area just below the umbilicus. In the colon, dyssynergic activity is rarely projected to the midline but usually is lateralized along the general course of the offending organ. Since the colon is large, festooning the abdomen, and full of fluid and partially compressible gas, contractions in one or another area of the bowel may force the contents back toward the cecum; a simultaneous dyssynergic contraction anywhere else in the colonic wall may trap gas in the area intervening, distending a relaxed but otherwise innocent portion of the bowel so that discomfort is referred to the distended site, often in the splenic or hepatic flexure. Excessive gas results entirely from air swallowed with food or drink or from such "tics" as sighing or forced belching. Sharp, unpleasant contrac-

tions in the left lower quadrant associated with straining at stool, and partially relieved by defecation, are called *tenesmus*. A sensation of urgent need to defecate—*rectal urgency*—is an extremely distressing symptom associated with irritability of the rectum. Sharp pain in the anal area is made worse by defecation and is usually associated with an inflammatory response in the skin of the anus—*anal pain.*

After establishing the presence or absence of these deviations, the physician must find out whether or not eating or defecation exacerbates or relieves them, whether the patient tries to mitigate the discomfort by moving about or lying still, or by holding the abdominal wall immobilized with his hands or against the mattress. Although the general topography of the area of distress may localize findings to large or small intestines, relief by defecation is a feature of disturbance of the left colon, as exacerbation by eating is a feature of malfunction of the small intestine or right colon. Restlessness occurs with colic; peritoneal irritation tends to immobilize the patient. All these disturbances originate as increases in the tone of the bowel wall, and pressure relationships between adjacent segments of intestine determine not only the tension exerted against the wall but also the speed and character of the flow of the fluid contents along the lumen. As increased tension may compress the vessels nourishing the gut wall, so disease or contraction of the nourishing vasculature may deprive the wall of its ability to contract, to absorb, or to secrete. Unabsorbed residue or unduly large volumes of secretions attract more fluid into the lumen, further distending the gut; if large volumes of swallowed air cannot be passed quickly along the small bowel to the cecum, as is usual, the movements of the air-fluid mixture in the small intestine become loud enough to be noticed by the patient; such *borborygmi* are heard normally in the colon. Sudden changes in volume of the abdomen—*distension*—occur when the intraluminal volume of small or large bowel increases, because of paralysis of neuromuscular elements, abnormal handling of gas, or mechanical obstruction behind which muscular contractile activity is greatly increased. Bowel sounds may be absent if the wall is paralyzed, faint if the injury is submaximal, or increased if a viable area is forced to raise its intraluminal pressure in order to drive fluid past an obstructed segment. Sudden changes in pain reference occurring during the course of an illness usually indicate that the peritoneal surfaces have become involved, with more accurate cerebral localization of the underlying disturbance, and perhaps with associated development of spasm or guarding of the overlying musculature.

DIARRHEA AND CONSTIPATION. *Diarrhea* and *constipation* are terms given to alterations in the normal pattern of human defecation habits. There is no standard definition by which patients or physicians may classify strictly the deviation from normal; the range of variation in bowel habits among apparently healthy persons is extraordinarily wide, so that the deviation must, in the last analysis, be compared with each patient's own previous habit pattern rather than with that characterizing the mean, the median, or the mode of the population. Such comparisons involve so many associated functions that it will suffice for the purposes of this discussion to define diarrhea as the frequent passage of unformed stools, and constipation as an undue delay in the evacuation of feces. It is the task of the physician to understand enough of the normal and disturbed physiology of digestion, absorption, and propulsive motility that he may ask pointed questions of the patient which serve to define more precisely the locus, the nature, and the severity of the disturbance. Since the gastrointestinal tract is a primitive organ upon which all manner of stimuli, from hunger to fear, rage, fever, and fatigue, from grossly infected or chemically toxic ingesta to the most subtly allergenic refined foods, exert effects that disturb function, this task is rarely simple.

ACUTE DIARRHEA. Acute disturbances of bowel function are relatively common and usually manifest themselves as diarrhea. The sudden onset of loose stools in a previously healthy person commonly is due to an active infection, and much less often to the ingestion of preformed toxins, poisonous chemicals or drugs, or to acute radiation sickness. When the patient is first seen, the history will usually point toward the source of the trouble: the eating of a particular meal or food in company with others who have also become similarly ill within 24 hr of eating the suspected food is *prima facie* evidence that a preformed toxin has been ingested; diarrhea developing in a number of patients within 28 to 72 hr after a common meal should make one suspect a salmonella infection. The presence of fever, malaise, muscle aching, and profound epigastric or periumbilical discomfort with severe anorexia suggests an inflammatory disease of the small intestine. The stools are characteristically watery, often accompanied by the explosive passage of gas; there is no rectal urgency or tenesmus and little hypogastric cramping. On physical examination one finds a generally tender abdomen without guarding, and one hears "whooshing" peristaltic sounds. A variant of the syndrome consists only of severe periumbilical pain and vomiting. The hemogram usually is within normal limits. Such an entity is commonly produced by infection with a virus, of which a number of species have been identified. The disease is called *viral gastroenteritis*, runs an acute course for 2 to 3 days, then gradually subsides.

The stool in viral gastroenteritis never contains recognizable exudate—it is singularly free of inflammatory cells, blood, or fibrin. Culture of the stool is usually nonproductive. By contrast, inflammatory diseases of the colon almost always result in leukocytic exudate and fibrin in the feces; stools may give cultures positive for organisms of the genus *Salmonella* or *Shigella* or may on microscopic examination show motile forms and/or cysts of various parasites, the most important of which in the United States is *Endamoeba histolytica*. Colonic infections usually are accompanied by hypogastric cramping, tenesmus, and

rectal urgency. The patient may not have true anorexia but may be afraid to eat because eating stimulates the urge to defecate. There is usually fever and leukocytosis.

The physician must remember that an acute diarrhea may be the presenting symptoms of any type of systemic infection or of a hitherto-silent chronic gastrointestinal disease, of which the most well-defined are regional enteritis and ulcerative colitis; the latter may occasionally begin with fulminant dysentery, the former more often presents as a tender mass in the right lower quadrant with mild diarrhea. Generalized cramping and diarrhea may follow use of a parasympathomimetic drug. Tenesmus, urgency, and left-sided hypogastric tenderness and cramping are classic symptoms of diverticulitis; the stool may contain pus, blood, or both, usually with much mucus. A fecal impaction may make a patient have rectal urgency, ask for a bedpan or visit the toilet often, but expel only a little watery exudate, or nothing. Short-circuiting operations on the intestine and stomach usually result in at least mild diarrhea for months after the operation.

Differential diagnosis of these varied entities is made by history, physical examination, gross and microscopic appearance of the stools, appropriate bacteriologic studies, and proctoscopy. It is important to see the excreta put out by the patient, not just to rely on his description or on that of a third party. Toilets are not distinguished for satisfactory lighting, nor upset patients for careful observation, and even trained personnel seldom display a curiosity sufficient to overcome the unpleasantness of a stool held close enough for accurate appraisal. Since fluid and electrolyte losses in diarrhea may be so great as to be life-threatening, the patient is given supportive care until studies indicate specific treatment. If no definitive etiologic agent can be identified, barium enema and upper gastrointestinal x-rays should be carried out. Upper gastrointestinal films may be very misleading when the barium meal is fed within the first few days of an acute enteritis or colitis, and should be reserved for a time when the whole disease has become more quiescent.

CHRONIC DIARRHEA. A history of bouts of loose stools extending over a period of months or years, usually intermittent in character, calls for painstaking investigation. One particularly wants to know the circumstances of the first such bout—did it follow an acute infection, an operation, an emotional upset of severe degree? The number of days or weeks lost by the patient from his daily occupation on account of the illness, changes in weight and strength, and the appearance of the patient give important leads as to the nature and severity of the underlying disease. By the time the patient sees a physician the presenting symptoms may not be diarrhea, but rather those of serious malnutrition, since any long-continued illness of this type may interfere with appetite, as well as with the absorptive and digestive functions of the gastrointestinal tract. Associated signs and symptoms may reveal that the diarrhea and malnutrition are due to a generalized disorder which may involve the intestines functionally or structurally—hyperthyroidism, tuberculosis, lymphosarcoma, to name a few. More often, no such disorder will be found, and the physician must consider another, more specifically gastrointestinal disease.

A long history of intermittent diarrhea unaccompanied by fever, weight loss, blood in the stools, or significant loss of working capacity suggests a disturbance of emotional or, less commonly, of allergic origin, and associated symptoms should be elicited (Chaps. 42, 260). A detailed dietary history is important in such cases, in order to establish the adequacy of the nutrient intake and to allow the patient a chance to ventilate his ideas on the relationship of food and eating to his symptoms. In such disordered functional states, the patient usually has a fairly formed stool on arising in the morning but then has one or two loose stools within the next hour. A similar pattern may occur after the evening meal. The stool caliber is usually small, and there may be mild discomfort, relieved by defecation, in the left lower quadrant of the abdomen. Such a triad of symptoms makes up the diarrheal component of the "irritable colon" syndrome, an extremely common disorder in anxious, nervous people, in which the symptoms result from exaggeration of normal colonic function.

When the history suggests that the diarrheal episodes have been characterized by blood in the stools, or by fever, malaise, anorexia, and weight loss in addition, one suspects a chronic inflammatory process involving either or both small bowel and colon. Regional enteritis may attack any portion of the intestine, producing an encroachment on the lumen and episodes of partial obstruction, ulcerations of the mucous membrane, or local abscesses and fistulas to the abdominal or anal skin, to the bladder, or to other loops of bowel. On proctoscopic examination the rectum is found to be uninvolved and the stools show little microscopic exudate although they are often positive for occult blood, gross bleeding being infrequently encountered. Tuberculosis and lymphosarcoma of the intestine can give similar symptoms and may be impossible to differentiate, although usually the roentgenologic appearances are dissimilar. The involvement may be primarily colonic, the most important disease entity being ulcerative colitis, whether idiopathic or due to amebic infestation, venereal lymphogranuloma, or chronic bacillary dysentery. Here the feces show pus cells and red cells when the disease is active, and proctoscopy is usually diagnostic. Stool cultures and examinations for parasites on numerous occasions are important aspects of the medical investigation.

When the patient presents with diarrhea of more than a few months' duration, without fever, blood in the stools, or cramping pain, but with weight loss, weakness, and symptoms of nutritional deficiency diseases (Chaps. 69, 197), one focuses attention on the small intestine. In children celiac disease and cystic fibrosis of the pancreas are the important disorders to be differentiated; in older patients the same distinction

between an absorptive defect and a digestive disorder must still be made in order to distinguish idiopathic steatorrhea from chronic pancreatitis. Whereas the stools in disease of the left colon are loose, often contain exudate on microscopic examination, and weigh less than 200 Gm per 24 hr, the stools associated with malabsorption are bulky, free of exudate, and weigh more than 300 Gm per 24 hr. Such a 24-hr collection, impounded in a collecting vessel, often has a shiny appearance and a foul odor which are almost diagnostic. See Chap. 197 for differential diagnosis of malabsorption.

A history of progressive disease characterized by arthritis, abdominal pain, diarrhea, and weight loss in middle-aged men suggests the diagnosis of intestinal lipodystrophy (Whipple's disease), in which abnormal deposits of glycoproteins accumulate in the lacteal system of the mesentery and small focal granulomas develop in the viscera and lymph nodes. Lymphosarcomas of low degrees of malignancy may produce malabsorption syndromes by blockage of lymphatic channels from the small bowel; loops of intestine made "blind" by surgery or by the healing of lesions of regional enteritis can produce syndromes of severe macrocytic anemia and diarrhea. Rarer causes of diarrhea are the enormous hypersecretion of gastric or intestinal juices due to endocrine tumors, the cramping diarrhea associated with high circulating levels of serotonin (see Chap. 90), and the painful wasting due to mesenteric vascular insufficiency.

Special techniques are often needed to define clearly all these abnormalities. Duodenal intubation and analysis of digestive juices for pancreatic enzymes is a procedure of considerable importance in ruling out primary disease of the pancreas. Nevertheless, the aid of the skilled radiologist is probably more useful than any test in interpreting all but the earliest manifestations of these syndromes. Pancreatic calcification, fistulas, distortions of the duodenal loop, diffuse granulomatous diseases of the small bowel, diverticula, polyps, ulcerated areas, stenosis, and obstruction—all these can be identified by modern radiologic techniques, which provide in addition base-line data for evaluating the natural history of the disease and response to therapy.

CONSTIPATION. Whereas diarrhea may be a dangerous symptom per se, with its accompaniment of dehydration and loss of cations, constipation of itself is not debilitating, although mild abdominal discomfort and straining at stool are not salutary and tend to increase the severity of preexisting anorectal lesions. The acute onset of severe obstipation in an apparently normal person signifies that something has disturbed the neural, vascular, or muscular integrity of the gut or associated defecatory reflexes and muscles. Such disturbances may result from severe infections, particularly of the central nervous system, from acute mesenteric circulatory catastrophes, from renal colic, from cerebrovascular accidents, from mechanical obstruction of large or small intestine, from painful anal lesions, from certain drugs, or from fecal impaction. Of these, the last is the most embarrassing to overlook, since the puttylike mass filling the rectum makes the patient try to move his bowels and often results in frequent calls for a bedpan or visits to the toilet; such fruitless attempts at defecations may be called diarrhea, and the poor patient may receive anti-diarrheal medications! Rapid but complete physical examination including a digital examinaton of the rectum and proctoscopy is called for in all cases of constipation of acute onset; if no other physical signs to explain the sudden constipation are elicited, a low-pressure barium enema should be given to establish the site of obstruction if present and appropriate measures taken.

A long history of intermittent bouts of constipation, accompanied by abdominal distress relieved by defecation and by passage of hard stools of small caliber, with or without much mucus, is characteristic of the *"irritable colon" syndrome*, one of the commonest forms of anxiety met by the physician. The abuse of laxatives over many years is frequently added to the underlying emotional disturbance to aggravate the clinical picture. The symptoms are essentially exaggerations of normal physiologic activity of the colon, and in mild degrees have probably been experienced by most healthy people as, for example, the constipation associated with travel. Extensive studies of sigmoid motility in patients with this syndrome have verified the clinical impression that disturbed motor function correlates closely with emotional conflicts. Proctoscopic examination of these patients demonstrates an unremarkable rectum and a rectosigmoid which is often spastic, the lumen smaller than normal, the veins prominent, and the mucus more abundant than usual. The stools are negative for blood, parasites, and pathogenic bacteria; the x-ray examination is usually not abnormal.

Another common form of constipation is also chronic and is not characterized by the triad of symptoms of the irritable colon syndrome. Whether as the result of childhood training or of a perverse understanding of the necessity for bowel movements occurring with chronometric precision, these patients have equated general health with "regularity." This leads to a dependence on laxatives or enemas to hasten the overdue evacuation, so that over the years they lose the sensitivity of the rectal defecatory reflexes. Consequently, they do not have a regular schedule for moving their bowels, which for most normal people is most easily accomplished after breakfast and, if needed, after the heaviest meal of the day; over the years they no longer demonstrate any rhythmicity in defecation, take laxatives whenever they feel "run down," and have stools which may be alternately voluminous and watery or small and hard. Lax abdominal muscles and a pelvic floor weakened by multiple deliveries may contribute to poor defecatory performance. On physical examination these patients often have a palpable colon filled with feces, and on rectal examination feces fill the ampulla, the patient being unaware of this. Such types of rectal insensitivity have been called *atonic constipation, dyschezia,* and *rectal constipation.*

In both the above types of constipation, it is obvious that a thorough analysis by the physician of dietary habits, defecatory habits, use of laxatives, mode of living, and emotional problems must be made before proper therapy can be instituted. At the same time it must be stressed that such patients are not immune to the development of neoplasms of the large bowel, and it is a most difficult task for the physician to decide how often complete studies should be carried out on patients with long-standing, apparently static, complaints. The simplest solution is to do repeated stool examinations for occult blood and digital and proctoscopic examinations, remembering also that in patients who have difficulty with evacuation, anal diseases—fissures, ulcers, and hemorrhoids—are commoner than in the general population.

A lifelong history of obstinate constipation may be associated with the enormous dilatation of the large bowel seen in idiopathic or acquired megacolon. In the former condition, the rectosigmoid is contracted and obstructing, because of its lack of the ganglionic cells necessary to pass on the propulsive waves of the proximal colon; in the latter condition, severe contraction of the voluntary anal sphincter produces enormous dilatation of the rectal ampulla and colon. Radiologic studies are usually very helpful in differentiating these two conditions.

When constipation is of recent onset and progressive, the investigation should be thorough and extremely comprehensive. This is the optimal time to detect a neoplasm of the large bowel. General physical and psychiatric examination may reveal a systemic disorder: hypothyroidism, hyperparathyroidism, tuberculosis, urinary tract disease, congestive heart failure; a major psychosis, profound depression, parkinsonism, or recent cerebrovascular accident may be responsible for progressive constipation. A careful history of drug ingestion may reveal that the patient received ganglionic-blocking agents or opiates prior to onset of symptoms or large amounts of sedation. A marked change in dietary regimen, particularly in combination with sedative drugs, may produce a marked decrease in frequency of bowel movements.

If the digital and proctoscopic findings fail to explain the constipation, a barium enema and upper gastrointestinal x-rays are indicated. Tumors of the gastrointestinal tract comprise nearly half of all cancer, and patients with colonic cancers have a better prognosis for survival after surgery than do those with gastric and esophageal lesions. A high index of suspicion for a neoplastic origin of changes in bowel habits, repeated tests for occult blood in the stools, and careful proctoscopy and x-ray studies will usually justify in salvaged lives the money and time spent.

PRURITUS ANI. See p. 137.
PROCTALGIA. See Chap. 185.

REFERENCES

Davenport, H. W.: "Physiology of the Digestive Tract," Chicago, Year Book Publishers, Inc., 1961.

Mendeloff, A. I.: Chronic Diarrhea, Am. J. Digest. Diseases. 3:801, 1958.

28 HEMATEMESIS AND MELENA
William H. Resnik

Hematemesis (vomiting of gross blood) and melena (passage of tarry stools) are with rare exceptions manifestations of hemorrhage in the upper digestive tract—esophagus, stomach, duodenum. In this discussion hematemesis may be used alone for the sake of brevity, although it is to be understood that both symptoms may occur as a result of the same hemorrhage, or either may appear alone. Whether hematemesis or melena takes place will depend on whether vomiting is aroused when the stomach or duodenum contains gross blood and how much blood gains access to the small intestine: melena may be the only symptom, even though the site is in the esophagus or the stomach; hematemesis may be the prominent symptom even though the bleeding originates in the duodenum. It has been demonstrated experimentally that at least 50 to 60 ml of blood is necessary to give the stool a tarry appearance.

There are no symptoms or signs that reveal accurately the size of the hemorrhage immediately after the event takes place. The statement of the patient regarding the amount of blood vomited is usually unreliable, and, in any case, a variable amount of blood has passed into the intestine. Blood counts and hematocrit determinations made shortly after the hemorrhage are of little value. Obviously, when signs of shock are clearly evident (pallor, cool moist skin, rapid thready pulse, hypotension, restlessness, cyanosis of finger tips, etc.), a serious loss of blood volume (40 per cent or more) has taken place. When the signs of shock are less apparent or absent, a fairly large hemorrhage may nevertheless have occurred and the patient may be in a compensated state. Despite the theoretic objections to the use of the Evans blue dye (T-1824) as a precise measure of plasma volume, for clinical purposes it can serve as a simple and rapid method of estimating the extent of the blood loss. After a number of hours has elased and time has been allowed for compensatory restoration of blood volume, the estimation of hemoglobin by an accurate method or, better still, of hematocrit levels, frequently repeated, affords additional information regarding the amount of blood lost and may indicate whether bleeding is continuous or recurrent. A well-marked decline in blood pressure in the sitting position may occur when the recumbent blood pressure is still normal. Decline in urine volume despite adequate fluid intake may also be a clue to onset of shock.

The severity of shock depends not only on the magnitude of the hemorrhage but also on the abruptness with which it takes place. Hemorrhage into the upper digestive tract is frequently associated with an elevation of the nonprotein nitrogen content of the blood, owing primarily to absorption of the digestion products of blood and enhanced in cases of extensive hemorrhage by the depression of renal function resulting from shock. The increase in urea nitrogen content of the blood usually reaches a peak in about 24 hr after a single hemorrhage, and its level serves as a measure of the severity of the hemorrhage. Preexisting renal disease leads to greater and more prolonged rises in urea nitrogen, so that one must include urinary findings in analyzing the situation. Elevation of temperature to 100°F is often manifest within 24 hr of the onset of the bleeding, and this may be due to the bleeding alone. Temperatures above 100°F and those lasting beyond the first 24 hr are usually due to the administered transfusions.

CAUSES OF HEMATEMESIS AND MELENA

PEPTIC ULCER. This is the commonest cause of hematemesis, accounting for about 50 per cent of the cases. Hemorrhage from duodenal ulcer comprises about 75 per cent of all bleeding ulcer cases. In most instances there is a history characteristic of ulcer, or the ulcer has been demonstrated by x-ray study. In a small percentage, hematemesis or melena may be the initial symptom. Bleeding usually results from the rupture of a small vessel in the ulcer or from an adjacent area of gastritis. More uncommonly, bleeding follows the erosion of a large sclerotic artery; it is in these latter cases that fatal hemorrhage is likely to ensue.

GASTRITIS AND ESOPHAGITIS. These must constitute a large group, although an accurate estimation is rarely possible, for the diagnosis is often a wastebasket for unexplained hematemesis. Not infrequently hemorrhage due to gastritis appears to be unquestionably related to excessive intake of alcohol and frequently of aspirin. Even when a peptic ulcer is known to be present, a gastritis at some distance from the ulcer may harbor the bleeding point.

CARCINOMA OF THE STOMACH. About 3 per cent of the cases of hematemesis are accounted for by carcinoma of the stomach. Although this is often responsible for a moderate or severe anemia, usually the loss of blood takes place as a persistent ooze; only relatively uncommonly is there eroded a blood vessel large enough to cause a brisk hemorrhage.

PORTAL HYPERTENSION. This is responsible for about 10 per cent of the cases, bleeding usually being due to an esophageal varix, but occasionally to a gastric varix. Of this group, cirrhosis of the liver (usually the Laennec type, and in certain regions liver disease due to schistosomiasis) is the most frequent cause. In the remainder, congestive splenomegaly without cirrhosis (splenic anemia or Banti's syndrome) is found.

MISCELLANEOUS CAUSES. In the miscellaneous group fall the rarer causes of hematemesis and melena: benign polyps and other uncommon tumors of the stomach, duodenum, and small intestine; hiatal hernia; tumors and inflammation of the biliary tract; hereditary hemorrhagic telangiectasia, which may cause bleeding from the esophagus as well as from the pharynx and stomach; laceration of the blood vessels of the gastroesophageal junction caused by vomiting after an alcoholic spree (Mallory-Weiss syndrome); neurofibromatosis, pseudoxanthoma elasticum, hereditary thrombopathic thrombocytopenia and other blood dyscrasias, etc.—in all, about 2 to 3 per cent of the total.

The figures regarding the frequency with which the various causes of hematemesis and melena occur are approximate and will vary widely in different reported series. They will depend partly upon the material studied by different observers. A population containing a large number of Puerto Ricans or persons originating in other areas of the Caribbean or South America or Africa where schistosomiasis is prevalent may show figures that are heavily weighted with cases due to cirrhosis caused by this disease. In part, the figures will depend on what criteria are used to define the extent of the hemorrhage. In the main, the variations can be attributed to the thoroughness with which the investigations were carried out. Formerly, and still in many institutions, careful study was instituted only after 2 or 3 weeks had elapsed after the bleeding had subsided. At this time careful study failed to reveal any adequate cause for the hemorrhage in a considerable number of cases. In some, a typical history of ulcer made it probable that the ulcer was healed before the diagnostic studies were carried out. When no lesion could be discovered by x-ray or gastroscopy, it was often assumed that an ulcer had already healed, even when there was no previous history to suggest ulcer. In others, when there was no suggestive history, it was assumed that the hemorrhage had been caused by an acute superficial ulceration or by gastritis. Nevertheless, careful follow-up studies of such cases of unexplained hematemesis have often subsequently revealed previously undetected lesions such as peptic ulcer, carcinoma of stomach, and tumors of small intestine. However, the more frequent employment of the esophagoscope and gastroscope within the first few days of bleeding has revealed sources of hemorrhage such as mucosal erosions, or ulceration due to esophagitis or gastritis, or uncommon lesions such as hereditary hemorrhagic telangiectasia that could not have been detected before. Moreover, even when peptic ulcer or cirrhosis was known to be present, a cause of bleeding unrelated to these disorders has not infrequently been uncovered. For example, peptic ulcer may be present in almost 20 per cent of patients with cirrhosis, and the ulcer, not the varices, may have caused the hemorrhage. Even now, when early and thorough diagnostic studies have been carried out, a small residual group of cases will almost invariably be present in every reported series in which no adequate cause for the bleeding has been revealed even at autopsy.

Hematemesis and melena may be due to a number of disorders. However, the problem of diagnosis is simplified if it is borne in mind that 90 per cent of all cases are due to primary intragastric or duodenal diseases such as peptic ulcer (including gastrojejunal ulcers), gastritis, superficial ulceration, and benign and malignant tumors of the stomach. Most of the remainder are due to bleeding from esophageal varices.

PROCEDURE

It should be mentioned that a red color in the toilet bowl does not necessarily signify blood; occasionally, a person who has eaten beets or has been given an injection of Bromsulphalein may exhibit a reddish discoloration in the stool. Moreover, bright red blood in the stool is not an invariable sign of lower-bowel bleeding. A hemorrhage from the upper gastrointestinal tract may be associated with the presence of relatively unaltered blood in the stool, if transit time is rapid. Finally, it is not always easy to distinguish between bleeding originating from the gastrointestinal tract and that from the respiratory tract.

If unmistakable evidences of shock are present, the first obligation is to replace the lost blood and then to exclude hemoptysis and bleeding from the nose and pharynx as possible sources of swallowed blood. If bleeding persists, gastric lavage with ice water, using a French 30 Ewald tube, is frequently effective in stopping the hemorrhage. If shock is not present, 500 to 1000 ml whole blood may be given, depending on one's estimation of the amount of blood lost. While these measures are being instituted, historical data regarding indigestion, alcoholism, previous episodes of bleeding or a familial bleeding tendency, recent medication with drugs, such as salicylates, cortisone, or phenylbutazone, or severe vomiting just prior to the hematemesis should be obtained from the patient or his family, and physical findings such as enlargement of the liver or spleen, jaundice, spider angiomas, a palpable supraclavicular node, Blumer's shelf, and telangiectases should be searched for. Hematologic studies should also be pursued if there is a suspicion that a blood dyscrasia is present.

What studies are then carried out, and when they are begun, vary with the facilities that are available. In some clinics early investigation within the first 24 to 48 hr is initiated—by esophagoscopy, gastroscopy, and x-ray examination. If these studies are carried out skillfully and with suitable caution, the reports thus far indicate that little or no additional risk is imposed on the patient, while the advantages of ascertaining the precise point of bleeding are obvious. It is generally believed that all such procedures should be deferred as long as shock persists, and most authorities prefer to delay these investigations until bleeding has probably ceased. Even when expert endoscopic examination is not at hand, pneumatic tamponade, combined with the intravenous injection of radioactive tagged red blood cells, may indicate whether the bleeding is occurring from the esophagus or from a site below the esophagus. Early or late x-ray examination will depend on the experience of the roentgenologist in handling such cases. Liver function tests are not of great value. There is no necessary correlation between impaired hepatic function and the degree of portal hypertension which is the basic cause of the development of varices.

A diagnostic approach, entirely different from that mentioned above, has also been advocated. In the vast majority of patients, the important problem hinges on whether the hemorrhage has been caused by an ulcerative lesion in the upper gastrointestinal tract or by a ruptured varix. Examination of the patient under emergency conditions by esophagoscopy, gastroscopy, x-ray must impose handicaps that may interfere with the accuracy of interpretation even in the most expert hands. The Sengstaken-Blakemore tube as a therapeutic test is not always reliable since a bleeding gastric varix may be distal to the gastric balloon. Besides, there are risks in using pneumatic tamponade, and these should be avoided when the balloon can do no good. Extensive experience has indicated that splenic pulp manometry can be employed with minimal risk and that pressures obtained by this method correlate very closely with portal pressures secured at operation. When a splenic pulp pressure of less than 250 mm H_2O is obtained, one can be assured that varices are not present and that bleeding is due to some other lesion. When the pressure is 290 or above, it is practically certain that varices are present and the probable cause of the hemorrhage. Values between 250 and 290 are indeterminate but still valuable. If the hemorrhage is caused by varices, the chances are good that tamponade will be effective. If active and persistent bleeding continues with the pulp pressure in the indeterminate range, it is then highly probable that the bleeding is caused by some other lesion than varices. Moreover, when it is important to resolve the doubt, portography will be decisive.

There is no unanimity regarding the criteria that determine when surgical intervention should be employed for bleeding not due to an esophageal lesion

or a blood dyscrasia. Hematemesis should first be managed as a medical problem, and in any case, the patient should not be subjected to operation until he represents a good operative risk, which means restoration of the blood volume to near-normal levels. A full discussion of this matter should be consulted in Chaps. 179 and 180.

REFERENCES

Ariel, I. M.: The Site of Upper Gastrointestinal Bleeding Detection by Radioactive-tagged Red Blood Cells, J.A.M.A., 180:213, 1962.

Brick, I. B., and H. J. Jeghers: Gastrointestinal Hemorrhage (Excluding Peptic Ulcer and Esophageal Varices), New England J. Med., 253:458, 511, 555, 1955.

Flatley, F. J., M. E. Atwell, and R. K. McEvoy: Pseudoxanthoma Elasticum with Gastric Hemorrhage, A.M.A. Arch. Int. Med., 112:352, 1963.

Ghrist, T. D.: Gastrointestinal Involvement in Neurofibromatosis, A.M.A. Arch. Int. Med., 112:357, 1963.

Grove, W. J.: Biliary Tract Hemorrhage as Cause of Hematemesis, A.M.A. Arch. Surg., 83:67, 1961.

Hood, R. H., and J. A. McChesney: Hiatus Hernia with Esophagitis and Acute Hemorrhage, J.A.M.A., 182:243, 1962.

Jones, F. A., A. E. Read, and J. L. Stubbe: Alimentary Bleeding of Obscure Origin. A Follow-up Study and Commentary, Brit. Med. J., 1:1138, 1959.

Panke, W. F., L. M. Rousselot, and A. H. Moreno: Splenic Pulp Manometry in Differential Diagnosis, Surg. Gynecol. Obstet., 109:270, 1959.

Weiss, A., E. R. Pitman, and E. C. Graham: Aspirin and Gastric Bleeding. Gastroscopic Observations, with Review of Literature, Am. J. Med., 31:266, 1961.

29 JAUNDICE AND HEPATOMEGALY
Frank L. Iber

JAUNDICE

Normally the bilirubin derived from the breakdown of hemoglobin in the reticuloendothelial system is discharged into the blood and excreted by the liver. When the rate of excretion fails to match that of pigment production, bilirubin accumulates in the serum and ultimately stains the tissues, giving rise to the characteristic yellow pigmentation known as *jaundice* or *icterus*.

Bilirubin may be found in the blood in two different forms. Free or unconjugated bilirubin (Fig. 29-1) is the form released from the breakdown of hemoglobin. It is relatively insoluble in water and circulates tightly bound to albumin. Conjugated bilirubin is esterified with two molecules of glucuronic acid on the propionic acid side chains and is more water-soluble. Normal concentrations of serum bilirubin range from 0.5 to 1.2 mg per 100 ml, and all the pigment is in the free form. The precise level at which icterus becomes clinically evident varies because the yellowness ob-

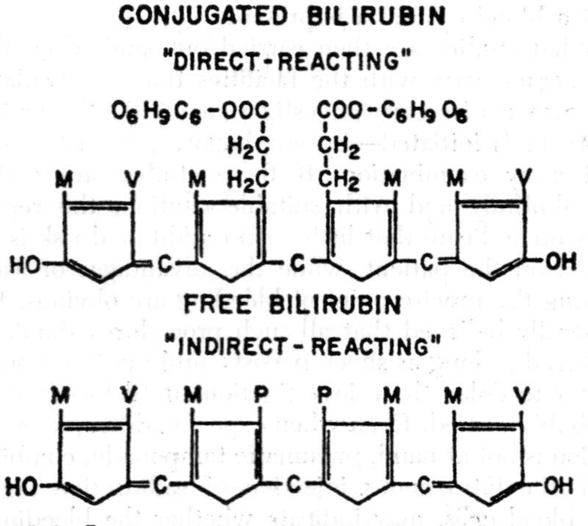

Fig. 29-1. Free or unconjugated bilirubin. (Adopted from Abraham Cantarow, Metabolism of Hemoglobin and Bile Pigments, chap. 27 in sec. V, of "Hemoglobin—Its Precursors and Metabolites," Sunderman and Sunderman (Eds.), Philadelphia, J B. Lippincott Company, 1964.)

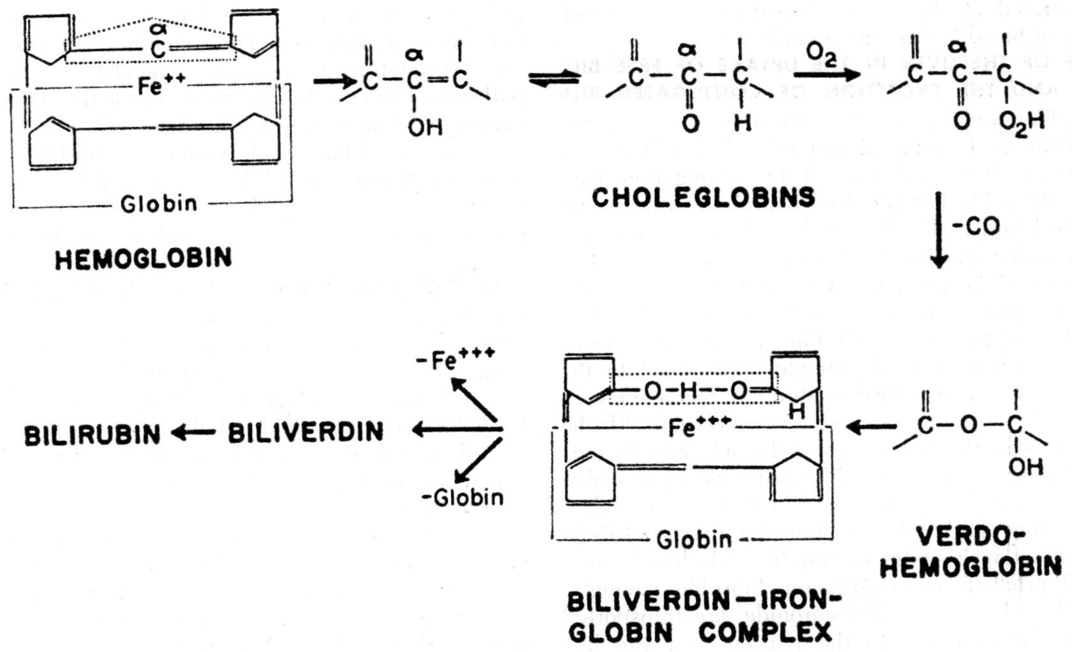

Fig. 29-2. Steps in the conversion of the haptoglobin-hemoglobin complex to free bilirubin, iron, globin, and haptoglobin. (*From Lester and Schmid, New Engl. J. Med., 270 (15): 780, 1964.*)

served depends on tissue staining rather than on the serum levels. The intensity of tissue staining depends on the type of bilirubin present in the serum and its level, the duration of elevation, and the nature of the tissue. When a high proportion of the pigment is conjugated, icterus is detectable at levels of 2 to 3 mg per 100 ml, for this form of the pigment stains the superficial tissues much more readily than free bilirubin. Most jaundice in adults results from predominantly conjugated bilirubin. This jaundice is more readily observed in tissues rich in elastic fibers, which accounts for the earlier appearance and greater intensity of the jaundice in the scleras and the skin of the face and upper trunk. Free bilirubin is more lipid-soluble and stains the fat depots more readily than the skin or elastic tissues; this accounts in part for the higher levels of serum bilirubin necessary to produce clinically apparent jaundice with this type of bilirubin. In jaundice predominantly due to free bilirubin the concentration must rise to 3 to 4 mg per 100 ml before it is clinically apparent. The skill of the examiner and the lighting determine whether or not minimal tissue staining is observed.

Early in the course of jaundice virtually all the pigment found in the serum is bilirubin. Later, however, small amounts of other unidentified pigments appear. Presumably these are bilirubin derivatives that arise in the bile-stained tissues, but their composition and origin are still uncertain.

PIGMENT METABOLISM—DEGRADATION OF HEMOGLOBIN TO BILIRUBIN. When a circulating erythrocyte reaches the end of its normal life span of approximately 120 days or is destroyed prematurely for any reason, it releases its hemoglobin into the blood stream, where it becomes attached to a globulin called *haptoglobin*. The haptoglobin-hemoglobin complex is taken up by the reticuloendothelial system and converted to free bilirubin, iron, globin, and heptoglobin. The known steps of this conversion are outlined in Fig. 29-2.

The normal pathway of hemoglobin degradation starts with the oxidative removal of the carbon atom in the alpha-methene bridge opening the porphyrin ring. The carbon leaves in the form of carbon monoxide, the only known reaction in human beings in which carbon monoxide is formed. Determination of the rate of CO production is a precise measurement of the conversion of hemoglobin to bilirubin. Biliverdin is a green-colored intermediate in this reaction and is rapidly and totally converted to bilirubin. The free bilirubin formed by this reaction is discharged into the plasma and becomes tightly bound to albumin.

Normally most of the bilirubin derived from hemoglobin appears to follow the pathway described, the principal sites of formation being the reticuloendothelial cells of the bone marrow, spleen, and liver. However, under pathologic conditions, and possibly to some extent under normal conditions, bilirubin may be derived from hematin, the trivalent iron hydroxide of protoporphyrin IX. Thus, in severe hemolytic states, such as erythroblastosis fetalis, blackwater fever, and *Clostridium perfringens* sepsis, intravascular hemolysis occurs with the release of free hematin. The latter combines with serum albumin to form methemalbumin, which in turn is converted to bilirubin, probably in the reticuloendothelial system by a mechanism similar to that involved in the degradation of heme. Similarly, the formation of bilirubin from hematin can be demonstrated at the site of hematomas and in collections of blood in the serosal cavities.

ROLE OF THE LIVER IN THE UPTAKE OF FREE BILIRUBIN AND THE EXCRETION OF CONJUGATED BILIRUBIN. The insolubility of free bilirubin in water poses a problem in its removal from the body. However, the normal liver solubilizes it by conjugation with glucuronic acid. Initially free bilirubin is taken up from the blood by the liver cells. Whether or not bilirubin remains attached to the albumin when it enters the liver cell is uncertain. Conjugation is an active enzymatic process occurring in the portion of the liver cells adjacent to the sinusoid. Glucuronic acid is transferred from uridine diphosphoglucuronic acid to the carboxyl groups of bilirubin through the agency of glucuronyl transferase, an enzyme associated with the microsomes of the hepatic parenchymal cells. In normal animals (and presumably man) no appreciable conjugation of bilirubin occurs in tissues other than the liver, but the kidney and intestine may contribute to this function in states of jaundice. The freely soluble end products of conjugation, bilirubin monoglucuronide and bilirubin diglucuronide, are transported through the liver cell to the portion near the bile canaliculus and are excreted into bile. Bilirubin monoglucuronide is an association complex between one molecule of free bilirubin and one of the diglucuronide. There is no convincing evidence that a single molecule of bilirubin with a single molecule of glucuronide exists. Small amounts of other water-soluble bilirubin conjugates, especially the sulfate conjugate, are demonstrable in bile. These also are the products of enzyme action. No free bilirubin is excreted into the bile, though the monoglucuronide is excreted.

The pathways of bilirubin metabolism through the blood stream and through the liver are shared by other substances. Thus, sulfa derivatives and other drugs have the identical binding sites on albumin as bilirubin and competitively interfere with its binding. Such competition for binding on albumin facilitates the movement of bilirubin into the liver and other tissues. Many substances with a phenolic —OH or a —COOH grouping are conjugated in ether or ester linkage with glucuronic acid by the same enzymes that conjugate bilirubin. Thus, menthol, chloramphenicol, tetrahydrocortisone, and salicylates share this pathway. The excretory mechanism for the removal of conjugated bilirubin from the liver cells into the bile seems identical for a wide variety of substances with an acidic group. Thus, bile salts, bilirubin, and sulfobromophthalein (BSP) share this pathway, and competitive inhibition with one another may be demonstrated.

FATE OF BILIRUBIN. On entering the intestinal tract bilirubin, as a consequence of bacterial action, undergoes a series of reductive reactions leading to the formation of two groups of compounds: (1) the colorless urobilinogens which characteristically react with Ehrlich's reagent to yield red aldehyde complexes, and (2) their colored oxidation products, the urobilins, which on mixing with Schlesinger's solution (zinc acetate in alcohol) yield zinc complexes with an intense green fluorescence. Since all these compounds have the same physiologic significance and are measured together in quantitative analyses (following preliminary reduction of the urobilins), it is customary to consider them collectively as urobilinogen, irrespective of their chemical structure or whether they are found in the urine, feces, or bile.

As shown in Fig. 29-3, bilirubin is reduced successively to mesobilirubin, dihydromesobilirubin, and finally to the two colorless urobilinogens, mesobilirubinogen and stercobilinogen. To a variable degree these are then oxidized to their respective urobilins: l-urobilin, which is optically inactive, and l-stercobilin, which is levorotatory.

It is to be emphasized that only conjugated bilirubin undergoes this bacterial conversion at a significant rate. Less than 5 per cent of duodenally administered free bilirubin undergoes these changes. Hemoglobin in the gastrointestinal tract does not give rise to either bilirubin or urobilinogen. Free bilirubin is absorbed in the small intestine to a greater degree than conjugated bilirubin. The majority of conjugated bilirubin passes with the fecal stream to the colon, where most of the bacterial changes occur. Only a small fraction

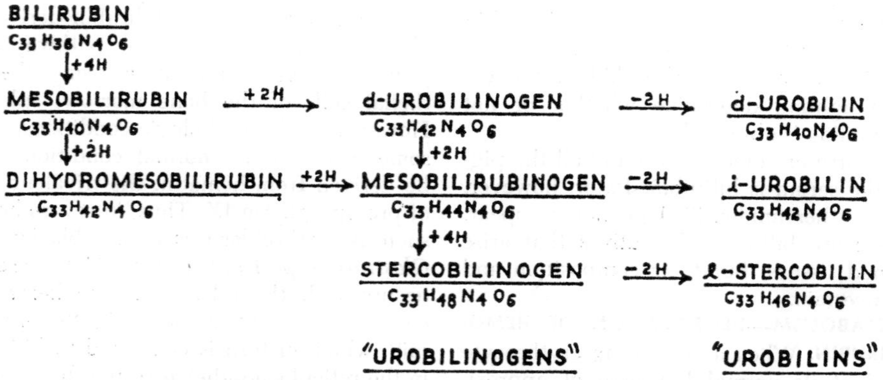

BILIRUBIN
$C_{33}H_{36}N_4O_6$
$\downarrow +4H$

MESOBILIRUBIN $\xrightarrow{+2H}$ d-UROBILINOGEN $\xrightarrow{-2H}$ d-UROBILIN
$C_{33}H_{40}N_4O_6$ $C_{33}H_{42}N_4O_6$ $C_{33}H_{40}N_4O_6$
$\downarrow +2H$ $\downarrow +2H$

DIHYDROMESOBILIRUBIN $\xrightarrow{+2H}$ MESOBILIRUBINOGEN $\xrightarrow{-2H}$ l-UROBILIN
$C_{33}H_{42}N_4O_6$ $C_{33}H_{44}N_4O_6$ $C_{33}H_{42}N_4O_6$
             $\downarrow +4H$

             STERCOBILINOGEN $\xrightarrow{-2H}$ l-STERCOBILIN
             $C_{33}H_{48}N_4O_6$ $C_{33}H_{46}N_4O_6$

             "UROBILINOGENS"   "UROBILINS"

Fig. 29-3. Reduction of bilirubin to mesobilirubin, dihydromesobilirubin, and the two urobilinogens, mesobilirubinogen and stercobilinogen. (*From Gerald Klatskin, Ann. Rev. Med., 12:228, 1961.*)

of conjugated bilirubin is converted to free bilirubin in the intestine. When the intestinal bacteria are suppressed with broad-spectrum antibiotics or by creating an ileostomy, unchanged bilirubin is excreted in the feces.

Normally about half (70 mg per day) of the urobilinogen formed in the intestine is reabsorbed and returned via the portal vein to the liver, where it is reexcreted into the bile (the enterohepatic circulation). Under normal conditions a small amount reaches the general circulation and is excreted by the kidneys, the amount excreted not exceeding 4 mg per day. However, if the liver is no longer able to clear the blood of reabsorbed urobilinogen, as in liver disease or when the bilirubin output is greatly increased, as in hemolytic jaundice, the urinary excretion of urobilinogen increases. In hemolytic jaundice the urinary urobilinogen may be increased two- or fourfold.

In a normal individual with a blood volume of 5 liters and a hemoglobin concentration of 15 Gm per 100 ml, the total circulating hemoglobin is 750 Gm. Since approximately one–one hundred and twentieth of the red cells are destroyed daily, 6.3 Gm hemoglobin is released for degradation. Assuming quantitative conversion of heme to bilirubin and thence to urobilinogen, the expected daily output of urobilinogen would be approximately 250 mg. Radioactive labeling experiments have indicated that a portion of the stool urobilinogen is derived from some source other than the hemoglobin of circulating erythrocytes. There is direct evidence that part of this fraction of bilirubin is produced directly by the liver and part as a by-product of hemoglobin synthesis in the bone marrow. In normal persons this pathway accounts for approximately 10 per cent of the total bilirubin production, so that the expected daily output of urobilinogen would be about 275 mg. However, the normal output of fecal urobilinogen ranges from 40 to 280 mg daily and is fairly constant when measured repeatedly in the same normal person. This discrepancy between the predicted and measured values for pigment production is not adequately accounted for by unreduced bilirubin or known further breakdown products of urobilinogen. It is likely, therefore, that there is an as yet undetermined pathway for the breakdown of bilirubin molecules in the intestine.

SPECIAL PROBLEMS OF BILIRUBIN METABOLISM. Urinary Excretion of Bilirubin. Free bilirubin cannot get into the urine, so that normally the urine contains no bilirubin. However, when conjugated bilirubin is present in the blood, it appears in the urine. The amount excreted in this way may be significant in bilirubin removal when normal hepatic or biliary pathways are blocked, and appears to be directly related to the glomerular filtration rate and the serum level of conjugated bilirubin.

Available studies indicate that bilirubin reaches the urine predominantly by filtration at the glomerulus. The rate of excretion does not correlate exactly with the level of circulating conjugated bilirubin, however,

indicating that other unknown factors play a role. At the onset of viral hepatitis, for example, bilirubin often appears in the urine at a time when the serum levels of conjugated bilirubin are only minimally elevated.

Extrahepatic Bilirubin Removal. Four circumstances exist in which paradoxic extrahepatic bilirubin removal seems to occur. (1) When the common bile duct is obstructed, the bilirubin level in the serum rises to a plateau, often at a level under 20 mg per 100 ml serum. At this time the rate of production of bilirubin is at least as fast as normal but further accumulation in the serum does not occur. Urinary excretion of conjugated bilirubin accounts for at least half the pigment produced under these conditions. (2) The Crigler-Najjar syndrome, a rare inborn error of metabolism, is associated with an inability of the liver to conjugate bilirubin, yet the bilirubin level reaches a plateau in such persons (see Chap. 194). Conversion of bilirubin to a water-soluble material excreted into the intestinal juices and urine seems to occur. (3) In jaundiced persons exposed to bright sunlight or ultraviolet irradiation there is a fall in the serum bilirubin level, unassociated with an increased excretion of any of the known products of bilirubin metabolism. (4) Similarly patients or animals treated with anti-inflammatory adrenal steroids show a decrease in serum bilirubin concentration that cannot be adequately accounted for by an increased excretion of known products of bilirubin or a decrease in hemoglobin breakdown. Observations such as these suggest that bilirubin may be degraded before it is excreted or that there may be an alternative pathway for the breakdown of hemoglobin that does not yield bilirubin.

Role of the Placenta in Bilirubin Metabolism in the Newborn. The mammalian placenta is capable of rapidly transporting free bilirubin from the fetal to the maternal circulation and thus serves to rid the fetus of bilirubin. In contrast, it is relatively impermeable to conjugated bilirubin, so that the pigment does not enter the fetal accumulation when there is maternal hyperbilirubinemia of the conjugated type.

Chemical Tests of Bilirubin Metabolism. The most widely employed chemical reaction for the determination of bilirubin in serum is the van den Bergh reaction. Water-soluble bilirubin (conjugated) reacts promptly with diazotized sulfanilic acid, with initial splitting of the bilirubin molecule at the middle methene bridge. Subsequently two colored molecules are produced from the dipyrrole fragments, and these may be readily determined by colorimetry. Free bilirubin reacts more slowly and incompletely unless made soluble by the addition of alcohol to the reaction mixture. Thus, the direct-reacting pigment, or the 1-min-reacting fraction parallels the conjugated bilirubin, and the indirect-reacting pigment (the difference between the color developing in 1 min and that which eventually develops on the addition of alcohol) parallels free bilirubin.

It should be recognized that the direct- and indirect-reacting pigments measured in the van den

Bergh reaction represent approximations of conjugated and free bilirubin, respectively. Even the laborious extraction and chromatographic techniques required to identify these two pigments precisely are relatively insensitive and lack quantitative precision.

The amount of bilirubin in the urine may be determined by either the Harrison spot test or the Ictotest[1] tablet test. The latter is more sensitive and more convenient to carry out.

Urobilinogen may be estimated in the urine by the semiquantitative Watson-Schwartz or the Diamond qualitative test.

Normally urobilinogen is found in a freshly voided urine at least 90 per cent of the time. An elevation in the level of urine urobilinogen is found most frequently in the presence of liver disease, increased production of bilirubin, or after a portacaval shunt. Absent urobilinogen in the urine suggests failure of bilirubin to reach the intestine. Occasionally total absence of urobilinogen in the urine is found in normal persons and patients on antibiotics. Patients with iliostomy frequently have no urobilinogen in the urine.

The estimate of fecal urobilinogen must be done quantitatively to be of value. The spot tests available on stool for bile salts or bilirubin pigments are too often misleading to be carried out with regularity. An increase in amount of pigment reaching the intestine may be the result of either increased breakdown of red cells or the resumption of bile flow following a period of biliary obstruction. Table 29-1 lists methods available for the detailed evaluation of bilirubin metabolism.

Table 29-1. SPECIAL TESTS TO EVALUATE
BILIRUBIN METABOLISM

1. Rate of conversion of hemoglobin to bilirubin
   a. Direct: rate of CO production
   b. Indirect: rate of red cell breakdown (Cr^{51} turnover); rate of labeling of fecal urobilinogen after C^{14} glycine
   c. Very indirect: indices of hemolysis: percentage saturation of circulating haptoglobin; reticulocyte count
2. Rate of bilirubin uptake: bilirubin tolerance test
3. Rate of conjugation of bilirubin by liver
   a. Direct: assay glucuronyl transferase in liver biopsy
   b. Indirect: rate of conjugation of menthol, N-acetyl-*p*-amino phenol, cortisone or cortisol
4. Rate of excretion of bilirubin conjugates by liver
   a. Direct: duodenal intubation and collection of bile
   b. Indirect: rate of biliary excretion of BSP (Chap. 188)
5. Conversion of bilirubin to urobilinogen: measurement of fecal urobilinogen

Jaundice may result from increased production of bilirubin, impairment in the capacity of the liver to take up, conjugate, transport, or excrete bilirubin, or obstruction of bile drainage (Table 29-2).

It is helpful in clinical diagnosis to subdivide the various forms of jaundice into those accompanied by predominantly *unconjugated* or *indirect-reacting bilirubin* in the serum (no bilirubin in urine) (1, 2, 3 of

[1] Trademark of Ames Company.

Table 29-2) and those with predominantly conjugated or direct-reacting bilirubin (4 and 5 of Table 29-2). The term "regurgitation" was applied to those forms of jaundice with mostly direct-reacting pigment (4 and 5 of Table 29-2), and the term "retention" applied to those forms with mostly indirect-reacting pigment (1, 2, and 3 of Table 29-2).

Table 29-2. CLASSIFICATION OF JAUNDICE BASED ON THE
UNDERLYING ALTERATION IN PIGMENT METABOLISM*

I. Increased production of bilirubin
   A. Increased breakdown of erythrocytes
   B. Increased "shunt" bilirubin
II. Impaired transfer of free bilirubin to liver cells: Gilbert's syndrome (some cases)
III. Impaired conjugation of bilirubin
   A. Failure of maturation of necessary enzymes—premature infants
   B. Inborn error of metabolism
      1. Crigler-Najjar syndrome
      2. Gilbert's syndrome (some cases)
   C. Inhibition of enzymes for conjugation—placental hormones
   D. Occasional cases of acquired liver disease
IV. Impaired transport and excretion of bilirubin conjugates
   A. Dubin-Johnson and Rotor syndrome
   B. Most cases of acquired liver disease
   C. Drug-induced cholestatic jaundice
   D. Idiopathic cholestatic jaundice
V. Obstruction to biliary drainage
   A. Extrahepatic biliary obstruction
   B. Intrahepatic biliary obstruction

*Note that several conditions appear under more than one classification.

(Margin annotations: "indirect serum" bracketing I–III; "Direct serum" bracketing IV–V)

JAUNDICE DUE TO INCREASED PRODUCTION OF BILIRUBIN (A Form of Unconjugated Hyperbilirubinemia). The amount of bilirubin produced depends primarily on the rate of red cell destruction. Normally the intact liver is capable of excreting all but a small fraction of this pigment, so that the concentration of bilirubin in the serum is maintained at a relatively constant low level. However, if bilirubin production is increased two- or threefold as a consequence of abnormally rapid hemolysis, it may exceed the excretory capacity of the liver and give rise to hyperbilirubinemia and jaundice.

The normal production of bilirubin is noted to be about 250 mg per day in a 70-kg man (see p. 121). The liver can excrete approximately 500 mg per day with only a slight rise in the level in the serum. As the concentration of pigment in the serum rises, the amount excreted by the liver increases. In addition, there is a limit to the amount of bilirubin that can be formed by the reticuloendothelial system of human beings from hemoglobin of approximately 1.5 Gm per day, irrespective of the amount of hemoglobin released for degradation. Because of these two limitations, a marked degree of hemolysis is required to raise the serum bilirubin to abnormal levels, and even maximal hemolysis will rarely raise it above 3 to 5 mg per

100 ml *unless complicated by* some degree of hepatocellular dysfunction.

Unconjugated bilirubin is the principal pigment found in the serum of patients with hemolytic jaundice. Small amounts of *direct-reacting pigment* also are often detectable, usually constituting less than 15 per cent of the total serum pigment. The explanation for this is unknown.

Increased production of bilirubin occurs in a variety of circumstances not always readily recognized. Table 29-3 outlines several of these.

Table 29-3. FREQUENT CAUSES OF INCREASED
PRODUCTION OF BILIRUBIN

I. Increased destruction of circulating red blood cells
   A. Inborn errors of metabolism
      1. Constant (sickle-cell disease)
      2. Intermittent (glucose 6-phosphate dehydrogenase deficiency)
   B. Acquired
      1. Lymphoma, lupus erythematosus
      2. Sepsis
      3. Hemolysins (snake bites, mushroom poisoning)
II. Increased destruction of sequestered red blood cells
   A. Absorption of hematomas and intraperitoneal blood
   B. Absorption of blood in massive infarctions
   C. Following burns
III. Increased destruction of transfused erythrocytes
   A. Mismatched transfusion
   B. Blood older than a few days
   C. Coombs-positive hemolytic anemia
IV. Other pathways: Thalassemia

The reserves of the normal liver are sufficient to prevent the onset of jaundice in many of these circumstances. However, increased production of bilirubin often raises the level of serum bilirubin in liver cell disease, in which case the rise in bilirubin is due to increased production of pigment rather than to additional hepatocellular damage.

JAUNDICE DUE TO IMPAIRED TRANSFER OF FREE BILIRUBIN TO LIVER CELLS (A Form of Unconjugated Hyperbilirubinemia). This mechanism for the production of jaundice has not been adequately studied in many conditions. However, specific studies indicate that many patients with Gilbert's familial hyperbilirubinemia have a defect in the transfer of bilirubin into the liver from serum albumin.

JAUNDICE DUE TO IMPAIRED CONJUGATION OF BILIRUBIN (A Form of Unconjugated Hyperbilirubinemia). Table 29-2 outlines circumstances in which impaired conjugation is found. By far, the most frequent is in the newborn. In vitro assays indicate that the normal liver can conjugate over twenty times the normal amount of bilirubin per day, suggesting huge amounts of this function.

Neonatal Jaundice. With few exceptions, newborn infants develop a transient hyperbilirubinemia within the first few days of life. All but a small fraction of the serum bilirubin is unconjugated. This accumulation of pigment is due primarily to a relative deficiency of glucuronyl transferase activity in the liver which limits

the excretion of bilirubin. In addition, the newborn infant may be further handicapped by a deficiency of uridine diphosphoglucose dehydrogenase, the enzyme required for the synthesis of uridine diphosphoglucuronic acid, the glucuronide donor essential for the conjugation of bilirubin. As the liver matures the activity of these two enzymes increases, ultimately attaining adult levels in a few weeks, which coincides with the return of the serum bilirubin level to normal.

The defect in bilirubin conjugation tends to be more severe in premature infants. When this defect is combined with increased breakdown of erythrocytes due to isoimmunization (Rh or other systems), the amount of serum bilirubin may exceed 20 mg per 100 ml, a level at which kernicterus, a serious neurologic disorder due to deposition of unconjugated bilirubin in the brain stem, becomes a threat. In such infants all the circulating bilirubin is unconjugated, the form of pigment responsible for the neurologic damage.

Occasionally, direct-reacting bilirubin in the serum rises to the high levels seen in obstructive jaundice. This has been termed the "inspissated bile syndrome" by those who attribute this type of jaundice to occlusion of the bile ducts by inspissated bile. However, histologic findings indicate hepatocellular disease rather than obstruction as the basis of this syndrome.

Congenital Familial Nonhemolytic Jaundice. (See Chap. 192.)

Jaundice predominantly due to unconjugated bilirubin and of less than 3.5 mg total per 100 ml is found in about 1 per cent of hospitalized patients. Increased production of bilirubin and hepatic disease sufficient to account for the jaundice are not found. The cause of the mild jaundice in such patients remains obscure (see Chap. 192).

JAUNDICE DUE TO IMPAIRED TRANSPORT AND EXCRETION OF BILIRUBIN CONJUGATES. The impaired excretion of conjugated bilirubin for any reason leads to its accumulation in the serum (direct-reacting pigment increases) and its excretion into the urine. The finding of bilirubin in the urine differentiates this and obstructive jaundice from the earlier three causes (Table 29-2).

Two known inborn errors of metabolism exist in which the excretion of conjugated bilirubin is impaired. The Dubin-Johnson syndrome and the Rotor syndrome are presented in Chap. 192.

Acquired hepatocellular disease may be associated with abnormalities in any of the hepatic phases of bilirubin metabolism. However, transport or excretion of conjugates is the most severely impaired of these and is the principal cause of jaundice in most such patients. Thus, the serum contains an excess not only of unconjugated bilirubin but also of its glucuronide, bilirubin, is excreted in the urine, and fecal urobilinogen is reduced. In contrast to obstructive jaundice, urine urobilinogen is increased since the parenchyma no longer is capable of completely clearing the portal blood of urobilinogen entering from the intestinal tract. However, the excretion of bile may be suppressed to such an extent that virtually no bilirubin reaches the intestine. Under these conditions the stools are clay-colored, production and reabsorption of urobilinogen in the intestine are diminished, and the urine urobilinogen falls to a low level or disappears. Hepatocellular jaundice cannot always be differentiated from obstructive jaundice solely on the basis of changes in pigment metabolism, and, indeed, there are instances in which the two are indistinguishable on the basis of any biochemical criteria.

The retention of unconjugated bilirubin in the serum probably reflects the combined effects of impaired uptake, transport, and conjugation of bilirubin by injured hepatic cells. Since the serum invariably contains conjugated bilirubin, it must be assumed that some pigment regurgitates from either the bile or the hepatic cells. Several possible mechanisms have been postulated to account for this phenomenon: (1) rupture of the canaliculi as a consequence of necrosis of the hepatic cells that constitute their walls; (2) occlusion of the canaliculi by inspissated bile or their compression by edema in the surrounding parenchymal cells; (3) obstruction of the terminal intrahepatic bile ducts, the cholangioles, by inflammatory cells; (4) injury to the hepatic cells which impairs their capacity to excrete to a greater extent than their ability to conjugate bilirubin so that the conjugate accumulates in the cells and ultimately diffuses out into the plasma; (5) altered permeability of the parenchymal cells, permitting reflux of the bile from the cell or the canaliculi. Although the escape of bile through rents in the walls of canaliculi in areas of necrosis can be seen occasionally in histologic sections and reflux of bile from the canaliculi into the sinusoids through injured but apparently viable cells has been demonstrated by fluorescent microscopy of the liver in rats injected with fluorescent dyes, the other mechanisms postulated to account for the regurgitation of bile in hepatocellular jaundice are purely speculative and open to question.

Though severe hepatocellular injury leads to a reduction in glucuronyl transferase activity in the liver, high levels of unconjugated bilirubin rarely accumulate. This seems reasonably explained by the observation that despite the reduced glucuronyl transferase activity, the capacity of the damaged liver is far greater for conjugation than for excretion of conjugates. Whether this is true for individual cells or represents the greater capacity of the uninjured cells for conjugation than excretion is uncertain.

Several agents used in clinical medicine interfere with the ability of the liver to excrete conjugates, including conjugated bilirubin. Norethandrolone is the best studied of these agents, and the effect seems the same for a large group of 17-alpha alkyl substituted testosterones. It is not fully agreed whether these agents produce solely an enzymatic change leading to a deficit in transport or anatomic changes. Electron microscopic observations indicate a loss of the microvilli of the smallest intracellular bile capillaries in animals and man exposed to these agents for a prolonged period. It is likely that one or more of the hormones associated with pregnancy produce similar changes,

for the excretion of bilirubin is impaired in the last trimester. This impairment is usually only sufficient to produce mild jaundice (mixed, conjugated and unconjugated) but assumes importance when there is underlying hepatocellular disease or a state or hemolysis is superimposed on the defect.

JAUNDICE DUE TO OBSTRUCTION TO BILIARY DRAINAGE. Complete obstruction of the extrahepatic bile ducts leads to an increase in amount of serum bilirubin, particularly of the direct-reacting type, the appearance of bilirubin in the urine, and the passage of clay-colored stools. As might be expected, the failure of bile to reach the intestine results in the virtual disappearance of urobilinogen from the urine and feces. The concentration of bilirubin in the serum rises progressively and then stabilizes at a level that rarely exceeds 25 mg per 100 ml. Since the rate of hemoglobin breakdown is not diminished, it must be assumed that when a plateau is reached the daily increment of bilirubin is excreted, diverted to the tissues, or degraded to other compounds.

Partial obstruction of the extrahepatic bile ducts may also give rise to jaundice, but only if the intrabiliary pressure is increased, since the excretion of bilirubin does not diminish until the intraductile pressure approaches the maximal secretory pressure of approximately 250 mm bile. Jaundice may occur at very much lower pressures if the obstruction is complicated by infection of the ducts or hepatocellular injury. Jaundice, bilirubinuria, and clay-colored stools are inconstant findings in *incomplete* biliary obstruction, and the amount of urobilinogen in the urine and stool varies with the degree of occlusion. Total obstruction of the bile duct complicated by heavy infection may lead to the production and urinary excretion of urobilinogen.

The functional reserve of the liver is so great that occlusion of the intrahepatic bile ducts does not give rise to jaundice unless the drainage of bile from a large segment of the parenchyma is interrupted. Thus, either of the two major hepatic ducts or a large number of secondary radicles may be occluded without production of jaundice. In experimental animals the ducts draining at least 75 per cent of the parenchyma must be occluded before jaundice appears. This is usually a result of recurrent sepsis of the liver or carcinoma of the bifurcation of the common bile duct.

Obstructive jaundice is a term widely used in clinical medicine and is *most typically represented* by patients in whom the common bile duct is occluded and the bile cannot reach the intestine. In such patients conjugated bilirubin accumulates in the bloodstream, no urobilinogen is formed in the intestine, the stools become white or gray, urobilinogen is totally absent from the urine, and the serum alkaline phosphatase level becomes elevated.

Cholestatic jaundice is the preferred term to describe those cases with the biochemical features of obstructive jaundice but in which no anatomic obstruction may be demonstrated. It occurs frequently in reactions to drugs, e.g., chlorpromazine, occasionally in viral hepatitis or alcoholic hepatitis, and rarely as a recurrent syndrome in otherwise normal persons or as a complication of the last trimester of pregnancy. The Dubin-Johnson syndrome and Rotor syndrome usually have the biochemical features of cholestasis in addition to others.

A few patients have normal bile passages anatomically, yet have the identical changes in bilirubin metabolism, alkaline phosphatase level, and stool color as those with complete obstruction; indeed, no bile reaches the intestine in either. Such patients invariably present problems in diagnosis because of these striking similarities. These patients are often said to have intrahepatic obstruction.

HEPATOMEGALY

The liver normally is almost completely covered on its surfaces accessible to palpation by the ribs or the rectus abdominis muscle. In a normal person who is examined at full inspiration in full relaxation the liver is frequently palpable. The liver is readily palpable when displaced by a low diaphragm on the right or by an abscess or tumor between the liver and the diaphragm. The liver enlarges in all directions except up toward the diaphragm and may be much more enlarged than its inferior displacement indicates. Thus, the detection of hepatomegaly by palpation has its limitations; but despite these limitations, it remains an important diagnostic sign.

The liver makes up about 2 per cent of the body weight; about two-thirds of its cells are hepatocytes and the remainder are reticuloendothelial cells (or Kupffer cells). The liver at rest receives about one-fifth of the output of the heart and produces about 2,000 ml per day of bile. Hepatomegaly may result from obstruction to the outflow of any of the fluids coming into the liver or produced there (blood, bile, lymph), infiltration of the liver with fat, glycogen, tumor, amyloid or other metabolic products, inflammation or regeneration. The cells of the reticuloendothelial system or the liver cells may be the predominant site of enlargement.

A patient with hepatomegaly should be examined carefully to ascertain that one is palpating the liver rather than other right upper quadrant masses and, if necessary, this should be confirmed by special studies such as a scintiscan of the liver or x-rays taken with the bile ducts or blood vessels of the liver opacified or with the surrounding structures made radio-apparent by perihepatic air injection or barium in the gastrointestinal tract.

The possible causes of hepatomegaly (Table 29-4) should be systematically reviewed and simple observa-

tions of the patient made to eliminate or support each of them. Thus, circulatory and biliary obstruction can often be ruled out by the absence of elevation of the venous pressure or obstructive jaundice. The specific methods for study of the liver are discussed in Chap. 188.

Table 29-4. CAUSES OF A PALPABLE LIVER AND HEPATOMEGALY

I. Palpable liver without hepatomegaly
    A. Right diaphragm displaced downward: asthma or emphysema
    B. Mass between liver and diaphragm: abscess or tumor
    C. Aberrant lobe of liver: Riedel's lobe
    D. Extremely thin or relaxed abdominal muscles: postpartum abdomen
    E. Thin persons well relaxed: 1 cm of liver is normal
II. Hepatomegaly with palpable liver
    A. Impaired drainage of blood from the liver: heart failure
    B. Impaired drainage of bile from the liver: obstructive jaundice
    C. Impaired drainage of lymph from the liver
    D. Infiltration of sinusoids or Kupffer's cells
        1. Glycogen storage disease
        2. Amyloid
        3. Tumor
        4. Extramedullary hematopoiesis
        5. Lymphoma and leukemia
        6. Gaucher's disease
    E. New growths: primary and secondary tumors, benign and malignant
    F. Inflammations
        1. Parasitic and bacterial
        2. Following liver injury, toxic
        3. With liver cell necrosis
    G. Regeneration of liver
III. Hepatomegaly without a palpable liver
    A. Very obese or muscular or uncooperative patient
    B. Enlargement predominantly in caudate lobe: pancreatic carcinoma
    C. Enlargement predominantly posteriorly or laterally, occasionally in cirrhosis

REFERENCES

Arias, I. M.: The Transport of Bilirubin in the Liver, in "Progress in Liver Disease," vol. 1, H. Popper and F. Schaffner (Eds.), New York, Grune & Stratton, Inc., 1961.

Klatskin, G.: Bile Pigment Metabolism, Ann. Rev. Med., 12:211, 1961.

Lester, Roger, and Rudi Schmid: Bilirubin Metabolism, New Engl. J. Med., 270:779, 1964.

Sherlock, S.: Jaundice, Brit. Med. J., 1:1359, 1962.

Section 6

Alterations in Body Weight

30 LOSS OF WEIGHT
George W. Thorn

Weight loss as elicited by history or detected by physical examination constitutes a cardinal manifestation of disease or disordered bodily function, unless an otherwise normal individual has imposed on himself caloric restriction in an effort to reduce.

Under normal circumstances decreased food intake or total starvation initiates a constellation of metabolic changes designed to reduce energy expenditure and heat loss. Chief among these are reduced basal metabolic rate, lowered body temperature, restricted physical activity, and reduced peripheral blood flow (vasoconstriction). By these means the body attempts to maintain the function of vital organs such as the heart, brain, kidneys, liver, and lungs. These mechanisms are seriously impaired when complications such as fever, vomiting, diarrhea, and dehydration supervene.

Anorexia is a frequent accompaniment of chronic as well as acute disease processes. In the absence of specific abnormalities of gastrointestinal function, loss of appetite may be due to toxic products liberated by microorganisms, by breakdown products of tumor tissue, or by retention of metabolic end products as occurs in late-stage renal and hepatic disease. Hypo-osmolarity of the body fluid compartment and increased cell water content may give rise to centrally mediated nausea and vomiting through its effect on specific hypothalamic centers. Thus, a patient with malignant hypertension may experience nausea as a consequence of vascular changes in the hypothalamic centers of brain or, later, as a result of retention of nitrogenous products with progressive renal failure.

In evaluating the implication of weight loss several considerations deserve special attention.

1. Is the patient's history concerning the magnitude and duration of weight loss reliable? Can it be documented by comparison with prior measurements or confirmed by physical examination?

2. Has there been a notable change in appetite or food intake?

3. Has there been evidence of disordered gastrointestinal function with a change in bowel habits?

4. Has there been evidence of polyuria, particularly nocturia?

The determination of the *magnitude of weight loss* is not always easy. Some patients follow changes in weight regularly on bathroom scales or weighing machines, or they have serial physical examinations.

Other patients may be quite vague or uninformed regarding actual changes in weight. Questions regarding a change in waist measurement or collar, suit, dress, or shoe size may provide helpful clues. Physical examination should then confirm this, with its opportunity to detect adipose tissue loss and the presence or absence of edema or dehydration. Special consideration should be given to the evaluation of overall weight loss in the presence of edema, as the actual tissue loss in such patients will, of course, greatly exceed the apparent decrease in total body weight.

Weight loss with anorexia and decreased food intake occurs in such a diversified range of acute and chronic diseases as not to be particularly helpful in differential diagnosis. The magnitude of weight loss may reflect either the *seriousness* or the *duration* of the underlying disorder. Thought should be given to the diagnosis of psychologic difficulties such as depression and anorexia nervosa, to generalized endocrine and metabolic disorders such as pituitary-adrenal insufficiency and hyperparathyroidism, and to hepatic and renal disease, as well as to chronic infection, neoplasm, and drug intoxication. Weight loss without a significant change in food consumption would suggest hypermetabolic states, such as thyrotoxicosis and anxiety or gastrointestinal hypermotility.

Of course, particular attention will be given in the history to any abnormality in gastrointestinal function as a cause of weight loss. Here again, one is concerned with *decreased food intake* such as might occur in partial intestinal obstruction; *decreased absorption*, which suggests pancreatic or hepatic disease, spruelike syndromes, regional enteritis, or severe food allergies; or *increased loss of food* and *fluids* through vomiting, diarrhea, or draining fistulas. Disorders of gastrointestinal function accompany systemic disorders so frequently that the physician must always maintain a high index of suspicion that what appears to be primarily a disorder of gastrointestinal function may actually reflect deep-seated infection, tumor, or renal, hepatic, cardiac, or pulmonary disease. On the other hand, *specific gastrointestinal disorders* may complicate systemic disease; thus, the patient with nausea, vomiting, and renal azotemia may have an associated peptic ulcer.

The presence of polyuria, and particularly nocturia, in association with anorexia and weight loss suggests diabetes mellitus, diabetes insipidus, chronic renal disease, and disorders giving rise to *hypercalcemia* or *hypokalemia*.

Physicians should encourage patients to weigh regularly and to maintain a lifelong record of changes in body weight, since alterations in weight so frequently mirror abnormalities in bodily function. Loss of weight may be the first indication of serious organic disease or psychologic disorder, the detection and significance of which may be measurably enhanced by carefully recorded changes in body weight.

31 GAIN IN WEIGHT
George W. Thorn

Gain in weight as a manifestation of disease or disordered function reflects an excessive accumulation of adipose tissue or fluid. In either instance, the excess may be generalized or local. However, a significant increase in total body weight usually reflects widespread accumulation of adipose tissue or edema fluid, although the distribution need not be uniform.

EXCESSIVE ACCUMULATION OF ADIPOSE TISSUE

NORMAL CALORIC INTAKE WITH REDUCED ENERGY EXPENDITURE. A decrease in basal metabolic rate and activity accompanies hypothyroidism and anterior pituitary deficiency. Some decrease in activity with an increased tendency for obesity occurs with primary gonadal failure—particularly in the female. Advancing age is characteristically attended by a progressive lowering of basal metabolic rate and, of course, in most instances with an appreciable reduction in physical activity. Disorders or diseases which limit ambulation, such as cardiac or pulmonary failure or bone and joint disease, will also predispose to weight gain unless caloric intake is appropriately readjusted.

Hypothyroidism may be suspected in an individual who has developed intolerance to cold, whose skin has become dry and coarse, and whose reflexes are hypoactive (see Chap. 82). Weight gain associated with a more severe degree of hypothyroidism or myxedema may be due to edema, ascites, and pleural effusion.

Anterior pituitary deficiency of a mild degree such as that described by Sheehan (Chap. 80) may be accompanied by weight gain. This syndrome is most frequently observed in women after childbirth. Hypopituitarism in males as well as in females may be caused by a chromaphobe adenoma or cyst of the pituitary. In such instances, a clue to the disorder may present as a result of local pressure, i.e., headache or visual disturbances. In all types of mild hypopituitarism one looks for signs of target gland deficiency, i.e., thyroid, adrenal, or gonadal. In the case of the latter, impotence in men and oligomenorrhea or amenorrhea in women may be important presenting evidence. The signs of secondary hypothyroidism do not differ ap-

preciably from those of primary, except that thyroid enlargement is not expected. Secondary adrenal cortical insufficiency is *not* associated with hyperpigmentation and rarely presents as severe mineral (aldosterone) deficiency. Hypoglycemic manifestations are frequently observed.

A decrease in physical activity secondary to a change in occupation, to traumatic injury, to heart disease, or to other incapacitating illnesses, will result in increased adiposity if normal caloric intake is maintained. In this instance there is no pathologic significance other than the generally unfavorable effect of obesity on weight-bearing joints.

INCREASED CALORIC INTAKE. Excessive food intake secondary to organic disease occurs most commonly in response to a hypoglycemic stimulus. When hypoglycemic symptoms occur under fasting conditions, one considers hyperinsulinism and pancreatic tumor. When hypoglycemic manifestations occur 3 to 5 hr after a meal, one may suspect the paradoxic hypoglycemic response of early diabetes mellitus (see Chap. 88). In the latter case it is thought that the prolonged elaboration of insulin represents an inappropriate response to the initial postprandial hyperglycemia. Occasionally traumatic injuries of the brain, localized encephalitis, and brain tumors appear to modify the satiety centers in the hypothalamus, with resulting stimulation of appetite over and above caloric needs.

Excessive food intake, or compulsive eating, may also reflect serious psychologic or emotional disorders. In this instance the ingestion of food has special significance for the patient. The importance of identifying major psychologic disturbances as a cause of weight gain cannot be overemphasized (see Chap. 78).

EXCESSIVE ACCUMULATION OF FLUID

Whereas a gradual increase in weight may be caused by increased adipose tissue or edema, a sudden increase in weight, i.e., in excess of 1 lb per day, must certainly indicate excess fluid retention. Excess fluid accumulation or edema (see Chap. 16) should suggest underlying renal, cardiac, or hepatic insufficiency. Hypoalbuminemia usually suggests renal disease, but it may reflect nutritional deficiency secondary to small-bowel pathology or inadequate protein intake. Occasionally, primary retention of water with hyponatremia will result from inappropriate antidiuretic hormone secretion. Excess salt intake, licorice, and drugs such as sex hormones, adrenal steroids, Dilantin, and reserpine may contribute to salt and water retention. The presence of edema and weight gain may mask a significant loss of body tissue. This is best exemplified by the cardiac or hypertensive patient who, following a brisk diuresis, becomes aware for the first time of the extent of body wasting.

Obese patients can retain rather large quantities of extracellular fluid without necessarily exhibiting edema. From a practical point of view, it should be assumed that a markedly obese patient has sequestered a significant volume of extracellular fluid. This can often be demonstrated by administering a diuretic agent, and, of course, this is the approach utilized by many "lose-weight-fast" schemes. Some appreciation of the salt- and water-retaining capacity of obese patients, or of patients with incipient edema, may be obtained by weighing the patient in the morning and again at night. It is not unusual for an obese individual, or a preedematous patient to gain 4 to 8 lb during the day, particularly if he is up and about.

CYCLIC EDEMA

This syndrome occurs almost exclusively in women and is characterized by heightened emotional tension with or without demonstrable organic disease, such as increased capillary permeability, hypoproteinemia, or renal, cardiac, or hepatic disorder. Patients frequently are obese and occasionally demonstrate rather marked postural hypotension. The increase in weight may occur suddenly and may amount to 10 to 20 lb in the course of a few days.

In summary, very few organic diseases are associated with a marked gain in adipose tissue. In most instances obesity results from excessive ingestion of food as a result of cultural influences, reduced physical activity, or psychologic and emotional disturbances. In contrast, the accumulation of excessive fluid (edema) should always suggest serious underlying organic disease, the single important exception being the syndrome of cyclic edema in middle-aged women.

Section 7

Alterations in the Integument

32 SKIN LESIONS
Donald M. Pillsbury and Walter B. Shelley

Inspection of the skin and mucous membranes is the simplest of all the procedures of physical examination. Nevertheless the examination of this organ system is frequently incomplete, and the description of presenting lesions inadequate. Sufficient exposure, proper illumination, and thoroughness are essential. Certain sites, such as the scalp, the folds of the skin, the buccal mucous membranes (not just the pharynx), the palms and soles, the anogenital region, and the vaginal membranes are often neglected. Gross diagnostic errors may result solely from insufficient illumination; in obsolescent hospital wards and clinic quarters the natural or artificial illumination available is frequently unsatisfactory. The routine use of a hand lens or a head loupe is essential for assessing many small lesions of the skin, especially moles and tumors.

The diagnosis of a disease affecting the skin often depends on accurate classification of the individual lesions. In diseases in which only the skin is involved, where there is no systemic disturbance, and no specific information is readily obtainable by laboratory studies, the morphologic characteristics furnish the only diagnostic clues. It is therefore important that they be described accurately. This can be done in straightforward, simple terms; there is no need to use an obsolescent or esoteric terminology. The essential facts to be noted are:

1. Distribution of the lesions. Many syndromes affecting the skin have characteristic distributions of lesions, which should be carefully noted, since they may be strongly suggestive of a particular diagnosis. Examples include psoriasis, scabies, syphilis, herpes zoster, variola, discoid lupus erythematosus, photosensitivity, reactions to contactants, and many others.

2. Physical characteristics:

a. Flat, raised, or containing fluid (serous, purulent, or sanguineous).

b. Size, shape, and color.

c. If palpable, any special characteristics.

Many conditions of the skin, especially chronic ones, present a variety of lesions. With few exceptions, however, a skin disease in the individual patient is characterized initially by predominance of a single type of lesion which may be pathognomonic. It is the mark of the expert in any field of medicine or surgery that he is able to sort out the presenting signs and symptoms in a complicated disorder and to determine which are most representative of the underlying disease. This faculty is particularly helpful in classifying diseases of the skin. Among the debris of a chronic dermatosis the characteristic primary or initial lesion represents true diagnostic treasure. From this it is ordinarily possible to determine the chain of secondary consequential lesions.

PRINCIPAL INITIAL LESIONS OF DISEASES AFFECTING THE SKIN. Macule. A macule represents simply a flat, circumscribed change in the color of the skin. The term ordinarily connotes relatively small lesions up to 1 or 2 cm in diameter. Larger lesions are ordinarily referred to as "patches" or "areas." Macular changes are of three general types: (1) those due to extrinsically derived colored materials, such as tattoo marks, or embedded material from lacerations or explosions; (2) those due to intrinsically derived pigment, i.e., flat moles, petechiae, and hemorrhages, or localized increase or decrease of melanin; (3) erythematous reactions to a wide variety of pathogenic agents. In the presence of constitutional symptoms or if there are purpuric changes in the lesion, macules must be regarded as probable evidence of systemic disease. Drug reactions are commonly macular, and this possibility must always be considered.

Papule. Papules are circumscribed elevations of the skin, varying roughly from a millimeter to a centimeter in size. Larger infiltrated areas are often called *plaques*. Nodules are circumscribed, usually solid, lesions which lie deeper in the skin or subcutaneous tissue. The term is frequently applied to inflammatory processes, e.g., erythema nodosum or subcutaneous fat necrosis, but it may be applied to tumors as well.

The majority of papular eruptions may be diagnosed accurately by clinical examination and appropriate laboratory studies, but in those which cannot be classified accurately, biopsy is usually mandatory. The histologic characteristics are, by and large, clear-cut. The most common dermatologic syndromes characterized by papules are tumors, psoriasis, lichen planus, warts, molluscum contagiosum, some drug eruptions, xanthoma, and certain lymphomas, though there are many others. The initial lesions of smallpox may be papular, and secondary syphilis is frequently so. The presence of atrophy or frank scarring immediately narrows the diagnostic considerations; uncomplicated psoriasis, for instance, never produces scarring.

Wheals (hives) are special types of papules. They may remain as small individual lesions but frequently enlarge to form large plaques, often with striking geographic outlines, or they may produce marked swelling of the face or an extremity (*angioderma*). Acute urticaria is most commonly produced by foods, drugs, and insect bites. The cause of chronic recurrent urticaria is usually difficult to determine; psychosomatic influences undoubtedly play a role. Wheals are frequently a component of the eruption of erythema multiforme. Wheals ordinarily respond to antihistaminics, though large doses may be necessary. Corticosteroid therapy is usually promptly effective, though the lesions may recur quickly, often in more severe form, if such treatment is discontinued without removal of the primary etiologic factor.

Vesicles and Bullae. These are sharply circumscribed collections of free fluid in the skin, principally in the outer layers. The most common representatives of vesicular dermatoses are contact dermatitis, dyshidrosis of the hands and feet, and herpes simplex. In most instances of acute vesicular eruptions the principal etiologic factor is readily determinable. Bullae, which are simply large vesicles, represent a very vigorous effort of the skin to counteract some noxious agent. Lesions may be bullous in a severe reaction to a contact allergen, and, of course, chemical irritants or physical agents frequently produce a bullous reaction. In extensive chronic bullous eruptions thorough study is indicated. The more important diseases char-

acterized by bullous lesions are pemphigus, dermatitis herpetiformis, and erythema multiforme (Stevens-Johnson type). Bullae do not occur in psoriasis, in most types of dermatitis other than reactions to contactants or drug eruptions, or in acquired syphilis in the adult.

Pustules. Pustules are simply circumscribed collections of free pus, i.e., very superficial abscesses of the skin. Dermatoses showing both vesicles and pustules are very common, and vesicles frequently become pustular even in the absence of overt bacterial infection. Pustular lesions of the skin cover a wide range of conditions. In pustular eruptions of more than a few days' duration pathogenic bacteria are frequently culturable, but it must not be assumed from this that all such organisms are necessarily acting as etiologic agents in the eruptions.

LESIONS WHICH REPRESENT SEQUENTIAL OR EVOLUTIONARY CHANGES. Scales. These are simply accumulations of loose, horny fragments of stratum corneum. Certain types of scales are quite characteristic, e.g., the greasy, rather yellowish scales of chronic seborrheic dermatitis, or the silvery, piled-up scales of psoriasis. Ichthyosis produces a distinctive type of scaling in which the dead cells of the stratum corneum are much more adherent than in normal skin. Any dermatitis terminates in a scaling phase. In chronic exfoliative dermatitis, the entire skin surface may scale profusely, and this may be a source of significant losses of protein.

Crusts (Scabs). These are the dried remains of exudate from oozing erosions or ulcers. They may consist of dried blood, serum, pus, or an admixture. Unless the diagnosis of a particular dermatosis is readily apparent, representative crusts should always be removed to see what lies underneath. One of the most characteristic of all crusts is that seen in diphtheria cutis, which produces a tenacious and adherent crust unlike that seen in any other infection.

Ulcers. Since ulcers represent a destructive process of the skin, they always require explanation. They may vary from small superficial erosions which heal without perceptible scarring, to deep, sometimes widespread, lesions which involve underlying tissues or even adjacent bone. If the etiologic factor concerned is not readily apparent, such lesions deserve the most thorough study. The factors concerned may sometimes be multiple and obscure. Ulcers may be factitial at times. Severe phagedenic ulcers may be associated with ulcerative colitis. Venereal diseases commonly produce ulcers, e.g., syphilis, chancroid, and lymphogranuloma venereum. In any long-standing ulcer, the possibility of neoplastic disease as a primary or secondary change must receive consideration.

Scars. Scars may, of course, follow ulcers or may result from conditions in which there is no previous ulceration, e.g., discoid lupus, atrophic lichen planus, stasis dermatitis, or circumscribed scleroderma. As with ulcers, if the cause of the scarring is not apparent, thorough and searching study from all standpoints is indicated. The differentiation between hypertrophic scars and keloids is sometimes difficult to make; temporary hypertrophy and elevation of scars after injury is by no means uncommon and may persist for several months. Scars are frequently slightly painful or itchy. Scars from ionizing irradiation are particularly vulnerable to trauma of all types, especially sunlight. Extensive scars from whatever cause, but most particularly those from thermal burns, tuberculosis, and x-ray therapy, are all prone to malignant changes.

CONFIGURATION OF LESIONS. Three characteristics of the configuration or arrangement of multiple lesions have considerable usefulness. They are:

Grouping. Characteristic grouped aggregations of vesicles occur in herpes simplex, zoster, and dermatitis herpetiformis. "Id" reactions in the skin to infections are sometimes grouped, e.g., in tuberculids or dermatophytids. The multicentric foci of epithelioma (*in situ* type) are frequently grouped and gradually coalesce to form a single tumor plaque.

Annularity. This is a striking feature of many dermatoses and reactions to systemic disease. Pityriasis rosea, lichen planus, superficial ringworm infections, bacterial infections, urticaria, erythema multiforme, sarcoidosis, discoid lupus, syphilis, deep fungal infections, and other processes may produce rather characteristic annular lesions.

Linearity. A linear arrangement of individual lesions may come about as part of the basic pattern of the disease, as in localized scleroderma, linear nevi, and herpes zoster. In some diseases the skin reacts to trauma in a characteristic linear pattern, as in lichen planus and psoriasis. Scars and keloids are frequently linear. Viral infections such as warts may be inoculated in the skin by a scratch.

THE PRIMARY INOCULATION OR CHANCRE COMPLEX. The association of a lesion at the site of inoculation with regional adenopathy or with a more or less linear development of subsequent lesions is most commonly seen in acute bacterial infections. Syphilis produces the best known of all the chancre complexes. Primary inoculations of tuberculosis and certain deep fungal infections such as blastomycosis, sporotrichosis, and coccidioidomycosis may follow a pattern of development of an inflammatory papule and ulcer at the site of inoculation. Regional adenopathy and the later development of inflammatory lesions along the areas of lymphatic drainage may occur. The recognition of such a mode of reaction is important in tuberculosis or deep fungal infections, as distinguished from spread of the lesions to the skin from a visceral focus, because the resistance displayed to the infection after inoculation in the skin is often high, and such infections may be self-limited.

DISTRIBUTION OF LESIONS. In some diseases the *pattern of distribution of skin lesions* over the body is so characteristic as to be almost pathognomonic; in others, though one distribution pattern may be most characteristic, variations from it are frequent. The following are diseases which tend to involve certain sites.

Acne. Since acne is a disease in which the follicular orifices and sebaceous glands are affected, the lesions are concentrated in areas where these structures are most abundant, large, and active. The face is the most frequently involved site, but lesions appear on the shoulders, chest, upper part of the back, neck, and upper arms in more extensive forms of the disease. The lack of involvement of the scalp is striking; even in the most severe cases only the scalp margins are invaded. An even more extensive distribution may be seen in so-called "tropical acne," in which the entire trunk may be affected, with lesions on the buttocks and thighs as well.

Rosacea. The lesions of rosacea occur in a highly characteristic pattern. In severe and long-standing examples, diffuse involvement of the face may be noted, but the flush areas are the sites affected initially. These are the malar prominences, the nose, the forehead, and the point of the chin. Rosacea is often seen in middle-aged persons who have had acne in adolescence. There is frequently an associated seborrheic dermatitis. In the more severe forms pustules are common, but these do not characteristically derive from blackheads, as does acne. The differentiation of rosacea from discoid lupus or systemic lupus erythematosus is ordinarily easily made, though, of course, the two conditions may coexist. The eyes should always be examined in rosacea, however mild, because of the infrequent but severe complication of rosacea keratitis.

Seborrheic Dermatitis. This is a third member of the common triad with acne and rosacea. In seborrheic dermatitis of moderate severity the scalp may be the only site involved, but the following areas are affected in approximate order of frequency in more extensive cases: eyebrows, skin above the bridge of the nose, sides of the nose, ears (especially the external auditory canals and retroauricular region), presternal and interscapular areas, eyelid margins (a frequent source of chronic blepharitis), intertriginous areas on any part of the body, especially the axillas, the anogenital region, and under the breasts in women. The skin of the involved areas is peculiarly susceptible to acute or chronic secondary bacterial infection; the intertriginous areas of the toes are rarely involved.

Psoriasis. A tendency to involve the scalp, knees, elbows, and back is characteristic of at least 75 per cent of all cases of psoriasis. The most common alternate distribution of psoriasis is to the seborrheic areas. Psoriasis is frequently misdiagnosed because of a failure to examine the skin carefully and to determine the presence of lesions elsewhere. This is likely if the nails are involved (which is common in psoriasis), when the condition may be wrongly diagnosed as a fungous infection; if the feet and hands are involved, when there may be confusion with ringworm infections and with syphilis; and if the genitalia are involved, when the condition may be taken for moniliasis.

Pityriasis Rosea. The individual lesion of pityriasis

rosea is annular and ovoid, often with a slight border and a characteristic narrow band of moderate scaling just inside this border. In the efflorescence which follows the appearance of the primary or mother plaque the lesions tend to involve principally the trunk and upper portions of the extremities, with the long axis of the lesions strikingly arranged along the lines of cleavage. Even in examples of the disease in which the lesions themselves are unusual, namely, urticarial or more inflammatory, this distribution pattern still holds. The most common alternate distribution is a tendency for the lesions to occur distally on the extremities with relatively no involvement of the trunk. Pityriasis rosea may involve the neck but rarely the face. It is a banal disease, though sometimes very worrisome to the patient. The course is that of a low-grade infection, though a causative organism has never been found. Second attacks occur in no more than 1 per cent of patients. Treatment is usually not necessary, but if the lesions are extensive, inflammatory, and pruritic, corticosteroid therapy for 3 to 4 days will usually give prompt relief.

Scabies. The female *Acarus* prefers the following sites for her burrows: the interdigital spaces of the fingers, the palms, the flexor surface of the wrists, the axillary folds, along the belt line, the buttocks, the genitalia in men, and about the areola of the breasts in women. The head is almost never involved in adults.

Atopic Dermatitis (Disseminated Neurodermatitis). The objective changes in this very chronic disease are principally the result of rubbing and excoriation; they involve the face, neck, antecubital spaces, popliteal fossae, wrists, and thighs. The condition commonly disappears after age twenty-five but sometimes persists in a more localized form such as a chronic dermatitis of the hands.

Contact Dermatitis. Reaction of the skin to external agents, which includes primary chemical irritant effects and true sensitization reactions, has a characteristic distribution involving the exposed sites in the case of industrial contactants, plants, and air-borne pollens and chemicals.

Lichen Planus. This chronic and pruritic disease is of little systemic significance. The milder forms involve the buccal surfaces of the cheek, the genitalia, the flexor surfaces of the wrists, and the trunk. In the hypertrophic form the most marked lesions may be found on the lower legs; this is the usual location of the lichen planus-like lesions of Atabrine dermatitis.

There are, of course, many other diseases with more or less characteristic patterns of distribution.

APPROACH THROUGH THE LABORATORY AND SKIN TESTING

The laboratory aids used in general medicine are, of course, necessary in arriving at a diagnosis of many diseases affecting the skin. Several special methods are also useful.

BIOPSY. Biopsy is an essential procedure in almost all chronic dermatoses, in all pigmented lesions which are excised, and in all lesions where there is a possibility of malignant change or serious systemic disease. The diagnosis of some lesions will require the services of a pathologist with special training in dermatopathology. Others present a clear-cut pathognomonic picture and are easily diagnosed by the general pathologist. A process involving the skin is seldom static. The skin is not bathed in a homeostatic milieu as are internal organs; it is subjected to numerous external influences which may disguise the primary process. It is the responsibility of the clinician to exercise care and judgment in selecting the lesion to be examined, in determining which technique shall be used in obtaining the biopsy, and in providing an informative protocol. The specimen should be typical of the process and least subject to secondary trauma. Generally this is the most recently evolved lesion. Occasionally more than one biopsy may be required before the exact nature of a disease can be determined. Multiple biopsies may be needed in large lesions such as chronic ulcers evolving at the site of an old burn or in granuloma inguinale.

Although consideration should be given to the cosmetic results in the procedure, it must be emphasized that an inadequate biopsy specimen is of no benefit to the pathologist, the physician, or the patient. The most satisfactory procedure is removal of small lesions *in toto* (excision biopsy), and, with larger lesions, the

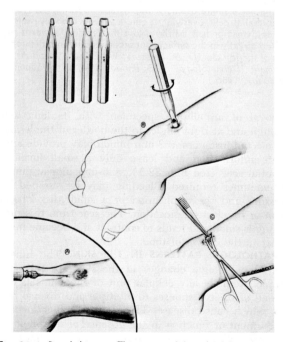

Fig. 32-1. Punch biopsy. This is a useful method for obtaining tissue from lesions in which complete excision is not feasible or when multiple biopsies may be desirable. The removal should extend to the subcutaneous fat. Punches of various diameters, 2 to 8 mm, are shown. (D. M. Pillsbury, W. B. Shelley, and A. M. Kligman: "Dermatology," p. 1331, Philadelphia, W. B. Saunders Company, 1956.)

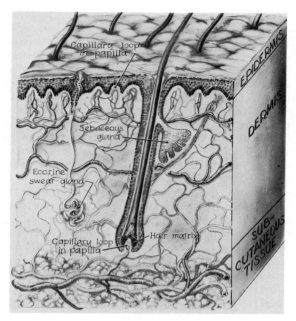

Fig. 32-2. The stratified organization of the skin. The top layer, the epidermis, is thin but solidly cellular, in contrast to the much thicker and largely fibrous corium, which acts mainly as a support for the appendages, vessels, and nerves. The hair is the deepest epidermal appendage, extending down to the subcutaneous tissue, 3 to 5 mm below the surface. Just as the hair papilla is an invagination of connective tissue into the cellular hair matrix, so the papillae of the upper corium extend upward as connective tissue intrusions into the epidermis. Each papilla has a single capillary loop which nourishes the "cap" of epithelial cells overlying it (there are no blood vessels in the epidermis or hair matrix). Note that eccrine sweat is delivered directly to the surface, but sebum empties into the upper part of the follicle. (D. M. Pillsbury, W. B. Shelley, and A. M. Kligman: "Dermatology," p. 3, Philadelphia, W. B. Saunders Company, 1956.)

removal of an elliptic specimen with its long axis through and at right angles to the border of the lesion. In selected instances, a 2-mm punch may provide adequate information and leave only a small inconsequential scar (see Fig. 32-1). A 5-mm biopsy punch is sometimes required. Bleeding may be stopped by pressure and the application of a small disk of gel foam or by electrodesiccation. The scar from this procedure is small and tends to contract and become more linear in the course of time.

PATHOLOGIC PATTERNS IN THE SKIN. The fundamental pathologic changes in the skin are few and simple. Actually any cellular unit of the skin has but a triad of basic responses to multiple and diverse factors which cause disease. These are (1) *functional*—impairment of function in the absence of morphologic changes; (2) *inflammatory*—degenerative changes following cellular injury; and (3) *proliferative*—increase in the number of cells of given type, namely, tumors, benign or malignant.

For purposes of analysis Table 32-1 presents the units of the skin which may undergo changes (see also Fig. 32-2).

Table 32-1. SKIN UNITS

Cells and layer		Epidermal appendages	Systems
Keratinocyte	Epidermis	Hair	Vascular
Melanocyte		Sebaceous gland	Neural
Fibrocyte			
Histiocyte	Dermis	Apocrine gland	Extraneous
Mastocyte			cells
Lipocyte	Subcutaneous	Eccrine sweat	Myeloid
		gland	Lymphoid

The clinician perceives three fundamental morphologic changes in the skin: in *color, mass,* or *fluid content.* The color changes (macules, plaques) usually involve the melanocyte or the vascular system. Changes in mass (papules, nodules, tumors) may result from hyperplasia of any of the units listed. Growths derived from the keratinocyte, melanocyte, and blood vessels are by far the most common. The change in free fluid of the epidermis (vesicle, bulla) is fundamentally a reaction of the keratinocyte to injury. In the dermis extravascular fluid masks itself clinically as a solid mass (urticaria).

EPIDERMIS. Keratinocyte. *Keratinization is the most important function of the epidermis.* Disturbances or lack of other functions are inconvenient but rarely of crucial importance. Complete failure of keratinization is incompatible with life. In addition to the hyperkeratinization which results from chronic injury, certain genetically influenced changes may be seen, an example being congenital hyperkeratosis of the palms and soles. Psoriasis is another disease in which keratinization is disturbed, with failure of the cycle to be completed. In ichthyosis the principal change appears to be a retarded exfoliation of the stratum corneum. This may reach severe degrees and be accompanied by atrophy or absence of eccrine and sebaceous glands.

Melanocyte. This is the second important cell of the epidermis. In the albino, a genetic flaw in enzyme systems (tyrosinase) results in complete failure of pigment formation. Negro skin contains an increased amount of melanin but the same number of melanocytes as white skin. Local areas in which the melanocyte elaborates too little melanin (vitiligo, leukoderma) or too much melanin (chloasma, freckles) are frequent.

The melanin-synthesizing capacity of the skin is regulated by the melanocyte-stimulating hormone (MSH) of the anterior pituitary gland. There is a balance between this hormone and those elaborated by the adrenal cortex which furnishes an explanation for the pigmentation seen in Addison's disease and, perhaps, in pregnancy.

The melanocyte reacts to injurious stimuli by producing less or more melanin. Certain superficial inflammatory processes, e.g., seborrheic dermatitis, may produce temporary depigmentation, but the ordinary response is increased pigment. This is useful in protecting the skin from acute or chronic changes. The incidence of epithelioma is directly related to the amount of sunlight to which the skin of the patient is exposed and to a lessened ability to lay down protective melanin in the epidermis. With aging, the activity of melanocytes varies and dyspigmentation results.

Neoplastic change in the melanocyte accounts for the most common of all skin lesions, the ordinary pigmented nevus, or mole, and is the origin of the most malignant of all skin tumors (malignant melanoma). Simple hyperplasia leads to hyperpigmented, flat macules (lentigo, junction nevus), or even palpable masses. Usually brown or black, nevi may be flesh-colored, indicating an absence of function in the hyperplastic cells. Not all melanocytic nevi are epidermal. Overgrowth of pigmented cells in the dermis gives a blue color (blue nevus, mongolian spot).

The interpretation of various types of pigmented lesions in the skin in terms of the possibility of malignant melanoma is a common and vexing clinical problem which is discussed in some detail later.

CORIUM (DERMIS). The master cell of the dermis is the *fibrocyte*, the source of collagen and ground substance. Normal functioning of this cell is essential to skin repair. Unrestrained reparative activity can lead to large deposits of collagen (keloid). This condition is due to a steady increase in scar tissue which may continue indefinitely in some individuals, principally Negroes. Benign overgrowth of the fibrocyte produces a simple fibroma. Malignant change is rare and produces fibrosarcoma or "spindle cell" sarcoma. Cortisone prevents the normal development of collagenous tissue, and vitamin C deficiency interferes with the elaboration of normal reticulum.

Histiocytes normally phagocytize particulate matter, including melanin (melanophore), lipids (foam cell), hemosiderin, some tattoo pigments, viruses, bacteria, fungi, and protozoa. When confronted with larger masses of material (uric acid crystals, petrolatum), histiocytes commonly fuse to form multinucleated foreign-body giant cells. In xanthomas, multinucleated histiocytes filled with lipid droplets appear (Touton giant cells). In granulomas, the histiocytes change into epithelioid cells, which divide into another form of giant cell (Langhans). These are phagocytic and are distinctive in the general group of granulomas of the skin (syphilis, tuberculosis, leprosy, sarcoidosis, and deep mycoses).

The third principal type of cell in the corium is the *mast cell*. This requires special histologic methods for its demonstration and is rarely seen in routine biopsy specimens. The mast cell granules contain both heparin and histamine. The mast cells are localized about the vascular system. The signal protective role of the mast cell is shown by the fact that it releases its granules in response to any injury, with production of immediate vascular changes and an outpouring of leukocytes and plasma from the bloodstream. This appears to be the mechanism involved in the production of the *triple response* and in dermographism.

LIPOCYTE. In this, the chief cell of subcutaneous fat tissue, inflammatory changes are common. Nonspecific fat necrosis manifests itself in subcutaneous nodules which may or may not be tender. There is often a preceding history of trauma, including the injection of various medicinal compounds, or reactions to insect bites, or thermal injury. Occlusive peripheral vascular changes may impair circulation to the subcutaneous tissue sufficiently to result in formation of localized areas of fat necrosis.

A striking specific syndrome which involves fatty tissue is Weber-Christian disease (relapsing febrile nodular nonsuppurative panniculitis, see p. 1378).

CYTOLOGIC SMEAR (TZANCK TEST). Cytologic examination of a fresh bulla is useful in the study of vesiculobullous eruptions. The youngest vesicular lesion present is swabbed with an alcohol sponge, the vesicle roof is split with a scalpel, and the fluid is sponged away with dry gauze. After the walls of the vesicle are reflected, the base of the lesion is scraped gently with a scalpel to remove the basal epidermal cells. The whitish material is smeared onto a clean glass slide, dried in air, fixed in methyl alcohol, and stained with a routine Giemsa stain. It may be mounted in balsam or examined directly after application of immersion oil to clear the cells. In pemphigus one sees numerous small, round epithelial cells, many in isolated form. No prickle cells are seen, and there is a basic acantholysis. The nucleus is large in relation to the cytoplasm, which may be condensed in a basophilic peripheral ring.

In herpes simplex, zoster, or varicella, the typical and significant cytologic findings are polymorphism and giant multinuclear epithelial cells.

DEMONSTRATION OF ORGANISMS. The most commonly employed procedure here is the study of scales, hair, and nails for the presence of fungi. Scales scraped from the periphery of a lesion are placed on a microscope slide in a drop of 10 per cent aqueous potassium hydroxide. Clearing occurs rapidly with warming, and under "high dry" magnification one may see the delicate hyphae of the organism. If the skin surface has been cleansed before making the scraping, any fungi demonstrated are significant and pathogenic. Cultures of the scales may also be made to determine the specific organism present. Such planting of scales on Sabouraud's agar is followed (in a few weeks of room-temperature incubation) by the appearance of a colony, often identifiable grossly to the mycologist.

Regular bacteriologic isolation techniques and antibiotic sensitivity testing of the pathogenic staphylococci should be employed in resistant pyodermas.

The dark-field examination of material from genital and other lesions suggesting infectious syphilis is a valuable procedure.

Likewise, at times, virologic isolation procedures may be carried out by specialized laboratories. Finally, smears from granulomatous lesions may be stained for the presence of Donovan bodies when granuloma inguinale is suspected.

SKIN TESTS. The accessibility of the skin offers an unrivaled opportunity for in vivo testing of the cutaneous effects of a wide variety of chemicals and biologic products. Nearly all these tests are done to detect the unusual or allergic response as an explanation for the appearance of disease. The universal response, such as irritation of the skin from acids and alkalies, can generally be recognized by the history without recourse to testing.

Patch Tests. The most commonly employed tests involve contact reactions to substances applied topically, e.g., under an adhesive patch for a period of up to 48 hr. The disease in miniature is thus produced in the sensitive person. The procedure is not so benign and simple as it might appear, since all substances must be applied in a concentration such as to be without primary irritancy. It should not be used indiscriminately; in exquisitely sensitive individuals it may lead to a bullous reaction so intense as to produce depigmentation, scarring, or even a generalized reaction. It has no value in predicting which persons may later become sensitized. However, intelligently used as an adjunct to a careful history, it is valuable in tracking the specific cause of a contact dermatitis.

Intradermal Tests. A wide array of commercially available extracts is available for scratch and intradermal skin testing. The *immediate* reaction is urticarial and erythematous, and it would seem to duplicate the disease; yet the method is of limited usefulness in clinical practice insofar as diseases of the skin are concerned.

The prototype of the *delayed* reaction is the tuberculin skin test, in which the inflammatory reaction occurs at 48 hr. This has considerable value in the assessment of lesions suspected to be allergic in nature (e.g., tuberculids). Many other biologic allergens are available, e.g., trichophytin, histoplasmin, and coccidioidin. All are used on occasion.

New agents for skin testing on cutaneous autoimmune states include erythrocytes and leukocytes. Here the reaction may be an immediate wheal type or a delayed inflammatory one.

Finally, attention is directed to the significance of the sarcoid skin test, which represents a 4- to 6-week delayed skin reaction. In this instance the material is introduced intradermally (Kveim antigen, lepromin, zirconium, beryllium). A positive reaction consists of the appearance of a papule which histologically is sarcoid in nature (pure epithelioid tubercles). This appears to represent a distinctive type of delayed allergic response which reduplicates the disease *in situ*. It should receive increasing attention in the study of sarcoidosis.

PHYSICAL ALLERGY. Abnormal reactions to sunlight may account for a great variety of cutaneous changes. This problem of *photosensitivity* is best attacked by specific light-testing procedures. Practical information can be obtained by exposing a small test site of the patient's skin to radiation from a carbon arc or hot quartz lamp. If marked photosensitivity is suspected, however, such tests should be considered very carefully. They are contraindicated in any patient suspected of having systemic lupus erythematosus.

Hypersensitivity to cold is easily demonstrated in some patients by contact of the skin with ice. Here the common reaction is an immediate urticarial one. In other individuals a general fall in skin temperature is the trigger mechanism, and testing in a cool room may be necessary.

Heat hypersensitivity likewise may be elicited by either a local or a general increase in the temperature. In the local type, heating produces a local wheal; in the generalized cholinergic type, exercise or a hot bath induces numerous small wheals with considerable axone reflex erythema.

SPECIAL TESTS FOR FUNCTION OF APPENDAGES OF SKIN. Sweating. Hyperhidrosis is obvious, but detection of anhidrosis requires actual observation of the patient under a heat stimulus. A regular heat cabinet offers the best tool, but too often improvised arrangements with infrared bulbs, blankets, and hot drinks have to suffice. The most satisfactory objective recording of the response is achieved with the starch paper iodine print method of Randall.

Sebum Formation. The secretion of the sebaceous gland is generally an invisible film of oil, but at times on the face and scalp one may see droplets of sebum which simulate eccrine sweat. These two secretions can be distinguished by making a contact print with a clean glass slide or paper. Sweat rapidly evaporates, and sebum does not.

Hair. In addition to biopsy and mycologic studies, examination of plucked hairs under the microscope gives a valuable assessment of general health changes in the patient during the past months. The shaft diameter quickly reflects general disturbances, including radiation damage. It is also possible to prognosticate in cases of alopecia by making a count of the relative number of hairs in a quiescent nongrowing state. The resting hair has an atrophic club ending quite unlike the ensheathed pigmented hair which is still growing. If the club hair percentage is above 20, this augurs further hair loss in the near future (see Fig. 34-2).

Nail. Using a small punch, biopsies may be secured of the nail plate and its underlying bed. If the matrix area is not entered, no deformity results. The most common examination, however, is of scrapings for fungi. It must not be forgotten that nail growth rates may be accurately observed by filing or cutting a transverse band at the base of the nail.

Blood Tests. Certain blood tests relate more specifically to skin disturbances. These include the serologic test for syphilis, lupus erythematosus test, demonstration of cryoglobulins, and detection of circulating cancer cells. In allergic studies, passive transfer tests may be employed occasionally.

Urine. The presence in the urine of porphyrins, melanin, or hemoglobin may herald the cutaneous signs of porphyria, malignant melanoma, or physical allergy, respectively.

33 ITCHING

Donald M. Pillsbury and Walter B. Shelley

Itching is the specific symptom of mild injury to the outermost frontier of the body. It is the cry of help, the "distant early warning" signal of the epidermis when attacked from either without or within. As such it evokes an immediate purposive motor response, namely, scratching. It is this primitive reflex which makes itching so very distinctive in the sensory modalities. It is not pain, for pain evokes reflex withdrawal, and yet it is allied, traveling much the same nervous pathway.

Itching is truly an epidermal sensation. Unlike pain, it is felt nowhere but in the skin and then only when the epidermis is present. Removing the epidermis removes the itch organ, for it is in the millions of fine free unmyelinated epidermal nerve endings that this sensation arises. Morphologically uninteresting, these endings make up the radar net of the peripheral nervous system. Lying between the epidermal cells, they at once are subject to the same trauma as the epidermis itself. On attack they initiate a train of impulses up the sensory nerve, along the lateral spinothalamic tract, to the thalamus, where afferent arcs induce reflex scratching with or without much sensory recognition.

Superficial damage is the *sine qua non* of pruritus, and thus many have searched for the mediator of itching. Actually any mechanical, thermal, electrical, or chemical stimulus may induce pruritus, if injury of a mild yet appropriate degree is produced. In clinical medicine, however, it would appear that chemical release of substances such as proteases, kinins, and histamine is the fundamental cause of pruritus. Thus, just as there is no single morphologically recognizable itch receptor, so no common single chemical mediator is known today. Histamine, however, is the classic agent for producing an itch experimentally. Apparently it is the cause of the itching associated with hives, since introduction of sufficient histamine into the skin to produce pruritus invariably induces an associated urticaria because of its effect on vascular permeability. Proteases as well as the products of protease activity, e.g., polypeptides and ammonia, are also effective pruritogens in extremely low concentrations. Such agents may be activated or released at times of epidermal injury.

The perception and response to peripheral injury is conditioned by the central nervous system. Invariably pruritus is associated with a lowering of the itch threshold in the general area, so that mere air currents may induce pruritus in this itchy skin area. This altered response of the body to tactile stimuli presumably results from central change. Conversely, pain may inhibit the itch sensation. It is for this reason that the scratch-tormented patient may learn to substitute pain for itch. Such an antipruritic state reflects changes in the central nervous system still beyond our understanding. Finally, it should be pointed out that itching

is no longer possible after an anterolateral cordotomy.

Itching is a capricious clinical symptom, varying in intensity from time to time. Even more remarkable is the variation among patients in itch sensitivity. Some individuals are truly "itchish." Others may experience little or no itch no matter what the stimulus may be.

Table 33-1. DISEASES WITH AND WITHOUT PRURITUS

Pruritus is Commonly Present:

Atopic dermatitis	Scabies
Contact dermatitis, allergic	Urticaria
Exfoliative dermatitis	Dermatitis herpetiformis
Localized neurodermatitis	Pediculosis
Nummular eczema	Diabetes mellitus
Varicella	Schistosomiasis
Insect bites	

Pruritus is Commonly Absent:

Epitheliomas	Hyperhidrosis
Hemangiomas	Lupus erythematosus
Nevi	Psoriasis
Keratoses	Erythema multiforme
Verruca	Pemphigus
Xanthomas	Rosacea
Impetigo	Acne
Furuncle	Tinea
Alopecia areata	Sarcoidosis
Scleroderma	Zoster
Vitiligo	

The variation in itch may also show circadian rhythm, usually being worse at night. The periodicity of pruritus is such that placebo therapy may be warmly endorsed by the patient. The enormous range of this subjective experience defies precise description and analysis. In some, scratching may be purely a mimicry phenomenon, in others it extends in severity to the point of exquisite torture and demands heroic measures for control. It is doubtful that the average physician ever carries enough sympathy for the patient with severe itching. Repeated paroxysms of generalized pruritus can turn the patient to thoughts of suicide.

Itch and scratch are the paired symptom and sign of disease. For the clinician they offer both diagnostic help and therapeutic challenge. First, let us consider the diagnostic help. Most obviously, itching reflects certain well-recognized skin diseases. Indeed, in some instances all the clinical signs result solely from incessant scratching. Such, for example, is the case in localized neurodermatitis. In this common skin disease the skin becomes thickened and lichenified in response to the ceaseless scratching and rubbing of a restricted patch of skin. No skin condition is more readily associated with pruritus than hives. Fortunately the pruritus of urticaria is limited in degree and duration. In the most extensive examples, itching may be a minor feature. In many instances drug or food intolerance is the cause, and appropriate elimination studies are indicated. All patients with allergic contact dermatitis experience a certain degree of pruritus since the epidermis itself is the site of antigen-antibody cytolysis.

Accordingly the epidermal itch receptor receives maximal stimulation, and rare is the patient who has not felt the rigors of a poison ivy itch. Likewise, bites, stings, and scratches initiate a train of pruritogenic impulses from the injured epidermis. Pediculosis, scabies, and mite infestations are among the more obvious causes. The itchy scalp is usually a sign of seborrheic dermatitis and will respond well to a variety of medicated shampoos. More commonly, pruritus results from overbathing. Dry, aging skin cannot sustain the abuse of frequent long showering and bathing. Detergents may play a role here in removing surface oils and in damaging the epidermal cuticle. In children and some adults the most common dermatologic explanation for persistent pruritus is atopic dematitis (infantile eczema). In these patients the skin becomes hyperalgesic and virtually any stimulus will be converted into pruritus. No skin disease brings more chronic itch than atopic dermatitis. In some patients scratching becomes a compulsive ritual, and in these persons deeply dug out scars may be the presenting sign. Such neurotic excoriations may represent a deep-seated psychosis—or at other times may reflect a tic-like habit of picking at acne. Finally, the clinician who is confronted with pruritus in association with skin disease should consider two unusual entities which are characterized by pruritus, namely, lichen planus and dermatitis herpetiformis (p. 593).

Turning to the significance of pruritus as a sign of internal disease, a number of conditions should be considered. The cutaneous picture is a nonspecific one of excoriations, lichenification, pigmentary change, eczematization, and at times secondary bacterial infection. Usually the pruritus is generalized, persistent, and disabling.

General medical study must be initially directed at the detection of one of four major causes: (1) obstructive jaundice, (2) lymphoblastoma, (3) malignancy, and (4) diabetes mellitus. Any interference with the free flow of bile induces jaundice. In the case of obstructive jaundice, surgery is usually remedial. Intrahepatic cholestasis, such as with drug intolerance hepatitis, is generally short-lived. However, it is in primary biliary cirrhosis that the unrelenting pruritus reduces the patient to a pitiful object. Fortunately this latter condition responds well to therapy with cholestyramine, a bile salt sequestrant ion exchange resin. Apparently the pruritus is due to an increase in bile salt levels in the blood. These salts may act as hastamine liberators.

Lymphoblastomas (p. 685) are notorious as causes of severe generalized pruritus in the absence of any primary skin change. Hodgkin's disease leads the list (p. 686), but leukemia and lymphosarcoma may also cause itching. In one particular example, mycosis fungoides, itching may precede recognizable cellular infiltrates in the skin for many years.

Other forms of malignancy, such as carcinoma, may also result in pruritus. Presumably the body becomes sensitized to the tumor and reacts to circulating extracts or fragments much as to a foreign drug. This is rare, but in any patient with unexplained widespread itching detailed studies must be done. As one could surmise, such a problem may explain the so-called "senile pruritus." Finally, in a few diabetics itching is a cardinal sign, alleviated only by control of the metabolic error.

Other internal medical problems rarely contribute to a persistent pruritus. However, one should exclude intestinal parasitism, hypothyroidism, renal failure, psychosis, and the paramedical problem of pregnancy. Itching is not associated with organic neural tumors, nor does it appear as a localized problem such as is seen with referred pain.

The *treatment* of pruritus calls for a direct attack on the cause. Elimination of an offending drug, parasite, or contact allergen places the patient squarely on the road to recovery. At times an admonition to reduce bathing to once a week does more than a score of medications. Today scabies is rare, but benzyl benzoate is still a modern miracle of complete therapeutic effectiveness, and should no more be forgotten than the disease itself. Atopic dermatitis calls for a manifold and skilled attack on the multiple allergens to which patients with this condition are sensitive. Steroids, topically as well as systemically, are often necessary. Secondary bacterial infection is eliminated with systemic antibiotics. Dermatitis herpetiformis (p. 593) often responds well to long-term low-dosage sulfapyridine, whereas lichen planus calls for rest and relaxation. The internal problems are likewise given appropriate treatment when recognized. In particular, cholestyramine therapy is gratifying. Within a week of oral dosage in the area of 10 Gm a day one can expect to see a significant reduction in the pruritus of primary biliary cirrhosis, whereas until recently little could be done to alleviate it.

When the causal factor cannot be directly eliminated, one has to fall back on symptomatic therapy. Here the armamentarium is less than desirable. There is no powerful specific antipruritic agent. However, inasmuch as a considerable part of pruritus is based on allergic mechanisms, antihistaminics and steroids are indicated. They alleviate the condition but are only crutches until more definitive measures can be instituted. Long-term high-dosage steroid therapy is not a recommended approach unless all else fails.

Barbiturates and analgesics have little or no effect on pruritus. Interestingly, salicylates may at times be helpful, by virtue of their anti-inflammatory activity.

Today the following four drugs enjoy the greatest popularity in the symptomatic attack on itching: (1) trimeprazine (Temaril), (2) dexachlorpheniramine (Polaramine), (3) methdilazine (Tacaryl), and (4) cyproheptadine (Periactin). None is specific, however, and after use of any of them one often finds the patient still begging for relief.

Topically, the use of menthol lotions, colloidal baths, and similar modalities may afford some relief in widespread pruritus. If the skin shows eczematous changes or excoriations, the patient generally benefits most from antibiotic and steroid creams. Furthermore, in such skin a degree of anesthesia may be attained by the application of antihistaminic creams.

PRURITUS ANI. The perianal area is richly endowed with an epidermal nerve network which magnifies all itch stimuli by virtue of the elevated skin temperature in this area. The threshold for itching in this area is so low that the sensation almost becomes physiologic. Persistent severe itching in this locale may reflect any one of the following:

1. Contact dermatitis. Many diverse allergens may be responsible, e.g., nail polish, colored toilet tissue, local treatment, or even food allergens.

2. Neurodermatitis. In some instances a virtually irreversible cycle of itching and scratching may be initiated.

3. Pinworm infestation.

4. Seborrheic dermatitis or psoriasis.

5. Reaction to broad-spectrum antibiotics. Oral administration of these agents may be followed by pruritus ani.

6. Hemorrhoidal tags or anal fissures.

Treatment should be specifically adapted to any causal factors. Scrupulous, bland hygiene coupled with the application of a steroid cream three times a day usually leads to considerable symptomatic relief.

PRURITUS VULVAE. The vulvar area is likewise richly endowed with a fine epidermal network which reduces the threshold for itching. The following are the common causes for a pathologic degree of itching in this area:

1. Contact dermatitis. Reactions may be observed to sanitary pads, douche materials, contraceptives, or local agents used in therapy.

2. Reactions following broad-spectrum antibiotics.

3. Diabetes mellitus.

4. Neurodermatitis, localized.

5. Conditions with an associated vaginal discharge. Monilial and trichomonal vaginitis must be considered.

Treatment centers on elimination of any contributory cause. Good local hygiene, coupled with topical corticosteroid creams, is often helpful. However, in recalcitrant cases systemic steroid administration is necessary.

34 ALOPECIA AND HIRSUTISM
Donald M. Pillsbury and Walter B. Shelley

Hair is made up of tightly fused horny cells which are of the "hard" keratin variety. Because sebaceous glands are invariably associated with the hair-bearing follicles, this appendageal unit is called the pilosebaceous apparatus. It originates from the epidermis at about the third month of fetal life. After birth the epidermis cannot generate new follicles; hence, loss by disease or trauma is permanent. An unimportant and singular exception to this is the regeneration of fine "fuzz" hairs on the face after dermabrasion.

The portion of the hair within the follicle beneath the surface is the root. The expanded lower part is the bulb which contains the matrix, from which the hair cells are formed. A connective tissue papilla with a capillary loop projects into the base of the bulb. A row of melanocytes is located over the top of the papilla. These furnish melanin for the horny cells coming up from below. Loss of melanocytic functioning, as in senile graying, has no effect on hair vitality. The matrix is physiologically one of the most active tissues in the body. Scalp hair grows at an average daily rate of about 0.35 mm, and this new growth consists almost entirely of protein (keratin). Hair growth takes place as a holocrine process by the continuous formation of new cells, which move upwards and cornify in a more gradual way than in the epidermis. Interference with cell division in the matrix is immediately reflected in inhibition of hair growth. The rate of cellular reproduction in hair growth is greater than that of any other tissue in the body, with the possible exception of the bone marrow. A highly active tissue of this kind is understandably susceptible to systemic stresses which compromise the general health.

Hair, like nails, grows more rapidly in summer, an expression of an overall enhancement of cutaneous activity. The hair matrix is a complex tissue which contains a variety of cell types. Its regenerative capacity is astonishing. Forceful manual plucking removes everything but a few torn clusters of matrix cells at the very base. Nonetheless, a perfectly normal hair re-forms from these surviving cells. Within limits, repeated hair plucking does not damage the follicle irreparably, luckily for women who make a lifelong practice of plucking their eyebrows.

A great reduction in hairiness is one of the distinctive features of the human animal, as compared to lower animals. The protection against cold and injury afforded by hair is no longer necessary for civilized man. Over most of the body's surface the hairs are fine and delicate, mere vestiges of their former selves. If hair has lost its biologic significance, its psychologic and cosmetic value have become so much the greater. Too much hair in women and not enough in men have become sensitive issues about which there is extraordinary concern, especially since beauty standards become more exacting and unrealistic with every passing day. As mankind has become more preoccupied with appearance, fictions about hair growth have proliferated.

All over the surface of the body, except the palms, soles, and a few other small regions, there are tiny light-colored vellus hairs which constitute "fuzz." They are barely visible, and most persons are unaware of their existence. They are the only hairs on the smooth glabrous skin. Even when an individual seems bald, vellus hairs are present. Terminal hairs, by contrast, are long, thick, coarse, and darker. They are well developed only in certain regions, such as the scalp, male beard, around the genitalia, etc. From the practical standpoint, terminal hairs are the ones of interest.

Terminal hairs have acquired special characteristics in different regions. This regional diversity is so great that generalizations about hair are not justifiable. For example, scalp and eyelash hairs are quite dissimilar. There are differences in growth rate, anatomic organization, and physiologic responsiveness. It is useful to classify hair into six morphologic types: (1) scalp, (2) eyebrow and eyelash, (3) beard, (4) axillary, (5) body, and (6) pubic.

Hair may also be divided into two types according to responsiveness to sex hormones. Androgens control the postpuberal development of hairs which make up the secondary sex characteristics, namely, axillary and pubic hair, beard and body hair. On the other hand, scalp hair, eyelashes, and hair of the extremities require no hormonal stimulus, although sex hormones may have modifying influences.

The relationship of sex hormones to hair growth has some curious features. Androgens govern sex hairs in women as in men. However, mustache and facial hair, which are hormone-dependent sexual hairs in men, often become prominent in postmenopausal women. Testosterone has completely opposite effects on different types of hairs. It stimulates beard hair, for instance, but conditions hair loss in male baldness. Male castrates never become bald. Neither do they have axillary, pubic, beard, or body hair. This situation is completely reversed when androgens are given. Eunuchs become "men" in respect to hair. They may lose scalp hair (if there is baldness in the family) and acquire normal hairy characteristics elsewhere. Hormones other than testosterone are generally of little account, either in excess or deficiency, in affecting hair. It is true that there may be some thinning of hair in hypothyroid myxedema, but this is probably secondary to mucinous infiltration of the skin. The effect of the pituitary is indirect through the production of male hormone by the adrenals and gonads. In rare feminizing disorders of males, excess estrogens may antagonize testosterone to the extent that secondary sex hair regresses.

Hair does not grow indefinitely, as do nails (Fig. 34-1). In every follicle, activity is cyclic—a resting period follows a growth period. The cycles are not synchronized in adjacent follicles. One has a population of independent individual units, each in its own particular phase of the cycle. Some are in infancy while others are in senescence. At the end of the growing phase the follicle involutes in a remarkable fashion, during which time the resting or club hair is formed. This remains passively in the quiescent follicle until it is expelled by the regenerating new hair. A certain number of club hairs is constantly being shed, but since this happens gradually, the loss is not perceptible. The situation is analogous to that in evergreen trees, which, though their liimbs are never bare like those of deciduous trees, nonetheless are continuously shedding needles.

Hairs in different regions have different cycles. The main difference is in the length of growing phase, which determines the final length of the hair. Short hairs obviously come from follicles with brief growing phases. It is roughly estimated that scalp hair grows for from 2 to 6 years. Actually, the hairs of certain persons may grow for much longer. If this were not true it would have been impossible in times past for some women to grow hair down to their knees, assuming an average daily growth rate of 0.35 mm. Resting hairs make up about 5 to 15 per cent of the terminal scalp hairs. Since the great majority of the approximately 100,000 hairs on the human scalp are growing at any

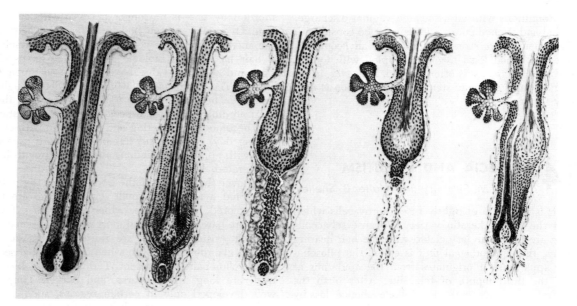

Fig. 34-1. Stages in hair cycle. Progressive changes from a growing (anagen) hair to a resting club hair (telogen)—second from right. In the normal human scalp, some 10 per cent of the hairs are in the resting phase. In various types of alopecia, this percentage rises sharply and may be easily determined by the number of hairs which are easily removed by gentle traction.

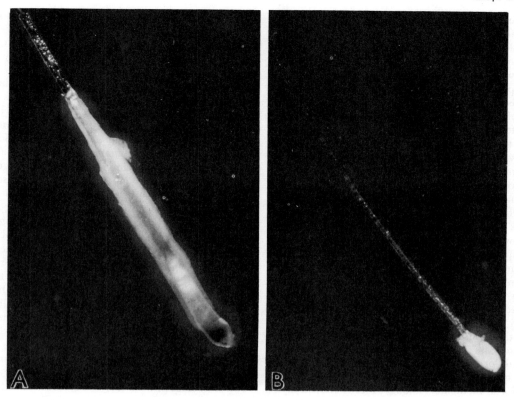

Fig. 34-2. Plucking the hair will show whether it is growing or resting (provided it does not break off). *A.* A growing hair. The hair root is surrounded by an extensive translucent sheath, and the proximal tip is deeply pigmented. The hair itself may be seen within the sheath. *B.* A resting or club hair. All that is seen is a bulbous, nonpigmented tip. There is no sheath save for an inconspicuous one limited to the very tip of the hair. Club hairs are also likely to be somewhat lighter and thinner, because pigment production and keratin synthesis diminish when the hair nears the end of the growth phase. (*D. M. Pillsbury, W. B. Shelley,* and *A. M. Kligman: "Dermatology," p. 42, Philadelphia, W. B. Saunders Company, 1956.*)

given time, the resting period must be short, perhaps a few months. The normal rate of scalp hair loss is in the range of 20 to 100 hairs daily. Most of the inconspicuous vellus hairs of the body will be found to be in the resting phase.

On the trunk, eyebrows, and extremities the growing period usually does not exceed 6 months and, hence, the hairs are not very long. These hairs rest for about the same length of time as they grow. Appreciation of the cyclic habit of hair growth has practical applications. Hair infection by the ringworm fungus, *Microsporum audouini,* is automatically cured when hairs enter the resting phase. It is easy to understand, then, why infections of the eyelashes and eyelids terminate spontaneously in a couple of months; such hairs are in a growing phase only for this long. In the scalp, however, the infection may last for years if treatment with griseofulvin is not instituted.

A variety of systemic stresses, especially acute febrile diseases, may interfere with hair growth and structure. It is scalp hair which is particularly vulnerable. A shortening of the life cycle, with premature formation of resting hairs, is one striking result. This may never become clinically apparent if gradual and limited, but if a majority of hairs is suddenly brought

into a synchronous resting phase, their loss shortly thereafter will be accompanied by signs of thinning and even baldness. This effect is generally temporary, since loss of normal resting hairs is regularly followed by regeneration of new hairs. More chronic stresses, by shortening the life cycles, cause more rapid turnover in the hair crop. More hairs are being lost and regenerated. As long as the birth rate of hairs equals the death rate, there may be thinning but not real baldness. It becomes important, therefore, to be able to recognize a club hair. In male baldness and in scarring diseases, the follicles shrivel and the hairs wither away so that regeneration is impossible.

A number of situations produce temporary partial baldness owing to the loss of an unusual number of resting hairs. This happens physiologically in infants within the first few months after birth. Post-partum hair loss is very common in mothers. The stress of the delivery and the physiologic drains of pregnancy are reflected in a goodly percentage of cases in the formation of a large number of club hairs. This premature shortening of the cycles may happen suddenly or over a period of months. Hair loss is very noticeable in the former case, but is merely an accentuation of a physiologic process. It abates spontaneously. Chronic emotional stress, debilitating disease of diverse origin, and, occasionally, profound malnutrition are responsible for similar phenomena.

The peculiar susceptibility of scalp hair is evident in other ways. Moderate doses of thallium acetate will cause depilation of scalp hair but not of other types of hair. This may be among the signs of accidental ingestion of thallium-containing rodenticides. Survivors of the atom bombings in Japan lost only their scalp hair (in the absence of scarring). The fact that scalp hair grows faster than other types may help to account for its sensitivity.

The scalp hair, like the nails, tends to reflect systemic illness and health-weakening stresses, again in no specific manner. The body has more important functions to perform at such times. Hair growth may slow down; the hairs may become thinner, more fragile, split, and in other ways poor in appearance.

Misconceptions about hair growth are legion. This simply reflects the tremendous psychologic significance of hair. One source of error has been the unwarranted application of results of animal researches. The skin and hair of the common laboratory animals such as the mouse, rabbit, and rat have unique properties. Procedures or drugs which will correct graying in animals or stimulate new hair growth, matters of concern to many human beings, have not proved useful in clinical medicine. Among widely believed myths are the following: shaving promotes the growth of dark, coarse hairs; singeing and cutting the hair weaken it; hair can turn gray overnight; hair "grows after death"; etc.

It should be realized that the hair shaft is a dead, inert structure. No force, chemical or physical, which is confined entirely to this structure can alter the hair-forming organ, which is situated well under the surface of the scalp and is, therefore, not easily harmed. As for massage, combing, brushing, oiling, and a thousand other practices thought to improve hair growth—none has established value. These activities are cosmetically satisfying but do not improve upon nature's capacity to produce healthy hair. Cleanliness is the only essential in maintaining scalp health. Everything else is for appearance.

The importance of vitamins in hair growth has been much exaggerated. No single vitamin has a pronounced influence. Nor is hair loss a particularly striking result of vitamin deficiency. It is only in advanced malnutrition, particularly with prolonged protein deprivation, that fragility or loss of hair becomes evident (p. 359).

ALOPECIA

Human hair becomes thinned or lost in a wide variety of conditions, a few of which are of general medical significance. The type of hair and its growth characteristics are the focus of an inordinate amount of attention and concern, particularly among women, and no physician can escape occasional or frequent questioning on hair of poor quality, too little hair, or too much hair.

Advancing age is always accompanied by some loss of scalp hair, more commonly and markedly among males than females. In some persons, this loss may be so moderate that they appear to have a luxuriant growth of hair even in advanced old age. Male-pattern baldness is so well known as to require little detailed description. It will suffice to say that it is genetically endowed and is dependent on androgenic stimuli. In some genetically unfortunate males, considerable loss of hair may be noted in the teens. This is generally first seen in the areas above the frontal bossae, producing an M-like outline of the frontal scalp margin. Coincident thinning of hair in the parietal region occurs. With early onset, the likelihood of significant baldness in the thirties is strong. No topical or systemic therapy has been shown to influence the inexorably advancing alopecia. Conversely, however, recent carefully controlled studies have shown that in males who have long been bald, prolonged application of a cream containing 1 per cent testosterone will induce transformation of residual fine vellus hairs into coarse terminal hairs. Creams containing estrogen have no effect.

It is not so generally realized that women frequently have female-pattern alopecia (Fig. 34-3A). This may begin in the late teens, but its onset is more commonly seen during or after middle age. It rarely progresses to complete baldness. The loss is confined to the frontal and parietal regions, growth on the sides and posterior scalp remaining normal. The only medical significance of this type of hair loss is psychic. Most women regard a full head of hair as a status symbol, and any threat to it may be very disturbing.

The factors controlling the long growing period of scalp hair and the involution into a resting period are largely unknown. In view of the complex chemistry involved, it is not surprising that a wide variety of local and systemic causes should upset the delicate synthesis of keratinous protein.

Acquired loss of hair from disease may be seen in skin which is normal in appearance, or as a result of inflammation and scarring, i.e., *nonscarring* and *scarring* alopecia.

Some of the diseases in which there is hair loss with or without gross visible changes in the skin are as follows:

ALOPECIA AREATA (Fig. 34-3F). This most commonly occurs in small to large round patches of the scalp. The sites of involvement are slightly though perceptibly depressed below the surrounding skin. On microscopic examination a very moderate lymphocytic infiltrate may be seen. If there are only a few areas, and if the hair loss begins in adult life, the outlook for hair regrowth is good. The defect in alopecia areata is probably determined genetically; a family history of the disease is not uncommon. Sometimes the disease may produce hair loss over the entire body; the outlook for regrowth in such cases is poor. The same may be said for alopecia areata beginning in

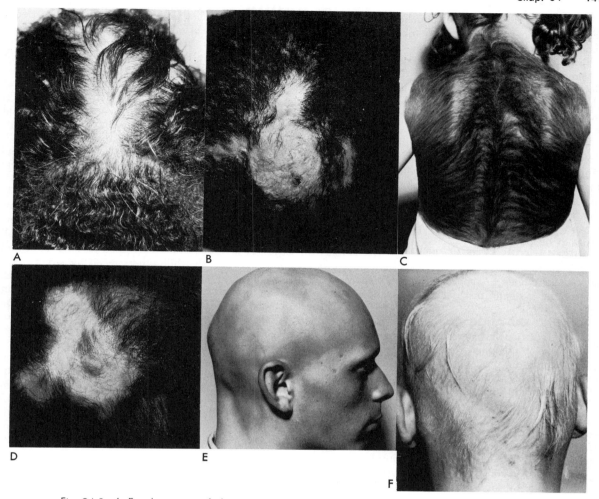

Fig. 34-3. *A.* Female pattern of alopecia. A common type of hair loss, confined to the frontal and parietal regions. Onset usually in middle age but not uncommon in the twenties. *B.* Scarring alopecia following overdose of x-rays for tinea capitis. Such areas are vulnerable to the development of epitheliomas. *C.* Extensive hairy nevus. Such lesions are ordinarily present full-blown at birth. *D.* Scarring and alopecia caused by discoid lupus erythematosus. *E.* Alopecia totalis. The outlook for regrowth in extensive involvement of this type is poor. *F.* Diffuse alopecia areata. Most of the hairs which have regrown are white, but a few have retained their original dark color.

childhood. Alopecia areata has been described as occurring after a severe nervous shock, but this is certainly not common.

A coincidental sign in alopecia areata is a variable dystrophy of the nails. In extreme cases the nails may be shed, but more commonly pits, ridges, or transverse furrows may be seen. The severity of the nail changes is roughly parallel to the extent of the alopecia.

Regrowth of hair may be stimulated by systemic corticosteroid therapy, but its effects are often transitory. It is difficult to justify long-term steroid administration for this disease, since it is of cosmetic significance only. Topical application of corticosteroid creams or intradermal injection of triamcinolone sometimes stimulates regrowth. Ultraviolet light exposures have no value in alopecia areata, nor does the application of irritants such as phenol. Treatment of alopecia areata by the administration of desiccated thyroid has no proved value. In fact, patients with this condition deserve examination for hyperthyroidism because this may be one of the precipitating factors in the loss of hair.

HAIR LOSS IN THE NEONATAL PERIOD AND DURING PREGNANCY. Physiologic shedding of scalp hair frequently occurs in infants during the neonatal period. Diffuse loss of hair in women is not uncommon during or shortly after pregnancy. The prognosis for regrowth in both instances is good.

FEVER. Marked diffuse loss of hair may be noted during or after any prolonged febrile illness. In presulfonamide and preantibiotic days, when many febrile infectious diseases could not be controlled promptly, this type of alopecia was seen with much greater frequency. Regrowth ordinarily occurs.

SYPHILIS. In the secondary spirochetemia of this infection, a typical moth-eaten type of alopecia is seen, though not commonly.

CHEMICALS AND DRUGS. Among compounds capable of producing moderate to marked alopecia are thallium, heparin, nitrogen mustard and other cancer chemotherapeutic agents, folic acid antagonists, chloroprene dimers, excessive prolonged intake of vitamin A, and triparanol.

PSYCHIC DISTURBANCES. Trichotillomania is occasionally seen in children and in disturbed or retarded adults. It is a habit tic similar to nail biting, in which the individual compulsively pulls hairs from an area of the scalp. The condition is easily recognized by the fact that the loss of hair is not complete; there are always some hairs which are regrowing but are too short to be pulled.

MISCELLANEOUS SYSTEMIC DISEASES. Dermatomyositis, systemic lupus erythematosus (LE), severe uncontrolled diabetes, cachexia, and lymphomas are among the systemic diseases that may cause loss of hair.

IONIZING RADIATION. The alopecia resulting from ionizing radiation is temporary and nonscarring with lower doses (400r plus), but permanent and scarring with large doses (probably 1,500r plus, depending on individual doses, intervals of treatment, and quality of the radiation) (see Fig. 34-3B).

SCARRING ALOPECIA. Any physical injury or disease capable of destroying the hair follicle will, of course, produce scarring and permanent hair loss. However, the scalp hairs are remarkably resistant and can survive rather severe temporary insults.

PHYSICAL AGENTS. Among the physical agents capable of causing loss of hair are third degree burns, excessive doses of ionizing irradiation, and deeply destructive contact with strong cauterants.

INFECTIONS. Those that cause significant hair loss are ordinarily deep, such as boils and carbuncles. Superficial ringworm infections and folliculitis rarely produce permanent alopecia.

VARIOUS CUTANEOUS AND SYSTEMIC SYNDROMES. Discoid lupus erythematosus invariably produces permanent scarring alopecia of the scalp and other areas in time (Fig. 34-3D). The clinical and pathologic features are highly characteristic.

Other conditions that may cause permanent loss of hair are localized or systemic scleroderma, tumors (late), certain nevi, herpes zoster, leprosy, cutaneous leishmaniasis, gumma of syphilis, sarcoid (occasionally), and, rarely, folliculitis decalvans, cicatricial lichen planus, pseudopelade.

In occlusive peripheral vascular disease of the lower extremities, hair loss from the dorsal surface of the toes and feet may be noted, though this is a comparatively late sign.

HIRSUTISM

Human hair varies greatly, both in its type and in the factors controlling its growth. This variation is seen among different individuals and in different areas of the same person. Genetic and racial factors determine the pattern of hair distribution and growth.

Hirsutism has two aspects, one unimportant in terms of systemic disease, the other of great significance. "Idiopathic" excessive growth of hair is quite common in girls and women, and may be a source of much concern, far out of proportion to the true significance of the problem. Women with this condition will go to remarkable lengths to modify or mask this cosmetic change. Far less common, but of much medical interest and importance, are those individuals who develop masculinizing syndromes as a result of tumors or hyperplasia of the pituitary, adrenals, or ovaries.

There is considerable reason to believe that persons who are apparently normal may differ greatly in responsiveness of the hair follicle to circulating hormones. As an example, some women receiving small doses of a corticosteroid compound note increased facial hair growth while others receiving larger doses for longer periods of time do not experience this. There may be an increased target response to ovarian or adrenal androgens in women. There may also be factors of delicate hormone balance, such as androgens becoming predominant in women whose estrogen levels are decreased at the menopause.

Although a good deal of information is available on patterns of hair growth which are racially or genetically endowed, such as moderate to marked hirsutism in young women of Mediterranean stock, few systematic surveys have been done on variations in hair growth among normal adults, particularly women. "Simple or idiopathic hirsutism" is not easy to define, but it is important that it be recognized in persons in whom the development of a masculinizing syndrome is suspected.

A survey of 400 young women was made at the University of Wales (McKnight). In this study, 60 per cent of the subjects were Welsh and 40 per cent were English. Non-European students were not included. Thirty-six of the 400 young women (9 per cent) were particularly hairy, only coarse terminal hairs being regarded as significant. Of these 36 with a hair distribution which was "masculine" in type, a further 16 had very marked hirsutism which was a social disadvantage. Such severely affected women have terminal hair on the breast, lumbosacral region, and upper part of the back, and a distribution of pubic hair which extends up toward the umbilicus in an inverted V. In these young women with severe hirsutism, menstrual disorders, minor anxiety states, and acne vulgaris were common. In the Welsh series 2 students had additional signs of virilism, such at clitoral enlargement and periods of amenorrhea, and on further investigation were found to have adrenal virilism.

From this study it is seen that almost 10 per cent of young Caucasian women will have noticeable hirsutism and in some 4 per cent it probably will be very marked. The percentage is almost certainly higher in persons of Mediterranean stock, though no precise figures are available.

In the markedly hirsute individuals, almost always with terminal hair on the breast, lumbosacral region, and upper part of the back, a small percentage will have evidence of pituitary, adrenal, or ovarian hyperplasia or tumor. The endocrinologic problems in such cases may be extremely complex.

Table 34-1. CAUSES OF HIRSUTISM

I. Genetic, racial, familial, and individual predisposition
II. Adrenal origin
   A. Cushing's syndrome (p. 458)
   B. Congenital adrenal hyperplasia (p. 469)
   C. Delayed onset of congenital adrenal hyperplasia
   D. Borderline adrenal dysfunction
   E. Virilizing adrenal tumors
III. Ovarian origin
   A. Stein-Leventhal syndrome (p. 525)
   B. Virilizing ovarian tumors (p. 528)
      1. Arrhenoblastoma
      2. Adrenal rest tumor
      3. Hilus cell tumor
IV. Associated with sexual abnormalities (p. 523)
   A. Male pseudohermaphroditism
   B. Gonadal dysgenesis with androgenic manifestations
V. Miscellaneous
   A. Iatrogenic
   B. Achard-Thiers syndrome

SOURCE: From S. Roy, "The Hirsute Female," p. 278, R. B. Greenblatt (Ed.), Springfield, Ill., Charles C Thomas, Publisher, 1963.

Hirsutism may be localized. It may be present in a particular area without any gross evidence of a nevus, but more commonly there is some macular hyperpigmentation, or a frank, fleshy pigmented nevus (Fig. 34-3C). Such lesions at times may be extensive and cosmetically disfiguring. The only reassuring aspect of such a lesion is that the possibility of malignant changes developing in the nevus is practically nil.

Localized hirsutism may occur as a result of prolonged severe repeated irritation. It is not uncommon among mental defectives who compulsively bite their forearms at one site. It may be seen on the shoulders of individuals whose work involves the daily carrying of heavy weights, such as sack bearers. It may occasionally be seen at the periphery of areas of localized neurodermatitis. It may occur in association with spina bifida.

Hirsutism may be noted after the prolonged administration of ACTH and, less commonly, after oral corticosteroid therapy. The excess hair growth usually disappears on suspension of treatment, but this may require many months. Increased growth of hair in women at the time of the menopause is by no means uncommon, and often quite conspicuous. There may be a rather heavy growth on the upper lip, or growth is scattered in rather profuse terminal hairs elsewhere on the face. The treatment of hirsutism, except in the very occasional case amenable to specific endocrinologic therapy, is unsatisfactory. Electrolysis is extremely tedious and is worthwhile only where the hairs are relatively few and scattered. Bleaching is commonly used, since it renders the hairs much less conspicuous, particularly if they are not especially coarse. Plucking is frequently employed and is not particularly dangerous except for the occasional case of folliculitis. Chemical depilatories containing sulfide salts are commonly used and are reasonably satisfactory unless they cause irritation. The most satisfactory and least hazardous method is shaving. Women commonly shave the legs and axillas, but they often have a psychologic aversion to removing hair on the face in this manner. Contrary to popular belief, there is no evidence to indicate that shaving stimulates hair growth.

REFERENCES

Brooksbank, B. W. L.: Endocrinological Aspects of Hirsutism, Physiol. Rev., 41(4):623, 1961.

McKnight, E.: The Prevalence of "Hirsutism" in Young Women, Lancet, I:410–413, 1964.

Pillsbury, D. M., W. B. Shelley, and A. M. Kligman: "Dermatology," Philadelphia, W. B. Saunders Company, 1956.

——, ——, and ——: "A Manual of Cutaneous Medicine," Philadelphia, W. B. Saunders Company, 1961.

Rogers, G. E.: pp. 179–232 in "Structural and Biochemical Features of the Hair Follicle in the Epidermis," W. Montagna and W. C. Lobitz, Jr. (Eds.), New York, Academic Press, Inc., 1964.

Rook, A.: Endocrine Influences on Hair Growth, Brit. Med. J., 1:609–614, 1965.

35 PIGMENTATION
Donald M. Pillsbury and Walter B. Shelley

The skin has a wide variety of pigmentation patterns, some of which are highly suggestive of certain systemic diseases. The principal endogenous sources of color in the skin are four in number, of which melanin is by far the most significant. The others are carotene, oxyhemoglobin, and reduced hemoglobin.

It is not surprising that the deposition of melanin in the skin varies greatly. Genetic factors are of obvious importance, controlling the type and degree of pigmentation at birth and, to some extent, the manner in which the skin pigment changes in response to a wide variety of local stresses, as well as to a number of metabolic and other systemic disturbances. In interpreting changes in melanin pigment, the racial background of the person must be considered. Areas of hyperpigmentation in a person of Mediterranean origin may be of no significance; similar changes in a Nordic blonde might justify searching study.

Another reason for variations in melanin pigmentation is the basic complexity of pigment formation. This is an extraordinarily intricate biochemical phenomenon, and a number of disturbances may occur in the progression from the basic substrate tyrosine to the end product of melanin granules in the epidermis.

Melanin pigmentation varies considerably in hue. If it is in the epidermis, the color ranges from light tan to jet black. This variation is due to the density of the melanin granules laid down; there is no change in the number of melanocytes. They vary in activity from a complete inability to form melanin, as in albinism or vitiligo, to a very high output, as in the Negro or in areas affected by acanthosis nigricans. There is no indication as to whether or not the chemical composition of melanin may vary with differences in color. The chemistry of melanin is not yet known.

If melanin is deposited in the dermis rather than the epidermis, a rather striking difference in color is seen. Because of the Tyndall light-scattering phenomenon, the color of the area is slate-gray or bluish. Such a color is seen in mongolian blue spots and in blue nevi in the corium. The pigment deposition occasionally seen in exposed areas in persons who have received phenothiazine in large doses for prolonged periods of time, usually years, is brownish blue.

The biochemistry of melanin formation, the known mechanisms which influence its synthesis, and the various syndromes associated with decreased or increased amounts of melanin in the skin are discussed in detail in Chap. 102. For a summary the reader is referred particularly to Table 102-1.

In addition to the disturbances of melanin pigmentation described in Chap. 102, two further characteristic syndromes may be included here.

ACANTHOSIS NIGRICANS

This easily recognized change may be entirely benign or may be associated with severe endocrine disease or with malignancy, the latter most frequently of the gastrointestinal tract or the breast.

Acanthosis nigricans is a symmetric, hyperpigmented verrucous and hyperkeratotic reaction of the folds of the skin. The most commonly involved sites are the axillas and anogenital region, but the process is sometimes more extensive. The surface of the skin has a velvety appearance, and the black color is often strikingly intense.

There has been some confusion about the classification of acanthosis nigricans in relation to systemic disease, but the following groups seem justified.

CONGENITAL. Seen in infancy, congenital acanthosis nigricans is of little or no systemic import.

JUVENILE. The juvenile type of this disease has its onset at puberty, with significant endocrine disease in about one-third of all cases. These endocrine disorders include pituitary adenoma of various types, Stein-Leventhal syndrome, Addison's disease, and diabetes mellitus.

ADULT MALIGNANT. When the skin changes develop in adult life they are highly significant in terms of associated malignancy, most commonly glandular in origin. Various series have shown such an associa-

tion in some 50 per cent of all cases. There may be a strong family history of malignancy in such patients.

PSEUDOACANTHOSIS NIGRICANS. The changes are confined to the skin and occur in obese individuals of any age. It is thought that they result from chronic irritation and maceration.

The gross and histologic features of the various types of acanthosis are similar, though there is considerable variation in the degree of pigmentation and keratinization.

PIGMENTATION DUE TO PHENOTHIAZINE

In 1964, the initial report of a peculiar type of pigmentation of the skin occurring in patients on longterm, high-dosage chlorpromazine therapy appeared. In many patients, this is associated with eye changes consisting of fine dotlike stippling of the anterior capsule of the lens and of the cornea, usually in the corneal endothelium. No better example of delayed recognition of an unwanted effect of a drug can be cited, since chlorpromazine was introduced into practice 10 years previously and has had very wide usage.

The pigmentation of the skin occurs after prolonged therapy in high doses, namely, between 2 to 10 years in doses of 400 to 1,500 mg a day or more. It develops in a variable small percentage of patients receiving such therapy. Its appearance on exposed portions of the skin indicates that sunlight plays a significant role. The condition is seen most frequently in female schizophrenics. Such treatment has ordinarily been given for patients in maximum security wards and has been continuous. The pigmentation is found primarily on the face, neck, and hands. It is brown to blue-gray in hue, with some patients showing almost a violet color.

The pigment is principally in the dermis, resulting in a bluish cast, though some pigment is noted in the epidermis as well. It is seen microscopically as brownish granules, chiefly about blood vessels and in macrophages. The pigment is positive with the Fontana stain and negative with iron stains. On this basis it is believed to be melanin, but this has not been established with absolute certainty. There is some indication that the pigment gradually fades with withdrawal of all phenothiazine compounds, but this has not been possible in many patients because of their return to a violent, disturbed schizophrenic state in the absence of phenothiazine therapy.

Of more importance are the eye lesions which have been observed in the patients with skin pigmentation. These occur with some frequency in the absence of any detectable skin changes, but only in patients who have had phenothiazine therapy over a long period and in a high dosage. The eye lesions occur almost equally in males and females. A brownish discoloration of the portions of the conjunctiva exposed to light is seen occasionally. The stippling of the cornea and lens is demonstrable by slit-lamp examination. There are no retinal changes. Significant visual impairment has been rare. There is some evidence that the eye lesions may regress after phenothiazine therapy is stopped, but this may require 6 months or more.

YELLOW PIGMENTATION

Carotene is normally present in the keratin of the skin. It is also found in subcutaneous fat. The amount of carotene may be greatly increased if excessive quantities of yellow vegetables or fruits (e.g., carrots and oranges) are ingested. The resultant yellow color may be striking, particularly in heavily keratinized areas such as the palms and soles. The sclerae are not involved. Carotenemia is occasionally seen in infants, but marked instances of it are not common in adults. It has been noted in male castrates, in panhypopituitarism, and in occasional diabetics. In combination with melanin deposition, it may be seen in myxedema.

Yellow pigmentation from exogenous chemicals may occur. It was an almost constant finding in military personnel receiving suppressive quinacrine (Atabrine) therapy during World War II. If such individuals developed dermatitis or the lichenoid syndrome from the drug, the range of colors produced could be remarkable. Pigmentation from quinacrine is slow to disappear, usually requiring several months.

Yellow pigmentation may be seen, though far less frequently than in the past, from absorption of dinitrophenol by workers in the explosive or dye industries. Tetryl, also used in the explosive industry, is capable of producing marked yellowing of the skin ("tetryl canary").

Jaundice is one of the best known of all discolorations of the skin (see Chap. 29). It varies greatly in its intensity, from a barely detectable light yellow to a greenish or even brownish color. The sclerae are involved.

Oxyhemoglobin imparts a redness to the skin which, in white individuals, is often very obvious. It varies from less apparent to indiscernible, however, in brown-to-black–skinned persons. Reduced hemoglobin is, of course, the source of the bluish color seen in cyanosis. Various abnormal hemoglobins may produce bizarre colorations (Chap. 119). These include carboxyhemoglobin—a cherry red (carbon monoxide), and nitric acid hemoglobin—bright red (fumes from explosives). Methemoglobin (a chocolate blue) and sulfhemoglobin (lead or mauve blue) may occur together and may arouse suspicion of cardiac or pulmonary disease. A number of drugs have been incriminated, including sulfonamides, phenacetin, acetanilid, trional, and sulfonal.

Hemosiderin is capable of producing slight to marked relatively permanent pigmentation of the skin. It is sometimes difficult to distinguish from melanin pigmentation, and, indeed, the two may coexist. Special stains for melanin (e.g., Fontana stain) and for iron may be necessary. The most striking example of combined hemosiderin and melanin hyperpigmentation is bronze diabetes (hemochromatosis) (see p. 555).

The most common example of hemosiderin deposition is that seen on the lower legs in persons above middle age. It is an almost invariable finding in persons who have chronic stasis and who have senile capillary fragility. The pigmentation may assume bizarre morphologic patterns; these patterns have received designation as separate syndromes in the older dermatologic literature but do not deserve this distinction.

Though purpura from any one of many sources is usually resorbed, in occasional instances the characteristic remains of hemosiderin deposits, ranging in appearance from cayenne pepper to brown stippling, persist. In older individuals, particularly, a somewhat guarded prognosis as to complete disappearance of marked purpura is often advisable.

METALLIC PIGMENTATION

The syndrome of argyria has almost disappeared from the medical scene. It was due largely to prolonged instillation of silver proteinate nose drops and to the administration of silver nitrate capsules for gastrointestinal ulcerative conditions, both types of therapy long discredited. Localized argyria may sometimes be produced by the application of silver salts to abraded skin. In diffuse argyria the skin becomes light to dark slate or blue gray in color, principally on exposed areas. The metal is permanently deposited in the dermis, principally about the sweat glands. Argyria is of cosmetic significance only.

Gold compounds may uncommonly produce skin pigmentation rather similar to that of argyria. This is related to the total dose, probably of the order of more than 100 mg per kg body weight.

Tattooing is of minor medical importance other than psychic. The chief danger is infection—principally infectious hepatitis and tuberculosis—transmitted from the "artist." Several cases of leprosy in Armed Forces personnel were apparently acquired from tattooing. Local dermatitic or granulomatous reactions may be seen, principally from sensitivity to the mercury component of cinnabar.

REFERENCES

Beerman, H., and H. Colburn: Some Aspects of Pigmentation of the Skin, Am. J. Med. Sci., 231:451, 1956.

Curth, H. O., and B. M. Aschner: Genetic Studies on Acanthosis Nigricans, A.M.A. Arch. Dermatol., 79:55–66, 1959.

Fitzpatrick, T. B., M. Seiji, and A. D. McGugan: Melanin Pigmentation, New England J. Med., 265:328, 1961.

Greiner, A. C., and K. Berry: Skin Pigmentation and Corneal and Lens Opacities with Prolonged Chlorpromazine Therapy, Can. Med. Assoc. J., 90:663, 1964.

Jeghers, H.: New England J. Med., 39:11, 1955.

Pillsbury, D. M., and W. R. Hill: "Argyria," Philadelphia, Williams & Wilkins Company, 1939.

Winkelmann, R. K., S. R. Scheen, Jr., and L. O. Underdahl: Acanthosis Nigricans and Endocrine Disease, J.A.M.A., 174:1145–1152, 1960.

36 SUNLIGHT AND PHOTOSENSITIVITY REACTIONS

Donald M. Pillsbury and Walter B. Shelley

Solar radiation, at once our prime source of vision, food, and fuel, may be also a source of disease. Ranging in wavelengths of from 2,900 to 18,500 Å, sunlight includes a spectrum of ultraviolet, visible, and infrared rays. The latter bands of visible and infrared rarely are responsible for disease; it is the pathogenic effects of the invisible ultraviolet (2,900 to 4,000 Å) light which usually account for the disturbances observed in the skin. Wavelengths below 2,900 Å do not reach the earth's surface.

By far the most common and familiar change is sunburn. Here, varying degrees of photochemical injury are induced by the absorption of rays between 2,900 and 3,200 Å. These rays penetrate into the superficial epidermis, where they act on unconjugated proteins to produce as yet unidentified initiators of the inflammatory response. Although the amount of radiation varies with the hour, day, latitude, altitude, atmospheric and surface conditions, most individuals can judge their tolerance. Once this is exceeded, the sunburn occurs after a 6- to 8-hr latent period, gradually subsiding after a course of 72 to 96 hr. Although the range of reaction extends from hyperesthesia and erythema to the formation of huge bullae, the primary process remains that of acute inflammation and is responsive to systemic corticosteroids. Following sunburn the skin may show evidence of occult vascular damage for over a year. With repeated episodes or prolonged excessive exposure to sunlight, dramatic premature localized aging of the skin ensues. Such thickened leathery skin shows histologic degeneration of the connective tissue. Comparison of the appearance of the skin of the neck and chest in any farmer rapidly convinces one of the deleterious effect of long-term solar radiation in large doses. Inevitably such sunlight induces premalignant actinic keratoses of the exposed areas and, later, carcinomas. Basal cell epitheliomas of the face may thus be the serious sequelae of indiscriminate and prolonged sun bathing. Significantly one finds a considerably greater incidence of cutaneous cancer in individuals living in areas where the sun's radiation is more intense. Negroes almost never develop actinic keratoses or epitheliomas.

What protection is afforded against this ultraviolet radiation? The body has three major constituents which partially absorb and nullify such noxious rays. The most obvious is melanin (acting as a stable free radical), produced by the melanocytes and then fed into the basal cells, where it forms supranuclear caps to protect the vital genetic code centers. The rate of formation of such melanin, i.e., tanning, is directly related to the ultraviolet dosage as well as to obvious genetic factors. Melanin formation is also stimulated by the longer wavelengths of visible blue light itself. Thickening of the dead absorbent stratum corneum is a second compensatory sun screen mechanism. This

regularly occurs following significant sun exposure. Finally, urocanic acid, a derivative of histidine, has been shown to be the component of sweat and thereby stratum corneum which strongly absorbs impinging ultraviolet radiation. To these may be added the innumerable synthetic screening agents that one may apply locally in the form of lotions, oils, and creams. At present, red veterinary petrolatum rides a wave of popularity for its protective topical effects. However, the most certain sunburn protective is window glass, since it absorbs all of the sunburn spectrum (below 3,200 Å).

In addition to the acute and chronic effects of solar ultraviolet light described above, there are certain altered reactions observed in patients which deserve note. All these may best be described as *photosensitivity* reactions. In other words, they are changes which reflect an abnormal sensitivity to a specific band of the sun rays. Usually drugs or chemicals are responsible for this altered state, and in some instances the photosensitizing substance is endogenous, as for example in porphyria. Such photosensitivity reactions may be either phototoxic or photoallergic in nature, just as the cutaneous reactions to a chemical may be toxic or allergic. Unfortunately it is often easier to dissociate these two types in concept than in practice.

In the *phototoxic* area the clinical response is an exaggerated sunburn. Apparently the photosensitizing compound absorbs light of a specific wavelength, thus exciting the formation of free radicals, with subsequent toxic damage to the superficial epidermis. No immunologic mechanisms are involved, oxygen being the only requirement. Thus, the drug or compound is the sole determinant—and the reaction occurs in nearly everyone exposed to both drug and the appropriate band of light.

By contrast, in the less common *photoallergic* process, immunologic mechanisms enter. In these, the reactions are polymorphic, appearing as papules, plaques urticaria, or eczema. The patient must be uniquely and specifically sensitized by previous exposure. However, the allergic process is triggered only by a specific band of solar radiation, possibly reflecting the formation of a light-induced allergen. The means of distinguishing phototoxic and photoallergic states are poor, so that often one must be content with a diagnosis of photosensitivity. Incidentally, if the sensitizer is topical, the result is described as contact photosensitization (ironically known to occur even as a result of sensitization to sun screen preparations).

Ideally, both the offending chemical and the solar wavelengths should be identified in these patients. As a practical reality much less is ordinarily achieved. Monochromator sources giving narrow bands of light of known energy levels should be ideal, but such instruments are still in the research class. Actually the sun may be employed for testing, but it is an inconstant and rather weak source. Hot quartz and carbon arc lamps are the best tools, but they must be used with selective filters, since they give a complete range of wavelengths. Cold quartz lamps are of no practical value, since they emit rays largely of the 2,537 Å band, a ray not present in terrestrial sunlight. Window glass is a most useful filter, permitting an answer to whether or not the sunburn rays are responsible. Only those rays above 3,200 Å are transmitted by such glass. Corning glass filter 7-38 permits transmission of rays between 3,200 and 3,800 Å, whereas filter 3-74 permits only those above 4,000 Å.

Two basic photo skin tests are usually employed, namely,

1. Determination of the 24-hr *minimal erythema dose* (M.E.D.) with a given lamp.

2. Determination of the 10-day *delayed erythema dose* (D.E.D.). In this instance one usually gives ten times the M.E.D. and watches for a delayed papular or eczematous response. Photo contact allergy is determined by coupling patch testing with exposure to specific radiation.

What are the suspect substances in a case of photosensitivity? Although dozens of drugs must be considered, as a matter of practical experience the following four groups account for most of the photosensitivity reactions observed clinically:

1. Sulfonamides, including sulfonyl ureas and chlorthiazides, are a common cause of photoallergic responses in exposed skin.

2. Phenothiazines may induce acute photosensitivity. High dosage over long periods leads to bizarre and extreme chronic pigmentation. Patients on such high doses should avoid sunlight.

3. Tetracyclines, especially demethyl chlortetracycline, which produces a phototoxic response coupled at times with onycholysis.

4. Furocoumarins. These plant derivatives include the psoralens prescribed for the purpose of inducing photosensitization to promote therapeutic melanization, as for example in vitiligo.

In the topical division, coal tar is the most powerful and regular sensitizer, but in many instances perfumes are found to be the offending agent.

Porphyria is associated with sunlight sensitivity because of the circulating porphyrins which act as sensitizers. This is an example of a phototoxic state produced by a metabolic or genetic fault. Congenital (erythropoietic) porphyria is often first recognized by the severe mutilating photosensitivity seen in children with this condition. In the hepatic type, low-grade blistering of the hands and face is characteristic only in the chronic form. Interestingly, the absorption spectrum of the photosensitizing porphyrins is in the 4,000 Å area so that it is this band which excites the response (see p. 560).

For certain conditions current knowledge does not permit any label other than idiopathic photosensitivity. This is also true in terms of the pathogenesis of the photosensitivity observed in patients with lupus erythematosus. Fortunately, chloroquine provides a rather specific and effective remedy for all persons with this idiopathic form. It must, however, be given in low dosage on a carefully regulated basis with suitable ophthalmologic consultation, since chloroquine may induce retinopathy.

REFERENCES

Baer, R. L., and L. C. Harber: Light Sensitivity in Biologic Systems, Fed. Proc., 24: No. 1, Part III, s15–s21, 1965.

Daniels, F.: The Physiological Effects of Sunlight, J. Invest. Dermatol., 32:147–155, 1959.

Kirshbaum, B. A., and H. Beerman: Photosensitization Due to Drugs: A Review of Some of the Recent Literature, Am. J. Med. Sci., 248:445–468, 1964.

Shelley, W. B.: Photosensitizers, pp. 88–103 in "Dermatoses Due to Environmental and Physical Factors," Rees B. Rees (Ed.), Springfield, Ill., Charles C Thomas, Publisher, 1962.

37 SWEATING DISORDERS

Donald M. Pillsbury and Walter B. Shelley

Although anatomically inapparent grossly, the eccrine sweat gland is the dominant appendage of the skin. Numbering some three million separate coiled tubules, the sweat gland organ has the critical task of assisting in man's thermoregulatory system. It does not perform any significant excretory function, although electrolytes, urea, and a few other substances may be eliminated by the gland in the process of secretion of water for cooling.

The distribution of sweat glands shows area differences, with the greatest density in the palms and soles. Indeed the upper arm and thigh show only one-fifth as many glands per unit area as the palms. Interestingly, the full complement of glands develops in the embryonic state and the variation noted in adults probably reflects the variable developmental growth rates of the various areas of skin. Thus, the twenty-four-week-old fetus has a sweat gland population twenty-five times as dense as that of the adult.

Anatomically the gland is a simple tubule extending down from the epidermis to the lower dermis. The lower portion is a tightly coiled secretory apparatus consisting of two types of cells. The one is a dark basophilic cell which secretes mucinous material; the other is a light acidophilic cell which is responsible for the passage of water and electrolytes. The duct plays an active part in the function of the gland, presumably a role of reabsorption.

The gland is excited to action by heat, being innervated by cholinergic fibers of the thoracolumbar sympathetic chain. Thus, all eccrine glands respond to cholinergic drugs, but it should be pointed out that they also secrete, in limited degree, following the introduction of adrenergic compounds. A rise in body temperature is accompanied by generalized sweating which reflects the central control mechanism of the hypothalamus. Psychic, emotional, or sensory stimulation may also activate the eccrine sweat glands. Here, the premotor area of the cerebral cortex serves as a control center, and usually the palms, soles, and axillas are the primary sites of response. The cortex may also have a center which inhibits sweating. Gustatory sweating is a response of the glands, especially on the face, to foods such as spices.

Sympathetic denervation is followed by failure of the gland in the affected area to respond to either fever or emotional strain, except in an abortive fashion to local heating. Atropine and its congeners are effective in producing a pharmacologic blockage of the sweat gland.

Axone reflex sweating can be induced as a local response to injury, or the intradermal injection of nicotine. The significance of this mechanism appears limited clinically to local hyperhidrosis seen at the margin of inflammatory dermatoses.

With repeated episodes of profuse sweating, the salt content of the sweat progressively declines. As part of the acclimatization process, this phenomenon probably reflects the appearance of salt-retaining corticosteroids as a result of thermal stress. Conversely, in disease the gland may function at a lower level of efficiency and the salt content is higher than normal. This is the case in mucoviscidosis (cystic fibrosis) and has been the basis for the diagnostic "sweat test" in these patients. Specifically, when the sweat chloride concentration exceeds 60 mEq per liter the test is positive. Normal values average 17 mEq per liter.

The apocrine sweat gland is still another gland distinctive from the eccrine sweat gland. Considerably larger, it is far more limited in distribution. Generally the apocrine glands of the skin are found in the axillas, ear canal, and to a limited extent in the nose and eyelid, as well as in the perineal, pubic, and mammary regions. A few ectopic glands may be found anywhere. The classic example is seen in the apocrine glands of the axilla. They are attached to the hair, forming an apopilosebaceous unit. Under hormonal development control they do not appear until puberty and begin to decrease in size and activity after the age of fifty. They appear to be an atavistic appendage with little real function except to pour small amounts of a milky white fluid onto the surface in response to emotional stress or adrenergic stimuli. This is attacked by the surface bacteria, resulting in a distinctive regional odor. Clinically, excessive secretion may be associated with an excessive odor. This can easily be erased by frequent bathing or the use of a topical bactericide. An additional clinical point is the fact that bacterial infection may occur down in the gland leading to an exquisitely chronic pyoderma which resembles furunculosis but is actually a distinctive apocrine disease, *hidradenitis suppurativa*. It demands intensive systemic antibacterial therapy coupled with surgery.

HYPERHIDROSIS

No clinical sign is more obvious than the outflow of sweat in hyperhidrosis. It can be viewed with the naked eye or under magnification. At times indirect methods such as use of starch iodine, quinizarin, or nitrozine paper may aid in its study.

LOCALIZED. Emotional hyperhidrosis is the most common cause of excessive sweating in restricted areas. Classically, it occurs in the axillas, palms, soles, and forehead in response to fear, excitement, or anxiety. Mental or physical effort, tension, or pain may cause these paroxysmal bursts of sweating. In a few instances medical help is necessary in the form of explanatory reassurance, tranquilizers, or anticholinergic compounds systemically. In the case of severe hyperhidrosis of the palms, which may interfere with every job or social opportunity, bilateral cervical sympathectomy has been a boon. Axillary hyperhidrosis can be combated by local surgical excision of many of the glands; more recently, the topical application of esters of scopolamine has been used. The average individual uses the commercially available astringent aluminum salts topically with varying degrees of success.

Any inflammatory process which causes discharge down the sympathetic fibers will induce local hyperhidrosis. Examples are seen in thrombophlebitis, Buerger's disease, causalgia, neuritis, and nerve injuries. Trench foot and immersion syndrome regularly show hyperhidrosis in some phases.

Neurologic diseases such as syringomyelia and encephalitis may be associated with localized hyperhidrosis, often of the gustatory type. This latter may also be associated with disease of the parotid gland, which initiates salivary reflexes.

GENERALIZED. The drenching sweats of a fever are the obvious example of this type of sweating. Warmth, alcohol, tea, coffee, and aspirin all serve to accentuate any tendency to sweating. Since sweat serves for evaporative cooling, any means of raising body temperature (hot bath, exercise) actually induces hyperhidrosis. Certain infectious diseases have long been associated with sweating, e.g., malaria, tuberculosis, brucellosis. Other examples are seen in association with diabetes mellitus and hyperthyroidism. An interesting and rare cause is pheochromocytoma. Cholinergic drugs, such as pilocarpine, physostigmine, or methacholine, may act directly. Drug allergies may also produce fever.

Neurologic disturbances which cause stimulation of the hypothalamus produce general hyperhidrosis. Encephalitis and diencephalic epilepsy have been reported in this connection. Compensatory hyperhidrosis is seen in the patient who has had so many glands denervated by extensive sympathectomy that the remainder have to function excessively to maintain homeostasis. This occurs, for example, if all four extremities are sympathectomized. Motion sickness and pain are two additional unusual causes of generalized hyperhidrosis.

ANHIDROSIS

Anhidrosis, i.e., the absence of the ability to sweat, is an "invisible" sign, one that calls for the positive approach of testing for sweat function. In its complete form it is the absence of sweating and, hence, the cause of heat intolerance which will manifest itself under thermal stress such as headache, fever, and asthenia. Hypohidrosis, i.e., diminished ability to sweat, may be a concomitant or cause of disease.

LOCALIZED. Inasmuch as the sweat gland is under sympathetic innervation, any interruption in the peripheral path will lead to localized anhidrosis. Thus, this condition may be seen in syringomyelia, transverse myelitis, tumors of the cord, multiple sclerosis, poliomyelitis, or sympathectomy. It may also follow trauma to the peripheral nerve, leprosy, or neuritis. The areas of anhidrosis will be evident and of diagnostic help only if tests for sweating are undertaken. Diverse diseases, especially gout and diabetes mellitus, are associated with degeneration of peripheral sympathetic fibers and hence with anhidrosis. Usually anhidrosis from this cause is most evident on the lower extremities.

Many skin diseases are associated with anhidrosis. In some instances the gland may be destroyed, as in atabrine or radiation dermatitis. Generally, however, the anhidrosis results from sweat retention occasioned by closure of the epidermal sweat pore. In its primary form, one sees miliaria (prickly heat) induced by the maceration of hyperhidrosis of hot environments. Depending on the depth of obstruction, anhidrosis may take on different forms. Secondary sweat retention anhidrosis is seen in patches of psoriasis, lichen planus, and atopic dermatitis, as well as in stasis dermatitis. Sweating still occurs, but none is delivered to the surface; hence the finding of anhidrosis.

GENERALIZED. The most significant area in sweat control is the hypothalamus. Injury to this area leads to generalized anhidrosis, as in tumor, vascular accident, heat stroke, surgery, or trauma.

Systemic disease such as myxedema, scurvy, or Simmonds' disease has also been known to produce anhidrosis. Finally, congenital absence of sweat glands accounts for some examples of anhidrosis which elude the casual observer. Erythroderma, such as may follow extensive psoriasis or atopic dermatitis, is another cause which may mask the sign.

Finally, generalized anhidrosis is found to occur in individuals in the Tropics. The affected person loses all sweat gland function except on the face, where a marked compensatory hyperhidrosis appears. Deep plugging of the sweat duct completely wipes out the person's defense against high temperatures. Exposure leads to fatigue, fever, vertigo, and collapse. Treatment centers on keeping the patient in a cool environment, where in the course of 2 weeks all the millions of closed sweat pores will spontaneously reopen and the patient will return to normal.

REFERENCES

Herxheimer, A.: Excessive Sweating: A Review, Trans. St. Johns Hosp. Dermatol. Soc., 40:20, 1958.

Hurley, H. J., and W. B. Shelley: "The Human Apocrine Sweat Gland in Health and Disease," Springfield, Ill., Charles C Thomas, Publisher, 1960.

Montagna, W., et al. (Eds.): "Eccrine Sweat Gland and Eccrine Sweating," New York, Pergamon Press, 1962.

Shelley, W. B., P. N. Horvath, and D. M. Pillsbury: Anhidrosis: An Etiologic Interpretation, Medicine, 29:195, 1950.

Sulzberger, M. B., and F. Herrmann: "The Clinical Significance of Disturbances in the Delivery of Sweat," Springfield, Ill., Charles C Thomas, Publisher, 1954.

Section 8

Anemia, Bleeding, Adenopathy, and Splenomegaly

38 PALLOR AND ANEMIA
M. M. Wintrobe

SIGNIFICANCE OF PALLOR. The color of the skin depends on many factors, which include the thickness of the epidermis, the quantity and type of pigment contained therein, and the number and degree of patency of the blood vessels, as well as the quantity and nature of the hemoglobin carried within them. Even the nature and fluid content of the subcutaneous tissue are significant factors. It is obvious, therefore, that pallor does not necessarily indicate that anemia is present.

A sallow complexion is present in certain individuals, as it was in their forebears before them, and may exist in the absence of any true anemia; the flush of excitement, on the other hand, or constant exposure to the sun and wind may produce an appearance which masks an underlying anemia. Physicians, at the turn of the present century, spoke of "rosy" chlorotics, as well as of green and pale ones. The number and pattern of distribution of the finer blood vessels vary in different individuals, and in the same person vasoconstriction may produce the appearance of pallor, whereas other factors, such as exercise, for example, may lead to the appearance of a "healthier" color. Certain disorders may affect the skin in such a way that

THE ERYTHRON

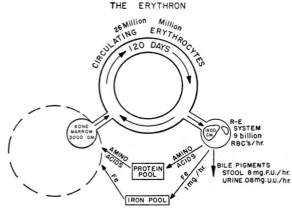

Fig. 38-1. The amount of blood in circulation represents the balance between production and destruction. In a 70-kg man the circulating red corpuscles carry approximately 770 Gm hemoglobin. Since the average life span of the red corpuscles normally is 120 days, the turnover rate per day is the total in the circulation divided by 120. In the average man this comes to approximately 2.16×10^{11} red corpuscles per day, or 9 billion per hour, and 6.4 Gm hemoglobin per day. From this are derived approximately 21 mg iron per day, 250 mg protoporphyrin, and 6.2 Gm globin. The iron and globin are reutilized. Of the protoporphyrin derived from the destroyed red corpuscles, somewhat less than 250 mg appears as fecal urobilinogen, since there are great variations in completeness of evacuation and also because of variations in the extent to which pigments giving this reaction are produced. Under normal conditions, through increased production and transformation of yellow marrow to red, the bone marrow is capable of approximately a seven- or eightfold increase in production capacity. Consequently, other things being equal, anemia will not develop as the result of increased blood destruction until the life span of the red corpuscles has been reduced to less than about 15 to 17 days.

a pallid appearance is produced, even though anemia is absent. These disorders include scleroderma, the various nephrotic states, and myxedema. The last two, however, may be accompanied by actual anemia.

ANEMIA

DEFINITION

THE ERYTHRON. The *erythron* refers to the circulating red corpuscles as well as to that part of·the hematopoietic system which is concerned with their production and destruction. As represented in Fig. 38-1, in the normal individual production is in equilibrium with destruction. Average wear and tear result in a "life span" of the red corpuscles which is approximately 120 days.

Hemoglobin, a compound of 67,000 mol wt, forms approximately 90 per cent of the red corpuscle (dry weight). It is made up of a colorless protein, globin, on the surface of which are four small prosthetic groups of heme molecules. Heme, which imparts the red color to the hemoglobin molecule, is a metal complex consisting of an iron atom in the center of a porphyrin structure (Fig. 38-2). The porphyrin has been designated protoporphyrin 9, type III. Like other

porphyrin rings, it consists of four pyrrole nuclei connected to one another by methene $\left(\begin{smallmatrix} H \\ =C- \end{smallmatrix}\right)$ bridges. The iron, which has the capacity of binding oxygen reversibly, is linked to the nitrogen atom in each of the pyrrole groups and also to the imidazole nitrogen of the histidine in globin.

The structure of heme is identical in all mammals, but the properties of hemoglobin with respect to electrophoretic mobility, solubility, and resistance to denaturation by alkali vary in different species, apparently because of subtle differences in the composition of globin. In addition, in man a number of different types of hemoglobin, dependent on genetically determined differences in globin structure, have been discovered which in some instances govern the development of hematologic abnormalities and certain clinical manifestations (p. 637).

FORMATION AND DESTRUCTION OF HEMOGLOBIN. The source material for the formation of porphyrin is a 4-carbon asymmetric compound arising in the tricarboxylic acid cycle. In vitro as well as in vivo studies have clarified the steps in the synthetic process (Fig. 38-3). Acetate is transformed into succinate and this, in the presence of magnesium ions, adenosine triphosphate, and coenzyme A, gives rise to "active" succinate (succinyl CoA). This is one of the sites at which pantothenic acid functions in erythropoiesis, since this vitamin is a component of CoA. The vitamin pyridoxine is involved in the next step. The activated form of succinate condenses with a pyridoxal phosphate-glycine-enzyme complex to form delta-aminolevulinic acid (Δ-ALA) and carbon dioxide via several intermediate compounds. Two molecules of Δ-ALA in the presence of glutathione and an appropriate enzyme condense to form a monopyrrole, porphobilinogen. The subsequent steps leading to the formation of protoporphyrin are shown in the diagram. Ultimately protoporphyrin is converted to hemoglobin in the presence

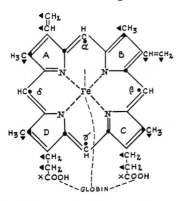

Fig. 38-2. Chemical structure of heme and its manner of union with globin to form hemoglobin. The carbon atoms derived from the alpha-carbon of glycine are represented by ●, those supplied from the methyl carbon of acetate by ▼, and those derived from the carboxyl group of acetate by ✗. The unmarked carbons are those derived either from the methyl carbon atom of acetate or from the carboxyl atom. (*Prepared by Dr. G. E. Cartwright.*)

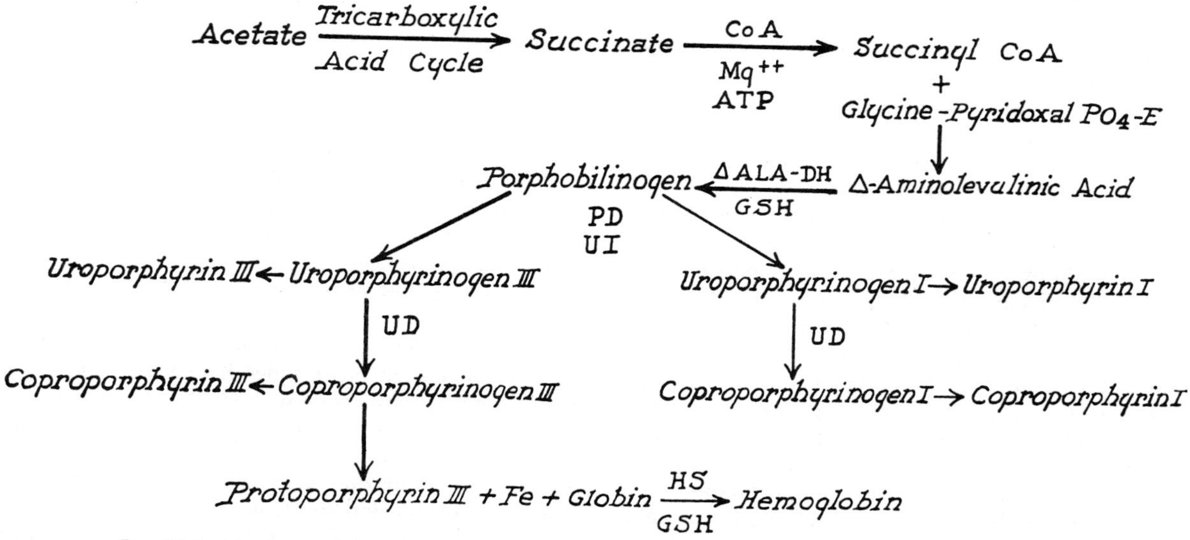

$$\text{Acetate} \xrightarrow[\text{Acid Cycle}]{\text{Tricarboxylic}} \text{Succinate} \xrightarrow[\substack{Mg^{++} \\ ATP}]{CoA} \text{Succinyl CoA}$$

+

$$\text{Glycine - Pyridoxal } PO_4\text{-}E$$

$$\text{Porphobilinogen} \xleftarrow[\substack{GSH}]{\Delta ALA\text{-}DH} \Delta\text{-Aminolevulinic Acid}$$

PD
UI

$$\text{Uroporphyrin } III \leftarrow \text{Uroporphyrinogen } III \qquad \text{Uroporphyrinogen } I \rightarrow \text{Uroporphyrin } I$$

$$\downarrow UD \qquad\qquad\qquad\qquad\qquad\qquad \downarrow UD$$

$$\text{Coproporphyrin } III \leftarrow \text{Coproporphyrinogen } III \qquad \text{Coproporphyrinogen } I \rightarrow \text{Coproporphyrin } I$$

$$\downarrow$$

$$\text{Protoporphyrin } III + Fe + Globin \xrightarrow[GSH]{HS} \text{Hemoglobin}$$

Fig. 38-3. The biosynthesis of hemoglobin and the by-products that are formed. (Prepared by Dr. G. E. Cartwright.) (M. M. Wintrobe: "Clinical Hematology," 5th ed., Philadelphia, Lea & Febiger 1961.)

of iron, glutathione, globin, and an enzyme, heme synthetase. Amino acids are the source materials for the independent process which results in the formation of globin.

In the breakdown of hemoglobin, the protoporphyrin ring is opened by an oxidative removal of the α-methene bridge, the iron remaining and the union with globin persisting to form a green iron-protein compound, choleglobin or verdohemoglobin. How the cleavage is achieved is not clear, nor is it understood how iron is ultimately split off and globin liberated to yield the bile pigment, biliverdin, a straight chain tetrapyrrole. It is known, however, that this takes place in the reticuloendothelial system and that the liberated iron is bound to protein in the tissues and then is transported as "plasma iron" via the transport protein, transferrin, a β_1 globulin, either to the bone marrow, where it is used in the synthesis of new hemoglobin, or to the storage depots where it is deposited as ferritin, a ferrous iron-protein complex, or as hemosiderin, a ferric hydroxide polymer. The liberated globin is degraded and is returned to the body pool of amino acids. Biliverdin, as discussed earlier (p. 119), is rapidly reduced to bilirubin, which is then transported from the site of hemoglobin breakdown to the liver via the blood plasma, where it is carried with albumin as a relatively stable protein-pigment complex. On reaching the liver, bilirubin is separated from albumin, conjugated with glucuronic acid, and excreted via the bile canaliculi and the bile ducts in the form of protein-free di- and monoglucuronides, the former predominating.

Under pathologic conditions, free hemoglobin may escape into the circulation. This colors the plasma faint pink to deep red, depending on the concentration. The latter can be measured quantitatively by the benzidine reaction. Hemoglobinemia occurs in severe hemolytic states when there is intravascular hemolysis, as in erythroblastosis fetalis, blackwater fever, and Clostridium welchii (C. perfringens) sepsis (p. 1601). Such hemoglobin is promptly bound by certain α_2 globulins with affinity for hemoglobin, the haptoglobins, and is carried to the reticuloendothelial system for breakdown there and conversion to bilirubin. The plasma haptoglobins can usually bind from 100 to 135 mg hemoglobin per 100 ml plasma. When this binding capacity is exceeded, hemoglobin is liberated in the plasma and escapes in the urine. In addition, some is converted in the plasma to a golden or brown pigment, methemalbumin. This represents a combination of the heme portion of the hemoglobin and the albumin of plasma. It reacts with benzidine and can be distinguished spectroscopically from other heme and pyrrole pigments. Demonstration of methemalbumin in plasma is pathognomonic for intravascular hemolysis. This compound may remain in the plasma for many hours or several days.

The so-called "renal threshold" for hemoglobin is probably not a true renal barrier but depends on the capacity of the binding proteins of the plasma and the reabsorptive capacity of the tubules. It is the free, unbound hemoglobin which appears in the urine. Hemoglobin usually appears in the urine if the plasma hemoglobin concentration rises to the range of 125 to 175 mg per 100 ml after acute hemolysis. Hemoglobinuria is then likely to continue until the plasma hemoglobin has fallen to 75 mg per 100 ml. Methemalbumin does not usually pass into the urine. However, the tubular epithelium of the kidney converts hemoglobin to hemosiderin, and hemosiderin occurs regularly in the urine of patients with low concentrations of heme pigments in their plasma. The passage of hemoglobin by the kidney is accompanied and also followed by proteinuria, hemoglobin casts, and precipitates of hemoglobin. The color of urine ranges from pink to deep red with oxyhemoglobin, from purple to black from reduced hemoglobin.

It has been held that bilirubin also can be derived from hematin, the trivalent iron complex of protoporphyrin 9. This may be formed in hematomas and collections of blood in serosal cavities.

It should be mentioned also that not all the bile pigment is derived from senescent erythrocytes. Studies of stercobilin excretion following the administration of N^{15}-labeled glycine indicate that normally at least 10 per cent, and in diseases like pernicious anemia and congenital porphyria as much as 30 to 40 per cent, is probably derived from heme or porphyrins produced in excess and not utilized in hemoglobin synthesis.

In the intestine, probably through the activity of the bacterial flora, bilirubin is converted to urobilinogen. Urobilinogen consists of three colorless chromogens, all of which are characterized by a strong Ehrlich aldehyde reaction, as well as by instability and ease of oxidation to three corresponding orange-yellow pigments which compose the urobilin group. The transition to urobilin can be hastened by mild oxidizing agents, such as iodine, and this is the basis of the Schlesinger (alcoholic zinc acetate) qualitative test for urobilin. Of the urobilinogen group, stercobilinogen is normally preponderant in the feces and urine. The remaining two substances are mesobilirubinogen and d-urobilinogen. Mesobilirubinogen is converted to stercobilinogen. d-Urobilinogen may be a precursor of mesobilirubinogen.

Although some investigators have maintained that the urobilinogens in urine come directly from bilirubin in the plasma, it is more generally held that they are derived from pigments absorbed from the colon into the portal circulation, most of which are returned to the liver and reexcreted in the bile but a small proportion of which escape into the general circulation and are excreted by the kidney.

The amount of urobilinogen excreted in the urine in 24 hr (UU) by the normal adult is 0 to 3.5 mg, most frequently 0.5 to 1.5 mg. The normal range for fecal urobilinogen (FU) as calculated from a 4-day period of collection is 40 to 280 mg per day, usually 100 to 200 mg. Lower values are found in young children. Mean values have been found to increase with age. The oral administration of chlortetracycline (Aureomycin) causes a marked decrease in the concentration of fecal urobilinogen, but this can be counteracted by the administration of aluminum hydroxide gel.

When the balance between the production and destruction of red corpuscles is altered in such a way that less than the normal quantity of red corpuscles is found in the circulation, anemia results. Anemia occurs, in other words, when production fails to keep up with demand. The latter may be normal, and yet anemia may develop because of (1) deficiency of materials required for the construction of the red corpuscles or (2) some defect in the metabolic processes concerned in erythropoiesis. On the other hand, anemia may occur in spite of vigorous production (3) because

of blood loss or (4) as the result of excessive blood destruction (Table 38-1).

PATHOGENESIS

The simplest mechanism by which anemia develops is blood loss. Anemia due to blood loss may be acute or chronic. In the former the cause of the anemia is usually obvious, although sometimes a large hemorrhage may have occurred under conditions which do not reveal themselves readily. Hemorrhage in the gastrointestinal tract, as from a peptic ulcer, may be dramatic in its symptomatology and may be so severe as to cause shock; at other times it may be insidious in character and may occur without the development of pain or of symptoms pointing clearly to the gastrointestinal tract. Hemorrhage into one of the serous cavities can cause puzzling symptoms and signs: profound anemia may develop suddenly and icterus may even eventually appear as the result of absorption of blood from a serous cavity.

Chronic loss of blood occurs most commonly from the pelvic organs in females and from the gastrointestinal tract in the male. A common cause of chronic posthemorrhagic anemia in certain parts of the world is infestation with the hookworm.

For the construction of red corpuscles, as already stated, amino acids and protein, iron, and the precursors of porphyrin, are required. Certain minerals such as copper and cobalt are concerned in erythropoiesis, and under experimental conditions in animals it can be shown that anemia will develop when they are lacking. Perhaps still other minerals are involved. Certain of the B vitamins are important in erythropoiesis. These include pantothenic acid, pyridoxine, folic acid (pteroylglutamic acid), and vitamin B_{12}; riboflavin and nicotinic acid are possibly concerned as well.

Without doubt, protein deficiency results in anemia in man, but since there exists in the body a "dynamic equilibrium" of the proteins, the deficiency of protein must be very great before hemoglobin production suffers. The role of the specific amino acids in erythropoiesis in man remains to be worked out.

It is clear that in man anemia can occur as the result of iron deficiency. Cobalt deficiency has never been demonstrated in man, but a form of copper deficiency associated with hypoproteinemia and microcytic hypochromic anemia has been described in infants. Of the B vitamins, deficiency in man has been demonstrated only in the case of folic acid and vitamin B_{12}. Deficiency of these substances is characterized by macrocytic anemia and megaloblastic bone marrow. Quite possibly the other B vitamins are available in sufficient amounts, even under the extraordinary circumstances under which man sometimes finds himself, so that anemia clearly attributable solely to lack of nicotinic acid, riboflavin, or pantothenic acid has not been demonstrated. Pyridoxine-deficiency anemia has only once been produced experimentally in the human infant, but anemia responding to the administration of pyri-

Table 38-1. ETIOLOGIC CLASSIFICATION OF ANEMIA

I. Loss of blood
   A. Acute posthemorrhagic anemia
   B. Chronic posthemorrhagic anemia
II. Deficiency of factors concerned in erythropoiesis
   A. Iron deficiency
      Experimentally, also copper and cobalt deficiencies
   B. Deficiency of various B vitamins
      Clinically B_{12} and folic acid deficiencies (pernicious anemia and related macrocytic, megaloblastic anemias) and "pyridoxine-responsive" anemia
      Experimentally pyridoxine, folic acid, B_{12}, and nicotinic acid deficiencies; possibly also riboflavin, pantothenic acid, and thiamine deficiencies
   C. Protein deficiency
   D. Possibly ascorbic acid deficiency
III. Excessive destruction of red corpuscles resulting from
   A. Extracorpuscular causes
   B. Intracorpuscular defects, congenital (see IV, A below) and acquired
IV. Faulty construction of red corpuscles
   A. Congenital or hereditary
      1. Sickle-cell anemia and related disorders (hemoglobin C disease, etc.)
      2. Thalassemia
      3. Hereditary spherocytosis and nonspherocytic hemolytic anemias
   B. Acquired
      1. Anemia associated with infection
      2. Anemia associated with various chronic diseases (renal, etc.)
      3. Anemia in plumbism; following irradiation; in drug sensitivity (aplastic anemia)
      4. Anemia in myxedema and in other endocrine deficiencies
      5. Myelophthisic anemias (leukemia, Hodgkin's disease, myelofibrosis, malignancy with metastases, etc.)
      6. Anemia associated with splenic disorders ("hypersplenism")
      7. Idiopathic bone marrow failure (aplastic, hypoplastic, or refractory anemias)
   C. Miscellaneous hypersideremic anemias (for additional details see Tables 112-1, 113-1, 114-1, pp. 620, 630, and 639, respectively.)

doxine has been reported in several adults in whom it may have developed as the consequence of some metabolic defect.

More frequently deficiencies which result in anemia in man are not due to lack of the substance in the diet but are "conditioned" by special circumstances. Thus lack of vitamin B_{12} in pernicious anemia results from an inability to absorb this vitamin because of lack of a gastric "intrinsic factor." Again, in sprue, vitamin B_{12} or folic acid deficiency may develop, presumably as the consequence of inadequate absorption. The same condition is occasionally encountered following extensive resection of the small bowel or in the case of a gastrocolic fistula. Excessive demands in pregnancy and greater needs for growth in childhood and adolescence may "condition" the development of various types of deficiency, and anemia will then ensue. (See Table 112-1, p. 620.)

The role of ascorbic acid in relation to anemia has not been established clearly; while anemia is seen in scurvy, it has not been shown that this is due directly to lack of vitamin C (see p. 626).

As already indicated, the whole red cell mass is replaced approximately every 4 months. Destruction at a more rapid rate is met by increased production of red corpuscles by the bone marrow, which is capable of approximately a sevenfold increase in activity. When destruction exceeds production, anemia develops. Such hemolytic anemias may be due to a large variety of causes which injure the red corpuscles (for extracorpuscular causes, see Table 113-1, p. 630), or they may be associated with intrinsic defects in the erythrocytes. The latter condition will be considered in brief below.

A number of anemias cannot be attributed to blood loss, impaired production as the consequence of deficiency of essential building stones, or increased blood destruction as the result of the action of injurious agents. It is plausible to consider that a fourth mechanism by which anemia may develop is impairment of the synthetic processes which normally result in the production of the red corpuscles. The fault may be qualitative or quantitative, or both. In the last case, less than the normal quantity of cells would be made, but those formed might conceivably be entirely normal or abnormal to only an insignificant degree. If the defect is qualitative, defective red corpuscles may be produced which are destroyed more readily than is usual. As already indicated, increased production may be expected to make up for losses resulting from increased destruction unless the latter exceeds the productive capacity of the hematopoietic system. If the metabolic defect is both qualitative and quantitative, anemia will develop. Its manifestations may be expected to be those of impaired production or of increased destruction or both, in different degrees, depending on the nature of the fault in erythropoiesis.

Considerable evidence is now accumulating which gives support to this concept. First in this category are several types of anemia which are hereditary in nature and hemolytic in their manifestations. These anemias are usually classified as hemolytic anemias due to intracorpuscular defects (Table 113-1, p. 630). It appears that they also belong in the category under discussion. Studies of the pathogenesis of sickle-cell anemia and certain related disorders have revealed that several different types of hemoglobin can be distinguished electrophoretically and that the production of an abnormal hemoglobin is the fundamental defect in these conditions. Thus it appears that a molecular abnormality in a simple protein may cause the sequence of events that characterize a single disease. There is evidence that a similar concept may apply to thalassemia. So far there is nothing to indicate that such a concept explains the pathogenesis of hereditary spherocytosis, but such an explanation seems plausible, since the abnormality in that disease has been shown to reside primarily in the red corpuscles. The pathogenesis of these disorders will be considered in more detail elsewhere (Chaps. 112 *et seq.*).

It seems likely that a fault in the construction of red corpuscles not only may be inherited but can also be acquired. It is possible that by one means or another, as will be mentioned below, the synthetic mechanisms by which red corpuscles are normally produced may become impaired. By interfering with erythropoiesis the metabolic disturbance may result in the production of fewer cells; or defective red corpuscles may be made which are destroyed more readily than is normal. Although the classic manifestations of hemolytic anemia are unusual in the types of anemia to be considered, it is conceivable that the rate of destruction, or perhaps even the manner of destruction, may be such that the classic manifestations of hemolytic anemia will be absent. In some instances, and even perhaps in all the types of anemia coming under this category, it is possible that both these mechanisms are involved; namely, fewer cells are produced, and many of those which are made are poorly constructed. The evidence to support this concept of the pathogenesis of the anemias, which will be mentioned below, is still only suggestive. However, it is a useful one for the present.

Thus, it has been observed that *infection* is associated with a profound disturbance in iron metabolism. This is manifested by a low plasma iron, reduced plasma iron–binding capacity, and decreased incorporation of iron into hemoglobin. The defect cannot be altered by iron administration, even if iron is given parenterally in large quantities. An increase in free erythrocyte protoporphyrin and in serum copper occurs at the same time. Whether the anemia associated with infection is due directly to these changes or is related to them more remotely is unknown. In any event, the profound metabolic defect caused by infection, of which these are presumably some of the manifestations, can be overcome by appropriate treatment of the infection. As this is accomplished, the anemia is also relieved. Various other forms of therapy directed toward relief of anemia, such as the administration of iron, are of no value.

The pathogenesis of the *anemia associated with chronic renal disease* is an enigma. Unlike the anemia associated with infection, anemia of renal insufficiency does not have hypoferremia as a constant feature. Like the anemia of infection, however, it is closely tied with the underlying disease and is uninfluenced by measures other than those which affect renal function. An exception to this statement is the influence of cobalt on both the anemia of renal disease and that associated with infection (p. 643). The nature of this effect is obscure, but it is probably not concerned with the fundamental cause of the anemia.

In association with renal insufficiency, erythropoiesis becomes depressed. Two patterns have been described, namely, one in which the arrest of erythropoiesis is almost complete and the red cell mass falls rapidly, and another in which moderate or considerable depression of red cell mass is present and persists over long periods of time. Only the second variety is related to the degree of uremia. In general severe anemia is observed when the creatinine rises above 2 mg per 100 ml and the blood urea nitrogen becomes greater than 70 mg per 100 ml. Concurrently with either form of depressed erythropoiesis, red cell survival is decreased, in part at least, as the consequence of an extracorpuscular factor. The nature of this factor is obscure; there is no evidence of an autoimmune mechanism, nor is there a clear relation with any of the products which are retained in renal insufficiency. The relationship of the anemia associated with renal insufficiency to the erythropoietic serum factors which may be produced in the kidney is obscure.

Inhibition of hemoglobin synthesis by toxic action on porphyrin-forming mechanisms appears to be a factor in the pathogenesis of the *anemia of plumbism*. Many of the red corpuscles that are formed are imperfect, and their accelerated removal from the circulation, as compared with the life span of normally formed cells, is probably another factor in the pathogenesis of this form of anemia. The *anemia which follows irradiation* is related to the inhibition of nucleic acid synthesis, but depending on such factors as dose and duration of exposure, other mechanisms may be involved as well, namely, accelerated breakdown, perhaps due to injury of the circulating red corpuscles, damage to capillary walls with resulting diversion of erythrocytes into tissue spaces and lymphatics, and hemorrhage. Individual susceptibility, perhaps based on an underlying abnormality in a detoxifying mechanism, or other unrecognized factors seem to be involved in the anemia which follows ingestion of certain drugs.

The pathogenesis of the *anemia* observed *in myxedema* is obscure. Defective absorption of vitamin B_{12}, uninfluenced by intrinsic factor, has been demonstrated in some cases. The anemia, which is usually only moderate in degree and is usually normocytic but may be macrocytic, disappears gradually as desiccated thyroid is given, but it seems unlikely that it is attributable directly to deficiency of the hormone. It has been suggested that it is brought about indirectly through the effect of the thyroid on the consumption of oxygen by the tissues. Moderate anemia is encountered in association with *adrenal cortical insufficiency* and in cases of *hypopituitarism*. The pathogenic mechanisms are not understood, but in view of what is now known concerning the functions of the hormones secreted by the adrenal glands and the pituitary gland, it is at least plausible that the anemia is the consequence of some metabolic disturbance resulting from deficiency of these hormones.

The pathogenesis of the *anemia in leukemia, Hodgkin's disease, malignancy with metastases* to bone marrow, *myelofibrosis*, and other similar conditions is as yet quite obscure. Such anemia has been classified as *myelophthisic*. The term implies wasting away of the marrow, but it is usually used to refer to encroachment on or replacement of the bone marrow by leukemia or metastases. There is little or no evidence, however, that the erythropoietic tissue is crowded out in these myelophthisic anemias. Measurements of red cell production rates have yielded normal or increased values. It has been suggested that in some cases erythrophagocytosis contributes to the anemia. A number of studies have shown the "life span" of the red corpuscles to be reduced, and occasionally frank hemolytic anemia develops. It is possible that no single explanation for the anemia associated with these diseases will be found, but it is plausible, at least, that a metabolic fault related to the underlying disease is an important factor.

The anemia accompanying certain *disorders involving the spleen* has been attributed to an exaggeration of the normal functional activities of this organ ("hypersplenism"), which include the removal of worn-out red corpuscles. Such anemia might therefore be regarded as hemolytic and resulting from extracorpuscular causes. That this is the sole cause of anemia accompanying various disorders of the spleen may be questioned, however. (See p. 678.)

It should not be overlooked that, in any given patient with a chronic ailment accompanied by anemia, more than one factor may play a role. Thus, in any long-standing illness there may be nutritional deficiency because of reduced intake and sometimes also because of faulty absorption from the gastrointestinal tract. Blood loss may be an added factor. In addition, as already discussed, a metabolic disturbance, like that which accompanies infection, may play a role as well. As noted already, in some instances excessive blood destruction complicates the picture still further.

SYMPTOMATOLOGY

Hemoglobin is the vehicle and the cardiovascular system the means of supply of oxygen to the tissues. Nevertheless, anemia may be present in severe degree and yet may be associated with few or no symptoms; on the other hand, mild grades of anemia may be found, and yet symptoms may be prominent. The development of symptoms in association with anemia depends on (1) the causative disorder; (2) the rapidity with which anemia has developed; (3) the degree of reduction in the oxygen-carrying power of the blood, as well as the extent of changes in total blood volume; and (4) the preexisting status of the cardiovascular system. The last factor is important because a defective cardiovascular system is less capable of adjustment to anemia than a normal one. The physiologic adjustments to anemia are represented diagrammatically in Fig. 38-4 and will be discussed shortly.

The nature of the condition which has led to the development of anemia is important, since disorders leading to anemia may—of themselves—cause pronounced symptoms which attract attention early; whereas other conditions are of such a nature that they are not likely to be detected until the effect of oxygen want, due to reduced oxygen-carrying power, becomes a factor. If anemia has developed so rapidly that there has been little or no time for physiologic adjustment, symptoms of oxygen want are likely to be prominent and to appear comparatively early; on the other hand, if the anemia has been insidious in onset, the adjustment may be so good that the volume of packed red cells may be even as low as 20 ml per 100 ml blood, or the hemoglobin as low as 6 Gm per 100 ml, without sufficient functional embarrassment occurring for the patient to appreciate his true condition.

When anemia is caused by the sudden loss of blood, the most prominent symptoms are those resulting from the reduction of the total blood volume, and they are relieved in large measure when the lost blood is replaced by absorption of fluid from the tissues or by the artificial introduction of fluid or red cells. When there is rapid destruction of blood, the chief symptoms are those connected with the disposal of the products of blood destruction—namely, hemoglobinuria and jaundice. There may also be fever and even abdominal pain. When the anemia is caused by faulty formation of blood, its onset is much more insidious than in the above circumstances, and the symptoms are referred chiefly to the respiratory, circulatory, neuromuscular, and gastrointestinal systems.

RESPIRATORY SYSTEM. Respiratory symptoms in patients suffering from anemia are often noticeable only after exertion or excitement, although when the anemia is profound there may be dyspnea and rapid breathing even at rest in bed. Respiratory complaints are also dependent on associated myocardial changes and alterations in the cardiovascular system in general.

CARDIOVASCULAR SYSTEM. Manifestations referable to the cardiovascular system depend on the severity of the anemia, the age of the patient, the rapidity of onset of the anemia, and the capacity of the cardiovascular system for adjustment. Anemia is one of the commonest causes of palpitation, shortness of breath, and pallor. If very severe, shock may develop. In chronic anemia, moderate dyspnea and palpitation may be the only symptoms related to the cardio-

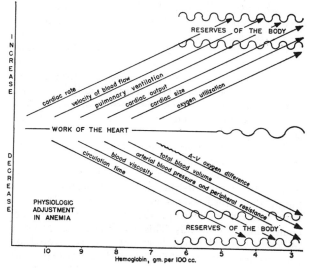

Fig. 38-4. Schematic diagram of physiologic adjustments to anemia. (M. M. Wintrobe: Blood, 1:121, 1946.)

vascular system, but, in certain cases, symptoms of congestive failure, angina pectoris, or intermittent claudication may be found as well.

Clinical evidences of an adjusting circulation in cases of anemia include a rapid heart rate, increased arterial pulsation, and increased pulse pressure; even capillary pulsation in the finger tips may be found, and still other signs of the "hyperkinetic syndrome" may be observed (p. 788). The heart may be dilated. These signs are due to increased venous return to the heart, with resulting increase in cardiac output. Thus the circulation time is shortened, and there may be a slight rise in right auricular pressure. Otherwise central venous and intracardiac pressures are not altered. The total circulating blood volume may decrease, although this is not always the case. Peripheral vascular resistance is lowered, and the oxygen dissociation curve is displaced to the right; that is, there is a reduction in the affinity of hemoglobin for oxygen. Extraction of oxygen by the tissues is therefore facilitated, and by this means tissue oxygen utilization can be maintained in spite of the narrowed arteriovenous oxygen difference and the rapid circulation time.

Coincidentally with the cardiovascular changes, the rate and depth of respiration often are increased and the vital capacity together with the reserve and complemental air volumes are lowered. The residual air is somewhat increased, and minute ventilation is increased.

These and other changes which have been demonstrated to occur in association with anemia may not take place in an orderly manner and naturally become more pronounced as the anemia becomes more severe. The deviations from the normal values vary from patient to patient but generally are definite when the hemoglobin is less than 7.5 Gm per 100 ml blood and are greatest at the lowest levels of hemoglobin concentration. However, even at low levels of hemoglobin, anemic individuals at rest are able to compensate satisfactorily in the delivery of oxygen and the transport of carbon dioxide. On the other hand, during exercise, depending on the degree of anemia, the various hemodynamic adjustments become insufficient.

Severe anemia may produce a systolic murmur, which is usually most marked at the pulmonic area but may be heard elsewhere over the precordium, especially at the apex. Very rarely, diastolic blows are heard at the base. Over the vessels of the neck a curious humming sound, the *bruit de diable*, may be heard.

When compensatory adjustments become imperfect or fail, the clinical picture of cardiac failure ensues. Lateral displacement of the left cardiac border, basal rales in the dependent portions of the lungs, downward extension of the liver edge, and liver tenderness develop. Edema is a frequent accompaniment of anemia. This may be the consequence of lowered renal blood flow but also is favored by such factors as hypoproteinemia and diminished tissue oxygen tension leading to increased capillary permeability. The reduction in the number of circulating red corpuscles is, of itself, of little importance in altering the osmotic pressure of the blood.

NEUROMUSCULAR SYSTEM. Headache, vertigo, faintness, increased sensitivity to cold, tinnitus or roaring in the ears, black spots before the eyes, muscular weakness, and easy fatigability and irritability are common symptoms associated with anemia. Restlessness is an important symptom of rapidly developing anemia. Drowsiness develops in severe anemia. Headache due to anemia may be so severe as to simulate that of meningitis. Delirium is seldom seen except in pernicious anemia and in the terminal stage of leukemia. Retinal hemorrhage is by no means infrequent.

Paresthesias are common in pernicious anemia, and they may be accompanied by signs and symptoms of extensive peripheral nerve and spinal cord degeneration. They may also be encountered in chronic hypochromic anemia, but in the latter, spinal cord degeneration is very rare. In leukemia, involvement of cranial and peripheral somatic nerves occurs, but it is then almost always due to pressure or infiltration.

ALIMENTARY SYSTEM. Loss of appetite is not unusual as an accompaniment of anemia. Nausea, flatulence, abdominal discomfort, constipation, diarrhea, vomiting, or abnormal appetite may also be found. In pernicious anemia and, less often, in chronic hypochromic anemia, glossitis and atrophy of the tongue and papillae are common. In the latter condition, in particular, dysphagia may be found. Necrotic lesions in the mouth and pharynx may develop in patients with aplastic anemia, in granulocytopenia, and in acute leukemia.

GENITOURINARY SYSTEM. Menstrual disturbances, most often amenorrhea, in the female and loss of libido in the male are frequently encountered in severe anemia. In other instances, excessive menstrual bleeding accompanies anemia. Slight proteinuria and even evidence of distinct renal function impairment may be seen in association with anemia.

NUTRITIONAL STATE. If the quantity of superficial fat is the criterion, the nutritional state may appear to be moderately or well preserved, in spite of the presence of anemia. When nutritional deficiency is present, the mucous membranes may be shiny and red, the tongue red and atrophic. Rarely there may also be fissures at the corners of the mouth, seborrheic accumulations about the nose, and erythematous lesions on the hands, face, neck, and elbows.

In severe anemia the basal metabolic rate may be moderately increased. Fever of mild degree is common when anemia is severe. A well-marked febrile reaction is characteristically found when there is rapid blood destruction.

SPLEEN. Enlargement of the spleen is rather frequent in various anemias of long standing. It is seen, in particular, in pernicious anemia, in chronic hypochromic anemia, and in the various hemolytic anemias, as well as in such conditions as leukemia, in which the spleen is specifically involved in the disease process. Moderate enlargement of the *liver* may be observed as well.

INTEGUMENTARY SYSTEM. The pallor which accompanies anemia has been discussed already. In addition, loss of normal skin elasticity and tone, thinning of the hair, and purpura and ecchymoses may develop in the chronic forms of anemia. When there is iron deficiency, the nails lose their luster, become brittle and break easily, and may become concave instead of convex (koilonychia).

So striking are its manifestations, and in certain parts of the country so common is the disorder, that special mention needs to be made of sickle-cell anemia. This condition exemplifies more than any other how varied the symptoms of anemia can be. The cardiac manifestations of sickle-cell anemia may be so pronounced as to be indistinguishable from those of rheumatic heart disease. Pain in the extremities may add to the confusion with rheumatic fever. Crises of abdominal pain have led to unnecessary operations many times, and the effects of thrombosis in the central nervous system have often raised the question of some neurologic disorder. Yet all these and still other bizarre symptoms and signs which are encountered in this disorder can be attributed to sickle-cell anemia alone.

DETECTION

The presence or absence of anemia is determined by the examination of the blood, but its existence may nevertheless be suspected and its degree even estimated with fair accuracy by proper examination of the patient. The skin itself, as already indicated, is an unreliable index of anemia; the mucous membranes (if not inflamed), the nail beds, and the palms of the hands are more dependable. The color of the conjunctiva may be very helpful, but one should not be misled by a coexistent conjunctivitis. The gums are not so useful as would be expected, for they may contain pigment or may be inflamed; furthermore, the pressure of the upper lip on the gums may produce some blanching if constriction of vessels results as the lip is retracted. Unless the hand has been held in an awkward position or has been exposed to cold or excessive heat, the nail beds and the palms of the hands will reveal anemia if much exists. In the palms the color of the creases is especially noteworthy, for they retain their red color even after the intervening skin of the palms has become definitely pale; when their color is lost, the hemoglobin may be judged as being below 7 Gm per 100 ml.

The presence or absence of anemia can be determined from the red cell count, the hemoglobin, or the volume of packed red cells as measured in the hematocrit. Of these procedures, the measurement of hemoglobin is the simplest, but the accuracy of various hemoglobinometers differs greatly. More accurate, as a rule, as an index of anemia (or polycythemia) is the measurement of the volume of packed red cells. When this is measured in the hematocrit, additional information becomes available which is extremely useful in the routine survey of a patient. This includes the sedimentation rate of the red corpuscles, the volume of packed white cells and platelets, and the icterus index. If 5 ml blood is collected from a vein in a mixture of ammonium and potassium oxalate (6 mg of the former and 4 mg of the latter per 5 ml blood), or in ethylenediamine tetracetate (Versene), blood is available for a number of quantitative determinations. The white cell count can be determined without the necessity of obtaining more blood from the patient. A clue as to their number can be gained from the thickness of the layer of white cells above the layer of packed red cells. If the volume of packed red cells is abnormal, red cell counts and hemoglobin can be determined and the average volume and hemoglobin content of the red cells calculated. If the volume of packed platelets is abnormal, they can be enumerated, and if the color of the plasma appears unusual, the icterus index can be measured or a clue is obtained which suggests the need for other chemical determinations. Blood smears must be made directly from the finger. They should be examined in all instances of suspected anemia, for the morphology of the cells can serve as a valuable clue to the nature of the anemia and may be used to check the calculated mean corpuscular constants.

The normal values of red corpuscles for people at various ages are presented in the Appendix. These data are for persons living at sea level. At higher altitudes, higher values are found, roughly in proportion to the elevation above sea level. In general, the blood of normal persons tends to approach the mean for the sex. Provided the measurements are accurate, a deviation below the mean of more than 10 per cent should be looked upon with suspicion as representing mild anemia.

STUDY OF A PATIENT WITH ANEMIA

Since anemia is a symptom, it is evident that the patient with anemia requires thorough examination. The *history* must be complete and must, in particular, give attention to the following details:

1. The possible occurrence of blood loss, either acute and in large amounts or chronic and long continued.

2. The diet, particularly with reference to the intake of foods rich in protein, vitamins, and minerals.

3. The presence or absence of symptoms suggesting an underlying disease such as chronic renal disease, chronic infection, or malignancy.

4. In the case of a child or adolescent, the rate of growth.

5. In the case of a woman, the nature of the catamenia (amount of flow, duration, and frequency); the number of pregnancies and abortions; the occurrence of excessive post-partum hemorrhage and the duration of lactation.

6. In certain cases, the possibility of exposure to poisons of various types should be investigated. In this last regard, attention must be given not only to the patient's occupation and its possible hazards but also to hobbies which may result in exposure to poisons, to possible exposure to insecticides, and to

the taking of drugs which may be harmful (chloramphenicol, sulfonamides, gold, etc.).

7. The family history is sometimes of great importance in the study of anemia. A history of splenectomy in some member of the family may be a valuable clue to the diagnosis. If a familial or hereditary disorder is suspected, other members of the family should be examined if possible, since the family may be unaware of the existence of any detectable abnormality.

The *physical examination* must likewise be thorough. The examination of the skin and mucous membranes has been referred to already. The fundi of the eyes should be examined, for they may reveal hemorrhages or the exudates characteristic of chronic renal disease or of leukemia. The tongue may be atrophic, and the mucous membranes may reveal purpuric spots. A thorough check needs to be made for evidence of glandular enlargement, and it is good practice to palpate the bones. If done systematically such palpation may reveal tenderness in the sternum or nodules or tenderness in the ribs. In any condition leading to bone marrow hyperplasia, localized tenderness over the sternum is usually encountered if systematically sought out. In cases of multiple myeloma one may find nodules or tenderness in the ribs. The heart cannot be ignored, for it may give evidence of hemic murmurs or may yield the first clue to the existence of a subacute bacterial endocarditis. The liver and spleen must also be examined carefully, and the kidneys must be given attention, for it is not unusual for hypernephroma to cause an obscure anemia. Neither the pelvic nor the rectal examination can be neglected, for they may yield the first indication as to the nature and cause of the anemia. The nervous system, particularly in cases of macrocytic anemia, is likely to reveal abnormalities of significance.

The physical examination may need to be supplemented by roentgenography. A roentgenographic film of the chest may reveal unsuspected mediastinal enlargement, while roentgenograms of the bones may lead to the discovery of tumors or of periosteal elevations suggesting leukemia.

The *laboratory examination* may well commence with the collection of 5 ml blood from a vein, as described already, together with a few blood smears. The discovery of anemia, as indicated by a reduced volume of packed red cells, should be followed by red cell counts and a hemoglobin determination; from them can be calculated the mean corpuscular volume, mean corpuscular hemoglobin, and mean corpuscular hemoglobin concentration. These findings should be checked by examination of the blood smear. In the latter may be found evidences of exaggerated erythropoiesis such as polychromatophilic red corpuscles, macrocytes, and even nucleated red cells. Evidences of disturbed red cell formation, such as poikilocytes, Cabot rings, and Howell-Jolly bodies, may also be found, or the smear may reveal an unsuspected protozoal parasite (e.g., that of malaria). An increased reticulocyte count gives evidence of physiologically stimulated red cell formation.

The fact should not be overlooked that the hematopoietic system functions as a physiologic unit. Consequently, when red cell formation is stimulated, it is found as a rule that there is, in addition, increased leukopoiesis and an increase in the quantity of platelets. Thus, following acute blood loss, there may be not only reticulocytosis but also moderate or even marked leukocytosis accompanied by an increase in the younger forms of leukocytes not ordinarily seen in such numbers in the blood ("shift to the left"). The quantity of platelets also is likely to be increased.

When erythropoiesis is impaired, owing to iron or to vitamin B_{12} deficiency or in aplastic anemia, one finds evidence of disturbed leukocyte and platelet formation as well. Thus, in pernicious anemia, leukopenia is a common accompaniment of the anemia and is usually associated with relative lymphocytosis and the presence of multisegmented polymorphonuclear leukocytes. Thrombocytopenia often exists as well.

Evidence of increased red cell destruction must also be sought out. The clue to this is generally given by the appearance of the plasma which, in cases of increased blood destruction, is distinctly icteric. The van den Bergh reaction reveals this to be of the "indirect" type, and examination of the urine in such cases reveals an increased quantity of urobilinogen (see p. 629). It is useful, where the facilities exist, to measure the quantity of urobilinogen excreted in the stool as well. Such measurements, however, have only limited usefulness as indices of increased blood destruction (p. 628). In relation to increased blood destruction, it is again important to look upon the hematopoietic system as a physiologic unit. Increased blood destruction, except in certain types of chronic hemolytic anemia, is accompanied not only by the chemical evidence just mentioned but also by reticulocytosis, leukocytosis, and thrombocytosis (see p. 629). If there is reason to believe that one is dealing with a hemolytic anemia, special procedures will aid in the differential diagnosis, such as a test of the osmotic fragility of the red corpuscles, the Coombs test, and the presumptive test for warm, cold, and acid hemolysins (see Chap. 113).

The anemia associated with chronic infection or with chronic renal disease, like aplastic anemia due to the action of a poison, is differentiated from the anemias due to nutritional deficiency and the anemias due to exaggerated blood destruction by the lack of evidence of hematopoietic activity. Thus the anemia is usually normocytic and is accompanied by relatively little poikilocytosis or anisocytosis; reticulocytes are normal in number, and nucleated red cells are not found in the blood smear; the leukocytes are not altered in number from the normal except in so far as they may represent a reaction to the underlying disorder.

The rapid growth of knowledge concerning the metabolism of the red cell and the chemical processes concerned in erythropoiesis has led to the introduction of a number of procedures which are useful in the recognition of certain anemias, particularly the less common varieties. These will be discussed in later chapters, but here the value of plasma iron determinations may be mentioned. The *plasma iron content* is reduced below normal in cases of iron deficiency, in association with the anemia of chronic infection, and in various types of anemia in which blood regeneration is active. An interesting difference between the findings in cases of iron deficiency and in those caused by infection is the fact that the iron-binding capacity of the plasma is greatly increased above normal when the hypoferremia is due to iron deficiency, whereas it is less than normal when the hypoferremia is associated with the anemia of chronic infection. The plasma iron content is increased in pernicious anemia in relapse and in hemolytic anemias. However, the increased plasma iron of pernicious anemia in relapse falls to values below normal during the time when blood regeneration is occurring as the result of specific therapy. In certain circumstances, particularly in the anemia of chronic infection, the content of *free protoporphyrin in the erythrocytes* is increased. In this type of anemia the *serum copper content* is also in excess of normal.

When the patient has been studied thoroughly in the manner indicated above, the number of instances in which *examination of the bone marrow* will be required is small. In Table 38-2 various types of

Table 38-2. CONDITIONS IN WHICH VARIOUS TYPES OF REACTION MAY BE OBSERVED, AS DEMONSTRATED BY BONE MARROW ASPIRATION

M/E (myeloid/erythroid) ratio increased

Myeloid forms of leukemia
The majority of infections
Leukemoid reaction
Decrease in nucleated red cells

Nonmyeloid cells increased

Other forms of leukemia
Multiple myeloma
Metastases from carcinoma, etc.
Gaucher's disease, Niemann-Pick disease
Aplastic anemia (usually relative increase only)
Infectious mononucleosis

Normoblastic hyperplasia

Hemorrhagic anemias
Iron-deficiency anemia
Hemolytic anemias
Thalassemia
Cirrhosis of the liver
Polycythemia vera
Plumbism
Anemia of chronic renal disease

Megaloblastic hyperplasia

Pernicious anemia
Sprue, idiopathic steatorrhea, resection of small intestine (certain cases)
Tropical macrocytic anemia
Nontropical nutritional macrocytic anemia
Macrocytic anemia with diphyllobothrium infestation
Megaloblastic anemia of infancy
Megaloblastic anemia of pregnancy
"Refractory megaloblastic" or "achrestic" anemia

reaction are listed which may be observed if differential counts on aspirated bone marrow are made. In the study of bone marrow as obtained by sternal, iliac crest, spinous process, or rib puncture, consideration should be given to the following:

1. What is the myeloid/erythroid (M/E) ratio? By this is meant the proportion of leukocytes of the myeloid series to nucleated red cells of all types.

2. If the M/E ratio is decreased—that is, if the proportion of nucleated red cells is greater than normal—this may be because of a decrease in the number of myeloid cells, or it may be the consequence of an increase in erythroid cells. In the latter event, one must differentiate between normoblastic and megaloblastic hyperplasia.

3. Is there an increased number of cells other than those of the myeloid or erythroid series? These include lymphocytes, plasma cells, reticulum cells, and other forms (myeloma cells, carcinoma cells, Gaucher cells, etc.).

4. Since megakaryocytes form so small a proportion of the cells of the bone marrow, specific attention should be given them and a number of preparations of marrow should be examined. Do they appear to be increased or greatly decreased in number? Is their morphology normal?

5. If little material has been obtained by puncture, is the bone marrow aplastic, fibrotic, or otherwise abnormal, the material obtained being essentially only blood? In such a case, surgical biopsy may be necessary.

In Table 38-3 are given normal values for the differential nucleated cell count of bone marrow obtained by puncture, and representative findings in a number of conditions are presented. These must be regarded only as examples of findings in typical cases and do not give the range of variation in disease. The latter obviously depends on the stage of the disease and the presence or absence of modifying factors and is difficult to present in tabular form.

Although in all cases the material obtained by sternal puncture is of interest, bone marrow examination is an essential aid in diagnosis only in a limited number of conditions. These include aleukemic leukemia, multiple myeloma, Gaucher's and Niemann-Pick diseases, and unusual cases of macrocytic anemia. In the last-mentioned condition the demonstration of megaloblasts is very useful, since it suggests vitamin B_{12} or folic acid deficiency. In "aleukemic" leukemia, the bone marrow reveals numerous immature forms, thus dispelling the doubt raised by their absence or scarcity in the blood. In addition to these disorders, it may be added that, in cases of parasitic diseases such as kala-azar, the causative organisms may be discovered in the bone marrow when they cannot be found in any other way. Again, the cells of metastatic lesions may be demonstrated by sternal puncture.

In aplastic anemia it is the negative character of the marrow material which may be helpful. In cases suspected of being instances of "atypical leukemia," "agnogenic myeloid metaplasia," or "hypersplenism," sternal puncture followed by surgical biopsy may sup-

Table 38-3. REPRESENTATIVE DIFFERENTIAL COUNTS OF BONE MARROW OBTAINED BY PUNCTURE

Types of cells	Normal[1] average and range	Leukemia, acute[2],[3]	Leukemia,[3] chronic myelocytic	Leukemia,[3] chronic lymphocytic	Multiple myeloma[4]	Pernicious anemia	Hemolytic anemias	Iron-deficiency anemia	I.T.P.[7]
Myeloblasts.........	2.0 (0.3–5.0)	50.0–.950[5]	4.0	...	0.5	0.8	0.8	0.5	
Promyelocytes......	5.0 (1.0–8.0)	....	10.0	0.8	1.8	2.7	3.0	2.0	1.5
Myelocytes									
Neutrophilic......	12.0 (5.0–19.0)	....	26.0	1.5	1.8	7.7	8.0	9.0	8.0
Eosinophilic......	1.5 (0.5–3.0)	....	2.0	0.7	...	0.8	2.0	0.8	
Basophilic......	0.3 (0.0–0.5)	....	0.4	0.2	...	0.3			
Metamyelocytes.....	22.0 (13.0–32.0)	....	22.0	8.0	3.3	14.5	18.0	15.0	15.3
Polymorphonuclear neutrophils.......	20.0 (7.0–30.0)	....	29.0	8.5	62.0	14.5	9.0	28.0	31.0
Polymorphonuclear eosinophils........	2.0 (0.5–4.0)	....	0.8	1.0	3.5	0.5	0.6	0.2	0.5
Polymorphonuclear basophils.........	0.2 (0.0–0.7)	....	0.4	3.0	1.2	0.2	...	...	0.2
Lymphocytes.......	10.0 (3.0–17.0)	....	1.4	60.0	13.0	9.5	10.0	1.0	2.5
Plasma cells........	0.4 (0.0–2.0)	....	...	...	4.5[4]	0.2	0.4	0.7	0.8
Monocytes..........	2.0 (0.5–5.0)	....	0.2	...	0.2	0.3			
Reticulum cells......	0.2 (0.1–2.0)	....	1.2	1.5	1.0	2.0	2.6	0.8	
Mitotic figures......	0	....	0.2	0.3	...	2.7	1.0		
Abnormal cells......	0	....							
Megakaryocytes.....	0.4 (0.03–3.0)		...	...	...	...	...	...	0.2[6]
Megaloblasts........	0	....	...	...	...	40.0			
Pronormoblasts.....	4.0 (1.0–8.0)	....	...	0.2	...	...	5.0	...	4.0
Normoblasts........	18.0 (7.0–32.0)	....	2.4	14.3	9.0	3.0	43.0	40.0	36.0
M/E ratio..........	4:1 (3–5:1)	....	40:1	1.5:1	8:1	1:1.5	1:1	1.4:1	1.5:1

[1] Adapted from M. M. Wintrobe: "Clinical Hematology," 5th ed., Philadelphia, Lea & Febiger, 1961.

[2] The immature forms are listed in the table as myeloblasts merely as a matter of convenience. In acute lymphoblastic leukemia the cells are lymphoblasts, not myeloblasts. Often it is difficult to distinguish the various immature abnormal cells seen in acute leukemia. The essential point is the great preponderance of very young forms.

[3] The bone marrow picture in *aleukemic leukemia* is similar to that of leukemia of the various types, whether or not changes can be demonstrated in the blood.

[4] The characteristic cells in multiple myeloma differ somewhat from typical plasma cells in that the nuclear chromatin is relatively fine and the wheel-spoke arrangement of the chromatin is not present; the cytoplasm is basophilic and bright blue, not blue-green as in the plasma cell. A perinuclear clear zone is unusual.

[5] The most significant changes are shown in *italics*.

[6] Although the number of megakaryocytes may not appear to be increased, in typical idiopathic thrombocytopenic purpura the majority (64 per cent in the case cited) have no platelets about them and most of the remainder (32 per cent) have very few.

[7] Idiopathic thrombocytopenic purpura.

port one of these diagnoses or, instead, may reveal myelosclerosis or myelofibrosis.

It is customary to think of the blood in relation to a unit of volume. It is not unusual to forget that the sample examined is only a portion of the whole mass of blood. Fortunately, the unit obtained by venipuncture or from the finger is reasonably representative, and it is rarely necessary to measure the total blood volume; nor is it often practicable to perform the latter determination. It is necessary, nevertheless, to bear in mind the concept of total blood volume and to recall that an increase in the fluid portion of the blood—that is, an increase in the total plasma volume —may give a false impression of anemia, the total red cell mass having been reduced little or not at all. Of even greater importance is the fact that extracellular fluid deficit (dehydration) may mask an underlying anemia.

ERYTHROKINETICS. The introduction of radioisotopes into the methodology of clinical medicine has made it possible to carry out quantitative measurements of hemoglobin production and destruction which have been helpful in gaining an understanding of the pathogenesis of various types of anemia. Thus, by tagging red corpuscles with Cr^{51} it is comparatively easy to measure their life span, and with the same isotope, an estimate of red cell mass can be made. Furthermore, by comparing counts over the heart, liver, and spleen, some estimate of the relative roles of the spleen and the liver in red cell breakdown is provided. A large stasis compartment in the spleen is suggested if two to three times more radioactivity is demonstrated there than over the liver 1 hr after injection; increased splenic destruction of red corpuscles is indicated when the radioactivity increases more over the spleen than over the liver during the subsequent 4 to 5 days.

By incubating Fe^{59} with the subject's plasma for 20 min to allow it to combine with the iron-binding globulin and then injecting the plasma intravenously, the plasma iron turnover rate can be measured. The rate of incorporation of the iron into new red cells can also be determined. Furthermore, by the use of a scintillation counter, the sites of red cell production and destruction can be outlined. When such data are available in addition to the reticulocyte count, the myeloid erythroid ratio of the bone marrow, and the fecal urobilinogen, a rough quantitative estimate of erythrocyte production and destruction can be made.

In diagnosis and for the successful treatment of the great majority of patients with anemia, such elaborate studies are unnecessary. Investigations by such methods, however, have provided two important concepts which are useful for the clinician. One concerns the balance between production and destruction. Reference has already been made to this, and the concept is illustrated in Fig. 38-1. It is conceivable that blood destruction might be greatly accelerated and yet no anemia would result, provided production is accelerated to an equal degree. This is known as *compensated hemolytic disease*. Again, destruction may be accelerated only slightly above the normal, and yet anemia may ensue if production fails to keep pace with even this moderate acceleration. However, production could not be reduced below the normal rate and yet anemia fail to develop, since there is a normal wear and tear for which production must make up if anemia is not to occur.

It is also important to distinguish between *total* erythropoiesis and *effective* erythropoiesis. The application of quantitative methods has revealed that in certain disease states a large gap exists between the effort of the marrow and the red cells which reach the circulation. Red cell proliferation and hemoglobin synthesis can take place which do not result in the production of viable circulating erythrocytes. Such "shunts" have been observed in thalassemia, in pernicious anemia, and in patients with bone marrow failure. It is now recognized that qualitatively defective red cells can be formed in the marrow and destroyed there without reaching the circulation. This knowledge has proved helpful in understanding the manifestations of certain types of anemia.

CLASSIFICATION

Anemia can be classified according to etiology, as outlined in Table 38-1. However, since more than one factor may be involved in the development of anemia, the various categories are not mutually exclusive. An alternative classification is based on morphology, according to the size and hemoglobin content of the red cells. According to the mean corpuscular volume and hemoglobin concentration, anemias may be (1) macrocytic, (2) normocytic, or (3) microcytic. The last category includes a well-defined group in which the hemoglobin concentration is reduced significantly—the microcytic hypochromic anemias—and a less distinct group, the simple microcytic variety, in which the reduction of corpuscular hemoglobin content corresponds to the decrease in volume, so that no significant reduction in hemoglobin concentration is present. Such a morphologic classification is presented in Table 38-4. This classification can serve as a guide in diagnosis and, thereby, in therapy as well.

Macrocytic anemias are characterized by an increase in the average volume (MCV) and weight of hemoglobin (MCH) in the red corpuscles. The concentration of hemoglobin in the red cells (MCHC) remains normal. The macrocytic anemias, in general, are of two types. The megaloblastic macrocytic anemias are characterized by the presence of megaloblasts in the bone marrow and are related to a lack of vitamin B_{12}, pteroylglutamic (folic) acid, and related substances, as will be outlined fully later (p. 619). To be distinguished from these are the nonmegaloblastic macrocytic anemias, which do not respond to administration of vitamin B_{12} or folic acid. These include cases of macrocytic anemia associated with hypothyroidism and with liver disease, some cases of aplastic anemia, and a number of conditions which ordinarily produce normocytic anemia. This macrocytosis depends on the fact that immature red cells, in general, are larger than their fellow mature corpuscles. Consequently, in conditions which ordinarily produce normocytic anemia, when there is an accompanying very intense activity of the bone marrow with liberation into the circulation of many immature cells, a temporarily macrocytic anemia develops.

The normocytic anemias are those characterized by red cells of normal average size and hemoglobin content. Theoretically and actually, they are due to (1) the sudden loss of blood; (2) the destruction of blood, acute or chronic; (3) lack of blood formation; or (4) hydremia, in which event there may be no true anemia (Table 38-5).

The simple microcytic anemias, as already mentioned, are characterized by a reduction in the size of the cells without a significant reduction in their hemoglobin concentration. This is the least well-defined of the morphologic groups of anemia and is found in association with subacute and chronic noninflammatory disease and in various chronic inflammatory conditions.

The hypochromic microcytic anemias are characterized by a reduction below normal in the average volume of the red cells, together with a marked reduction in the concentration of hemoglobin. Excepting a congenital and hereditary disorder known as *thalassemia* and combinations of thalassemia with certain abnormal hemoglobinopathies, and rare conditions such as *pyridoxine-responsive anemia*, a *hypocupremic syndrome* in infants, and a variety of uncommon *hypersideremic anemias*, the hypochromic

Table 38-4. MORPHOLOGIC CLASSIFICATION OF ANEMIAS

Class and severity	Number of red corpuscles	Mean corpuscular volume, vol/RBC	Mean corpuscular hemoglobin, Hb/RBC	Mean corpuscular hemoglobin concentration, Hb/vol	Summary
Macrocytic					Red cells increased in volume; *mean corpuscular hemoglobin proportionately increased;* increase in size and hemoglobin content of red cells roughly inversely proportional to number of cells; mean corpuscular hemoglobin concentration remains normal throughout or may be slightly reduced
Slight...............	−	+	+	0	
Moderate............	− −	+ +	+ +	0 −	
Severe..............	− − −	+ + +	+ + +	0 −	
Normocytic					Reduction in the number of red cells without any, or at most only slight, increase in mean corpuscular volume and mean corpuscular hemoglobin; mean corpuscular hemoglobin concentration normal throughout
Slight...............	−	0	0	0	
Moderate............	− −	+0	+0	0	
Severe..............	− − −	+0	+0	0	
Simple microcytic					Reduction in volume and hemoglobin content characteristically less marked than reduction in number of red cells; mean corpuscular hemoglobin concentration normal or only slightly reduced
Slight...............	−	0	0	0	
Moderate............	− −	−	−	0 −	
Severe..............	− − −	− −	− −	0 −	
Hypochromic microcytic					*Reduction in volume and hemoglobin content characteristically more marked than reduction in number of red cells;* mean corpuscular hemoglobin concentration characteristically reduced
Slight...............	0	−	− −	−	
Moderate............	−	− −	− − −	− −	
Severe..............	− −	− − −	− − − −	− − −	

Hb indicates the quantity of hemoglobin in grams per 1,000 ml blood; vol = volume of packed red cells in milliliters per 1,000 ml blood; RBC, the number of red cells in millions per cubic millimeter; +, increase; −, decrease; 0, no change from the normal; 0−, no, or only slight, decrease; +0, slight or no increase. The amount of increase or decrease is indicated by the number of plus or minus signs, respectively.

microcytic anemias are due to iron deficiency. This deficiency may be the result of a lack of iron in the diet, defective absorption, chronic loss of blood, or excessive demands for iron (growth, repeated pregnancies), but it is most often produced by chronic blood loss (gastrointestinal tract, uterus), aggravated by several of the other factors operating in various degrees and combinations. These anemias respond to the administration of iron.

The morphologic classification of anemia is useful because, as outlined above, it offers a clue to the cause of the anemia as well as for its treatment. However, the determination of the corpuscular constants requires exacting care; without this, the results can be misleading. The simultaneous examination of a blood smear is essential in interpreting the results.

As is so common in clinical medicine, no single procedure and no classification of anemia is ideal. The competent clinician is one who is a keen observer, takes exacting care, and is able to integrate the facts so gathered to reach a reasonable conclusion.

MANAGEMENT

In the sense that by their administration a specific deficiency is corrected, vitamin B₁₂, folic acid, and iron may be considered to be specific agents for the treatment of certain types of anemia. In macrocytic anemias characterized by megaloblastic bone marrow, of which pernicious anemia is the commonest example, the administration of vitamin B₁₂ corrects the deficiency and the anemia is relieved. In certain rare instances of macrocytic megaloblastic anemia, folic acid rather than vitamin B₁₂ or purified liver extract relieves the anemia. Examples are the megaloblastic anemia of infancy, "refractory megaloblastic" or "achrestic" anemia, many cases of "pernicious anemia of pregnancy," and some cases of sprue. These agents

Table 38-5. MORPHOLOGIC AND CLINICAL CLASSIFICATION
OF ANEMIA

I. Macrocytic anemias (MCV* 94–160 cu μ, MCH† 32–50
   γγ, MCHC‡ 32–36%)
   A. Those related to deficiency of vitamin B_{12} and folic
      acid (*megaloblastic macrocytic anemias*)
      1. Pernicious anemia
      2. Sprue and other conditions in which intestinal
         absorption is impaired
      3. Megaloblastic anemia of infancy
      4. Megaloblastic anemia of pregnancy
      5. Nutritional macrocytic anemias, refractory
         megaloblastic anemia, etc.
      6. Antimetabolites and increased demands for
         hematopoietic factors
   B. Where there is intense activity of the bone marrow
      and in other circumstances (*nonmegaloblastic macro-
      cytic anemias*)
      1. Reticulocytosis (acute posthemorrhagic anemia,
         hemolytic anemias, and other conditions usually
         associated with normocytic anemia)
      2. Some cases of hypothyroidism, liver disease,
         aplastic anemia
         (For details, see Table 112-1, p. 620)
II. Normocytic anemias (MCV 82–92 cu μ, MCH 28–32
    γγ, MCHC 32–36%)
    A. Sudden loss of blood
    B. Destruction of blood—acute and chronic hemolytic
       anemias (see Table 113-1, p. 630)
    C. Lack of blood formation—hypoplastic and aplastic
       or refractory anemias due to poisons, infection,
       metastases, etc.
    D. Hydremia—not a true anemia
III. Simple microcytic anemias (MCV 72–82 cu μ, MCH
     21–27 γγ, MCHC 30–36%)
     Anemia associated with chronic infection, chronic renal
     disease, etc.
IV. Hypochromic microcytic anemias (MCV 50–82 cu μ,
    MCH 12–27 γγ, MCHC 24–32%)
    A. Iron deficiency due to
       1. Chronic blood loss
       2. Inadequate intake of iron together with
       3. Faulty absorption (achlorhydria, sprue, etc.) and
       4. Excessive demands for iron (growth, menstrua-
          tion, pregnancies)
    B. Thalassemia and combinations with abnormal hemo-
       globinopathies
    C. Rare miscellaneous causes (pyridoxine-responsive
       anemia, hypocupremic syndrome of infants, miscel-
       laneous hypersideremic anemias)

* MCV refers to mean corpuscular volume.
† MCH refers to mean corpuscular hemoglobin.
‡ MCHC refers to mean corpuscular hemoglobin concen-
tration.

are valueless in anemias other than those in which the
bone marrow is megaloblastic.

Likewise iron therapy is effective in iron-deficiency
anemias and is useless in all other types of anemia.
Such therapy is almost always effective by mouth, and
only in the rare instances of severe gastrointestinal intolerance and in cases of chronic ulcerative colitis with
iron deficiency is it justifiable to give iron parenter-

ally. The parenteral administration of iron may be
associated with a sense of warmth and palpitation,
nausea, vomiting, hyperpnea, and even precordial
pressure.

Whether or not desiccated thyroid and ascorbic acid
should be classed as specific therapeutic agents, as
they are in Table 38-6, is debatable. It is clear that the
anemia accompanying hypothyroidism is relieved only
by the administration of thyroid, but whether this is
the direct consequence of the relief of a deficiency is
less certain. The relationship of ascorbic acid therapy
to the anemia of scurvy is even less apparent, as already discussed in this chapter.

Anemias which are neither due to deficiency of iron
nor caused by lack of vitamin B_{12} or folic acid are
most difficult to manage. Iron or liver therapy, vitamins, or combinations of these, given orally or parenterally, are useless and wasteful of the patient's funds
and the physician's time. These anemias cannot, in
the present state of our knowledge, be relieved without the elimination of the underlying cause. Thus, the
anemia of chronic renal disease is difficult to treat because the renal disease itself is usually so unremittent
in character. Likewise, the anemia of chronic infection
persists as long as the underlying infection continues.
Aplastic anemias in which the bone marrow has been
damaged in general carry a very poor prognosis. In
some instances the destruction of hematopoietic tissue
may not be complete, and in such cases the maintenance of life by transfusion may ultimately be followed by some, or even occasionally by complete,
regeneration of bone marrow. The anemia of leukemia
is relieved if the leukemic process can be checked by
irradiation or chemotherapy. The same is true of the
anemia of Hodgkin's disease and other disorders of
the lymphoid tissue. In all these conditions the administration of iron, vitamin B_{12}, and folic acid or
liver is valueless, and the giving of transfusions is but
a temporary measure of limited value.

The use of blood transfusions in the treatment of
anemia and other hemopoietic disorders is discussed
in a separate chapter (p. 647).

Adrenocorticosteroids and corticotropin may be very
useful in the management of acquired hemolytic
anemias, and indirectly, when they affect the leukemic
process, they serve to relieve anemia temporarily in
acute lymphoblastic leukemia. The corticosteroids and
androgens also have some value in other instances of
anemia, for example, certain aplastic anemias.

Splenectomy produces permanent relief of the anemia of hereditary spherocytosis and may be valuable
in some cases of hemolytic anemia of the acquired

Table 38-6. THERAPEUTIC AGENTS FOR ANEMIA

I. Specific: Vitamin B_{12}, folic acid, iron
   Desiccated thyroid (?), ascorbic acid (?)
II. Nonspecific: Blood transfusions
    Irradiation and chemotherapy (in leukemia, etc.)
    ACTH, adrenocorticosteroids, and androgens
    Splenectomy

type. This is especially true in the more chronic cases and when leukopenia and thrombocytopenia are also present. This operation is effective in the treatment of many instances of thrombocytopenic purpura, and it can be helpful, together with venous shunt operations, in the management of Banti's disease. It is also valuable in certain cases characterized by "hypersplenism" (p. 678). However, splenectomy should not be undertaken without a thorough diagnostic study and full knowledge of the risks involved—the operative mortality, the possibility of postoperative atelectasis or other complications, such as thrombosis in association with the marked thrombocytosis which may develop after operation, and the likelihood of failure to achieve the result desired by this operation.

Details of the management of anemia will be discussed in later chapters in connection with the various types of anemia. In dealing with cases of anemia, the value of a diet containing food factors especially useful in blood regeneration, such as animal protein, the B vitamins, and iron, should not be overlooked. Such a diet offers much more than can be gained from vitamin capsules. The diet should also include all other nutritional essentials, such as ascorbic acid. In addition, the physician should ensure a reasonable balance between rest and activity, and attention should be given to the need for reassurance and understanding concerning the patient's illness. Palliative measures may also be required for various complaints as they arise.

It should be apparent from what has been said already that adequate management of anemia is impossible without a thorough study of the patient and discovery of the nature and cause of the anemia.

REFERENCES

Finch, C. A.: Quantitative Aspects of Erythropoiesis, Ann. N. Y. Acad. Sci., 77:410, 1959.

Laurell, C. B., and M. Nyman: Studies on the Serum Haptoglobin Level in Hemoglobinemia and Its Influence on Renal Excretion of Hemoglobin, Blood, 12:493, 1957.

Lester, R., and R. Schmid: Bilirubin Metabolism, New England J. Med., 270:779, 1964.

Sproule, B. J., J. H. Mitchell, and W. F. Miller: Cardiopulmonary Physiological Responses to Heavy Exercise in Patients with Anemia, J. Clin. Invest., 39:378, 1960.

Wintrobe, M. M.: "Clinical Hematology," 5th ed., Philadelphia, Lea & Febiger, 1961.

39 BLEEDING
M. M. Wintrobe

Except for that which occurs during menstruation or after injury to blood vessels, the loss of blood is abnormal, and this symptom, therefore, is a definite indication to search for disease. The commonest cause

Table 39-1. CAUSES OF HEMORRHAGE OR PURPURA

I. Vascular abnormalities
   A. Congenital and familial
      1. Hereditary hemorrhagic telangiectasia
      2. Poorly defined syndromes (vascular pseudohemophilia, hereditary familial purpura simplex)
   B. Acquired ("nonthrombocytopenic purpuras")
      1. Trauma; erosion of blood vessels by pathologic processes (Table 39-3); mechanical obstruction; purpura factitia; orthostatic purpura
      2. Symptomatic purpuras: infections; purpura fulminans; diabetes; uremia; hypertension; arteriosclerosis; neoplastic diseases; scurvy
      3. Immunologic disorders: Henoch-Schönlein (allergic) purpura; serum sickness; polyarteritis and other forms of vasculitis; drug sensitivity; autoerythrocyte sensitization; DNA hypersensitivity
      4. Toxins, venoms

II. Extravascular abnormalities
   A. Congenital and familial
      1. Ehlers-Danlos syndrome
      2. Pseudoxanthoma elasticum
      3. Hereditary hypoplasia of the mesenchyme (osteogenesis imperfecta, Marfan's syndrome)
   B. Acquired
      1. Atrophy of subcutaneous tissues (purpura senilis, purpura cachectica)
      2. Cushing's syndrome

III. Intravascular abnormalities
   A. Platelet abnormalities
      1. Quantitative deficiencies: symptomatic and idiopathic thrombocytopenic purpuras (Table 120-1)
      2. Qualitative abnormalities
         a. Congenital and familial: with defective clot retraction (Glanzmann's thrombasthenia); other thrombocytasthenias and thrombocytopathies
         b. Acquired: hemorrhagic thrombocythemia; thrombocytasthenia in uremia and in paraproteinemias; following infusion of synthetic macromolecules
   B. Coagulation defects
      1. Deficiency of factor VIII (hemophilia A, AHF deficiency)
      2. Vascular hemophilia (von Willebrand's disease)
      3. Deficiency of factor IX (hemophilia B, PTC deficiency, Christmas disease)
      4. Deficiency of factor XI (PTA deficiency)
      5. Congenital "hypoprothrombinemias"
         a. Congenital factor II deficiency (hypoprothrombinemia)
         b. Congenital factor V deficiency (parahemophilia)
         c. Congenital factor VII (SPCA) deficiency (hypoproconvertinemia)
         d. Congenital factor X (Stuart-Prower) deficiency
      6. Acquired "hypoprothrombinemias"
         a. Newborn (hemorrhagic disease of the newborn)
         b. Vitamin K deficiency (obstructive jaundice, biliary fistula, impaired intestinal absorption, impaired bacterial growth in bowel)
         c. Miscellaneous diseases (liver disease, leukemia, etc.)

Table 39-1. CAUSES OF HEMORRHAGE OR PURPURA
(Continued)

      d. Anticoagulant drugs (coumarin and indan-
         dione compounds)
  7. Hypofibrinogenemias
     a. Congenital
     b. Acquired: fibrinolytic purpuras or disorders of
        intravascular clotting; complications of preg-
        nancy (abruptio placentae, retention of dead
        fetus, amniotic fluid emboli, self-induced abor-
        tion), pulmonary manipulation, neoplastic
        diseases, disorders of bone marrow, severe
        liver damage, shock, snake bite
  8. Circulating anticoagulants
     a. In association with coagulation defects (espe-
        cially factors VIII and IX)
     b. Idiopathic and in association with pregnancy
        and various diseases, especially systemic lupus
     c. Administration of excessive heparin
  9. Congenital deficiency of fibrin-stabilizing factor
 10. Coagulation defect in disorders associated with
     qualitative and quantitative protein abnormali-
     ties (multiple myeloma, cryoglobulinemia, cryo-
     fibrinogenemia, macroglobulinemia, purpura hy-
     perglobulinemica)

of hemorrhage is injury of large vessels by trauma or by erosion from pathologic processes, but, as indicated in Table 39-1, bleeding may arise from a great variety of other causes, which may involve any of the systems of the body. The table represents a systematic and logical classification rather than one based primarily on frequency.

Less common is bleeding attributable to some form of generalized vascular disorder. Very rare are instances of hemorrhage that occurs as a result of fragility of the skin and its blood vessels. Defects in the factors concerned in blood coagulation represented a comparatively infrequent cause of bleeding until bishydroxycoumarin (Dicumarol) and heparin were introduced as therapeutic agents.

COAGULATION AND HEMOSTASIS

Before discussing the causes of hemorrhage it will be useful to consider first what is known about the process of coagulation and the mechanisms for hemostasis.

Hemostasis is the arrest of the escape of blood from a vessel and is effected through the combined actions of three fundamental groups of factors: (1) *extravascular*, such as subcutaneous tissue, muscle, and skin, which qualitatively depend upon age, mass, tonicity, tautness, and resiliency; (2) *vascular*, comprising the blood vessels, which vary with age, type, size, tone, location, and nutritional state; and (3) *intravascular*, which includes all the factors concerned with coagulation, including the blood platelets.

When bleeding from a vessel occurs, these factors normally function in a coordinated manner. Although many details of the hemostatic mechanism have yet to be clarified, the course of events may be pictured as follows. After injury, prompt vasoconstriction and retraction of the vessels occur. Egress of blood from the vessel into the surrounding tissues results in increased hydrostatic pressure in the tissues, while that in the vessel falls. These adjustments, in combination with normal tissue tone, tend to halt the escape of blood temporarily. Initial vasoconstriction is maintained for 3 to 4 min, during which time blood platelets, partly through the action of adenosine diphosphate (ADP), agglutinate and adhere to the area of broken intima. Disintegrating platelets release a vasoconstrictor substance (serotonin) and other factors, while fibrin is deposited about them to form a plug at the interface of the open blood vessel and its tissue milieu. Coagulation of the escaped blood, markedly enhanced by tissue thromboplastin, extends to include the platelet plug. Vasoconstriction of vascular origin ceases, but narrowing of the vessel is maintained through the cohesive and vasoconstrictor properties of the platelet plug and its interlacing network of fibrin. Blood coagulation within the vessel, initiated at the time of bleeding, continues, and fibrin reinforces the vascular side of the plug. Although intravascular coagulation soon ceases, permanent hemostasis occurs as the result of contraction and organization of the clot.

THEORY OF COAGULATION. The classic theory of Morawitz, which regarded coagulation as involving four essential components—thromboplastin, calcium, prothrombin, and fibrinogen—reacting in two stages, now appears to have been an oversimplification. Although there is disagreement concerning details, newer observations indicate clearly that in the intravascular process of coagulation generation of intrinsic or blood thromboplastin is a preliminary phase and that blood coagulation is a stepwise process consisting of (1) formation of thromboplastin, (2) conversion of pro-

Table 39-2. SYNONYMS FOR VARIOUS COAGULATION FACTORS

International nomenclature	Synonyms
Factor I	Fibrinogen
Factor II	Prothrombin
Factor III	Thromboplastin
Factor IV	Calcium
Factor V	Proaccelerin, labile factor, accelerator globulin (AcG), thrombogen
(Factor VI)	Accelerin)
Factor VII	Proconvertin (→ convertin), stable factor, serum prothrombin conversion accelerator (SPCA), autoprothrombin I
Factor VIII	Antihemophilic factor (AHF), antihemophilic globulin (AHG), thromboplastinogen, platelet cofactor I, plasma thromboplastic factor A, *facteur antihémophilique* A
Factor IX	Plasma thromboplastin component (PTC), Christmas factor, platelet cofactor II, autoprothrombin II, plasma thromboplastic factor B, *facteur antihémophilique* B
Factor X	Stuart-Prower factor
Factor XI	PTA (plasma thromboplastin antecedent)
Factor XII	Hageman factor

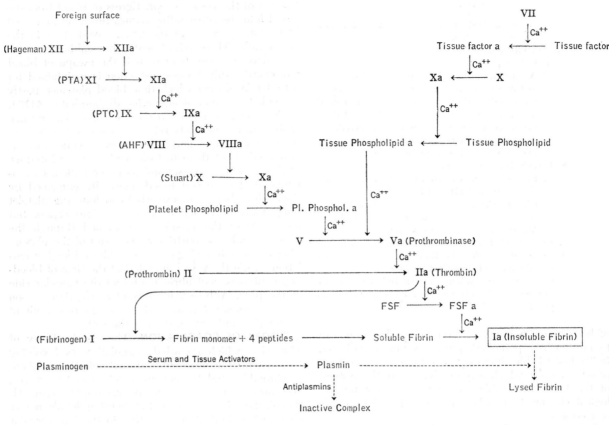

Fig. 39-1. Outline of the process of coagulation and of the counterforces. The various factors are indicated according to international nomenclature. The letter a denotes the activated form of each factor. FSF = fibrin-stabilizing factor. The process of coagulation is visualized as an "enzyme cascade" consisting of a series of steps, each dependent on the preceding one. (Prepared with the aid of Dr. Paul Didisheim.)

thrombin to thrombin, and (3) formation of fibrin. MacFarlane visualizes the process as a cascade of pro-enzyme-enzyme transformations, each enzyme activating the next until the final substrate, fibrinogen, is reached. This is illustrated in Fig. 39-1. Only the supposed activation of factor V has not been demonstrated to date. Hageman factor (XII) deficiency was discovered in a man of that name in whom coagulation time was found to be greatly prolonged, although no hemorrhagic tendency was associated. Contact with foreign surfaces initiates intravascular coagulation by activating factor XII. Platelets provide platelet factor 3, which is equivalent to certain phosphatides, principally phosphatidyl ethanolamine and phosphatidyl serine. The role of these phospholipids is still undefined, but it is thought that they act as surface catalysts. The role of calcium is unclear.

Blood clotting is thought of as a dynamic process in which positive forces leading to coagulation are antagonized by negative forces, which include natural anticoagulants and agents that remove the formed clot.

In addition to supplying phospholipids, platelets are important in hemostasis because, by their adhesiveness and agglutination, they serve directly in sealing an injured blood vessel, and by liberating the vasoconstrictor, serotonin, they play a part in the vasoconstrictive response observed when vessels are injured. Before coagulation of the blood, platelets undergo a change called *viscous metamorphosis*. This consists first in clumping of the platelets, then swelling of the mass, and finally release of granular material, probably phospholipids, into the surrounding plasma. At the same time a change in permeability occurs so that the platelet plug, at first permeable to blood, soon becomes impermeable and bleeding ceases.

The extravascular process of coagulation is simpler. The substance, tissue thromboplastin, is a high molecular weight lipoprotein, which is released from tissues directly after injury and is widely distributed in the body as an intracellular compound. It is found in highest concentration in the brain, lungs, placenta, thymus, and testes. Factors X and V and calcium are concerned in the extravascular process of coagulation, as well as in the intravascular, and an additional factor (VII) is also required to form, with tissue thromboplastin, a product (prothrombinase) which causes prothrombin to be converted to thrombin.

All the events which have been described have the purpose of causing prothrombin to be converted to thrombin. As indicated in Fig. 39-1, the final prothrombin-converting factor (Va, prothrombinase) is generated in both intravascular and extravascular systems. Whether prothrombin, a glycoprotein, is converted to thrombin by an enzymatic or an autocatalytic process is unsettled, but it appears that a carbohydrate fragment is lost and that thrombin is a compound of half the molecular weight of prothrombin, or less. The activity of thrombin is that of a proteolytic enzyme. It leads to polymerization of fibrinogen, a protein of large molecular weight, with the result that needle-shaped crystal-like protofibrils are ultimately produced. These then become aligned into fiber strands by lateral association, and insoluble fibrin is formed.

The formation of fibrin, the end point of the process of clotting, is followed by clot retraction, a process that makes the seal firm and strong. Here, again, the platelets are involved. Soon after fibrin has been laid down, *intact* platelets in the interior of the mass are found around the fibrin needles, adhere to them, and form large knots at their intersections. As the knots are being formed, the fibrin becomes bent, twisted, and shortened. Retraction of the clot is more complete, the higher the number of platelets, and the greater the concentration of thrombin in relation to the quantity of fibrinogen. In this process an actomyosinlike protein present in platelets is involved, and ATP is consumed. By these steps the *thrombus* is formed.

Coagulation is conceived to be like a chain reaction that develops at an ever-accelerating pace. The first phase is a relatively slow reaction, particularly the intravascular process. Once a small amount of thrombin has been formed, the velocity accelerates. To some extent the process of coagulation is such that it may compensate for a limited deficiency of the individual coagulation factors; only when severe deficiencies exist do clinical manifestations develop.

Negative forces exist which serve to oppose the solidification of the blood and favor the fluid state. One of the safeguards is the slowness of thrombin production. Another is the unbroken continuity of the vascular endothelium. In addition, certain anticoagulant factors exist in the circulating blood, namely, antithrombin and antithromboplastin. Furthermore, thrombin has an affinity for fibrin surface, which makes for a ready means whereby dangerous extension of a thrombus is prevented. There is also a mechanism for dissolution of the blood clot. This is achieved by the action of leukocytes, as well as by means of a specific proteolytic enzyme, plasmin. The last is derived from a precursor, plasminogen, which is carried in the globulin fraction of the plasma. Plasminogen activation occurs spontaneously or as a result of contact with activators of tissue, body fluid, or bacterial origin.

HEMORRHAGE AS THE RESULT OF INJURY OF LARGE VESSELS BY TRAUMA OR BY EROSION FROM PATHOLOGIC PROCESSES

Trauma is one of the chief causes of this type of bleeding. It may lead to external bleeding, in which event the cause and source are usually apparent. When bleeding is internal, the true nature of the condition may not be discovered so readily. Different systems of the body may be affected. Intracranial hemorrhage is not uncommon following injury. The symptoms depend on the location of the hemorrhage. Injury to the chest may lead to the fracture of ribs, and this, in turn, by damaging the pleura, may lead to hemothorax. Abdominal injury may lead to rupture of viscera, with which some blood loss is associated. Rupture of the spleen in particular is accompanied by great loss of blood, since this is so vascular an organ. In fracture of the pelvis, severe retroperitoneal hemorrhage may occur.

Hemorrhage in the absence of trauma or of a disorder in the process of coagulation suggests some pathologic process or congenital abnormality as the cause of the bleeding. Occasionally, trauma is the precipitating factor, inducing hemorrhage from vessels which are congenitally abnormal or are already damaged by disease.

Some of the possible causes of hemorrhage resulting from pathologic processes are listed in Table 39-3. A few comments may be added. In younger persons bleeding in the *nervous system* suggests rupture of a thin-walled and saccular congenital aneurysm in the circle of Willis. Inflammatory disease of the nervous system rarely causes significant hemorrhage. Tumors, likewise, are not commonly associated with hemorrhage, although bleeding into a tumor is by no means unusual.

Inflammatory processes involving the *nasal mucous*

Table 39-3. COMMON CAUSES OF HEMORRHAGE

I. Trauma to any part of the body
II. Congenital abnormalities or pathologic processes
    A. Nervous system: hypertension, arteriosclerosis, aneurysm in circle of Willis
    B. Nose, ears, and throat: local irritation, hypertension, skull fracture
    C. Lungs: mitral stenosis, tuberculosis, lung abscess, bronchiectasis, tumor
    D. Gastrointestinal tract: peptic ulcer, esophageal varices, carcinoma of the stomach, ulcerative colitis, hemorrhoids
    E. Urinary tract: glomerulonephritis, stone, tumor
    F. Genital apparatus: uterine fibroids, ruptured ectopic gestation
III. Generalized vascular disorders
    A. Hereditary hemorrhagic telangiectasia
    B. Allergic purpuras
    C. Symptomatic purpuras (Tables 120-1, 120-2)
IV. Defects in the factors concerned in coagulation
    A. Thrombocytopenic purpuras
    B. Hemophilia and PTC deficiency
    C. Induced hypoprothrombinemia (Table 39-1)

membrane (e.g., diphtheria, streptococcal infections) may cause such engorgement of Kiesselbach's (Little's) area that a varix may develop which is readily made to bleed by mechanical factors. Epistaxis due to increased hydrostatic pressure is not unusual in hypertension. This symptom frequently is the initial and even the sole complaint in cases of multiple hereditary telangiectasia.

Bloody mucus, rather than free bleeding, is associated with perforation of the cartilaginous portion of the nasal septum, which may be produced by syphilis or by chromium poisoning or may be encountered in typhoid fever. Tuberculous perforation of the bony portion of the septum is not associated with bleeding. Only one type of nasal polyp leads to epistaxis. This is a fibroepithelioma which possesses a wide base and is situated on the septum.

Diseases of the nasal passages and sinuses other than those mentioned above are rarely a cause of hemorrhage. Trauma and severe streptococcal infections are the commonest causes of bleeding from the *throat*. Hemorrhage from the *ear*, if not due to a direct blow, suggests fracture of the skull.

Hemorrhage from the *lungs* may arise in association with inflammatory, neoplastic, and vascular processes in the respiratory tract. Common causes of hemoptysis include tuberculosis, bronchiectasis, bronchogenic carcinoma, mitral stenosis, pulmonary infarction, and lung abscess. In pulmonary tuberculosis, arteriobronchial fistula may cause alarming hemorrhage from the lung which at times stops as abruptly as it begins, without the characteristic "tailing off" seen in bleeding from polyps and bronchial adenomas. When there is consolidation of the lung, as in pneumonia, the sputum may contain blood, but rarely is there much blood. Less common causes of bleeding from the respiratory passages include atypical pneumonia, coccidioidomycosis, broncholithiasis, and erosion of the respiratory passages by conditions affecting the mediastinum, such as aneurysm of the aorta and disease of the lymph nodes.

It is not always easy to determine whether the patient has coughed up or vomited the blood which has been expelled. Blood coming from the lungs is usually bright red in color and is often frothy, since it has been mixed with air. However, blood coming from the respiratory tract does not always present this classic appearance. Thus, if it comes from an area which is inflamed or congested, aeration may not be good and the blood may be somewhat dark, suggesting material obtained from the stomach. Furthermore, blood from the respiratory passages may be swallowed first and then vomited, with the result that it has all the characteristics of blood coming from the stomach. Blood coming from the stomach is generally dark because of the formation of acid hematin by mixture of hemoglobin with hydrochloric acid. It may be mixed with stomach contents.

By far the commonest cause of massive *gastrointestinal bleeding* is peptic ulcer. Ruptured esophageal varices and carcinoma of the stomach cause less than 10 per cent of such bleeding. A hemorrhagic diathesis is the cause of gastric hemorrhage less than once in 100 cases.

Hematemesis and melena are discussed in a separate chapter (Chap. 28) and will not be considered in detail here. It should be mentioned, however, that a cause of hemorrhage hitherto little recognized is hiatus or diaphragmatic hernia. Massive bleeding may also be due to gastric polyps. Although malignant neoplasms of the stomach of the usual type rather infrequently cause severe hemorrhage, rhabdoleiomyomas have a definite tendency to cause free bleeding, but these are exceedingly rare. A phytobezoar in the stomach may cause ulceration and so lead to hemorrhage.

Meckel's diverticulum may cause massive hemorrhage from the *intestinal tract*. Benign polyps of the intestine may lead to blood loss, but this is rarely dramatic or large in amount. Ulcerative malignant processes will likewise cause hemorrhage, but this again is usually of a chronic character. The blood loss associated with inflammatory processes, except in the case of nonspecific ulcerative colitis or typhoid fever, is rarely of significant amount. When intussusception, volvulus, or mesenteric thrombosis is present, a bloody discharge rather than true hemorrhage is found. The rarer forms of tumor of the intestine, such as lymphosarcoma, sometimes cause bleeding. Hemorrhoids, of course, are an important source of blood loss. Large hemorrhages are rare in tuberculosis of the colon, but they do occur and then are likely to prove fatal. Of the parasites which may be found in the intestine, the hookworm, *Ancylostoma duodenale*, is an important cause of chronic blood loss. Hemorrhage from the *alimentary tract* may also be encountered in uremia.

Bleeding from the *urinary tract* (hematuria) is seen in glomerulonephritis or with stones or tumors in the bladder or kidney pelvis, such as benign or malignant papilloma of the bladder and hypernephroma of the kidney. A polycystic kidney sometimes produces this symptom. Severe bleeding, even with the production of clots in the bladder, may occur when only prostatic hypertrophy is present, perhaps because of the rupture of a varicose vein on the middle lobe. Of inflammatory processes, tuberculosis is the commonest cause of hemorrhage.

When cystitis is severe, much bleeding may occur. The urinary tract is the commonest site of bleeding complicating coumarin therapy.

Uterine fibroids are a common cause of abnormal bleeding from the *female genital tract*, while ruptured ectopic gestation is a common cause of internal bleeding. Much rarer is hemorrhage due to the rupture of an ovarian cyst.

BLEEDING DUE TO GENERALIZED VASCULAR DISORDERS

These include some well-defined, as well as certain vaguely differentiated, conditions associated with bleeding. *Hereditary hemorrhagic telangiectasia* is a vascular anomaly characterized clinically by hemorrhage and anatomically by multiple dilatations of capillaries and venules which are found in the skin and mucous membranes (Chap. 122). Trivial trauma sustained by these abnormal, relatively exposed vessels results in unusual bleeding. Although these telangiectases are usually quite evident when attention is called to them, not infrequently they are overlooked.

In addition to this well-defined disorder, from time to time individuals with a bleeding diathesis have been described with such manifestations as excessive bleeding following tonsillectomy or excessive and unexplained uterine bleeding. In some the bleeding time was prolonged. Out of this poorly defined group of cases, better defined entities are being drawn; e.g., von Willebrand's disease (p. 660) and Glanzmann's disease (p. 660). Poorly differentiated is *vascular pseudohemophilia*, a condition transmitted as a dominant to both sexes, in which the blood vessels are thought to be incapable of response to vasoconstrictor influences. Careful study of some patients thought to have this condition, however, has revealed them to have one of the more clearly defined disorders mentioned above.

The so-called "nonthrombocytopenic purpuras" comprise a poorly defined group of conditions associated with bleeding. Bleeding is due to direct alteration of the vessel wall, such as may occur in heart failure and shock (possibly on the basis of hypoxia), ascorbic acid deficiency, senility, allergic states, or collagen diseases, or from the effects of toxins of bacterial, chemical, vegetable, or animal origin.

Purpura simplex is a term generally applied to instances of mild purpuric skin manifestations unassociated with well-defined abnormalities in the blood. A hereditary, familial form has been reported. "Devil's pinches" may be included here.

Mechanical purpura refers to purpuric manifestations associated with violent muscular contractions such as occur in whooping cough or convulsions, with the result that capillaries are ruptured.

Purpura accompanying a large variety of disorders is termed *symptomatic*. Thus, *infectious processes* too numerous to list may result in increased capillary permeability, with bleeding presumably on the basis of capillary damage produced by toxins. Important examples include meningococcemia, staphylococcemia, rheumatic fever, subacute bacterial endocarditis, scarlet fever, smallpox, measles, diphtheria, and certain chronic infectious states. The purpuric manifestations of capillary permeability in these disorders are to be sharply distinguished from the embolic phenomena that also occur in some of these conditions. A multiplicity of *drugs* have been cited in isolated instances as causing purpura of a vascular nature. Although considered the result of idiosyncrasy, the mechanism that produces increased capillary permeability in such cases is not clear. It may be that endothelial cellular enzymes, necessary for the growth and integrity of the vessel wall, are actually inhibited by the antigen-

antibody reaction or by specific toxic substances. Certainly, the hemorrhagic effects of certain snake venoms appear to be due to direct toxic injury of the endothelial lining of the capillaries and small veins.

Purpura fulminans is a term applied to a very rare form of purpura observed in association with infections, such as scarlet fever, and with pregnancy. It is characterized by sudden onset, fever, symmetric ecchymoses in the skin without hemorrhage from the mucous membranes, and often a fatal course of 1 to 4 days. The same term has been used in relation to an extreme state of vascular collapse due to adrenal hemorrhage or necrosis in meningococcemia (Waterhouse-Friderichsen syndrome). In most instances no abnormality in coagulation has been demonstrated, but factor V deficiency, excess antithrombin, and hypofibrinogenemia have been reported.

Advanced *renal disease* and acute glomerulonephritis are sometimes associated with purpura. In chronic renal disease with azotemia, purpura of the skin and mucous membranes as well as large subcutaneous extravasations or hemorrhages into the internal organs may be found. Purpura in acute glomerulonephritis, on the other hand, is usually discrete and petechial and is likely to involve only the skin of dependent portions of the body. The purpura of renal disease may be due to the qualitative platelet defect (thrombocytopathia) that is frequently present.

Purpura of the skin and mucous membranes and large subcutaneous extravasations or hemorrhages into the internal organs may be found when there has been acute destruction of the *liver*. The purpura of liver disease may be associated with deficiencies of prothrombin, factors VII, IX, X, V, and fibrinogen, increased fibrinolytic activity, and qualitative abnormality of platelets. Hemorrhagic manifestations have been noted also in a number of cases of hemochromatosis, primary amyloidosis, and polycythemia.

Prolonged *deficiency of vitamin C* may result in unusual hemorrhage, which characteristically is perifollicular, gingival, and subperiosteal in location but also occurs in the skin, subcutaneous tissues, and muscles. The bleeding may be extensive and is attributed to increased capillary permeability due to lack of intercellular cement or ground substance. Bleeding ceases after the administration of lemon juice and similar antiscorbutic substances (ascorbic acid).

Allergic purpuras (Chap. 120) include a wide variety of conditions characterized clinically by bleeding into the skin, joints, and viscera and associated with one or more of the common manifestations of allergy such as erythema, urticaria, or effusion of serum into subcutaneous tissues or viscera. These and certain rare hemorrhagic disorders such as *von Willebrand's disease* and *Glanzmann's thrombasthenia* will be discussed later (Chap. 120).

Autoerythrocyte sensitization refers to patients in whom tender ecchymoses with surrounding erythema and edema occurred. These manifestations could be reproduced by means of trauma or by subcutaneous injections into the patient of a small volume of autologous red cells or their stroma. Observed only in women, the condition is thought to be psychosomatic in nature. Similar manifestations have been shown to be due to localized hypersensitivity to deoxyribonucleic acid.

BLEEDING DUE TO ALTERATION OF EXTRAVASCULAR FACTORS OF HEMOSTASIS

Occasionally hemorrhage results from fragility and hyperlaxity of the skin or atrophy of the subcutaneous tissue. This is seen most commonly in purpura senilis and purpura cachectica, where it is characterized by purplish ecchymoses of varying size that appear in the skin after trauma. The hemorrhagic manifestations seen in Cushing's syndrome are attributed to skin fragility, while those in the very rare Ehlers-Danlos syndrome are attributed to hyperlaxity of the skin. Degeneration of elastic tissue or collagen is thought to be the basic lesion in pseudoxanthoma elasticum, a disorder in which bleeding may occur from any organ. In the skin, firm discrete waxy papules appear, and the surrounding thickened skin may contain telangiectases. Other diseases associated with cutaneous hemorrhagic manifestations include annular telangiectatic purpura (Majocchi's disease), angioma serpiginosum, Schamberg's disease, and pigmented purpuric lichenoid dermatitis.

BLEEDING DUE TO ALTERATIONS OF INTRAVASCULAR FACTORS OF HEMOSTASIS

As outlined in Table 39-1, bleeding due to disturbances of blood coagulation may be related to (1) platelet abnormalities or (2) a defect in one of the factors concerned in coagulation.

Platelet abnormalities may be of two kinds: (1) quantitative deficiencies of platelets or (2) qualitative abnormalities. The latter are rare, the former relatively common. Thrombocytopenic purpura, which will be discussed in detail later (p. 656), may be associated with and symptomatic of a large variety of disorders and can be produced by a number of chemical, physical, animal, and vegetable agents, but an "idiopathic" form of unknown etiology is also well recognized. Disorders associated with qualitative platelet abnormalities, the "thrombocytopathies," are becoming more clearly defined than they once were and will also be discussed later.

The number of recognized coagulation defects has increased as knowledge has been extended concerning the various factors involved in the clotting mechanism. Thus, instead of the single entity hemophilia, a number of bleeding disorders are now recognized, one of which resembles the classic disease even in its mode of inheritance, while others present a very similar clinical picture and can be differentiated only by more sensitive techniques than those which once served as the sole criterion, namely, the coagulation time and the bleeding time. It is also clear that disorders such as hemophilia may be inherited as comparatively mild defects which can be quite troublesome under certain circumstances but which cannot be recognized as due to a defect in coagulation by such crude procedures as the measurement of coagulation time. Again, the measurement of prothrombin time, when used by itself, is not a sufficiently sensitive or specific technique for the study of hemorrhagic diatheses. The term *hypoprothrombinemia* was originally used to refer to a delayed reaction in certain tests which were assumed to measure prothrombin. It is now recognized that these are influenced by a number of factors in addition to prothrombin, including factors V, VII, and X. Prothrombin has been isolated from plasma in highly purified form, and it appears that true hypoprothrombinemia is a very rare condition. However, hypoprothrombinemia, as demonstrated by the commonly used Quick test or by one of its modifications, is encountered frequently, both as an acquired condition and, much less often, as one of a number of congenital disorders.

Hemophilia and certain very closely related conditions will be discussed in a later chapter (p. 660), but the hypoprothrombinemias and various other forms of bleeding due to alterations of intravascular factors of hemostasis may be considered here.

DIMINUTION OF THE "PROTHROMBIN" CONTENT OF THE BLOOD. If the "prothrombin" time (Quick one-stage) is more than $2\frac{1}{2}$ times the control value, hemorrhage may occur, since the blood will not clot properly. Such hypoprothrombinemia may arise in various ways (Table 39-1).

Toxins. The toxic principle in spoiled sweet clover hay, which produces a hemorrhagic disease when fed to cattle, was found to be a coumarin compound. This, under the trade name Dicumarol, has become a widely used anticoagulant. Hypoprothrombinemia develops whenever this drug or a related compound, such as ethyl biscoumacetate (Tromexan), is administered. These agents produce low levels of true prothrombin and of factor VII, as well as IX and X. Bleeding due to Dicumarol- or Tromexan-induced hypoprothrombinemia usually occurs into the genitourinary and gastrointestinal tracts as well as in localized areas of the skin and subcutaneous tissue.

Administration of Salicylates. When salicylates are given in very large quantities, the prothrombin content of the blood plasma may be reduced. The mechanism of this action is thought to be through metabolic antagonism to vitamin K.

Lack of Vitamin K. The liver is concerned in the formation of true prothrombin and factors VII, IX and X. The fat-soluble vitamin K, a naphthoquinone, is essential for the synthesis of all four of these factors. It is found abundantly in alfalfa, spinach, cauliflower, cabbage, and kale. Since it is fat-soluble, bile salts are required for its absorption. Consequently, vitamin K deficiency may be found when there is complete obstruction of the flow of bile into the intestinal tract or when a biliary fistula exists. Deficiency may also develop where absorption from the bowel is impaired, as in sprue, the steatorrheas, gastrocolic fistulas, or after extensive surgical removal of much of the intestinal tract. Vitamin K is produced in abundance by bacteria growing in the intestinal tract, and for this reason lack of vitamin K in the diet is an extremely rare cause of vitamin K deficiency. However, in cases where prolonged use of drugs inhibits the growth of organisms in the gastrointestinal tract, vitamin K deficiency may ensue.

When vitamin K is deficient, prothrombin and factors VII, IX and X are depressed. These defects can all be corrected by the intramuscular, or cautiously slow intravenous administration of fat-soluble vitamin K. Synthetic water-soluble vitamin K preparations are usually less effective.

Hemorrhagic Disease of the Newborn. The fetus and the newborn infant receive their store of prothrombin from the mother. After food has been taken by the infant and bacteria begin to grow in the intestinal tract, these serve to provide vitamin K. Occasionally an infant may be born with a poor supply of prothrombin and may suffer severe hemorrhage before it can produce vitamin K for itself. It is thought that this is the result of an accentuation of the hypoprothrombinemia which is normally observed in the newborn, perhaps as a consequence of functional immaturity of the liver. In some instances, trauma to the child at birth with hemorrhage and loss of coagulation factors may also play a role.

Liver Disease. Multiple serious plasma clotting factor defects develop in the patient with decompensated hepatocellular disease, as mentioned earlier (p. 169). These defects are not corrected by the administration of vitamin K. The treatment of the hemorrhagic state associated with severe liver disease requires the administration of blood. To ensure the administration of the necessary coagulation factors, this must be fresh, or at least less than a week old.

Congenital and Idiopathic Hypoprothrombinemias. A hemorrhagic diathesis is occasionally encountered characterized by hypoprothrombinemia and yet not attributable to the recognized causes, mentioned above. The clinical manifestations in such patients resemble those of hemophilia. The commonest symptom is epistaxis. Other frequent symptoms are bleeding from the gums, spontaneous bruising, menorrhagia, and severe bleeding from injuries. Hematuria is moderately common, and hemarthroses have been recorded. Prothrombin time as measured by the one-stage method is prolonged, and when the defect is sufficiently severe, coagulation time is lengthened as well. Several forms have been differentiated.

True congenital hypoprothrombinemia is exceedingly rare; only three cases are known. Less rare is *congenital factor V deficiency* (parahemophilia), which appears to be inherited as an autosomal recessive (see p. 286) and has been observed in both sexes. The condition varies greatly in severity as does the degree of prolongation of prothrombin time and coagulation time and the decrease in prothrombin

consumption. *Congenital factor VII (SPCA) deficiency* probably is the commonest of the congenital hypoprothrombinemias and is thought to be inherited as an incompletely recessive autosomal characteristic with variable penetrance. By means of the prothrombin consumption and thromboplastin generation tests, factor VII deficiency has been distinguished from *factor X (Stuart-Prower) deficiency,* a condition thought to be inherited as a highly penetrant but incompletely recessive autosomal characteristic.

Recognition of the various types of congenital hypoprothrombinemia has been important because it has led to a better understanding of the clotting process through identification of the various factors involved. From a clinical standpoint, the idiopathic hypoprothrombinemias need to be differentiated from the much commoner disorder, hemophilia, and from the various forms of purpura. Their treatment depends on supplying the missing factor. Vitamin K does not correct the prolonged prothrombin time. Fresh whole blood or plasma is necessary to correct factor V deficiency and serum or plasma to correct factor VII or X deficiency. Fresh or stored blood or plasma, but not serum, corrects the defect in hypoprothrombinemia. The observation that factor X increases during pregnancy suggests the possible value of progestational agents in the treatment of this deficiency.

Decreased Fibrinogen. Afibrinogenemia and fibrinogenopenia are extremely rare causes of bleeding. A *congenital* disorder has been described in which hemorrhagic manifestations begin in infancy. Congenital hypofibrinogenemia is inherited as an autosomal recessive characteristic. *Acquired hypofibrinogenemia* develops under a variety of circumstances and as the effect of different mechanisms. Since it is formed in the liver, plasma fibrinogen may be reduced when severe destructive changes occur in this organ, as in acute yellow atrophy. Severe liver damage, however, produces impairment of prothrombin production before fibrinogen deficiency occurs, the latter being essentially a terminal event. In clinical practice, hypofibrinogenemia is often the consequence of a pathologic fibrinolytic state.

In certain pathologic states, such as those mentioned below, abnormal amounts of plasminogen activator may be released from the tissues into the circulation. This activator then transforms the inactive plasminogen into the fibrinolytic enzyme, plasmin. In others, thromboplastic material may gain access to the circulation and, by bringing about intravascular clotting, may consume fibrinogen and other clotting factors and induce a secondary fibrinolytic response. The clinical problem is usually complex, however, and a complete analysis of the events which take place is not yet available. The end result, in any event, is fibrinogenopenia. Other plasma coagulation factors, such as prothrombin and factors V and VIII, are often depleted as well, and thrombocytopenia may be found also, but these usually are not the primary factors involved in the development of the bleeding diathesis. In occasional instances, evidence of inhibition of the fibrinogen-to-fibrin reaction has been obtained, but this appears to be an unusual cause for apparent fibrinogenopenia.

Clinically, fibrinolysis has been observed in five main conditions: (1) under conditions of stress and in association with severe and extensive physical trauma and following extensive burns; (2) following surgery, particularly pulmonary surgery; (3) as a result of obstetric complications of abruptio placentae, intrauterine retention of a dead fetus, and amniotic fluid embolism, or of self-induced abortion; (4) during the course of neoplastic disease, especially if the prostate or, less often, the lung, pancreas, or stomach is involved; and (5) in a variety of miscellaneous disorders, such as polycythemia vera, leukemia, sarcoidosis, and hepatic cirrhosis. The clinical picture may develop with great suddenness and be characterized by the appearance of extensive ecchymoses and severe bleeding from mucous membranes; or the symptoms may be of lesser severity and magnitude (*purpura thrombolytica, fibrinolytic purpura*).

The bleeding in cases of acquired fibrinogenopenia is often of extreme gravity and requires the prompt administration of whole, preferably fresh, blood and fibrinogen (4 to 10 Gm, occasionally even 15 to 20 Gm). Certain inhibitors of plasminogen activation to plasmin, such as ε-aminocaproic acid may be helpful in these cases.

Circulating Anticoagulants. A hemorrhagic diathesis may occur as the result of the action of inhibitors of any of the factors concerned with coagulation, since they prevent clot formation. Heparin and Dicumarol are used therapeutically as anticoagulants in the management of thrombosis, and in clinical practice this is the commonest manner in which excess anticoagulant produces hemorrhage. Strictly speaking, the coumarin compounds are not anticoagulants, but they inhibit the synthesis of certain clotting factors in the liver. Ingestion of a coumarin derivative used as a rat poison or surreptitious ingestion of coumarin may cause bleeding.

In addition to the anticoagulants which may be given deliberately or those which appear in various circumstances as described above, there are circulating anticoagulants that may cause hemorrhagic disorders. These may interfere with any phase of coagulation and can be classified in accordance with their mechanism of action. The type of anticoagulant frequently encountered has been antithromboplastic in action; in some cases, however, it appears to inhibit prothrombin directly. A significant number of reported cases represent hemophilia in which an anticoagulant opposing the action of antihemophilic globulin developed after repeated transfusions. Other cases have occurred in women, usually in the childbearing period, the hemorrhagic manifestations developing some time after delivery. In a few cases a circulating antithromboplastin has been observed in association with some disease, especially disseminated lupus erythematosus, while in others the hemorrhagic disorder was of entirely obscure etiology.

Various forms of paraproteinemia, whatever their cause, may be associated with purpura. These forms include the purpura sometimes encountered in multiple myeloma and in association with other instances of hyperglobulinemia and cryoglobulinemia (p. 694). Under the title *purpura hyperglobulinemica*, a miscellaneous group of cases have been described characterized by innumerable acute episodes of purpura, especially after unusual exertion, prolonged standing, or excessive pressure from garments. In these cases a considerable increase in gamma-globulin and in the 7 S component in the ultracentrifuge was observed. This probably does not constitute a diagnostic entity.

SYMPTOMS PRODUCED BY HEMORRHAGE

The symptoms associated with blood loss differ according to whether the loss is large and rapid or relatively slow and long continued. They also depend on the site of the hemorrhage and on whether the bleeding occurs into a relatively nonexpansile space, such as a synovial joint, or in loose connective tissue. Acute and severe blood loss occurring within a matter of a few minutes results in syncope, but when the loss occurs over a period of hours the picture of shock is induced. The classic examples are seen in hemorrhage from peptic ulcer or ruptured ectopic pregnancy. The clinical picture and the pathogenesis of peripheral circulatory failure are discussed on pp. 728–732.

The acute loss of blood stimulates the hematopoietic system, with the result that the reticulocytes are increased in number, and if the hemorrhage is very severe, even occasional nucleated red cells of the normoblastic type may be found in the circulating blood. At the same time, the leukopoietic tissues are stimulated and a marked leukocytosis occurs. This leukocytosis is due to the liberation of cells formed in the bone marrow, with the result that the juvenile neutrophils are increased and even some myelocytes may appear. At the same time the number of blood platelets increases. Their number may be increased twofold, or even more. When the hemorrhage is entirely within the body, the absorption of the blood may produce hyperbilirubinemia. This, in turn, may result in an increase in the quantity of urobilinogen in the urine and may even be accompanied by noticeable jaundice.

Slow *chronic blood loss* ultimately produces anemia and the symptoms characteristic of anemia, which have been described elsewhere (Chaps. 38 and 111). The anemia eventually becomes hypochromic and microcytic in type, and instead of leukocytosis and thrombocytosis, one finds leukopenia with relative lymphocytosis, often accompanied by the presence of multisegmented polymorphonuclear neutrophils. At the same time there may be a somewhat reduced number of platelets. However, in spite of this "hypoplastic" blood picture, if the anemia is severe, occasional small nucleated red cells ("microblasts") will be found.

STUDY OF A PATIENT WITH HEMORRHAGE

Hemorrhage, if severe, first requires treatment by blood replacement. Rational treatment beyond this, however, depends on a clear understanding of the cause of the hemorrhage. This entails recognition of whether or not the bleeding results from a fault in the coagulation process, dysfunction of the blood vessels, or trauma or pathologic processes unrelated to disorders of the blood. As is always the case, there is no short cut to an accurate history and a complete and thorough physical examination. Differential diagnosis of the causes of hemorrhage other than those concerned with disorders of the blood is beyond the scope of this section, for it entails consideration of disorders that include all the systems of the body. These are dealt with in other sections.

The history may reveal a story of trauma or the symptoms of some disorder of which the hemorrhage may be a manifestation; or one may learn about exposure to agents associated with the patient's occupation or hobby that may have caused bleeding, or the ingestion of drugs, which the patient may have been taking from time to time for a number of years. A family history of bleeding should arouse suspicion of such conditions as hemophilia or of the various disorders which resemble classic hemophilia, thrombocytopenic purpura, or hereditary hemorrhagic telangiectasia (see pp. 656–663). The physical examination may reveal vascular anomalies, as in the case of hereditary telangiectasia, and may indicate the site of hemorrhage.

The examination of the blood should include the determination by reliable methods of coagulation time, clot retraction, prothrombin time, partial thromboplastin time, bleeding time, and the platelet count. A tourniquet test should be done as well. Some of these procedures are relatively crude, but if carefully performed they are useful, nevertheless. In special cases, other laboratory procedures are needed, as will be outlined below. Circumstances in which changes in these tests take place are summarized in Table 39-4.

The *coagulation time* is a measure of the capacity of the blood to clot after it has been removed from the body and, thus, in the absence of tissue factors. It can be carried out in siliconized as well as in uncoated test tubes. The latter measures the coagulation of blood after it has come into contact with a surface that can initiate the process. The coagulation time should be measured in test tubes of uniform size, and a control determination on the blood of a normal person should be made at the same time. In the determination of *prothrombin time*, it is important that a potent thromboplastin be used and that a determination be made on a normal person at the same time. It is important to recognize that by the one-stage technique a prolonged prothrombin time does not specifically indicate reduction of prothrombin, since prolongation also occurs with deficiencies of factor V, VII, X and fibrinogen, and in the presence of heparin and other anticoagulants of the anti-thrombin or anti-tissue-thromboplastin type. These conditions are differentiated from true hypoprothrombinemia by certain special tests, which depend on the use of fresh and stored plasma, normal serum, aluminum hydroxide–treated plasma, and Russell viper venom (corrects factor VII but not X deficiency), or by means of the serum prothrombin time (normal in factor VII but not in X deficiency).

More sensitive than the coagulation time is the *partial thromboplastin time*. The test is simple and is sensitive to all the factors to which coagulation time is sensitive (prothrombin, V, VIII, IX, X, XI, XII, fibrinogen, antithrombins). It detects minor abnormalities of these factors more readily than does the coagulation time. Only in the regulation of heparin therapy is the coagulation time superior to the "P.T.T." For this, the latter is too sensitive.

The test for *bleeding time* is simple but crude, and unless it is done carefully, a false normal result may be obtained. The test depends on the effect of a skin puncture in producing bleeding and is a measure of the hemostatic integrity of vascular and extravascular factors as well as the strength of the platelet plug. The bleeding time is characteristically prolonged in the thrombocytopenic purpuras because there is inadequate platelet activity. As arbitrarily defined, the bleeding time is normal in hemophilia, but subsequent oozing after the initial factors of hemostasis have ceased to function may occur for days because of imperfect coagulation. Bleeding-time measurements, therefore, should be avoided in hemophiliac patients.

Platelet counts are notoriously difficult to perform accurately and should always be verified by examination of the blood smear, which should reveal gross discrepancies if they exist. Since *clot retraction* depends chiefly on an adequate supply of platelets, delayed retraction suggests thrombocytopenia, but it has also been observed in Glanzmann's thrombasthenia (p. 660).

The *tourniquet test* is useful in demonstrating decreased capacity of the capillaries to withstand the effects of increased pressure. It depends primarily on the integrity of the capillary endothelial cells, the availability of intercellular cement substances, and the quantity of platelets. The tourniquet test is usually positive whenever there is severe thrombocytopenia and also, for a different reason, in many instances of nonthrombocytopenic purpura. It is negative as a rule in hemophilia and in other nonthrombocytopenic conditions involving the coagulation mechanism. It is noteworthy that a positive test result is encountered also in a high proportion of patients with diabetes complicated by vascular disease and in hypertension, in scurvy, in Weil's disease and other infections, and occasionally in apparently normal individuals.

It is important that several determinations be carried out simultaneously. In a classic case of thrombocytopenic purpura the bleeding time is prolonged, the platelet count is reduced, partial thromboplastin or coagulation time is normal, but clot retraction is

Table 39-4. CAUSES OF ALTERATIONS IN COMMONEST MEASURES OF COAGULATION

Laboratory finding	Condition	Mechanism
I. *Coagulation time* and *partial thromboplastin time* prolonged	A. Hemophilia	Deficiency of factor VIII (AHF)
	B. Factor IX deficiency	Deficiency of factor IX (PTC)
	C. PTA deficiency	Deficiency of PTA
	D. Hageman trait	Deficiency of Hageman factor
	E. "Hypoprothrombinemia"	When prothrombin time is greatly prolonged, deficiency of prothrombin or of factor V, or X
	F. Afibrinogenemia or hypofibrinogenemia	Decreased synthesis, rapid utilization, or destruction of fibrinogen
	G. Hyperheparinemia	Excess heparin or heparinoid substances (heparin therapy, anaphylactic and peptone shock)
	H. Circulating anticoagulants	Anti-VIII, anti-IX, anti-V, etc.
II. *Prothrombin time* (one-stage) prolonged	A. Excess Dicumarol or related therapeutic anticoagulant	Deficiency of prothrombin, factors VII and X
	B. "Parahemophilia"	Factor V deficiency
	C. "SPCA" deficiency	Factor VII deficiency
	D. Vitamin K deficiency	In newborn (hemorrhagic disease of newborn) and whenever absorption of vitamin K is impaired
	E. Liver disease	Reduction in prothrombin, factors V, VII, IX, X and fibrinogen
	F. Circulating anticoagulants	Antiprothrombin, antithromboplastin
III. *Prothrombin consumption* or *thromboplastin generation* reduced	A. Thrombocytopenia	Impaired thromboplastin formation
	B. Thrombocytopathia	Diminished platelet factor 3
	C. Hemophilias	Deficiency of factor VIII, IX, or PTA
	D. Other deficiencies	Deficiency of factor V, X or Hageman factor
	E. Circulating antithromboplastin	Anti-VIII, anti-IX, anti-V, etc.
IV. *Bleeding time* prolonged	A. Thrombocytopenic purpura	Lack of platelets
	B. Any of the causes under I or II if sufficiently severe	Extreme deficiency of blood coagulation factors
	C. Vascular hemophilia (angiohemophilia, von Willebrand's disease)	Deficiency of plasma factor necessary for normal bleeding time
	D. Thrombocytopathia	Diminished platelet factor 3
V. *Tourniquet test* positive	A. Nonthrombocytopenic purpuras	Damage to capillary endothelium
	B. Thrombocytopenic purpuras	Platelets too few to support capillaries under pressure
	C. Scurvy	Deficiency of intercellular cement substance
	D. Thrombocytopathia	Diminished platelet factor 3
VI. *Thrombocytopenia*	Thrombocytopenic purpuras, primary and secondary	Platelet antibodies, megakaryocyte damage, etc.
VII. *Clot retraction* poor	A. Thrombocytopenias of various types	Insufficient platelets to induce fibrin contraction
	B. Thrombasthenia	Impaired platelet aggregation

SOURCE: From M. M. Wintrobe: "Clinical Hematology," 5th ed., Philadelphia, Lea & Febiger, 1961.

delayed and the tourniquet test is positive. When these are the findings, one has confidence in the results of each of the tests. When there is a discrepancy between them, they should be repeated to seek out possible sources of error.

Of the more specialized procedures employed in the study of bleeding disorders, the *prothrombin consumption test* is a relatively simple one. This test is based on the principle that, by determining the prothrombin before and after coagulation is complete, a measure of the blood thromboplastin that converts prothrombin to thrombin is obtained. The same reagents are required as in Quick's method for determining prothrombin. Another simple procedure that can be employed when there is a demonstrable defect in coagulation is to attempt to correct the defect by adding blood or plasma of known composition; for example, stored plasma is deficient in factors V and VIII, serum contains factors VII, IX, X, XI and XII but little prothrombin, factor V, VIII or fibrinogen, etc. When the bloods of patients with hemorrhagic disorders are available, they can be tested for their ability to correct the defect in the unanalyzed sample.

Simple screening tests for abnormal coagulation of blood are available, and there are special tests for circulating anticoagulants. Another valuable procedure is the *thromboplastin generation test,* a most useful method for differentiating abnormalities in coagulation in which there is impaired formation of blood thromboplastin, such as hemophilia and factor IX deficiency, and conditions in which there is abnormal platelet function. The procedure, however, requires training and some technical skill and, therefore, is not available in the average laboratory.

In any case of bleeding it is desirable to study the morphology of the red cells and the leukocytes and to determine the reticulocyte count. An increase of reticulocytes is the response of a normal bone marrow to hemorrhage, and its degree gives a rough index of the severity of the hemorrhage. The lack of reticulocytosis would mean either inability of the bone marrow to respond, as in aplastic anemia, or less severe hemorrhage than other indications had suggested. The degree of leukocytosis likewise is an index of the severity of the hemorrhage and the capacity of the bone marrow to react. A low leukocyte count, in the face of a severe hemorrhage, would suggest some abnormality of the marrow, as might be the case in "aleukemic" leukemia or in aplastic anemia. The presence of very immature leukocytes suggests "aleukemic" leukemia, but it must be borne in mind that a few myelocytes form part of the picture of a vigorous response to hemorrhage.

REFERENCES

Biggs, Rosemary, and R. G. MacFarlane: "Human Blood Coagulation," 3d ed., Philadelphia, F. A. Davis Co., 1962.

Cartwright, G. E.: "Diagnostic Laboratory Hematology," 3d ed., New York, Grune & Stratton, Inc., 1963.

Hougie, C.: "Fundamentals of Blood Coagulation in Clinical Medicine," New York, McGraw-Hill Book Company, Inc., 1963.

Ratnoff, O. D.: "Bleeding Syndromes. A Clinical Manual," Springfield, Ill., Charles C Thomas, Publisher, 1960.

Wintrobe, M. M.: "Clinical Hematology," 5th ed., Philadelphia, Lea & Febiger, 1961.

40 ENLARGEMENT OF LYMPH NODES AND SPLEEN

M. M. Wintrobe

There are some 500 to 600 lymph nodes in the body, varying from less than 1 mm to 1 to 2 cm in size. These structures afford mechanical filtration for the lymph stream, removing cellular debris, foreign particles, and bacteria which may have gained access to the lymph from the various structures drained by the lymph channels. In the normal individual very few lymph nodes are palpable, even on careful physical examination. However, the access of disease-producing bacteria and certain viruses sets up an inflammatory reaction in the nodes, and various types of malignant cells can proliferate there. It has been aptly stated that in the exercise of their function the lymph nodes may sacrifice their own integrity for the welfare of the organism as a whole. One may wonder whether they do not mistakenly also nourish neoplastic tissue at their own expense.

These structures are also the site of formation of lymphocytes and of antibodies. Furthermore, the cells of the reticuloendothelial system contained within the nodes can revert to the task of blood formation. This is known as *myeloid metaplasia* and is a reflection of embryonal hematopoietic potentialities. This reaction is also accompanied by lymph node enlargement.

CAUSES OF LYMPH NODE ENLARGEMENT

Enlargement of the lymph nodes may be purely local, or it may be widespread. Such enlargement may be accompanied by all the signs of acute inflammation, such as heat, reddening of overlying skin, and tenderness; and the glands, instead of remaining discrete, may fuse with one another as the result of the perilymphangitis which occurs. Necrosis may even ensue and may be followed by rupture of the nodes and the formation of a sinus. On the other hand, very great enlargement of the lymph nodes may take place in the absence of any signs of inflammation whatever, and the glands may remain discrete at the same time. Enlarged lymph nodes may be extremely hard, or only moderately so, or may even be soft or feel cystic. When mediastinal, abdominal, or other deeply placed lymph nodes are affected, their enlargement may be first discovered as the result of the pressure such enlargement may produce. Thus acute mediastinal lymphadenitis in young children may lead to stridor, cyanosis, and dysphagia. Noninflammatory enlargement of the nodes in this region may lead to one or more of these signs. Again, if the condition is inflammatory in character, fever and leukocytosis and other signs of systemic involvement may be the first evidences of disease. When it is not due to infection, the glandular enlargement may be huge and evidences of systemic involvement may be wholly lacking; or, instead, wasting, anemia, and even fever may be more prominent than the glandular swelling.

The chief causes of lymph node enlargement are listed in Table 40-1. The strategic location of lymph nodes along the lymph channels makes them likely to be involved in a variety of infections, both acute and chronic. The enlargement of the anterior cervical nodes in association with streptococcal sore throat, and enlargement of the epitrochlear node draining a digit

Table 40-1. CHIEF CAUSES OF LYMPH NODE ENLARGEMENT

I. Infections
  A. Acute, regional: etiologic agents include strepto-
     coccus, staphylococcus, Ducrey's bacillus, *Pasteur-
     ella tularensis*, *Treponema pallidum*, virus of lymph-
     ogranuloma venereum, *Pasteurella pestis* (plague)
  B. Acute, systemic: infectious mononucleosis, measles,
     rubella, chickenpox, etc.
  C. Chronic: tuberculosis, syphilis, fungous infections;
     sarcoid
II. Allergic reactions: serum sickness
III. Congenital abnormalities (lymphangiomas)
IV. Primary lymph node diseases: Hodgkin's disease,
    lymphosarcoma, reticulum cell sarcoma, etc.
V. Leukemia
VI. Metastases from malignant disease in breast, stomach,
    etc.

which is infected are well-known examples of a regional reaction to local infection. The satellite node of
tularemia is another example, as are the buboes of
lymphogranuloma venereum and of plague. Many
types of acute generalized infection are accompanied
by lymphadenopathy which may be local or widespread. Lymph node enlargement frequently accompanies measles, rubella, mumps, and chickenpox. This
is usually most prominent in the anterior cervical chain.
In infectious mononucleosis, generalized lymph node
enlargement is characteristic, but cervical glandular enlargement is often more striking than that found elsewhere in the body. Lymphadenopathy may be encountered in acute anterior poliomyelitis, especially in
infants and children, in whom, in particular, the development of an acute infection of almost any variety
is frequently accompanied by some degree of lymph
node enlargement. Other acute infections are accompanied by adenopathy, but this may not be easily dis-
cernible (for example, the mesenteric lymph node enlargement which is seen in typhoid fever).

Of the chronic infections, tuberculosis and syphilis
are the commonest causes of lymphadenopathy. In
tuberculosis the cervical, mediastinal, or mesenteric
glands are most often involved. The enlargement usually is slowly progressive and is easily confused with
that caused by Hodgkin's disease. However, tuberculous glands frequently are tender and firm and adhere
to one another. Sometimes breakdown of the overlying
skin occurs, leading to the production of a stubborn
draining sinus. Rarely the lymph node enlargement is
acute and rapidly developing, and in such cases the
glands may remain discrete and freely movable. In
relation to syphilis, mention may be made of the firm,
painless swelling in the regional lymph nodes draining
the primary lesions; the generalized, firm, shotty, nontender nodes which accompany the secondary stage;
and the glandular swelling of various degrees which
may accompany the late stages or the congenital form.
Other chronic infections in which glandular swelling
may be prominent include fungous infections and filariasis. Sarcoidosis often must also be considered. In
sarcoidosis the pre- and postauricular lymph nodes, the
submaxillary, submental, epitrochlear, and paratra-

cheal glands are more often affected than in Hodgkin's
disease. A history of involvement of the eyes and of
the parotid glands (uveoparotid fever) suggests sarcoid, and punched-out areas in the small bones of the
hands and feet may be demonstrable by roentgenography (see Chap. 385).

Serum sickness should not be overlooked as a cause
of lymphadenopathy, particularly since it is usually
accompanied by fever. Again, it may be noted that
trauma, caused by running and jumping, has been
known to lead to painful swelling of the inguinal and
femoral lymph nodes. Of congenital abnormalities
which may lead to lymphoid enlargement, simple or
capillary lymphangiomas, cavernous lymphangiomas,
and the cystic form (cystic hygroma) may be mentioned. Treatment of convulsive disorders with various
hydantoin or hydantoinlike drugs may produce a clinical and pathologic syndrome which closely mimics the
"lymphomas."

Hodgkin's disease, lymphosarcoma, reticulum cell
sarcoma, and giant follicular lymphoma are frequently
classed under the single heading of primary lymph
node diseases or lymphomas because, clinically, they
are usually indistinguishable. In these conditions the
lymph node enlargement is characteristically localized
at first; only as the disease progresses does wide dissemination occur. The glandular enlargement usually
is discrete and firm and ranges greatly in degree. When
the adenopathy becomes widespread, nodes may be
discovered in locations where the presence of lymphoid
tissue may not have been suspected. Such cases of
lymph node enlargement are distinguished from those
due to leukemia chiefly by the changes in the blood
characteristically seen in the latter condition, but also
by the asymmetry of the swellings which is often seen
in the "lymphomas." In leukemia, lymph node enlargement is usually generalized and symmetric, although,
especially in acute leukemia, adenopathy may be much
more prominent in the neck than elsewhere.

Metastatic enlargement of lymph nodes, as a rule,
is distinctly localized, and the glandular swelling ordinarily is very hard. Such enlargement may involve
nodes which are easily discovered, such as those of
the axilla in cases of carcinoma of the breast. It may
be more often heard about than seen, such as Virchow's
sentinel node above the clavicle in cases of carcinoma
of the stomach or other abdominal organs. Or the
adenopathy may exist in some region of the body inaccessible to physical examination but discoverable
only by roentgenography or through the indirect effects
of pressure produced by enlargement of the nodes. A
very useful procedure for the differential diagnosis of
certain diseases involving the lungs, such as sarcoidosis,
is the biopsy of lymph nodes which are not palpable
because they are situated deeply in the lower neck and
upper mediastinum but which can be found by adequate exploration of the scalenus fat pad. This lies
between the clavicle and the scalenus anticus and
sternocleidomastoid muscles. It is easily removed under
local anesthesia through a small incision in the supraclavicular fossa.

Lymph node hyperplasia is encountered in Addison's disease, hyperthyroidism, and hypopituitarism, in which conditions the adenopathy is noteworthy since it contrasts with the tendency for lymph node atrophy found in association with inanition due to other causes.

DIFFERENTIAL DIAGNOSIS OF LYMPH NODE ENLARGEMENT

It should be evident, from this discussion, that the discovery of the cause of glandular enlargement requires a thorough examination of the patient. It is important, of course, to determine the extent of the adenopathy. The systematic examination should especially include careful palpation of the cervical regions, the epitrochlear regions, the arms (for swelling of brachial nodes), the axillas, the lateral borders of the chest, the inguinal and femoral regions, and the popliteal spaces. Tenderness of lymph nodes suggests infection rather than one of the lymphomas, leukemia, or metastatic involvement. However, some degree of tenderness, as well as pain, may be encountered when the glands have enlarged rapidly, especially in Hodgkin's disease. A resilient firmness, somewhat like that of uncured gum rubber, is characteristic of lymphosarcoma and reticulum cell sarcoma and may be found in Hodgkin's disease. In the last condition, the presence of connective and fibrous tissue in the nodes may cause them to be harder than usual; they may have the consistency of cartilage. In carcinoma the glands are usually stony hard.

The location of the glandular enlargement may suggest the site of origin of the disease and sometimes may give some clue as to its nature. Acute cervical adenitis should direct attention to the mouth and pharynx, mastoid adenitis to scalp infections, axillary adenitis to the upper extremity and the breast, epitrochlear enlargement to involvement of the ulnar side of the hand or forearm, and inguinal swelling to the lower extremities and genitalia. Supraclavicular gland enlargement, it may be noted, may result from infection in the thumb and index finger as well as in the neck. If the gland is hard and not tender, it may be the seat of tumor. Lymph drainage to this node is such that, if the right node is enlarged, some primary process in the chest should be suspected; whereas enlargement of the left supraclavicular node should direct attention to the abdomen. Enlargement of the inferior deep cervical glands in the posterior triangle of the neck is more often due to Hodgkin's disease, or secondary to malignancy, than due to an infection arising in the throat. The occipital glands are not infrequently affected in rubella and in secondary syphilis. The finding of discrete, nontender nodes in regions where lymph nodes are rarely palpated, as along the brachial artery or in the femoral (as distinguished from the inguinal) region, should arouse suspicion of the existence of a systemic disorder involving the lymphatic system, such as leukemia.

The general examination of the patient must also be painstaking, for sometimes secondary glandular enlargement may be much more prominent than the primary cause. Thus, for example, cervical metastases from a nasopharyngeal tumor usually overshadow the primary growth, which is characteristically small and easily overlooked unless a careful nasopharyngoscopic examination is made. The study of the patient should include careful palpation of the sternum for tenderness and of the abdomen for splenic enlargement, as well as examination of the chest for evidence of mediastinal tumor. Rectal and pelvic examination must not be overlooked.

Important laboratory procedures include the serologic test for syphilis, examination of the blood for agglutination reactions, blood culture and culture of the throat, sputum, and other possible sources which might reveal infection, as well as examination of the blood and sometimes of the bone marrow for morphologic evidences of disease. Skin tests, such as tuberculin, histoplasmin, and coccidioidin, may also need to be performed; culture of the lymph nodes may be helpful occasionally; and roentgenograms may have to be taken of the lungs, the gastrointestinal system, the kidneys, or other structures. In chronic forms of lymph node enlargement, biopsy of a node is often necessary, especially when it is a matter of differentiating the various types of primary lymph node disease.

THE SPLEEN

It is rare that one can palpate the spleen in a person who is entirely normal, although it must be admitted that very occasionally a person is encountered in whom the spleen is palpable and in whom even prolonged observation fails to reveal any evidence of disease. How often this may occur is difficult to state.

The pulp of the spleen is composed of (1) anastomosing strands of lymphoid tissue, (2) a reticular network and branching multipolar cells which are placed about blood sinuses and intermingle with the strands of lymphoid tissue, and (3) lymphocytes, granulocytes, and erythrocytes. The spleen is a very vascular organ and is capable of changing substantially in size, depending on its content of blood. It is also contractile; its capsule contains a small amount of elastic tissue. The circulation of the spleen is unique and blood flows from the arterioles into pulp spaces and possibly into other poorly defined channels. In the sense that blood flow may proceed rapidly as in most other tissues, or cells may bypass the main stream of circulation and enter more stagnant areas, the circulation may be considered partly open and partly closed. Normally only a small proportion of the blood, perhaps 20 ml, is present outside the main channel of blood flow.

FUNCTIONS OF THE SPLEEN. The spleen serves as a reservoir for blood and is concerned with blood destruction. There is good evidence that the spleen is the chief graveyard of the red cell. In man, in contrast to certain other mammalian species, the reservoir function does not seem to be very important. However, sequestration of red corpuscles takes place in the spleen, and this probably plays a role in the detection and removal of effete worn-out corpuscles and undoubtedly is important in the blood destruction which occurs in certain disorders of the blood (p. 627). This organ, in contrast to the lungs and the kidneys, is able to dispose of the iron derived from red cell destruction and makes it available for the formation of new cells.

During embryonic life the spleen plays an important part in blood formation, and the potentialities of this organ for blood formation persist even in adult life. Lymphocytes are normally produced in the mature animal by the malpighian corpuscles of the spleen, and monocytes may also arise in that organ. In certain circumstances, foci of extramedullary blood formation can be found in the spleen; thus, when the functional activity of the bone marrow is impaired, the hematopoietic potentiality of the spleen may become an important asset. In this connection the interesting observation was made that the recovery of hematopoietic tissue following whole body radiation was significantly hastened by lead shielding of the exteriorized spleen. Other tissues have a similar though less striking influence. The protective factor was at first thought to be noncellular in nature, but it is now believed that recovery depends on the seeding or colonization of cells from the spleen.

Following splenectomy, certain characteristic alterations in the blood occur. Nucleated red cells appear, as well as corpuscles with Howell-Jolly bodies, and diffusely basophilic cells, target cells, and siderocytes are found, while the percentage of reticulocytes is increased. Leukocytosis occurs, and the number of platelets increases. These changes have been cited as evidence that the spleen exerts an inhibitory action on the bone marrow. In so far as the red cell changes are concerned, there is experimental evidence to support the view that the spleen normally *removes* the forms which are not usually seen in the blood in the absence of splenectomy or of hematopoietic disorders such as pernicious anemia or thalassemia. No evidence has been provided that the spleen exercises control over erythropoiesis in any other way. In relation to the leukocytes and platelets, however, there is at least some evidence to support the possibility that their production and liberation from the marrow may be influenced by the spleen. In addition, in certain situations the spleen appears to destroy these structures, especially the platelets, as, for example, when they are coated with antibodies.

In view of the large collection of reticuloendothelial cells and lymphoid tissue in the spleen, and for other reasons, it seems likely that the spleen plays a role in the defense mechanism of the body, perhaps through antibody production. In certain species, such as the dog and the rat, the spleen is important in maintaining natural resistance to certain bacterial, protozoal, and hematozoic infections. However, in man, at least, the spleen does not appear to be essential for these purposes, and little evidence has been found for the suggestion that the predisposition to infection is significantly greater in splenectomized persons, even in young children, than in otherwise normal individuals.

ENLARGEMENT OF THE SPLEEN. This may occur under a great variety of circumstances. The chief ones are listed in Table 40-2.

Of greatest frequency is the enlargement of the spleen which occurs in association with infections. The *"acute splenic tumor"* accompanying various systemic infections such as typhoid fever and septicemia are examples. Like lymph node enlargement, splenic enlargement is frequently encountered in various contagious diseases and is often seen in infectious mononucleosis. Likewise, various subacute infections, notably bacterial endocarditis, are characteristically accompanied by enlargement of the spleen. *Abscess* of the spleen is rare and is usually secondary to pyemia arising from some other site. Frequently multiple and unrecognized, it is unusual for a splenic abscess to achieve prominence and produce local symptoms such as pain, elevation of the left leaf of the diaphragm, or rupture into the peritoneal cavity.

Malaria is, perhaps, the commonest cause of splenic enlargement when the world population is considered. Infection with other parasites which leads to splenic enlargement includes leishmaniasis, trypanosomiasis, and schistosomiasis. In kala-azar the spleen may be huge.

Table 40-2. CHIEF CAUSES OF SPLENOMEGALY

I. Inflammatory splenomegaly
   A. "Acute splenic tumor": many acute and subacute infections
      1. Bacterial (typhoid, septicemias, subacute bacterial endocarditis, abscess, etc.)
      2. Viral and miscellaneous (contagious diseases, infectious mononucleosis)
   B. Chronic infections (tuberculosis, syphilis, brucellosis, histoplasmosis, malaria, schistosomiasis, leishmaniasis, trypanosomiasis, etc.)
   C. Miscellaneous diseases (lupus erythematosus, rheumatoid arthritis, sarcoidosis, histiocytosis X, etc.)
II. Congestive splenomegaly (Banti's syndrome)
   A. Cirrhosis of liver
   B. Thrombosis or stenosis, portal or splenic veins
III. Hyperplastic splenomegaly
   A. Hemolytic anemias, congenital and acquired
   B. Thalassemia and certain hemoglobinopathies
   C. Myelofibrosis, myelophthisic anemias
   D. Polycythemia vera
   E. Miscellaneous chronic anemias (pernicious anemia, chronic iron deficiency, "pyridoxine-responsive anemia," etc.)
   F. Thrombocytopenic purpura
   G. Obscure disorders ("big spleen syndrome," "primary splenic neutropenia," and "panhematopenia")
IV. Infiltrative splenomegaly
   A. Gaucher's disease, Niemann-Pick disease
   B. Amyloidosis, hemosiderosis
V. Neoplasms and cysts
   A. True cysts (dermoid, echinococcus, etc.)
   B. False cysts (hemorrhagic, serous, inflammatory, degenerative)
   C. Benign tumors (lymphangioma, hemangioma, etc.)
   D. Leukemia, lymphomas
   E. Malignant tumors (direct invasion or metastatic)

Primary tuberculous splenomegaly is extremely rare, but slight enlargement of the spleen accompanying a widespread tuberculous infection is by no means unusual. Splenomegaly may occur in connection with syphilis, especially congenital syphilis. Enlargement of this organ may also accompany the late stages of syphilis in association with gummas or amyloidosis. Rheumatoid arthritis, brucellosis, and sarcoidosis are other chronic diseases which may be accompanied by splenic enlargement. Splenic enlargement has been observed in about 25 per cent of cases of disseminated lupus erythematosus.

The vascularity of the spleen and its location in the portal bed make this organ liable to swelling as the result of increased venous pressure in that region. Such types of enlargement of the spleen can be classed under the general heading of "congestive splenomegaly" and include the syndromes known as *Banti's disease* and *splenic anemia,* as well as the splenic enlargement which accompanies cirrhosis of the liver and thrombosis of the splenic or portal vein (p. 677) and that which may be associated with cardiac failure.

The functions of the spleen in relation to the hematopoietic system result in enlargement of this organ when there is increased blood destruction (acute and chronic hemolytic anemias) or in the presence of chronic anemia of various types such as pernicious anemia, chronic hypochromic anemia, myelophthisic anemia, thalassemia, hemoglobin-C disease, and other hemoglobinopathies. Again, the spleen is enlarged, as a rule, in leukemia. In polycythemia vera splenomegaly is often encountered, and this finding helps to distinguish the primary disorder from secondary forms of polycythemia, where splenic enlargement is rare. The lymphatic hyperplasia which is associated with hyperthyroidism may be accompanied by splenomegaly. The spleen is also enlarged in myelofibrosis, primary splenic neutropenia (p. 678), and primary splenic panhematopenia (p. 679).

Certain rare diseases such as Gaucher's disease and Niemann-Pick disease are characterized by splenic enlargement. In these conditions the swelling of the organ is probably due to the excessive storage of normal and abnormal metabolic products in the cells of the spleen (see pp. 680 and 681).

Like other organs, the spleen may be enlarged as the consequence of the presence of neoplasms of various types. Hodgkin's disease, lymphosarcoma, reticulum cell sarcoma, and giant follicular lymphoma, however, are far commoner causes of splenomegaly than other types of new growth. Carcinoma is the most frequent type of metastatic tumor, but even this is extremely rare. Direct extension from carcinoma of the stomach and hematogenous spread from the stomach, lung, pancreas, and breast and from malignant melanoma may occur. Other tumors that may involve the spleen include lymphangioma, hemangioma and endothelial sarcoma (lymphangiosarcoma), fibrosarcoma, leiomyosarcoma, and myoma. A subcapsular cavernous hemangioma may rupture into the peritoneal cavity and produce acute hemorrhagic shock.

Cysts of the spleen may be of parasitic origin or nonparasitic. Of the latter, those containing serous or hemorrhagic fluid and due to trauma are commonest. They can sometimes be identified roentgenographically because of calcification of the wall. Echinococcus cysts occur more rarely in the spleen than in the liver. "True" cysts are formed from embryonal defects or rests and include dermoids and mesenchymal inclusion cysts.

DIFFERENTIAL DIAGNOSIS OF SPLENOMEGALY

A thorough physical examination, together with the history and examination of the blood, will serve to differentiate many of the causes of splenomegaly which have been outlined. Sometimes additional procedures may be required, such as blood culture, sternal puncture, a roentgenogram of the chest, serologic tests including those for syphilis, liver function tests, and spleen or lymph node biopsy.

The absence of fever is more helpful in differential diagnosis here than is its presence, since most of the conditions which have been mentioned may be accompanied by fever. However, at times, as in malaria and in undulant fever, the characteristic temperature curve is very helpful in making the diagnosis. In the septicemias the splenic enlargement is, as a rule, obviously only a minor feature of the whole clinical picture. The exanthemas are recognized by the respective characteristic changes in the skin. In their absence the skin should be inspected carefully for evidence of the petechiae which may accompany acute leukemia, thrombocytopenic purpura, or other hematopoietic disorders; the red petechiae occurring in crops together with the larger, slightly nodular and tender Osler nodes so characteristic of subacute bacterial endocarditis; or the spider telangiectases which accompany longstanding liver diseases. The plum-red "cyanosis" of polycythemia vera can hardly be overlooked.

Moderate lymph node enlargement accompanying splenomegaly is seen in many infectious diseases as well as in leukemia, but an asymmetric enlargement should arouse suspicion of Hodgkin's disease or lymphosarcoma. Great enlargement of the lymph nodes is seen in the last-named conditions as well as in chronic leukemia, especially in the lymphocytic form. The discovery of icterus suggests hemolytic anemia as a cause or, if there is little or no anemia and the splenic enlargement is only slight, infectious hepatitis. The splenomegaly associated with the Banti syndrome (congestive splenomegaly) and with cirrhosis of the liver is usually substantial in degree, and jaundice is not the rule under these circumstances. Malaria must be kept in mind among the causes of hemolytic anemia.

Lesions in the mucous membranes accompanying splenic enlargement are seen in measles (Koplik's spots), secondary syphilis (mucous patches), infectious mononucleosis (infection of the throat, tonsillar enlargement, sometimes signs of Vincent's angina), and acute leukemia (swollen, thickened gums which may be bleeding or purplish in color). In the leukemias, sternal tenderness may be quite pronounced.

The discovery of very great enlargement of the spleen tends to rule out the acute splenic tumor of various systemic infections, although sometimes the spleen may extend 4 to 6 cm below the costal margin in septicemia and in subacute bacterial endocarditis. Huge spleens are encountered in the chronic leukemias, in the Banti syndrome, in kala-azar, in schistosomiasis, in Gaucher's disease, in Hodgkin's disease and lymphosarcoma, in myelofibrosis, and in many instances of chronic hemolytic anemia.

Examination of the blood may indicate at once the nature of the disorder, as in malaria, the frank leukemias, or infectious mononucleosis. The discovery of icterus will lead to a reticulocyte count, examination of the stools and urine for the products of blood destruction, an erythrocyte fragility test, and other studies (see p. 630) to rule out the various hemolytic anemias. The discovery of leukopenia should lead to the consideration of malaria, "aleukemic" leukemia, the Banti syndrome, typhoid fever, histoplasmosis, and leishmaniasis, but it must be kept in mind that the white cell count may sometimes be low also in infectious mononucleosis and in some cases of chronic hemolytic anemia. The demonstration of thrombocytopenia, as well as prolonged bleeding time, poor clot retraction, and positive tourniquet test, is an important finding, for it suggests acute leukemia. In that condition immature leukocytes will be found in the blood. In the "aleukemic" form, immature cells are absent from the blood or very scarce, but they are readily demonstrated by sternal puncture. In idiopathic thrombocytopenic purpura, the spleen is barely palpable in about 33 per cent of cases, but it is never very large. Thrombocytopenia only very rarely accompanies infectious mononucleosis and, while present in other conditions such as pernicious anemia, chronic hypochromic anemia, chronic hemolytic anemias, myelophthisic anemia, the Banti syndrome, Hodgkin's disease, and the related lymph node disorders, it is rarely severe in these diseases.

Sternal puncture may be very helpful if "aleukemic" leukemia, leishmaniasis, or Gaucher's disease is being considered seriously, for the characteristic cells or causative organisms may be demonstrated in this way. Sternal puncture does not often reveal malaria when the parasites have eluded careful study of the blood, but sometimes positive blood cultures for bacteria are obtained by this means when the usual method has failed. Splenic puncture is helpful when parasites, storage cells, signs of myeloid metaplasia, or granulomas are found, but this procedure should not be undertaken when hemorrhagic manifestations are present or in the absence of evidence of distinct splenic enlargement.

Various disorders of the spleen are discussed in a later chapter (Chap. 125).

REFERENCES

Saltzstein, S. L., and L. V. Ackerman: Lymphadenopathy Induced by Anticonvulsant Drugs, Cancer, 12:164, 1959.

Wintrobe, M. M.: "Clinical Hematology," 5th ed., Philadelphia, Lea & Febiger, 1961.

Section 9

Alterations in Nervous Function

41 GENERAL CONSIDERATIONS
Raymond D. Adams

The symptoms and signs of nervous disease, which comprise the subject material of this section, are probably the most frequent and at the same time the most complex in all of medicine. Naturally, they interest students of neurology and psychiatry, but they are so often found in patients who do not have classifiable diseases of the nervous system that they inevitably become the concern of every physician.

A lucid exposition of the diverse and complex manifestations of nervous disease is difficult, and a certain bias, which will be apparent at once to specialists in this field, is almost unavoidable. The method chosen here is somewhat unconventional and requires a few words of explanation. The aim has been to bring together all the expressions of disordered nervous function. They are described in some detail, and the most generally accepted explanations from anatomy, biochemistry, physiology, and psychology are offered. No distinction is drawn between relatively simple phenomena such as motor and sensory paralysis, which are usually based on an easily demonstrated structural change, and the most complex ones such as anxiety, depression, or paranoia, to which at present no gross or microscopic pathologic changes can be assigned.

An attempt has been made, wherever indicated, to present both the neurologic and the psychologic conceptions of the more complex phenomena, but the emphasis is on the neurologic, for it is more understandable to physicians and surgeons, as the approach is the same as that to all other medical diseases.

NEUROLOGIC AND PSYCHOLOGIC CONCEPTIONS OF NERVOUS DISEASE

An understanding of these two conceptions of nervous disease is necessary in order to appreciate current trends in neurology and psychiatry. At the very beginning of this brief exposition of methodology and clinical approach, it should be stated that the terms *neurologic* and *psychologic* do not denote the respective activities of neurologists and psychiatrists. Neurologic means the concepts of medicine applied to the study of nervous disease. They may be and are used by physicians, psychiatrists, and neurologists. Psychologic means another set of ideas, largely nonmedical and used by many psychiatrists as well as by neurologists and physicians. In other words, the conception, the method, or the subject matter does not strictly pertain to any one discipline.

The *neurologic conception* starts with the assumption that all the phenomena of nervous disease are related to a pathologic process within the nervous system. This process may be obvious, like a cerebral infarct or tumor; or it may be impossible to see even with an ordinary light microscope, like the encephalopathy of delirium tremens. In all instances the pathologic process is the result of some physical or chemical change, and the visible lesion may represent only its most advanced and often irreversible stage. The symptoms and clinical signs of nervous disease are the expressions of the activity of the pathologically altered nervous system. These clinical manifestations vary widely and include, on the one hand, the relatively simple, easily elicited, stereotyped objective signs, such as motor paralysis or ataxia, and, on the other, the most complex, difficult to evoke, highly individualized, subjective signs, such as hallucination, delusion, or obsessive thoughts. This is perhaps the most difficult idea for the student to grasp—that there is no necessary difference between "physical" and "mental" or "organic" and "functional" symptoms. To the neurologist, as to other physicians, all these symptoms have their objective as well as their "conscious" or subjective aspects, and the prominence of one or the other should not change our way of looking at them. In either the paralyzed or the delirious patient, something of normal behavior has been lost as a consequence of nervous disease, and often something new in his behavior has emerged, presumably because of the unbalanced or unrestrained action of the undamaged parts of the brain. Some symptoms, like the dementia of general paresis, are understandable largely through the structural alteration of the brain, and the clinical picture is a combination of deficits of function and the activity of intact parts of it. The patient still exhibits behavior and thinking and still responds to his environment. No doubt previous personality structure, educational level, etc., modify the clinical state. Other symptoms, such as a paranoid idea, though believed

to be based on a neuropathologic process, are more difficult to analyze, for we cannot easily identify the primary defect nor trace its effects in the patient's reaction. Such symptoms and reactions become more comprehensible when viewed against the background of all previous life experiences of which they may be a part. The previous life experiences thus become part of the present illness; but though possibly explaining the content of the nervous symptom and its mode of evolution, they do not explain its occurrence. The neurologic examination becomes merely a device which permits one to sample systematically the activities of the altered nervous system at one moment; and special techniques, particularly refined psychologic methods, may be needed to supplement it. Also, special laboratory procedures, such as biochemical tests of the blood, the electroencephalogram (EEG), the examination of the cerebrospinal fluid, and x-rays, yield additional objective data that cannot be obtained by observation. Pathologic study provides the final confirmation of the disease. The goal of the neurologic method, or of neuropathology (the laboratory study of nervous disease), is to define the essential pathologic processes underlying disease and to determine their cause and mechanism. A complete theory of a nervous disease should embrace all aspects of it, the anatomic, pathologic, biochemical, and physiologic, as well as psychologic. The method is that of the medical sciences and of medicine itself.

The *psychologic conception of disease* rests on many of the same assumptions as the neurologic concept. For example, it is assumed that in many patients psychologic difficulties are caused by structural changes at the molecular, chemical, or tissue level. They may be due to a genetic or developmental defect, and a lesion may be visualized. The main premise, however, is that the nervous disorder, like the content of the mind, is determined within broad limits by previous life experiences. Certain features of personality, the degree of emotional maturity, and the capacity to adjust adequately to a social situation are thought to depend to a considerable extent on learned patterns of reaction. Aberrations of mental function are regarded as immature and unstable reactions to environmental circumstances, derived, it is believed, from personality inadequacy or traceable to unfortunate experiences in early life. Some of these experiences are easily remembered, i.e., "conscious"; others are forgotten, i.e., "unconscious," and can be recalled with difficulty and sometimes only through the free-association method of psychoanalysis. In either case the principal method of approach is to review the patient's autobiography and determine the relationship of the present symptoms to past experiences. The symptoms and signs of mental disease, whether the grandiose delusion of the general paretic or the phobia of a neurotic person, are regarded as responses to a number of stimulus situations acting upon individuals who differ from normal mainly in that they have learned to think and to react emotionally in an abnormal manner. Since their symptoms are often traced to psychic conflicts that have arisen in their personal life, they are in this sense psychogenic. By interview and frank discussion, the physician endeavors to demonstrate these relationships to the patient and thereby to assist him to adjust to them satisfactorily. The ultimate aim of the psychologic study of disease or of psychopathology, which is the scientific study of the psychologic origins of symptoms, is to discover abnormal mental processes and to find their psychologic cause and mechanism. Examples of some of the established mechanisms are conflict, projection, repression, conditioning, and arrest of libido. It is held, particularly by some of the more narrowly trained psychoanalysts, that all psychologic theories of mental disorder must be couched in psychologic terms and that anatomic, biochemical, physiologic, and pathologic terms have no place in such a formulation. The method is that of psychology, and the conception is in line with rationalistic philosophy.

Each method and each conception of disease has its place in medicine. The two methods operate at entirely different levels. In the *diagnosis* of nervous disease the physician's first responsibility is to record accurately all the symptoms and signs obtained in a single examination or a series of them. Here the neurologic method is the only sound system. It permits the problem of nervous disease to be approached as any other medical problem. The psychologic method is not of great diagnostic value, because eliciting the patient's biography and finding psychologic explanations for his symptoms is a time-consuming procedure and commits one prematurely to a formula of his present illness that may be totally erroneous. In *therapy* and in the *management* of many diseases, including those for which there is no known treatment, a detailed knowledge of the patient's personality and his general reactions are, on the other hand, quite indispensable. Success in all fields of medicine depends on the ability to deal with the patient as a troubled individual. Here the psychologic method is of practical value, and the neurologic one often has relatively less to offer. This is a province of medicine where trained psychiatrists may function with great skill. In *theorizing* about disease and in doing *medical research*, however, the neurologic method and concept provide the soundest approach, for they embrace all the methods of medicine and the medical sciences, anatomic, physiologic, biochemical, and neuropathologic, as well as psychologic. Here the psychologic method has limited application, and though it yields useful data about the evolution of symptoms and their content or form, it will probably never explain completely a disease of the nervous system.

Thus, from the very beginning, we are confronted by one of the crucial problems of neurology—defining nervous diseases. Failure to do this has resulted in great confusion and has been an obstacle to research. The authors propose to define nervous disease as *disease in which there is a lesion in the nervous tissue or in which there is reasonable evidence of an anatomic abnormality or a consistent physical or biochemical disturbance.* This should be distinguished from an abnormal psychologic reaction, which is defined as *a disorder of behavior caused apparently by maladjustment in social relations.* Worry over the loss of a job or the ill health of a child, with all its potential visceral reverberations, would not be classified as a disease. These and countless other daily problems are better looked upon as natural psychologic and physiologic reactions to social problems and dealt with at a psychologic level. A persistent anxiety state without obvious cause in a previously healthy young housewife, on the other hand, would be viewed differently. Most psychiatrists would consider it a reaction to some unconscious conflict, whereas many neurologists might consider it an unexplained, socially evoked disorder as mysterious as was hyperthyroidism a century ago. Anyone who essays to investigate it should do so with a completely open mind and be prepared to review critically any apparently satisfactory explanation, whether psychologic or neurologic. Mania, depression, paranoia, and the several varieties of schizophrenia, which are the major problems of psychiatry, have, unfortunately, an uncertain status. Many experienced psychiatrists would probably agree that they are diseases, rather than deviate ways of living or abnormal psychologic reactions, and that the more comprehensive methods of medicine and the medical sciences offer a more promising approach than does psychology. To the neurologist the major deficiencies in the study of these latter disorders of the nervous system in the past few years have been the relative overemphasis on psychopathology and the neglect of neuropathology, using this term in its broadest sense.

NEUROLOGY AND PSYCHIATRY

All that has been said is to explain the different ways in which neurologists and psychiatrists conceptualize the problems of nervous disease. Actually the fields of neurology and psychiatry are broad and touch every medical and surgical specialty. Both are concerned with disturbances of behavior, conduct, thinking, and emotional control due to diseases of the brain. In addition, neurology is concerned with many diseases of the nervous system that do not alter the mind, and psychiatry is occupied with countless problems of adjustment in daily life, which are sources of much unhappiness and disability and yet cannot be defined as nervous diseases.

A comprehensive account of the major psychiatric and neurologic diseases will be presented in the second half of this book in their appropriate place, with diseases of the nervous system. Certain major manifestations of mental illness and of neurologic disease, those most likely to be encountered by general practitioners and internists, will be discussed in the first half of this book, and an attempt will be made to explain them in terms of current anatomic, physiologic and psychologic theory. A systematic discussion of normal personality development is desirable, but space is too limited. Neurologic disorders will be discussed in order, ranging from the most frequent and general symptoms and signs to the most specific.

THE IMPORTANCE OF PSYCHOLOGIC MEDICINE

The magnitude of the field of psychologic medicine can hardly be overestimated, and emphasis on the neurologic method is not intended to depreciate the importance of the psychologic approach. Every physician would agree that illness invariably creates problems for the patient and his family. Some, such as the temporary loss of employment or interruption of normal activities, are relatively minor. Others, such as fear of disability or death, may be so overwhelming as to demand the most thoughtful treatment. The need to understand the patient and his reactions must be taken into account in every medical procedure, even in history taking, where the reliability and validity of symptoms must be evaluated against the background of the patient's personality and his cultural environment. The group of illnesses called the *psychoneuroses* or *neuroses* manifest a wide variety of symptoms that may be confused with those of medical disease.

Of even greater significance is the large category of diseases of unknown origin (peptic ulcer, mucous colitis, ulcerative colitis, bronchial asthma, atopic dermatitis, urticaria, angioneurotic edema, hay fever, Raynaud's disease, hypertension, hyperthyroidism, amenorrhea and other disturbances of menstruation, enuresis, dysuria, rheumatoid and other forms of arthritis, headache, syncope, and epilepsy) in which a stressful personal problem appears often associated with initial development, exacerbation, or prolongation of symptoms. Three lines of evidence tend to set these *psychosomatic diseases* apart from all others. (1) A large series of observations, made by Cannon, Wolff, Mittelman, Wolf, Cobb, Finesinger, White, Jones and others, have established the fact that the function of the offending organ is excited and possibly deranged by strong emotions and assuaged by feelings of security and relaxation. (2) A careful analysis of the biographies of patients with these diseases has shown what is believed to be an inordinately high incidence of resentment, hostility, dependence or independence, suppressed emotionality, inability to communicate matters of emotional concern or to differentiate between reality and subjective falsification (cf. studies of Lindemann, Dunbar, French, and Alexander). (Preliminary studies of personality promised at first to show a special group of personality traits to be operating in each disease, but subsequent inquiry indicates that this is not the case.) (3) A search through the biographic data of patients with these diseases has related exacerbations of symptoms with the occurrence of frustrating or disturbing incidents, and unsuccessful medical therapy has seemed to result when emotional factors were neglected.

In the field of psychosomatic disease, despite intensive investigation by psychiatrists in the last 20 years, the reports of which make up an enormous literature,

very few facts have been established. Surely it can be said that, like the psychoneuroses, they are "part disturbances" of the personality. But they differ from the psychoneuroses in that (1) they have different symptoms; (2) as a rule, they last longer; (3) they have in most instances a known and demonstrable pathologic basis and often a known cause, e.g., allergy in asthma and atopic dermatitis; (4) treatment has been concerned more directly with the relief of symptoms and has tended to be directed by different groups of specialists; (5) the incidence of frank psychoneuroses in this group of patients is no greater than in the population at large, and these psychosomatic disorders are not more frequent in neurotic individuals. No complete proof has thus far been adduced that psychic factors are the primary cause of any of these psychosomatic diseases, any more than they are the cause of angina pectoris or exophthalmic goiter. Moreover, the concepts formed about these diseases in recent years, although educationally useful, have not been of great theoretical value. There is no evidence that the therapeutic results obtained by a thoughtful understanding physician, unsophisticated in psychologic theory, are less good than those of the most experienced psychiatrists.

The basic fault in this field of psychologic medicine, as it was in the "somatic medicine" that flourished before and after the First World War, is that one aspect is stressed with too little reference to the other. As pointed out by Wolff in his scholarly exposition of the mind-body relationship, the logical fallacy of such ideas as "psychogenic," "psychosomatic," and "emotional causes of disease" is that they imply a mind acting in opposition to a body.

An ancient approach to this broad area of medicine, first suggested by Claude Bernard and ably espoused by Adolph Meyer, regards man as a psychobiologic unit functioning in relationship to his physical and his uniquely social environment. Disease represents a faulty or inadequate adaptation of the organism to the environment. Sometimes the maladaptation can be traced to a single agent in the environment such as the tubercle bacillus, without which the disease tuberculosis could not develop. In other instances, a recurrent infection is much more complex, manifesting a primary physical defect in the individual, as in agammaglobulinemia. Again, exhaustion from a prolonged, stressful situation or malnutrition may render the patient susceptible to an infectious agent. Seldom, however, even in straightforward disease such as tuberculosis or delirium tremens, can one reduce the problem to a single physical or psychic factor. Hence, a rigid and narrow physical or psychologic approach must be supplanted by this broader, more biologic one, which attempts to weigh each of several factors that make up the equation of disease. At present this is difficult, for all the factors, particularly in psychosomatic diseases, have not been isolated and studied. Until such time as new facts are obtained, the physician must cope with a huge population of patients, as many as 50 per cent, with inadequate methods of diagnosis and treatment.

Fortunately, most of these patients suffer from relatively minor ailments which time and kindly reassurance alleviate or from psychoneuroses that are not disabling. The physician and student must acquire a sensitivity to psychologic problems without becoming so mindful of them that every illness is reduced to a naive psychologic formula. Above all, an open mind should be adopted, one that will permit critical review of all hypotheses in this field and acceptance of only those based on the valid data of controlled clinical observation and scientific experiment.

REFERENCES

Cobb, S.: "Emotions and Clinical Medicine," New York, W. W. Norton & Company, 1950.

Finesinger, J. E.: Psychiatric Components in Medical Disease: Psychosomatic Medicine, New England J. Med., 227:578, 1942.

Masserman, J. H.: "Behavior and Neurosis: An Experimental Psychoanalytic Approach to Psychobiologic Principles," Chicago, University of Chicago Press, 1943.

Wolf, S., and H. G. Wolff: "Human Gastric Function: An Experimental Study of a Man and His Stomach," New York, Oxford University Press, 1947.

42 NERVOUSNESS, ANXIETY, AND DEPRESSION

Raymond D. Adams and Justin Hope

Upon close questioning the majority of patients who enter a physician's office or a hospital will admit to being nervous, anxious, or depressed. Evidently the natural human reactions to the prospect of real or imaginary disease or to the stresses of contemporary social environment are being experienced. If they stand in clear relationship to a stresssful situation, e.g., anxiety over pressing economic reverses or grief over the death of a loved one, these states may be accepted as normal, and they become the basis of medical consultation only when excessively intense and uncontrollable or when accompanying derangements of visceral function are excessive. The problem increases in complexity when similar symptoms occur in individuals whose immediate environment appears to be entirely innocuous; any threatening situation, if it exists, is either unknown to the conscious mind of the patient, or has been suppressed. The relationship between social stimulus and the prevailing alteration of mood can then be discovered only by the gentle probings of the psychologically sophisticated physician. Once the connection is established and the problem dealt with realistically, the symptoms become understandable and often disappear.

There is still another broad category of nervousness, anxiety, and depression, the significance of which we cannot fully comprehend. These are states in which the individual suffers profound and prolonged anxiety and depression without obvious explanation. Delving into the unconscious mind fails to reveal a plausible psychogenesis. In many such instances a genetic factor appears to operate, and the principal features of the illness and its natural cause are so stereotyped as to indicate a fundamental derangement of the emotional apparatus of the nervous system. These latter states are categorized as diseases even though they do not possess an established pathology.

The problem confronting every physician is to recognize these nervous disorders in all their variations and decide whether they constitute the nervous reactions of a normal person, a pathologic reaction the psychologic antecedents of which are veiled in the obscurities of the unconscious mind, or a grave disease of the nervous system demanding the attention of specialists in psychologic medicine.

In this chapter the cardinal features of these conditions will be described along with current views of their psychologic and physiologic origins; and lines of inquiry that might help determine their significance will be suggested.

NERVOUSNESS

By this rather vague term the lay person usually refers to a state of restlessness and overactivity, tension, uneasy apprehension, or hyperexcitability. But it may also mean other things, such as thoughts of suicide, fear of killing one's child or spouse, a distressing hallucination or paranoid idea, or frank hysterical behavior. Careful questioning as to its exact nature is always necessary.

In its usual signification a period of nervousness may represent no more than one of the variations to which many otherwise normal individuals are subject. For example, adolescence rarely passes without its period of turmoil, as the young person attempts to emancipate himself from his family and to adjust to school, work, and the opposite sex. In the female the menses are accompanied by increased tension and moodiness, and, of course, the menopause is another critical period. Some individuals claim they have been nervous throughout life, and one should then suspect a psychoneurosis or psychosis even though adjustment to school, family, and work seem to have been adequate. Others come to the physician because of a recent development of nervousness; in this instance one must consider a variety of conditions such as psychoneurosis, psychosis, endocrine disease (e.g., hyperthyroidism), a drug reaction (corticosteroid therapy), or withdrawal reaction from a drug (alcoholic or barbiturate delirium). Some patients complain of nervousness that attends the development of a medical disease; it would appear to be secondary, occasioned by fear of disability, dependency, or death.

Nervousness even in its simplest form is reflected in many important activities of the human organism. When it is present, there is often a mild somberness of mood and increased emotionality. Fatigue that bears no proper relationship to sleep and rest is frequent; and sleep is often troubled, as are eating and drinking habits. The patient subject to headaches often reports these to have increased in frequency and intensity. All these symptoms, along with sweating, awareness of cardiac action, queer sensations in the head or giddiness, upset stomach, and frequency of micturition, indicate that the nervous state is inducing some of the same visceral changes that occur with anxiety. Thus, it would appear that nervousness and anxiety constitute a graded series of reactions, anxiety being usually a more intense and protracted nervousness; the underlying cause and mechanisms appear to be essentially the same for both conditions (see p. 1266).

THE ANXIETY STATE

Anxiety is "the fundamental phenomenon and central problem of neurosis . . . a nodal point, linking up all kinds of most important questions, a riddle of which the solution must cast a flood of light upon our whole mental life." (Freud) From the viewpoint of the social historian, anxiety is said to be "the most prominent mental characteristic of Occidental civilization." (Willoughby) In these contexts anxiety has a broad meaning, more or less equivalent to social and psychologic unrest. In more general psychologic terms it has been defined as "an emotional state arising when a continuing strong desire seems likely to miss its goal." (McDougall)

The more strictly medical meaning of the word *anxiety*, and the one used in this chapter, designates a state characterized by a subjective feeling of fear and uneasy anticipation (apprehension), usually with a definite topical content and associated with the physiologic accompaniments of fear, i.e., breathlessness, choking sensation, palpitation, restlessness, increased muscular tension, tightness in the chest, giddiness, trembling, sweating, flushing, and broken sleep. By topical content is meant the idea, the person, or the object about which the person is anxious. The several vasomotor, visceral, and chemical changes that underlie many of the symptoms and signs are mediated through the autonomic nervous system, particularly the sympathetic part of it, and involve the thyroid and adrenal glands.

Forms of Anxiety

Anxiety manifests itself in acute episodes, lasting a few minutes, or a protracted state continuing for weeks, months, or even years. In the acute attacks, called *anxiety attacks* or *panics*, breathlessness, palpitation, choking, sweating, and trembling accompany an intense fear of dying, losing one's reason, or committing a horrid crime. In states of chronic anxiety, nervousness, restlessness, irritability, excitability, fatigue, pressure or tension headaches, and insomnia again are the major symptoms, but they tend to be milder and less frightening but by no means less disabling. Discrete anxiety attacks and protracted states of anxiety are not mutually exclusive, though they often occur separately. Episodic anxiety occurring in attacks, without any major disorder of mood and of thinking, is usually classified as an *anxiety neurosis;* the prolonged state of anxiety is called *neurocirculatory asthenia*. These two conditions will be discussed in greater detail in Chap. 213.

PHYSIOLOGIC AND PSYCHOLOGIC BASIS

The cause, mechanism, and biologic meaning of anxiety have been the subjects of much speculation. The psychologist has come to regard anxiety as anticipatory behavior, i.e., a state of uneasiness concerning something which may or will happen in the future. It is believed to be based on an inherited instinctual pattern (fear); and the occurrence of this emotional state in situations that would not be expected to provoke it could be an example of a conditioned or learned response.

The only well-systematized psychologic theory is that put forth by psychoanalysts, who look upon anxiety as a response to a situation which in some manner threatens the security of the individual. Anxiety is a response to danger, the topical content of which lies in the unconscious mind. It is pointed out that the somatic symptoms of anxiety are similar to those of fear. The postulated danger is internal rather than external; a primitive drive that is not compatible with current social practices has been aroused and can be satisfied only at risk to the individual.

Most psychiatrists accept this theory and believe that psychotherapeutic interviews will disclose the anxiety-provoking stimulus of which the patient is himself unaware. Once insight is gained into the psychodynamic mechanism, the anxiety symptoms are said to subside.

A search for evidences of visceral disease in patients with anxiety has thus far been unrewarding. A reduced capacity for physical work and strong effort has suggested the possibility of a defect in aerobic metabolism, as evidenced by increased oxygen consumption and an excessive rise in blood acetate. Moreover, such patients seem unable to tolerate the physiologic and biochemical effects of work as well as does the average person. Whether these differences are of primary significance or are due merely to lack of training and poor physical condition has not been settled.

A number of endocrinologic studies have been done and have yielded interesting data. The urinary excretion of epinephrine has been found elevated in some individuals; in others, an increase in the urinary excretion of norepinephrine has been noted; in still a third group normal values for both epinephrine and norepinephrine were obtained. Elmadjian and his associates have observed that aldosterone excretion in patients with anxiety neurosis is two to three times that of normal control subjects. This work has been in part corroborated by Venning who demonstrated an increase in aldosterone excretion in medical students experiencing fear and anxiety while preparing for examinations. The interpretation of these observations is not certain.

CLINICAL SIGNIFICANCE OF ANXIETY

Clinical diagnosis of the anxiety state depends upon recognition of (1) the implicit or subjective disturbance, i.e., the uneasiness and apprehension, and (2) the more objective vasomotor or visceral changes. The presence of diffuse or more or less circumscribed attacks of autonomic or thyroid and adrenal excitation, without psychic counterpart, does not establish the diagnosis of anxiety. Similar autonomic and endocrine discharges may occur with thyrotoxicosis, pheochromocytoma, corticosteroid therapy (usually in large doses), hypoglycemia, and menopause. Penfield has described them as a manifestation of tumors of the third ventricle (diencephalic autonomic epilepsy), and they have occasionally occurred as a prelude (aura) to a frank convulsive state. When the psychic components of anxiety are fully described by a patient who admits to having the visceral manifestations, one must consider as diagnostic possibilities anxiety neurosis, depression, hysteria, psychasthenia, schizophrenia, or a drug or endocrine psychosis. The differential diagnosis of the anxiety state will be discussed more fully in Chap. 213. The history and physical examination, if analyzed carefully, usually permit distinction between pure derangements of autonomic nervous and endocrine systems and true anxiety. One of the commonest sources of error is to mistake an anxious depression for an anxiety neurosis.

DEPRESSION

There are few individuals who do not experience periods of discouragement and despair, and these become manifestly more frequent as modern society increases in complexity, demanding ever greater inhibition of one's impulses and greater conformity to a group. As with anxiety, depression of mood that is appropriate to a given situation in life seldom becomes the basis of medical complaint. The patient seeks help only when he cannot overcome or control his grief or unhappiness or does not fully recognize its cause. Thus, depression, like anxiety, may be either a normal reaction or a pathologic state, and the distinction may require searching analysis of the medical data by a discerning physician.

Information about depressions, like knowledge of all psychiatric syndromes, is gained from three sources: the history obtained from the patient; the history obtained from the family or a friend in close contact with the patient; and the findings on examination.

The majority of patients who suffer from depression "give a history" of "not feeling well," of being "low in spirits," "blue," "glum," "unhappy," or "morbid." They are vaguely aware that their emotional reactions have changed; activities that were formerly pleasant are no longer so. But it often happens that these patients do not perceive their unhappiness and instead complain of being nervous, worried, fatigued, or unable to think with accustomed efficiency. Pain of obscure origin may be the predominant topic of their conversation, or any other symptom common in adult life, e.g., tinnitus, dry mouth, burning tongue, arthritis, constipation, pruritus. Multiplicity and persistence of complaint has led to many of these persons being classed as hypochondriacs; and, indeed, the most typical examples of excessive preoccupation with symptoms in middle-aged and elderly persons are depressed individuals. Since these associated symptoms are so conspicuous a feature of depression, they will be presented in further detail.

LASSITUDE, FATIGUE, LACK OF ENERGY. A decrease in energy output is a common symptom. The patient complains of being continuously without energy and of tiring out of proportion to the amount of work done. The appetite is usually poor; the patient derives no real enjoyment from eating and may comment, "I only eat to live," "I only eat because I have to." Weight loss is common and probably due to decreased food intake; and the majority of severely depressed patients are constipated.

LOSS OF INTEREST AND INCAPACITY FOR ENJOYMENT. These are noted by both the patient and his family. Where formerly the patient found pleasure in his work and was quite capable of doing it well, even the simplest tasks now demand great effort. He feels that he lacks his former efficiency in his work and often ascribes this to forgetfulness. However, when one questions his employer, one learns that there has been no impairment of memory or judgment but only a lack of the usual interest in and enthusiasm for work. Also, when the patient's memory is systematically tested, the deficit in memory of which he complains appears as a difficulty in concentration rather than a true memory deficit. This lack of interest and enthusiasm extends also to other activities. Absorbing recreational pursuits now give no pleasure. Cherished friendships are abandoned simply because it is too much of an effort to see people. Waning of libidinal interests or complete loss of libido is common. Irritability is also frequent, and patients who formerly were quite placid and imperturbable find themselves easily irritated by trivial happenings. The noises of children playing about the house are intolerable. However, if the patient is overcritical or harsh with them, he feels guilty and reproaches himself.

WORRY AND DIFFUSE CONCERN. These symptoms are prominent in most cases of depression. Patients find themselves worrying about things that have not happened or feeling apprehensive and fearful about the outcome of some ordinary activity. Incidents that occurred years before may be the objects of concern. For example, the patient may become very much upset and unhappy and may cry about the death of a relative that occurred many years before. He is assailed by pessimistic thoughts and by feelings of inadequacy and unworthiness and is often preoccupied with the possibility of suicide.

INSOMNIA. Almost always present, insomnia manifests itself in several ways. The patient may find it difficult to fall asleep; or he may fall asleep quickly but soon awaken and be unable to return to sleep. Some patients state that they do not awaken during the night but their sleep is restless and unsatisfactory. Usually when unable to sleep, they cannot remain quietly in bed. Plagued by pessimistic thoughts, they arise, walk about the house, smoke a cigarette, get something to eat, and resort to various measures to induce sleep. Bad dreams or nightmares are common. Occasionally there is excessive sleep, and the patient finds relief from his worries in slumber.

A closely related complaint is that of not feeling rested upon awakening in the morning. Patients frequently state, "I feel more tired upon awakening than I did before I went to sleep." A diurnal variation in mood swing is characteristic. In most patients all symptoms are worse in the morning and improve as the day progresses. Occasionally the reverse is true, and the symptoms are worst in the afternoon or evening.

ANXIETY. A large proportion of depressed patients experience anxiety. There may be anxiety attacks in which the patient becomes tense and apprehensive, perspires freely, and experiences palpitation and labored respiration. These symptoms may occur in discrete attacks or may continue in milder form over a long period of time. There may be crying spells in association with attacks of tenseness and palpitation for reasons not apparent to the patient or to an observer.

NERVOUSNESS. This is another common symptom. Very often depressed patients and psychoneurotic patients state that nervousness is their chief complaint. They may mean by this term a vague, ineffable psychologic state or a feeling of uneasy expectancy or impending doom, the precise nature of which is uncertain. Again, nervousness may mean tenseness, inner tremulousness, or a diffuse uneasiness. Depressed patients also use "nervousness" to mean a feeling of sadness, with outbreaks of spontaneous weeping.

PAIN. Though it is not generally appreciated, pain may occasionally be one of the earliest, if not the first, manifestations of depression, occurring before other obvious depressive symptoms appear. The pain is often described as "tearing," "pulling," "twisting," "burning," "clamping" and may be localized or migratory. In one patient it appeared first in the right external auditory canal and then successively in the right chest and shoulder, the left pudendal region, and both lower extremities, starting in the left instep and radiating upward to the left groin, then in the right instep radiating to the right groin. The pain is usually constant from the time of onset. There may, however, be fluctuations in severity, with exacerbations which the patient associates with fatigue and emotional disturbances.

The family, in relating the story of the illness, usually can do more than just verify many of the patient's symptoms. They can give a clearer idea of the degree of worry, the extent of disability, the depth of the alteration of emotional reaction, and the distressing effect of the patient's disturbed behavior on others. Moreover, they are often helpful in documenting the time of onset of the illness, the natural fluctuations, and the response to therapy.

SIGNS OF DEPRESSION. Before considering the objective signs on examination, it should be pointed out that the chief abnormalities occur in three domains of psychic function: emotion, ideation, and psychomotor activity. Abnormalities in these three spheres are designated by some psychiatrists as the cardinal signs or "unit symptoms" of the disorder.

The *facial expression* is often plaintive, troubled, pained, or anguished. The patient's attitude and manner betray the prevailing mood of depression, discouragement, and despondency. In other words, the affective response, which is the outward expression of feeling, is consistent with the depressed mood. The patient's eyes during the course of the interview may become tearful, or he may cry openly. At times the immobility of the face will mimic the facies of parkinsonism.

The stream of speech, from which the ideational content is determined, is slow. At times the patient is mute and speaks neither spontaneously nor in response to questions. Again, he may speak very slowly with a long period between his spontaneous utterances, or there may be a long delay between the questions posed by the examiner and the answers given by the patient. The retardation is present regardless of the topic of conversation and is not restricted to certain subjects as it is in the case of emotional blocking (selective retardation) seen in other psychiatric illnesses. At times the flow of speech is accelerated rather than retarded, but still the topical content tends to be restricted to a few subjects such as the patient's symptoms and his personal problems.

The motor activity may be decreased in varying degrees, from slow and deliberate movement even to the point of stupor. Frequently the patient will sit for hours in one place without moving; the slightest movement appears to require great effort. Again, motor activity may be increased to the point of restlessness and agitation, the patient pacing the floor, wringing his hands, and loudly bemoaning his fate.

The *content of speech* varies and is largely conditioned by the past experiences of the patient. Conversation is replete with pessimistic thoughts and fears of cancer or other serious diseases. Expressions of self-depreciation, self-accusation, feelings of unworthiness, inferiority, guilt, a belief that life is not worthwhile, and suicidal preoccupation are frequent. Although systematized ideas of persecution are not common in depression, the patient often believes he is not liked by his relatives or friends. The patient's reaction to these ideas is usually one of agreement, since he himself feels unworthy and sees no reason for people wanting him around or enjoying his company. In severe depressions some of the ideas expressed by the patient are bizarre and assume the form of somatic and nihilistic delusions. Various parts of the body are said to be "rotting"; there have been "no normal bowel movements for weeks or months"; "all my blood is dried up," "I am dead," etc. In severe depressions auditory, visual, tactile, or olfactory hallucinations occur, and as a rule their salient features are consistent with the depressed mood.

Personal and abstract judgment is often pessimistically tinged by the depressed mood. The patient evaluates his illness as a hopeless one and his business as destined for certain failure. His outlook toward the future is pessimistic and hopeless. Insight may be entirely lacking. The patient may feel that he is suffering from malignancy or some incurable disease despite repeated reassurance to the contrary. However, some patients do realize that they are depressed and that their feelings are for the most part dictated by this depression.

ETIOLOGY AND MECHANISM. Psychiatrists are not in complete agreement concerning the cause of the depressive syndrome. There are two schools of thought, one of which contends that the depressive reaction has its genesis in hereditary factors; the other, based largely on psychoanalytic theory, considers it to be a psychogenic disturbance brought about by the inability of a rigid personality to adjust its instinctual drives to the demands of the environment. The latter theory, while interesting, has not been substantiated and has not resulted in the development of effective psychotherapeutic measures. Rauwolfia compounds and other agents used to treat nervousness and anxiety may induce a depressive mood, a fact of considerable theoretical importance.

CLINICAL SIGNIFICANCE. All these symptoms and signs comprise a clinical syndrome of importance because of its frequency and gravity. Errors in diagnosis in our best hospitals are frequent and at times serious. Large numbers of such patients tend to accumulate in the various medical clinics, taking up the time of the medical staff which attempts to give them symptomatic therapy. Here the serious consequences of misdiagnosis lie mainly in the fact that the patient does not receive the appropriate treatment for his depression (see p. 1281). When anxiety symptoms are prominent, an incorrect diagnosis of anxiety neurosis may be made. This mistake, or the false attribution of depression to some environmental circumstance, may obscure the fact that the illness is in reality an endogenous psychosis, and the patient may unexpectedly commit suicide even while receiving psychotherapy.

Depression may occur intermittently in conjunction with all the psychoneuroses, and persistently in manic-depressive psychosis, and in association with medical and neurologic diseases. Chronic infection, endocrine disorders (hyperparathyroidism, hypothyroidism, or Addison's disease), or neoplasia may at times produce chronic fatigue that is difficult to distinguish from depression.

Thus, if a patient presents any one of the above symptoms, it is incumbent on the physician to take a complete history and to examine the mental status in some detail in an effort to determine the existence of a depressive state. Once it is established, since it is but one cardial manifestation of several psychiatric illnesses, the physician must then undertake a differential diagnosis along the lines suggested in Chap. 204.

43   LASSITUDE AND ASTHENIA
Raymond D. Adams

The term *weakness* is used by patients to describe a variety of subjective complaints which vary in their import and prognostic significance. Most subjective disorders embraced by this term will be found, on careful questioning, to fall within the following classification:

I. Lassitude, fatigue, lack of energy, listlessness, and languor. These terms, while not synonymous, shade into each other; all refer to weariness and a loss of that sense of well-being typically found in persons who are healthy in body and mind. Symptoms of this type are present in a large majority of all patients and have little diagnostic specificity. For the sake of brevity this group of complaints will be considered together under Lassitude and Fatigue.
II. Weakness, loss of muscular strength, and asthenia. These may be either persistent or episodic.
   A. Persistent weakness: This may be (1) restricted to certain muscles or groups of muscles (paresis, palsy, paralysis) or (2) general, involving the entire musculature, in which instance the term *asthenia* or *myasthenia* is used. Paralysis is discussed on pp. 199–200. The generalized type of weakness will be considered below under Asthenia. It is far less common than lassitude and more likely to indicate serious disease.
   B. Recurrent weakness: Many patients complain of "attacks of weakness," and careful questioning reveals that a diminished sense of alertness, a feeling of lightheadedness, or a sensation of faintness is the actual symptom. These complaints are subjectively different from lassitude and asthenia, and the causes are likewise different; such recurrent attacks of weakness are discussed in Chap. 44.

It should be restated that the unqualified term weakness is so vague as to be almost useless and that a sound clinical approach to this problem entails, as the initial step, an analysis of what the patient himself means when he uses this and similar terms.

LASSITUDE AND FATIGUE (Lack of Energy, Languor, Listlessness, Weariness, and Neurasthenia)

Of all symptoms these are among the most frequent and at the same time the most abstruse. More than half of all patients make direct complaint of this group of symptoms or admit their presence when questioned. During the Second World War they figured so prominently in military medicine that the term *combat fatigue* was applied to all acute psychiatric illnesses on the battlefield. Therefore, it behooves every student of medicine to learn as much as possible about these symptoms and their physiologic and psychologic antecedents.

Lassitude or fatigue most commonly refers to a feeling of weariness or tiredness. Patients who complain of this symptom have a more or less characteristic way of describing it. They speak of being "all in," "without pep," having "no ambition," "no interest," or "being fed up." They are inclined to lie down. On close analysis there is a difficulty in initiating activity, and also in sustaining it.

This condition is the familiar aftermath of prolonged labor or great physical exertion, and under such circumstances it is accepted as a physiologic reaction. When, however, the same symptoms or similar ones appear in no relation to such antecedents, they are recognized as being unnatural, and the patient rightly suspects some recently acquired disease.

The physician's first task then is to determine whether his patient is merely suffering from the physical and mental effects of overwork without realizing it. Overworked and overwrought people are everywhere observable in our society. Their actions are both instructive and pathetic. They seem to be impelled by notions of duty and refuse to think of themselves. Or, as is often the case, some personal inadequacy prevents them from deriving pleasure from any activity except their work, in which they indulge as a defense mechanism. Such individuals often experience a variety of symptoms such as weariness, irritability, nervousness, and sleeplessness. The behavior of these individuals and their varied symptomatology are best understood by referring to psychologic studies of the effect of fatigue on normal individuals.

THE EFFECT OF FATIGUE ON THE NORMAL PERSON

According to the most authoritative sources, fatigue has several effects, some explicit, others implicit. These are (1) a series of physiologic changes in many organs of the body, (2) an overt disorder of behavior in form of reduced output of work, known as *work decrement,* and (3) an expression of dissatisfaction and a subjective feeling of tiredness or weariness in association with a variety of psychologic changes.

Fatigue indicates the presence of changes in the physiologic balance of the body. Continuous muscular work results in depletion of muscle glycogen and accumulation of lactic acid and probably other metabolites which reduce the contractility and the recovery of active muscle. It is said that the injection of blood of a fatigued animal into a rested one will produce the overt manifestations of fatigue in the latter. During fatigue states muscle action is tremulous, and movements become clumsy and cannot be

sustained for long without increasing effort. The rate of breathing increases; the pulse quickens; the blood pressure rises and the pulse pressure widens; and the white blood count and the metabolic rate are increased. These reactions bear out the hypothesis that fatigue is in part a manifestation of altered metabolism.

The decreased capacity for work or productivity which is the direct consequence of fatigue has been investigated by industrial psychologists. Their findings show clearly the importance of the motivational factor on work output, whether it be in the operation of an ergograph or the performance of heavy manual labor. Also it appears that there are individual differences in the energy potential of human beings, just as there are differences in physique and temperament. Some people are strong and vigorous from birth, whereas others are weak and lacking in energy.

The subjective feelings of fatigue have been carefully recorded. Aside from weariness the tired person complains of nervousness, restlessness, inability to deal effectively with complex problems, and a tendency to be upset by trivialities. The number and quality of his associations in tests of mental functions are reduced. Behavior tends to be less rational than normal, and the capacity to deliberate and to reach judgments is impaired. The worker physically exhausted after a long, hard day is unable to perform adequately his duties as head of a household, and the example of the tired businessman who becomes the proverbial tyrant of the family circle is well known. A disinclination to try and the appearance of ideas of inferiority are other characteristics of the fatigued mind.

Instances of fatigue and lassitude resulting from overwork are not difficult to recognize. A description of the patient's daily routine will usually suffice; and if he can be persuaded to live at a more reasonable pace, his symptoms promptly subside. Errors in diagnosis are usually in the direction of ascribing fatigue to overwork, chronic infection, or anemia when it actually reflects a psychoneurosis or depression.

FATIGUE AS A MANIFESTATION OF PSYCHIATRIC DISORDER. The great majority of patients who enter a hospital because of unexplained chronic fatigue and lassitude have been found to have some type of psychiatric illness. In former times the term *neurasthenia* was applied to this group of patients, but since fatigue rarely exists as an isolated phenomenon, the current practice is to label such cases according to the total clinical picture. The usual associated symptoms are nervousness, anxiety, irritability, depression, insomnia, palpitation, headaches, breathlessness, inability to concentrate, sexual disorders, and disturbances of appetite. In one series of cases of severe fatigue in a general hospital, 75 per cent were diagnosed as anxiety neurosis or tension state. Depression and "psychosomatic disease" accounted for another 10 per cent, and the remainder had miscellaneous illnesses with hysterical, obsessive, or phobic symptoms.

Several features are common to the psychiatric group. The fatigue is frequently worse in the morning. The patient often desires to lie down but finds himself unable to sleep when he does. The feeling of fatigue relates more to some activities than to others; at times certain affairs are prosecuted with great vigor; while even the thought of other activities completely exhausts the patient. A careful inquiry into the circumstances under which the fatigue first occurred or recurs often reveals a specific relationship to certain events. Instances of an acute episode of fatigue coming on during an unpleasant emotional experience, in connection with a grief reaction, or after a surgical operation have been noted. And, finally, the feeling of tiredness extends to mental as well as physical activities. The individual's capacity for sustained mental effort, as in solving problems or carrying on a difficult conversation, is impaired.

Depressing emotion, whether grief from bereavement or a phase of manic-depressive or involutional psychosis, has its characteristic effect on the impulse life and energy of the individual. The initiation of activity is difficult, and the capacity for work is reduced. Lassitude and fatigue are a more prominent feature in many mild depressive illnesses than is the depression of mood. Patients typically complain that everything they do, whether mental or physical, requires great effort, and all their accustomed activities no longer give the usual satisfaction and enjoyment. Sleep is poor, with a tendency to early morning waking. Such individuals are at their worst, both in spirit and in energy output, in the morning and tend to improve as the day wears on. It is difficult to decide whether their fatigue is a primary effect of disease or is secondary to lack of interest.

Many physicians may question whether all patients with chronic fatigue as seen in everday practice deviate far enough from normal to justify a diagnosis of psychoneurosis or depressive psychosis. Some people because of circumstances beyond their control have no purpose in life and much idle time. They become bored with the monotony of their daily routine. Such conditions are conducive to fatigue, just as optimism or enthusiasm for a new enterprise dispels fatigue. There are other patients who, as far as one can tell, were reasonably healthy and well-adjusted until they met some adversity which aroused fear and worry. They then develop a state which may be classified as simple nervousness or reactive anxiety with the usual lassitude and fatigue, sleeplessness, and difficulty in concentration. Reactions such as these are understandable to everyone who has had "stage fright" or "buck fever." The sense of physical weakness, the utter incapacity to act, the sudden transformation of a normally well-ordered mind into intellectual chaos, and the exhaustion which follows the episode are indelible experiences in the minds of most of us.

PSYCHOLOGIC THEORIES. The significance of lassitude and fatigue in these different life situations and psychiatric illnesses has been the subject of much speculation. Physiologists have remarked on the enervating effect of strong emotion and have argued that a simple prolongation of the emotional experience would provide a rational explanation for all the symptoms of chronic anxiety. This, however, only takes the explanation one step further back and does not account for the patient's being emotionally aroused at a time when there is no overt stimulus to emotion.

The dynamic schools of psychiatry, particularly the psychoanalytic, have postulated that chronic fatigue, like the anxiety from which it derives, is a danger signal that something is wrong; some activity or attitude has been persisted in too intensely or too long. The purpose of fatigue may be regarded as self-preservation, not merely as a protection against physical injury but also to preserve the individual's self-esteem, his concept of himself. Another hypothesis is that the fatigue is the result of the exhaustion of one's store of energy by the demands of repression. The characteristic situation in which the fatigued patient finds himself is said to be one in which effective behavior is of a type forbidden by the patient's own idea of what is permissible to him as a member of society. Fatigue then is not a negative quality, a lack of energy, but an unconscious desire for inactivity. A reciprocal relationship is believed to exist between fatigue and anxiety. Both are believed to be protective devices, but anxiety is the more imperative. It calls the individual to take some positive action to extricate himself from a predicament, whereas fatigue calls for inactivity. Both fatigue and anxiety operate blindly. The individual does not perceive what it is that must be done or stopped. All this happens at an unconscious level.

Other psychiatrists are not satisfied with the psychoanalytic hypothesis, especially for cases of lifelong weakness and fatigability. They point out that individuals differ basically in energy potential. Certain persons, it is believed, seem endowed with a limited store of energy. The physiologic or psychologic basis for this deficiency is unknown. Eugene Kahn regards it as a constitutional inadequacy and states that at present it cannot be decided whether this is inborn or acquired. Under the heading "Psychopath Weak in Impulse," he describes the individual who has an evident physical inferiority. He is a weakling; his vitality is low. He is unusually susceptible to disease and requires longer to convalesce than the average. Such a person may spend half his life recuperating from illnesses that would not bother a normal person. Vigorous games tire him, and his performance is usually so poor that he takes no interest in sports. Unless born in favorable economic circumstances he earns a meager livelihood. He seeks and accepts subordinate positions and usually cannot establish an independent social position of his own. He gives the impression of weakness of will, dullness, or nervousness, though many such individuals possess an average or superior intellectual endowment. His success is limited by his lack of drive and industry. Sexual impulse is also weak and he may find marriage impossible. He requires medical attention throughout life and whenever subjected to any unusual stress is apt to break down and complain of nervousness, lassitude, insomnia, and many other vague symptoms. The physical inferiority and lack of sexual impulse bring to mind that dwarfs of endocrine origin often show this same deficiency in impulse life. This weakness in impulse is found in the chronic invalid seen in everyday practice.

It is perfectly obvious that these various psychologic theories are not mutually exclusive. Undoubtedly there are certain individuals whose impulse to activity is weak throughout life, and this deficiency probably is largely, if not exclusively, determined by genetic factors. It is equally clear that boredom, lack of interest, depression of mood, and strong emotion, regardless of the conditions under which they arise, are usually accompanied by fatigue and lassitude. The more chronic varieties of fatigue are probably in most instances related to psychiatric illnesses, and here the proposition that fatigue, like anxiety, is part of a psychologic defense mechanism seems most applicable.

LASSITUDE AND FATIGUE IN CHRONIC INFECTION AND ENDOCRINE DISEASES.

Chronic infection is another cause of chronic fatigue, though a much less frequent one. Everyone has at some time or other sensed the abrupt onset of a tired ache in all the muscles of the body as an acute infection develops, or the listlessness that accompanies an afternoon fever. In chronic infections the patient has lassitude, fatigue, mental depression, and vague aches and pains. Also, there is often a period of easy fatigability, irritability, and inability to work effectively after a protracted febrile illness. Some diseases, e.g., influenza and hepatitis, are more likely to be followed by these convalescent symptoms than others. If symptoms of this type are prolonged, it is often difficult if not impossible to decide whether they are due to the disease in question or to the presence of chronic anxiety or depression. In many chronic diseases such as infectious hepatitis and brucellosis, neurotic symptoms are often added to those of the original disease.

Metabolic and *endocrine disturbances* (see pp. 401 and 1301) of various types may produce lassitude or fatigue. The symptom is likely to be extremely marked and to be associated with true muscular weakness. In Addison's disease and Simmonds's disease it dominates the clinical picture. In persons with hypothyroidism with or without frank myxedema, lassitude is usually pronounced. It is also present in many patients with hyperthyroidism, although often less troublesome than the associated nervousness. Uncontrolled diabetes may be accompanied by excessive fatigability. Hyperparathyroidism, Cushing's disease, and hypogonadism are other instances of endocrine diseases in which lassitude may be prominent. Any type of nutritional deficiency may, when severe,

cause lassitude, and in the early stages of the disease this may be the only complaint. Weight loss and the dietary history may be the only objective clues as to the nature of the illness.

DIFFERENTIAL DIAGNOSIS. Since a large variety of physical and emotional disorders may be accompanied by lassitude, the following discussion is limited to causes likely to be obscure.

When chronic fatigue and lassitude are the presenting symptoms, the commonest cause is a psychoneurosis or depressive psychosis. The basis of diagnosis is the nature of the symptom and its pervasive effect on both mental and physical function, the associated psychiatric symptoms, usually of anxiety or depression, and the absence of signs of somatic disease. However, since psychic and somatic disorders frequently coexist, it is wise to search for organic disease before concluding that the illness is entirely psychogenic. The clinical examination should be thorough and prompt; unnecessary prolongation of the procedure may aggravate an anxiety state, if present. A careful inquiry should be made for situational factors in the patient's life which could possibly be related to the psychiatric symptoms. If found, measures should be taken to assist the patient to understand how these factors are affecting him. If reassurance that no somatic disease is present and discussion of the patient's problems do not afford relief, a psychiatric consultation is desirable. If the diagnosis is obscure, psychiatric appraisal should be part of the initial examination. Common errors are to mistake a depressive illness in which the leading symptom is chronic fatigue for a psychoneurosis; to fail to recognize the basic energy lack in an "asthenic psychopath" and to attempt to treat him as an individual with a chronic somatic disease or a recently acquired neurotic illness; and to misjudge the relative importance of psychic and somatic factors in a chronic medical disease.

Obscure infections and surgical operations may cause symptoms which closely resemble those of psychoneurosis. Indeed, individuals who have suffered from all three conditions report that the "nuclear" emotional state is similar. As a rule, aches and pains, weight loss, and low-grade fever are more prominent in chronic infection, and anxiety is in the foreground of the neurotic illness. In the United States tuberculosis, subacute bacterial endocarditis, chronic brucellosis, chronic pyelonephritis, subacute infectious hepatitis, or certain parasitic infections such as malaria and hookworm should be considered as a cause of an illness of this type. The status of chronic brucellosis has been especially difficult to evaluate. Unfortunately there is no reliable method (other than blood culture, which is rarely positive in chronic cases) of diagnosing this condition.

Anemia (Chap. 38), when moderate to severe, and regardless of the cause, is likewise frequently responsible for lassitude. The severity of the symptom is more likely to parallel the hemoglobin level of the blood than the number of erythrocytes. It is the author's impression that mild grades of anemia are usually asymptomatic and that lassitude is ascribed to anemia much too often. *Nutritional deficiency* in many parts of the world is a source of lassitude and fatigability; it is often combined with anemia.

The diagnosis of the fatigue and lassitude which accompany endocrine diseases may be difficult. These conditions are relatively rare in comparison to the psychiatric diseases which cause chronic fatigue. One of the most helpful points to keep in mind is that many of these patients are actually experiencing some degree of asthenia as well as fatigue. Details as to the most reliable methods of diagnosis of these rare diseases will be found in later chapters of the book.

Almost any type of chronic *exogenous* or *endogenous intoxication* is likely to be associated with lassitude, which, however, is only rarely the chief complaint. Among the commoner examples are alcoholism, bromism, prolonged ingestion of barbiturates, morphine addiction, and uremia. In these the clue to diagnosis is usually provided by the more troublesome complaints. In persons with acute infections, in patients with malignant tumors, and in many individuals with almost any type of serious disease, the other symptoms are in the foreground and are much more likely to have diagnostic significance than the associated lassitude.

Lassitude of sudden onset is likely to be due to (1) an acute infection, (2) a disturbance of fluid balance, especially one producing extracellular fluid deficit, or (3) rapidly developing circulatory failure of either peripheral or cardiac origin. In these various disorders, discussed in detail in later chapters, the subjective manifestation—lassitude—is likely to be accompanied by outspoken objective phenomena, i.e., fever, tachycardia, etc.

GENERALIZED MUSCULAR WEAKNESS, DEBILITY, ASTHENIA

This symptom is relatively uncommon, as compared with the great frequency of lassitude. True asthenia is probably never due to psychogenic disorders alone and is not likely to result from anemia or from the chronic infections, except in their advanced stages. It is observed in the terminal phases of most wasting diseases and throughout the course of severe acute fevers. Its commonest causes are senility and prolonged confinement to bed, regardless of the underlying disease process. When asthenia is the presenting symptom in a patient who is not senile and has not been at bed rest, one should think of the severe forms of the common anemias, of nutritional deficiencies, of the diffuse disorders of the motor system, and of the diseases of the pituitary, adrenal, thyroid, and parathyroid glands, such as Addison's disease and Simmonds's disease, which may give rise to both fatigability and asthenia.

The distinction between lassitude and asthenia is not a sharp one; the former symptom shades into the latter. All patients with asthenia also have lassitude, but most patients with lassitude do not have genuine asthenia. Before concluding that a person has true loss of strength rather than the more common and less serious loss of energy, one either should be able to demonstrate the muscular weakness objectively, or should obtain a story from the patient that he is no longer able to perform specific muscular acts which previously could be done readily.

One not extremely rare cause of asthenia merits special attention—namely, myasthenia gravis. In this remarkable disorder the patient may have nearly normal muscular strength following prolonged rest, but quickly develops weakness of the affected muscles following repeated contraction. The muscles supplied by the cranial nerves, ocular movement, swallowing, and speech are especially involved (see pp. 1322–1325).

When more than one member of the family is subject to recurrent attacks of weakness proceeding to the point of actual paralysis, but without loss of consciousness, and when such attacks are separated by intervals of good health, one should be suspicious of a rare disorder—familial periodic paralysis (see pp. 1325–1326). Recurrent and persistent weakness and aching of muscles after exercise should suggest McArdle's disease (see pp. 1316 and 1321). Persistent weakness is a common feature of polymyositis and cortisone myopathy (see p. 1315).

There are probably several mechanisms of asthenia, but only a few are known. In myasthenia gravis it has been said that a toxic substance with an action very similar to that of curare interferes with the neuromuscular transmission of nerve impulses. It can be inhibited by cholinergic drugs such as neostigmine, which are of great therapeutic value. (See p. 1323 for other theories.) Familial periodic paralysis is believed to be intimately linked to potassium metabolism; and low serum potassium levels, found in some but not all cases at the time of the paralysis, interfere with the contractility of muscle fibers. McArdle's syndrome was recently shown to be due to a deficiency of the enzyme phosphorylase, normally present in the striated muscle fibers. Thyrotoxic myopathy is associated with a reduced creatine tolerance and an impairment of muscle metabolism. Probably the asthenia of senility, cachexia, and other metabolic diseases will ultimately be traced to metabolic changes in muscle.

DIFFERENTIAL DIAGNOSIS. Procedure in a Patient with Obscure Persistent Weakness as the Presenting Symptom.

The decision as to whether an obscure but active chronic infection exists is made largely on the basis of measurements of *temperature* (preferably taken at 2-hr intervals and under conditions of activity if the resting temperatures are normal), *leukocyte count*, and *sedimentation rate*. If any of these are persistently elevated, there is strong likelihood that the patient has either an infection or some other process such as neoplasm, thrombosis with infarction, or arteritis, which is causing tissue injury. These tests are not infallible, for individuals otherwise healthy may have a slight elevation of temperature or an elevated sedimentation rate. (The procedures utilized in differentiating these various conditions are discussed in Chap. 266.) The presence of persistently normal values for these functions makes it unlikely that a bacterial infection exists at a sufficiently active level to cause weakness, but it does not exclude parasitic and other infections that may produce weakness by causing anemia or by interfering with nutrition.

The presence of a persistent tachycardia (greater than can be accounted for by the level of the temperature) suggests thyrotoxicosis, subacute rheumatic fever, or a psychogenic disorder. In the last condition, unlike the other two, the *sleeping pulse rate* is likely to be normal, and the hands, though moist, are usually cold.

The decision whether anemia, from whatever cause, is of sufficient severity to cause weakness can be made readily by measurement of the hematocrit. Measurements of the number of red blood corpuscles and the quantity of hemoglobin are often inaccurate, so that whenever these values are low they must be checked in order to determine their accuracy. There is no absolute level of anemia at which weakness may be expected. Its rate of development is important; acute blood loss has a much greater effect than a chronic one. Minor degrees of anemia are usually not the correct explanation of weakness. Once anemia of significant degree has been demonstrated, the problem becomes one of determining its nature and cause (Chap. 38).

In deciding whether advanced nutritional deficiency is responsible for weakness, one can depend upon objective methods; but *in the earlier states of deficiency diseases reliance has to be placed on the dietary history,* supplemented, in certain instances, by vitamin saturation tests, etc. (see Chap. 66).

Concerning the possible causative role of the commoner endocrine and metabolic factors, a few simple clinical observations and laboratory tests will usually suffice. The rarer types require more elaborate tests for diagnosis. These are discussed in the chapters on endocrinology.

The history as regards habits (alcohol), *occupation* (lead, etc.), and *drugs* offers the main clue for the diagnosis of exogenous intoxication as the cause of weakness.

The social history as regards the patient's adjustment to his family and friends, his happiness, and the existence of personal problems in relation to his home and work is helpful in deciding whether lassitude and possible weakness are of emotional origin.

The considerations mentioned will lead to an accurate evaluation of the cause of weakness in many patients. Even so, there will remain a group of subjects (unfortunately, not rare) in whom the most exhaustive investigation fails to uncover the cause. In some such individuals time will furnish the answer, but in others recovery will eventually occur without the cause being known.

44 FAINTNESS, SYNCOPE, AND EPISODIC WEAKNESS

Raymond D. Adams and T. R. Harrison

Episodic faintness, lightheadedness or giddiness, and reduced alertness are frequent and vexatious symptoms. The patient may refer to these symptoms as "weak spells" when he actually means loss of vigor, weakness of limbs, or impaired alertness. Any difference between faintness and syncope appears to be only quantitative. Since syncope, though less common, is more definite, it will be considered in greater detail. Those types of episodic weakness, such as myasthenia gravis and familial periodic paralysis, which are associated with striking reduction of muscular strength but not with impairment of consciousness, are discussed in other chapters. Epilepsy, which is also associated with episodic unconsciousness, differs from syncope in most other respects. It is discussed in Chap. 52.

CARDINAL FEATURES OF SYNCOPE

The term *syncope* literally means a "cutting short," "cessation," or "pause," and it is synonymous with swoon or faint. Syncope comprises a generalized weakness of muscles, with inability to stand upright and impairment of consciousness. Abrupt onset, brief duration, and complete recovery within a few minutes are other distinguishing features. Faintness, in contrast, refers to lack of strength, with a sensation of impending faint; it is an incomplete faint. Both faintness and syncope vary somewhat according to their mechanism, but both conform roughly to the following pattern.

The syncopal attack develops rapidly, but it is doubtful whether consciousness is ever terminated with the absolute suddenness of an epileptic seizure. At the beginning of the attack, the patient is nearly always in the upright position, either sitting or standing (the Stokes-Adams attack [cf. p. 773] is exceptional in this respect). Usually the warning of the impending faint is a sense of "feeling badly." The patient is assailed by giddiness, the floor seems to move, and surrounding objects begin to sway. His senses become confused, he yawns or gapes, there are spots before his eyes, or vision may dim, and his ears may ring. Nausea and sometimes actual vomiting accompany these symptoms. If the patient can lie down promptly, the attack may be averted without complete loss of consciousness. If he cannot, there is "loss of senses" and falling to the ground. What is most noticeable, even at the beginning of the attack, is a striking pallor or ashen-gray color of the face, and very often the face and body are bathed in cold perspiration. As a rule, the deliberate onset enables the patient to lie down or at least protect himself as he slumps. A hurtful fall is exceptional.

The depth and duration of the unconsciousness vary. Sometimes the patient is not completely oblivious of his surroundings. His senses are confused, but he may still be able to hear the voices or see the blurred outlines of people around him. Again, unconsciousness may be profound, and there may be complete lack of awareness and of capacity to respond. The patient may remain in this state for seconds to minutes or even as long as half an hour.

Shortly after the beginning of unconsciousness, convulsive movements occur in some instances. These usually consist of several clonic jerks of the arms and twitchings of the face. Rarely is there a generalized tonic-clonic convulsion. Usually the person who has fainted lies motionless, with skeletal muscles completely relaxed. Sphincter control is usually maintained. The pulse is feeble or cannot be felt; the blood pressure is low, and breathing is almost imperceptible. The reduction in vital functions, the striking pallor, and unconsciousness simulate death.

Once the patient is in a horizontal position, perhaps from having fallen, gravitation no longer hinders the flow of blood to the brain. The strength of the pulse improves, and color begins to return to the face. Breathing becomes quicker and deeper. Then the eyelids flutter, and consciousness is quickly regained. There is from this moment onward a correct perception of the environment. The patient is nevertheless keenly aware of physical weakness; and if he rises too soon, another faint may be precipitated. Headache and drowsiness, which, with mental confusion, are the usual sequelae of a convulsion, do not follow a syncopal attack.

CLASSIFICATION OF CAUSES OF RECURRENT WEAKNESS, FAINTNESS, AND DISTURBANCES OF CONSCIOUSNESS

The following list is based on established or assumed physiologic mechanisms. Some of the disorders frequently cause episodic weakness but rarely cause syncope. A few are especially apt to cause syncope associated with convulsions. These features are indicated in accompanying parentheses. Unless this specific notation is made, it may be assumed that the disorder in question is likely to cause faintness (when mild) and syncope (when severe).

I. Circulatory (deficient *quantity* of blood to the brain—common causes of either faintness or syncope)
  A. Peripheral
    1. Psychogenic (vasovagal) syncope
    2. Postural hypotension
    3. Increased intrathoracic pressure, e.g., tussive syncope
    4. Other causes of peripheral circulatory failure (Chap. 135)
  B. Cardiac (acute cardiac failure, see Chap. 143)
    1. Alterations in rate or rhythm
      a. Bradycardia
      b. Ectopic tachycardias (Chap. 140)
        (1) Myogenic (heart block, see Chap. 140, convulsions frequently occur and syncope common during recumbency)

        (2) Neurogenic (reflex bradycardia)
          (a) Hypersensitive carotid sinus
          (b) Rarer causes of reflex bradycardia
    2. Acute myocardial injury (especially infarction, see Chap. 148)
    3. Mechanical hindrance
      a. Aortic stenosis
      b. Disorders of pulmonary vessels, e.g., embolism
II. Other causes of weakness and episodic disturbances of consciousness
  A. Chemical (defective *quality* of blood to the brain)
    1. Hyperventilation (faintness common; syncope seldom occurs)
    2. Hypoglycemia (episodic weakness common, faintness occasional, syncope rare)
  B. Cerebral
    1. Epilepsy (akinetic, see Chap. 52, other convulsive disorders common)
    2. Cerebral vascular disturbances (cerebral ischemic attacks, see Chap. 204)
    3. Emotional disturbances, anxiety attacks, and hysterical seizures (see Chap. 214)

This list of conditions which cause weakness, faintness, and disturbances of consciousness is deceptively long and involved. Close study, however, reveals that the commoner types of faint are reducible to a few simple mechanisms. In order not to obscure the central problem of fainting by too many details, only a few of the commoner varieties likely to be encountered in clinical practice are discussed below.

COMMON TYPES OF SYNCOPE

VASOVAGAL, VASODEPRESSOR (PSYCHOGENIC) SYNCOPE. This is the ordinary faint, and the description already given applies most perfectly to this form of it. The loss of consciousness usually takes place when the systolic pressure falls to 70 mm Hg or below. The pulse is weak or imperceptible, and its rate may be either slowed or slightly increased. Sudden vasodilatation, particularly of intramuscular vessels, is responsible for the fainting. It has been thought to represent a response to an emotional or physical stimulus which would ordinarily call for immediate strenuous physical activity. In the absence of such activity, there is sudden pooling of blood in the muscles, with inadequate venous return, decline in cerebral blood flow, and loss of consciousness. These considerations explain the rarity of vasovagal syncope in the recumbent position or during active muscular exercise, which increases the venous return. However, this explanation is somewhat speculative, and there are surprisingly few studies of this type of syncope.

Vasovagal or vasodepressor faints occur (1) in normal health as a consequence of a strong emotional experience or in conditions that favor vasodilatation, e.g., hot crowded rooms, especially if the person is tired, hungry, or ill; (2) in anxiety states and neurocirculatory asthenia; (3) during pain; (4) after injury to tissues as a consequence of shock, pain, and psychologic factors.

POSTURAL HYPOTENSION WITH SYNCOPE. This type of syncope affects persons who have a chronic defect in, or a variable instability of, vasomotor reflexes. The character of the syncopal attack differs little from that of the vasovagal or vasodepressor type. The effect of posture is the cardinal feature of it. Sudden arising from a recumbent position or standing still is the condition under which it usually occurs.

Nature has provided man with several mechanisms by which his circulation adjusts to the upright posture. The pooling of blood in the lower parts of the body is prevented by (1) pressor reflexes which induce constriction of peripheral arteries and arterioles; (2) reflex acceleration of the heart by means of aortic and carotid reflexes; (3) improvement of venous return to the heart by activity of the muscles of the limbs and by increased rate of respiration. A normal individual placed on a tilt table to relax his muscles and tilted upright has a slightly diminished cardiac output, and blood accumulates in the legs to a slight degree. This is followed by a slight transitory fall in systolic blood pressure and then, within a few seconds, by a compensatory rise. Some normal individuals, if tilted on a table, will faint. In them it has been found that at first the blood pressure falls slightly and then stabilizes at a *lower* level. Shortly thereafter these compensatory reflexes suddenly fail, and the blood pressure falls precipitously. This also happens in some of the conditions listed below. In others, e.g., after surgical sympathectomy and in the unusual condition of chronic orthostatic hypotension, the blood pressure never stabilizes after tilting but falls steadily to a level at which cerebral circulation cannot be maintained.

Postural syncope tends to occur under the following conditions: (1) in otherwise normal individuals who for some unknown reason have defective postural reflexes (chronic orthostatic hypotension); (2) rarely, as part of a syndrome which comprises orthostatic hypertension and symptoms and signs of pyramidal and extrapyramidal nervous disorders; (3) after prolonged illness with recumbency, especially in elderly individuals with flabby muscles; (4) after a sympathectomy that abolishes vasopressor reflexes; (5) in diabetic neuropathy, tabes dorsalis, and other diseases of the nervous system which cause flabby, weak muscles and paralysis of vasopressor reflexes; (6) in persons with varicose veins because of pooling of blood in the abnormal venous channels; (7) in patients receiving antihypertensive and certain sedative drugs.

In *chronic orthostatic hypotension,* a special form of this type of syncope and a relatively rare condition, the hypotension differs from that already described in that the systolic and diastolic blood pressures fall rapidly as soon as the patient assumes an upright position but without compensatory tachycardia, pallor, sweating, nausea, or other symptoms. The loss of consciousness is usually abrupt and may be attended by confusion. Recumbency restores the circulation of the brain, with a prompt return to consciousness. The pooling of blood in the abdomen and legs does not excite vasoconstriction of peripheral vessels. This is apparently because of an abnormality in the autonomic nervous system. There is also evidence that patients with this type of postural hypotension are deficient in release of norepinephrine and epinephrine. Repeated attacks may result in mental confusion, slurred speech, and other neurologic signs.

SYNCOPE OF CARDIAC ORIGIN (CARDIAC SYNCOPE). The occurrence of fainting in patients with a permanently slow pulse was first described by Morgagni and subsequently by Adams and by Stokes. It is today known as the Stokes-Adams syndrome. The heart rate is usually less than 40, and the electrocardiogram shows a transient or permanent atrioventricular block. Rarely this may be present only during the attack. Usually without more than a momentary sense of weakness, the patient suddenly loses consciousness. This may occur at any time of the day or night regardless of the position of the body. When the patient is upright, the unconsciousness will develop after a briefer period of asystole than with the recumbent position. According to Engel, 4 to 8 sec of asystole produce coma in the erect position, and 12 to 15 sec are required in recumbency. If cardiac standstill is more than 12 sec, the patient turns pale, falls unconscious, and may exhibit a few clonic jerks. The blood pressure falls rapidly during the period of asystole. With the resumption of the heartbeat the face and neck become flushed. Longer periods of asystole, up to 5 min, result in coma, ashen-gray pallor giving way to cyanosis, stertorous breathing, fixed pupils, incontinence, and bilateral Babinski signs. Prolonged confusion and neurologic signs due to the relative ischemia of parts of the brain supplied by narrowed, arteriosclerotic arteries may persist in some patients, and permanent impairment of mental function is not unknown. Cardiac faints of this type may recur several times a day. Occasionally the heart block is transitory, and the electrocardiogram taken later shows only evidence of myocardial disease. Another form is that in which the heart block is reflex and due to irritation of the vagus nerves. Examples of this phenomenon have been observed with esophageal diverticula, mediastinal tumors, carotid sinus disease, glossopharyngeal neuralgia, and pleural and pulmonary irritation. However, reflex bradycardia is more commonly of the sinoatrial type than of the atrioventricular type.

Aortic stenosis and, less often, insufficiency dispose to fainting attacks. In rare instances it is due to heart block but the more frequent mechanism appears to be diversion of blood from the brain to the exercising muscles in a patient who is unable to increase his cardiac output because of the mechanical hindrance. A characteristic clinical feature is that the faint occurs during or immediately after exertion. There may be an initial pallor, weakness, or lightheadedness, or no warning whatsoever. Unconsciousness may last as long as half an hour, and convulsions sometimes occur.

Paroxysmal atrial and ventricular tachycardia cause unconsciousness by interfering with cardiac filling and output. Bigeminal rhythm (p. 764) may rarely have the same effect. Most patients who faint because of paroxysmal ectopic tachycardia are aware of the preliminary rapid heart action. Otherwise, the syncopal attack does not differ from the aforementioned types.

A cardiac faint, sometimes fatal, may occur in patients with disease of the coronary arteries. No explanation for death is found at autopsy. Such faints as well as those occurring during myocardial infarction may be due to ventricular tachycardia, ventricular fibrillation, heart block, or, rarely, to severe pain alone.

CAROTID SINUS SYNCOPE. The carotid sinus is normally sensitive to stretch and gives rise to sensory impulses carried via the intercarotid nerve of Hering (branch of the glossopharyngeal nerve) to the medulla oblongata. Massage of one or both carotid sinuses, particularly in elderly persons, causes a reflex slowing of the heart or even heart block, a fall of blood pressure without cardiac slowing, or an interference with the circulation of the ipsilateral cerebral hemisphere.

Syncope due to carotid sinus sensitivity may be initiated by turning of the head to one side, by a tight collar, or, as in one reported case, by shaving over the region of the sinus. The absence of such stimuli is of no aid in diagnosis, since spontaneous attacks may occur. The attack nearly always begins when the patient is in an upright position, usually when he is standing. The onset is sudden, often with falling. Clonic convulsive movements are not infrequent in the vagal and depressor type of carotid sinus syncope. Unilateral paresthesias or convulsions have been reported in the central type. The period of unconsciousness seldom lasts longer than a few minutes. The sensorium is immediately clear when consciousness is regained. The majority of the reported cases have been in males.

In a patient displaying faintness on compression of one carotid sinus, it is important to distinguish between the benign disorder, hypersensitivity of one carotid sinus, and a much more serious condition, atheromatous narrowing of the opposite carotid or of the basilar artery (see Chap. 204).

TUSSIVE SYNCOPE ("LARYNGEAL VERTIGO"). This condition is rare, but it should be mentioned because it illustrates another mechanism of fainting—that resulting from a paroxysm of coughing. The few patients that the authors have observed have been men with chronic bronchitis. After hard coughing the patient suddenly becomes weak and loses consciousness momentarily. The unconsciousness that results from breath holding in infants is probably similar. Not all the underlying physiologic changes are known. It is said that the intrathoracic pressure becomes elevated and interferes with the venous return to the heart. The Valsalva maneuver of trying to exhale against a closed glottis is believed to produce an identical effect. Episodes of faintness and lightheadedness are not infrequent in pertussis and chronic laryngitis.

Pathophysiology of Syncope

In the final analysis the loss of consciousness in these different types of syncope must be caused by a change in the nervous elements in those parts of the brain which subserve consciousness. Syncope resembles epilepsy in this respect; yet there is an important difference. In epilepsy, whether major or minor, the arrest in mental function is almost instantaneous and, as revealed by the electroencephalogram, is accompanied by a paroxysm of activity in certain groups of cerebral neurones. Syncope, on the other hand, is not so sudden. The difference relates to the essential pathophysiology—a sudden spread of an electric discharge in epilepsy, and the more gradual failure of cerebral circulation in syncope.

During syncopal attacks, measurements of cerebral circulation (Schmidt-Kety and Gibbs's methods) demonstrate a significant degree of reduction in cerebral blood flow and of cerebral oxygen utilization (cerebral metabolism). Cerebral vascular resistance is decreased. The electroencephalogram reveals high-voltage slow waves 2 to 5 per sec coincident with the loss of consciousness. Hyperventilation results in hypocapnia, alkalosis, increased cerebrovascular resistance, and decreased cerebral blood flow.

Conditions Often Associated with Episodic Weakness and Faintness but Not with Syncope

ANXIETY ATTACKS AND THE HYPERVENTILATION SYNDROME. This condition is discussed in detail in Chaps. 42 and 213, and it is necessary here only to state that this disorder is one of the commonest causes of recurrent faintness without actual loss of consciousness, the symptoms *are not relieved by recumbency*, and the diagnosis depends in large measure on reproducing the symptoms by hyperventilation. Two mechanisms are involved in the attacks; the loss of carbon dioxide as the result of hyperventilation and the release of epinephrine. Both mechanisms are said to be initiated by anxiety or allied emotional disturbances.

Of aid in diagnosis, as well as in therapy, is the demonstration to the patient of many of the symptoms of anxiety attack by voluntary hyperventilation for a period of 2 to 3 min and the cautious, slow, intravenous injection, during a period of several minutes, of 0.01 to 0.1 mg epinephrine. However, it must be admitted that the initial symptoms of the attack are not usually reproduced and that in some cases such measures are entirely without demonstrable effect.

HYPOGLYCEMIA. Another frequent cause of obscure episodic weakness is spontaneous hypoglycemia. When severe, the condition is likely to be due to a serious disease such as a tumor of the islets of Langerhans or advanced adrenal, pituitary, or hepatic disease, in which instances there may be a confusion or even a loss of consciousness. When mild, as is usually the case, hypoglycemia is of the reactive type (Chap. 88) and occurs 2 to 5 hr after eating. The fasting blood glucose is normal. The diagnosis depends largely upon the history and the reproduction by the injection of insulin of a symptom complex exactly similar to that occurring in the spontaneous attacks.

ACUTE INTERNAL HEMORRHAGE. This condition, usually within the gastrointestinal tract, is an occasional cause of syncope. Peptic ulcer is the commonest source of the hemorrhage. When pain is absent, as it often is, and when there is no hematemesis, the cause of the weakness, faintness, or even unconsciousness may remain obscure until the passage of a black stool.

CEREBRAL ISCHEMIC ATTACKS. Some patients with arteriosclerotic narrowing or occlusion of the major arteries of the brain may have repeated attacks, all of identical pattern, in which there is a temporary focal deficit in cerebral function. The main symptoms vary from patient to patient and include dim vision, hemiparesis, numbness of one side of the body, dizziness, and thick speech; and to those may be added an impairment of consciousness. The mechanism of this vascular syndrome has not been fully elucidated. Some physicians hold that localized vasospasm is responsible; others ascribe the attacks to small focal vascular lesions. The author's own investigations suggest some other mechanism than either of these. The condition is discussed in Chap. 204.

HYSTERICAL FAINTING. Fainting, which is rather frequent, usually occurs under dramatic circumstances. These are described in Chap. 214. The attack is unattended by any outward display of anxiety. The evident lack of change in pulse and blood pressure or color of the skin and mucous membranes distinguishes it from the vasodepressor faint induced by a shocking emotional experience. The diagnosis is based on the bizarre nature of the attack in a person who exhibits the general personality and behavior characteristics of hysteria (see Chap. 214).

Differential Diagnosis

OF SYNCOPE FROM OTHER TRANSITORY NERVOUS DISORDERS. More typical varieties of syncope must be distinguished from other disturbances of cerebral function, the most frequent of which is akinetic epilepsy (see Chap. 52). Epilepsy may occur day or night, regardless of the position of the patient; syncope rarely appears when the patient is recumbent, the only common exception being the Stokes-Adams attack. The patient's color does not usually change in epilepsy; pallor is an early and invariable finding in all types of syncope, except chronic orthostatic hypotension and hysteria, and it precedes unconsciousness. Epilepsy is more sudden in onset, and if an aura is present, it rarely lasts longer than a few seconds before consciousness is abolished. The onset of syncope is usually more deliberate.

Injury from falling is frequent in epilepsy and rare in syncope for the reason that only in the former are protective reflexes instantaneously abolished. Tonic convulsive movements with upturning eyes are frequent in epilepsy in contrast to syncope, though the same cannot be said of clonic movements of the arms. The period of unconsciousness tends to be longer in epilepsy than in syncope. Urinary incontinence is frequent in epilepsy and rare in syncope; but since it may be observed occasionally in syncope, it cannot be used as a means of excluding this condition. The return of consciousness is prompt in syncope and slow in epilepsy. Mental confusion, headache, and drowsiness are the common sequelae of epilepsy, whereas physical weakness with clear sensorium characterizes the postsyncopal state. Repeated spells of unconsciousness in a young person at a rate of several per day or month are much more suggestive of epilepsy than syncope. It should be emphasized that no one of these points will absolutely differentiate epilepsy from syncope, but taken as a group and supplemented by electroencephalograms (see p. 200), they provide a means of distinguishing the two conditions.

OF THE DIFFERENT TYPES OF SYNCOPE. Differentiation of the several conditions that diminish cerebral blood flow is discussed in some detail in Chap. 50, and only a few points need to be repeated here.

When faintness is related to reduced cerebral blood flow resulting directly from a disorder of cardiac function, there is likely to be a combination of pallor and cyanosis, pronounced dyspnea, and distension of the veins. When, on the other hand, the peripheral circulation is at fault, pallor is usually striking but not accompanied by cyanosis or respiratory disturbances, and the veins are collapsed. When the primary disturbance lies in the cerebral circulation, the face is likely to be florid and the breathing slow and stertorous. During the attack a heart rate faster than 150 per min indicates an ectopic cardiac rhythm, while a striking bradycardia (rate less than 40) suggests the presence of complete heart block. In a patient with faintness or syncope attended by bradycardia, one has to distinguish between the neurogenic reflex and the myogenic (Stokes-Adams) types. Occasionally electrocardiographic tracings will be needed, but as a rule the Stokes-Adams seizures can be recognized by their longer duration, by the greater constancy of the heart rate, by the presence of audible sounds synchronous with atrial contraction, and by marked variation in intensity of the first sound, despite the regular rhythm (Chap. 140). Clinical diagnosis may at times be difficult or impossible.

The color of the skin, the character of the breathing, the appearance of the veins, and the rate of the heart are therefore valuable data in diagnosis *if the patient is seen during the attack.* Unfortunately, the physician does not have the opportunity to see most of the patients during their "spells" of weakness. Hence he must obtain the proper clues from the patient's story. It is therefore of primary importance that the physician be familiar with the *circumstances* and the *precipitating* and *alleviating* factors in a given episode of weakness or fainting.

Type of Onset. When the attack begins with relative suddenness, i.e., over the period of a few seconds, carotid sinus syncope or postural hypotension is likely. When the symptoms develop gradually during a period of several minutes, hyperventilation or hypoglycemia (spontaneous or induced by insulin) is to be considered. Onset of syncope during or immediately after exertion suggests aortic stenosis and, in elderly subjects, postural hypotension. Exertional syncope is likewise occasionally seen in persons with aortic insufficiency.

Position at Onset of Attack. Attacks due to hypoglycemia, hyperventilation, hypertensive encephalopathy, or heart block are likely to be independent of posture. Faintness associated with a decline in blood pressure (including carotid sinus attacks) and with ectopic tachycardia usually occurs only in the sitting or standing position, whereas faintness resulting from orthostatic hypotension or orthostatic tachycardia is apt to set in shortly after change from the recumbent to the standing position.

Associated Symptoms. The associated symptoms during the attack are important, for palpitation is likely to be present when the attack is due to anxiety or hyperventilation, to ectopic tachycardia, or to hypoglycemia. Numbness and tingling in the hands and face are frequent accompaniments of hyperventilation. Irregular jerking movements and generalized spasms without loss of consciousness or change in the electroencephalogram are typical of the hysterical faint. Genuine convulsions during the attack, although characteristic of epilepsy, may occasionally occur with heart block and with hypertensive encephalopathy.

Duration of Attack. When the duration of the seizure is very brief, i.e., a few seconds to a few minutes, one thinks particularly of carotid sinus syncope or one of the several forms of postural hypertension. A duration of more than a few minutes but less than an hour particularly suggests hypoglycemia or hyperventilation.

SPECIAL METHODS OF EXAMINATION

In many patients who complain of recurrent weakness or syncope but do not have a spontaneous attack while under the observation of the physician, an attempt to *reproduce* attacks is of great assistance in diagnosis. In order to avoid the effects of suggestion, rigid controls must be adopted. Thus, if one wishes to determine whether the attacks in a given subject are hypoglycemic in type and may be reproduced by insulin injection, it is necessary to control the observations by injecting other drugs such as atropine, nitroglycerin, or histamine which evoke subjective symptoms of a different type. When properly controlled, the insulin test is of great value in the diagnosis of spontaneous hypoglycemia. Without such controls the procedure is useless.

When hyperventilation is accompanied by faintness, the pattern of symptoms can be reproduced readily by having the subject breathe rapidly and deeply for 2 or 3 min. This test is often of therapeutic value also because the underlying anxiety tends to be lessened when the patient learns that he can produce and alleviate the symptoms at will simply by controlling his breathing.

Among other conditions in which the diagnosis is commonly clarified by reproducing the attacks are

carotid sinus hypersensitivity (massage of one or the other carotid sinus), orthostatic hypotension, and orthostatic tachycardia (observations of pulse rate, blood pressure, and symptoms in the recumbent and standing positions). In all such instances one should remember that the *crucial point is not whether symptoms are produced* (the procedures mentioned frequently induce symptoms in healthy persons) but whether the exact pattern of symptoms that occurs in the spontaneous attacks is reproduced in the artificial seizures.

Multiple mechanisms of syncope frequently coexist. Combinations of hypoglycemia, hyperventilation, and postural hypotension, or any two of them, are frequent. In order to reproduce exactly the spontaneous symptoms, it may be necessary to have the patient stand and hyperventilate at a time when the blood sugar has been reduced by insulin administration. When tremor, palpitation, and fright are present in the spontaneous attacks, it may be necessary to carry out these procedures in association with the administration of epinephrine. There is great psychotherapeutic value to the patient in *knowing* that the physician can turn his "spells" on and off at will and, therefore, is not guessing about their cause and significance.

Lastly, the electroencephalogram is helpful in diagnosis. In the interval between epileptic seizures it may show some degree of abnormality in 40 to 80 per cent of cases. In the interval between syncopal attacks it should be normal.

TREATMENT

Fainting in most instances is due to a relatively innocent cause. In dealing with patients who have fainted the physician should think first of those causes of fainting that constitute a therapeutic emergency. Among them are massive internal hemorrhage and myocardial infarction, which may be painless. In an elderly person a sudden faint, without obvious cause, should arouse the suspicion of complete heart block, even though all findings are negative when the physician sees the patient.

If the patient is seen during the preliminary stages of fainting or after he has lost consciousness, one should make sure that he is in a position which permits maximal cerebral blood flow, i.e., with head lowered between the knees, if sitting, or lying supine. All tight clothing and other constrictions should be loosened and the head turned so that the tongue does not fall back into the throat, blocking the airway. Peripheral irritation such as sprinkling or dashing cold water on the face and neck or the application of cold towels is helpful. If the temperature is subnormal, the body should be covered with a warm blanket. If available, aromatic spirit of ammonia may be given cautiously by inhalation. One should be prepared for a possible emesis. Nothing should be given by mouth until the patient has regained consciousness. Then ½ tsp aromatic spirit of ammonia in a half glass of cold water or a sip of brandy or whisky may be given. The patient should not be permitted to rise until his sense of physical weakness has passed, and he should be watched carefully for a few minutes after rising.

As a rule, the physician sees the patient after the faint has occurred, and he is asked to explain why it happened and how it can be prevented in the future. The prevention of fainting depends on the mechanism involved. In the usual vasovagal faint of adolescents, which tends to occur in periods of emotional excitement, fatigue, hunger, etc., it is enough to advise the patient to avoid such circumstances. If the patient is sickly, measures to improve general health and circulatory efficiency are useful. In postural hypotension the patient should be cautioned against arising suddenly from bed. Instead, he should first exercise his legs for a few seconds, then sit on the edge of the bed and make sure he is not lightheaded or dizzy before he starts to walk. He should sleep with the headposts of the bed elevated on wooden blocks 8 to 12 in. high. A snug elastic abdominal binder and elastic stockings are often helpful. Drugs of the ephedrine group (ephedrine sulfate, 8 to 16 mg) may be useful if they do not cause insomnia. If there are no contraindications, a high intake of sodium chloride, which expands the extracellular fluid volume, may be beneficial.

In the syndrome of chronic orthostatic hypotension, oxytocin (Pitocin) has been reported to give relief in some cases.

The treatment of carotid sinus syncope involves first of all instructing the patient in measures that minimize the hazards of a fall (see below). Loose collars should be worn, and the patient should learn to turn the whole body, rather than the head alone, when looking to one side. Atropine or the ephedrine group of drugs should be used, respectively, in patients with pronounced bradycardia or hypotension during the attacks. Radiation or surgical denervation of the carotid sinus has apparently yielded favorable results in some patients, but it is rarely necessary. Once the possibility has been excluded that the attacks are due to a narrowing of major cerebral arteries, emphatic reassurance is essential for such patients, the majority of whom are under the mistaken impression that strokes or cardiac disease are responsible for the episodes.

The treatment of the various cardiac arrhythmias which may induce syncope is discussed in Chap. 140. The treatment of hypoglycemia will be found on p. 509 and of the hyperventilation syndrome and hysterical fainting on pp. 329 and 197.

The chief hazard of a faint in most elderly persons is not the underlying disease but rather fracture or other trauma due to the fall. Therefore, patients subject to recurrent syncope should cover the bathroom floor and bathtub with rubber mats and should have as much of their home carpeted as is feasible. Especially important is the floor space between the bed and the bathroom, because faints are common in elderly persons when walking from bed to toilet. Outdoor walking should be on soft ground rather than hard surfaces, when possible, and the patient should avoid standing still, which is more likely than walking to induce an attack.

SUMMARY

In conclusion, it should be emphasized that the majority of conditions which produce recurrent weakness and syncope are not serious. When the less frequent conditions, such as heart block, ventricular arrhythmias, myocardial infarction, aortic stenosis, internal hemorrhage, cerebral vascular disease, and organic lesions of the brain, have been excluded, the assumption of a relatively benign disorder is usually justified. The same may be said of the chemical disorders that usually induce episodic weakness rather than syncope.

Attacks of both types are likely to be interpreted by the patient, and occasionally by the physician, as due to serious disease of the circulatory apparatus or of the nervous system. Many of these patients therefore are worried and anxious, often out of all proportion to the seriousness of the condition. Once the mystery has been solved by careful study, and its exact significance has been explained to the patient, his fears are usually allayed.

A number of the topics considered in this chapter are discussed elsewhere in this book. The mechanisms of the circulatory disorders which may cause syncope are considered in Chap. 44. Epilepsy as a cause of recurrent unconsciousness is discussed in Chap. 52. The hyperventilation syndrome is considered in Chap. 61.

REFERENCES

Engel, G. L.: "Fainting," Springfield, Ill., Charles C Thomas, Publisher, 1950.

Gowers, W. R.: "The Borderland of Epilepsy," London, J. A. Churchill, 1907.

45 MOTOR PARALYSIS
Raymond D. Adams

The motor system may undergo dissolution in several ways during the course of disease. In diffuse disorders of the cerebrum there may be disintegration first of the highest nervous integrations and then of the lower ones. Concepts or memories of specialized movement patterns may be lost while less complicated volitional and automatic movements are retained. Later there may be a paralysis of all volitional movements, without change or even with exaggeration of reflex activities. In lesions of the spinal cord all movements, both volitional and reflex, may be abolished. The resulting impairments may be subdivided into (1) paralysis due to affection of lower motor neurones, (2) paralysis due to a disorder of upper motor neurones, (3) apraxic or nonparalytic disturbances of purposive movement, and (4) abnormalities of movement and posture due to disease of the extrapyramidal motor systems. The first three types of motor disorder will be discussed briefly here, and the fourth type will be explained in Chap. 46.

DEFINITIONS. The term *paralysis* is derived from two Greek words, *para,* beside, and *lysis,* a loosening. In medicine it has come to refer to an abolition of function, either sensory or motor. When applied to voluntary muscles, paralysis means loss of contraction due to interruption of some part of the motor pathway from the cerebrum to the muscle fiber. Lesser degrees of paralysis are sometimes spoken of as *paresis,* but in everyday medical parlance motor paralysis usually stands for either partial or complete loss of function. The word *plegia* comes from the Greek word meaning stroke; and the word *palsy,* from an old French word, has the same meaning as paralysis. All these words are used interchangeably in medical practice, though it is preferable to use paresis for slight and paralysis or plegia for severe loss of motor function.

Paralysis Due to Disease of the Lower Motor Neurones

The essential facts concerning the anatomy and physiology of this system of motor nerve cells are well known. A few points, however, deserve brief comment because they explain important clinical phenomena.

Each motor nerve cell through the extensive arborization of the terminal part of its fiber comes into contact with 100 or 200 or more muscle fibers; altogether they constitute "the motor unit." All the variations in force, range, and type of movement are determined by differences in the number and size of motor units called into activity and the frequency of their action. Feeble movements involve only a few small motor units; powerful movements recruit many more units of increasing size. When a motor neurone becomes diseased, as in progressive muscular atrophy, it may manifest increased irritability and all the muscle fibers that it controls may discharge sporadically in isolation from other units. The result of the contraction of one or several such units is a visible twitch, or *fasciculation,* which can be recorded in the electromyogram as a large diphasic or multiphasic action potential. If the motor neurone is destroyed, all the muscle fibers to which it is attached undergo a profound atrophy, namely, denervation atrophy. For some unknown reason the individual denervated muscle fibers now begin to contract spontaneously, though they can no longer do so in response to a nerve impulse or as a part of a motor unit. This isolated activity of individual muscle fibers is called *fibrillation* and is so fine that it cannot be seen through the intact skin but can be recorded only as a repetitive short-duration spike potential in the electromyogram (see Chap. 221).

The motor nerve fibers of each ventral root intermingle as the roots join to form plexuses; and although the innervation of the muscles is roughly metameric, or according to segments of the spinal cord, each large

muscle comes to be supplied by two or more roots. For this reason the distribution of paralysis due to disease of the anterior horn cells or anterior roots differs from that which follows a lesion of a peripheral nerve.

All motor activity, even of the most elementary reflex type, requires the cooperation of several muscles. The analysis of a relatively simple movement such as clenching the fist affords some idea of the complexity of the underlying neural arrangements. In this act the primary movement is a contraction of the flexor muscles of the fingers, the flexor digitorum sublimis and profundus, the flexor pollicis longus and brevis, and the abductor pollicis brevis. In the terminology of Beevor, these muscles act as *agonists* or *prime movers* in this act. In order that flexion may be smooth and forceful the extensor muscles (*antagonists*) must relax at the same rate as the flexors contract. The muscles which flex the fingers also flex the wrist; and since it is desired that only the fingers flex, the muscles which extend the wrist must be brought into play to prevent its flexion. The action of the wrist extensors is *synergic,* and these muscles are called *synergists* in this particular act. Lastly the wrist, elbow, and shoulder must be stabilized by appropriate flexor and extensor muscles, which serve as *fixators.* The coordination of agonists, antagonists, synergists, and fixators involves reciprocal innervation and is managed by segmental spinal reflexes under the guidance of proprioceptive sensory stimuli. Only the agonist movement in a voluntary act is believed to be initiated at a cortical level.

If all or practically all peripheral motor nerves supplying a muscle are destroyed, both voluntary and reflex movements are abolished. The muscle becomes soft and yields to passive stretching, a condition known as *flaccidity.* Muscle tone—the slight resistance that normal relaxed muscle offers to passive movement—is reduced (*hypotonia* or *atonia*). The denervated muscles undergo extreme atrophy, usually being reduced to 20 or 30 per cent of their original bulk within 3 months. The reaction of the muscle to sudden stretch, as by tapping its tendon, is lost. And, finally, it may be demonstrated that the muscle will no longer respond to electric stimuli of short duration, i.e., faradic stimuli, but still does respond to currents of long duration, galvanic stimuli. This alteration of electric response is known as *Erb's reaction of degeneration.* If only a part of the motor units in the muscles are affected, only partial paralysis or paresis will ensue. The atrophy will be less, the tendon reflexes weakened instead of lost, and the reaction of degeneration may not be obtained. Quantitative testing by determination of strength-duration curves is a means of showing partial denervation, but electromyographic evidence of fibrillations and fasciculations may also be obtained.

The tonus of muscle and the tendon reflexes are now known to depend on the muscle spindles and the afferent fibers to which they give origin and on the small anterior horn cells whose axones terminate on the small muscle fibers within the spindles. These small spinal motor neurones are called *gamma neurones* in contrast to the large *alpha neurones*. A tap on a tendon, by stretching the spindle muscle fibers, activates afferent neurones which terminate in alpha motor neurones. The result is the familiar muscle contraction or tendon reflex. The spindle muscle fibers are relaxed by an inhibitory mechanism, which terminates the reflex. Thus the setting of the spindle fibers and state of excitability of the gamma neurones (normally inhibited by the corticospinal fibers and other supranuclear neurones) determines the level of activity of the tendon reflexes and the responsiveness of muscle to stretch.

Lower motor neurone paralysis is the direct result of physiologic arrest or destruction of anterior horn cells or their axones in anterior roots and nerves. The signs and symptoms of a lower motor neurone lesion vary according to the location of the lesion. Probably the most important question for clinical purposes is whether sensory changes coexist. The combination of flaccid, areflexic paralysis and sensory changes usually indicate involvement of a mixed motor and sensory nerve or affection of both anterior and posterior roots. If sensory changes are absent, the lesion must be situated in the gray matter of the spinal cord, in the anterior roots, or in a purely motor branch of a peripheral nerve. The distinction between nuclear (spinal) and anterior root (radicular) lesions may at times be impossible to make. The coexistence of spastic weakness in muscles innervated by segments below the level of the lesion points to intraspinal disease.

Paralysis Due to Disease of the Upper Motor Neurones

Several anatomic and physiologic facts concerning the upper motor neurones are worthy of note. It was formerly believed that the corticospinal tract originated from the large motor cell of Betz in the fifth layer of the precentral convolution. However, there are only about 25,000 to 30,000 Betz cells, whereas the pyramidal tract at the level of the medulla contains approximately 1 million axones. This tract must, therefore, contain many fibers that arise not from the Betz cells of the motor cortex (area 4 of Brodmann) but rather from the smaller cells of area 4 and the cells of the adjacent precentral (area 6) and postcentral cortex (areas 1, 3, 5). Furthermore, since about half the fibers in the pyramid remain intact after removal of the precentral and postcentral convolutions (i.e., hemispherectomy), these must originate in subcortical structures and descend to the spinal cord or ascend from spinal levels, as recently shown by Brodal and his associates. The pyramidal tract is the only long fiber connection between the cerebrum and the spinal cord. At the level of the internal capsule these corticospinal fibers are intermingled with many others destined to end in the globus pallidus, substantia pallidus, substantia nigra, and reticular substance. The fibers to the cranial nerve nuclei become

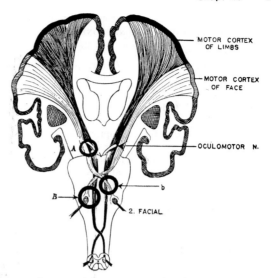

Fig. 45-1. Diagram of the corticospinal and corticobulbar tracts. Lesion at (A) produces ipsilateral oculomotor palsy and contralateral paralysis involving face, arm, and leg. Lesion at (B) causes ipsilateral facial paralysis of peripheral type and contralateral paralysis of arm and leg. Lesion at (b) results in ipsilateral facial weakness of upper motor neurone of central type and contralateral paralysis of arm and leg. (Bergmann and Staeheln: "Krankheiten des Nervensystems," Berlin, Springer-Verlag, 1939.)

separated at about the level of the midbrain and cross the midline to the contralateral cranial nerve nuclei (Fig. 45-1). These fibers form the corticopontine and corticobulbar tracts. The decussation of the pyramidal tract at the lower end of the medulla is variable in different individuals. A small number of fibers, 10 to 20 per cent, do not cross but descend ipsilaterally as the uncrossed pyramidal tract. The termination of the corticospinal tract is in relation to nerve cells in the intermediate zone of gray matter, and not more than 10 to 15 per cent establish direct synaptic connection with anterior horn cells. These facts must of necessity modify current views of the anatomy of the pyramidal tract and suggest new interpretations of symptoms that result from the interruption of this tract.

The motor area of the cerebral cortex is difficult to define. It includes that part of the precentral convolution which contains Betz cells, but, as already mentioned, it probably extends anteriorly into area 6 and posteriorly into the parietal lobe, where it overlaps the sensory areas. Physiologically it is defined as the region of the cortex from which isolated movements can be evoked by stimuli of minimal intensity. The muscle groups of the contralateral face, arm, trunk, and leg are represented in the motor cortex, those of the face being at the lower end of the precentral convolution and those of the leg in the paracentral lobule on the medial surface of the cerebral hemisphere. These motor points are not fixed but vary somewhat with the conditions of previous stimulation. The parts of the body capable of the most delicate movements have, in general, the largest cortical representation.

Table 45-1. DIFFERENCES BETWEEN PARALYSIS OF
UPPER AND LOWER NEURONE TYPES

Upper, supranuclear, or corticospinal (pyramidal) paralysis	Lower, spinomuscular, or infranuclear paralysis
Muscle groups affected diffusely, never individual muscles	Individual muscles may be affected
Atrophy slight and due to disuse	Atrophy pronounced, 70 to 80 per cent of total bulk
Spasticity with hyperactivity of the tendon reflexes	Flaccidity and hypotonia of affected muscles with loss of tendon reflexes
Babinski sign +	Plantar reflex, if present, is of normal flexor type
Fascicular twitches never present	Fascicular twitches may be present
Normal reactions to galvanic and faradic current	Loss of faradic reaction, retention of galvanic reaction (reaction of degeneration)

Area 6, the premotor area, is also electrically excitable but requires more intense stimuli to evoke movements, and the movements produced are more complex than those evoked from area 4. Very strong stimuli elicit movements from a wide area of premotor frontal and parietal cortex, and the same movements may be obtained from several points. From this it may be assumed that one of the functions of the motor cortex is to synthesize simple movements into an infinite variety of finely graded, highly differentiated patterns.

Thus upper motor neurone paralysis may be due to lesions in the cerebral cortex, subcortical white matter, internal capsule, brain stem, or spinal cord. The distribution of the paralysis varies with the locale of the lesion, but there are also other typical features. Paralysis due to a lesion of the upper motor neurones always involves a group of muscles, never individual muscles, and the proper relationships between antagonists, synergists, and fixators are always preserved. The paralysis never involves all the muscles on one side of the body.[1] Movements that are invariably bilateral, such as movements of the eyes, jaw, pharynx, larynx, neck, thorax, and abdomen, are little if at all affected. The hand and arm muscles suffer most severely, the leg muscles next, and of the cranial musculature only the muscles of the lower face and tongue are involved to any significant degree. Broadbent was the first to call attention to this distribution of paralysis, and this predilection of certain muscles to paralysis with pyramidal tract disease is referred to as *Broadbent's law.* Paralysis of pyramidal type is rarely complete for any long period of time, and in this respect it differs from the total and absolute paralysis due to a lesion of the lower motor neurones. The paralyzed arm may suddenly move during yawning or stretching, and various reflex activities can be elicited at all times. However, acute disorders may abolish function

[1] Even in the hemiplegia resulting from a complete lesion of the corticospinal tract.

in parts of the nervous system distant from the site of the lesion. For example, a sudden lesion of the pyramidal tract in the cervical spinal cord may not only cause paralysis of voluntary movements but also abolish all of the spinal reflexes. This is known as *spinal shock.* It usually lasts but a few days or weeks and is replaced by spasticity of the paralyzed muscles. This phenomenon of *spasticity* is another characteristic of lesions of the upper motor neurones and is due to a release of spinal reflex mechanisms or the release of a "normal component in movement from its natural competitor" (Denny-Brown). Spasticity does not appear immediately after the onset of a sudden lesion but develops gradually over several weeks. In exceptional cases the paralyzed limbs remain flaccid. The spasticity affects some muscle groups more than others. The arm is usually held in a flexed position, and any attempts to extend it encounter resistance, which is maximal at the beginning and then yields (clasp-knife phenomenon). The leg is maintained in an extended position, and passive flexion is resisted. If the limbs are moved to a new position, either flexion or extension, that position is maintained (lengthening and shortening reaction). If patients have suffered paresis due to a lesion of the pyramidal tract, they not infrequently display associated movements upon attempting to carry out a voluntary movement with the weak limb. Attempts to flex the arm may result in involuntary pronation (the pronation phenomenon); or when the hemiplegic leg is flexed, the foot may automatically dorsiflex and evert (Strümpell's tibialis phenomenon). When the patient is asked alternately to pronate and supinate the paretic limb, the healthy limb may mimic these movements (i.e., *mirror movements*).

Table 45-1, modified from Stewart, shows the main differences between paralyses of the lower and those of the upper motor neurones.

APRAXIC OR NONPARALYTIC DISORDERS OF MOTOR FUNCTION

Aside from upper and lower motor neurone paralysis there may be loss of purposive movement without paralysis or loss of movement. This is called *apraxia* and may be explained as follows. Many simple actions are acquired by learning or practice. Movement patterns, particularly those which involve manufacture, i.e., the use of tools and instruments as well as gestures, once established, are remembered and may be reproduced under the proper circumstances. Any purposive act may be conceived as occurring in several stages. First, the idea of an act must be aroused in the mind of the patient by an appropriate stimulus situation, perhaps by a spoken command to do something. This idea or concept is then translated by excitation of the premotor or motor cortex and thence by the corticospinal tracts, which not only initiate particular movements of individual muscle groups but also modify or suppress the subcortical mechanisms that control the basic attitudes and postures of the body. In right-handed and most left-handed individuals the neural mechanisms for the formulation of an idea of an act and its reproduction are believed to be centered in the posterior and inferior part of the left parietal lobe, near the angular gyrus; these are connected with the left premotor regions for the control of the right hand and the motor areas of the right cerebral hemisphere through the corpus callosum for the control of the left side. Complex skills called forth by spoken commands involve connections from the auditory perception area to frontal regions.

A failure to execute certain acts in the correct context while retaining the individual movements upon which such acts depend is the main feature of *apraxia*. The most adequate clinical test of motor deficits of this type is to observe a series of actions such as using a comb, a razor, a toothbrush, or a common tool or gesturing, i.e., waving goodbye, saluting, shaking the fist as though angry, or blowing a kiss. These may be initiated by the patient or be done in response to a command or as an attempt to imitate the examiner. Of course, failure to follow a spoken request may be due to aphasia that prevents understanding of the spoken or written word or agnosia that prevents recognition of a tool or object to be used. But aside from these sources of difficulty there remains a peculiar motor deficit in which the patient appears to have lost his memory of how to perform a given act, especially if called upon for it in an unnatural setting. The maximal degree of it is called *ideomotor apraxia* and implies an inability to translate the idea of the movement into a precise well-executed movement. The failure is evident both after spoken command and in attempts to imitate the examiner. The least degree of it, bordering upon paralysis of willed movement, involves only one group of muscles such as tongue or lips. Confused or demented patients also may fail entirely to understand what the examiner requests and be unable to perform certain acts. Only if this deficit is out of proportion to all others, thus reflecting a specific loss of certain learned patterns of movement (a "specific amnesia," so to speak, analogous to the amnesia of words in aphasia), can one recognize the condition in such patients. An added element of mental confusion imparts to it the form of ideational apraxia, a bilateral disorder; and the addition of voluntary motor paralysis converts it to a motor apraxia. Apraxia becomes manifest only with cortical, subcortical, and corpus callosal lesions. In the latter it involves only the left side. If the lesion is in the left dominant cerebral hemisphere, the apraxia is usually bilateral; if in the right hemisphere, the apraxia is in the left arm and leg.

Lesions of areas 6 and 8 which leave the more posterior part of the motor and the sensory cortex intact may produce a curious syndrome in which many voluntary movements are retained but are slow and awkward. Moreover, grasping and sucking reflexes are manifest. The tendon reflexes are lively, and the

plantar reflexes are flexor. In some cases there is a persistence of hand and foot flexion on tactile stimulation of the palmar and plantar surfaces, so that the patient is unable to release his grip or dorsiflex his foot (tonic innervation) voluntarily as long as the stimulus is present. In lesions of the parietal lobe a whole series of aversion or avoidance reactions to sensory stimuli become manifest. For a more complete discussion of the several types of apraxia, see Chap. 54.

Examination Scheme for Motor Paralysis and Apraxia

The first step is to inspect the paralyzed limb, taking note first of its posture and of the presence or absence of muscle atrophy, hypertrophy, and fascicular twitchings. The patient is then called upon to move each muscle group, and the power and facility of movement are graded and recorded. The range of passive movement is then determined by moving all the joints. This provides information concerning alterations of muscle tone, i.e., hypotonia, spasticity, and rigidity. Dislocations, disease of joints, and ankyloses may also be revealed by these same maneuvers. Enlargement of muscles with increased strength denotes true hypertrophy, which may be either physiologic or a manifestation of myotonia congenita. Slight atrophy may be due to disuse from any cause, i.e., pain, fixation as the result of a cast, or any type of paralysis. However, a pronounced atrophy usually occurs only with denervation of several weeks' or months' standing.

The tendon reflexes are then tested. The usual routine is to try to elicit the jaw jerk (increased in pseudobulbar palsy) and the supinator, biceps, triceps, quadriceps, and Achilles tendon reflexes. Two cutaneous reflexes are then tested, the abdominal and the plantar reflexes. (The extensor plantar reflex is Babinski's sign.)

If there is no evidence of upper or lower motor neurone disease but certain acts are nonetheless imperfectly performed, one should look for a disorder of postural sensibility or of cerebellar coordination or rigidity with abnormality of posture and movement due to disease of the basal ganglions. In the absence of these disorders, the possibility of a hysterical disorder of motor function should be investigated.

Hysterical paralysis is easily distinguished from chronic lower motor neurone disease by the areflexia and severe atrophy that are so characteristic of the latter condition. Diagnostic difficulty arises only in certain acute cases of upper motor neurone disease that lack all the usual changes in reflexes and muscle tone. In hysterical paralysis one arm or one leg or all one side of the body may be affected. The hysterical gait is sometimes diagnostic in itself (see Chap. 47). Often there is loss of sensation in the paralyzed parts and sometimes loss of sight in the eye, of hearing in the ear, and of smell in the nostril on the paralyzed side, a group of sensory changes that is never seen in organic brain disease. The patient should be asked to move the affected limbs; as he does so, the movement is seen to be slow and jerky, often with contraction of both agonist and antagonist muscles simultaneously or intermittently. Hoover's sign and Babinski's combined leg flexion test are helpful in distinguishing hysterical from organic hemiplegia. To elicit Hoover's sign the patient, lying on his back, is asked to raise one leg from the bed; in a normal individual the back of the heel of the contralateral leg is pressed firmly down, and the same is true when the patient with organic hemiplegia attempts to lift the paralyzed leg. To carry out Babinski's combined leg flexion test, a patient with an organic hemiplegia is asked to sit up without using his arms; when he does so, the paralyzed or weak leg flexes at the hip, and the heel is lifted from the bed while the heel of the sound leg is pressed into the bed. Both these signs are absent in hysterical hemiplegia.

If there is no definite paralysis except in the performance of certain specific acts, then the possibility of apraxia must be considered. This defect is best demonstrated by asking the patient to carry out certain commands such as to make a fist, to put out his tongue, to stamp his foot, to touch his nose, to place one heel on the opposite knee, to brush his hair, to light a cigarette, or to drink a glass of water; he is then asked to imitate the examiner in these acts. One must also take note of the state of mentation and the speed of comprehension. Confusion and aphasia interfere with the understanding of spoken commands.

DIFFERENTIAL DIAGNOSIS OF PARALYSIS

The diagnostic consideration of paralysis may be simplified by the following subdivisions, which relate to the location and distribution of weakness.

1. *Monoplegia* refers to weakness or paralysis of all the muscles in one limb, whether leg or arm. It should not be applied to paralysis of isolated muscles or groups of muscles supplied by a single nerve or motor root.

2. *Hemiplegia* is the commonest distribution of paralysis—loss of strength in arm, leg, and sometimes face on one side of the body.

3. *Paraplegia* indicates weakness or paralysis of both legs. It is most commonly found in spinal cord disease.

4. *Quadriplegia* indicates weakness of all four extremities. It may result from lesions involving peripheral nerves, gray matter of the spinal cord, or corticospinal tracts bilaterally in the cervical cord, upper brain stem, or cerebrum. *Diplegia* is a special form of quadriplegia in which the legs are affected more than the arms.

5. *Isolated paralyses* refer to weakness localized to one or more muscle groups.

MONOPLEGIA

The physical examination of patients who complain of weakness of one extremity often discloses an un-

noticed weakness in another limb, and the condition is actually hemiplegia or paraplegia. Or instead of weakness of all the muscles in a limb, only isolated groups are found to be affected. Ataxia, sensory disturbances, or pain in an extremity will often be interpreted by the patient as weakness, as will the mechanical limitation resulting from arthritis or the rigidity of parkinsonism.

In general, the presence or absence of atrophy of muscles in a monoplegic limb can be of diagnostic help.

PARALYSIS WITHOUT MUSCULAR ATROPHY. Long-continued disuse of a limb may lead to atrophy, but this is usually not so marked as in diseases that denervate muscles; the tendon reflexes are normal, and the response of the muscles to electric stimulation and electromyogram are unaltered.

The most frequent cause of monoplegia without muscular wasting is a lesion of the cerebral cortex. Only occasionally does it occur in diseases which interrupt the corticospinal tract at the level of the internal capsule, brain stem, or spinal cord. A vascular lesion (thrombosis or embolus) is commonest, but, of course, a tumor or abscess may have the same effect. Multiple sclerosis and spinal cord tumor, early in their course, may cause weakness of one extremity, usually the leg. As indicated above, weakness due to damage to the corticospinal system is usually accompanied by spasticity, increased reflexes, and an extensor plantar reflex (Babinski's sign), and the electric reactions and electromyogram are normal. However, acute diseases that destroy the motor tracts in the spinal cord may at first (for several days) reduce or leave unaltered the tendon reflexes and cause hypotonia (the condition known as *spinal shock*). This does not occur in partial or slowly evolving lesions. In acute diseases affecting the lower motor neurones the tendon reflexes are always reduced or abolished, but atrophy may not appear for several weeks. Hence one must take into account the mode of onset and the duration of the disease in evaluating the tendon reflexes, muscle tone, and degree of atrophy before reaching an anatomic diagnosis.

PARALYSIS WITH MUSCULAR ATROPHY. This condition is more frequent than paralysis without muscular atrophy. In addition to the paralysis and reduced or abolished tendon reflexes, there may be visible fasciculations. If completely paralyzed, the muscles exhibit an electric reaction of degeneration and the electromyogram shows reduced numbers of motor units (often of large size), fasciculations at rest, and fibrillations. The lesion may be in the spinal cord, spinal roots, or peripheral nerves. Its location can usually be decided by the distribution of the palsied muscles (whether the pattern is one of nerve, spinal root, or spinal cord involvement), by the associated neurologic symptoms and signs, and by special tests (cerebrospinal fluid examination, x-ray of spine, and myelogram).

Brachial atrophic monoplegia is relatively rare, and

when present, it should suggest in an infant a brachial plexus trauma, in a child poliomyelitis, in an adult poliomyelitis, syringomyelia, amyotrophic lateral sclerosis, or brachial plexus lesions. Crural monoplegia is more frequent and may be caused by any lesion of thoracic or lumbar cord, i.e., trauma, tumor, myelitis, multiple sclerosis, etc. It should be noted that multiple sclerosis almost never causes atrophy and that ruptured intervertebral disk and the many varieties of neuritis rarely paralyze all or most of the muscles of a limb. Muscle dystrophy may begin in one limb, but by the time the patient is seen the typical more or less symmetric pattern of proximal limb and trunk involvement is evident.

HEMIPLEGIA

This is the most frequent distribution of paralysis in man. With rare exceptions (a few unusual cases of poliomyelitis or motor system disease) this pattern of paralysis is due to involvement of the corticospinal tract.

LOCATION OF LESION PRODUCING HEMIPLEGIA. The site or level of the lesion, i.e., cerebral, capsular, brain stem, or spinal cord, can usually be deduced from the associated neurologic findings. Diseases localized in the cerebral cortex, cerebral white matter (corona radiata), and internal capsule usually evoke weakness or paralysis of the face, arm, and leg on the opposite side. The occurrence of convulsive seizures or the presence of a defect in speech (aphasia), a cortical type of sensory loss (astereognosis, loss of two-point discrimination, etc.), anosognosia, or defects in the visual fields suggest a cortical or subcortical location.

Damage to the corticospinal tract in the upper portion of the brain stem (see Fig. 45-1) may cause paralysis of the face, arm, and leg on the opposite side. The lesion in such cases is localized by the presence of a paralysis of the muscles supplied by the oculomotor nerve on the same side as the lesion (Weber's syndrome) or other neurologic findings. With low pontine lesions a unilateral abducens or facial palsy is combined with a contralateral weakness or paralysis of the arm and leg (Millard-Gubler syndrome). Lesions of the lowermost part of the brain stem, i.e., in the medulla, affect the tongue and sometimes the pharynx and larynx on one side and arm and leg on the other side. These "crossed paralyses," so common in brain stem diseases, are described in Chap. 202.

Rarely, a homolateral hemiplegia may be caused by a lesion in the lateral column of the cervical spinal cord. At this level, however, the pathologic process often induces bilateral signs, with resulting quadriparesis or quadriplegia. If one side of the spinal cord is extensively damaged, the homolateral paralysis is combined with a loss of vibratory and position sense on the same side and a contralateral loss of pain and temperature (Brown-Séquard syndrome).

Muscle atrophy of minor degree often follows lesions of the corticospinal system but never reaches the proportions seen in diseases of the lower motor neurones. The atrophy is due to disuse. When the motor cortex and adjacent parts of the parietal lobe are damaged in infancy or childhood, the normal development of the muscles and the skeletal system in the affected limbs is retarded. The palsied limbs and even the trunk on one side are small. This does not occur if the paralysis begins after skeletal growth is attained. In the hemiplegia due to spinal cord injury muscles at the level of the lesion atrophy as a result of damage to anterior horn cells or ventral roots.

CAUSES OF HEMIPLEGIA. In this condition vascular diseases of the cerebrum and brain stem exceed all others in frequency. Trauma (brain contusion, epidural and subdural hemorrhage) ranks second, and other diseases such as brain tumor, brain abscess and encephalitis, demyelinative diseases, complications of meningitis, tuberculosis, and syphilis are of decreasing order of importance. Most of these diseases can be diagnosed by the mode of evolution and the conjoined clinical and laboratory data presented in the chapters on neurologic diseases.

PARAPLEGIA

Paralysis of both lower extremities may occur in diseases of the spinal cord and the spinal roots or of the peripheral nerves. If onset is acute, it may be difficult to distinguish spinal from neural paralysis, for in any acute myelopathy spinal shock may result in abolition of reflexes and flaccidity. As a rule in acute spinal cord diseases with involvement of corticospinal tracts, the paralysis affects all muscles below a given level; and often, if the white matter is extensively damaged, sensory loss below a particular level (loss of pain and temperature with lateral spinothalamic tracts and loss of vibratory and position sense with posterior columns) is conjoined. Also, in bilateral disease of the spinal cord, the bladder and bowel sphincters are paralyzed. Alterations of cerebrospinal fluid (dynamic block, increase in protein or cells) are frequent. In peripheral nerve diseases both sensory and motor loss tend to involve the distal muscles of the legs more than the proximal ones (an exception is acute idiopathic polyneuritis), and the sphincters are often spared or only briefly deranged in function. Sensory loss, if present, is more likely to consist in distal impairment of touch, vibration, and position sense, with pain and temperature spared in many instances. The cerebrospinal fluid protein may be normal or elevated.

For clinical purposes it is helpful to consider separately the acute and the chronic paraplegias and to divide the chronic ones into two groups, those which occur in infancy and those which begin in adult life.

Acute paraplegia, beginning at any age, is relatively infrequent. Fracture dislocation of the spine with traumatic necrosis of the spinal cord, spontaneous hematomyelia with bleeding from a vascular malformation (angioma, telangiectasis), thrombosis of a spinal artery with infarction (myelomalacia), and dissecting aortic aneurysm or atherosclerotic occlusion of nutrient spinal arteries arising from the aorta with resulting infarction (myelomalacia) are the commonest varieties of sudden paraplegia (or quadriplegia, if the cervical cord is involved). Postinfectious or postvaccinal myelitis, acute demyelinative myelitis (Devic's disease if the optic nerves are affected), necrotizing myelitis, and epidural abscess or tumor with spinal cord compression tend to develop somewhat more slowly, over a period of hours or days, or they may have a subacute onset. Poliomyelitis and acute idiopathic polyneuritis, the former a purely motor disorder with meningitis, the latter predominantly motor but often with minimal sensory disturbances (paresthesias or objectively demonstrated impairment), must be distinguished from the other acute myelopathies and from one another.

In pediatric practice, delay in starting to walk and difficulty in walking are common problems. These conditions may be associated with a systemic disease such as rickets or may indicate mental deficiency or, more commonly, some muscular or neurologic disease. Congenital cerebral disease accounts for a majority of cases of infantile diplegia (weakness predominant in the legs, with the arms minimally affected). Present at birth or manifest in the first months of life, it may appear to progress; but actually it is stationary and only becomes apparent as the motor system develops. Later there may seem to be slow improvement as a result of the normal maturation processes of childhood. Congenital malformation of the spinal cord or birth injury of the spinal cord are other possibilities. Friedreich's ataxia and familial paraplegia, progressive muscular dystrophy, and the chronic varieties of polyneuritis tend to appear later during childhood and adolescence and are slowly progressive.

In adult life multiple sclerosis, subacute combined degeneration, spinal cord tumor, ruptured cervical disk and cervical spondylosis, syphilitic meningomyelitis, chronic epidural infections (fungous and other granulomatous diseases), Erb's spastic paraplegia and motor system disease, and syringomyelia represent the most frequently encountered forms of spinal cord disease. The several varieties of polyneuritis and polymyositis must be considered in their differential diagnosis, for they, too, may cause paraplegia.

QUADRIPLEGIA

All that has been written about the common causes of paraplegia applies to quadriplegia. The lesion is usually in the cervical rather than the thoracic or lumbar segments of the spinal cord. If it is situated in the low cervical segments and involves the anterior half of the spinal cord, as in occlusion of the anterior spinal artery, the arm paralysis may be flaccid and areflexic and the leg paralysis spastic (anterior spinal syndrome). There are only a few points of difference between the common paraplegic and quadriplegic

syndromes. In infants, aside from developmental abnormalities and anoxia of birth, an inherited cerebral disease (Schilder's disease, metachromatic leukoencephalopathy, lipid storage disease) may be responsible for a quadriparesis or quadriplegia. Congenital forms of muscular dystrophy may be recognized soon after birth and also infantile muscular atrophy (Hoffmann-Werdnig disease).

In adults repeated cerebral vascular accidents may lead to bilateral hemiplegia, usually accompanied by pseudobulbar palsy.

ISOLATED PARALYSIS

Paralysis of isolated muscle groups usually indicates a lesion of one or more peripheral nerves. The diagnosis of a lesion of an individual peripheral nerve is made on the presence of weakness or paralysis of the muscle or group of muscles and impairment or loss of sensation in the distribution of the nerve in question. Complete transection or severe injury to a peripheral nerve is usually followed by atrophy of the muscles it innervates and by loss of their tendon reflexes. Trophic changes in the skin, nails, and subcutaneous tissue may also occur.

Knowledge of the muscular and sensory function of each individual nerve is needed for a satisfactory diagnosis. Since lesions of the peripheral nerves are relatively uncommon in civil life, it is not practical for the general physician to keep all these facts in his memory, and a textbook of anatomy or Chap. 201, the Section on mononeuropathies, should be consulted. It is, however, of considerable importance to decide whether the lesion is a temporary one of conduction only (neuropraxia) or whether there has been a pathologic dissolution of continuity, requiring nerve regeneration for recovery. Electromyography may be of value here.

All the diseases mentioned in the differential diagnosis of monoplegia, hemiplegia, paraplegia, and quadriplegia will be discussed in the chapters on neurologic diseases.

MUSCULAR PARALYSIS AND SPASM UNATTENDED BY VISIBLE CHANGE IN NERVE OR MUSCLE

A discussion of motor paralysis would not be complete without some reference to a group of diseases that appear to have no basis in visible structural change in motor nerve cells, nerve fibers, motor endplates, and muscular fibers. This group is comprised of myasthenia gravis, myotonia congenita (Thomsen's disease), familial periodic paralysis, disorders of potassium, sodium, calcium, and magnesium metabolism, tetany, tetanus, botulinus poisoning, black widow spider bite, and the thyroid myopathies. In these diseases, each of which possesses a fairly distinctive clinical picture, the abnormality is purely biochemical, and even if the patient survives for a long time, no visible microscopic changes develop. An understanding of these diseases requires knowledge of the processes involved in nerve and muscle excitation and in the contraction of muscle. They will be discussed in Chap. 221.

46 TREMOR, CHOREA, AND OTHER ABNORMALITIES OF MOVEMENT AND POSTURE

Raymond D. Adams

In this chapter are discussed the automatic, static, and less modifiable postural activities of the human nervous system. These are believed, on good evidence, to be an expression of the activity of the *older motor system*, meaning, according to S. A. K. Wilson, who introduced this term, the extrapyramidal motor structures in the basal ganglions and brain stem.

In health, the activities of both the old (extrapyramidal) and the new (pyramidal) motor system are blended. The static postural activities are indispensable to voluntary, or willed, movement.

This close association of the pyramidal and extrapyramidal is shown by disease of the human nervous system. Lesions of the pyramidal tract result not only in paralysis of volitional movements of the contralateral half of the body but in the appearance of a fixed posture or attitude in which the arm is maintained in flexion and the leg in extension (predilection type of Wernicke-Mann). Similarly, decerebration from a lesion in the upper pons or midbrain releases another posture in which all four extremities are extended and the cervical and thoracolumbar spine dorsiflexed. In these released action patterns one has evidence of the postural and righting reflexes which are mediated through bulbospinal and other brain stem structures.

If an oversimplification may be permitted for clarity of exposition, the extrapyramidal motor system may be subdivided into two parts: (1) the striatopallidonigral and (2) the cerebellar. Disease in either of these parts will result in disturbances of movement and posture without significant paralysis. These two major systems and the symptoms that result when they are diseased are reviewed on the following pages.

EXTRAPYRAMIDAL MOTOR DISTURBANCES DUE PRIMARILY TO DISEASES OF THE BASAL GANGLIONS

Probably no area of neuroanatomy and neurophysiology has been developed more rapidly in the past 50 years than that of the basal ganglions; but despite immense research activity and a rapidly accumulating literature, it is not possible to write on this subject with any degree of finality.

Human clinicopathologic studies have yielded some of the most significant facts concerning the role of the basal ganglions in behavior. In 1912 S. A. K. Wilson delineated the syndrome of chronic lenticular degeneration, and in 1920 Oskar and Cecil Vogt described a number of other motor disturbances associated with lesions limited to the striatum. Lewy was one of the first to describe the pathology of paralysis agitans, and Tretiakoff (in postencephalitic forms) and Hassler (in paralysis agitans) have established the localization of at least part of the lesions in the substantia nigra. A long series of observations, the most recent ones being those of J. Purdon Martin, have demonstrated the relationship between a hemiballismus and hemichorea and lesions in the subthalamic nucleus of Luys. Unfortunately, many of the classic cases left much to be desired. In some instances the disease process was of diffuse type, and many other parts of the brain were affected, as in Wilson's hepatolenticular degeneration; even now the topography of the pathologic findings in several of these diseases (e.g., dystonia musculorum deformans) has not been fully determined.

Table 46-1 presents clinicopathologic correlations accepted by many neurologists; however, there is still much uncertainty as to finer details.

The symptoms that lend themselves best to clinical

Table 46-1. CLINICOPATHOLOGIC CORRELATIONS

Symptoms	Principal location of morbid anatomy
Unilateral plastic rigidity with static tremor (Parkinson's syndrome)	Contralateral substantia nigra plus (?) other structures
Unilateral hemiballismus and hemichorea	Contralateral subthalamic nucleus of Luys, prerubral area, and Forel's fields
Chronic chorea (Huntington's chorea)	Caudate nucleus, putamen, pallidum (?), and corpus Luysi
Athetosis and dystonia	Striatum and pallidum (?), thalami (?)
Cerebellar ataxia, i.e., intention tremor, slowness in starting and stopping, alternating, voluntary movements, hypotonia, rebound phenomenon	Homolateral cerebellar hemisphere or middle and inferior cerebellar peduncles, superior brachium conjunctivum (ipsilateral if below, contralateral if above the decussation)
Decerebrate rigidity, i.e., opisthotonos, extension of arms and legs, modification of these postures by turning of head and neck (increased extensor and decreased flexor tone on side toward which head is turned	Lesion usually bilateral in tegmentum involving red nuclei or structures between red nuclei and vestibular nuclei
Palatal and facial myoclonus (rhythmic)	Lesion in the central tegmental tract, inferior olivary nucleus, and olivodentate connections

analysis are rigidity, chorea, athetosis, dystonia, and tremor.

RIGIDITY, SPASTICITY, AND ALTERATIONS OF MUSCLE TONE IN ATHETOSIS

Already it has been pointed out that muscle tone (the small resistance to muscle stretch offered by healthy muscle) is enhanced in the many conditions that cause a paralysis of voluntary movement by interrupting the corticospinal tract. The special distribution of the increased tone, i.e., greater in antigravity muscles (extensors of leg and flexors of the arm in man), the sudden augmentation of tone with gradual yielding (the lengthening reaction or clasp-knife phenomenon) upon quick movement and the absence of resistance upon slow movement, and its disappearance in relaxed muscle with "electromyographic silence," and exaggerated tendon reflexes are the identifying characteristics of this spasticity. This type of hypertonus is believed in some instances to be due to hyperactivity of the small gamma motor neurones, with increase in the sensitivity of the spindle muscle fibers to stretch; in other instances it seems related to excessive activity of the larger alpha motor neurones. The "gamma spasticity" is abolished by procaine injection of the motor nerve (procaine paralyzes the small motor and sensory fibers, leaving the larger ones intact) without weakening the willed contractions of the muscle, whereas the "alpha spasticity" is not affected.

In the state known as *rigidity* the muscles are continuously or intermittently firm, tense, and prominent; and the resistance to passive movement is intense and even, like that noted in bending a lead pipe or in stretching a strand of toffee. Although present in all muscle groups, both flexor and extensor, on the whole, it tends to be more prominent in those which maintain a flexed posture, i.e., flexor muscles of trunk and limbs. It appears to be somewhat greater in the large muscle groups, but this may be merely a question of muscle mass. The smaller muscles of the face and tongue and even those of the larynx are often affected. The tendon reflexes are not enhanced. Nevertheless, like "gamma spasticity," this rigidity is said to be abolished by procaine (Rushworth and Walshe) and later Foerster had demonstrated that it is eradicated by posterior root section. In the electromyographic tracing, motor unit activity is more continuous than in spasticity, persisting even after relaxation.

A special type of rigidity, first noted by Negro in 1901, is the *cogwheel phenomenon*. When the hypertonic muscle is passively stretched, the resistance may be rhythmically jerky, as though the resistance of the limb were controlled by a ratchet. A number of different explanations of this phenomenon have been suggested. Wilson postulated it might be due to a minor form of the lengthening-shortening reaction, but a more likely explanation is an associated static tremor that is masked by rigidity during an attitude of repose but emerges faintly during manipulation.

Rigidity is prominent in paralysis agitans, postencephalitic Parkinson's syndrome, and some cases of athetosis and cerebral palsy.

The *tension hypertonus of athetosis* differs from both spasticity and rigidity. Strictly speaking, it takes two forms, one which occurs during the involuntary athetotic movement, the other which appears in the absence of any involuntary motion. Clinically these forms of hypertonus are variable from one moment to the next and are paradoxic in that they sometimes disappear during a rapid passive movement or when the limb is passively shaken. The tendon reflexes may be normal or brisk. The lengthening and shortening reactions are absent. This form of variable hypertonus is found in cases of double athetosis and choreoathetosis and in some cases of dystonia musculorum deformans. Usually in Sydenham's and Huntington's chorea a state of hypotonia prevails.

INVOLUNTARY MOVEMENTS

CHOREA. Derived from the Greek word meaning "dance," chorea refers to widespread arrhythmic movements of forcible, rapid, jerky type. These movements are involuntary and are noted for their irregularity, variability, relative speed, and brief duration. They are quite elaborate and of variable distribution. In some respects they resemble a voluntary movement; yet they never combine into a coordinated act. The patient may, however, incorporate them into a deliberate movement, as if to make them less noticeable. They may be limited to a limb or to an arm and leg on one side (hemichorea), or they may involve all parts of the body. They may cause grimacing or peculiar respiratory sounds; they may be superimposed on voluntary movements, giving to these a grotesque and exaggerated character. Usually they are discrete, but if very numerous, they may flow into one another; the resultant picture then resembles athetosis. Normal volitional movements are, of course, possible for there is usually no paralysis, but they too may be excessively quick and poorly sustained. The limbs are often unusually slack or hypotonic. A choreic movement may be superimposed on a tendon reflex, giving the "hung-up reflex." The tendon reflexes tend to be pendular; when the knee jerk is elicited with the patient sitting, the leg swings back and forth four or five times, like a pendulum, rather than one or two times as in a normal person.

Chorea appears in typical form in Sydenham's chorea and was noted also in the acute stages of epidemic encephalitis lethargica. In Huntington's chorea (chronic chorea) the movements are more typically choreoathetotic. Vascular lesions in the subthalamus, particularly those in and near the subthalamic nucleus of Luys, may result in wild flinging movements of the opposite arm and leg (hemiballismus). As these subside they become indistinguishable from chorea.

ATHETOSIS. This term is from a Greek word meaning "unfixed" or "changeable." The condition is characterized by an inability to sustain the fingers and toes in any one position in which they are placed and by continuous, slow, sinuous, purposeless movements. They are most pronounced in the digits and the hands but often involve the tongue, throat, and face. Basic patterns of movement, such as extension and pronation of the arm alternating with flexion and supination, and an alternate flexion and extension of the fingers, are evident in most cases. They may be unilateral, especially in children who have suffered a hemiplegia at some previous date (posthemiplegic athetosis). The movements are slower than those of chorea, but in many cases gradations between the two (choreoathetosis) are seen. Most athetotic patients exhibit variable degrees of motor deficit owing in some instances to associated pyramidal tract disease. Discrete individual movements of the tongue, lips, and hand are often impossible, and attempts to perform such voluntary movements result in a contraction of all the muscles in the limb (an intention spasm). Variable degrees of rigidity are generally associated, and these may account for the slow quality of athetosis in contrast to chorea. It must be admitted, however, that in some cases it is almost impossible to distinguish between chorea and athetosis.

Athetosis or choreoathetosis of all four limbs is a cardinal feature of a curious state known as double athetosis, which begins in childhood or adolescence. Athetosis appearing in the first months of life usually represents a congenital or postnatal condition such as hypoxia, kernicterus, or birth injury. Postmortem examination in some of the cases has disclosed a peculiar pathologic change of unknown etiology, a status marmoratus in the striatum; in others there has been a loss of medullated fibers, a status dysmyelinisatus, in the same regions.

TORSION SPASM, OR DYSTONIA. This is closely allied to athetosis, and the two may coexist. Dystonia is chiefly distinguished by the fact that it affects preponderantly the trunk musculature and proximal segment of the limbs. It results in fixed postures such as retraction of the head, excessive lordosis, and twisting of the trunk, as well as a variety of contortions. If it is mild, the dystonic movements cease at rest and the limbs are then quite flaccid. Involuntary spasm may return with voluntary movement.

Dystonia may be seen in the condition of double athetosis after hypoxic damage to the brain, in kernicterus, and rarely in Wilson's hepatolenticular degeneration. It is most characteristic in the syndrome designated dystonia musculorum deformans (Chap. 211). The etiology of this disorder is unknown.

Chorea, athetosis, and dystonia are all closely related. The movements are elaborate and depend for their expression on cortical mechanisms. Paralytic lesions involving the pyramidal tract abolish the involuntary movements. The hypotonia in chorea and some cases of athetosis, the pendular reflexes, and some degree of incoordination of movement are also reminiscent of the syndrome that follows disease of the cerebellum.

TREMOR. This consists of a more or less regular rhythmic oscillation of a part of the body around a fixed point, owing to alternate contractions of agonist and antagonist muscles. The rate is usually 3 to 6 beats per sec, but faster frequencies do occur; in any one individual the rate is fairly constant in all affected parts, regardless of the size of the involved muscle mass. It is generally most pronounced in the distal parts of the limb but may involve the head, tongue, face, and trunk.

There are many different types of tremor, and only a few are recognized as related to disease of the extrapyramidal motor system; but since tremors have not been discussed elsewhere, all the different types will be considered here.

Tremors can be classified in several ways. They may be subdivided according to their distribution, amplitude, regularity, and relationship to volitional movement. The following tremors should be familiar to every physician.

Static (Parkinsonian) Tremor. This is a coarse rhythmic tremor, with an average rate of 4 to 5 beats per sec, most often localized to one or both hands, the feet, or occasionally the jaw or tongue. Its most characteristic feature is that it occurs when the limb is in repose and is at least temporarily suppressed by willed movement. If the tremulous limb is completely relaxed, the tremor usually disappears but the average patient rarely achieves this degree of relaxation. In some cases the tremor is constant; in others it varies from time to time and may move from one group of muscles to another. It may be rather gentle and more or less limited to the distal muscles, as in paralysis agitans, or may be of wider range and involve proximal muscles as in postencephalitic Parkinson's disease and hepatolenticular degeneration. In many cases there is an associated rigidity of plastic type. The tremor interferes with voluntary movements surprisingly little; it is not uncommon to see a patient who has been trembling violently raise a full glass of water to his lips and drain the contents without spilling a drop. The handwriting of these patients is often small and cramped (micrographia). The gait may be of a festinating type (see Chap. 47, Disturbances of Gait). The combination of static tremor, slowness of movement, rigidity, and flexed postures without true paralysis constitutes Parkinson's syndrome. The exact pathologic anatomy of static tremor is unknown. In paralysis agitans and postencephalitic Parkinson's syndrome, the visible lesions are predominantly in the substantia nigra. In hepatocerebral degeneration, where this syndrome mixed with cerebellar ataxia occurs, the lesions are more diffuse. A similar tremor, without rigidity, slowness of movement, flexed postures, or masked facies, is seen in senile individuals. Unlike Parkinson's disease it does not progress.

Action Tremor. This term refers to a tremor present

when the limbs are actively maintained in a certain position, as when outstretched, and throughout voluntary movement. It may increase slightly as the action of the limbs becomes more precise, but it never approaches the degree of intention tremor. It disappears completely when the limbs are relaxed. Probably the *action tremor* is but an exaggeration of normal or physiologic tremor, which ranges from 6 to 8 per sec, being slower in childhood and old age. More particularly, it is a fine, 8 per sec tremor, somewhat irregular and involving the outstretched hand, head, and less often the lips and tongue, and it interferes little with voluntary movements such as handwriting and speech. This type of tremor is seen in numerous medical, neurologic, and psychiatric diseases and is therefore more difficult to interpret than static tremor. It may occur as the only neurologic abnormality in several members of a family and is then known as *familial* or *hereditary tremor*. Familial tremor persists throughout adult life and is worse when the patient is under observation. It is a source of embarrassment because it suggests to the onlooker that the patient is nervous. A curious fact about familial tremors is that one or two drinks of an alcoholic beverage may abolish them, and they may become worse after the effects of the alcohol have worn off. Similar tremors are seen in delirious states such as delirium tremens, in the chronic alcoholic patient as an isolated symptom, and in general paretics. An action tremor, usually more rapid than the above, is also characteristic of hyperthyroidism and other toxic states, and a similar tremor is frequently observed in patients suffering intense anxiety.

Intention Tremor. The word *intention* is ambiguous in this context because the tremor itself is not intentional. The tremor requires for its full expression the performance of an exacting, precise, willed movement. The term *ataxic tremor* is suggested by Mettler, for it is always combined with cerebellar ataxia. The tremor is absent when the limbs are in repose and during the first part of a voluntary movement, but as the action continues and greater precision of movement is demanded (e.g., in touching a target such as the patient's nose or the examiner's finger), a jerky, more or less rhythmic interruption of forward progression, with side-to-side oscillation, appears. It continues for a fraction of a second or so after the act is completed. The tremor may seriously interfere with the patient's performance of skilled acts. Sometimes the head is involved (*titubation*). This type of tremor invariably indicates disease of the cerebellum and of its connections. When the disease is very severe, every movement of the limb results in a wide-ranging tremor, a condition often seen in multiple sclerosis, Wilson's disease, and vascular lesions of midbrain and subthalamus.

Hysterical Tremor. Hysterical tremors may simulate any of the aforementioned varieties and are difficult to diagnose. One notable feature is that they usually do not correspond to any of the better known types of organic tremor. Most often they are restricted to a limb and are seldom as regular as the static tremors of paralysis agitans. If the affected limb is restrained by the examiner, the tremor may move to another part of the body. It persists during movement and at rest and is less subject to the modifying influences of posture and willed movement than are organic tremors. In the author's experience this manifestation of hysteria is exceedingly rare.

OTHER INVOLUNTARY MOVEMENTS. There are other abnormalities of movement, about which only a few words can be said. They vary from simple irritative phenomena to complex psychologic phenomena such as compulsions. Many have no particular relation to the extrapyramidal motor system but may be conveniently discussed here. The reader should consult a standard text on neurology for further details.

Spasmodic Torticollis. This is an intermittent or continuous spasm of sternomastoid, trapezius, and other neck muscles, usually on one side, with turning or tipping of the head. It is involuntary and cannot be inhibited and differs from habit spasm or tic. The author thinks that this condition should be considered a form of dystonia. It is worse when the patient sits, stands, or walks, and contactual stimulation of the chin or of the back of the head partially alleviates the muscle imbalance. Psychiatric treatment is ineffectual. In severe cases muscle sectioning, neurectomy, section of the anterior cervical roots, or cryothalamotomy have given favorable results.

Tics and Habit Spasms. Many individuals throughout life are prone to habitual movements such as sniffing, clearing the throat, protruding the chin, or blinking whenever tense. The patient will admit that the movements are voluntary and that he feels compelled to make them in order to relieve tension; they can be inhibited by effort of will. In certain cases they become so ingrained that the person is unaware of them and unable to control them. Children between five and ten years of age are especially liable to habit spasms. The movements are often purposive coordinated acts, originally provoked by some physical or emotional stimulus and continued as a habit. They are arrhythmic and stereotyped. Multiple convulsive tics (*Gilles de la Tourette's disease*) is a more severe form of the same condition. In children it is best to ignore the habit spasm and at the same time to arrange for more rest and a calmer environment. In adults relief of nervous tension by tranquilizing drugs and psychotherapy is helpful, but the disposition to tic formation persists.

Myoclonus. Several different motor phenomena are included under this term. Some neurologists use it to denote a brief contraction of a single muscle or part of a muscle. Again, it has been applied to a sudden abrupt contraction of a group of muscles, regardless of their functional state. The latter contractions may be arrhythmic and diffuse or rhythmic and confined to one part of the body. An example of the latter phenomenon is nystagmus of the palate, or *palatal myoclonus* (rhythmic contractions of the soft palate and pharyngeal muscles and sometimes of the vocal cords, diaphragm, or facial muscles, at the rate of 10 to 50 or more per min). The lesions producing this sign, whether vascular, neoplastic, or encephalitic, have been situated in all instances in the central tegmental tract, in the inferior olivary nucleus, or in the olivocerebellar tracts. Diffuse arrhythmic myoclonus is sometimes associated with dementia and epilepsy and has been referred to as the *familial myoclonic epilepsy of Unverricht and Lundborg*. In the author's opinion, this myoclonus is a form of epilepsy, a disseminate form of epilepsia partialis continua. Other familial and nonfamilial forms in childhood are due to inclusion-body encephalitis or lipid-storage diseases and in adulthood to a degenerative cerebral disease of unknown etiology, associated with dementia, i.e., Jakob-Creutzfeldt disease, and as a sequel to hypoxic encephalopathy. Isolated myoclonic jerks occur in epileptic patients, particularly in children with petit mal. This is the most frequent form of arrhythmic myoclonus.

One of the most remarkable discoveries of recent years, to be credited largely to the pioneering efforts of Meyer and Cooper, has been the abolition of tremors, rigidity, and involuntary movements of the limbs by a surgical lesion in the medial segment of the globus pallidus or the ventrolateral nucleus of the thalamus. The effects are contralateral. Usually the lesion has been made by the injection first of procaine (Novocain) and then alcohol, by cooling and freezing (Cooper), by electrocoagulation (White and Sweet and Leksell), by ultrasound (Meyer), or by a proton beam (Leksell). The operation has been successful in temporarily alleviating tremor or rigidity in a high percentage of cases of unilateral paralysis agitans and the postural abnormality in dystonia musculorum deformans and double athetosis. It has been perfected to the point where the mortality is relatively low, less than 1 per cent, and the risk of hemiplegia or some other sequel is less than 10 per cent. The therapeutic effect indicates that the pallidum and ventrolateral nucleus, possibly through their connections with the cerebral cortex (motor cortex and its pyramidal pathway), are essential for the expression of these extrapyramidal syndromes. The indications for these surgical procedures are discussed in Chap. 211.

EXTRAPYRAMIDAL MOTOR DISTURBANCES DUE PRIMARILY TO DISEASES OF THE CEREBELLUM

Isolated lesions in the midline flocculonodular lobe result in grave disturbances of equilibrium. Often the symptoms are exhibited only when the patient attempts to stand and walk. He sways, staggers, titubates, and reels (see under Cerebellar Gait, Chap. 47). There may be no disturbance in coordination and no intention tremor of the limbs. A midline tumor of the cerebellum, such as a medulloblastoma, usually produces this syndrome.

Extensive lesions of one cerebellar hemisphere, especially the anterior lobe, cause disturbances of volitional movements of the ipsilateral arm and leg. This is known as *ataxia*. The movements "are characterized by an inappropriate range, rate and strength of each of the various components of the motor act and by an improper sequence of those components." Electromyographic analysis has shown that ataxia is manifested as a decomposition of movement consisting of abnormal duration and sequences of bursts of contraction and relaxation of agonists and antagonists of a joint, usually a large joint (Carrera and Mettler). This incoordination is also called an *asynergia*. The defects are particularly noticeable in acts that require rapid alternation of movements. Slowness in acceleration and deceleration, which is almost invariably present, impedes the performance. The direction of purposive movement is frequently inaccurate. Owing to delay in arresting the movement, it may overshoot its mark. The antagonist muscles do not come into play at the proper time, possibly because of the hypotonia that is almost always present. This may be demonstrated by having the patient flex his arm against a resistance that is suddenly released. The patient with cerebellar disease will sometimes strike his face because he fails to check the flexion movement (Holmes rebound phenomenon). In movements requiring accurate direction, as the limb approaches its destination it may stop short and then advance by a more or less rhythmic series of jerks. In addition to hypotonia, there may be, in acute cerebellar lesions, some slight weakness. Bilateral lesions of the cerebellar hemispheres and midline flocculonodular lobe lead to such a severe disturbance in all movements that the patient may be unable to stand or walk or use his limbs effectively. In addition, there are ocular and speech disturbances, namely, nystagmus, skew deviation of the eyes, and dysarthria. Lesions of the cerebellar peduncles have the same effect as extensive hemispheral lesions. This syndrome of one cerebellar hemisphere (neocerebellum) may be observed in a tumor or abscess of the cerebellar hemisphere or in vascular lesions of the brain stem and cerebellar peduncles. It tends to be bilateral and symmetric in primary atrophy or degeneration of the cerebellum.

EXAMINATION AND DIFFERENTIAL DIAGNOSIS

In Chap. 45 the methods of examining the motor system were described at some length, so only a few additional remarks concerning extrapyramidal disorders need to be made here. These abnormalities are best demonstrated by seeing the patient in action. If he complains of a limp after walking a distance or of difficulty in climbing stairs, he should be observed under these conditions. Tests of rate, regularity, and coordination of voluntary movement must be sufficiently varied and demanding of the patient's motor coordination to bring out the defect. The physician must cultivate the habit of accurately observing and describing abnormalities of movement and not be content merely to give the condition a name or force it into some category such as chorea or tic or myoclonus. The main postures of the body in all common acts should be noted. Aside from the assessment of muscle power and of gait, the usual test applied to the upper limb is to ask the patient to touch the examiner's finger tip and then the tip of his own nose repeatedly (finger-to-nose test). In testing the leg the patient is asked to place his heel on one knee and then to run it down his shin and back to the knee (heel-to-knee-to-shin test). Finer movements of the hand may be tested by having the patient successively touch each finger to his thumb or pat his thigh rapidly or by having him use tools or handle objects. The performance of rapidly alternating movements such as pronation and supination of the hands is another valuable test.

The fully developed extrapyramidal motor syndromes can be recognized without difficulty once the physician has become familiar with the typical pictures. He should form a mental picture of Parkinson's syndrome with its slowness of movement, poverty of facial expression, static tremor and rigidity, and absence of true paralysis or reflex changes. Similarly, the gross distortions and postural abnormalities of dystonia, whether widespread in trunk muscles or involving only neck muscles, as in spasmodic torticollis, should be familiar. Athetosis with its instability of postures and ceaseless movements of fingers and hands, intention spasm, and chorea with its abrupt and complicated movements that flit over the body are other standard syndromes. Characteristic of all are the lack of pyramidal signs (i.e., motor paralysis, spasticity, increased tendon reflexes, and Babinski's sign), the effects of emotional stimuli (which invariably exaggerate the symptoms), the quieting effect of relaxation and sleep, and the presence of a mild defect in voluntary movement.

The clinical differences between pyramidal and extrapyramidal disorders are summarized in Table 46-2.

Early or mild forms of these conditions, like all medical diseases, may offer special difficulties in diagnosis. Cases of paralysis agitans, seen before the appearance of tremor, are often overlooked. The patient may complain of being nervous and restless or may have experienced an indescribable stiffness and aching in certain parts of the body. Because of the absence of weakness or of reflex changes, the case may be considered psychogenic or rheumatic. It is well to remember that Parkinson's syndrome often begins in a hemiplegic distribution, and the case may be misdiagnosed as cerebral thrombosis. A slight masking of the face, a suggestion of a limp, blepharoclonus (uninhibited blinking of eyes when the bridge of the nose is tapped), a mild rigidity, failure of an arm to swing naturally in walking, or loss of certain movements of cooperation will help in diagnosis at this time. Every case presenting the syndrome of Parkinson or other abnormality of movement and posture in adolescence or early adult life should be surveyed for hepatolenticular degeneration by tests of liver function, slit-lamp examination for corneal pigmentation (Kayser-Fleischer ring); if facilities are available, urinary amino-nitrogen excretion and copper excretion should be determined.

Mild or early chorea is often mistaken for simple nervousness. If one sits for a time and watches the patient, the diagnosis will often become evident. There are cases, nonetheless, in which it is impossible to distinguish simple nervousness from early Sydenham's chorea, especially in children, and there is no laboratory test that one can depend upon. The first postural manifestation of dystonia may suggest hysteria, and it is only later, when the fixity of the postural abnormality, the lack of the usual psychologic picture of hysteria, and the relentlessly progressive character of the illness become evident, that accurate diagnosis is reached. Another common error is to assume that a bedfast patient who has complained of dizziness, staggering, and headaches and exhibits no other neurologic abnormality is suffering from hysteria. The flocculonodular cerebellar syndrome is demonstrable only when the patient attempts to stand and walk.

Table 46-2. CLINICAL DIFFERENCES BETWEEN PYRAMIDAL AND EXTRAPYRAMIDAL SYNDROMES

	Pyramidal	Extrapyramidal
Character of rigidity	Clasp-knife effect	Plastic, equal throughout passive movement or intermittent (cogwheel rigidity)
Distribution of rigidity	Flexors of arms, extensors of legs	Flexors of all four limbs and trunk
Shortening and lengthening reaction	Present	Absent
Involuntary movements	Absent	Presence of tremors, chorea, athetosis, dystonia
Tendon reflexes	Increased	Normal or slightly increased
Babinski's sign	Present	Absent
Paralysis of voluntary movement	Present	Absent or slight

REFERENCES

Carrera, R. M. E., and F. A. Mettler: Function of the Primate Brachium Conjunctivum and Related Structures, J. Comp. Neurol., 102:151, 1955.

Denny-Brown, D.: "Diseases of the Basal Ganglia and Subthalamic Nuclei," New York, Oxford University Press, 1945.

Martin, J. Purdon and Ian R. McCaul: Acute Hemiballismus Treated by Ventrolateral Thalamolysis, Brain, 82:104, 1959.

47   VERTIGO AND DISORDERS OF EQUILIBRIUM AND GAIT

Maurice Victor and Raymond D. Adams

The terms to describe sensations of unbalance are often rather ambiguous, and the patient must be carefully questioned. He often uses *dizziness* to indicate not only a sense of rotation but also vague sensory experiences such as unsteadiness, insecurity, weakness, faintness, and light-headedness. *Giddiness* has almost the same significance, with perhaps more implication of altered consciousness and swaying sensation. *Vertigo* literally means "sense of turning" either of one's body or of the surroundings, a definition which, with a few important qualifications to be mentioned below, is used throughout this chapter. *Equilibrium* refers simply to a state of balance or equipoise in which opposing forces such as gravity and postural reflexes exactly counteract each other.

Disorders of equilibrium are suitably considered in connection with dizziness and vertigo because of their frequent conjunction (vertiginous ataxia). However, there are other disorders of equilibrium quite independent of vertigo, e.g., those due to a loss of joint and muscle sense (sensory ataxia) or cerebellar disease (cerebellar ataxia). These are also considered briefly in this chapter.

ANATOMIC, PHYSIOLOGIC, AND PSYCHOLOGIC CONSIDERATIONS

Several mechanisms are responsible for the maintenance of a balanced posture and make us aware of the body's position in relation to its surroundings—afferent impulses from the eyes, labyrinths, muscles, and joints inform us of the position of the body in space. In response to these impulses the organism makes fine and rapid adjustments to maintain equilibrium. Normally we are unaware of these adaptive movements, since they operate for the most part at a reflex level. The most important of the afferent impulses are the following:

1. Impulses from the retina and possibly proprioceptive impulses from the ocular muscles.

2. Impulses from the labyrinths, which are highly specialized spatial proprioceptors. The primary function of the semicircular canals and the vestibule is to register changes in direction of motion (either acceleration or deceleration) and in the position of the body. The semicircular canals respond to movement and angular momentum, and the otoliths—the sense organs of the utricle and saccule—are mainly concerned with orienting the organism in reference to gravity.

3. Impulses from the proprioceptors of the joints and muscles. Those from the neck are of special importance in relating the position of the head to the rest of the body.

All the afferent nerve fibers from these sense organs are connected with the cerebellum, the vestibular nuclei, the red nuclei, and other brain stem ganglionic centers. These are the central structures concerned with regulating posture.

Important psychologic phenomena are also involved in the maintenance of equilibrium, namely, those which deal with the relationship between ourselves and the external world. We learn to perceive that portion of space occupied by our body and construct from sensory data a general concept, called by some neurologists the *body schema*. The space around our body, i.e., the external world, is then said to be represented by another schema. These two schemas are neither static nor independent: they are constantly being modified and adapted to one another; their interdependence is ascribed to the fact that the various sense organs which supply the information on which the two schemas are based are usually simultaneously activated by any movement of our bodies. By a process of learning we see objects as having motion or being still, when we are either moving or stationary. Motion of an object in space is always relative. At times, especially when our own sensory experience is incomplete, we mistake movement of our surroundings for movements of our own body as, for example, the feeling of movement which is experienced in a stationary train when a neighboring train is moving. Hence, in this frame of reference, orientation of the body in space is possible only by the maintenance of an orderly relationship between the body schema and the schema of the external world. As a corollary, disorientation in space, or disequilibrium, occurs when this relationship is upset.

On clinical grounds, disorders of equilibrium may be divided into three groups: (1) true vertigo; (2) pseudovertigo, or giddiness; and (3) abnormalities of equilibrium without either vertigo or giddiness.

VERTIGO

CHARACTERISTICS. In disorders in which vertigo is a leading symptom, the patient's history assumes special importance in diagnosis, for this symptom may be accompanied by no objective signs. The diagnosis of vertigo is an easy matter when the patient reports that objects in his environment spun around, or his body was turning, or his head was spinning. Very often, however, he is not so explicit. He may state that there was a feeling of to-and-fro or up-and-down movement of the body, usually the head; or he may relate that objects in his environment suddenly sank or rose up toward him or that he was pulled strongly to one side or to the ground. The feeling of impulsion is particularly characteristic of vertigo; the patient feels that he is impelled or moved by some force acting outside his body. In walking he may feel unsteady, tending to veer to one side. In exceptionally severe attacks the patient may without warning be thrown violently to the ground and only then experience vertigo, nausea, and vomiting. If vertigo is at all severe, equilibrium is almost invariably affected and the patient usually notes that his symptoms are especially troublesome when he attempts to sit, stand, and walk. With intense vertigo it may be impossible for him to do so. This type of gait disturbance, which depends on an abnormality of labyrinthine or vestibular function, may be called *vertiginous ataxia*. It is noteworthy that under these circumstances the coordination of individual movements of the limbs is never impaired. With milder degrees of vertigo, the patient may have difficulty in describing his symptoms. It may help to ask him whether his present symptoms are similar to the feelings of movement one experiences when coming to a halt after being rapidly rotated.

The symptoms of vertigo are usually paroxysmal and of short duration, but at times they may linger for weeks or even months. The chronic state may or may not follow an acute attack; in this latter instance the patient complains of a continuous state of imbalance, swaying, or a vague sense of movement in the environment. Characteristically the vertigo is made worse or may only become manifest when the patient assumes a certain posture, stands upright, or moves. For these reasons and because of fear of falling he must walk carefully.

DISTINCTION BETWEEN TRUE AND FALSE VERTIGO. It is important to distinguish clearly between true vertigo and a second group of symptoms, which do not have the same significance (*pseudovertigo*). In the latter condition the patient may describe a feeling of uncertainty, light-headedness, or a swimming sensation; or he may feel as though he is going to fall or is walking on air. These sensory phenomena are particularly common in psychoneurotic states and in introspective individuals with an overawareness of various body parts. Other peculiar aberrations, such as, for example, a feeling of lengthening of the legs or a sensation as if the ground were receding, are remarked upon. A feeling of light-headedness is frequently brought about by hyperventilation, and similar symptoms often occur in patients with anemia, hypertension, and pulmonary disease, particularly emphysema. In anemia, mild hypoxia is the probable mechanism, and ischemia is probably the cause in emphysematous patients, in whom an attack of coughing may lead to dizziness or even fainting, owing to impaired venous return to the heart (tussive syncope). The dizziness that so often accompanies hypertension is more difficult to evaluate. In some cases it may be due to associated nervousness; in others, one cannot be sure that it does not depend upon transient changes in the

intracranial vasculature. *Postural* dizziness is a closely related complaint. Poorly conditioned individuals and many elderly persons, especially if they have cerebrovascular disease, are troubled upon arising from a recumbent position or after stooping with a momentary giddiness or a swaying type of dizziness with dimming of vision or spots before the eyes. In the elderly arteriosclerotic person there need be no fall in brachial blood pressure at the time of symptom production. The condition is probably due to a momentary failure of reflex vasoconstriction in overcoming the "pooling" effect of gravity upon the circulating blood. This type of dizziness may occur in normal individuals on arising and is more pronounced after a hot bath; it is frequent in patients convalescing from debilitating illness. A mild syncopal reaction of any type may give rise to similar symptoms and may be described by the patient as "dizziness." Finally, petit mal epilepsy may be referred to as a "dizzy spell."

In practice it is not difficult to separate these symptoms from true vertigo; there is not the feeling of rotation nor of impulsion so characteristic of the latter. In addition, a number of ancillary symptoms accompany true vertigo, including varying degrees of nausea, vomiting, headache, pallor, and sweating. Actual loss of consciousness may occur as part of a vertiginous attack, but it is very rare and usually signifies another category of disorder such as syncope or convulsion. Both the vertigo and the nausea and vomiting are made worse by movement, so that characteristically the vertiginous patient remains immobile with eyes closed during an attack.

NEUROLOGIC SIGNIFICANCE. A disorder of any of the following structures may give rise to vertigo.

1. Cerebral cortex
2. Ocular muscles
3. Cerebellum
4. Labyrinthine-vestibular apparatus
5. Brain stem

Vertigo may constitute the aura of an epileptic seizure, which gives support to the view that a *cortical lesion* can produce vertigo. This usually occurs with lesions of the temporal lobe, mainly on the lateral aspect of the middle and posterior portions or at the parietotemporal junction. The patients experience a sensation of movement, either of their body away from the side of stimulation or of the environment in the opposite direction. This observation also supports the concept that the sensation of vertigo depends largely on the perception of relative movement between the body and the external world. Vertiginous seizures may occur very rarely as a reflex phenomenon, the result of vestibular (e.g., caloric) stimulation.

Ocular disturbances may give rise to vertigo and may even be accompanied by staggering and nausea; this occurs most frequently at the outset of an ocular muscle paralysis when the patient looks in the direction of action of the paralyzed muscle. The vertigo is apparently due to a faulty projection of the visual field, the patient being presented with two conflicting images. Some people experience a type of giddiness or uncertainty when wearing bifocal lenses for the first time. The necessity of adapting to an unusual visual environment, as in looking down from a height, may result in a similar sensation.

Whether *lesions of the cerebellum* can produce vertigo seems to depend on what portion of this structure is involved. Thus vertigo may be absent despite large lesions of the cerebellar hemispheres but present if the vestibulocerebellar connections are damaged.

Although cortical, ocular, and cerebellar causes should all be considered in the differential diagnosis of vertigo, they are clinically uncommon. Usually the problem resolves itself into deciding whether vertigo has its origin in the labyrinth, in the vestibular division of the eighth cranial nerve, or in the vestibular nuclei and their immediate connections with other structures in the brain stem. A number of features, especially the form of the attack and the associated symptoms, help in this decision.

Vertigo of labyrinthine origin (aural vertigo) tends to occur in paroxysmal attacks. It has an abrupt onset, is maximal at the beginning, and subsides in a matter of minutes or in an hour or two. Similarly, the nausea, vomiting, pallor, immobility, and ataxia associated with the attack are short-lived. The accompanying nystagmus tends also to be transient and characteristically is rather fine, rotatory, and most pronounced when the eyes are turned away from the offending labyrinth. Occasionally, patients with labyrinthine disease may have a more chronic form of vertigo. However, it seldom continues for more than a few days or weeks, the central mechanisms apparently compensating for the peripheral lesion. Labyrinthine vertigo is frequently associated with deafness and tinnitus, since the pathologic process in the inner ear encroaches on the cochlear apparatus.

Vertigo of brain stem origin usually lasts much longer than aural vertigo and may disorganize the patient's equilibrium for several weeks or even longer. In these cases, auditory function is usually spared, since vestibular and cochlear fibers become separated soon after entering the brain stem. It is a fairly reliable clinical rule that the combination of auditory and vestibular symptoms occurs only in diseases that involve the inner ear or eighth cranial nerve. The nystagmus accompanying central lesions tends to be coarse and protracted, is more marked on lateral gaze to one side than the other, and may have a vertical component, particularly on upward gaze. Vertical nystagmus nearly always indicates disease of the brain stem. A small plaque of multiple sclerosis may affect vestibular connections, and this diagnosis should always be considered when a young person has a severe and protracted attack of vertigo without auditory symptoms. Vascular and neoplastic lesions may also give rise to vertigo through involvement of the vestibular nuclei and their immediate connections. In addition, there may be signs of interference with the long sensory and motor tracts that pass through the brain

stem. This feature clearly points to a brain stem location of the lesion and is, in the final analysis, the most important point in differentiation from aural vertigo.

DIAGNOSIS

When the patient's complaint is dizziness, it is first necessary to obtain a clear description of the symptoms. The element of rotation or a similar sensation, the sense of impulsion, and the accompanying nausea and vomiting, if present, usually distinguish the case of true vertigo from one of giddiness. The latter has no element of rotation or impulsion, and nausea, vomiting, tinnitus, and deafness are absent. Although fearful of falling or swooning, the patient can nonetheless walk without difficulty if forced to do so. Blurred vision, smothering and choking feelings, palpitation, trembling, sweating, and a sense of fear or apprehension complete the usual clinical picture of neurotic dizziness. Frequently in cases of recurrent aural vertigo i.e., Ménière's syndrome, symptoms of anxiety and depression may be added to the total clinical picture, which adds to the difficulty of interpretation.

If the physician is uncertain whether the patient has vertigo or dizziness, it is sometimes helpful to induce these sensations in order that the patient may compare them with his usual attacks. This can be done by having the patient breathe deeply for 3 min (which causes giddiness in most persons), stoop over for a minute and then straighten up (postural giddiness), and, while standing, turn rapidly in one direction ten times in order to provoke vertigo. If the patient fails to distinguish these sensations, his history is probably inaccurate and he should be asked to take careful note of his sensations during his next spontaneous attack.

In some cases the attack may be so abrupt and severe that the patient falls immediately to the ground without loss of consciousness. Here the diagnosis may be clarified by nausea, vomiting, and dizziness, which almost invariably follow such a fall. If the vertigo has been very mild in degree, it is helpful to elicit a history of disinclination to walk during the attack, a tendency to list to one side, discomfort in sitting or riding in a vehicle, and a preference for maintaining one position fixedly.

A neurologic examination, including tests of ocular movements and nystagmus, cranial nerve function, gait, and coordination of limbs, should be carried out on all patients with dizziness as the presenting complaint. The eardrums should be inspected and hearing tested by the methods indicated in Chap. 48. Vestibular function should also be tested. This is usually done by irrigating the ear with 5 ml ice water, the head being tilted back 30° from the vertical, since in this position the horizontal canal is stimulated maximally. The normal labyrinthine responses consist of falling to the side of the vestibular lesion, past-pointing to that side, and rotary nystagmus on gaze to the opposite side. The nystagmus begins about 20 sec after the irrigation and persists for 90 to 120 sec. The duration of these periods is variable, however, and comparison of the affected and normal labyrinths is more important.

DISTURBANCES OF GAIT

Probably no aspect of neurology is more interesting or affords greater opportunity for brilliant diagnosis than the study and analysis of gait.

The normal gait seldom attracts attention. The body is erect, the head straight, and the arms hang loosely and gracefully at the sides, each moving rhythmically forward with the opposite leg. The feet are slightly everted, and the steps are of moderate length and approximately equal. With each step there is coordinated flexion of hip and knee and dorsiflexion of foot and a barely perceptible elevation of the hip so that the foot clears the ground. The heel strikes the ground first, and inspection of shoes will show that this part is most subject to wear. In the erect posture, the muscles of greatest importance in maintaining equilibrium are the erector spinae and the extensors of the hips and knees.

There are many individual variations of gait, and it is a commonplace observation that the sound of an individual's footsteps, notably his pace and heaviness of tread, may identify him. The manner of walking and the carriage of the body provide clues to character and personality and sometimes indicate occupation. Furthermore, the gaits of the male and the female differ, the steps of the latter being quicker and shorter and the movement of the trunk and hips more graceful and delicate. Certain female characteristics of gait, if observed in the male, immediately impart an impression of femininity; or male characteristics in the female, one of masculinity.

When confronted with a disorder of gait, the examiner must observe the patient's natural stance and the attitude and dominant positions of the legs, trunk, and arms. It is good practice to watch the patient as he walks into the examining room, because he is apt to walk more naturally then than during special tests. He should be asked to stand with his feet together, head erect, with eyes first open and then closed. Swaying due to nervousness may be overcome by asking that he touch the tip of his nose with the finger of first one hand and then the other. Next the patient should be asked to walk forward and backward, with his eyes first open and then closed. Any tendency to reel to one side, as in cerebellar disease, can be checked by having him walk around a chair. When the affected side is toward the chair, the patient tends to walk into it; and when it is away from the chair, he veers outward in ever-widening circles. More delicate tests of gait are walking a straight line heel to toe (Frenkel's test) or having the patient arise quickly from a chair and walk briskly, and then stop or turn suddenly (Fournier's tests). If all these tests are successfully executed, it may be assumed that any difficulty in locomotion is not due to disease of the proprioceptive mechanisms

or cerebellum. Detailed neurologic examination is then necessary in order to determine which of the many other possible diseases is responsible for the patient's disorder of gait.

The following abnormal gaits are so distinctive that with a little practice they can be recognized at a glance.

CEREBELLAR GAIT. The main features of this gait are *wide base* (separation of legs), *unsteadiness, irregularity,* and *lateral reeling.* Steps are short and uncertain, with sudden lurching to one side or the other. The unsteadiness is more prominent on quickly arising from a chair and walking, on stopping suddenly while walking, or on turning abruptly. If the ataxia is severe, the patient cannot stand without assistance. Standing with feet together and head erect, with eyes either opened or closed, may be difficult. In its mildest form the ataxia is best demonstrated by having the patient walk a line heel to toe. After two or three steps he loses his balance and must step to one side to avoid falling. Romberg's sign, i.e., marked swaying or falling with the eyes closed but not with the eyes open, is not a feature of cerebellar disease. The abnormality of gait may or may not be accompanied by other signs of cerebellar incoordination and intention tremor of the arms and legs. The presence of the latter signs depends on involvement of the cerebellar hemispheres as distinct from anterior and midline structures; if the lesion is unilateral, they are always on the same side. Cerebellar gait is most commonly seen in multiple sclerosis, medulloblastoma of the cerebellar vermis, and the cerebellar atrophies.

GAIT OF SENSORY ATAXIA. This is due to an impairment of kinesthetic sensation resulting from interruption of afferent nerve fibers in the peripheral nerves, posterior roots, posterior columns of the spinal cord, or medial lemnisci; it may also be produced by a lesion of both parietal lobes. Whatever the location of the lesion, the patient is deprived of knowledge of the position of his limbs. The principal features of the resulting gait disorder are the *uncertainty,* the *irregularity,* and the *stamp* of the feet. Hunt characterized this type of gait very well when he said that the ataxic patient is recognized by "his stamp and his stick." There is great difficulty in standing and walking, and in advanced cases there is a complete failure of locomotion, although muscular power is retained. The legs are kept far apart to correct the instability, and the patient carefully watches the ground and his legs. As he steps out, the legs are flung brusquely forward and outward, often lifted higher than necessary. The steps are of variable length, and many are attended by an audible stamp as the foot is banged down on the floor. The body is held in a slightly flexed position, and the weight may be supported on the cane the severely ataxic patient so often carries. The incoordination is greatly exaggerated when the patient is deprived of visual cues, as in walking in the dark. When asked to stand with feet together and eyes closed, he shows increased swaying or actual falling (Romberg's sign).

It has been said that a lame man whose shoes are not worn in any one place is probably suffering from sensory ataxia. There is almost invariably a loss of vibratory and position sense in the feet and legs. Gaits of this type are observed in tabes dorsalis, Friedreich's ataxia, subacute combined degeneration, syphilitic meningomyelitis, chronic polyneuritis, and those cases of multiple sclerosis in which posterior column disease predominates.

HEMIPLEGIC AND PARAPLEGIC (SPASTIC) GAITS. In hemiplegia the leg is held rigidly and does not swing freely and gracefully at the knee and hip. It tends to rotate outward and describes a semicircle, first away from and then toward the trunk (circumduction). The foot scrapes along the floor, and the outer side of the sole of the shoe is worn. One can diagnose the hemiplegic gait by hearing the slow rhythmic scuff of the foot along the floor. The other muscles of the body on the affected side are weak and stiff to a variable degree, particularly the arm, which is carried in a flexed position and does not swing naturally. This type of gait disorder is most frequent after vascular disease of the brain.

The spastic paraplegic gait is entirely different from the gait of sensory ataxia, though the two may be combined. Each leg is advanced slowly and stiffly with restricted motion at the knee and hip. The patient looks as though he were wading in water. The legs are extended or slightly bent at the knees and may be strongly adducted at the hips, tending almost to cross ("scissors" gait). The steps are regular and short. The forepart of the shoe becomes worn because there is a tendency for the advancing foot not to clear the ground. Movements are generally slow, and the patient may be able to advance only with great effort. The laity have referred to this state as "creeping palsy." An easy way to remember the main features of this gait is by the letter S, which begins each of its descriptive adjectives—spastic, slow, scuffing. Cerebral spastic diplegia, multiple sclerosis, syringomyelia, spinal syphilis, combined system disease, and spinal cord compression are the common causes of spastic paraparesis.

FESTINATING GAIT. This term comes from the Latin word *festinatio*, haste, and is appropriate for the gait disorder of both paralysis agitans and postencephalitic Parkinson's syndrome. The general attitude is one of flexion. Rigidity or immobility of the body is another conspicuous feature. The trunk is bent forward, and the arms are carried ahead of the body. There is a paucity of the automatic movements made in sitting, standing, and walking. The arms do not swing; the head does not turn on looking to one side; the arms are seldom folded, and the legs are rarely crossed. The hands are held stiffly as though in preparation for writing, and the facial expression is unblinking and mask-like. The legs are stiff and bent at knee and hip. The steps are short, and the feet barely clear the ground as the patient shuffles along. Once forward or backward locomotion is started, the upper part of the body advances ahead of the lower part, as though the patient were chasing his center of gravity. His steps become more and more rapid, and he may fall if not assisted. This is the festination, and it may occur when the patient is walking forward or backward, taking the form of either propulsion or retropulsion. *Rigidity, shuffling, and festination* are the cardinal features of this gait; and when they are joined to typical tremors, generalized rigidity, and slowness of movement, there can be no doubt as to the diagnosis. Other unusual gaits are sometimes observed in the postencephalitic patient. For example, he may be unable to take his first step forward until he hops or takes one step backward; or walking may be initiated by a series of short steps that give way to a more normal gait; occasionally such a patient may run better than he walks.

ATHETOTIC, DYSTONIC, AND CHOREIC GAITS. These are less common than the preceding gait disorders. The athetotic patient is rigid, and his body often assumes the most grotesque postures. One arm may be held aloft and the other one behind the body with wrist and fingers alternately undergoing slow flexion, extension, and rotation. The head may be inclined in one direction, the lips alternately retract and then purse, and the tongue intermittently protrudes from the mouth. The legs advance slowly and awkwardly. Sometimes the foot is plantar flexed at the ankle, and the weight is carried on the toes; or it may be dorsiflexed or inverted. This type of gait is typical of congenital athetosis.

In dystonia musculorum deformans the first symptom may be a limp due to inversion or plantar flexion of the foot or a distortion of the pelvis. The patient stands with one leg rigidly extended or one shoulder elevated. The trunk may be in a position of exaggerated lordosis and the hips are partly flexed, with a tilting forward of the pelvis. Because of the muscle spasms that deform the body in this manner, the patient may have to walk with knees flexed. The gait may seem normal as the first steps are taken, but as the patient walks, one or both legs become flexed, giving rise to the "dromedary" gait. In the more advanced stages walking becomes impossible, owing to torsion of the trunk or the continuous flexion of one leg.

In *chorea* the gait is often bizarre. As the patient stands or walks there is a continuous play of irregular "choreic" movements affecting the face, neck, and hands and, in the advanced stages, the large proximal joints and trunk. The positions of the trunk and upper parts of the body vary with each step. There are jerks of the head, grimacing, squirming, twisting movements of the trunk and limbs, and peculiar respiratory noises. The general features of these conditions are described more fully in Chaps. 46 and 211.

STEPPAGE, DROP-FOOT, OR EQUINE GAIT. This is caused by paralysis of the pretibial and peroneal muscles. The legs must be lifted abnormally high in order to clear the ground. There is a flapping noise as the foot strikes the floor. The anterior and lateral border of the sole becomes worn. The steps are regular and even; otherwise, walking is not remarkable. The steppage gait may be unilateral or bilateral and occurs in diseases that affect the peripheral nerves of the legs or motor neurones in the spinal cord, such as poliomyelitis, progressive muscular atrophy, and Charcot-Marie-Tooth disease (peroneal muscular atrophy). It is also observed in patients with peripheral types of muscular dystrophy.

WADDLING GAIT. This gait is characteristic of progressive muscular dystrophy. The attitude of the body may be straight, but more often the lumbar lordosis is accentuated. The steps are regular but a little uncertain. With each step there is an exaggerated elevation of the hip, and once the weight is on this hip, it yields to an abnormal degree so that the upper trunk then inclines to that side. This alternation of lateral trunk movements results in the rolling gait, or *waddle,* a term suggested by Oppenheim. The gluteal musculature is weak and inefficient, although leg muscles may appear well developed. Muscular contractures may lead to an equinovarus position of the foot, particularly in childhood cases, so that the waddle is combined with circumduction of the legs and "walking on the toes."

STAGGERING OR DRUNKEN GAIT. In the drunken gait the patient totters, reels, tips forward and then backward, threatening each moment to lose his balance and fall. Control over trunk and legs is greatly impaired. The steps are irregular and uncertain. There is a wide diversity of excursions of all parts of the body. The reeling is in many different directions, unlike the cerebellar gait, and no effort is made to correct it by watching the legs or the ground, as in sensory ataxia. The patient appears stupefied and indifferent to the quality of his performance, but under certain circumstances he can momentarily correct his defect. A staggering gait is characteristic of alcoholic and barbiturate intoxication. The gait in severe disease of the cerebellum may be similar, but it is not so irregular and bizarre.

HYSTERICAL GAIT. This may take any one of several forms. The patient may have a hysterical monoplegia, paraplegia, or hemiplegia; the muscles may be rigid with contracture or may be flaccid. The paralysis is usually of sudden onset and complete, though under unexpected stress the patient may move the affected part. The monoplegic or hemiplegic patient does not lift the foot from the floor while walking; instead, he drags it as a useless member or pushes it ahead of him as though it were a skate. The characteristic circumduction is absent in hysterical hemiplegia, and the typical hemiplegic posture, hyperactive tendon reflexes, and Babinski's signs are missing. The hysterical paraplegic cannot very well drag both legs, and usually he depends on a crutch or remains helpless in bed, sometimes with severe contractures. The gait may be quite dramatic. Some patients look as though they were walking on stilts, and others lurch wildly in all directions, actually demonstrating by their gyrations

the most remarkable ability to make rapid postural adjustments.

Astasia-abasia, in which the patient, though unable to either stand or walk, retains normal use of his legs while in bed, is nearly always hysterical. When such a patient is placed on his feet, he takes a few normal steps and then becomes unable to advance his feet; he lurches wildly and crumples to the floor if not assisted.

SENILE GAIT. Elderly persons often complain of difficulty in walking, and examination may disclose no abnormality other than the slightly flexed posture of the senile and the short uncertain steps, *marche à petits pas.* At times the patient halts, unable to advance without great effort, but with a little assistance he does much better. Speed, balance, and all the graceful, adaptive movements are lost.

FRONTAL LOBE ATAXIA. Equilibrium and the capacity to stand and walk may be severely disturbed by diseases that affect the frontal lobes, particularly their medial parts. Although this disorder is spoken of as an ataxia, it really represents an *apraxia* of gait, since the difficulty in walking cannot be accounted for by weakness or loss of sensation alone. The movements become slow, hesitant, and poorly directed. At the same time dementia may develop. Grasping, groping, hyperactive tendon reflexes, and bilateral Babinski signs may or may not be present. A unique feature of this disorder is failure to perform certain skilled movements, even though the capacity for crude movement is retained. In some of the reported examples of this disorder, however, all movements of the legs are slow, hesitant, and awkward, and the limbs when passively moved offer variable resistance (*gegenhalten*). Such cases have characteristics of both extrapyramidal (Parkinsonian) and premotor cortical disorder (magnetic apraxia of Denny-Brown). Pronounced degrees of this disorder interfere with locomotion. There is difficulty in standing and walking and even in turning in bed. The end result is a "cerebral paraplegia in flexion." If one frontal lobe is affected, awkwardness of movement appears in the oppoite arm and leg, simulating cerebellar ataxia at times except for the absence of intention tremor, pendular reflexes, Holmes's rebound sign, etc. This apractic motor defect is discussed further in Chap. 54.

REFERENCES

Alpers, B. J.: "Vertigo and Dizziness," Modern Medical Monographs, New York, Grune & Stratton, Inc., 1958.
Brain, W. R.: Vertigo, Brit. Med. J., p. 605, Sept. 17, 1938.
Citron, L., and C. S. Hallpike: Observations upon the Mechanism of Positional Nystagmus of the so-called "Benign Paroxysmal Type," J. Laryngol. & Otol., 70:253, 1956.
Symonds, C.: The Significance of Vertigo in Neurological Diagnosis, J. Laryngol. & Otol., 66:295, 1952.

48 COMMON DISTURBANCES OF VISION, OCULAR MOVEMENT, AND HEARING

Raymond D. Adams and Maurice Victor

Disturbances of vision and hearing are sufficiently frequent to be of concern to the general physician, for often he is the first to be consulted by patients with such complaints. Of the many patients who recognize the nature of their trouble and seek out directly the ophthalmologist or otologist, a certain number are found to have an abnormality that lies not in the eye or ear, but in the central nervous system. Such patients are referred back to the physician, internist, or neurologist for further study. Although perhaps more properly considered under diseases of cranial-nerves, the eye and ear present so many special problems that they will be dealt with in a separate chapter.

DISORDERS OF VISION

Here the most frequent complaint is blurred, impaired, or distorted vision and less often diplopia, ocular pain, irritation of eyes, or inability to keep the eyelids open. It is to be noted that patients do not always distinguish between mild diplopia and a true impairment or diminution of vision in one or both eyes; both conditions may be described as blurring or dimming, and there may be also surprising inaccuracy in stating whether one or both eyes are affected. In adolescents increasing difficulty in focusing eyes and in seeing clearly usually can be traced to developing myopia, though one must rule out ocular or suprasellar tumors. In the middle years (forty-five to fifty) presbyopia, an almost invariable accompaniment of age, is the usual explanation of this phenomenon; and still later in life glaucoma and cataract are the most frequent causes of this symptom.

Episodic blindness in one or both eyes merits separate consideration. When it is bilateral and the blind spots are bordered by bright lines and then followed by unilateral headache and nausea, classic migraine is almost invariably the diagnosis. Episodic blindness limited to one eye, lasting a few minutes only but usually recurring (amblyopia fugax), usually indicates atherosclerosis of the carotid artery with impending thrombosis, but it may happen over the period of a few days in cranial or temporal arteritis or Takayasu's disease. Obscurations of vision of minutes' duration attend increased intracranial pressure and papilledema; they often herald permanent blindness and secondary optic atrophy.

Distortions of vision take several forms. The perceived objects may appear too small (micropsia), too large (macropsia), or they may seem to be askew. Such phenomena always suggest a lesion of the temporal lobes. The latter may also be accompanied by complex visual hallucinations (of landscapes, of peo-

ple, etc.), which actually represent a sensory seizure (see Chap. 52).

ANATOMIC AND PHYSIOLOGIC CONSIDERATIONS

The first neuronal elements in the visual pathway are the rod and cone cells situated in the deepest layer of the retina. The cones are responsible for sharp vision and color discrimination, and they alone are present in the fovea. The rods, which are more sensitive to low intensities of light, predominate in the rest of the retina. Visual impulses are transmitted through the second system of neurones, the bipolar cells, to the ganglion cells, the axons of which form the optic nerve by perforating the sclera at the optic disk, creating a sievelike structure, the *lamina cribrosa*. The absence of visual end organs at this point accounts for the blind spot in the field of vision. Thus, the optic nerve is actually a part of the central nervous system, with glial cells between its fibers but no Schwann cells as in the other cranial and spinal nerves. The optic nerves extend from the disk to the optic chiasm, where their fibers undergo partial decussation (Fig. 48-1). The rearranged optic fibers continue as

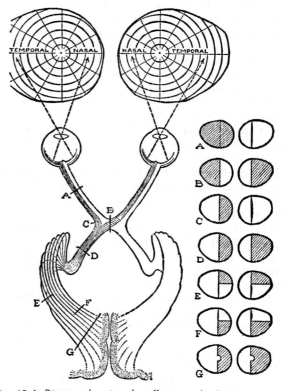

Fig. 48-1. Diagram showing the effects on the fields of vision produced by lesions at various points along the optic pathway. *A*, complete blindness in left eye; *B*, bitemporal hemianopsia; *C*, nasal hemianopsia of left eye; *D*, right homonymous hemianopsia; *E* and *F*, right upper and lower quadrant hemianopsias; *G*, right homonymous hemianopsia with preservation of central vision. (Homans: "A Textbook of Surgery," Springfield, Ill., Charles C Thomas, Publisher, 1945.)

the optic tract, which partially encircles the cerebral peduncles and synapses with cells in the lateral geniculate body. From these cells arises the fourth system of neurones, the final visual pathway, comprising the geniculocalcarine tract and the optic radiations. These fibers lie close to the wall of the temporal horn of the lateral ventricle. The upper ones take a direct course posteriorly, the lower ones loop forward over the temporal horn of the lateral ventricle into the temporal lobe (Meyer's loop) before they pass posteriorly and join the upper fibers on their way to the calcarine cortex.

The types of visual field defect resulting from lesions in different parts of the visual pathways are shown in Fig. 48-1. A prechiasmal lesion causes either a scotoma (an island of impaired vision within the visual field) or a cut in the peripheral part of the visual field. A small scotoma in the macular part of the visual field may seriously impair visual acuity. Demyelinative diseases, toxic (methyl alcohol, quinine, and certain of the phenathiazine tranquilizing drugs) or nutritional disorders, and vascular disease involving the papillomacular bundle in the optic nerve are the usual causes of central scotomas. The toxic and nutritional states cause bilateral and more or less symmetric scotomas; the vascular lesions cause unilateral scotomas; demyelinative diseases give unilateral or asymmetric bilateral scotomas. If the lesion is near the optic disk, there may be swelling of the optic nerve head, i.e., papillitis, which can usually be distinguished from papilledema by the marked impairment of vision it produces.

Another common defect encountered on visual field examination is concentric constriction. This may be due to papilledema, in which case it is usually accompanied by an enlargement of the blind spot. A concentric constriction of the visual field, at first unilateral and later bilateral, and pallor of the optic disks (optic atrophy) should suggest chronic syphilitic optic neuritis. Glaucoma is another cause of this type of field defect. Tubular vision, i.e., constriction of the visual field to the same degree regardless of the distance of the visual test stimulus from the eye, is a sign of hysteria. In organic disease the area of the constricted visual field enlarges as the distance between the patient and the stimulus increases.

Hemianopsia means blindness in one-half the visual field. *Bitemporal hemianopsia*, indicating a lesion of the decussating fibers of the optic chiasm, is usually due to tumor of the pituitary gland or of the infundibulum or third ventricle, to meningioma of the diaphragm of the sella, or occasionally to a large suprasellar aneurysm of the circle of Willis. *Homonymous hemianopsia* (a loss of vision in corresponding halves of the visual fields) indicates a lesion of the visual pathway behind the chiasm and, if *complete*, gives no more information than that. *Incomplete homonymous hemianopsia*, however, has more localizing value: if the field defects in the two eyes are similar (*congruous*), the lesion is in the calcarine cortex; if *incon-*

gruous, the visual fibers in the parietal or temporal lobe are more likely to be implicated. Since the fibers from the peripheral lower quadrants of the retina extend for a variable distance into the temporal lobe, lesions of this lobe may be accompanied by a homonymous upper quadrantic field defect. Parietal lobe lesions may affect the lower quadrants more than the upper.

If the entire optic tract or calcarine cortex on one side is destroyed, there is complete homonymous hemianopsia, including half the field that represents the macula. Incomplete lesions of the optic tract and radiation usually spare central (macular) vision. It must be kept in mind that apparent macular sparing is frequently due to imperfect fixation of gaze. A lesion of the tip of one occipital lobe produces central homonymous hemianopsia, because half the macular fibers of both eyes terminate there. Lesions of both occipital poles result in bilateral central scotomas; and if all the calcarine cortex on each side is destroyed, there is complete "cortical" blindness. Altitudinal or horizontal hemianopsias are nearly always due to lesions of the occipital lobes below or above the calcarine cortex.

In addition to blindness, i.e., visual anesthesia, there is another category of visual impairment, which consists of a defect of visual perception, i.e., *visual agnosia*. The patient can see but cannot recognize objects unless he hears, smells, tastes, or palpates them. The failure of visual recognition of words is called *alexia*. Lesions that produce visual object agnosia are usually bilateral in the parieto-occipital regions and the white matter beneath the angular gyri; those producing alexia are in the region of the major angular gyrus and include fibers from the right occipital lobe crossing in the corpus callosum. These subjects are discussed further in Chaps. 49 and 54.

The optic nerves also contain the afferent fibers for the pupillary reflexes. These fibers leave the optic tract and terminate in the superior colliculi. A lesion of the optic nerve or tracts may abolish the pupillary light reflex; the pupil is dilated and unreactive. Cerebral lesions, on the other hand, leave the pupillary light reflex unaltered. The lack of direct reflex in the blind eye and of consensual reflex in the sound one means that the afferent limb of the reflex arc (optic nerve) is the site of the lesion. A lack of direct light reflex with retention of the consensual reflex places the lesion in the efferent limb of the reflex arc (the homolateral oculomotor nucleus or nerve). Loss of light reflex without visual impairment or ocular palsy (Argyll Robertson pupillary phenomenon) is thought to be due to a lesion in the superior colliculi or periaqueductal region (see below).

Amaurosis refers to blindness from any cause. *Amblyopia* refers to a dimness of vision not due to an error of refraction or some other disease of the eye. *Nyctalopia*, or night blindness, means poor twilight or night vision and is associated with vitamin A deficiency.

DIPLOPIA AND STRABISMUS AND DISORDERS OF THE THIRD, FOURTH, AND SIXTH NERVES

Strabismus (*squint*) refers to an ocular imbalance that results in improper alignment of the two eyes. It may be due to paralysis of an eye muscle; the ocular deviation results from the unrestrained activity of the opposing muscle. It may be due to inequality of tone in the muscles that hold the two eyes in a central position. The former is called *paralytic strabismus* and is primarily a neurologic problem; the latter is *concomitant* or *nonparalytic strabismus* and is an ophthalmologic problem. Any type of ocular imbalance causes diplopia, for the reason that images then fall on disparate or noncorresponding parts of the two retinas. After a time, however, the patient learns to suppress the image of one eye. This almost invariably happens early in concomitant strabismus of congenital nature, and the individual grows up with a weak eye (amyblyopia ex anopsia).

The oculomotor, trochlear, and abducens nerves innervate the extrinsic and intrinsic musculature of the eye. A knowledge of their origin and anatomic relationships is essential to an understanding of the various paralytic ocular syndromes, and the interested reader should consult an anatomy textbook.

The oculomotor nucleus consists of several groups of nerve cells ventral to the aqueduct of Sylvius, at the level of the superior colliculi. The nerve cells that innervate the iris and ciliary body are situated anteriorly in the so-called "Edinger-Westphal nucleus." Below this nucleus are the cells for the superior rectus, inferior oblique, internal rectus, and inferior rectus, in that order from above downward. Convergence is under the control of the medial groups of cells, the nuclei of Perlia. The cells of origin of the trochlear nerves are just inferior to those of the oculomotor nerves. The sixth nerve arises at a considerably lower level, from a paired group of cells in the floor of the fourth ventricle at the level of the lower pons. The intrapontine portion of the facial nerve loops around the sixth nerve nucleus before it turns anterolaterally to make its exit; a lesion in this locality usually causes a homolateral paralysis of both lateral rectus and facial muscles.

All three nerves, after leaving the brain stem, course anteriorly and pass through the cavernous sinus, where they come into close proximity with the ophthalmic division of the fifth nerve, and together they enter the orbit through the superior orbital fissure. The oculomotor nerve supplies all the extrinsic ocular muscles except two—the superior oblique and the external rectus—which are innervated by the trochlear and abducens nerves, respectively. The voluntary part of the levator palpebrae muscle is also supplied by the oculomotor nerve, the involuntary part being under the control of autonomic fibers which also supply the sphincter pupillae and the ciliary muscles (muscles of accommodation).

Although all the extraocular muscles probably participate in every movement of the eyes, particular muscles move the eye in certain fields. The lateral rectus rotates the eye outward; the medial rectus, inward. The function of the vertical recti and the obliques varies according to the position of the eye. When the eye is turned outward, the elevators and depressors of the eye are the superior and inferior recti; when the eye is turned inward, they are the inferior and superior obliques, respectively. In contrast, torsion of the eyeball is effected by the oblique muscles when the eye is turned outward and by the recti when it is turned inward.

Accurate binocular vision is achieved by the associated action of the ocular muscles, which allows a visual stimulus to fall on exactly corresponding parts of the two retinas. Conjugate movement of the eyes is controlled by centers in the cerebral cortex and brain stem. Area 8 in the frontal lobe is the center for voluntary conjugate movements of the eyes to the opposite side. In addition, there is a center in the occipital lobe concerned with contralateral following movements. Fibers from these centers pass to the opposite sides of the brain stem, where they connect with lower centers for conjugate movements: those for right lateral gaze are in the proximity of the right abducens nucleus; those for the left lateral gaze are near the left abducens. Simultaneous innervation of one internal rectus with the other external rectus during lateral gaze is a function of the medial longitudinal fasciculus. The arrangements of nerve cells and fibers for vertical gaze and convergence are situated in the superior colliculi and tegmental parts of the midbrain, respectively.

OCULAR MUSCLE AND GAZE PALSIES

There are three types of paralysis of extraocular muscles: (1) paralysis of isolated ocular muscles, (2) paralysis of conjugate movements (gaze), and (3) syndromes of mixed gaze and ocular muscle paralysis.

Characteristic clinical disturbances result from single lesions of the third, fourth, or sixth cranial nerves. A complete third nerve lesion causes ptosis (since the levator palpebrae is supplied mainly by the third nerve), an inability to rotate the eye upward, downward, or inward, a divergent strabismus due to unopposed action of the lateral rectus muscle, a dilated nonreactive pupil (iridoplegia), and paralysis of accommodation (cycloplegia). When only the muscles of the iris and ciliary body are paralyzed, the condition is termed *internal ophthalmoplegia*. Fourth nerve lesions result in an extorsion of the eye and a weakness of downward gaze, so that patients commonly complain of special difficulty in going downstairs. Head tilting, to the opposite shoulder, is especially characteristic of fourth nerve lesions. This maneuver causes a compensatory intorsion of the lower eye, enabling the patient to obtain binocular vision. Lesions of the sixth nerve result in paralysis

Table 48-1. COMPARISON OF LESIONS WITHIN AND
OUTSIDE THE BRAIN STEM

Effect	Lesions within the brain stem	Lesions external to the brain stem
Involvement of multiple contiguous nerves	±	+
Involvement of sensorimotor tracts	+, often "alternating" or crossed sensory or motor palsies	±
Disturbance of consciousness	+	0 (+ late)
Evidence of other segmental disturbances of the brain stem such as decerebrate rigidity, tonic neck reflexes, pseudobulbar palsy	+	0 (+ late)
X-ray evidence of erosion of cranial bones or enlargement of foramens	0	+

of abduction and a convergent strabismus owing to the unopposed action of the internal rectus muscles. With incomplete sixth nerve palsies, turning the head toward the side of the paretic muscle may overcome diplopia. The foregoing signs may occur with various degrees of completeness, depending on the severity and site of the lesion or lesions.

Ocular palsies may be central, i.e., due to a lesion of the nucleus or the intramedullary portion of the cranial nerve, or peripheral. Ophthalmoplegia due to lesions in the brain stem is usually accompanied by involvement of other cranial nerves or long tracts. Peripheral lesions, which may or may not be solitary, have a great variety of causes; the most common are aneurysm of the circle of Willis, tumors of the base of the brain, carcinomatosis of the meninges, herpes zoster, and syphilitic meningitis. The third-nerve palsy that occurs with diabetes is probably due to infarction of the third nerve, and the prognosis for recovery in such cases, as with other nonprogressive diseases of the peripheral nerve, is usually excellent. The points of difference between lesions within and outside of the brain stem are tabulated in Table 48-1, and the various intramedullary and extramedullary cranial nerve syndromes are described in Tables 202-1 and 202-2.

When the ocular palsy is slight, there may be no obvious squint or defect in ocular movement; yet the patient experiences diplopia. Study of the relative positions of the images of the two eyes then becomes the most accurate way of determining which muscle is involved. The image seen by the affected eye is usually less distinct, but the most reliable way of distinguishing the two images is by the red glass test. *A red glass is placed in front of the patient's right eye.* He is then asked to look at a flashlight, held at a

distance of a meter, to turn his eyes in various segments of his visual fields, and to state the position of the red (right) and white (left) images. The relative positions of the two images are plotted as indicated in Fig. 48-2.

Three rules aid in the analysis of ocular movements by the red glass test. (1) The direction in which the distance between the images is at a maximum is the direction of action of the paretic muscle. For example, if the greatest separation is in looking to the right, either the right abductor or the left adductor muscle is weak. (2) The image projected farther to the side belongs to the paretic eye. If the patient looks to the right and the red image is farther to the right, then the right abducens muscle is weak. If the white image is to the right of the red, then the left internal rectus muscle is weak. (3) In testing vertical movements, again the image of the eye with the paretic muscle is the one projected most peripherally in the direction of eye movement. One ignores lateral separation at this time. It must be remembered that there are two elevator and two depressor muscles. The responsible muscle may be either one of the obliques or vertical recti muscles. For example, if the maximum separation of images occurs on looking downward and to the left, and the white image is projected farther down than the red, the paretic muscle is the left inferior rectus. If the maximum separation occurs on looking down and to the right and the white image is lower than the red, the paretic muscle is the left superior oblique. Separation of images on looking up and to the right or left will similarly distinguish paresis of the inferior oblique and superior rectus muscles.

Monocular diplopia may occur and is related to diseases of the lens and refractive media of the eye. Also paresis of accommodation may produce diplopia for near vision; its cause is unknown.

PARALYSIS OF CONJUGATE MOVEMENT (GAZE). The term *conjugate gaze*, or *conjugate movement*, refers to the simultaneous movement of the two eyes in the same direction. An acute lesion in one frontal lobe may cause paralysis of contralateral gaze. The eyes turn toward the side of the lesion. The ocular disorder is temporary (several days' duration). In bilateral frontal lesions the patient may be unable to turn his eyes voluntarily (oculomotor apraxia) in any direction—up, down, or to the side—but retains fixation and following movements, which are believed to be occipital lobe functions. Gaze paralysis of cerebral origin is not attended by strabismus or diplopia. The usual causes are vascular occlusion with infarction, hemorrhage, and abscess or tumor of the frontal lobe. With diseases of the basal ganglions, e.g., postencephalitic Parkinsonism or Huntington's chorea, ocular movements may be limited in all directions, especially upward. Lesions of the superior colliculus, near the posterior commissure, interfere with voluntary reflex upward gaze, and often movements of convergence as well as the pupillary light reflexes are abolished (Parinaud's syndrome). There also exists a pontine center for conjugate lateral gaze, probably in the vicinity of the abducens nuclei. A lesion here causes ipsilateral gaze palsy, with the eyes turning to the opposite side. The palsy tends to last longer than with cerebral lesions and is frequently accompanied by other signs of pontine disease. Fully developed forms of gaze paralysis are readily discerned, but lesser degrees may be overlooked unless one pays special attention to the predominant position of the eyes and tests the ability to sustain conjugate movement.

Skew deviation is a poorly understood disorder of gaze, characterized by a maintained deviation of one eye above the other. The deviation differs from peripheral muscle palsy in being constant in all fields of gaze. It may occur with any lesion of the posterior fossa but particularly with a lesion of the cerebellum.

MIXED GAZE AND OCULAR PARALYSES. These are always a sign of intrapontine or mesencephalic disease. With a lesion of the lower pons in or near the sixth-nerve nucleus, there is a homolateral paralysis of the lateral rectus muscle and a failure of adduction of the opposite eye, i.e., a combined paralysis of the sixth nerve and of conjugate lateral gaze. Lesions of the medial longitudinal fasciculi interfere with lateral conjugate gaze in another way. On looking to the right, the left eye fails to adduct; on looking to the left, the right eye fails to adduct. The abducting eye shows nystagmus. This condition is referred to as *internuclear ophthalmoplegia* and should always be suspected when the medial recti alone are affected. If the lesion is in the lower part of the medial longitudinal fasciculi, convergence is intact; if the lesion is in the higher part, i.e., near the oculomotor nuclei, convergence may be lost.

NYSTAGMUS. This refers to involuntary rhythmic movements of the eyes; it is of two types, oscillating or pendular and rhythmic or jerk. In jerk nystagmus, the movements are distinctly faster in one direction than the other; in pendular nystagmus, the oscillations are roughly equal in rate for the two directions, although on conjugate lateral gaze, the pendular type may convert to a jerk type with the fast component to the side of the gaze.

In testing for nystagmus, the eyes should first be examined in the central position and then during upward, downward, and lateral movements. If nystagmus is monocular (as described below), each eye should be tested separately, with the other one covered. Labyrinthine nystagmus is most obvious when visual fixation is prevented by shielding the eyes; brain stem and cerebellar nystagmus are brought out best by having the patient fixate on a finger. Labyrinthine nystagmus may vary with the position of the head; hence these various tests should be performed with the head in several different positions. In particular, the postural nystagmus of Barány is evoked by hyperextension of the neck, with the patient in the supine position. Opticokinetic nystagmus should be tested by asking the patient to look at a rotating

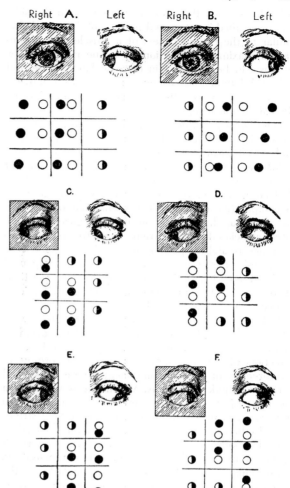

Fig. 48-2. Diplopia fields with individual muscle paralyses. The dark glass is in front of the right eye, and the fields are projected as the patient sees the images. *A.* Paralysis of right external rectus. Characteristic: right eye does not move to the right. Field: horizontal homonymous diplopia increasing on looking to the right. *B.* Paralysis of right internal rectus. Characteristic: right eye does not move to the left. Field: horizontal crossed diplopia increasing on looking to the left. *C.* Paralysis of right inferior rectus. Characteristic: right eye does not move downward when eyes are turned to the right. Field: vertical diplopia (image of right eye lowermost) increasing on looking to the right and down. *D.* Paralysis of right superior rectus. Characteristic: right eye does not move upward when eyes are turned to the right. Field: vertical diplopia (image of right eye uppermost) increasing on looking to the right and up. *E.* Paralysis of right superior oblique. Characteristic: right eye does not move downward when eyes are turned to the left. Field: vertical diplopia (image of right eye lowermost) increasing on looking to left and down. *F.* Paralysis of right inferior oblique. Characteristic: right eye does not move upward when eyes are turned to the left. Field: vertical diplopia (image of right eye uppermost) increasing on looking to left and up. (Cogan: "Neurology of the Ocular Muscles," 2d ed., Springfield, Ill., Charles C Thomas, Publisher, 1956.)

cylinder on which several stripes have been painted or a striped cloth moved across the field of vision.

A few irregular jerks are observed in many normal

individuals when the eyes are turned far to the side. These so-called "nystagmoid movements" are probably similar to the tremulousness of a muscle that is contracted maximally. Occasionally a fine rhythmic nystagmus can be obtained in extreme lateral gaze, but if it is bilateral and disappears as the eyes move a few degrees toward the midline, it usually has no clinical significance.

Pendular nystagmus is found in a variety of conditions in which central vision is lost early in life, such as albinism and in various other diseases of the retina and refractive mediums. The syndrome of miners' nystagmus, formerly a common cause of industrial disability, occurs after many years of work in comparative darkness. The oscillations of the eyes are very rapid, increase on upward gaze, and are often associated with vertigo, head tremor, and intolerance of light. *Spasmus nutans* is a specific type of pendular nystagmus of infancy and is accompanied by head nodding and occasionally by wry positions of the neck. The prognosis is good; most patients recover within a few months.

Jerk nystagmus is the commoner type. It may be lateral or vertical, particularly on ocular movement in these planes, or it may be rotary. By custom, the direction of the nystagmus is named according to the direction of the fast component. There are several varieties of jerk nystagmus. When one is watching a moving object—e.g., the passing landscape from a train window or a rotating drum with vertical stripes—a rhythmic jerk nystagmus, *opticokinetic nystagmus*, normally appears. The slow phase is a result of visual fixation; the quick phase is compensatory. With unilateral cerebral lesions, particularly in the parietooccipital region, there is loss of opticokinetic nystagmus when the moving stimulus, e.g., the drum, moves toward the side of the lesion.

Aside from opticokinetic nystagmus, in the hospital lateral and vertical nystagmus are most frequently due to barbiturate intoxication. Jerk nystagmus may signify disease of the labyrinthine-vestibular apparatus. Labyrinthine stimulation or irritation produces a nystagmus with the fast phase to the opposite side. The slow component reflects the effect of impulses derived from the semicircular canals, and the fast component is a corrective movement. Vestibular-labyrinthine nystagmus may be horizontal, vertical, or, most characteristically, rotary. Vertigo, nausea, vomiting, and staggering are the usual accompaniments, as in Ménière's syndrome or labyrinthitis (see Chap. 47). Brain stem lesions often cause a coarse unidirectional nystagmus, which may be horizontal or vertical; the latter is usually brought out on upward gaze and rarely on downward gaze. The presence of vertical nystagmus is pathognomonic of disease in the tegmentum of the brain stem. Vertigo is inconstant, and signs of disease of other nuclear structures and tracts in the brain stem are frequent. Jerk nystagmus of this type is frequent in demyelinative or vascular disease, in tumors, and syringobulbia. The Arnold-Chiari mal-

formation is often manifested by a vertical nystagmus on looking downward. Cerebellopontine angle tumors cause bilateral horizontal nystagmus that is coarser and with the fast component to the side of the lesion. Nystagmus probably does not occur with cerebellar disease unless the fastigial nuclei and their connections with the vestibular nuclei are involved. The nystagmus that occurs only in the abducting eye and is said to be a pathognomonic sign of multiple sclerosis probably represents an incompletely developed form of internuclear ophthalmoplegia. The movement of the adducting eye (which does not show nystagmus) is impaired.

Convergence nystagmus is a rhythmic oscillation in which a slow abduction of the eyes in respect of each other is followed by a quick movement of adduction. It is usually accompanied by other types of nystagmus and by one or more features of Parinaud's syndrome. Occasionally there is also a jerky retraction movement of the eyes (*nystagmus retractorius*) or a maintained spasm of convergence, best brought out on attempted elevation of the eyes to command. These unusual phenomena all point to a lesion of the upper midbrain tegmentum and are usually manifestations of vascular disease or of pinealoma.

Oscillopsia refers to illusory movement of the environment, which may or may not occur with turning of the eyes and consequent displacement of the image on the retina. When the eyes are turned voluntarily, the environment is interpreted as being stationary, whereas passive displacement of the eye or nystagmus from stimulation of the labyrinth results in oscillopsia during the slow phase of movement.

ALTERATIONS OF PUPILS

Pupil size is determined by the balance of innervation between the dilator and constrictor fibers. The pupillodilator fibers arise in the posterior part of the hypothalamus, descend in the lateral tegmentum of the midbrain, pons, medulla, and cervical spinal cord to the eighth cervical and first thoracic segments, where they synapse with the lateral horn cells. The latter give rise to preganglionic fibers that synapse in the superior cervical ganglion; the postganglionic fibers course along the internal carotid artery and traverse the cavernous sinus to join the first division of the trigeminal nerve, finally reaching the eyes as the long ciliary nerves. The pupilloconstrictor fibers arise in the nucleus of Edinger-Westphal, join the oculomotor nerve, and synapse in the ciliary ganglion with the postganglionic neurones that innervate the iris and ciliary body.

The pupils are usually equal in size, though if the eyes are turned to one side the pupil of the abducting eye dilates slightly. Pupil size varies with light intensity; as one pupil constricts under a bright light (direct reflex), the other unexposed pupil does likewise (consensual reflex). Pupillary constriction is also part of the act of convergence and accommodation for near objects.

Interruption of the sympathetic fibers either centrally, between the hypothalamus and their point of exit from the spinal cord, or peripherally, in the neck or along the carotid artery, results in miosis and ptosis (due to paralysis of the levator palpebrae), with loss of sweating of the face, and occasionally enophthalmos (Bernard-Horner syndrome). Stimulation or irritation of the pupillodilator fibers has the opposite effect, i.e., lid retraction, slight proptosis, and dilatation of the pupil. The ciliospinal pupillary reflex, evoked by pinching the neck, is effected through these efferent sympathetic fibers. Abnormal dilatation of the pupils (mydriasis), often with loss of pupillary light reflexes, may result from midbrain lesions and is a frequent finding in cases of deep coma. Extreme constriction of the pupils (miosis) is commonly observed in pontine hemorrhage, presumably because of bilateral interruption of the pupillodilator fibers.

The functional integrity of the sympathetic and parasympathetic nerve endings in the iris may be determined by the use of certain drugs. Atropine and homatropine dilate the pupils by paralyzing the parasympathetic nerve endings, while physostigmine and pilocarpine constrict them, the former by inhibiting cholinesterase activity at the neuromuscular junction and the latter by direct stimulation of the sphincter muscle of the iris. Cocaine dilates the pupils by stimulating the sympathetic nerve endings. Morphine acts centrally to constrict the pupils.

In chronic syphilitic meningitis and other forms of late syphilis, particularly tabes dorsalis, the pupils are usually small, irregular, and unequal, they do not dilate properly in response to mydriatic drugs, and they fail to react to light, although they do constrict on accommodation. This is known as the *Argyll Robertson pupil*. The exact locality of the lesion is not known; it is generally believed to be in the tectum of the midbrain proximal to the oculomotor nuclei, where the descending pupillodilator fibers are in close proximity to the light-reflex fibers. The possibility of a partial third-nerve lesion or a lesion of the ciliary ganglion has not been excluded. A dissociation of the light reflex from the accommodation-convergence reaction is sometimes observed with other midbrain lesions, e.g., pinealoma and multiple sclerosis, and also in diabetes mellitus. In these diseases miosis, irregularity of pupils, and failure to respond to a mydriatic are not constantly present. Another interesting pupillary abnormality is the myotonic reaction, sometimes referred to as *Adie's pupil*. The patient may complain of blurring of vision or may have suddenly noticed that one pupil is larger than the other. The reaction to light and convergence are absent if tested in the customary manner, although the size of the pupil will change slowly on prolonged stimulation. Once contracted or dilated, the pupils remain in that state for some minutes. The affected pupil reacts promptly to the usual mydriatic and miotic

drugs but is unusually sensitive to 2.5 per cent solution of mecholyl, a strength that will not affect a normal pupil. The myotonic pupil usually appears during the third or fourth decade and may be associated with absence of knee jerks, and hence be mistaken for tabes dorsalis.

DISTURBANCES OF HEARING

Tinnitus and *deafness*, which are frequent symptoms, always mean disease of cochlea or the auditory nerve and its central connections.

Tinnitus, or ringing in the ears, is a purely subjective phenomenon and may also be reported as a buzzing, whistling, hissing, or roaring sound. It is a very common symptom in adults and may be of no significance, as, for example, the hissing sound due to wax in the external auditory canal or a blocked eustachian tube. On the other hand, it is regularly associated with disease of the eighth nerve, inner ear, or ossicles, and severe and prolonged tinnitus in the presence of normal hearing is very rare. If tinnitus is localized to one ear and is described as having a tonal character, such as ringing or a bell-like tone, and particularly if the recruitment phenomenon (see below) is present, it is probably cochlear in origin. Noises described as rushing water or escaping steam point to disease of the nerve or even the brain stem. Clinking sounds are caused by intermittent contraction of the tensor tympani. A pulsating tinnitus synchronous with the pulse may be related to an intracranial vascular malformation; however, this symptom must be carefully judged, since introspective individuals often report hearing their pulse when lying down with one ear on a pillow. Certain drugs such as salicylates and quinine produce tinnitus and transient deafness. Nervous individuals are less tolerant of tinnitus than are more stable persons; depressed or anxious patients may demand relief from tinnitus that has existed for years.

Examination of hearing should always begin with inspection of the external auditory canal and the tympanic membrane. A watch or whispered words are suitable means of testing hearing at the bedside, the opposite ear being closed by the finger. If there is any suspicion of deafness or a complaint of tinnitus or vertigo, or if the patient is a child with a speech defect, then hearing must be tested further. This can be done with the use of tuning forks of different frequencies, but the most accurate results are obtained by the use of an electric audiometer and the construction of an audiogram, which reveals the entire range of hearing at a glance. An auditory recruitment test may also be helpful: the difference in hearing between the two ears is estimated, and the loudness of the stimulus delivered to each ear is then increased by regular increments. In nonrecruiting deafness (characteristic of a nerve trunk lesion) the original difference in hearing persists in comparisons above threshold. In recruiting deafness (as occurs in Ménière's disease) the bad ear gains in loudness and finally is equal to the good ear.

Deafness is of two types: (1) nerve deafness, due to interruption of cochlear fibers, and (2) conduction deafness, due to disease of the middle ear (or occlusion of the external auditory canal or eustachian tube). In differentiating these two types, the tuning fork tests are of value. When the vibrating fork is held several inches from the ear (the test for air conduction), sound waves can be appreciated only as they are transmitted through the middle ear and will be reduced with disease in this location. When the fork is applied to the skull (test for bone conduction), the sound waves are conveyed directly to the cochlea, without the intervention of the middle ear apparatus and will therefore not be reduced when the disease is confined to the middle ear. With affection of the cochlea or eighth nerve, both air and bone conduction will be reduced or lost. Normally air conduction is better than bone conduction. These principles form the basis for several tests of auditory function.

In *Weber's test,* the vibrating fork is applied to the forehead in the midline. In middle ear deafness the sound is localized in the affected ear, in nerve deafness in the normal ear. In *Rinne's test* the fork is applied to the mastoid process, the other ear being closed by the observer's finger. At the moment the sound ceases, the fork is held at the auditory meatus. In middle ear deafness the sound cannot be heard by air conduction after bone conduction has ceased (abnormal or negative Rinne test). In nerve deafness the reverse is true (normal or positive Rinne test), although both air and bone conduction may be quantitatively decreased. In *Schwabach's test,* the patient's bone conduction is compared with that of a normal observer. In general, high-pitched tones are lost in nerve deafness and low-pitched ones in middle ear deafness, but there are frequent exceptions to this rule.

The common causes of middle ear deafness are otitis media, otosclerosis, and rupture of the eardrum. Nerve deafness has many causes. The internal ear may be aplastic from birth (hereditary deaf-mutism), or it may be damaged by rubella in the pregnant mother. Acute purulent meningitides or chronic infections spreading from the middle ear are common causes of nerve deafness in childhood. The auditory nerve may be involved by tumors of the cerebellopontine angle or by syphilis. Deafness may also result from a demyelinative plaque in the brain stem. Hysterical deafness may be difficult to distinguish from organic disease. In the case of bilateral deafness, the distinction can be made by observing a blink (cochleoorbicular reflex) or an alteration in skin sweating (psychogalvanic skin reflex) in response to a loud sound. Unilateral hysterical deafness may be detected by an audiometer, with both ears connected, or by whispering into the bell of a stethoscope

attached to the patient's ears, closing first one and then the other tube without the patient's knowledge.

49 DISORDERS OF SENSATION
Maurice Victor and Raymond D. Adams

Loss or perversion of somatic sensation not infrequently represents the principal manifestation of a disease of the nervous system. The logic of this is clear enough, since the major anatomic pathways of the sensory system are distinct from those of the motor system and may be selectively disturbed by disease. The clinical analysis of these functions involves special tests designed to indicate the nature of the sensory disorder and its locality.

ANATOMIC AND PHYSIOLOGIC CONSIDERATIONS

An understanding of these sensory disorders depends on a knowledge of applied anatomy. Ideally one should be familiar with the sensory organs in the skin and deep structures, the distribution of the peripheral nerves and the spinal roots, and the pathways by which the sensory impulses are conveyed

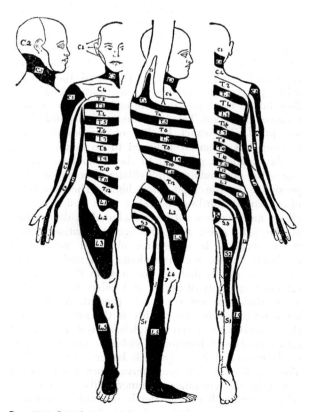

Fig. 49-1. Distribution of the sensory spinal roots on the surface of the body. (Holmes: "Introduction to Clinical Neurology," Edinburgh, E. & S. Livingstone, Ltd., 1946.)

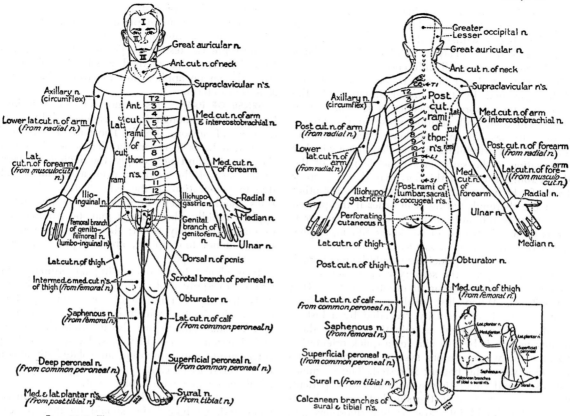

Fig. 49-2. The cutaneous fields of peripheral nerves. (Haymaker and Woodhall: "Peripheral Nerve Injuries," Philadelphia, W. B. Saunders Company, 1945.)

through the spinal cord and brain stem to the thalamus and parietal lobe cortex. These topics were introduced in Chap. 4, General Considerations of Pain. Unfortunately, space does not permit a detailed review here of the anatomy of the sensory system, nor of its physiology. A final statement on the physiology of the sensory system is not possible, because of the radical revision resulting from the recent experiments of Bishop, Weddell, and their associates and others. We have, nevertheless, included sensory charts of the main nerves and roots for the convenience of the reader (see Figs. 49-1 and 49-2).

Disorders of the somatic sensory apparatus pose special problems for the patient. He is confronted with derangements of sensation unlike anything he has previously experienced. And he has few words in his vocabulary to describe what he feels. He may say that a limb feels "numb" and "dead" when in fact he means weakness or paralysis and not a sensory disturbance. Nevertheless, observant individuals may discover a loss of sensation, for example, inability to feel discomfort on touching an object hot enough to blister the skin or unawareness of articles of clothing and other objects in contact with the skin. Even more strange, the disease may induce a new and unnatural series of sensory experiences, which are as often a source of complaint as loss of

sensation. If nerves, spinal roots, or spinal tracts are only partially interrupted, a touch may arouse tingling or prickling, meaning presumably that the remaining touch and pain fibers are acting abnormally. Similarly, burning and pain may represent overactivity of surviving thermal and pain fibers. Tightness, drawing and pulling sensations, a feeling of a band or girdle around the limb or trunk are common with partial involvement of pressure fibers. These abnormal sensations are called *paresthesias*, or *dysesthesias*, if they are unpleasant; and their character and distribution inform us of the anatomy of the lesion involving the sensory system.

EXAMINATION OF SENSATION

The examination of sensation is the most difficult part of the neurologic examination. For one thing, test procedures are relatively crude and inadequate, and at times no objective sensory loss can be demonstrated despite symptoms that clearly indicate the presence of such a deficit. Also, a response to a sensory stimulus is difficult to evaluate objectively, and the examiner's conclusions depend on the patient's interpretation and editing of sensory stimuli. This, in turn, depends on his general awareness and responsiveness, his desire to cooperate, and his fatigability, as well as his intelligence, education, and suggestibility. At times, children and relatively uneducated persons are better witnesses than more sophisticated individuals who are likely to analyze their feelings minutely and report small differences.

The degree of detail in which sensation is tested will be governed by the clinical situation. If the patient has no sensory complaints, it is sufficient to examine vibration and position sense in the fingers and toes, to test the appreciation of pain over the face, trunk, and extremities, and to determine whether this sensation is the same in symmetric parts of the body. A rough survey of this sort may detect sensory defects of which the patient is unaware. On the other hand, more thorough testing is in order if the patient has complaints referable to the sensory system, or if there is localized atrophy or weakness, ataxia, trophic changes of joints, or painless ulcers.

A few other general principles should be mentioned. One should not press the sensory examination in the presence of fatigue, for an inattentive patient is a poor witness. When first dealing with a patient, sensory testing is of necessity preceded by a history and often by a general examination; under these circumstances it is best to aim for a quick orientation regarding the whole sensory system and to return to the details when the patient is rested. The examiner must also avoid suggesting symptoms to the patient. After having explained in the simplest terms what is required, he should interpose as few questions and remarks as possible. Consequently, the patient must not be asked "Do you feel that?" each time he is touched but simply told to say "yes" or "sharp" every time he has been touched or feels pain. The patient should not be permitted to see the part under examination. For short tests it is sufficient that he close his eyes; during more detailed testing it is preferable to interpose a screen between his eyes and the part examined. Finally, all the findings of the sensory examination should be accurately recorded on a chart.

Sensation is frequently classified as *superficial* (cutaneous, exteroceptive) and *deep* (proprioceptive); these are convenient terms for examination and reporting. The former comprises the modalities of light touch, pain, and temperature; the latter includes the sense of position, passive motion, vibration, and deep pain.

SENSE OF TOUCH. This is usually tested with a wisp of cotton. The patient is first acquainted with the nature of the stimulus by applying it to a normal part of the body. Then he is asked to say "yes" each time he is touched in various other parts. A patient simulating sensory loss may say "no" in response to a tactile stimulus. Cornified areas of skin, such as the soles and palms, will require heavier stimulus, whereas the hair-clad parts are sensitive to a lighter stimulus because of the numerous nerve endings around the follicle. A moving stimulus of any kind is more effective than a stationary one. The application of the examiner's or preferably the patient's finger tips is

a useful method of testing, particularly, as Trotter originally showed, in mapping out an area of tactile loss following peripheral nerve injury.

More precise testing is possible by using a von Frey hair. By this method a stimulus of constant strength can be applied and the threshold for touch sensation determined.

SENSE OF PAIN. This is most efficiently estimated by pinprick, although it can be evoked by a great diversity of noxious stimuli. The patient must understand that he is to report the degree of sharpness of the pinprick and not simply the feeling of contact or pressure of the point or even a special sensation due to penetration of the skin. A few other simple rules should be kept in mind. If the pinpricks are applied rapidly, their effects may be summated and excessive pain may result; therefore they should be delivered not too rapidly, about 1 per sec, and not over the same spot.

It is almost impossible, using an ordinary pin or needle, to apply each stimulus with equal intensity. This difficulty can be largely overcome by the use of an algesimeter, which enables one not only to give constant stimuli but also to grade their intensity and determine threshold values. Even when the pinpricks are of equal intensity, an isolated stimulus may be reported as excessively sharp, apparently because of direct contact with a pain spot.

If an area of diminished or absent sensation is encountered, its boundaries should be demarcated, to determine whether it has a segmental or peripheral nerve distribution or whether sensation is lost below a certain level. Such areas are best delineated by proceeding from the region of impaired sensation toward the normal, and the changes may be confirmed by dragging a pin lightly over the skin.

DEEP PRESSURE SENSE. One can estimate this sense simply by pinching or pressing deeply on the tendons and muscles; no special virtue is attached to the traditional and somewhat sadistic use of the testicle for this test. Pain can often be elicited by heavy pressure even when superficial sensation is diminished; conversely, in some diseases, such as tabetic neurosyphilis, the loss of deep pressure sense may be more prominent.

THERMAL SENSE. The proper evaluation of this sensation requires attention to certain details of procedure. One may fail consistently to evoke thermal stimuli if small test objects are used. The perception of heat and cold is relatively delayed, especially if the test objects are applied only lightly and momentarily against the skin. At a temperature below 10°C or above 50°C, sensations of cold or warmth become confused with pain. As the temperature of the test object approaches that of the skin, the patient's response will be modified by the temperature of the skin itself.

The following procedure for testing thermal sensation is therefore suggested. The areas of skin to be tested should be exposed for some time before the examination. The test objects should be large, preferably Erlenmeyer flasks containing hot and cold water. Thermometers, which extend into the water through the flask stoppers, indicate the temperature of the water at the moment of testing. At first, extreme degrees of heat and cold (e.g., 5 and 50°C) may be employed, to delineate roughly an area of thermal sensory disturbance; over such an area the patient will report that the flask feels "less hot" or "less cold" than over a normal part. If areas of deficit are found, the borders may be more accurately determined by moving the flask along the skin from the insensitive region to the normal one than by applying the flask at intervals. The qualitative change should then be quantitated as far as possible by estimating the *differences in temperature* the patient can recognize. The patient is asked to report whether one stimulus is *warmer or colder* than another. The patient should not simply be asked whether a given stimulus is warm or cold, since the cooler to him may be interpreted as warm. The range of temperature difference between the two flasks is gradually narrowed by mixing their contents. A normal person is capable of detecting 1° of difference when the temperature of the flasks is in the range of 28 to 32°C. In the warm range he should readily recognize differences between 35 and 40°C and in the cold range between 10 and 20°C. In many older persons and in others with poor peripheral circulation (especially in cold weather), the responses may be modified in an otherwise normal patient.

The sensation of heat or cold depends not only on the temperature of the stimulus but also on the time and area over which it is applied. This principle may be employed to detect slight impairment of sensation; the patient may be able to distinguish small differences in temperature when the bottom of the flask is applied for 3 sec but unable to do so if only the side of the flask is applied for 1 sec. Throughout the test procedure, especially when small temperature differences are involved, the area of sensory disturbance should be continually checked against perception in normal parts.

POSTURAL SENSE AND THE APPRECIATION OF PASSIVE MOVEMENT. These modalities are usually lost together, although in any particular case one may be disproportionately affected.

Abnormalities of postural sensation may be revealed in any of several ways. When the patient extends his upper limbs in front of him and closes his eyes, the affected arm will wander from its original position; if the fingers are spread apart, they may undergo a series of slow changing postures ("piano-playing" movements, or *pseudoathetosis*).

The lack of position sense in a lower limb may be demonstrated by displacing the limb from its original position and asking the patient to point to his large toe. If postural sensation is defective in both lower limbs, the patient will be unable to maintain his balance with feet together and eyes closed (Romberg's

sign). This sign should be interpreted with caution. Even a normal person in the Romberg position will sway slightly more with his eyes closed than open. A patient with lack of balance due to motor weakness or cerebellar disease will also sway more if visual cues are removed. Only if there is a marked discrepancy between the state of balance with eyes open and closed can one confidently state that the patient shows Romberg's sign, i.e., loss of proprioceptive sensation. Mild degrees of unsteadiness in nervous or suggestible patients may be overcome by diverting their attention, as by having them alternately touch the index finger of each hand to their nose while standing with their eyes closed.

The appreciation of passive movement is first tested in the fingers and toes, and the defect, when present, is reflected maximally in these parts. It is important to grasp the digit firmly at the sides opposite the plane of movement from the source of pressure of the examiner's fingers. This applies as well to the testing of the more proximal segments of the limb. The patient should be instructed to report each movement as "up" or "down" in relation to the previous stationary position, and not in relation to the neutral position. It is useful to demonstrate the test with a large and easily identified movement, but once the idea is clear to the patient, the smallest detectable changes in position should be tested. The range of movement normally appreciated in the digits is said to be as little as 1°. Clinically, however, defective appreciation of passive movement is judged by comparison with a normal limb or, if bilaterally defective, on the basis of what the examiner has through experience learned to regard as normal. Slight impairment may be disclosed by a slow response or, if the digit is displaced very slowly, by a relative unawareness that movement has occurred; or after the digit has been displaced in the same direction several times, the patient may misjudge only the first movement in the opposite direction; or after the examiner has moved the toe, he may detect that the patient is trying to determine the position of the part by making small voluntary movements of the digit, a sign probably of uncertainty.

THE SENSE OF VIBRATION. This is a composite sensation comprising touch and rapid alterations of deep pressure sense. It depends for its conduction on both cutaneous and deep afferent fibers, which ascend in the dorsal columns of the cord. It is therefore rarely affected in lesions of single nerves but will be disturbed in polyneuritis and disease of the dorsal columns, medial lemniscus, and thalamus. Except in cases of cortical lesions, vibration and position sense are usually lost together. There are exceptions to this statement, however, for in some instances the loss of vibration sense is more severe than loss of position sense (e.g., combined system disease). With advancing age, vibration sense may be diminished at the toes and ankles.

Vibration sense is tested by using a tuning fork with

a low rate of vibration (128 d.v.) placed over the bony prominences. The examiner must make sure that the patient responds to the vibration and not to just the contact stimulus. Although there are mechanical devices to quantitate the intensity of vibration sense, it is sufficient for clinical purposes to compare the point tested with a normal part of the patient or of the examiner. A 256-d.v. fork can be used for finer testing. The level of vibration-sense loss due to spinal lesions can be estimated by placing the fork over successive vertebral spines.

DISCRIMINATIVE SENSORY FUNCTIONS. Damage to the sensory cortex or to the sensory projections from thalamus to cortex results in a special type of disturbance that affects mainly the patient's ability to make sensory discriminations. Lesions in these structures may disturb postural sense but leave the primary modalities (touch, pain, temperature, and vibration sense) relatively little affected. In such a situation, or if a cerebral lesion is suspected on other grounds, discriminative function should be tested further by the following tests.

Two-point Discrimination. The ability to distinguish two points from one point is tested by using a compass, the points of which should be blunt and applied simultaneously and painlessly. The distance at which such a stimulus can be recognized as double varies greatly; 1 mm at the tip of the tongue, 3 to 6 mm at the finger tips, 1.5 to 2 cm on the palms and soles, 3 cm on the dorsa of the hands and feet, and 4 to 7 cm on the body surface. It is characteristic of the patient with a lesion of the sensory cortex to mistake two points for one, although occasionally the opposite is true.

Cutaneous Localization and Number Writing. Cutaneous localization is tested by touching various parts of the patient's body and asking him to point to the part touched or to a corresponding part of the examiner's limb. Recognition of *number writing*, or of the direction of lines drawn on the skin, also depends on the localization of tactile stimuli.

Appreciation of Texture, Size, and Shape. Appreciation of *texture* depends mainly on cutaneous impressions, but the recognition of *shape and size* of objects is based on impressions from deeper receptors as well. The lack of recognition of shape and form, therefore, though frequently found with cortical lesions, may also be present with lesions of the spinal cord and brain stem, due to interruption of tracts transmitting postural and tactile sensation. Such a sensory defect, called *stereoanesthesia*, should be distinguished from *astereognosis*, which connotes an inability to identify an object by palpation, the primary sense data being intact. The latter defect is essentially a tactile agnosia and is associated with lesions lying posterior to the postcentral gyrus. In practice, a pure astereognosis is rarely encountered, and the term is employed where the impairment of tactile and joint sense is of such slight degree that it could not account for the difficulty.

Extinction of Sensory Stimuli and Sensory Inattention. In response to bilateral simultaneous testing of symmetric parts, the patient may acknowledge only the stimulus on the sound side, or he may improperly localize the stimulus on the affected side, whereas those applied individually are properly appreciated. This phenomenon of *extinction* or cortical *inattention* is characteristic of parietal lobe lesions, the symptomatology of which is considered on pp. 275 and 276.

A few other terms require definition, since they may be encountered in reading about sensation. Most of them are pedantic, and it is recommended that the simplest terms possible be used. *Anesthesia* refers to a loss and *hypesthesia* to a diminution of all forms of sensation. Loss or impairment of specific cutaneous sensations is indicated by an appropriate prefix or suffix, e.g., *thermoanesthesia* or *thermohypesthesia*, *analgesia* (loss of pain) or *hypalgesia*, *tactile anesthesia* (loss of sense of touch), and *pallanesthesia* (loss of vibratory sense). The term *hyperesthesia* requires special mention; although it implies a heightened receptiveness of the nervous system, careful testing will usually demonstrate an underlying sensory defect, i.e., an elevated threshold to tactile, painful, or thermal stimuli; once the stimulus is perceived, however, it may have a severely painful or unpleasant quality (*hyperpathia*).

SENSORY SYNDROMES

SENSORY CHANGES DUE TO INTERRUPTION OF A SINGLE PERIPHERAL NERVE

These changes will vary with the composition of the nerve involved, depending on whether it is predominantly muscular, cutaneous, or mixed. Since proprioceptive fibers run for a time at least with the muscular (mainly motor) nerves, and cutaneous sensibility is carried in sensory nerves, each of these sensory systems may be affected separately. In lesions of cutaneous nerves, it is said that the area of tactile anesthesia is more extensive than the one for pain, but there is no general agreement on this point.

Because of the overlap from adjacent nerves, the area of sensory loss following division of a cutaneous nerve is always less than its anatomic distribution. If a large area of skin is involved, the sensory impairment characteristically consists of a central portion, in which all forms of cutaneous sensation are lost, surrounded by a zone of partial loss, which becomes less marked as one proceeds from the center to the periphery. The sense of deep pressure and passive movement is intact, as it is carried by muscular nerves. Along the margin of the hypesthetic zone the skin soon becomes excessively sensitive. A light contact may be felt as a smarting, mildly painful sensation. According to Weddell, this is due to collateral regeneration from surrounding healthy nerves into the denervated region.

In lesions involving the brachial and lumbosacral plexuses, the sensory disturbance is no longer confined to the territory of a single nerve and is accompanied by muscle weakness and reflex change.

SENSORY CHANGES DUE TO MULTIPLE NERVE INVOLVEMENT (POLYNEUROPATHY)

In most instances of polyneuropathy the sensory changes are accompanied by varying degrees of motor and reflex loss. Usually the sensory impairment is symmetric, with notable exceptions in some instances of diabetic and periarteritic neuropathy. Since the longest and largest fibers are most often affected, the sensory loss is most severe over the feet and legs and less severe over the hands. The abdomen, thorax, and face are spared except in the most severe cases. The sensory loss usually involves all the modalities, and although it is manifestly difficult to equate the degrees of impairment of pain, touch, temperature, vibration, and position sense, one of these may seemingly be impaired out of proportion to the others. One cannot accurately predict, from the patient's symptoms, which mode of sensation may be disproportionately affected. The term *glove and stocking anesthesia* is frequently employed to describe the sensory loss of polyneuropathy. Although this term draws attention to the predominantly distal pattern of sensory involvement, it is incorrect in that no sharp border exists between normal and impaired sensation. The sensory loss shades off gradually, and the transition to normal sensation occurs over a variable vertical extent of the limb. In hysteria, by contrast, the border between normal and absent sensation is usually sharp.

SENSORY CHANGES DUE TO INVOLVEMENT OF MULTIPLE SPINAL NERVE ROOTS

Because of considerable overlap from adjacent roots, division of a single sensory root does not produce complete loss of sensation in any area of skin. Compression of a single sensory cervical or lumbar root (in herniated intervertebral disks, for example) causes varying degrees of impairment of cutaneous sensation. When two or more roots have been completely divided, a segmental zone of sensory loss can be found, in which reduction of touch and pain perception are about equal in extent. A narrow zone of partial loss surrounds the area of anesthesia in which a raised threshold may or may not be present and accompanied by overreaction (*hyperesthesia*). The presence of muscle paralysis, atrophy, and reflex loss indicates involvement of ventral roots as well.

THE TABETIC SYNDROME. This results from damage to the large proprioceptive fibers of the posterior lumbosacral roots. It is usually caused by neurosyphilis, less often by diabetic or other types of neuritis. Numbness or paresthesias and lightning pains are frequent complaints, and areflexia, atonicity of the bladder, abnormalities of gait (Chap. 47), and hypotonia without muscle weakness are found on examination. The sensory loss may consist only of loss of vibration and position sense in the lower extremities, but in severe cases some loss or impair-

ment of superficial or deep pain sense or of touch may be added. The feet and legs are most affected, less often the arms and trunk.

COMPLETE SPINAL SENSORY SYNDROMES. In a complete transverse lesion of the spinal cord, all forms of sensation are abolished below a level that corresponds with the lesion. There may be a narrow zone of "hyperesthesia" at the upper margin of the anesthetic zone. It is important to remember that during the evolution of such a lesion there may be a discrepancy between the level of the lesion and the level of the sensory loss, the latter ascending as the lesion progresses. This can be understood if one conceives of a lesion evolving from the periphery to the center of the cord, affecting first the outermost fibers carrying pain and temperature sensation from the legs. Conversely, a lesion advancing from the center of the cord may effect these modalities in the reverse order.

PARTIAL SPINAL SENSORY SYNDROMES. Hemisection of the Spinal Cord (Brown-Séquard Syndrome). In rare instances disease is confined to one side of the spinal cord. Provided that the lesion is above the level where pain and temperature fibers have completely decussated (about the tenth thoracic segment), there will result a loss of pain and temperature sensation on the opposite side and of proprioceptive sensation on the same side as the lesion. The loss of pain and temperature sensation begins two or three segments below the lesion. An associated motor paralysis on the side of the lesion completes the syndrome. Touch is not affected, since the fibers from one side of the body are distributed in tracts (posterior columns and anterior spinothalamic) on both sides of the cord.

LESIONS OF THE CENTRAL GRAY MATTER (SYRINGOMYELIC SYNDROME). Since fibers conducting pain and temperature cross the cord in the anterior commissure, a lesion in this location will characteristically abolish these modalities on one or both sides but tactile sensation is spared. The commonest cause of such a lesion is syringomyelia, less often tumor and hemorrhage. The sensory loss usually occurs in a segmental distribution, and since the lesion frequently involves other parts of the gray matter, varying degrees of amyotrophy, loss of reflexes, and of touch sensation may be added.

POSTERIOR COLUMN SYNDROME (SUBACUTE COMBINED DEGENERATION OF THE CORD). There is loss of vibratory and position sense below the lesion, but the sense of pain, temperature, and touch are relatively little affected. This may be difficult to distinguish from the tabetic syndrome. In some diseases, as mentioned earlier, vibratory sensation may be selectively involved, whereas in others position sense is more affected. It is important to remember that a lack of proprioceptive impulses may interfere with discriminative sensory function, such as two-point discrimination and recognition of size, shape, and weight, and that impairment of this function may occur solely with posterior column disease. Paresthesias in the form of tingling and "pins-and-needles" sensations or girdle sensations are a common complaint with posterior column disease, and pain stimuli may also produce unpleasant sensations.

THE ANTERIOR AND LATERAL COLUMN SYNDROME. With occlusion of the anterior spinal artery or other destructive lesions that predominantly affect the ventral portion of the cord, there is a relative or absolute sparing of proprioceptive sensation and loss of pain and temperature sensation below the level of the lesion. Since the corticospinal tracts and the ventral gray matter also fall within the area of distribution of the anterior spinal artery, paralysis of motor function forms a prominent part of this syndrome.

DISTURBANCES OF SENSATION DUE TO LESIONS OF THE BRAIN STEM. A characteristic feature of lesions of the medulla and lower pons is that in many instances the sensory disturbance is crossed; i.e., there is loss of pain and temperature sensation of one side of the face and of the opposite side of the body. This is accounted for by involvement of the trigeminal tract or nucleus and the lateral spinothalamic tract on one side of the brain stem. In the upper pons and midbrain, where the spinothalamic tracts and the medial lemniscus become confluent, an appropriately placed lesion may cause a loss of all superficial and deep sensation over the contralateral side of the body. Cranial nerve palsies, cerebellar ataxia, or motor paralysis is often associated, as indicated in Chap. 48.

SENSORY LOSS DUE TO A LESION OF THE OPTIC THALAMUS (SYNDROME OF DEJÉRINE-ROUSSY)

Involvement of the nucleus ventralis posterolateralis of the thalamus, usually due to a vascular lesion or tumor, causes loss or diminution of all forms of sensation on the opposite side of the body. Position sense is affected more frequently than any other sensory function, and deep sensory loss is usually, but not always, more profound than cutaneous loss. There may be spontaneous pain or discomfort ("thalamic pain") on the affected side, and any form of stimulus may have a diffuse, unpleasant, lingering quality. Interestingly, this overresponse is usually associated with an elevated threshold; i.e., a stronger stimulus is necessary to produce a sensation, in spite of the greater discomfort experienced by the patient once the sensation had been evoked.

SENSORY LOSS DUE TO LESIONS IN THE PARIETAL LOBE

There is a disturbance mainly of discriminative sensory functions on the opposite side of the body, particularly the face, arm, and leg. Astereognosis, loss of position sense, impaired tactile localization, elevation of two-point threshold, and a general inattentiveness to sensory stimuli on one side of the body are the most prominent findings. Although pain and temperature, touch, and vibratory sense are stated to be intact in cortical lesions, this is only relatively true and impairment of these latter modalities may take a form other than elevation of threshold. Thus, on one examination sensation may appear almost normal and on a second examination the patient's responses may be inconstant and irregular. This type of response is often attributed to hysteria. Other features of parietal lobe symptomatology and the differences between dominant and nondominant parietal lobe syndromes will be considered in Chap. 54.

SENSORY LOSS DUE TO SUGGESTION AND HYSTERIA

The possibility of suggesting sensory loss to a patient has already been mentioned. In fact, hysterical patients almost never complain spontaneously of cutaneous sensory loss, although they may use the term *numbness* to indicate a paralysis of a limb. Complete hemianesthesia, often with reduced hearing, sight, smell, and taste, as well as impaired vibration sense over only half the skull, is a common finding in hysteria. Anesthesia of one entire limb or a sharply defined sensory loss over part of a limb, not conforming to the distribution of root or cutaneous nerve, is also frequently observed. Postural sensation is rarely affected. The diagnosis of hysterical hemianesthesia is best made by eliciting the other relevant symptoms of hysteria or, if this is not possible, by noting the discrepancies between this type of sensory loss and that which occurs as part of the usual sensory syndromes.

REFERENCES

Holmes, Gordon: "Introduction to Clinical Neurology," 2d ed., chaps. 8 and 9, Baltimore, The Williams & Wilkins Company, 1952.

Kibler, R. F., and P. W. Nathan: A Note on Warm and Cold Spots, Neurology, 10:874, 1960.

Mayo Clinic: "Clinical Examinations in Neurology," Philadelphia, W. B. Saunders Company, 1956.

Oppenheimer, D. R., E. Palmer, and G. Weddell: Nerve Endings in the Conjunctiva, J. Anat., 92:322, 1958.

Walshe, F. M. R.: "Critical Essays in Neurology," Baltimore, The Williams & Wilkins Company, 1948.

50 COMA AND RELATED DISTURBANCES OF CONSCIOUSNESS

Raymond D. Adams

The practitioner of medicine is frequently called upon to treat patients whose principal abnormality is an impairment of consciousness, which varies from simple confusion to coma. In large municipal hospitals it is estimated that as many as 3 per cent of total admissions are due to diseases that have caused coma, and although this figure seems high, it serves to emphasize the importance of this class of neurologic diseases and the necessity for every student of medicine to acquire a theoretic as well as a practical knowledge of them.

The terms *consciousness, confusion, stupor, uncon-*

sciousness, and *coma* have been endowed with so many different meanings that it is almost impossible to avoid ambiguity in their usage. They are not strictly medical terms, but literary, philosophic, and psychologic ones as well. The word *consciousness* is the most difficult of all. William James once remarked that everyone knew what consciousness was until he attempted to define it. To the psychologist consciousness denotes a state of awareness of one's self and one's environment. Knowledge of one's self, of course, includes all "feeling attitudes and emotions, impulses, volitions, and the active or striving aspects of conduct" (English)—in short, an awareness of all one's own mental functioning, particularly the cognitive processes. These can be judged only by the patient's verbal account of his introspections and indirectly by his actions. Physicians, being practical men for the most part, have learned to place greater confidence in their observations of the patient's general behavior and his reactions to overt stimuli than in what he says. For this reason when they employ the term *consciousness* they usually do so in its commonest and simplest signification, namely, a state of awareness of the environment. This narrow definition has another advantage in that the word *unconsciousness* is its exact opposite —a state of unawareness of environment or a suspension of those mental activities by which man is made aware of his environment. However, it must be pointed out that in psychoanalysis the word *unconscious* has a different meaning, standing for that repository of memories of previous experiences that cannot be immediately recalled to the conscious mind.

DESCRIPTION OF STATES OF NORMAL AND IMPAIRED CONSCIOUSNESS

The following definitions, while admittedly unacceptable to most psychologists, are of service to medicine, and they will provide the student with a convenient grammar for describing the mental states of his patients.

NORMAL CONSCIOUSNESS. This is the condition of the normal individual when fully awake, in which he is responsive to psychologic stimuli and "indicates by his behavior and speech that he has the same awareness of himself and his environment as ourselves." This normal state may fluctuate during the course of the day from keen alertness or deep concentration with a marked constriction of the field of attention to general inattentiveness and drowsiness.

SLEEP. Sleep is a state of physical and mental inactivity from which the patient may be aroused to normal consciousness. A person in sleep gives little evidence of being aware of himself or his environment, and in this respect he is unconscious. Yet he differs from a comatose patient in that he may still respond to unaccustomed stimuli and at times is capable of some mental activity in the form of dreams, which leave their traces in memory. And, of course, he can be recalled to a state of normal consciousness when stimulated.

COMA. The patient who appears to be asleep and is at the same time incapable of sensing or responding adequately to either external stimuli or inner needs is in a state of coma. Coma may vary in degree, and in its deepest stages no reaction of any kind is obtainable. Corneal, pupillary, pharyngeal, tendon, and plantar reflexes are all absent. There may or may not be extensor rigidity of the limbs and opisthotonos, signs which, Sherrington showed, indicate decerebration. Respirations are often slow and may be periodic, i.e., Cheyne-Stokes breathing. In lighter stages, referred to as *semicoma,* most of the above reflexes can be elicited, and the plantar reflexes may be either flexor or extensor (Babinski's sign). Moreover, pricking or pinching the skin, shaking and shouting at the patient, or an uncomfortable distension of the bladder may cause the patient to stir or moan and his respirations to quicken.

STUPOR. In stupor mental and physical activity are reduced to a minimum. Although inaccessible to many stimuli, the patient opens his eyes, looks at the examiner, and does not appear to be unconscious. Response to spoken commands is either absent or slow and inadequate. As a rule tendon or plantar reflexes are not altered. On the other hand, tremulousness of movement, coarse twitching of muscles, restless or stereotyped motor activity, and grasping and sucking reflexes are not infrequent. In psychiatry the term *stupor* means a state in which impressions of the external world are normally received, but activity is marked by negativism, e.g., catatonic schizophrenia.

CONFUSION. A state in which the patient cannot take into account all elements of his immediate environment. Like delirium it always implies an element of sensorial clouding. The term lacks precision, however, for often it signifies an inability to think with customary speed and coherence. Here the difficulty is in defining thinking.

A severely confused person is usually unable to do more than carry out a few simple commands. His capacity for speech may be limited to a few words or phrases, or he may be voluble. He is unaware of much that goes on around him and does not grasp his immediate situation. A moderately confused individual can carry on a simple conversation for short periods of time, but his thinking is slow and incoherent and he is disoriented in time and place. In mild degrees of confusion the disorder may be so slight that it is overlooked unless the examiner is objective in his analysis of the patient's behavior and conversation. The patient may be roughly oriented as to time and place and able to speak freely on almost any subject. Only occasional irrelevant remarks betray an incoherence of thinking. Patients with mild or moderately severe confusion may be submitted to psychologic testing. The degree of confusion often varies from one time of day to another and tends to be least pronounced in the early morning. Severe confusion or stupor may resemble semicoma during periods when the patient is drowsy or asleep. Many events that happen to the confused patient leave no trace in memory; in fact, capacity to recall later events that transpired in any given period is one of the most delicate tests of mental clarity.

Some neurologists regard *delirium* as a state of confusion with excitement and hyperactivity, and in some medical writings delirium and confusion are used interchangeably. It is undoubtedly true that the delirious patient is nearly always confused. However, the vivid hallucinations which characterize delirious states, the relative inaccessibility of the patient to other events than those to which he is reacting at any one moment, his extreme agitation and tremulousness, and the tendency to convulse suggest a cerebral disorder of a somewhat different type. The clearest evidence of the relationship of confusion, stupor, and coma is that the patient may pass through all three states as he becomes comatose or emerges from coma. The author has not observed any such relationship between coma and delirium, and the latter is discussed as a separate entity (Chap. 54).

At times a patient with certain types of aphasia, especially jargon aphasia, may create the impression of confusion, but close observation will reveal that the disorder is confined to the sphere of language and that behavior is otherwise natural.

THE ELECTROENCEPHALOGRAM AND DISTURBANCES OF CONSCIOUSNESS

One of the most delicate confirmations of the fact that these states of altered consciousness are expressions of neurophysiologic changes is the electroencephalogram. In the normal waking state the electrical potentials of the cortical neurones are integrated into regular waves of two frequency ranges, from 8 to 15 (alpha rhythm) and 16 to 25 (beta rhythm). These wave forms are established by adolescence, but certain individual differences in general pattern and dominance of alpha waves are maintained throughout adult life. With sleep these cortical potentials slow down and amplitude (voltage) of the individual waves increases. At one stage in light sleep characteristic bursts of 14 to 16 per sec waves appear, the so-called "sleep spindles," and in deep sleep all the waves of normal frequency and amplitude are replaced by slow ones of high voltage (1½ to 3 per sec). Similarly, some alteration in brain waves occurs in all disturbances of consciousness except the milder degrees of confusion. This alteration usually consists of a disorganization of the electroencephalographic pattern, which shows random, slow waves of high voltage in stages of confusion; more regular, slow, 2 to 3 per sec waves of high voltage in stupor and semicoma; and slow waves or even suppression of all organized electrical activity in deep coma (see Chap. 200). The electroencephalograms of deep sleep and light coma resemble one another. Not all diseases that cause confusion and coma have the same effect on the electroencephalogram. Some, such as barbiturate intoxication, may cause an increase in frequency and amplitude of the brain waves. In epilepsy the disturbance of consciousness is usually attended by paroxysms of "spikes"

(fast waves of high amplitude) or by the characteristic alternating slow waves and spikes of petit mal. Other diseases such as hepatic coma characteristically cause a slowing in frequency and an increasing amplitude of "brain waves" and special triphasic waves. Whether all metabolic diseases of the brain induce similar changes in the electroencephalogram has not been determined. Probably there are differences between them, some of which may be significant.

MORBID ANATOMY OF COMA

For a long time it has been known to neuropathologists that lesions situated in the upper midbrain and diencephalon are most likely to be accompanied by prolonged disturbances of consciousness. This was anticipated by Herbert Spencer in his *Principles of Psychology,* when he suggested that the seat of consciousness would be found to reside where there is a confluence of sensory pathways. His idea was based on sound psychologic reasoning and not on mystical speculations, as was Galen's localization of consciousness in the lateral ventricles or Descartes' in the pineal gland.

Since the time of Hughlings Jackson it has been suggested that both the cerebral cortex and diencephalon provide the anatomic substratum of consciousness. After observation of pathologic coma in some cases of pituitary tumor and the hypersomnia of encephalitis lethargica, attention turned to the hypothalamus. Research on this part of the brain has done much to elucidate the neural mechanisms of wakefulness and sleep. It was discovered that the reticular nuclei of the midbrain and the intralaminar and anterior nuclei of the thalami are part of a diffuse recruiting or activating system that influences large parts of the cerebral cortex. Lesions in this system of neurones diffusely alter the electrical activity of the cortex and produce coma. Collaterals from the medial and lateral lemnisci, i.e., the main sensory afferents, terminate in this region. Thus it would appear that stimulation of sensory neurones has a double effect, conveying to the body information of the outside world and also providing some of the energy for activating those parts of the nervous system on which consciousness depends.

MECHANISMS WHEREBY CONSCIOUSNESS IS DISTURBED IN DISEASE

Knowledge of diseases of the nervous system is so limited that it is not possible to identify all the different mechanisms by means of which consciousness is disturbed. Already several ways are known in which the mesencephalic-diencephalic-cortical systems are deranged, and there are probably many others.

In a number of disease processes there is direct interference with the metabolic activities of the nerve cells in the cerebral cortex and the cerebral nuclear masses of the brain. Hypoxia, hypoglycemia, and deficiencies of thiamine, nicotinic acid, vitamin B_{12}, pantothenic acid, and pyridoxine are well-known examples. The intimate details of these underlying bio-chemical changes have not yet been fully elucidated, but methods are becoming available for their study. The rate of cerebral blood flow can now be determined in human beings with considerable accuracy (Schmidt-Kety method) by measuring the rate of diffusion of inert gases such as N_2O or krypton into the brain, namely, the time required for the gas to reach the same degree of concentration in the jugular venous blood as in arterial blood after 10 min inhalation of the gas. The normal value of cerebral blood flow (CBF) is 700 to 800 ml per min. The cerebral meta-bolic rate (CMR = oxygen consumption per minute) is determined at the same time by measuring the oxy-gen difference between arterial and jugular blood and multiplying this difference by the rate of cerebral blood flow. The normal value of the cerebral metabolic rate is 46 ml per min. In hypoglycemia the cerebral blood flow is normal or above normal, whereas the cerebral metabolic rate is diminished owing to defi-ciency of substrate. In thiamine and vitamin B_{12} de-ficiency the cerebral blood flow is normal or slightly diminished, and the cerebral metabolic rate is dimin-ished, presumably because of insufficiency of coen-zymes. Extremes of body temperature, either hyper-thermia (temperature over 106°F) or hypothermia (temperature below 97°F), probably induce coma by exerting a nonspecific effect on the metabolic activity of neurones.

Diabetic acidosis, uremia, hepatic coma, and the coma of systemic infections are examples of endoge-nous intoxications. The identity of the toxic agents is not known. In diabetes acetone bodies (acetoacetic acid, β-hydroxybutyric acid, and acetone) are present in high concentration, and in uremia there is probably accumulation of phenolic derivatives of the aromatic amino acids. In both conditions "dehydration" and acidosis may also play an important role. In many cases of hepatic coma elevation of blood NH_3 to levels five to six times normal has been found. The mode of action of bacterial toxins is unknown. In all these conditions the cerebral metabolic rate is reduced, whereas cerebral blood flow remains normal.

In toxic and metabolic diseases the patient usually approaches coma through a state of drowsiness, con-fusion, and stupor, and the reverse sequence occurs as he emerges from it. Each disease probably manifests itself by a characteristic clinical picture, which will be described in a later section of the book.

A critical decline in blood pressure, usually to a systolic level below 70 mm Hg, affects neural struc-tures by causing a decrease in cerebral blood flow and, secondarily, a diminution in cerebral metabolic rate. If decline in blood pressure is episodic, the corre-sponding clinical picture is syncope (see Chap. 44). Here the clinical picture is one of physical weakness usually preceding and following the loss of conscious-ness, the whole process being acute and promptly reversible.

The sudden, violent, and excessive discharge of epi-lepsy is another mechanism. Usually a Jacksonian con-vulsion has little effect on consciousness until it spreads from one side of the body to the other. Coma immediately ensues, presumably because the spread-ing of the seizure discharge to central neuronal struc-tures paralyzes their function. Other types of seizure in which consciousness is interrupted from the very beginning are believed to originate in the diencepha-lon. Concussion exemplifies still another special patho-physiologic mechanism. In "blunt" head injury it has been shown that there is an enormous increase in intracranial pressure of the order of 200 to 700 lb per sq in., lasting a few thousandths of a second. Either the vibration set up in the skull and transmitted to the brain or this sudden high intracranial pressure is believed to be the basis of the sudden paralysis of the nervous system that follows head injury. That the in-creased pressure itself may be the main factor has been suggested by experiments in which raising the intraventricular pressure to a level approaching dias-tolic blood pressure has abolished all vital functions.

Large, destructive, and space-consuming lesions of the brain such as hemorrhage, tumor, or abscess inter-fere with consciousness in two ways. One is by direct destruction of the midbrain and diencephalon; the other, far more frequent, is by producing herniation of the medial part of the temporal lobe through the opening of the tentorium and crushing the upper brain against the opposite free edge of the tentorium. The latter, usually referred to as the *tentorial pressure cone*, is responsible for the dilated (Hutchinson's) pupil on the side of a large cerebral lesion or bilater-ally, the ipsilateral hemiparesis and bilateral Babin-ski signs, the coma, and the slowing or irregularity of respirations.

CLINICAL APPROACH TO THE COMATOSE PATIENT

Coma is not an independent disease entity but is always a symptomatic expression of disease. Some-times the underlying disease is perfectly obvious, as when a healthy individual is struck on the head and rendered unconscious. All too often, however, the pa-tient is brought to the hospital in a state of coma, and little or no information about him is immediately available. The physician must then subject the clinical problem to careful scrutiny from many directions. To do this efficiently he must have a broad knowledge of disease and a methodical approach to the problem that leaves none of the common and treatable causes of coma unexplored.

It should be pointed out that when the comatose patient is seen for the first time, simple therapeutic measures take precedence over diagnostic procedures. A quick survey should make sure that the comatose patient has a clear airway and is not in shock (cir-culatory collapse) or, if trauma has occurred, that he is not bleeding from a wound. In patients who have suffered a head injury there may be a fracture of the cervical vertebras, and therefore one must be cau-tious about moving the head and neck lest the spinal cord be inadvertently crushed. There must be an immediate inquiry as to the previous health of the patient: whether the patient had suffered a head injury or had been seen in a convulsion, and the circumstances in which he was found. The persons who accompany the comatose patient to the hospital should not be permitted to leave until they have been questioned.

DIAGNOSTIC PROCEDURES. The temperature, pulse, respiratory rate, and blood pressure are of aid in diagnosis. Fever suggests a severe systemic infection such as pneumonia, bacterial meningitis, or a brain lesion that has disturbed the temperature-regulating centers. An excessively high body temperature, 107 to 110°F, associated with dry skin should arouse the suspicion of heat stroke. Hypothermia is frequently observed in alcoholic or barbiturate intoxication, extracellular fluid deficit, or peripheral circulatory failure. Slow breathing points to morphine or barbiturate intoxication, whereas deep rapid breathing (Kussmaul's respiration) suggests diabetic or uremic acidosis but may also occur in intracranial diseases. Rapid breathing accompanied by an expiratory grunt and associated with fever is a frequent finding in lobar pneumonia. Diseases that elevate the intracranial pressure or damage the brain, especially the brain stem, often cause slow, irregular, or periodic (Cheyne-Stokes) breathing. The pulse rate is less helpful, but if exceptionally slow, it should suggest heart block or, if combined with periodic breathing and hypertension, an increase in intracranial pressure. A tachycardia of 160 or above calls attention to the possibility of an ectopic cardiac rhythm with insufficiency of cerebral circulation. Marked hypertension occurs in patients with cerebral hemorrhage and hypertensive encephalopathy and, at times, those with increased intracranial pressure; whereas hypotension is the usual finding in the coma of diabetes, alcohol or barbiturate intoxication, or internal hemorrhage.

Inspection of the skin may also yield valuable information. Multiple bruises, and in particular a bruise or boggy area in the scalp, favor cranial trauma. Bleeding from an ear or nose or orbital hemorrhage also raises the possibility of trauma. Puffiness and hyperemia of face and conjunctivas and telangiectasia are the usual stigmas of alcoholism; marked pallor suggests internal hemorrhage. The presence of a maculohemorrhagic rash indicates the possibility of meningococcal infection, staphylococcus endocarditis, typhus, or Rocky Mountain spotted fever. Pellagra may be diagnosed from the typical skin lesions on face and hands.

The odor of the breath may provide clues to the nature of a disease causing coma. The odor of alcohol is easily recognized. The spoiled-fruit odor of diabetic coma, the uriniferous odor of uremia, and the musty fetor of hepatic coma are distinctive enough to be identified by physicians who possess a keen sense of smell.

PHYSICAL EXAMINATION. The next step is a careful physical examination with special attention to the neurologic function. Although limited in many ways, careful observation of the stuporous or comatose patient may yield considerable information concerning the function of different parts of the nervous system. One of the most helpful procedures is to sit at the patient's bedside for 5 to 10 min and observe what he does. The predominant postures of the body, the position of the head and eyes, the rate, depth, and rhythm of respiration, and the pulse should be noted. The state of responsiveness should then be estimated by noting the patient's reaction when his name is called, his capacity to execute a simple command, or to respond to painful stimuli.

Usually it is possible to determine whether or not the coma is accompanied by meningeal irritation or focal disease in the cerebrum or brain stem. With meningeal irritation from either bacterial meningitis or subarachnoid hemorrhage, there is resistance to active and passive flexion of the neck but not to extension, turning, or tipping the head. Resistance to movement of the neck in all directions indicates disease of the cervical spine or is part of generalized rigidity. In infants, bulging of the anterior fontanel is at times a more reliable sign of meningeal irritation than stiff neck. A cerebellar pressure cone or decerebrate rigidity may also limit passive flexion of the neck and may be confused with meningeal irritation.

Evidence of disease of midbrain, pons, or medulla can be obtained even though the patient is comatose by noting the prevailing posture of the body and by examining the cranial nerves. Decerebrate rigidity is indicated by extension of all four extremities and opisthotonos, and it may be continuous or intermittent; if intermittent, it is sometimes referred to as a *tonic cerebellar fit*. Tonic neck reflexes, i.e., extension of the right arm and leg and flexion of the left arm and leg upon turning of the head to the right, and the opposite movements when the head is turned to the left, may be demonstrated in some cases of decerebration. These attitudes and postures signify a disorder of upper pons and midbrain, and although it may be due to a functional derangement, as in a toxic or metabolic disorder, more often it points to a gross structural lesion such as a hemorrhage, basilar artery occlusion, or temporal lobe pressure cone. In contrast, the decorticate patient lies with arms rigidly flexed and legs extended, or at times with diagonal postures, i.e., one arm and the opposite leg flexed and other limbs extended. By decorticate is usually meant a lesion not of the cerebral cortex but of the motor parts of the cerebral hemispheres or the internal capsules.

Lesions of the oculomotor and abducens nerves can be detected by pupillary inequality, unequal width of palpebral fissures, or strabismus. It must be remembered that in coma the eyes tend to diverge slightly owing to relaxation of the effort of accommodation. In light coma the eyes can often be induced to move to either side by turning the head; e.g., when the head is turned to the right, the eyes move conjugately to the left, and when the head is turned to the left, the eyes move to the right. In deep coma irrigation of each ear separately with 10 to 15 ml ice water causes the eyes to turn to the side stimulated, thus proving the integrity of the pontine and brain tegmentum. A sustained conjugate deviation of both eyes in one direction indicates either a paralysis of gaze in the opposite direction or a contralateral homonymous hemianopia. Loss of the pupillary light reflex on one side means either blindness of that eye or a lesion in midbrain or oculomotor nerve and its nucleus. A loss of consensual reflex places the lesion in the efferent limb of the reflex arc (i.e., oculomotor nucleus or nerve). Bilateral constriction of the pupils may occur in pontine hemorrhage or in opiate intoxication. Absent corneal reflex on one side implicates the trigeminal nerve or its spinal nucleus in the pons or medulla. The same may be said of failure to wince or avert the head when one side of the face is pricked. Hemianesthesia of cerebral origin may also weaken or abolish the corneal and pharyngeal reflexes on one side. Severe pressure exerted upon the supraorbital ridges makes the patient grimace, and drooping and flacidity on one side of the face when in repose indicate a facial paralysis. Also the cheek on the paralyzed side may puff out with each expiration.

Integrity of the auditory nerve is sometimes shown by blinking of the eyes at a loud sound. Persistent nystagmus, especially when unidirectional, suggests disease of the vestibular nuclei. Nystagmus in all directions of eye movement in a drowsy or confused patient raises suspicion of barbiturate intoxication. Swallowing movements can be observed, and a few drops of water in the mouth will test their adequacy. They may be abolished in deep coma or in diseases that cause lesions in both cerebral hemispheres or upper brain stem. Gag reflexes are evoked by stimulating each side of the pharyngeal wall. Facility of movement of the tongue may be determined by stroking the lips and observing spontaneous licking, vocalizing, and masticatory movements. In stupor or coma the patient may be unable to inhibit closing the eyes when in a bright light or closing the mouth and clenching the jaw when an object such as a throat stick is placed in the mouth. This may be mistaken for negativism or voluntary resistance.

Paralysis of the arms and legs can be discovered, if the patient is restless, by the lack of movement in certain parts. Another useful maneuver is to lift the limbs from the bed, feel the muscle tone on passive movement, and permit them to fall. Paralyzed limbs fall more heavily, remain in uncomfortable positions, and flatten out on the bed more than nonparalyzed ones. Pinprick may provoke movements of the limbs. Failure to heed a painful stimulus on one side, and a response such as quickening of respirations or groaning or grimacing or restless movement on the other, suggest hemianesthesia. If sensation is intact but one arm and leg are paralyzed, a grimace, a groan, and restless movements may occur when a painful stimulus is applied to either side. Of course, the voluntary withdrawal of one arm and leg from the stimulus or complex avoidance reactions are prevented by the hem-

iplegia. The tendon reflexes are often unequal on the two sides, tending to be diminished on the side of a recent acute hemiplegia and increased on the side of a chronic hemiplegia. The plantar reflexes may be bilaterally extensor, but they may be absent or more definitely extensor on the paralyzed side.

A history of headache before or at the onset of coma, recurrent vomiting, and papilledema afford the best clues to increased intracranial pressure. This can be confirmed by lumbar puncture, which is usually safe unless there is a herniation of the temporal lobe through the tentorium or of the cerebellum through the foramen magnum. In the latter instance the cerebrospinal fluid pressure may not reflect intracranial pressure. Papilledema may develop within 12 to 24 hr in brain trauma and brain hemorrhage but, if pronounced, usually signifies brain tumor or abscess of longer duration. Multiple retinal or large subhyaloid hemorrhages are usually associated with ruptured saccular aneurysm or hemorrhage from an angioma. Papilledema, with widespread retinal exudates, hemorrhages, and arteriolar changes, is an almost invariable accompaniment of hypertensive encephalopathy. In patients with evidence of increased intracranial pressure, lumbar puncture, although admittedly dangerous because it may promote further herniation, is nevertheless necessary in some instances. See Chap. 109 for further discussion of retinal changes.

LABORATORY PROCEDURES. Unless the diagnosis is established at once by history and physical examination, it is necessary to carry out a number of laboratory procedures. If poisoning is suspected, the gastric contents must be aspirated and saved for later chemical analysis. A catheter is passed into the urinary bladder, and a specimen of urine is obtained for determination of specific gravity, sugar, acetone, and albumin content. Urine of low specific gravity and high protein content is nearly always found in uremia, but proteinuria may also occur for 2 or 3 days after a subarachnoid hemorrhage or with fever. Urine of high specific gravity, glycosuria, and acetonuria are almost invariable in diabetic coma; but glycosuria and hyperglycemia may result from a massive cerebral lesion. If bromide or barbiturate intoxication is suspected, it can be verified by special tests for these substances. A blood count is made, and in malarial districts a blood smear is examined for malarial parasites. Neutrophilic leukocytosis occurs in bacterial infections and also with brain hemorrhage and softening. Venous blood should be examined for glucose, nonprotein nitrogen, CO_2, sodium, potassium, and chlorides. The cerebrospinal fluid must be drawn, and the pressure, presence of blood, white cell count, and results of Pandy's test should be recorded. Bloody cerebrospinal fluid occurs in cerebral contusion, subarachnoid hemorrhage, brain hemorrhage, and occasionally with hemorrhagic infarcts due to thrombophlebitis or embolism. If there is pleocytosis, a stained smear of the sediment should be searched for bacteria and a rough quantitative sugar determination should be done. The standard cerebrospinal fluid formula in bacterial meningitis is elevated pressure, high white cell count (5,000/ 20,000), elevated protein, and subnormal sugar values. The fluid should be saved for quantitative tests for sugar and protein, and a bacterial culture and Wassermann reaction should be performed. If the pressure is suspected of being elevated, a No. 20 needle should be used. A very high pressure must be slowly reduced by removal of 10 to 15 ml over a period of 15 to 20 min, and urea or other hypertonic solutions should be given intravenously. Afterward the foot of the bed should be elevated. Jugular compression tests are obviously contraindicated. X-rays of the skull should be obtained as soon as possible after these procedures, preferably on the way from the emergency ward to the hospital room.

CLASSIFICATION OF COMA AND DIFFERENTIAL DIAGNOSIS

The demonstration of focal brain disease or meningeal irritation, with cerebrospinal fluid abnormality, helps in differential diagnosis. The diseases that frequently cause coma can be conveniently divided into three classes, as follows:

CLASSIFICATION OF COMA

I. Diseases that cause no focal or lateralizing neurologic signs or alteration of the cellular content of the cerebrospinal fluid
   A. Intoxications (alcohol, barbiturates, opiates, etc.)
   B. Metabolic disturbances (diabetic acidosis, uremia, Addisonian crisis, hepatic coma, hypoglycemia, hypoxia)
   C. Severe systemic infections (pneumonia, typhoid fever, malaria, Waterhouse-Friderichsen syndrome)
   D. Circulatory collapse (shock) from any cause, cardiac decompensation in the aged
   E. Epilepsy
   F. Hypertensive encephalopathy and eclampsia
   G. Hyperthermia or hypothermia
II. Diseases that cause meningeal irritation, with either blood or an excess of white cells in the cerebrospinal fluid, usually without focal or lateralizing signs
   A. Subarachnoid hemorrhage from ruptured aneurysm, occasionally trauma
   B. Acute bacterial meningitis
   C. Some forms of virus encephalitis
   D. Acute hemorrhagic leukoencephalitis
III. Diseases that cause focal or lateralizing neurologic signs, with or without changes in the cerebrospinal fluid
   A. Brain hemorrhage (Chap. 204)
   B. Brain softening due to thrombosis or embolism (Chap. 204)
   C. Brain abscess (Chap. 207)
   D. Epidural and subdural hemorrhage and brain contusion (Chap. 205)
   E. Brain tumor (Chap. 206)
   F. Miscellaneous, i.e., thrombophlebitis, some forms of virus encephalomyelitis (Chap. 208)

If the history and the examination of the comatose patient and the accessory laboratory procedures enable the physician to decide which of these three classes of neurologic disease his patient has, the differential diagnosis is greatly simplified. Class I includes essentially the toxic and metabolic encephalopathies, and usually any definite sign of localized lesion in one cerebral hemisphere, the brain stem, or cerebellum, or a cellular change in the cerebrospinal fluid, is sufficient to exclude these diseases.

It must be conceded that clinical cases are complex and that even the most careful analysis will not always yield the correct diagnosis. If the patient has had a focal brain lesion before the onset of his present illness, the signs of it could become more pronounced during coma from toxic or metabolic diseases and this may at times be a source of error. Or a difficult lumbar puncture resulting in a "bloody tap" may also cause an erroneous diagnosis. Finally, certain rare diseases like lead encephalopathy in infants may induce a mild pleocytosis and elevation in the protein content of the cerebrospinal fluid. Another difficulty sometimes encountered in dealing with the comatose patient is that the level of unconsciousness is so deep that it is impossible to detect focal or lateralizing signs. Often, however, such an illness is so completely beyond control of the physician that diagnosis becomes unimportant.

It must be remembered that diagnosis has as its prime purpose the direction of therapy, and it matters little to the patient whether or not we diagnose a disease for which we have no treatment. The treatable forms of coma are drug intoxications, toxemia from systemic infections, epidural and subdural hematoma, brain abscess, bacterial and tuberculous meningitis, diabetic acidosis, and hypoglycemia.

Incidence of Diseases That Cause Coma

There have been only a few attempts to determine the relative incidence of diseases that lead to coma. A report from the Boston City Hospital (Solomon and Aring) includes the largest series of clinical cases but was heavily skewed by the large local problem of chronic alcoholics, which made up 60 per cent of all admissions in coma. Trauma (13 per cent), cerebral vascular disease (10 per cent), poisonings (3 per cent), epilepsy (2.4 per cent), diabetes, bacterial meningitis, pneumonia, uremia, and eclampsia followed in that order. In the series of fatal cases studied at the Cook County Hospital (Holcomb), accuracy of clinical diagnosis was not more than 50 per cent and did not improve with increasing length of survival (in half the fatal cases the patient died in the first 24 hr and in two-thirds, within 48 hr). Again, trauma, cerebrovascular disease, meningitis, and alcoholism accounted for the majority of cases.

Of course, figures like these do not provide information concerning coma caused by multiple factors. For example, a patient with a cerebral vascular lesion, old or recent, and diabetes mellitus may lapse into coma during an insulin reaction at a time when there is still sugar in the urine. Only by appreciating the interplay of these several common factors is one likely to reach the correct diagnosis.

The differential diagnosis of diseases that cause focal or lateralizing signs and meningitis will be taken up under the discussions of traumatic, neoplastic, vascular, and infective diseases of the brain.

CARE OF THE COMATOSE PATIENT

Impaired states of consciousness, regardless of their cause, are often fatal because they not only represent an advanced stage of many diseases but also add their own characteristic burden to the primary disease. The main objective of therapy is, of course, to find the cause of the coma, according to the procedures already outlined, and to remove it. It often happens, however, that the disease process is one for which there is no specific therapy; or as in hypoxia or hypoglycemia, the disease process may already have expended itself before the patient comes to the attention of the physician. Again, the problem may be infinitely complex, for the disturbance may be attributable not to a single cause but rather to several possible factors acting in unison, no one of which could account for the total clinical picture. In lieu of direct therapy, supportive measures must be used, and, indeed, it may be said that the patient's chances of surviving the original disease often depend in large measure on their effectiveness.

The physician must give attention to every vital function in the insensate patient. The following is a brief outline of the more important procedures. In order for them to be carried out successfully a well-coordinated team of nurses under constant guidance of a physician is needed.

1. If the patient is in shock, this takes precedence over all other abnormalities. The treatment of shock is discussed in Chap. 135.

2. Shallow and irregular respirations and cyanosis require the establishment of a clear airway and oxygen. The patient should be placed in a semiprone position so that secretions and vomitus do not enter the tracheobronchial tree. Pharyngeal reflexes are usually suppressed, and therefore an endotracheal tube can be inserted without difficulty. Stagnant secretions should be removed with a suction apparatus as soon as they accumulate, since they will lead to atelectasis and bronchopneumonia. Oxygen can be administered by mask in a 100 per cent concentration for 6 to 12 hr, alternating with 50 per cent concentration for 4 hr. The depth of respiration can be increased by the use of 5 to 10 per cent carbon dioxide for periods of 3 to 5 min every hour. Atropine should not be given; edema of the lungs and fluid in the tracheobronchial passages are not glandular secretions. Furthermore, atropine thickens this fluid and also may disturb temperature regulation of the body. Amino-

phylline is helpful in controlling Cheyne-Stokes breathing. Respiratory paralysis dictates the use of a positive-pressure respirator or electrophrenic stimulator, but in the author's experience neither has been effective in comatose states in which there is disorganization of respiratory centers.

3. The temperature-regulating mechanisms may be disturbed, and extreme hypothermia, hyperthermia, or an unrecognized poikilothermia may occur. In hyperthermia, removal of blankets and use of alcohol sponges and cooling solutions are indicated.

4. The bladder should not be permitted to become distended. If the patient does not void, a retention catheter should be inserted. If more than 500 ml urine is found in the bladder, decompression must be carried out slowly over a period of hours. Urine excretion should be kept above 800 to 1,000 ml per day. The patient should not be permitted to lie in a wet or soiled bed.

5. Diseases of the central nervous system may upset the control of water, glucose, and salt. The unconscious patient can no longer adjust his intake of food and fluids by hunger and thirst. Salt-losing and salt-retaining syndromes have both been described with brain disease. Water intoxication and severe hyponatremia may of themselves prove fatal. The maintenance of water and electrolytes will be discussed in Chap. 60. If coma is prolonged, the insertion of a stomach tube will ease the problem of feeding the patient and maintaining fluid and electrolyte balance.

6. One should not attempt to forestall the development of bronchopneumonia by the prophylactic use of penicillin and streptomycin or some other broad-spectrum antibiotics; instead, appropriate ones should be administered when the infection occurs. The legs should be examined each day for signs of phlebothrombosis.

7. If the patient is capable of moving, suitable restraints should be used to prevent a possible fall out of bed.

8. Convulsions should be controlled by measures outlined in Chap. 219.

REFERENCES

Holcomb, B.: Causes and Diagnosis of Various Forms of Coma, J.A.M.A., 77:2112, 1921.

Munro, D.: "Craniocerebral Injuries, Their Diagnosis and Treatment," New York, Oxford University Press, 1938.

Purdon-Martin, J.: Consciousness and Its Disturbances, Brit. Med. J. (Lancet), I:48, 1946.

Solomon, P., and C. D. Aring: The Causes of Coma in Patients Entering a General Hospital, Am. J. Med. Sci., 188:805, 1938.

——, and ——: Differential Diagnosis in Patients Entering a General Hospital in Coma, J.A.M.A., 105:7, 1935.

51 SLEEP AND ITS ABNORMALITIES
Raymond D. Adams

Sleep, that familiar yet inexplicable condition of repose in which consciousness is in abeyance, is obviously not abnormal; yet there is no absurdity in considering it in connection with abnormal phenomena. There are no doubt irregularities of sleep which approach serious extremes, just as there are unnatural forms of waking consciousness.

Everyone has had much personal experience of sleep, or the lack of it, and has observed others in sleep; so it requires no special knowledge of medicine to know something about this condition or to appreciate its importance to health and well-being. Nearly all the great writers of the past have expressed their views on the psychologic and physical benefits of sleep but probably none with more feeling than Sterne, who has Tristram Shandy remark: " 'Tis the refuge of the unfortunate—the enfranchisement of the prisoner—the downy lap of the hopeless, the weary, the broken-hearted; of all the soft, delicious functions of nature this is the chiefest; what a happiness it is to man, when anxieties and passions of the day are over. . . ."

Physicians are often sought by individuals who suffer an illness caused by or accompanied by some derangement of sleep. Most often the problem is one of sleeplessness, but sometimes it concerns peculiar phenomena occurring in connection with sleep.

THE EFFECTS OF LOSS OF SLEEP

Of the conditions making for human efficiency, sleep is one of the most important. Sleep is absolutely essential to normal body metabolism. Experimental animals deprived of sleep will die within a few days, no matter how well they are fed, watered, and housed.

Despite the many studies of the effect of sleeplessness on human beings and animals, we still do not know as much as we should about it. Experiments on human beings have taken the form of enforced abstention from sleep for several days, with tests administered before, during, and after. One group of psychologists succeeded in keeping their subjects going in a state of apparent wakefulness for 90 hr. The surprising result was that on tests such as tapping, aiming at targets, reading letters, and calculation there was no failure of performance even after the loss of two nights' sleep. The sleepless subjects did fail, however, in tasks requiring sustained attention. They could do as well as they normally would on short tests, but on longer ones of the same degree of difficulty they became slow and inaccurate. Another characteristic was sluggishness of attention in shifting from one task or one test item to another. It was difficult for the subjects to redirect their activity; once started on a given line, they could hardly be diverted from it. Whatever their achievement on the tests, all subjects reported numerous symptoms such

as burning eyes, headache, dazed feeling, nervousness, emotional instability, loss of motor power and coordination, and distressing visual hallucinations. In general deportment they were alternately irritable and silly, tending to laugh at anything said to them.

The reason for the relatively good test performance in the face of these bodily sensations is the ability of the normal individual to compensate. He can "shake himself out of it" and apply himself with an effort that overcomes his deficiencies. The extra effort put forth to remain oriented to the task cannot be maintained without cost. The energy consumed during an arithmetic test, as measured by the metabolic rate, is about three times greater in persons who have lost sleep.

Another surprising finding was that the subjects recovered on less than 35 per cent of the sleep that had been lost. In other words, the amount of sleep required after the experiment is not equal to the number of hours that they were kept awake. Probably the explanation is that the subjects were not fully awake at all times, and in the latter part of the experiment they may have been half asleep.

A corollary of this hypothesis is that persons who sleep for long periods do not necessarily obtain the maximum benefits from sleep. Sleep may be sound and restful or light and fitful. In sound sleep the psychogalvanic test of skin resistance of the palm is raised, and in poor sleep it remains the same as in the waking state. It has also been found that only in sound sleep does the blood pressure fall. From these fragmentary studies it must be concluded that the value of sleep to the metabolism of the human organism is a function of its depth multiplied by its length and that long hours spent in bed are no substitute for sound sleep.

Recent work by Aserinsky and Kleitman has shown that the sleep pattern of normal man and many mammals is characterized by four or five periods each night during which the electroencephalogram reveals fast waves. At the same time there is ocular movement, cessation of muscular tone, fluctuations of pulse and respiration, and penile erection. When subjects are awakened during these periods, they almost always report that they had been dreaming. This constellation of electric and physiologic changes has been called the "D" or "dream state," and the experiments of Jouvet indicate that it depends on a positive mechanism.

DERANGEMENTS OF SLEEP

INSOMNIA. The word *insomnia* signifies want of sleep and is used popularly to indicate any interference with the duration or depth of sleep. As every physician knows from practical experience, this is not a disease but a symptom of many diseases, which differ widely in their nature and gravity. It is associated equally with trivial ailments and with conditions which jeopardize life. The persistence and severity of insomnia are no guide to the diagnosis of the condition on which it depends.

Since insomnia is often a symptom of a minor illness, there is a tendency for the physician to make light of it. Yet few common conditions cause more misery and discomfort to the patient. When deprived of the nightly restoration of his energies, he grows weary and his whole mental and physical vigor is impaired. He seems to exhaust his fund of reserve force. His tolerance of pain, noise, and the countless irritations of everyday life is reduced. This, in turn, reflects itself in his psychologic reaction to all the ordinary symptoms of disease. Also, the capacity for effective work is intimately related to the ability to sleep; in fact, this is one of the most reliable measures of sound health.

Once there was a tendency to formulate elaborate classifications of insomnia according to the nature of the diseases in each of the different organ systems of the body. This approach has little to offer, because in the final analysis the factors operating in all these diseases are relatively few. Most instances of unyielding insomnia are due to (1) the presence of pain and discomfort or (2) anxiety and other nervous disorders.

Several types of sensory disorder may cause abnormal wakefulness. The pain of spine and root or peripheral nerve disease may be particularly troublesome at night, and the same is true of abdominal discomfort in a number of gastrointestinal diseases such as pancreatic carcinoma. Tired, aching, restless legs, which has been described as the "restless leg syndrome" (anxietas tibialis) may regularly delay the onset of natural sleep. Excessive fatigue may give rise to many abnormal muscular sensations of a similar nature. Acroparesthesia, that peculiar nocturnal tingling numbness of the hands which is so common in women, may awaken the patient nightly.

Insomnia is a frequent complaint of patients suffering from psychiatric disease. Its simplest form is that of a reactive nervous state in which domestic and business worries keep the patient in a turmoil. Also, vigorous mental activity late at night or excitement counteracts drowsiness and sleep. Under these circumstances there is difficulty in falling asleep and a tendency to sleep late in the morning. Sleeplessness is also commonly recorded in the histories of patients suffering from psychoneuroses and psychoses. In a valuable study of the character of sleep in psychiatric patients Muncie informs us that in illnesses in which anxiety and fear are prominent symptoms there is usually difficulty in falling asleep and light, fitful, or intermittent sleep. Also, disturbing dreams, so common in such conditions, may awaken the patient, and he may even try to stay awake in order to avoid them. In contrast, the depressive illnesses, particularly manic-depressive or involutional depression, cause early morning waking and inability to return to sleep. If anxiety is combined with depression, both the above patterns are observed. In states of mania all types of sleep disorder are known to occur. The sleep rhythm may be totally deranged in acute confusional states and delirium. In the latter the patient may only doze for short periods both day and night. The total amount and depth of sleep in a 24-hr period is reduced. Frightening hallucinations may prevent sleep. The senile and arteriosclerotic patient tends to catnap during the day and then refuse to go to bed at night; his nocturnal sleep is intermittent, and the total amount may be either increased or decreased.

Finally, there are patients who are convinced of the absolute necessity of obtaining sleep of a certain ideal quantity or quality. These are the "sleep pedants" and the "sleep hypochondriacs" of Laudenheimer. They become obsessed with the importance of sleep. Every night they are in a panic lest they remain awake; they cannot sleep because of their anxiety over it. Often they claim to be sleepless the night through, when in fact they are seen fast asleep on more than one occasion. They demonstrate the truth of William McDougall's statement that "peace of mind is an essential preliminary to sleep." Especially interesting is that group for whom insomnia becomes the excuse for all inadequacies and failures in adjustment to the everyday problems of living. Such individuals, although they want to sleep, worry about the loss, and their mental agitation actually opposes sleep.

Whatever the cause may be, the physician should always be on his guard when listening to reports of the amount of sleep lost by sufferers from insomnia, because they are usually exaggerated. Every individual who has lain awake at night will recall how much longer the time seemed than it actually was. This is an example of an illusion in the perception of unfilled time.

DISTURBANCES IN THE TRANSITIONAL PERIOD OF SLEEP (SOMNOLESCENT STARTS, SENSORY PAROXYSMS, AND NOCTURNAL PARALYSIS). As sleep comes on, it would appear that certain nervous centers may be excited to a burst of insubordinate activity. The result is a sudden start that rouses the incipient sleeper. It may involve one or both legs or the trunk, less often, the arms. If the start occurs repeatedly during the process of falling asleep and is a nightly event, it may become a matter of great concern to the patient. These starts are more apt to occur in individuals in whom the sleep process develops slowly, and it has been observed that they are especially frequent in tense, nervous persons. It is probable that some relationship exists between these nocturnal starts and the sudden isolated jerk of a leg, or arm and leg, which may occur in healthy, fully conscious individuals. It does not appear to be related to epilepsy despite certain superficial resemblances. Disturbances of this nature may be the stimulus for night terrors. These somnolescent starts must be distinguished from flexor spasms of the legs, which occur in individuals who have suffered disease of the pyramidal tracts and a rare condition known as nocturnal myoclonus.

Sensory centers may be disturbed in a similar way, either as an isolated phenomenon or in association with phenomena that induce motion. As the patient drops off to sleep he may be roused by a sensation that darts through his body. Such sensory symptoms are often in the domain of one of the special senses, especially hearing. A sudden clang or crashing sound disturbs commencing sleep. Sometimes a sudden flash of light occurs as sleep is coming on. A sensation of being lifted and dashed to earth or of being turned is probably a similar sensory paroxysm involving the labyrinthine mechanism.

Curious paralytic phenomena, so distressing to a patient as to cause him to seek medical advice, may also occur in the transition from the sleeping to the waking state. Sometimes in an otherwise healthy individual a state supervenes in the morning in which, although awake, conscious, and fully oriented, he is unable to innervate a single muscle. He lies as though still asleep with eyes closed and is all the while engaged in a struggle for movement. He has the impression that if he could move a single muscle, the spell would instantly vanish and he would regain full power. It has been reported that the slightest cutaneous stimulus such as the touch of a hand may abolish the paralysis. Such attacks are usually transient and of no special significance. They have also been reported to occur during the development of sleep. They may be related to narcolepsy.

NIGHTMARES AND NIGHT TERRORS. Awakening in a state of terror has happened to nearly everyone. Children and nervous adults are especially prone to it. Fevers dispose to it, and it has been said that any upsetting condition of the body, such as a disturbance of digestion, may have a similar effect. Bad dreams, stimulated directly by recent memory of bloodcurdling television programs before going to bed, may account for night terrors in children. Some psychologists have drawn a distinction between the nightmare which is merely a terrifying dream and that in which there are visual hallucinations and motor activity. Considering the predominantly visual nature of dreams, it is doubtful if such a separation is valid. Probably any difference is only one of degree.

A night terror is probably always connected with an alarming dream. The victim sits up or jumps out of bed, shouts, or rushes frantically from his room. He is at first unconscious of his surroundings, but usually the intensity of emotional disturbance and the physical activity awaken him. The following morning he may have only a hazy recollection of the experience.

Such phenomena are of little significance as isolated events in childhood but must be distinguished from nocturnal epilepsy. They seldom persist beyond adolescence. If they occur with excessive frequency and continue very long, a relationship to other disturbances, such as psychoneurosis, usually exists.

SOMNAMBULISM AND SLEEP AUTOMATISM. Examples of sleepwalking come to the attention of the practicing physician not infrequently. This condition likewise occurs more often in children than in adults. After being asleep for a time, the patient arises from his bed and walks about the house. He may turn on a light or perform some other familiar act. There is no outward sign of emotion; the eyes are open, and the sleeper is guided by vision, thus avoiding familiar objects. The sight of an unfamiliar object may awaken him. If spoken to, he makes no response; if told to return to bed, he may do so but more often must be led back to it. Sometimes he will mutter wrong phrases or sentences over and over. The following morning he usually has no memory of the episode.

Most psychiatrists hold that these are dissociated mental states similar to the hysterical trance and fugue, except that they begin during sleep. Undoubtedly this is true, and sleepwalking may be accepted as evidence of a nervous disorder, probably of the psychoneurotic variety. There are nonetheless examples of this in adults who have no other signs of mental illness. One can only regard such a case as an isolated disorder of sleep-waking mechanism. It is probably allied to talking in one's sleep, though the two conditions seldom occur together.

Half-waking somnambulism, or sleep automatism, is a state in which an adult patient, half-roused from sleep, goes through a fairly complex routine such as going to a window, opening it, and looking out, but afterward recalling only a part of the episode. The patient may injure himself during sleepwalking.

NOCTURNAL EPILEPSY. Paroxysmal abnormalities of the brain waves of the type seen in epilepsy tend to occur in epileptic patients during or shortly after the onset of sleep. This characteristic electroencephalographic pattern has been found so frequently in the epileptic patient that the practice of artificially inducing sleep in order to obtain confirmation of epilepsy has been adopted in many laboratories. Of course, it has long been known that epilepsy occurs during sleep.

The sleeping epileptic patient attracts attention by a cry, violent motor activity, or labored breathing. As in the diurnal seizure, after the tonic-clonic phase the patient becomes quiet and falls into a state resembling sleep but from which he cannot be aroused. His appearance depends on the phase of the seizure he happens to be in when first observed. Seizures of this type may occur at any time during the night, and some patients may have all their seizures at night. If the seizure during the night is unobserved, the only indicaton of it may be a few drops of blood on the pillow, wet bed linen from urinary incontinence, a bitten tongue, or sore muscles.[1] Rarely, a patient may die in an epileptic seizure during sleep, presumably from being smothered by bedclothes or for some other obscure reason.

Other less well-defined types of seizure occur at night. The patient may arise as though in a night

---

[1] In some children the occurrence of a seizure is betrayed only by incoherent behavior or a headache, the common aftermaths of a convulsive disorder that was unnoticed.

terror and perform complex acts. He may be excited and overactive and, if restrained, become combative. After some minutes he is subdued and returns to sleep. The following morning he disclaims all memory of the episode. Whether this represents a psychomotor seizure or a night terror is difficult to decide. An electroencephalographic study is helpful in such cases.

Nocturnal jerks of the legs, also called *nocturnal myoclonus,* is another troublesome symptom for it interferes with sleep night after night. Only recently has it been classified as a myoclonic form of epilepsy. It is unaccompanied by all other epileptic manifestations. Anticonvulsant drugs are said to control the condition, though in two cases the author has had better success with an occasional dose of Pantopon. It differs from the restless leg syndrome in that involuntary movements occur.

Epilepsy may occur in conjunction with both night terrors and somnambulism, and the question then arises whether the latter is in the nature of postepileptic automatism. Usually no such relationship is established.

PROLONGED STATES OF SLEEP AND REVERSAL OF SLEEP-WAKING RHYTHM. Encephalitis lethargica, or "epidemic encephalitis," that remarkable illness which appeared on the medical horizon during the great pandemic of influenza following the First World War, has provided some of the most dramatic instances of prolonged somnolence. In fact, protracted sleep lasting days to weeks was such a prominent symptom that the disease was called the "sleeping sickness." The patient appeared to be in a state of continuous sleep, or "somnosis," and remained awake only while stimulated. Although the infective agent was never isolated, the pathologic anatomy was fully divulged by many excellent studies, all of which demonstrated a destruction of neurones in the midbrain, subthalamus and hypothalamus. Patients surviving the acute phases of the illness often had difficulty in reestablishing the normal sleep-waking rhythm. As the somnolence disappeared, some patients exhibited a reversal of sleep rhythm, tending to sleep by day and stay awake at night.

Other diseases localized to the floor and walls of the third ventricle are known to produce continuous somnolence. Small tumors in the posterior hypothalamus and midbrain have been associated with arterial hypotension, diabetes insipidus, and a somnolence lasting many weeks. Such patients can be aroused, but if left alone, they immediately fall asleep. Traumatic brain lesions and other diseases have been found to produce similar clinical pictures.

NARCOLEPSY AND CATAPLEXY. The term *narcolepsy* has been used rather loosely. According to most authorities, it should refer to peculiar brief recurrent attacks of sleep and not to prolonged or continuous sleep. *Cataplexy* is a sudden brief loss of muscular power evoked by strong emotion, usually laughter. Although a few of the reported cases are doubtless

examples of hysteria, there is unquestionably a well-defined clinical entity which bears no relationship to neurosis or any other known psychiatric condition. This will be discussed further in Chap. 217.

SLEEP PALSIES AND ACROPARESTHESIAS. Curious and at times distressing paresthetic disturbances develop during sleep. Everyone is familiar with the phenomenon of an arm or leg falling asleep. The immobility of the limbs and the maintenance of uncomfortable postures without being aware of them permits pressure to be applied to exposed nerves. The ulnar, radial, and peroneal nerves are quite superficial in places; pressure of the nerve against an underlying bone may interfere with intraneural circulation of the compressed segment. If this lasts for half an hour or longer, a sensory and motor paralysis sometimes referred to as *sleep palsy* may develop. This condition usually lasts only a few hours or days, but if the compression is prolonged, the nerve may be severely damaged so that functional recovery awaits regeneration. Unusually deep sleep, as in alcoholic intoxication, or anesthesia renders the patient especially liable to sleep palsies merely because he does not heed the discomfort of an unnatural posture.

Acroparesthesias are frequent in adult women and are not unknown in men. The patient will say that after being asleep for a few hours she is awakened by an intense numbness, tingling, prickling, or "pins-and-needles" feeling in fingers and hands. There are also aching, burning pains, or tightness and other unpleasant sensations. At first there is a suspicion of having slept on the arm, but the usual bilaterality and the occurrence regardless of the position of the arms dispel this notion. Usually the paresthesias are in the distribution of the median nerves. Vigorous rubbing of the hands restores normal sensation, and the paresthesias subside within a few minutes, only to return later or upon first awakening in the morning. The condition never occurs during the daytime unless the patient is lying down or sitting with the arms and hands in one position. It may be unilateral but is more often bilateral. It never occurs in the feet. When acroparesthesias are frequent, the hands may at all times feel swollen, stiff, clumsy, and slightly numb. Careful examination discloses little or no objective sensory loss, though in some cases touch and pain sensation have been slightly altered in parts supplied by the median nerves. Slight atrophy and weakness of the abductor pollicis brevis and opponens pollicis have been noted, and in a few cases it has been marked. The use of the hands for heavy manual work during the day seems to aggravate the condition, and a holiday or a period of hospitalization may relieve it. It often occurs in young housewives with a new baby or in factory workers who perform a routine skill. Recently it has been demonstrated that there is a compression of the median nerves in the carpal tunnel of the wrist. The injection of 50 mg hydrocortisone beneath the carpal ligament and the use of diuril or one of its analogs has given immediate relief in a respectable number of cases. The section of the flexor retinaculum has nearly always cured the condition.

DIAGNOSIS OF DISORDERS OF SLEEP

The diagnosis of the cause of insomnia may be troublesome. The difficulty is usually not with the severe case of insomnia as much as with the chronic one. A common source of error is failure to recognize an underlying psychiatric illness such as anxiety neurosis or depressive psychosis. This failure can be avoided only by having the main symptoms of these illnesses clearly in mind and making particular inquiry concerning them in every case.

Somnolescent starts, somnolescent sensory paroxysms, and night terrors may all be confused with nocturnal epilepsy, but actually the only real problem here is to distinguish between night terrors and epilepsy. This may at times be difficult if not impossible. The occurrence of other types of seizures, especially if they occur during the daytime, the lack of any display of terrifying emotion, and the presence of urinary incontinence and tongue biting all indicate epilepsy. Often electroencephalographic confirmation can be obtained.

In the diagnosis of diseases that cause protracted somnolence, a thorough neurologic study with x-rays of skull, electroencephalogram, and lumbar puncture must be employed. Diabetes insipidus, signs of pituitary insufficiency, blindness in parts of visual fields, ophthalmoplegia, and sometimes extrapyramidal motor disturbances are helpful in that they indicate disease in areas adjacent to the posterior hypothalamus and midbrain.

Sleep palsies must be distinguished from other diseases affecting the peripheral nerves. The onset during sleep, maximal functional disturbance immediately afterward, and steady improvement are the main characteristics. A delay in the appearance of muscular atrophy may be perplexing unless it is remembered that it takes 2 to 3 months for denervation atrophy to develop fully. The syndrome of acroparesthesias is often mistaken for ruptured cervical disk, anterior scalene and cervical rib syndrome, peripheral neuritis, or multiple sclerosis. The nocturnal incidence, the localization to the fingers and hands in the median nerve distribution, and the lack of other neurologic signs are diagnostic. A tourniquet around the arm just above the elbow may reproduce the acroparesthetic syndrome.

TREATMENT

In general, there are three varieties of wakefulness. For best management, treatment should be based on the type exhibited by the patient. In younger patients the most frequently observed type of insomnia is the inability to fall asleep. These individuals have become more and more tense during the day and are unable to relax. This type of insomnia usually lasts from 1 to 3 hr, and then the individual sinks into an exhausted, deep sleep which continues through the night. For these patients a quick-acting, fairly rapidly destroyed hypnotic such as secobarbital (Seconal), 0.1 Gm given 15 to 20 min before going to bed, is useful.

The second group consists of patients who are able to go to sleep but who awaken in 1 or 2 hr and lose sleep in the middle of the night. Some are alternately awake and asleep all night. Often these are sick persons with a debilitating or painful illness which generates more pain and restlessness as muscles relax and leave painful areas unsplinted. In others, fever, sweats, dyspnea, or other distressful symptoms develop and demand attention. Frequently, these patients secure relief from pentobarbital (Nembutal), 0.1 Gm given at bedtime. For cardiac patients who have Cheyne-Stokes respiration or moderate orthopnea, a rectal suppository of aminophylline, 0.5 Gm given at bedtime, will frequently relieve the respiratory distress and promote sleep. When pain is a factor in insomnia, acetylsalicylic acid, 0.3 to 0.6 Gm, should be given with the sedative. Occasionally codeine phosphate, 30 mg, may be required when pain is severe.

The third group of insomnia patients consists of those who go to sleep promptly and sleep well most of the night only to awaken too early in the morning. Most of these individuals are older persons who turn night into day. They go to bed and get up earlier and earlier so that soon they are sleeping during the day and are alert during the night. Into this category also fall those individuals who are under great tension, worry, or anxiety or are overworked and exhausted. These people sink into bed and sleep through sheer exhaustion, but around 4 or 5 A.M. they awake with their worries and are unable to get back to sleep. Most of these patients are benefited by barbital, 0.3 Gm given with fruit juice or milk at bedtime. For debilitated patients the compressed tablets of insoluble material should be crushed to ensure proper absorption, or sodium barbital should be substituted. Chloral hydrate, 1.0 Gm given with fruit juice at bedtime, is also effective and may be substituted for barbital if desired.

Patients with serious mental agitation, delirium, or excitement who require prompt, easily controlled, relatively safe sedation should receive whisky, 30 to 60 ml by mouth, or paraldehyde, 15 to 30 ml by mouth in iced fruit juice, or the same dose by rectum but diluted with 200 ml physiologic saline solution or 120 ml olive oil. Generally, it is wise to avoid barbiturates with highly agitated patients, since occasionally they may precipitate serious mental confusion, excitement, or even manic tendencies. Chloral hydrate, 1.0 to 2.0 Gm by mouth or rectum, is useful in the management of these individuals and frequently proves more satisfactory than the barbiturates.

A word of caution about oversedation is wise in any discussion of sedative drugs. All too frequently they are abused in that they are given when not needed, the dosage is too great, or the wrong preparation is used. These drugs are a common source of constipation, lead to fatigue and lack of energy and strength, and interfere with the patient's recovery from his illness.

When large dosages of quicker-acting barbiturates, 0.4 to 0.6 Gm daily, are given for more than a week or two, there is real danger of habituation, which once developed, is pernicious in character. Withdrawal, unless accomplished skillfully and in graded steps, may cause serious mental disturbance or precipitate convulsions. The patient should not be encouraged to use sedative drugs as a crutch on which to limp through life. One should search out and correct the underlying difficulty, using sedation when necessary, as a temporary helpful tool.

Barbiturate sedatives may be of value in treating night terrors, and if their differentiation from nocturnal epilepsy is impossible, a trial on diphenylhydantoin sodium (Dilantin Sodium) and phenobarbital is indicated. (See Chap. 219 for further information concerning anticonvulsant medication.)

REFERENCES

Kremer, M., R. W. Gilliatt, J. S. R. Golding, and T. G. Wilson: Acroparesthesiae in the Carpal-tunnel Syndrome, Brit. Med. J. (Lancet), II:590, 1953.

Miller, H. R.: "Central Autonomic Regulations in Health and Disease," p. 260, New York, Grune & Stratton, Inc., 1942.

Muncie, W.: "Psychobiology and Psychiatry," p. 104, St. Louis, The C. V. Mosby Company, 1939.

52 RECURRENT CONVULSIONS
Raymond D. Adams

The magnitude of the problem of epilepsy and its importance in our society can hardly be overstated. The statistics of Lennox and Lennox show that at least 500,000 persons in the United States are or have been subject to seizures. After apoplexy, epilepsy is the most frequent neurologic disorder. Therefore, the physician must know something of the nature and etiology of this common disorder and of the mechanism that produces symptoms.

Epilepsy is an intermittent disorder of the nervous system due presumably to a sudden, excessive, disorderly discharge of cerebral neurones. This was the postulation of Hughlings Jackson, the eminent British neurologist of the nineteenth century, and modern electrophysiology offers no evidence to the contrary. This discharge results in an almost instantaneous disturbance of sensation, loss of consciousness, convulsive movements, or some combination thereof. A terminologic difficulty arises from the diversity of the clinical manifestations. It seems improper to call a condition a convulsion when only an alteration of sensation or of consciousness takes place. The word *seizure* is preferable as a generic term and also lends itself to qualification. Motor or convulsive seizure is therefore not tautologic, and one may speak also of sensory seizures. The word *epilepsy*, which in times past meant the "falling evil," has many unpleasant connotations, and although it is a useful medical term, probably it is best avoided in open discussions until the general public becomes more enlightened.

Epilepsy may begin at any age. It may occur once in the lifetime of an individual or several times a day. Sometimes it is an obvious symptom of a brain disease that also manifests itself in other ways, and at times it is the solitary expression of deranged cerebral function in an individual who otherwise maintains perfect health. The latter is the more frequent circumstance and explains why the convulsive state has for so long been looked upon as a disease entity. However, it is illogical to suppose that a convulsion occurring by itself represents a disease, whereas one occurring in combination with other symptoms is only a manifestation of a disease. The convulsive state must always be looked upon as symptomatic. Use of such epithets as "genuine" or "essential" or "idiopathic" in no sense changes its status.

THE COMMON TYPES OF CONVULSIVE DISORDERS

In a statistical survey of nearly 2,000 patients it was reported that 51 per cent of all epileptic patients had had *generalized convulsions;* 8 per cent, minor seizures referred to as *petit mal;* 1 per cent, *psychic* or *psychomotor seizures;* and the remaining 40 per cent, two or even all three types, the most prominent form being psychomotor. Thus psychomotor epilepsy, as pointed out by Singh, is probably as frequent as grand mal. Although the total number of seizures that had a focal onset was not determined, these data give some notion of the principal forms of the convulsive state in the majority of patients.

THE GENERALIZED CONVULSION (GRAND MAL, MAJOR EPILEPSY)

The term *convulsion* is most applicable to this form of seizure. The patient may sense its possible approach by any of several subjective sensations. For some hours he may feel apathetic, depressed, irritable, or the opposite—unusually alert or even ecstatic. Flatulence, constipation, and headache are other prodromal symptoms, and myoclonic twitches, i.e., sudden movements that affect one or another limb or the trunk, may precede the convulsion by some hours. In approximately half the cases there is some type of sensation or movement of one part of the body before the loss of consciousness or the generalized convulsion. This is called the *aura*, and as will be developed later, it provides the most reliable clue to the location of the underlying disease. The most frequent aura is an epigastric sensation, a sinking or gripping feeling, a strangulation or palpitation. A tingling numbness of the fingers or lips or some other part of the body, a flashing light or panorama, and disagreeable taste or odor are other well-known sensory auras. Clonic twitches, tonic contraction of the muscles of a limb, and turning of the head and eyes are somatic motor auras. These may spread from one part of the body to another in an orderly, predictable sequence. Usually by the time all one side of the body is affected there is a loss of consciousness. The aura, though truly a warning of the oncoming seizure, is actually the first part of the seizure and not a prodrome. It seldom lasts more than a few seconds.

The generalized convulsion, or *fit*, as it is often called, begins with a sudden loss of consciousness and falling to the ground. The whole musculature is seized in a violent spasm. The contraction of the diaphragm and chest muscles produces a characteristic cry. The eyes turn up or to one side, the face is contorted, the jaw is set, often with biting of the tongue and oozing of saliva or blood from the lips, and the limbs may assume any of several positions. With continued spasm of the respiratory muscles breathing is impossible, and the color of the skin and mucous membranes becomes dusky or cyanotic. After a fraction of a minute the rigid or tonic state of the muscles gives way to a series of clonic jerking movements. Air begins to enter the lungs in short convulsive gasps, and a bloody froth, a mixture of saliva and blood from a bitten tongue or cheek, forms on the lips. The arms, legs, face, and head jerk violently. After a minute or two the movements become slower, then irregular, and finally cease. The patient then lies relaxed, breathing rather deeply and sweating profusely. There may have been loss of control of urine and occasionally of feces. The state is now one of deep coma, and even the most intense pain evokes no response. After a few minutes the patient stirs and then opens his eyes. His first remarks or questions usually betray mental confusion. For the next several minutes or even hours there is a tendency toward incoherence of thought and drowsiness. Often the patient falls into a deep sleep. Headache is another frequent postseizure or postictal symptom. The patient himself is completely unaware of what has happened or at most remembers only the aura. He may come to his senses in a hospital or other strange place, and his only way of telling that something has happened is by the hiatus in his memory, his disheveled appearance, the sore tongue, and a soreness of the vigorously exercised muscles. Injury may be sustained during the fall and as a consequence of violent muscular contraction; one or several vertebras may be crushed. Periorbital subcutaneous hemorrhages may reflect the violence of the exertion during the seizures.

Convulsions of this type ordinarily come singly or in groups of two or three and may occur when the patient is awake or when he is asleep. About 5 to 8 per cent of patients at some time have a series of seizures without regaining consciousness between times. This is known as *status epilepticus* and demands urgent treatment. Instead of the whole sequence of changes described above, only one part of the seizure may occur; for example, there may be only the aura without loss of consciousness, or the entire spell may consist of a brief loss of consciousness and momentary spasm of the limbs.

PETIT MAL (MINOR EPILEPSY, AND SMALL ILLNESS, L'ABSENCE)

In contrast to the generalized seizure, these attacks are so brief that they are often overlooked. In fact, many patients may have them for years before their true nature is recognized.

The attack comes without warning and consists of sudden loss of consciousness. The person is motionless, and a staring expression of the face and failure to speak or to respond to commands are the only signs of abnormality. In contrast to grand mal, motor disturbances are conspicuously absent, and at most only a few flickering contractions of the eyelids and facial muscles and jerking of the arms at a rate of three contractions per second are seen. The patient does not fall, as a rule, and he may continue such complex acts as walking or even riding a bicycle during an attack. After 2 to 15 sec more consciousness is regained abruptly and fully, and the patient promptly resumes whatever action he was performing before the seizure. To the patient there is only a blank place, an "absence" in his stream of consciousness.

Closely related to petit mal are the *akinetic seizures*, in which the patient suddenly loses consciousness and falls motionless to the ground, and the myoclonic seizure, which consists of a sudden violent contraction of some part or all of the body, often followed by a lapse of posture with falling and loss of consciousness of a few seconds' duration (*generalized myoclonus*). Because of frequent association with petit mal and the similarity of the electroencephalographic pattern, Lennox groups petit mal, the akinetic seizure, and myoclonic seizure into a single entity called the *petit mal triad*.

Episodes of this type are much more frequent in childhood and adolescence. Another characteristic is their great frequency. As many as several hundred may occur in one day. Although benign, they may, if frequent, derange the mental processes so that the patient does poorly in school. Rarely, a series of them in close succession will interrupt consciousness for a longer period of time. This is known as *petit mal status*. *Pyknolepsy* is an almost obsolete term for frequent petit mal during childhood, terminating at puberty. When present as the only type of seizure during childhood, petit mal may, as the patient grows older, give way to or be combined with grand mal.

PSYCHOMOTOR EPILEPSY (EPILEPTIC EQUIVALENTS, PSYCHIC VARIANTS, EPILEPTIC MANIA OR DELIRIUM, EPILEPSIA PROCURSIVA)

This differs in several ways from the two types of seizure discussed above. (1) The aura, if it occurs, is often a complex hallucination or perceptual illusion. There may be an unpleasant smell or taste or the revival of a complicated visual scene involving people, dwellings, etc., usually taken from past experiences and resembling a dream. Furthermore, the patient's perception of what is seen and heard and his relationship to the outside world are altered. Objects appear to be far away or unreal (*jamais vu*); or strange objects or persons may seem familiar (*déjà vu phenomenon*). Hughlings Jackson applied the term *dreamy state* to these psychic disturbances. (2) Instead of losing all control of his thoughts and actions, the patient behaves as though he were partially conscious during the attack. He may get up and walk about, unbutton or remove his clothes, attempt to speak, or even continue such habitual acts as driving a car. If he is asked a specific question or given a command, it is evident that he is out of contact with the examiner and does not understand. When restrained, he may resist with great energy and at times can be violent. This type of behavior is said to be *automatic,* presumably because the patient behaves like an automaton. (3) Convulsive movements, when present, are likely to consist of chewing, smacking and licking of the lips, and, less often, tonic spasms of the limbs or turning of the head and eyes to one side.

In any given case one or several of these phenomena may be observed. In the series studied by Lennox and Lennox, which numbered 414 cases, 43 per cent of patients displayed some of these motor or psychomotor phenomena; 32 per cent, the automatic state; and 25 per cent, the psychic changes. Because of the concurrence of these three symptom complexes they have referred to the whole group as the *psychomotor triad.* These types of seizure vary in frequency and duration. Some are very brief, lasting only for seconds, and others continue for hours or days. This calls to mind that the duration of the seizure is an unsatisfactory criterion for classification. Two-thirds of the patients have generalized convulsions at some time in their lives.

In addition to these three major types, the clinicians of the nineteenth century recognized many other special forms of epilepsy, some of which were given descriptive names. The term *tonic seizure* referred to tonic muscle contractions, to the exclusion of phasic qualities. *Epilepsia partialis continua* specified a repetitive clonic contraction of one group of muscles. The terms *focal motor* or *focal sensory epilepsy* were applied to a tonic or clonic movement or a sensation restricted to one portion of the body. *Myoclonic epilepsy* referred to a syndrome of epilepsy and isolated twitches of a muscle or group of muscles, called *myoclonus* (see Chap. 46). Random, arrhythmic myoclonus in a sense might be designated as *epilepsia partialis discontinua et disseminata.* It is usually caused by a more or less diffuse disease of the cerebral and cerebellar cortex and possibly of other parts of the nervous system such as the thalamus.

It is obvious that the traditional division of seizures into three general types leaves much to be desired. Petit mal is a more or less homogeneous type, whereas grand mal represents a phase of generalization of the seizure discharge, regardless of its origin or the initial symptoms of the seizure. Psychomotor epilepsy, as will be evident upon further analysis, is not a uniform syndrome but encompasses a diversity of clinical phenomena. Moreover, careful study of the first symptoms of the seizure and the use of the electroencephalogram have given us a new means of subdividing seizures according to other more significant attributes. The seizure pattern provides information that not only is of great value in determining the topography of the disease causing the convulsive disorder but affords a new basis of classification that will serve until the etiology is discovered.

Other Common Focal Seizure Patterns

A number of seizure patterns have been identified; they are so helpful in the localization of cerebral lesions that every student of medicine should be familiar with them. These types of epilepsy are often termed *focal* because they can be traced to a circumscript lesion of the brain. Many cases of this type come under the surveillance of neurosurgeons, and their contributions to this field have been of great value.

MOTOR SEIZURES (GENERALIZED, CONTRAVERSIVE, FOCAL MOTOR, AND JACKSONIAN SEIZURES)

A lesion in one or other frontal lobe may give rise to a generalized or major convulsive seizure of the type described above, without introductory sensory aura. In some cases there is a turning movement of the head and eyes to one side, simultaneously with loss of consciousness, and in others there are no turning movements. It has been postulated that in both types of seizure, the one with and the one without contraversive movements, the discharge from the frontal lobe spreads immediately into an integrating center such as the thalamus, with immediate loss of consciousness. In cases with head and eye turning, the discharge is believed to reach area 8 (area for contralateral turning of head and eyes), although it has been found that contralateral turning of the head and eyes can be induced in the experimental animal by stimulation of temporal or occipital as well as of the premotor cortex.

Do most cases of generalized motor seizures (grand mal) of idiopathic type have a frontal focus? Unfortunately, this question cannot be answered at the moment. Such a focus has been found in only a small number of such cases, and these may not be representative of the whole group.

The characteristics of the *Jacksonian motor seizure* are well known. It begins usually with a twitching of the fingers of one hand, the face on one side, or one foot. The movements are clonic and rhythmic; their speed varies. They may occur in bursts, or paroxysms. The disorder then spreads or marches from the part first affected to other muscles on the same side of the body—from the face to the neck, hand, forearm, arm, trunk, and leg; if the first movement is in the foot, the order is reversed. The high incidence of onset in the lips, fingers, and toes probably is related to the greater cortical representation of these parts of the body. The disease process or focus of excitation is usually the Rolandic cortex, area 4 (Fig. 54-1) on the opposite side; in a few cases it has been found in the post-Rolandic convolution. Lesions confined to the premotor cortex (area 6) are said to induce contractions of an arm, face, neck, or all of one side of the body. Perspiration and piloerection, sometimes of the parts of the body involved in a focal motor seizure, suggest that these autonomic functions have cortical representation in the Rolandic area. Some neurologists distinguish focal motor and Jacksonian motor seizures by the absence of a characteristic march in the former, but both have essentially the same localizing significance.

Another type of focal motor epilepsy, the previously mentioned *epilepsia partialis continua,* consists of rhythmic clonic movements of one group of muscles, usually in the face, arm, or leg. These may continue for a variable period of time, minutes to weeks or months. The seizure usually does not march to other parts of the body. Its localizing value has not been settled. Some cases have a lesion in the opposite sensorimotor areas of the cerebral cortex.

SOMATIC, VISUAL, AND OTHER SENSORY SEIZURES

Somatic sensory seizures, either focal or "marching" to other parts of the body on one side, nearly always indicate a parietal lobe lesion. The usual sensory disorder is described as a numbness or a tingling or "pins-and-needles" feeling. Other variations are sensations of crawling (formication), buzzing, electricity, or vibration. Pain and thermal sensations are infrequent. The onset is in the lips, fingers, and toes in the majority of cases, and the spread to adjacent parts of the body follows a pattern determined by sensory arrangements in the postcentral (post-Rolandic) convolution of the parietal lobe. In Kristiansen and Penfield's series the seizure focus was found in the postcentral convolution in 24 of 55 cases; it was central, either pre- or post-Rolandic, in 18, and precentral in 7 cases. One may conclude that this type of sensory phenomenon always indicates a focus in or near the post-Rolandic convolution of the opposite cerebral hemisphere; if localized in the head, the locus is in the lowest part of the convolution, near the Sylvian fissure; if in the foot or leg, the upper part near the superior sagittal sinus is involved.

Visual seizures are also of localizing significance. Lesions in or near the striate cortex of the occipital lobe usually produce a sensation of lights, of darkness, or of color. According to Gowers, red is the most frequent color, followed by blue, green, and yellow. The patient may tell of seeing stars or moving lights in the visual field on the side opposite the lesion. Sometimes they appear to be straight ahead of the patient. Often, if they occur on only one side of the visual field, he believes only one eye to be affected, the one opposite the lesion, probably because the average person is unaware that he has two corresponding visual

fields. It is curious that a lesion arising in one occipital lobe may cause momentary blindness in both eyes. It has been noted that lesions on the lateral surface of the occipital lobes (Brodmann's areas 18 and 19) are more likely to cause twinkling or pulsating lights. Complex visual hallucinations are usually due to a focus in the posterior part of the temporal lobe, near its junction with the parietal, and may be associated with auditory hallucinations. Often the visual images, either those of the hallucination or of objects seen, are distorted and seem too small (*micropsia*) or unnaturally arranged.

Auditory hallucinations are rather infrequent as an initial manifestation of a seizure. Occasionally a patient with a focus in the superior temporal convolution on one side will report a buzzing or a roaring in his ears. A human voice sometimes repeating recognizable words has been noted a few times in patients with lesions in the more posterior part of the dominant temporal lobe.

Vertiginous sensations of a type suggesting vestibular stimulation may be the first symptom of a seizure. The lesion is usually localized in the superior posterior temporal region or at the junction between parietal and temporal lobes. Foerster is said to have evoked a sensation of vertigo by stimulating the parietal lobe, and in one of Penfield's cases the lesion was here. Occasionally with a temporal focus vertigo is followed by an auditory sensation. Giddiness is also a frequent prelude to a seizure, but this has so many different meanings that it is of little diagnostic import.

Olfactory hallucinations are often associated with disease of the inferior and medial parts of the temporal lobe, usually in the region of the hippocampal convolution or the uncus (hence the term *uncinate seizures,* after Jackson). Usually the smell is exteriorized, i.e., projected to someplace in the environment, and is of a disagreeable nature. Gustatory hallucinations have also been recorded in approved cases of temporal lobe disease. Sensations of thirst and salivation may be associated. Stimulation of the upper surface of the temporal lobe in the depths of the Sylvian fissure during neurosurgical operations has reproduced peculiar sensations of taste.

Visceral sensations arising in the thorax, epigastrium, and abdomen are among the most frequent of the auras. They are described as a vague, indefinable feeling, a sinking sensation in the pit of the stomach, and a weakness in the epigastrium or substernal area that rises to the throat and head. In several such cases the seizure discharge has been localized to the upper bank of the Sylvian fissure, but in a few cases lesions were in the upper intermediate or medial frontal areas near the cingulate gyrus. Palpitation and acceleration of pulse at the beginning of the attack have also been related to a temporal lobe focus.

PSYCHIC PHENOMENA

The studies of many neurologists have served to establish the close relationship between psychic changes and the temporal lobe. Disease of either temporal lobe may be accompanied by seizures that have many of the characteristics outlined under Psychomotor Epilepsy. In addition to olfactory and gustatory hallucinations, there are often others of more complex visual and auditory perception and feelings of unreality, and partial or complete interruption of consciousness may be observed. Compulsive thoughts or actions may recur in a fixed pattern during each seizure. Automatic behavior or even frank psychoses of many different types, lasting for hours or days, may be induced by seizure discharges or electrical stimulation of the temporal lobe. Masticatory movements are also frequent.

LOSS OF CONSCIOUSNESS

A lapse of consciousness is the initial event in petit mal, which is believed now to represent a disorder of the diencephalon, the so-called "centrencephalic epilepsy." Lesions in the prefrontal regions have been observed to abolish consciousness at the very beginning of the seizure, presumably through the effects on the diencephalon and midbrain structures.

The various motor, sensory, or psychic phenomena may be combined in many different sequences. These presumably indicate the spread of a seizure discharge from one cortical area to another. A flash of light followed by tingling of one side of the body suggests that the epileptic discharge began in the occipital lobe and extended to the somatic sensory areas in the parietal lobe. A smell of something burning, followed by chewing and smacking movements, and then loss of speech would be interpreted as a spread of the seizure discharge from the region of the uncus to the upper parts of the temporal and the inferior frontal lobe. A focal motor seizure followed by a tonic contraction of one side of the body and then turning of the head and eyes contralaterally would indicate a successive involvement of the motor, premotor, and contraversive cortical field for head and eyes. Little is known about the factors that facilitate or inhibit the spread of seizure discharges from one part of the brain to another.

THE EVOCATION OF SEIZURES (Reflex Epilepsy)

For a long time it has been known that seizures could be evoked in certain epileptic individuals by a physiologic or psychologic stimulus. Approximately 1 in every 15 patients will have remarked that their seizures occur under special circumstances, such as being exposed to flickering light, passing from darkness to light or the reverse, being startled by a loud noise, hearing a series of monotonous sounds or music, touching, rubbing, or hurting a particular part of the body, making certain movements, eating a large meal or experiencing digestive changes, or being subjected to fright or other strong emotion. The evoked seizure may be focal (beginning often in the part of the body that has been stimulated) or generalized and may take the form of one or a series of myoclonic jerks, a petit mal, or a grand mal. In a few instances such as *reflex epilepsy*, as it is called, it has been due to a focal cerebral disease, such as a tumor, but more often its

cause cannot be ascertained. W. Watson has discovered a strong tendency to familial incidence in a variety of myoclonic jerking elicited by photic stimulation, and some patients in whom this phenomenon had been noted were unaware of ever having had a seizure. Also of interest in these cases of evoked seizure has been the phenomenon of willfully averting the seizure by undertaking some mental task, e.g., thinking about some distracting subject or counting, or by initiating some physical activity.

Patients of this type suggest to us that epilepsy is a natural state, a physiologic event resulting from excitation and subsequent inhibition of an injured part of the cerebrum.

PATHOPHYSIOLOGY AND BIOCHEMISTRY OF EPILEPSY

From what has been said about epilepsy it is obvious that a satisfactory theory must account for the following clinical and pathologic data. (1) The majority of demonstrable epileptogenic lesions are situated in or near the cerebral cortex, which suggests that some property of the neural organization of the cortex disposes to this condition. (2) The foci induced by any given disease may or may not give rise to epilepsy; some peculiarity of the lesion must, therefore, determine this phenomenon. (3) The epileptic focus, once present, is known to become active, i.e., to discharge, only on occasion, or at least the electrical discharge which attends it may be detected in the electroencephalogram and the seizure occurs only from time to time. (4) Several events appear to activate the focus, some of physiologic or psychologic nature and others biochemical. The former include photic and other sensory stimuli; the latter pentylenetetrazol (Metrazol), picrotoxin, and acetylcholine. (5) The seizure discharges upon reaching a certain magnitude spread along preformed pathways from their site of origin to other cortical areas and to the diencephalon. (6) Some inhibitory process counteracts and ultimately terminates the seizure discharge. (7) In many cases in human beings no cortical lesion has been demonstrated by current neuropathologic methods, and in this group there may be a genetic factor. The evidence on this latter point is not altogether convincing. Certainly, epilepsy and paroxysmal disturbances in the electroencephalogram have been observed in a large series of identical twins. However, the incidence of convulsions among blood relatives of epileptic patients is only two or three times that in the public at large.

Much experimental work has been done to explain these phenomena, but limitations of space permit no more than a condensed review of it here. Investigators have centered their attention on human cases of focal epilepsy and on focal epileptic lesions in the mammalian cortex. In both man and animal the neurophysiologic analog to the convulsive seizure in human beings has been the repetitive, self-sustained discharge of electrical activity akin to posttetanic potentiation, which continues after a stimulus to a circumscript cortical area has terminated. The neurosurgeon has found this so consistently in or near epileptic foci and has so frequently observed a seizure discharge to accompany it that he has accepted it as the electrical sign of the epileptic lesion. As pointed out by Symonds, the afterdischarge, once started, continues at a regular frequency of 10 to 14 per sec. Within a short time (seconds to minutes), the intervals between spikes increase; they tend then to be grouped, and their voltage rises. When the pauses between bursts reach ½ sec or more, the afterdischarge ceases altogether and the area of cortex becomes electrically inactive and inexcitable. Adrian in his study of this state interprets cessation to indicate a rivalry between two opposing processes, the initial one excitatory, the final one inhibitory. A possible physiologic basis of these two processes has been demonstrated by Eccles. Each motor anterior horn cell, when activated, stimulates through a collateral branch another cell, the Renshaw cell, which is inhibitory in its action and imposes this inhibition on the anterior horn itself. Similarly, Phillips has noted an arrangement between the Betz cells in the cerebral cortex and other interneurones that inhibit the Betz cells. Thus both anterior horn cells and Betz cells can initiate excitation in another cell via their main axone and have their own activity inhibited by an adjacent inhibitory nerve cell. Moreover, on the afferent side of nervous activity all recent physiologic work has shown that each sensory neurone from the end organ to the cerebral cortex is monitored by a central descending inhibitory system.

A convulsive seizure could be conceived, therefore, either as an excessive excitation resulting from narrowly focused afferent stimulation on the injured cerebral cortex or as a deficiency of suppressive influences from either the afferent neurones or the special inhibitory neurones of the cortex. It is of interest that strychnine, one of the most potent agents for discharging neurones and producing seizures, does not facilitate the excitatory postsynaptic potential of motor neurones but rather diminishes their inhibitory postsynaptic potentials. Furthermore, it has been shown that solutions of strychnine, by themselves too weak to have any effect on the cortex, condition it in such a fashion that sensory stimuli conveyed to it could discharge the altered neurones and thus produce convulsive activity. This state of affairs resembles that which prevails in epileptic patients, where a silent, subliminal epileptic focus is discharged by a particular type of sensory stimulus and is restored to its quiescent state by inhibitory neurones.

Since electrical activity is believed to depend on chemical changes (flux of Na, K, Ca, Mg), it is rather to be expected that a search would have been made for special excitatory and inhibitory substances in the brain. Acetylcholine is known to be an effective convulsive agent when applied to the animal cortex, and cholinesterase inhibitors such as isopropylfluorophosphate also produce seizures. Cortical lesions in epileptic patients have been found to contain an increased amount of acetylcholinesterase and in a test

tube are unable to "bind" acetylcholine. After a seizure there are increased amounts of acetylcholine in human cerebrospinal fluid. Barbiturates and diphenylhydantoin (Dilantin) are said to act as anticonvulsants because they enhance the acetylcholine-binding power of the cerebral cortex.

With respect to inhibitory substances Florey found that cerebral and spinal cord tissue contain an agent identified as gamma aminobutyric acid (GABA), which if applied to the cortex, blocks excitation of the superficial layer and augments inhibition—an action opposite to that of strychnine. It is formed from glutamic acid, and one of the coenzymes which catalyzes its synthesis is pyridoxine (vitamin B_6), lack of which is known to produce seizures in animals and man. Metrazol and picrotoxin prevent the inhibitory effect of GABA. The action of GABA as an intrinsic anticonvulsant has not been fully explored. Given intravenously, it is said to protect animals against chemically induced seizures. There is disagreement on this point, however, for others have found it to be ineffective when given by this route and have noted that it fails to cross the blood-brain barrier. If this is true, only a lesion which destroys this barrier would be expected to permit the entrance of GABA into the discharging focus. This subject is still under investigation.

Whatever the basic chemistry of the process, it is reasonably well established that changes in the blood such as oxygen supply, acid-base equilibrium, calcium, magnesium, glucose, chloride, and fluid balance alter the seizure threshold. Lennox and Lennox have depicted the relationship of these many factors to epilepsy by drawing the analogy of a reservoir. Water enters a reservoir from various underground springs, each of which represents one cause of seizures. As the reservoir fills, it periodically overflows the restraining dam and a seizure results. The height of the restraining dam indicates the seizure threshold, and the amount of water in the reservoir stands for the force of the influences that cause seizures. The restraining dam is lowered by alkalosis, decreased oxygenation, hydration, hypoglycemia, and elevation of the intracranial pressure and raised by the opposite conditions. This metaphorical reservoir stresses the importance of the factors operating to prevent seizures in any given patient.

Although high-amplitude activity of a group of neurones represents the "functional unit of epilepsy," it is the spread of this electrical potential to other parts of the nervous system that characterizes the whole convulsive seizure both clinically and electroencephalographically. The spread of these discharges proceeds along preformed pathways, i.e., via the uncinate fibers to adjacent cortical fields, via the corpus callosum to corresponding parts of the contralateral cerebral hemisphere, or along corticothalamic and thalamocortical pathways to the diencephalon and reticular formation. Little is known about factors that interfere with the spread of the seizure discharge. The corpus callosum has been sectioned in animals and human beings for this purpose, and although the results were not conclusive, the seizures usually remained unilateral. The anticonvulsant activity of phenobarbital and diphenylhydantoin is believed to be mainly in preventing the spread of seizure discharges, and these drugs are said to have rather little suppressive action on the epileptic focus.

These many investigations raise more new questions than they answer, but one fact is certain—scientists are now searching out the basic facts concerning the epileptic discharge and are coming to view it in both its biochemical and its neurophysiologic aspects. Approximate explanations are no longer acceptable. The observation that a lesion in the motor cortex causes focal or Jacksonian seizures does no more than center attention on one link in a chain of causal events. It enables us to say only that such a lesion provides suitable conditions for the development of a convulsion.

Certain occurrences in the seizure, such as the cry, the motor activity, and the sensory experience, may be regarded as the direct manifestations of the seizure discharge in the brain. Some of these immediate effects, when regarded from the more general neurophysiologic point of view, are excitatory and others, like the lapse of consciousness of petit mal, are inhibitory. Electrical stimulation of the brain through the intact skull, as in electroshock convulsions for the treatment of depression, or by the application of electrodes on the surface of the brain is observed to produce the same changes. This initial outburst lasts for only a brief period of time and is often followed by a total or subtotal paralysis or inhibition of cerebral function. A focal motor seizure, for example, may result in suppression of activity in motor areas and a temporary paralysis of the involved muscles (Todd's postepileptic or exhaustion paralysis). The loss of consciousness that follows a generalized motor seizure, in contradistinction to that of petit mal, is probably due to a postexcitatory paralysis of either diencephalic or midbrain structures. Vital functions may also be arrested, but usually for only a few seconds. In rare instances, however, death may occur owing to a cessation of respiration, derangement, cardiac action, or some unknown cause. The automatic behavior so characteristic of psychomotor epilepsy appears in some instances to be a direct stimulatory effect in the temporal lobe and in others is a postexcitatory, inhibitory, or paralytic effect.

The electroencephalogram provides a delicate proof of Hughlings Jackson's theory of epilepsy—that it is an excessive, disorderly discharge of cortical neurones. At the onset of the focal seizure this is registered in or near the focus as a series of spikes or sharp waves interrupting the normal alpha and beta waves. The clinical spread of the seizure has its electroencephalographic equivalent in the extension of the abnormal electrical waves; and with generalization of the seizure (grand mal) the entire electroencephalographic recording surface of the brain exhibits spikes of high voltage. Petit mal is accompanied by a characteristic

cold wave–spike complex occurring simultaneously in all cortical leads and presumably taking origin from a diencephalic focus. At first there was thought to be a characteristic electroencephalographic picture for psychomotor epilepsy, but further studies have not confirmed this. The postseizure state, sometimes called *postictal disturbance of cerebral function*, also has its electroencephalographic correlate in random generalized slow waves; with recovery the electroencephalogram returns to normal. If the electroencephalographic tracing is obtained during the interval between seizures, it is abnormal to some degree in approximately 40 per cent of fully conscious and 75 per cent of sleeping patients.

The electroencephalographic changes are discussed in Chap. 200.

DISEASES CAUSING SYMPTOMATIC EPILEPSY

In the list of diseases of the nervous system with which every physician must be familiar, a few stand apart by reason of their tendency to produce recurrent convulsions. The seizures are said to be symptomatic in contrast to the large majority of cases in which epilepsy is idiopathic. The physician must distinguish by the usual clinical and laboratory methods the different diseases that may cause, accompany, or precipitate convulsions.

DISEASES LOCALIZED IN THE CEREBRAL HEMISPHERES

Almost any type of cerebral lesion may cause seizures; on the other hand, no cerebral lesion is invariably accompanied by them. In patients with cerebral lesions the seizures are usually focal, leading in most instances to a generalized convulsion of grand mal type; less commonly they are of the petit mal type.

CEREBRAL TUMORS. They give rise to seizures in 35 to 60 per cent of cases; in approximately 10 per cent of all cases of tumor the seizure is the initial symptom. The nearer the tumor is to the excitable motor cortex, the greater is the likelihood of seizures. Tumors of the cerebellum and brain stem are seldom associated with any of the types of seizures described above, but they may cause episodes of decerebrate rigidity, i.e., opisthotonos and extension of all four extremities, sometimes called *tonic cerebellar fits*.

CEREBRAL TRAUMA. Trauma may cause seizures immediately after the injury, i.e., within hours or days, or after an interval of several months or years. In the former case seizures are rare; in the latter they vary in incidence, being more frequent in the severer grades of head injury. Uncomplicated concussion results in epilepsy in only about 0.5 per cent of cases, which is about the expected frequency in the population at large, whereas with penetrating injuries, the incidence rises to approximately 20 per cent and some figures have been as high as 40 per cent. The average interval between the head injury and the first seizure is about 9 months, with a range of 6 months to 2 years or longer. The frequency of seizures varies from patient to patient; as years pass they tend to become less frequent.

CEREBROVASCULAR DISEASES. It has been said that, although seizures occur at the time of the hemorrhage or infarction in a small percentage of cases, vascular disease is rarely responsible for recurrent convulsions. Recently, however, analysis of our own material showed that cases of vascular disease of the cerebral cortex, particularly of infarction due to embolism, showed recurrent convulsions in about the same frequency as traumatic disease of the cerebral cortex. Hypertensive encephalopathy is often attended by convulsions. Venous thrombosis and infarction are a notable cause of focal epilepsy, and the same is true of vascular lesions in infancy and childhood, which may be either arterial or venous in nature. Seizures are also a frequent manifestation of vascular malformations.

CEREBRAL INFECTIONS. All types of cerebral infection may lead to epilepsy. Brain abscess is accompanied by seizures in about 50 per cent of cases, and they may continue after the abscess has been drained or removed surgically. The seizures that accompany viral encephalitis, dementia paralytica, and other inflammatory diseases of the brain are related to cortical lesions. Inclusion-body encephalitis and subacute sclerosing encephalitis give rise to arrhythmic myoclonus, which is often combined with progressive dementia. In diseases that do not involve the cerebral cortex, such as encephalitis lethargica, there is little or no disposition to epilepsy.

DEGENERATIVE DISEASES. All types of degenerative diseases, if they affect the cerebral cortex, may be associated with recurrent seizures. Lipid-storage diseases and Jakob-Creutzfeldt disease must be added to the list of myoclonic dementias. Tuberous sclerosis almost invariably gives rise to seizures. They occur but are infrequent in Alzheimer's disease and Pick's disease. About 3 per cent of multiple sclerosis patients have convulsions in some phase of their illness.

CONGENITAL MALDEVELOPMENT OF THE BRAIN. This is frequently associated with epilepsy, which may be part of the syndrome of mental retardation, spastic diplegia, and other disturbances of motor function. The seizures usually develop in the first weeks or months of life. Special types of infantile and childhood seizures are discussed later in Chap. 212.

METABOLIC DISEASES

Conditions that disturb the metabolism of the brain may induce recurrent seizures. With hypoxia of whatever cause that damages the cerebral cortex, a series of seizures may begin within a few hours to days and continue intermittently for a variable period of time, usually a few days. Many of the author's surviving patients usually have not been subject to epilepsy, but a small group has developed intention myoclonus. Cerebral edema, resulting from excess ingestion of water or large infusions of glucose and water, may be attended by one or several generalized convulsions followed by headache and mental confusion. Uremia is accompanied by muscular twitching and occasionally

by one or more terminal convulsions. Low blood calcium due to rickets or hypoparathyroidism often results in both tetany and seizures. Hypoglycemia caused by an overdose of insulin or an insulin-secreting islet cell tumor often induce seizures, but they invariably follow an initial period of mental confusion, stupor, or coma. The usual history is for the attack to occur several hours after a meal or following a period of fasting. Seizures occur frequently in alcoholic patients and in those who have become addicted to barbiturates, during the period of withdrawal.

DRUG INTOXICATION. The classic examples of direct seizure evocation by drugs are camphor, Metrazol, and picrotoxin. Withdrawal from barbiturates and alcohol in addicted individuals also gives rise to generalized convulsions.

APPROACH TO THE CLINICAL PROBLEM OF RECURRENT SEIZURES

A history of recurrent attacks of loss of consciousness or awareness associated with abnormal movements or confusion is usually sufficient to establish a diagnosis of epilepsy. With such patients a very thorough history, a complete physical and neurologic examination, examination of the visual fields, and laboratory study, including x-ray examination of the skull and an electroencephalogram, should be done. The results of these essential procedures will determine to which of the categories in the above classification the case belongs and whether it should be labeled idiopathic epilepsy.

The history should be particularly searching in regard to epilepsy in the family history and occurrence of head trauma or infections in the past; and careful description of the disease itself, including prodromata, aura, manifestations during the seizure, and the postictal period, must be obtained. Seizures in the family history favor the diagnosis of idiopathic epilepsy. Signs of pulmonary or ear infection or of congenital heart disease with a right-to-left shunt should suggest, in a patient with recently acquired seizures, the possibility of a brain abscess. The presence of a heart murmur and fever or of atrial fibrillation favor embolism. Head trauma of a serious nature, followed by seizures at an interval of several weeks to 2 years, indicates that an injury may have given rise to convulsions. A regularly recurring aura, especially of a focal nature, may indicate the presence of a localized lesion in the brain. Similarly, a focal convulsive movement at the onset of the seizure probably indicates a localized cerebral lesion. A transient monoplegia or hemiplegia (Todd's paralysis) in the postictal period also has considerable significance in localizing a lesion. In fact, its presence may provide the best clue to a focal brain lesion. A history of other neurologic symptoms such as headache, localized paralysis, or mental changes often indicates the need for special diagnostic studies.

A complete physical examination, including a careful survey of nervous function, is mandatory for each epileptic patient. The findings can be clues to the legion of conditions associated with epilepsy. The presence of protuberances over the skull may suggest an underlying pathologic condition. Vascular nevi over the body, especially over the face and in the retina, may be associated with vascular abnormalities within the skull. Small tumors, often pedunculated, distributed over the body surface bring to mind the diagnosis of von Recklinghausen's disease and, when associated with seizures, may indicate an intracranial glioma or neurofibroma. Sebaceous adenomas of the face in the typical butterfly distribution point to the diagnosis of tuberous sclerosis. Cranial nerve disturbances are also helpful in diagnosis; thus, a sixth nerve paralysis is often associated with increased intracranial pressure. Localized weakness, differences in reflexes, or the presence of abnormal reflexes, such as Babinski's response, all have potential localizing value. Coupled with the history, such findings in the examination will often yield a localizing as well as an etiologic diagnosis.

The question of what laboratory procedures should be done in cases of epilepsy can be answered only on the basis of the clinical findings. With generalized convulsions simple blood chemistries are among the first things to do. The determination of blood glucose helps orient the examiner in instances of hypoglycemia and hyperglycemia; the calcium level provides the main clue to hypocalcemia, the blood urea nitrogen (BUN) to kidney disease, and sodium and potassium levels to multiple metabolic disturbances including dilutional hyponatremia. X-rays of the skull should be taken in all cases. Significant findings related to increased intracranial pressure include erosion of the clinoid markings and, in infants and children, separation of the sutures. Hyperostoses, erosions of the skull, abnormal vascular markings, and intracranial calcifications are other findings of importance that may appear in skull x-rays. Because of the frequency of cerebral metastases from primary carcinoma of the lung, chest films should be made in all patients suspected of having intracranial neoplasm.

Lumbar puncture can be of considerable value in elucidating the causes of epilepsy. If the history, neurologic examination, or skull x-rays show any abnormality, especially if it suggests a focal lesion in the brain, then a lumbar puncture is mandatory. Of special importance are determination of the pressure, cell count, total protein, and serologic tests. Increased pressure points to an expanding intracranial lesion. An abnormal cell count often indicates an infectious process. An elevation in total protein (greater than 100 mg per 100 ml) favors the diagnosis of a tumor. If the pressure is normal, but other symptoms or signs point to a recently acquired, localized brain lesion, an arteriogram or pneumoencephalogram may be needed. If, in addition to localizing signs, the patient shows signs of increased intracranial pressure, whether by papilledema or high cerebrospinal fluid pressure, then a ventriculogram may be preferred to a pneumoencephalogram, although arteriography is now used

Table 52-1. CAUSES OF RECURRENT CONVULSIONS IN DIFFERENT AGE GROUPS

Age of onset, yr	Probable cause
Infancy, 0–2	Congenital maldevelopment, birth injury; metabolic (hypocalcemia, hypoglycemia), B$_6$ deficiency
Childhood, 2–10	Birth injury, trauma, infections, thrombosis of cerebral arteries or veins, idiopathy
Adolescence, 10–18	Idiopathy, trauma, congenital defects
Early adulthood, 18–35	Trauma, neoplasm, idiopathy, alcoholism, drug addiction
Middle age, 35–60	Neoplasm, trauma, vascular disease, alcoholism, drug addiction
Late life, over 60	Vascular disease, degeneration, tumor

more frequently than air visualization because of its greater safety. The visualization of the cerebral hemisphere by these procedures may be of particular help to the neurosurgeon in localizing the lesion and in planning a surgical approach to it.

The electroencephalogram, although now routinely employed in the definitive diagnosis of cases with epilepsy, is not absolutely conclusive, since it may be normal in some patients, particularly if the seizures are relatively infrequent, or abnormal in diseases that do not cause epilepsy. The test is of particular value in diagnosing petit mal, for here clinical or subclinical attacks are apt to be frequent enough to register during the electroencephalographic test. Abnormal electrical waves may manifest themselves in other types of epilepsy as well, and the electroencephalogram may be abnormal during the interseizure period, demonstrating either focal or generalized abnormalities of cortical activity. Activation of the electroencephalogram by photic stimulation, drug-induced sleep, or Metrazol injection is now standard procedure in many laboratories.

The type of clinical study in any given case is dictated to some extent by the age of the patient. Up until early adulthood the plan should be outlined as above. Most patients in this age group turn out to have idiopathic epilepsy. With increasing age, the incidence of idiopathic epilepsy becomes less and symptomatic epilepsy increases. Thus the appearance of convulsions for the first time at a period past middle age should be presumptive evidence of brain tumor until every effort has been made to rule it out. However, in the last analysis each case must be dealt with on an individual basis, subsequent procedures depending on the previous findings.

The most frequent causes of recurrent convulsions in different age groups are presented in Table 52-1.

DIFFERENTIAL DIAGNOSIS

The clinical differences between a seizure and a syncopal attack were presented in Chap. 44 and need not be repeated here. It must be emphasized once again that there is no single criterion for distinguishing between them. The author has erred in calling akinetic seizures simple faints and in mistaking cardiac or carotid sinus faints for seizures. Petit mal may be difficult to identify because of the brevity of attacks. One helpful maneuver is to have the patient count for 5 to 10 min. If he is having petit mal, he will blink or stare, pause in counting, or skip one or two numbers. Psychomotor seizures are most difficult of all to diagnose. These attacks are so variable in character and so likely to induce minor disturbances in conduct rather than obvious interruptions of consciousness that they may be diagnosed as temper tantrums, hysteria, psychopathic behavior, or acute psychosis.

A special problem in diagnosis is offered by states of mental dullness and confusion. Epileptic patients as seen in hospital and office practice usually show no mental deterioration, regardless of the type of seizure. Therefore, the appearance of dementia, confusion, or some other derangement of mental function should suggest the possibility of recurrent subclinical seizures not controlled by medication, drug intoxication, postseizure psychosis, or a brain disease that has caused both dementia and seizures. To distinguish these clinical states may require careful observation, along the lines suggested in Chap. 54, and electroencephalography.

REFERENCES

Lennox, W., and M. Lennox: "Epilepsy," Boston, Little, Brown & Company, 1960.

Penfield, W., and H. Jasper: 'Epilepsy and the Functional Anatomy of the Brain," Boston, Little, Brown & Company, 1954.

53 AFFECTIONS OF SPEECH
Raymond D. Adams

Language or speech functions are of fundamental significance to man, in both his social intercourse and his private intellectual life; and when they are disordered as a consequence of developmental anomaly or disease of the brain, the resultant physiologic loss exceeds all others in gravity—even blindness, deafness, and lameness.

The physician is concerned with all derangements of language function, including those of reading and writing, because they are the source of much unhappiness and disability and are almost invariably manifestations of disease of the brain. Furthermore, language is the means whereby the patient communicates his complaints and his feelings to his physician and, at the same time, the medium for that interpersonal transaction between physician and patient which we call psychotherapy. Thus, any disease process that interferes with speech or the understanding of spoken words touches the very core of the patient-physician relationship. Finally, the clinical study of language

disorders serves to illuminate the abstruse relationship between psychologic functions and the anatomy and physiology of the cerebrum. Language mechanisms fall halfway between the well-localized sensorimotor functions and the complex mental functions, such as imagination and thinking, which cannot be localized.

GENERAL CONSIDERATIONS

It has often been remarked that man's commanding position in the world rests on the possession of two faculties: (1) the ability to employ verbal symbols as a "background for his own ideation" and as a means of transmitting his thoughts to others of his kind; and (2) the remarkable facility of his hands. One curious and provocative fact is that the evolution of both speech and manual dexterity occurs in relationship to neurophysiologic pathways located in one cerebral hemisphere. This is a departure from nearly all other localizable neurophysiologic patterns, which are organized according to a bilateral and symmetric plan. The dominance of one cerebral hemisphere, usually the left, emerges with speech and the preference for the right hand, especially in writing; and a lack of development or loss of cerebral dominance as a result of disease disturbs both these traits.

There is abundant evidence that higher animals are able to communicate with each other by vocalization and gestures. However, the content of their communications is their feeling tone at the moment. This *emotional language,* as it is called, was studied by Charles Darwin, who noted that it underwent increasing differentiation in the animal kingdom. Similar instinctual patterns of emotional expression are observed in man. In fact, they are the earliest type of speech to appear (in infancy) and may have been the first to develop in primitive man. Moreover, the language we use to express joy, anger, and fear is retained even after destructive lesions of the dominant cerebral hemisphere; i.e., the neural arrangements that subserve emotional expression are bilateral and symmetric and do not even depend exclusively on the cerebrum. The experiments of Cannon and Bard have amply demonstrated that emotional expression is possible in animals after the removal of both cerebral hemispheres, provided the diencephalon, and particularly the hypothalamus and lower parts of the neuraxis, remain undamaged. In the human infant emotional expression is well developed at a time when the cerebral cortex is still immature.

Propositional, or *symbolic, speech* differs from emotional speech in several ways. Instead of communicating feeling, it transmits ideas from one person to another and requires in its development the substitution of a series of sounds or marks for objects or concepts. This type of speech is not found in animals nor in the human infant. It is not instinctive but learned and is therefore subject to all the modifying influences of social and cultural environments. However, the learning process becomes possible only after the nervous system has reached a certain degree of maturity. The units of propositional language, i.e., words and phrases, have acquired symbolic value and have become the medium of our thought processes. Facility in symbolic language, which is acquired over a period of 15 to 20 years, depends on both maturation of the nervous system and education.

THE DEVELOPMENT OF LANGUAGE

The acquisition of symbolic language by the infant and child has been observed methodically by a number of eminent scientists, and their findings provide a basis for understanding the various derangements of speech.

First, there is the *babbling* and *lalling stage* during which the infant a few weeks of age emits a variety of sounds in combinations of vowel and labial or nasoguttural consonants. This predominantly motor speech activity is no doubt stimulated and reinforced by auditory sensations, which become linked to the kinesthetic ones arising from the speech musculature. It is not clear whether the capacity to hear and understand the spoken word precedes or follows the first motor speech. Possibly it varies from one infant to another, but certainly both speaking and auditory perception of words develop very early in life. Soon babbling merges with *echo speech,* in which the infant repeats parrotlike whatever he hears. Thereafter, auditory, visual, and kinesthetic sensations are gradually combined, and a sound comes to stand for or symbolize an object. Nouns are learned first, then verbs and other parts of speech. Single words and groups of words are used meaningfully in thinking and talking. They form propositions, which, according to Hughlings Jackson, are the very essence of speech. By the age of eighteen to twenty-four months the average infant can construct a phrase; in the months and years that follow, he learns to speak in full sentences. A six-year-old child has a speaking vocabulary of several thousand words and an even larger understanding vocabulary.

The child is now ready for the next stage, reading. This involves the association of graphic visual symbols with the auditory and kinesthetic images of words that have already been acquired. Writing is learned soon after reading, and word auditory-visual symbols now must become linked to cursive movements of the hand. Only those destined to become literate learn to read and write; and to be a complete master of the art of writing is an attainment of only a few select members of our society.

Language development appears to proceed in an orderly manner, but there are individual variations in the actual time at which each successive stage is reached and, to a limited extent, in the order of the different stages. The pattern appears to be set by the neurologic equipment of the individual at any given age. Psychologic factors are of minor importance, at least in the beginning. There is, therefore, good reason why educators have found it unprofitable to teach reading and writing before the sixth year.

Anthropologists have suggested that the individual merely recapitulates the language development of his race. It is supposed that gestures and the utterance of simple meaningful sounds first occurred in primitive man as a differentiation of emotional speech. Gradually these movements and sounds became the conventional signs and verbal symbols of concrete objects, then of the abstract qualities of objects. Signs and spoken language were the first means of human communication; graphic records appeared much later. The American Indian, for instance, never attained a written language. Writing began as pictorial representation, and only much later were alphabets devised. The reading and writing of words and propositions have been relatively recent developments.

The increasing importance of language in contemporary society may be overlooked unless we reflect on the proportion of man's time devoted to purely verbal pursuits. *External speech,* by which we mean the expression of thoughts by spoken and written words and reception of the thoughts of others, is an almost continuous activity when human beings are gathered together; and *internal speech,* or the formation in our minds of unuttered words, is the "coin of mental commerce." It goes on even during a state of preoccupation, when a man is apt to think in words and may, in doing so, subconsciously utter words.

THE ANATOMY OF THE LANGUAGE FUNCTIONS

The conventional teaching is that there are four language areas, situated, in the majority of individuals, in the left hemisphere (Fig. 54-1). Two are receptive and two are executive. One of the former, an area where the neural mechanisms for auditory memory images of words are said to be located, is situated in the posterior part of the first and second temporal convolutions (areas 41 and 42) near the auditory receptive area in Heschl's convolution; the other is for the visual memory, i.e., images of words, and occupies the angular convolution (area 39) in the inferior parietal lobule, near the areas concerned with vision. The intervening area between auditory and visual word centers (area 37), which includes the posterior part of the temporal lobe and the supramarginal convolution, is believed also to be concerned with language formation. Of the executive areas, one at the posterior end of the third frontal convolution (usually referred to as Broca's convolution, or area 44) is for motor speech and the other, situated at the foot of the second frontal convolution above Broca's area, is for writing. These sensory and motor areas are connected by the arcuate bundle of nerve fibers which pass through the isthmus of the temporal lobe, and the same connections may traverse the external capsule of the lenticular nucleus. These areas are also connected with the thalamus and to corresponding areas in the minor cerebral hemisphere through the corpus callosum and anterior commissure.

There has been much difference of opinion concerning these cortical areas, and objection has been made to calling them centers, for they do not represent circumscribed neural structures of constant function and fixed localization. Actually there is relatively little information concerning the anatomy and physiology of these areas. A competent neuroanatomist could not distinguish under the microscope some of these cortical speech areas from other parts of the cerebral cortex. Crude electrical stimulation of the parts of the cortex concerned with speech while the patient is alert and talking (during craniotomy under local anesthesia) causes only an arrest of speech. Knowledge of the location of speech functions has come almost exclusively from the study of human beings who have succumbed to focal brain diseases. From the available information it seems almost certain that the whole language mechanism is not divisible into a number of parts, each depending on a certain fixed group of neurones. Instead, speech must be regarded as a sensorimotor process roughly localized in the opercular or peri-Sylvian region of the left cerebral hemisphere, and the more complex elaborations of speech probably depend on the entire cerebrum.

Carl Wernicke, more than any other person, must be credited with the anatomic-psychologic scheme upon which contemporary ideas of *aphasia* rest. Paul Broca, of Paris, had made the fundamental observation that a lesion of the posterior part of the left inferior frontal convolution deprived man of speech. But Wernicke's article showed that a lesion in the posterior part of the left superior temporal convolution, near the termination of the acoustic pathway would result not in loss of speech but in a paraphasia (sometimes jargon) in which words are used incorrectly, and there is a failure to comprehend what is said and written, an inability to repeat what is said, and an inability to write. The rapid, fluent paraphasic quality of the speech he ascribed to a loss of the internal correction by the receptive speech zone of the activities of the motor speech area of Broca. The occurrence of *alexia* with lesions in the auditory perceptive field he explained as a consequence of the fact that one learns to read by associating written symbols with previously learned auditory ones. Similarly, *agraphia* would be expected because one learns to write by linking visual word symbols with kinesthetic ones for hand movement. Wernicke and his pupils, Lichtheim, Liepmann, Bonhoeffer, Foerster, Kleist, and Goldstein, went on to define auditory conduction aphasia (a triad of paraphasia, inability to repeat what was heard, and intact comprehension of written and spoken words), showing that it was due to a lesion of the arcuate superior longitudinal fasciculus, which separated the auditory association area from the frontal area of Broca. They described pure word deafness, a syndrome based anatomically on disconnection of Wernicke's auditory association area from the auditory receptive area; and they later showed that bilateral lesions in the temporal gyri of Heschl caused cortical deafness. Déjerine, one of Charcot's successors in Paris, reported the first case of pure alexia with a lesion of left occipital lobe and splenium of the corpus callosum.

All these syndromes and their anatomic substructure have withstood severe criticism from Pierre Marie, Henry Head, Von Monakow, Arnold Pick, and Kurt Goldstein, who had attacked the work of Wernicke as being too strictly anatomic. Indeed, diagrams probably are much oversimplified, yet they serve as a theory that integrates a series of observations into a workable concept and has permitted the prediction of new syndromes.

Henschen, the most extreme of the "localizers," in a monograph consisting of three large volumes, collected the clinical and pathologic findings in all the 1,500 cases of aphasia in the literature published prior to 1920, and included 60 of his own. These and other concepts of speech have recently been reviewed by Brain in "Neurology," the monograph originally edited by Wilson and Bruce.

From the available clinical and pathologic data it may be concluded that the locus of the anatomic lesion is more significant than the extent of brain damage. Localization of the lesion is in most instances predictable from the clinical symptomatology, but there are variations. For example, patients with lesions in Broca's area do not always suffer the same disturbance of speech. This lack of consistency in the anatomy of any given speech disorder has engaged the attention of many students of aphasia, and several different hypotheses have been proposed to explain it. The "classic" one has been that the net effect of any lesion depends not only on locus and extent of lesion but on the degree of cerebral dominance. If cerebral dominance is poorly established, a left-sided lesion has less effect on speech than if dominance is strong. Unfortunately, handedness and cerebral dominance are not recorded in many of Henschen's cases. Another factor which imparts an element of unpredictability to the anatomy of speech is that no two individuals acquire language in the same way; some depend more on auditory sense, others on the visual. Lastly, clinical analyses of speech disorders may fail to identify a biologically meaningful functional deficit. We then try to correlate a phenomenon of secondary importance to the anatomy of the lesion.

CEREBRAL DOMINANCE AND ITS RELATIONSHIP TO SPEECH AND HANDEDNESS

The functional supremacy of one cerebral hemisphere is so crucial to language function that it must be considered in greater detail. There are three ways of determining that the left side of the brain is dominant: (1) the loss of speech when disease occurs in certain parts of the left hemisphere and its preservation in diseases involving the right hemisphere; (2) the greater facility in the use of the right hand, foot, and eye; (3) the arrest of speech immediately after the injection of amobarbital (Sodium Amytal) or some other drug in one of the internal carotid arteries. Only (2) and (3) are of use in deciding the cerebral dominance of a living and healthy patient.

Of the general population approximately 90 to 95 per cent are right-handed; the remainder prefer the left hand. A person is said to be right-handed if he chooses the right hand for intricate, skilled acts and is more skillful with it. The preference is more complete in some than others. Most individuals are neither completely right-handed nor completely left-handed but favor one hand for more complicated tasks. Orton refers to this as *intergrading*. The manner in which dextrality and sinistrality are acquired is of interest. Most infants and small children are ambidextrous in their first actions. Writing may be carried out with either hand at first, and "mirror writing" at this early stage is frequent. Between the ages of two and six years one hand and one foot are selected for throwing and kicking a ball, sawing a board, cutting bread, etc. By middle childhood there is usually no doubt as to the dominant side. The reason for hand preference is still controversial. There is strong evidence of a hereditary factor, but the mode of inheritance is uncertain. Learning is also a factor; for many children are shifted at an early age from left to right (shifted sinistrals) because it is a handicap to be left-handed in a right-handed world. Many right-handed persons sight with the right eye, and it has been said that eye preference determines hand preference. Even if true, this still does not account for eye dominance. It is noteworthy that handedness develops simultaneously with language, and the most that can be said at the present is that speech localization and the preference for one eye, one hand, and one foot are all manifestations of some fundamental and inherited tendency not yet defined. There is no observable anatomic difference between the dominant and the minor cerebral hemispheres except that the occipital horn of the left lateral ventricle is usually larger than the right, and the left sulcus lunatus more prominent. No consistent differences in the electroencephalogram between the two hemispheres have been found.

Left-handedness may result from disease of the left cerebral hemisphere in early life, and this probably accounts for its higher incidence among the feeble-minded and brain-injured. Presumably the neural mechanisms for language become centered in the right cerebral hemisphere. Handedness and cerebral dominance may fail to develop in some individuals, and this is particularly true in certain families. Developmental defects in speech and reading, stuttering, "mirror writing," and general clumsiness are much more frequent in these families.

Differences in degree of cerebral dominance do unquestionably account for some of the inconsistency in the cerebral localization of speech in different individuals. In studies of groups of left-handed individuals who suffer cerebral derangements of speech it has been noted that approximately 75 per cent of them have had lesions in the left cerebral hemisphere. Further, in those aphasias due to the right cerebral lesions, the patient is always left-handed and the speech disorder tends to be less severe and enduring. The latter tends to take the form of an expressive disturbance rather than alexia or amnestic aphasias; and visuoconstructive troubles are prominent, as are also faults in calculation and recognition of one's neurologic deficits (anosognosia).

TYPES OF LANGUAGE DISORDER ENCOUNTERED IN MEDICINE

These can be divided into four categories:

1. Disturbances of speech that occur with diseases affecting the higher nervous integrations, namely, delirium and dementia. Speech is seldom lost in these conditions but is instead merely deranged as part of a general impairment of intellectual functions. *Palilalia* and *echolalia,* in which the patient repeats, parrot-like, the syllables and words which he hears, are special abnormalities usually observed in states of dementia with extrapyramidal signs.

2. The loss or disturbance of speech due to a cerebral lesion that does not deprive a man of his reason or paralyze other motor or sensory functions. This condition has been termed *aphasia;* milder degrees of it have been called *dysphasia.*

3. A defect in articulation with intact mental functions and normal comprehension and memory of words. This is a pure motor disorder of the muscles of articulation and may be due to flaccid or spastic paralysis, rigidity, repetitive spasms (stuttering), or ataxia. The term *anarthria* or *dysarthria* has been applied to some of these conditions.

4. Loss of voice due to a disease of the larynx or its innervation, with resulting *aphonia* or *dysphonia.* Articulation and internal language are unaffected.

In the practice of medicine the most frequent and troublesome disorders of speech are aphasia, stuttering, dysarthria, and aphonia. The remainder of this chapter will be devoted to these clinical problems and their diagnostic significance.

Types of Aphasia

The following tests will usually make it possible to decide whether the patient has a *global aphasia* (with loss of all or nearly all speech functions), a *motor* or *expressive aphasia* (sometimes called *verbal,* or *executive,* or *Broca's aphasia*), or a *receptive aphasia* (*Wernicke's aphasia*) predominantly of auditory and visual type, *auditory verbal aphasia* (word deafness), and *alexia* (inability to read). Writing is disturbed to some extent in the majority of cases of aphasia and is rarely deranged alone.

GLOBAL APHASIA. This is due to a lesion that destroys a large part of the speech areas of the major cerebral hemispheres. It is most commonly due to the occlusion of the left internal carotid or middle cerebral artery, but a massive hemorrhage (hypertensive or traumatic), an infiltrative tumor, or other lesion may also cause this syndrome. The middle cerebral artery nourishes all the speech areas, and nearly all the aphasic disorders due to vascular occlusion are caused by involvement of this artery or its branches. The only exceptions are (1) Heubner's recurrent branch of the left anterior cerebral artery, which supplies the subcortical white matter of the frontal lobe; occlusion of it is said to cause subcortical motor aphasia; and (2) the temporal and calcarine branches of the posterior cerebral artery, which supplies part of area 37, the medial occipital lobe and splenium of corpus callosum. Occlusion of this may rarely cause a difficulty in the visual recognition of words and amnestic aphasia, i.e., an inability to name objects seen, or an alexia. Left hemispherectomy for glioma or epilepsy has had a similar effect. Most patients with global amnesia are speechless or can say at most a few words; they cannot read or write and can understand only a few simple spoken words and phrases. Recovery depends on the nature and extent of the disease and whether or not the right cerebral hemisphere had previously engaged in language formulation and expression. If the left hemisphere was strongly dominant, there will usually be little or no recovery, which casts doubt on the popular notion that the right hemisphere can take over speech function.

MOTOR OR EXPRESSIVE APHASIA. This condition is due to a lesion in the posterior part of the inferior or third frontal convolution, the subcortical white matter of the insula, or the external capsule of the lenticular nucleus. Softening due to occlusion of anterior, superior branches of the middle cerebral artery is a more frequent cause than neoplasm or trauma. The patient loses the power of expressing himself by spoken words. He is unable to speak spontaneously, to read aloud, or to repeat what he hears or sees. And yet he is not dumb. He can usually say "yes" or "no" and a few other words previously habitual with him. One may mistake this difficulty for an anarthria until it is observed that the patient has no difficulty in other acts, such as chewing and swallowing, which require movement of the tongue, lips, palate, and larynx. A weakness of the muscles of the lower part of the right side of the face and a deviation of the tongue to the right may be present. For a time there may be an inability to purse the lips properly, to blow out a candle, or to make other purposeful lip movements. The motor incapacity for certain acts in the absence of paralysis of the necessary muscles or groups of muscles is called *apraxia*, and it has been contended that expressive aphasia is actually a verbal apraxia. The patient repeats his few words over and over again as if compelled to do so. Words in a well-known song may be sung and others uttered as expletives when the patient is angered or excited, illustrating the point that the patient, though "speechless" under ordinary conditions, has not become "wordless." Usually he can recognize some of his own mistakes and may manifest signs of exasperation or despair over them. Most patients are unable to write, and even though hemiplegic and so denied the use of their right hand,

they are unable to write recognizable words with the left hand. An occasional patient with Broca's aphasia has been observed to be able to repeat some words spoken by the examiner, to read aloud, and to copy words; this condition is called *transcortical motor aphasia*. The area involved in initiating motor speech is damaged, but the motor mechanism can still be activated via the temporoparietal speech areas. Sometimes the ability to write is retained with a severe Broca's aphasia, and the ability to read and understand spoken language is faultless, showing that inner language is undisturbed. This is called *subcortical motor aphasia*. Alajouanine has traced the regression of expressive aphasia along two lines: (1) through stereotyped obligatory verbal utterance to *agrammatism*, in which only a skeleton of nouns and verbs is spoken; (2) from anarthria through dysarthria with various degrees of residual phonetic disintegration.

THE MAJOR SYNDROME OF RECEPTIVE OR SENSORY APHASIA. Sensory aphasia is more difficult to define than expressive aphasia. It usually appears as a rather complex syndrome consisting essentially of a loss of comprehension of spoken language and of written words and an inability to write. The patient is able to speak, often volubly, but misuses words. According to present terminology, the defects are, respectively, auditory verbal agnosia; visual verbal agnosia, or alexia; agraphia; and paraphasia. The term *agnosia* was first introduced by Sigmund Freud and means a disturbance of recognition or identification with relatively intact sensation. In word deafness hearing is not reduced, but there is an inability to comprehend spoken words (i.e., word deafness with intact hearing). All these elements were noted by Wernicke, and it is now customary, when the entire syndrome is present, to refer to it as *Wernicke's aphasia*. The lesion is variable in its extent but usually involves the posterior part of the upper temporal convolutions and the supramarginal convolution and white matter beneath it. Left temporal lobectomy has had a similar effect if the incision extends posteriorly and superiorly. Special interest attaches to the patient's manner of speech. His articulation is normal, unless there is an associated expressive aphasia. He often pauses or gropes for a word, substitutes an incorrect word, omits words, and is unable at times to construct a sentence. When he begins to speak, the first sentence or two is well composed; but as he continues, the difficulty becomes increasingly evident. When the speech is severely disorganized, it gives way to *jargon aphasia*, also called *choreatic aphasia* (Kussmaul) and *syntactical aphasia* (Head). During recovery one may observe progress from an undifferentiated through an asemantic and then paraphasic jargon. The patient does not seem to notice his own errors and is not much disturbed by them; i.e., he has lost insight.

The basic disorder in paraphasia has been disputed. Some investigators believe that the patient has merely lost the ability to understand his own spoken words; i.e., he has an auditory verbal agnosia. This simple explanation does not seem to account for all the facts. Head's explanation is more likely the correct one, that internal language mechanisms are deranged; i.e., the mental processes by which visual and auditory word memories are evoked in response to certain ideas are disordered.

Many aphasic patients present only part of the syndrome. The term *transcortical sensory aphasia* is applied to the state in which the patient can repeat what he hears but without comprehension; he also reads aloud without understanding the words. *Amnestic* or *nominal aphasia* is almost invariably present in Wernicke's aphasia, but it may occur as a solitary symptom. The patient is unable to affix a name to many common objects when they are visually presented. He tells instead the use of the object, and if the auditory receptive centers are intact, he can immediately recognize the name when it is spoken by the examiner. The question of location of the responsible lesion is still debated. Nielsen believes it to be in area 37 or near the isthmus of the temporal lobe, and he has observed this type of aphasia in cases with temporal lobe abscess, tumors, or vascular lesions. *Visual aphasia, word blindness,* or *alexia* may dominate the picture but seldom occurs in pure form; usually there is some paraphasic fault in the patient's utterance and some degree of *agraphia* owing to a loss of memories of written or printed words. If capacity to write is conserved, the defect is called *subcortical visual aphasia,* and the lesion is believed to be in the subcortical white matter deep in the inferior parietal lobe. As pointed out by Osler, it is often associated with a contralateral homonymous hemianopia.

WORD DEAFNESS. This may occur in pure form in lesions (usually small infarcts of a superior temporal branch of the left middle cerebral artery) that separate the left and right auditory receptive areas from Wernicke's auditory verbal association area in the posterior part of the superior temporal gyrus. The patient cannot understand anything said to him nor can he repeat words or write from dictation, yet he reads with excellent comprehension and speaks and writes fluently. There is no paraphasia. Auditory perception of musical notes and sounds is intact. Many of the published examples of this syndrome have shown bilateral temporal lobe lesions. Liepmann and Storch, however, observed it in a patient with a single lesion in the left temporal lobe.

WORD BLINDNESS (ALEXIA). In this condition the ability to recognize written symbols is lost, but the patient can understand what he hears, speak normally, and may or may not write. Usually he cannot name colors. The common lesions are infarct, hemorrhage, or tumor that separate the angular gyrus from the left and right visual receptive areas. Often an infarct has been present in the left occipital lobe, causing a right homonymous hemianopia and another in the splenium of corpus callosum or subcortical white matter of left parietal lobe.

Pure agraphia, i.e., inability to write with preservation of all other elements of speech and good

strength and sensation in the hand, has not been reported. This is one of the reasons for doubting the existence of a writing center.

APPROACH TO THE CLINICAL PROBLEM OF APHASIA. In investigating a case of aphasia it is first necessary to inquire into the patient's native language, his handedness, and his previous education. Many naturally left-handed children are trained to use their right hand for writing; therefore, in determining this point we must ask which hand is used for throwing a ball, threading a needle, or using a spoon or common tools such as hammer, saw, or bread knife. One should quickly ascertain whether the patient has other signs of a gross cerebral lesion such as hemiplegia, facial weakness, homonymous hemianopia, or cortical sensory loss.

It is important before the beginning of the examination to determine whether the patient is alert and mentally clear or suffering from confusion, because this may prevent accurate assessment of language. One must also avoid the effects of fatigue as far as possible by making the interview short. Explanation of the purpose of the tests, sympathy, and encouragement are often necessary to assure full cooperation.

Many elaborate examination schemes have been devised for testing the language functions, and some of them lead to refinements that are of little physiologic or clinical significance. The following procedure will yield sufficient data for diagnosis.

1. Can the patient spontaneously utter intelligible words in proper sequence and well-constructed phrases and sentences? The fluency of speech, the extent of vocabulary, the grammatical construction of sentences, the accuracy of word usage, and clarity of enunciation should all be observed and examples incorporated into the record of the interview. Wrong choice of words, misplacement of words or syllables, omission of essential words, and use of disjointed phrases may be slight in degree and take the form of paraphasia; if severe, they may result in an unintelligible jabbering or jargon. Can the patient repeat or copy what he hears or reads?

2. Can the patient understand what he hears? If he is unable to speak, give him a series of commands of increasing complexity. Ask him to close his eyes, open his mouth, hold up his left hand, place the index finger of the left hand to the right ear, etc. Often the patient will execute the first one or two simple commands correctly and will fail on all others, sometimes repeating the first act over and over (perseveration).

3. Can the patient read? Written questions or commands should be presented and the responses observed.

4. Can the patient write spontaneously? If his right hand is paralyzed, he should be encouraged to try with his left. It must also be determined whether or not he can write from dictation or can copy words or sentences.

5. If he is able to speak, can he name common objects shown visually, such as a penny, button, pencil, fountain pen, handkerchief, the various parts of a

wrist watch, safety pin, key, flashlight, matches? If not, does he recognize the correct name when he hears it? Can he repeat the words that he hears? Can he read aloud from a newspaper or magazine? Are his gestures appropriate?

Disorders in the Development of Language in Children

A close parallelism exists between the symptoms observed in adults who have suffered a loss in language functions as a result of brain injury and those seen during the development of language skills. This reminds us that there may be faulty development of language and of cerebral dominance. It has been found that a high percentage of these patients have a strong family background of speech disorders and that strong preference for the right or the left hand is not present. Males are affected much more frequently than females (ratio, 10:1).

Developmental disorders of language and congenital deafness are far more frequent than aphasia. These include developmental alexia (special reading disability, congenital word blindness), developmental agraphia (special writing disability), developmental word deafness, developmental motor aphasia (motor speech delay), and developmental apraxia (abnormal clumsiness of the limbs). The development of language, instead of proceeding in the manner outlined in the early part of this chapter, is arrested or delayed. These conditions are often misunderstood by parents, teachers, and physicians. Sometimes the unfortunate child is judged to be feebleminded or lazy. Another frequent error is to assume the condition is due to psychologic factors.

CONGENITAL WORD DEAFNESS. If an individual is born deaf, he never learns to talk without special training; he is "deaf and dumb." Should deafness develop within the first few years of life, after speech has been acquired, the child gradually loses speech but can be retaught by the lip-reading method. His speech is harsh, poorly modulated, and unpleasant, and he is apt to make many peculiar throat noises of a snorting or grunting kind. Such patients are bright and alert and clever at pantomime and gesturing. They are inattentive to household noises and do not appear to understand what is said to them. The deafness can be demonstrated at an early age by careful observations of the child's responses to sounds, but it cannot be accurately tested before the age of three or four years. The psychogalvanic reflex technique for testing reaction to sounds and tests of the labyrinths, which are usually unresponsive in the deaf-mute, may be helpful. In contrast the idiot or moron is stupid in all his actions and talks little because he has nothing to say. Developmental word deafness may be difficult to distinguish from true deafness. Usually the parents have noted that the word-deaf child responds to loud noises and music, though obviously this does not assure perfect hearing, particu-

larly for high tones. The word-deaf child does not understand what is said, and there is delay and distortion of speech. These children are alert, active, and inquisitive and may chatter incessantly. They adopt a language of their own design, and attentive parents come to understand it. This peculiar type of speech is known as *idioglossia*. It is also observed in children who have marked difficulty in the articulation of certain consonants. They learn to lip-read very quickly and are clever at acting out their own ideas.

CONGENITAL WORD BLINDNESS (ALEXIA). In this unusual condition the patient has good eyesight, is able to see the word but not to grasp its meaning. There is no loss of the ability to recognize the meaning of objects, pictures, and diagrams. Usually with assiduous training, the patient, who is otherwise bright and intelligent, can learn to read individual letters and a few simple words. Spelling is impossible. Often the patient cannot write anything of his own composition but can copy skillfully. Lesser degrees of congenital alexia are commoner than the severe forms and pose serious problems in the classroom. The problem is a complex one, for difficulty in learning to read well is unquestionably influenced by the teaching techniques used in the school. Only a few of the severely handicapped children have a right homonymous hemianopia or a right-sided sensory loss; most of them show no other abnormality.

ABNORMALITIES OF ARTICULATION AND PHONATION (LISPING, DYSLALIA). A number of odd varieties of deficient articulation may come to the notice of the physician. One is *lisping*, in which the s sound is replaced by *th;* e.g., "thister" for "sister." Another condition, called *lallation* or *dyslalia*, a common speech disorder observed in early childhood, is characterized by multiple substitutions or omissions of consonants. In severe forms, speech may be almost unintelligible. These children are unaware that their speech differs from that of other persons and are distressed at not being understood. Milder degrees consist of the failure to pronounce only one or two consonants. For example, there may be imperfect enunciation of the sound r so that it sounds like w. "Running a race" becomes "wunning a wace." The nature of this disorder is not known. It has been suggested that the development of language in some children is so rapid that there is a partial failure of both perceptive and imitative speech. The patient usually recovers spontaneously from this disorder or responds promptly to speech therapy, which is best carried out at about the age of five years. These abnormalities are more frequent among feebleminded than normal children, and mental defect should always be suspected if numerous consonants are mispronounced and the condition persists beyond the age of twelve or thirteen years. The speech disorder resulting from *cleft palate* is easily recognized. Many of these patients also have a harelip, and the two abnormalities together interfere with suckling and later in life with the enunciation of labial and guttural consonants. The voice has an unpleasant nasality and often, if the defect is severe, there is an audible escape of air through the nose.

STAMMERING AND STUTTERING. Stammering and stuttering are difficult to classify. In some respects they belong to the developmental disorders, but they differ from them in being largely centered in articulation. They consist of a spasm of the muscles of articulation when an attempt is made to speak. The spasm may be tonic and result in a complete block of speech, sometimes called stammering, or a repetitive spasm that leads to repeated utterance of the first syllable, i.e., a stutter. Certain syllables offer greater difficulty than others. The patient falters on an initial consonant or syllable, which he repeats over and over again before he finally succeeds in enunciating the rest of the word, e.g., p-p-paper, b-b-b-boy. The severity of the stutter is increased by excitement, as in speaking before strangers or a group of people. The spasms may overflow into other muscle groups not directly concerned with speech. Males are affected three times as often as females. The time of onset may be when the child first begins to talk, i.e., at two or three years of age, or between the ages of six and eight years. These are the two critical periods of language development. Many of these children also have some degree of reading and writing disability. Slowness in developing hand preference or enforced change from left- to right-handedness are noted in many cases. If mild, the condition tends to develop or to be present only during periods of emotional distress; and it usually disappears spontaneously during adolescent or early adult years. If severe, it persists all through life, regardless of treatment, but tends to improve as the patient grows older.

The essential character of stuttering is difficult to define. There is no detectable paralysis or incoordination of speech musculature, which seems to function normally in other commonplace acts and when the patient is alone and relaxed or singing. Stuttering differs from apraxia in that the muscles, when called upon to perform the specific act, go into voluntary spasm; but since the spasm does not occur during other movements in which these muscles are involved, it differs from the intention spasm of athetosis. It appears to represent a special category of movement disorder and is much like writer's cramp, another motor disorder of unknown etiology.

Everyone who has studied stuttering and stammering has been impressed with the high incidence of similar disabilities in other members of the same family, sometimes going back several generations. This and the preponderance in males suggest a sex-linked characteristic, but the inheritance does not follow a simple pattern.

Many of the patients, probably as a natural result of this impediment to free social intercourse, become increasingly fearful of speaking and have feelings of inferiority after a few years. By the time adolescence and adulthood are reached, emotional factors are so prominent that many physicians have mistaken stuttering for neurosis. Usually there is little or no evidence of any personality deviation before the onset of stuttering, and psychotherapy by competent psychiatrists, though unquestionably helpful in relieving emotional tension and assisting a satisfactory adjustment to the condition, has not significantly modified the underlying defect. Occasionally stuttering will develop during adult life as a consequence of brain disease.

Disorders of Articulation and Phonation

The third group of speech abnormalities are the disorders of articulation. In simple dysarthria there is no abnormality of the cortical centers. The dysarthric patient is able to understand perfectly what he hears, and if literate, he reads and has no difficulty in writing, even though unable to utter a single intelligible word. This is the strict meaning of being inarticulate.

The act of speaking is a highly coordinated sequence of contractions of the larynx, pharynx, palate, tongue, lips, and respiratory musculature. These are innervated by the hypoglossal, vagal, facial, and phrenic nerves. The nuclei of these nerves are controlled through the corticobulbar tracts by both motor cortices. As with all movements, there is also an extrapyramidal influence from the cerebellum and basal ganglions. A current of air is produced by expiration, and the force of it is finely regulated and coordinated with the activity of other muscles engaged in speech. *Phonation*, or the production of vocal sounds, is a function of the larynx. Changes in the size and shape of the glottis and in the length and tension of the vocal cords are affected by the action of the laryngeal muscles. Vibrations are set up and transmitted to the column of air passing over the vocal cords. Sounds thus formed are modified as they pass through the nasopharynx and mouth, which act as resonators. Articulation consists of contractions of the tongue, lips, pharynx, and palate, which interrupt or alter the vocal sounds. Vowels are of laryngeal origin, as are some consonants; but the latter are formed for the most part during articulation. For instance, the consonants *m*, *b*, and *p* are labial, *l* and *t* are lingual, and *nk* and *ng* are nasoguttural.

Defective articulation and phonation are best observed by listening to the patient during ordinary conversation or while reading aloud from a newspaper or a book. Test phrases or the rapid repetition of lingual, labial, and guttural consonants may bring out the particular abnormality. Disorders of phonation call for an examination of the apparatus of voice. The movements of the vocal cords should be inspected with the aid of a hand mirror or, even better, a laryngoscope, and those of the tongue, palate, and pharynx by direct observation.

Defects in articulation may be subdivided into several types: paralytic dysarthria, spastic and rigid dysarthria, and ataxic dysarthria.

PARALYTIC DYSARTHRIA. This is due to a neural or bulbar (medullary) paralysis of the articulatory muscles (lower motor neurone paralysis). Bulbar poliomyelitis and "progressive bulbar palsy" are examples of diseases that may produce partial or complete anarthria. In the latter the shriveled tongue lies inert on the floor of the mouth, and the lips are relaxed and trembling. Saliva constantly collects in the mouth because of dysphagia, and drooling is troublesome. Speech becomes less and less distinct. There is special difficulty in the correct utterance of vibratives such as *r:* and as the paralysis becomes more complete, lingual and labial consonants are finally not pronounced at all. Lesser degrees of this abnormality are observed in myasthenia gravis. Bilateral paralysis of the palate, which may occur with diphtheria, poliomyelitis, or involvement of the tenth cranial nerve by tumor, produces a disorder of articulation similar to that of the cleft palate. The voice has a nasal quality, since the posterior nares are not closed during phonation, and certain consonants such as *n*, *b*, and *k* are altered. The abnormality is sometimes less pronounced in recumbency and increased when the head is thrown forward. Bilateral paralysis of the lips interferes with enunciation of labial consonants; *p* and *b* are slurred and sound more like *f* and *v*.

SPASTIC AND RIGID DYSARTHRIA. These are more frequent than the paralytic variety. Diseases that involve the corticobulbar tracts, usually vascular disease or motor system disease, result in the syndrome of pseudobulbar palsy. The patient may have had a minor stroke some time in the past affecting the corticobulbar fibers on one side; but since the bulbar muscles are probably represented in both motor cortices, there is no impairment in speech or swallowing from a unilateral lesion. If another stroke occurs involving the other corticobulbar tract and possibly the corticospinal tract at the pontine, midbrain, or capsular level, immediately the patient becomes anarthric or dysarthric and dysphagic. Unlike bulbar paralysis due to lower motor neurone involvement, there is no atrophy or fasciculation of the paralyzed muscles, the jaw jerk is exaggerated, the palatal reflexes are retained, emotional control is poor (pathologic laughter and crying), and sometimes breathing becomes periodic (Cheyne-Stokes). The patient may be anarthric and aphonic for a time, but as he improves, or in mild degrees of the same condition, speech is thick and indistinct, much like that of partial bulbar paralysis.

In paralysis agitans, or postencephalitic Parkinson's syndrome, one observes an extrapyramidal disturbance of articulation. The patient speaks slowly and articulates poorly, slurring over many syllables and trailing off the end of sentences. The voice is low-pitched, monotonous, and lacking inflection. The words are pronounced hastily. In advanced cases speech is almost unintelligible; now only whispering may be possible. It may happen that the patient finds it impossible to talk while walking but can speak if he sits or lies down.

In chorea and myoclonus speech may also be severely affected, and the defect is distinguished from the speech of pseudobulbar palsy or paralysis agitans by the interruptions of the abnormal movements. Grimac-

ing and other characteristic motor signs must be depended upon for diagnosis. Pyramidal and extrapyramidal disturbances of speech may be combined in generalized cerebral diseases such as general paresis, in which slurred speech is one of the cardinal signs.

In many cases of capsular hemiplegia or partially recovered Broca's aphasia the patient is left with a dysarthria that may be difficult to distinguish from a pure articulatory defect. Careful testing of other language functions, especially writing, may bring out the aphasic quality.

ATAXIC DYSARTHRIA. This is characteristic of acute and chronic cerebellar lesions. It may be observed in multiple sclerosis, Friedreich's ataxia, cerebellar atrophy, and heat stroke. The principal speech abnormality is slowness; precise enunciation, monotony, and unnatural separation of the syllables of words (scanning) are other features. Coordination of speech and respiration are poor. There may not be enough breath to utter certain words, and others may be ejaculated explosively. *Scanning dysarthria* is distinctive, but in some cases, especially if there is some possibility of spastic weakness of the tongue from corticobulbar tract involvement, it is impossible to predict the anatomy of the disease from analysis of speech alone. Myoclonic jerks involving the speech musculature may be superimposed on cerebellar ataxia in a number of diseases.

APHONIA AND DYSPHONIA. Lastly, a few points should be made concerning disturbances of voice. In adolescence and early adult life there may be a persistence of the unstable "change of voice" normally seen in boys soon after puberty. As though by habit, the patient speaks part of the time in a falsetto voice. This can usually be overcome by training.

Paresis of the respiratory movements, as in poliomyelitis and acute infectious polyneuritis, may affect voice because insufficient air is provided for phonation and speech. Also, disturbances in the rhythm of respiration may interfere with the fluency of speech. This is particularly noticeable in so-called "extrapyramidal diseases," and one may note that the patient tries to talk upon inspiration. Reduced volume of speech due to limited excursion of the breathing muscles is another common feature; the patient is unable to speak loudly or to shout.

Paresis of both vocal cords causes complete aphonia. There is no voice, and the patient can speak only in whispers. Since the vocal cords normally separate during inspiration, their failure to do so when paralyzed may result in an inspiratory stridor. If one vocal cord is paralyzed, the voice becomes hoarse, low-pitched, and rasping.

Another curious condition about which little is known is *spastic dysphonia*. The author has seen several cases, middle-aged or elderly men and women, otherwise healthy, who gradually lost the ability to speak quietly and fluently. Any effort to speak resulted in contraction of all the speech musculature so that the patient's voice was strained and articulation was labored. Apparently this is a neurologic disorder of undetermined kind. The patients are not neurotic, and psychotherapy has been ineffective. This condition differs from the stridor caused by spasm of the laryngeal muscles in tetany.

Instability or changeableness of voice, a common problem for adolescent boys, may persist into adult life. Its basis is not known. Voice training has been helpful in many patients.

DIAGNOSIS

Speech is such a complex act that it has not been possible to present all its facets. Nothing, for example, has been said here about speech changes during various psychiatric illnesses. This does not mean that the psychiatric syndromes are unimportant, for there is no doubt that hysterical aphonia, the various tics that interrupt the speech of tense individuals, and the altered rate, fluency, and content of speech in the psychoses pose formidable problems.

In diagnosing disorders of speech the physician must attempt in every case to decide first whether the problem is one of aphasia, dysarthria, or dysphonia. The examination procedure outlined above will, if carried out systematically, permit this first and important step to be made.

If the patient is aphasic, *it should be determined whether his aphasia is global, expressive, or sensory in type,* and whether it is a *restricted motor disorder, alexia,* or *word deafness.* Global aphasia signifies a disease involving the posterior frontal, the superior temporal, or inferior parietal and intervening insula and external capsular parts of the left cerebral hemisphere in a right-handed person, or, rarely, the right cerebral hemisphere in a left-handed person. Expressive aphasia indicates a lesion in the insular region and frontal lobe; sensory aphasia points to disease more posteriorly, in the temporoparietal region. Contralateral hemiplegia, hemianesthesia, and hemianopia with sensory aphasia are frequently associated with motor aphasia.

The general physician is frequently called upon to examine children who show some disorder of speech or delay in language development. From the above remarks it will be seen that these disorders fall into several broad categories, of which stuttering, delay in onset of speech, dyslalia, partial or complete deafness, word deafness, cleft palate, lisping, and word blindness are the most frequent. When faced with problems of this type, the physician must ask several questions. *Is the child partially or completely deaf? Does he have a more generalized mental or neuromuscular defect— is he feebleminded or suffering from an infantile hemiplegia or spastic diplegia? Does he stammer, stutter, or show dyslalia?* In attempting to answer these questions, the parents' account of the child's development and his behavior at home is most helpful. Failure to respond to noise of any kind suggests deafness. An interest in sounds and music but not in stories or conversation, together with slow development of understanding and use of speech are indicative of high-tone deafness or word deafness (auditory verbal ag-

nosia). Delayed onset of suckling, head control, sitting, standing, walking, etc., deserve a neurologic examination; one should look particularly for spastic weakness or rigidity of the limbs and poor motor control of the tongue, as well as mental retardation. The latter can be assessed at an early age by intelligence tests such as the performance part of the Stanford-Binet test. If the child is otherwise normal, recitation of a nursery rhyme will disclose a stammering, stuttering lallation of cleft palate speech. Disturbances of articulation point to involvement of a different set of neural structures, such as the motor cortices, the corticobulbar pathways, the seventh, ninth, and tenth nuclei, the brain stem, and extrapyramidal nuclei and tracts. Often it is necessary to use other neurologic findings to decide which of these are implicated in any given case. The important distinction between the pseudobulbar or supranuclear palsies and the bulbar palsies is grasped only with difficulty by the average student. The information obtained by localizing these two major types of dysarthria is extremely helpful in differential diagnosis. Dysphonia should lead to an investigation of laryngeal disease either primary or secondary to an abnormality of innervation.

TREATMENT

The sudden loss of speech would be expected to cause great apprehension, but except for almost pure motor defects, most patients show remarkably little concern. It appears that the very lesion that deprives them of speech also causes at least a partial loss of insight into their own disability. This reaches almost a ludicrous extreme in some cases of Wernicke's aphasia, in which the patient becomes indignant when others cannot understand his jargon. Nonetheless, as improvement occurs, many patients do become discouraged. Reassurance and a positive program of speech rehabilitation are the best ways of helping the patient at this stage.

The contemporary methods of training and reeducation in overcoming an aphasic defect have never been critically evaluated. Most aphasic difficulty is due to vascular disease of the brain, and nearly always this is accompanied by some degree of spontaneous improvement in the days, weeks, and months that follow the stroke. Sometimes recovery is complete within hours or days; at times not more than a few words are regained after a year or two of assiduous speech training. Nevertheless, it is the opinion of many experts in the field that speech training is worthwhile.

One must decide for each patient whether speech training is needed and when it should be started. As a rule, therapy is not advisable in the first few days of an aphasic illness, because one does not know how lasting it will be. Also, if the patient suffers a severe global aphasia and can neither speak nor understand spoken and written words, the speech therapist is helpless. Under such circumstances, one does well to wait a few weeks until some one of the language functions has begun to return. Then the physician may begin to encourage and help the patient to use the function to a maximum degree. In milder aphasic disorders the patient may be sent to the speech therapist as soon as the illness has stabilized.

The methods of speech training are specialized, and it is advisable to call in a person who has been trained in this field. However, inasmuch as the benefit is largely psychologic, an interested member of the family or a schoolteacher can be used if a speech therapist is not available in the community.

The language problems of children are serious, demand skillful diagnosis and treatment, and often show excellent results. Most of the well-organized urban school systems have remedial reading teachers who will take over the problem once it has been evaluated medically. The emotional problems that often accompany the developmental disturbances of language and of cerebral dominance must be dealt with gently and firmly.

The physician should by wise counseling help the patient understand the nature of this problem and try to avoid some of the secondary emotional problems that the speech disorder creates. Prolonged psychotherapy helps with the emotional problems but has not, in the author's experience, corrected the underlying speech defect. Fortunately, the natural course of mild stuttering is toward improvement during adolescence, and many patients recover spontaneously by adult life. In severe cases a lifelong problem must be faced, and none of the present methods of therapy, including psychoanalysis, have corrected the defect.

There is no special treatment for the dysarthric disturbance of speech.

REFERENCES

Alajouanine, T.: Verbal Realization in Aphasia, Brain, 79:1–29, 1956.

Brain, R.: Aphasia, Apraxia, Agnosia, chap. 83 in "Neurology," 2d ed., vol. 3, S. A. K. Wilson and N. Bruce (Eds.), Baltimore, The Williams & Wilkins Company, 1955.

Nielsen, J. M.: "Agnosia, Apraxia, Aphasia; Their Value in Cerebral Localization," 2d ed., New York, Hafner Publishing Company, Inc., 1962.

Orton, S. T.: "Reading, Writing and Speech Problems in Children," New York, W. W. Norton and Company, Inc., 1937.

54 DERANGEMENTS OF INTELLECT AND BEHAVIOR INCLUDING DELIRIUM AND OTHER CONFUSIONAL STATES, KORSAKOFF'S AMNESTIC SYNDROME, AND DEMENTIA

Raymond D. Adams and Maurice Victor

Every physician sooner or later discovers through clinical experience the need for special competence in assessing the mental faculties of his patients. He must be able to observe with detachment and complete objectivity their character, intelligence, mood, memory, judgment and other attributes of personality in much the same fashion as he observes the nutritional state and color of the mucous membranes. The systematic examination of these affective and cognitive functions permits him to reach certain conclusions regarding mental status, and these are also of value in understanding the patient and his illness. Without the data obtained from the study of the mental status, errors will be made in evaluating the reliability of the patient's history, in diagnosing the neurologic or psychiatric disease from which he suffers, and in conducting any proposed therapeutic program.

Perhaps the content of this chapter will be more clearly understood if we repeat a few of the introductory remarks of Chap. 41. The main thesis of the neurologic physician is that mental and physical functions of the nervous system are simply two aspects of the same basic vital process. The mind is no more or less than the highest and most complex expression of the self-regulating, goal-seeking quality manifest in the activities of all living things. It is only because of the prodigious complexity of man's brain, his high capacity for memory, imagination, and reasoning, his opportunity to make conscious choice and to reflect on the working of his own psychic processes that the illusion of separation of mind and body was created. Biologists and psychologists have reached the modern monistic view by placing all protoplasmic activities of the nervous system (growth, development, behavior, and mental function) in a continuum and noting the inherent purposiveness and creativity common to all of them. The physician is persuaded of its truth by his daily experiences with disease, in which every known aberration of behavior, intellect, and personality appear as expressions of diseases of the cerebrum.

In this chapter we are concerned with common disturbances of behavior and intellection that have not been previously discussed and which stand as cardinal manifestations of cerebral disease. The most frequent of these are confusion, disturbances of memory, and abnormalities of thinking or reasoning. For completeness a resumé of clinical phenomena resulting from diseases of the different lobes of the cerebrum will be appended.

DEFINITION OF TERMS

The following nomenclature, though tentative, is useful and will be employed throughout this textbook:

Confusion, as stated in Chap. 50, is a term that has two meanings. The commonest refers to a general reduction in alertness and an inattentiveness to environmental stimuli, an inability to take notice of all elements of a situation within a short period of time. It is often associated with misinterpretations of stimuli, and hallucinations and drowsiness may be prominent. The other usage designates slowness and inefficiency in thinking, often with impairment of subsequent recall. Thus, in the first sense it is aligned with disorders of consciousness, attention, and perception; as was pointed out in Chap. 50, confusion may represent one stage on the way to coma or emergence therefrom. *Delirium* also specifies a disorder of consciousness, perception, and attention, but always on the side of excessive alertness, sleeplessness, and frenzied excitement. Mental activity may be interrupted by the abrupt intrusion of hallucinations, which are frequent. We believe that confusion and delirium represent essentially different types of cerebral disorder. In many textbooks of psychiatry, however, confusion and delirium are grouped together and called toxic-exhaustive psychosis or "organic reaction type," indicating their postulated cause and pathologic basis. Confusion as an impairment of thinking, on the other hand, is related to derangements of intellect, i.e., dementia.

The term *amnesia* means loss of the ability to form memories despite an alert state of mind. It presupposes an ability to grasp the problem, to use language normally, and to maintain adequate motivation. The failure is mainly one of retention, recall, and reproduction, and it should be distinguished from that which attends drowsiness and confusion, where the learned material seems never to have been adequately assimilated. *Dementia* means loss of reason or, more particularly, a deterioration of intellect. Implied in the word is the idea of a general enfeeblement of mental powers in a person who formerly possessed a normal mind. *Amentia* by contrast indicates a *congenital* feeblemindedness.

OBSERVABLE ASPECTS OF BEHAVIOR AND THEIR RELATION TO CONFUSION, DELIRIUM, AMNESIA, AND DEMENTIA

In the strict sense the intellectual, emotional, volitional, and behavioral activities of the human organism are so complex and varied that one may question the possibility of using derangements of them as reliable guides to cerebral disease. Certainly they have not the same reliability and ease of anatomic and physiologic interpretation as sensory and motor paralysis or aphasia. Yet one observes certain of these higher cerebral disturbances recurring with such regularity in certain diseases as to be useful in clinical medicine; and some of them gain in specificity because they are often combined in certain ways to form syndromes, which are essentially what states of confusion, delirium, amnesia, and dementia are. Of course, we do not always know the value of certain elements of these syndromes, i.e., which are of primary or secondary importance.

The components of mentation and behavior that lend themselves to bedside examination are (1) the processes of sensation and perception; (2) the capacity for memorizing; (3) the ability to think, reason, and form logical conclusions; (4) temperament, mood, and emotion; (5) initiative, impulse, and drive; (6) insight. Of these (1), (2), and (3) may be grouped as cognitive, (4) as affective, and (5) as conative or volitional. Insight includes essentially all introspective observations made by the patient concerning his own normal or disordered functioning. Each component of behavior and intellection has its objective side, expressed in the manifest effects of certain stimulus conditions on the patient and his behavioral responses, and its subjective side, expressed in what the patient says he thinks and feels.

Disturbances of Perception

Perception, i.e., the processes involved in acquiring through the senses a knowledge of the "world about" or of one's own body, undergoes certain predictable types of derangements in disease. Most often there is quantitative reduction in the number of perceptions in a given unit of time and failure properly to synthesize them and relate them to the ongoing activities of the mind. One must appreciate that the perception of an object or person involves many things, aside from the simple sensory process of being aware of the attributes of a stimulus; it includes the selective focusing and maintaining of attention, elimination of all other extraneous stimuli, and recognition of the stimulus by knowing its relationship to past personal remembered experience. Perceptual disturbances are manifested in inattentiveness, fluctuations of attention, distractibility (pertinent and irrelevant stimuli having acquired equal value), inability to persist in an assigned task, and in the reporting and reacting to only a small part of a complex of stimuli. Qualitative changes also appear, mainly in the form of misinterpretation and misidentification of objects and persons; and these, at least in part, form the basis of hallucinatory experience in which the patient reports and reacts to stimuli not present in his environment. The loss of ability to perceive simultaneously all elements of a large complex of stimuli is sometimes explained as a "failure of subjective reorganization." Major disturbances in the perceptual sphere, sometimes called "clouding of the sensorium," occur most often in confusional states and deliriums, but quantitative deficiency may become evident in the advanced stages of amentia and dementia.

Disturbances of Memory

Memory, i.e., the retention of learned experiences, is involved in all mental activities. It may be arbitrarily subdivided into several parts, namely, (1) *registration*, which includes all that was mentioned under perception; (2) *mnemonic integration*, and *retention*; (3) *recall*; and (4) *reproduction*. As was stated above, in disturbances of perception and attention there may be a complete failure of learning and memory for the reason that the material to be learned was never assimilated. In Korsakoff's amnestic syndrome newly presented material appears to be temporarily registered but cannot be retained for more than a few minutes, and there is nearly always an associated defect in the recall and reproduction of memories formed before the onset of the illness (retrograde amnesia). Dislocation of events in time and the fabrication of stories, called *confabulation,* constitutes a third feature of the syndrome. Sound retention with failure of recall is at times a normal state; but when it is severe and extends to all events over a given period of time, it is usually due to hysteria or malingering. Proof that the processes of registration and recall are intact under these circumstances comes from hypnosis and suggestion, by means of which the lost items are fully recalled and reproduced. In Korsakoff's amnestic state the patient fails on all tests of learning and recent memory and his behavior accords with his deficiencies of information. Since memory is involved to some extent in all mental processes, it becomes the most testable component of mentation and behavior.

Disturbances of Thinking

Thinking, which is central to so many important intellectual activities, remains one of the most elusive of all mental operations. If by thinking we mean problem solving and capacity to reason and form sound judgments (the usual definition), obviously the working units of most complex experiences of this type are words and numbers. The activity of substituting word and number symbols for the objects for which they stand (symbolization) is a fundamental part of the process. These symbols are formed into ideas, and the arrangement of new and remembered ideas into certain orders or relationships, according to the rules of logic, constitute another intricate part of thought, presently beyond the scope of analysis. In a general way one may examine thinking for ideational content, the coherence and logical relationships of ideas, the quantity and quality of associations to a given idea, and the propriety of the feeling and behavior engendered by an idea.

Information concerning the thought processes and associative functions is best obtained by analyzing the patient's spontaneous verbal productions and by engaging him in conversation. If he is taciturn or mute, one may then have to depend on his responses to direct questions or upon written material, i.e., letters, etc. One notes the prevailing trends of the patient's thoughts, whether his ideas are reasonable or precise and coherent or vague, circumstantial, tangential, and irrelevant, and whether his thought processes are shallow and completely fragmented. Disorders of thought are frequent in degenerative and other types of cerebral disease. The patient may be excessively critical, rationalizing, and hairsplitting; this is a type of thinking often manifest in depressive psychoses. Derangements of thinking may also take the form of a virtual flight of ideas. The patient moves nimbly from one idea to another, and his associations are numerous and haphazard. This is a common feature in hypomanic or manic states. The opposite condition, poverty of ideas (the more frequent condition), is characteristic both of depression, where it is combined with gloomy thoughts, and of dementing diseases, where it is part of a general reduction in all intellectual activity. Thinking may be distorted in such a way that the patient fails to check his ideas against reality. When a false belief is maintained in spite of normally convincing contradictory evidence, the patient is said to have a *delusion.* Delusion is common to many illnesses, particularly manic-depressive and schizophrenic states. Ideas may seem to have been implanted in the patient's mind by some outside agency such as radio, television, or atomic energy. These reflect the passive feelings characteristic of manic-depressive and schizophrenic psychoses. Other distortions of logical thought such as gaps or condensations of logical associations are typical of schizophrenia, of which they constitute a diagnostic feature.

Disturbances of Emotion, Mood, and Affect

The emotional life of the patient is expressed in a variety of ways, and there are several points to be made about it. In the first place, rather marked individual differences in basic temperament are to be observed in the normal population; some persons are throughout their life cheerful, gregarious, optimistic, and free from worry, whereas others are just the opposite. In fact, the unusually volatile, cyclothymic person is believed to be liable to manic-depressive psychosis and the suspicious, withdrawn, introverted person to schizophrenia and paranoia. Strong, persistent emotional states such as fear and anxiety may occur as reaction to life situations and may be accompanied by derangements of visceral function. If excessive and disproportionate to the stimulus, they have medical significance; they are usually manifestations of anxiety, neurosis, or depression. Variations in the degree of responsiveness to emotional stimuli are also frequent and, when excessive and persistent, are important. In depression all stimuli tend to enhance the somber mood of unhappiness. Emotional response that is excessively labile, variable from moment to moment, and poorly controlled or uninhibited is a condition common to many diseases of the cerebrum, particularly those involving the corticopontine and corticobulbar pathways. It may constitute a part of the syndrome of pseudobulbar palsy. All emotional expression may be lacking, as in apathetic states or severe depressions. Or the patient may be a victim of every trivial problem in daily life; i.e., he cannot control his worries. Finally, the emotional response may be inappropriate to the stimulus, e.g., a depressing thought is attended by a smile, as in schizophrenia.

Since there are relatively few overt manifestations of temperament, mood, and other emotional experiences described above, the physician must evaluate these states by the appearance of the patient and by verbalized accounts of his feelings. For these purposes it is convenient to divide emotionality into mood and feeling or affect. By *mood* is meant the prevailing emotional state of the individual without reference to the stimuli impinging upon him, i.e., his immediate environmental circumstances. It may be pleasant and cheerful or melancholic. The language, e.g., the adjectives used, and the facial expressions, attitudes, and postures, and speed of movement most reliably betray the patient's mood.

By contrast, *feelings* or *affects* are emotional experiences evoked by environmental stimuli. According to some psychiatrists, feeling is the subjective component and affect the overt manifestation. Others apply either word to the subjective state. The difference between mood as a prevailing emotional state and feeling and affect as emotional reactions to stimuli may seem rather tenuous, but these distinctions are considered valuable by psychiatrists.

Impulse, that basic biologic urge, driving force, or purpose, by which every organism is directed to reach its full potentialities, appears to be another extremely important and observable but neglected dimension of behavior. Again, one notes wide normal variations from one person to another in strength of impulse to action and thought, and these individual differences are present throughout life. One of the most conspicuous pathologic deviations is an apparent constitutional weakness in impulse in certain neurotic individuals. Moreover, with many types of cerebral disease, particularly those which involve the posterior orbital parts of the frontal lobes, a reduction in impulse is coupled with an indifference or lack of concern about the consequences of actions. In such cases all other measurable aspects of psychic function may be normal. Extreme degrees of lack of impulse, or *abulia,* take the form of mutism and immobility, called *akinetic mutism.* Psychomotor retardation is a lesser degree of the same state and is also a feature of depression, in which instance mood alteration and extreme fatigability are conjoined, or of cerebral disease.

Lastly, *insight,* the state of being fully aware of the nature and degree of one's deficits, becomes manifestly impaired or abolished in relation to all types of cerebral disease that cause disorders of behavior. Rarely does the patient himself with any of the aforementioned states seek advice or help for his illness. Instead, his family usually brings him to the physician. Thus, it appears that the diseases which produce all these abnormalities not only evoke observable changes in behavior but also alter or reduce the capacity of the patient to make accurate introspections of his own psychic function. This fact stands as one of the most incontrovertible proofs that the cerebrum is the organ both of behavior and of all inner psychic experiences; that is to say, behavior and mind are but two inseparable aspects of the function of the nervous system.

COMMON SYNDROMES

This entire group of confusional states is characterized principally by clouding of consciousness with prominent disorders of attention and perception that interfere with clarity of thinking and the formation of memories. One syndrome, here called *delirium,* includes overactivity, sleeplessness, tremulousness, and hallucinations. Convulsions often precede the delirium. In a second syndrome, here called *primary mental confusion,* drowsiness, reduced awareness and responsiveness are the principal abnormalities. All these illnesses tend to develop acutely, to have multiple causes, and to terminate within a relatively short period of time (days to weeks) leaving the patient without residual damage. These two syndromes will be described separately.

Delirium

CLINICAL FEATURES. These are most perfectly depicted in the alcoholic patient. The symptoms usually develop over a period of 2 or 3 days. The first indications of the approaching attack are restless irritability, tremulousness, insomnia, and poor appetite. One or several generalized convulsions are the initial major symptom in 30 per cent of the cases. The patient's rest becomes troubled by unpleasant and terrifying dreams. There may be momentary disorientation or an occasional irrational remark. These initial symptoms rapidly give way to a clinical picture that, in severe cases, is one of the most colorful and dramatic in medicine. The patient talks incessantly and incoherently and looks distressed or perplexed; his expression is in keeping with his vague notions of being pursued by someone who seeks to injure him. From his manner and from the content of his speech it is evident that he misinterprets the meaning of ordinary objects and sounds around him and has vivid visual, auditory, and tactile hallucinations, often of a most unpleasant type. At first he can be brought momentarily into touch with reality and may in fact answer questions correctly; but almost at once he relapses into his preoccupied, confused state. Before long he is unable to shake off his hallucinations even for a second and does not recognize his family or his physician. Tremor and restless movements are usually present and may be violent. The countenance is flushed, and the conjunctivas are injected; the pulse is rapid and soft, and the temperature may be raised. There is much sweating, and the urine is scanty and of high specific gravity. The symptoms abate, either suddenly or gradually, after 2 or 3 days, although in exceptional cases they may persist for several weeks. The most certain indication of the end of the attack is the occurrence of sound sleep and of lucid intervals of increasing length. Recovery is usually complete.

Delirium is subject to all degrees of variability, not only from patient to patient but in the same patient from day to day and hour to hour. The entire syndrome may be observed in one patient and only one or two symptoms in another. In its mildest form, as so often occurs in febrile diseases, it consists of an occasional wandering of the mind and incoherence of expression interrupted by periods of lucidity. This form, shorn of motor and autonomic overactivity, is sometimes referred to as a *quiet delirium* and is difficult to distinguish from other confusional states. The more severe form, sometimes called *active delirium* and best exemplified by delirium tremens, is characterized by a great excess of motor activity and marked confusion, which may progress to a "muttering stupor" and which in about 10 per cent of patients ends fatally.

MORBID ANATOMY AND PATHOPHYSIOLOGY. The brains of patients who have died in delirium tremens usually show no pathologic changes of significance. A number of diseases, however, may cause delirium and also give rise to focal lesions in the brain, such as focal embolic encephalitis, viral encephalitis, Wernicke's disease, or trauma. The topography of these lesions is of particular interest. They tend to be localized in certain parts of the brain, particularly in the midbrain and subthalamus and in the temporal lobes.

Penfield's studies of the human cortex during surgical exploration clearly indicate the importance of the temporal lobe in producing visual, auditory, and olfactory hallucinations. With subthalamic and midbrain lesions, there may occur visual hallucinations of a pleasurable type accompanied by good insight, namely, the peduncular hallucinosis of Lhermitte.

The electroencephalogram in delirium shows nonfocal slow activity in the 5 to 7 per sec range, a state that rapidly returns to normal as the delirium clears. However, in other cases only activity in the fast beta frequency is seen, and in milder degrees of delirium there is usually no abnormality at all.

An analysis of the several conditions conducive to delirium suggests at least two different physiologic mechanisms. In alcoholism and barbiturate intoxication the clinical manifestations appear after the withdrawal of drugs known to have a strong inhibitory effect on the central nervous system. In the case of bacterial infections and poisoning by certain drugs, such as atropine and scopolamine, the delirious state probably results from the direct action of the toxin or chemical.

Psychophysiologic mechanisms have also been postulated. It has long been suggested that some individuals are much more liable to delirium than others. There is much reason to doubt this hypothesis, for it has been shown that all of a group of randomly selected persons would develop delirium if the causative mechanisms were strongly operative. This is to be expected, for any healthy person under certain circumstances may experience phenomena akin to those found in delirium. Thus after repeated auditory and visual stimulation the same impressions may continue to be perceived even though the stimuli are no longer present. Moreover, it has been shown that a healthy individual can be induced to hallucinate by placing him in an environment as free as possible of sensory stimulation. A relation between delirium and dream states has been postulated because in both there is a loss of appreciation of time, a richness of visual imagery, and indifference to inconsistencies. Moreover, patients may refer to some of these delirious symptoms as a "bad dream"; and normal persons may hallucinate in the so-called "hypnagogic state," the short period between sleeping and waking. In general, however, formulations in the field of dynamic psychology seem more reasonably to account for the topical content of delirium than to explain its occurrence. Wolff and Curran, having observed the same content in repeated attacks of delirium due to different causes, concluded that the content depends more on age, sex, intellectual endowment, occupation, personality traits, and past experience of the patient than on the cause or mechanism of the delirium.

The main difficulty in understanding delirium arises from the fact that it has not been possible from clinical studies to ascertain which of the many symptoms have physiologic significance. What is the basis of this lack of harmony between actual sensory impressions of the present and memory of those in the past? Obviously, there is something missing from total behavior, something that leaves the patient at the mercy of certain sensory stimuli and unable to attend to others, yet at the same time incapable of discriminating between sense impression and fantasy. There appears to be some lack of inhibition of sensory processes, which may also be the basis of the sleep disturbance (insomnia) and the convulsive tendency.

Confusional States Associated with Reduced Mental Alertness and Responsiveness (Primary Mental Confusion)

CLINICAL FEATURES. In the most typical examples of this syndrome all mental functions are reduced to some degree, but alertness, attentiveness, and the ability to grasp all elements of the immediate situation suffer most. In its mildest form the patient may pass for normal, and only failure to recollect and reproduce happenings of the past few hours or days reveals the inadequacy of mental function. The more obviously confused patient spends much of his time in idleness, but what he does do may be inappropriate and annoying to others. Only the more automatic acts and verbal responses are properly performed, but these may permit the examiner to obtain from the patient a number of relevant and accurate replies to questions about age, occupation, and residence. Reactions are slow and indecisive, and it is difficult for the patient to sustain a conversation. He may doze during the interview and is observed to sleep more hours each day than is natural. Responses tend to be rather abrupt, brief, and mechanical. Perceptual difficulties are frequent, and voices, common objects, and the actions of other persons are frequently misinterpreted. Often one cannot discern whether the patient hears voices and sees things that do not exist, i.e., whether he is actively hallucinating, or is merely misinterpreting stimuli in the environment. Inadequate perception and forgetfulness results in a constant state of bewilderment. Failing to recognize his surroundings and having lost all sense of time, he repeats the same questions and makes the same remarks over and over again.

As the confusion deepens, conversation becomes

more difficult, and at a certain stage the patient no longer notices or responds to much of what is going on around him. Replies to questions may be a single word or a short phrase spoken in a soft tremulous voice or whisper. The patient may be mute. Irritability may or may not be present. Some patients are extremely suspicious; in fact, a paranoid trend may be the most pronounced and troublesome feature of the illness.

In its most advanced stages confusion gives way to stupor and finally to coma. As the patient improves, he may pass again through the stage of stupor and confusion in the reverse order. All this informs us that at least this category of confusion is but a manifestation of the same disease processes that in their severest form cause coma.

In some instances the mental aberration never exceeds that of confusion with stupor; in others, with more than the usual degree of irritability and restlessness, one cannot fail to notice the striking resemblance to delirium. In both there is a clouding of consciousness, impairment of attention, slowness, and disordered perception and association of ideas. Indeed, if the delirious state were shorn of its tremor, vivid hallucinations, vigilant excited attitude, insomnia, and the low convulsive threshold, the differentiation would be impossible. Actually typical cases showing one or the other of these two syndromes are easily distinguished, but it must also be admitted that in numerous patients with an acute confusional state the differentiation is impossible.

MORBID ANATOMY AND PATHOPHYSIOLOGY. All that has been said on this subject in Chap. 50 is applicable to at least one subgroup of the confusional states. In the others no consistent pathologic change has been found. The electroencephalogram is of interest because it is almost invariably abnormal in more severe forms of this syndrome, in contrast to delirium, where the changes are relatively minor. High-voltage slow waves in the 2 to 3 per sec (delta) range or the 5 to 7 per sec (theta) range are the usual finding.

Senile and Other Dementing Brain Diseases Complicated by Medical Diseases (Beclouded Dementia)

Many elderly patients who enter the hospital with medical or surgical illness are mentally confused. Presumably the liability to this state is determined by preexisting brain disease, in this instance senile dementia, which may or may not have been obvious to the family before the onset of the complicating illness.

All the clinical features of confusion described in the previous sections may be present. The severity may vary greatly. The confusion may be reflected only in the patient's inability to relate sequentially the history of his illness, or it may be so severe that he is virtually *non compos mentis*.

Although almost any complicating illness may bring

out this confusion, it is particularly frequent with infectious disease, especially in those cases which resist the effects of antibiotic medication; with post-traumatic and postoperative states, notably after concussive brain injuries and removal of cataracts (in which case the confusion is probably related to being temporarily deprived of vision); with congestive heart failure, chronic respiratory disease, and severe anemia, especially pernicious anemia. Often it is difficult to determine which of several possible factors is responsible for the confusion in this heterogeneous group of illnesses. There may be more than one factor. A cardiac patient with a confusional psychosis may be febrile, have marginally reduced cerebral blood flow, be intoxicated by one or more drugs, or be in electrolyte imbalance. The same is true of postoperative confusional states, where a number of factors such as fever, infection, dehydration, and drug intoxication may be incriminated. The presence of alcoholism may further complicate the matter.

When he recovers from the medical or surgical illness, the patient usually returns to his premorbid state, though his shortcomings, now drawn to the attention of the family and physician, may be more obvious than before.

Coincidental Development of Schizophrenia or Manic-depressive Psychosis during a Medical or Surgical Illness

A certain proportion of psychoses of the schizophrenic or manic-depressive type first become manifest during an acute medical illness or following an operation or parturition. A causal relationship between the two is usually sought but cannot be established. Usually the psychosis began long before but was not recognized. The diagnosis of the psychiatric illness must proceed along the lines suggested in Chaps. 215 and 216. Close observation will usually reveal a clear sensorium and relatively intact memory, which permits differentiation from the acute confusional states.

KORSAKOFF'S AMNESTIC SYNDROMES AND THE RESIDUAL MENTAL STATES FOLLOWING DELIRIUM AND CONFUSION

The majority of patients suffering from delirium and confusion recover completely after a few days or weeks. Afterward one can detect no evidence of damage to the nervous system. In contrast, in cases of beclouded dementia, as the sensorial disturbance subsides, the patient is left with the same mental weakness that existed before the onset of the confusional state. Sometimes the dementia seems more pronounced afterward, and the family will later remark that the patient's mind failed at the time of the acute illness. However, one has the impression that they merely became aware of the insidiously developing dementia at this time.

There is another group of cases, by no means small or insignificant, in which the acutely delirious or confused patient is left with a severe deficit. The inattentiveness, hallucinations, and sleep disorder disappear. The patient is alert, easily engaged in conversation, and quite proper in his general deportment. Nevertheless, he is incompetent to look after himself. A careful evaluation of his mental status will reveal a severe memory deficit of the type found in Korsakoff's psychosis. The distinguishing feature of this latter illness is not memory loss alone but the disproportionate affection of memory in relation to the patient's alertness and the integrity of other faculties. It is further characterized by the inability to learn new facts and, in its early stages, by confabulation. This state, once fully developed, may be permanent, though often there is some improvement in learning capacity and memory as the months pass. It represents a special type of dementia.

The clinical features of Korsakoff's psychosis are presented in detail in Chap. 210. Although frequently observed in patients who suffer from alcoholism and malnutrition, the same clinical picture may occur with other diseases, such as ruptured saccular aneurysm and subarachnoid hemorrhage, tuberculous meningitis, and tumors in the walls of the third ventricle.

Since the confusional states may accompany many types of cerebral disease, other residual states may occur, as would be expected. The author has several times seen severe and permanent dementia after acute inclusion-body encephalitis. Extreme hyperpyrexia may leave a patient mentally altered with cerebellar ataxia and pyramidal tract signs.

Classification of the Acute Confusional States and Korsakoff's Amnestic Syndrome

The syndrome itself and its main clinical relationships are the only satisfactory basis for classification until such time as the actual cause and pathophysiology are discovered. The tendency in the past to subdivide the syndromes according to their most prominent symptom or degree of severity, e.g., "picking delirium," "microptic delirium," "acute delirious mania," "muttering delirium," has no fundamental value.

I. Delirium
  A. In a medical or surgical illness (no focal or lateralizing neurologic signs; cerebrospinal fluid usually clear)
    1. Typhoid fever
    2. Pneumonia
    3. Septicemia, particularly erysipelas and other streptococcal infections
    4. Rheumatic fever
    5. Thyrotoxicosis and ACTH intoxication (rare)
    6. Postoperative and posttraumatic states
  B. In neurologic disease that causes focal or lateralizing signs or changes in the cerebrospinal fluid
    1. Vascular, neoplastic, or other diseases, particularly those involving the temporal lobes and upper brain stem
    2. Cerebral contusion and laceration (traumatic delirium)
    3. Acute purulent and tuberculous meningitis
    4. Subarachnoid hemorrhage
    5. Encephalitis due to viral causes and to unknown causes, e.g., infectious mononucleosis
  C. The abstinence states (after drug intoxications), postconvulsive states, or intoxications; signs of other medical, surgical, and neurologic illnesses absent or coincidental
    1. Delirium tremens and chronic barbiturate intoxication
    2. Drug intoxications: camphor, caffeine, ergot, bromides, scopolamine, atropine, amphetamine
    3. Postconvulsive delirium
II. Confusion associated with psychomotor underactivity
  A. Associated with a medical or surgical disease (no focal or lateralizing neurologic signs; cerebrospinal fluid clear)
    1. Metabolic disorders: hepatic stupor, uremia, hypoxia, hypercapnia, hypoglycemia, porphyria
    2. Infective fevers, especially typhoid
    3. Congestive heart failure
    4. Postoperative, posttraumatic, and puerperal psychoses
  B. Associated with drug intoxication (no focal or lateralizing signs; cerebrospinal fluid clear): opiates, barbiturates, bromides, Artane, etc.
  C. Associated with diseases of the nervous system (the focal or lateralizing neurologic signs and cerebrospinal fluid changes of this condition are commoner than in delirium)
    1. Cerebral vascular disease, tumor, abscess
    2. Subdural hematoma
    3. Meningitis
    4. Encephalitis
    5. Preexisting neurologic disease (e.g., senile dementia) complicated by a medical or surgical disease
  D. Beclouded dementia, i.e., senile brain disease in combination with infective fevers, drug reactions, heart failure, etc.
III. Korsakoff's amnestic syndrome
  A. Deficiency of thiamine
    1. Alcoholic disorders with peculiar dietary habits, gastrointestinal diseases, etc.
  B. Subarachnoid hemorrhage from ruptured aneurysms
  C. Tumors and infective granulomas in walls of the third ventricle

THE CLINICAL SYNDROME OF DEMENTIA

In current neurologic parlance the term *dementia* usually denotes a clinical state comprised of failing memory and loss of intellectual functions due to chronic progressive degenerative disease of the brain.

It may or may not be associated with signs of disease in one or more of the so-called "projection areas" of the cerebrum. The chronicity of the process is ordinarily emphasized, but the illogic of setting apart any one constellation of cerebral symptoms on the basis of their speed of onset or duration is obvious.

The earliest signs of dementia may be so subtle as to escape the notice of even the most discerning physician. Often an observant relative of the patient or an employer is the first to become aware of a certain lack of initiative, of irritability, of loss of interest, and of inability to perform up to the usual standard. Later there is distractibility, inability to think with accustomed clarity, reduced general comprehension, perseveration in speech, action, and thought, and defective memory, especially for recent events. Frequently a change in mood becomes apparent, deviating more often toward depression than elation. The direction of this deviation is said to depend on the previous personality of the patient rather than upon the character of the disease. Excessive lability of mood may also be observed, i.e., an easy fluctuation from laughter to tears on slight provocation. Moral and ethical standards are lost, early in some cases and late in others. Paranoid ideas and delusions may develop. As a rule, the patient has little or no realization of these changes in himself; he lacks insight. As the condition progresses, there is loss of almost all intellectual faculties, with mental retardation and extreme incoherence and irrationality. Mutism, unresponsiveness, dysarthria, aphasia, and sphincteric incontinence may be added to the clinical picture. In a late state a secondary physical deterioration also takes place. Food intake, which may be increased in the beginning of the illness, is in the end usually limited, with resulting emaciation. Finally the patient remains in bed most of the time and dies of pneumonia or some other intercurrent infection. This whole process may evolve over a period of months or years.

Many of these alterations of behavior are the direct result of disease of the nervous system; expressed in another way, the symptoms are the primary manifestations of neurologic disease. others are secondary; they are reactions to the catastrophe of losing one's mind. For example, the dement is said to seek solitude to hide his affliction and may thus appear asocial or apathetic. Again, excessive orderliness may be an attempt to compensate for failing memory; apprehension, gloom, or irritability may express general dissatisfaction with a necessarily restricted life. Even in a state of fairly advanced deterioration the patient is still capable of reacting to his illness and to the individuals who care for him.

Attempts to relate loss of memory and failing intellectual function to lesions in certain parts of the brain have been eminently unsuccessful. Two types of difficulty have obstructed progress in this field. (1) There is the problem of defining, analyzing, and determining the significance of the so-called "intellectual" functions. (2) The morbid anatomy of these diseases is so complex that it cannot be fully defined and quantitated.

In the most careful analyses of the intellectual functions, certain general and certain specific factors have been isolated. The general factors are not localized at the moment to any one area of the brain, whereas the specific ones do have at least a regional localization in the cerebrum. Spearman, Thurstone, and others have been able to single out a number of specific factors such as verbal capacity, ability to appreciate spatial relationships, ability to learn and to reason inductively and deductively, facility in the use of numbers and in numerical calculation, and retentive memory. All these qualities are tested in standard intelligence and achievement tests. Memory correlates poorly with all the other factors and seems to be an independent item. There is an intercorrelation between all the other factors. In other words, a person who performs well in tests of verbal capacity tends to do well on tests of spatial orientation, numerical relationships, learning, and reasoning tests. Some general factor, ?G factor of Spearman, is being measured by each test and determines in part the level of performance. In addition, there are special aptitudes or factors, S. factors of Spearman, that account for individual superiorities or (in disease) inferiorities in one or another test.

In dementia the memory impairment that is a constant feature may occur with extensive disease in any part of the cerebrum. Yet it is interesting to note that the function of certain parts of the diencephalon and of the hippocampi may be more fundamental to retentive memory than integrity of the cortex, and, as will be pointed out below, it may be the cortico-thalamic connections that are particularly concerned with this function. Failure in tests of verbal function (the most advanced degree is aphasia) is closely associated with disease of the dominant cerebral hemisphere, and particularly the speech areas in the frontal, temporal, and parietal lobes and insula. Loss of capacity for arithmetic, reading, and numerical calculation (acalculia) is related to lesions in the posterior part of the left (dominant) cerebral hemisphere. Impairment in drawing or constructing simple and complex figures with blocks, sticks, picture arrangement, etc., as shown by tests of visual construction, is most pronounced in right (nondominant) parietal lobe lesions, as will be pointed out below. Thus, the clinical picture resulting from cerebral disease depends in part on the extent of the lesion, i.e., the amount of cerebral tissue destroyed, and on the specific locality of the lesion.

Morbid Anatomy and Pathologic Physiology of Dementia

Dementia is related usually to obvious structural disease of the cerebrum and the diencephalon. Knowledge of the detailed anatomy of the diencephalic nuclei and their connections with one another and with the various parts of the cerebral cortex is so limited that it has thus far been impossible to define either the topography of many of the diseases with which we are concerned or the nature of the lesion. In some diseases, such as Alzheimer's and Pick's presenile or senile dementia, the main process appears to be a degeneration of nerve cells in the association areas, with secondary changes in the cerebral white matter. In others, such as Huntington's chorea, Jakob-Creutzfeldt pseudosclerosis, and the cerebrocerebellar degenerations, loss of neurones in the cerebral cortex is accompanied by a similar degeneration of neurones in the putamen and caudate nuclei, and the cerebellum, respectively. Arteriosclerotic vascular disease results in multiple foci of infarction all through the thalami, basal ganglions, brain stem, and cerebrum and, in the latter, in the motor, sensory, or visual projection areas as well as in the association areas. Severe trauma may cause contusions of cerebral convolutions and degeneration of the central white matter (Strich), with the resulting protracted stupor or dementia (rare). Most diseases that produce dementia are quite extensive, and the frontal lobes are affected more often than other parts of the cerebrum.

Other mechanisms than the destruction of brain tissue may operate in some cases. Chronic increased intracranial pressure or chronic hydrocephalus (with large ventricles the pressure may not exceed 180 mm), regardless of cause, is often associated with a general impairment of mental function. The compression of one or both cerebral hemispheres by chronic subdural hematomas may cause a widespread disturbance of cortical function. A diffuse inflammatory process is at least in part the basis for dementia in syphilis and in neurotropic virus infections. Lastly, several of the toxic and metabolic diseases discussed in Chap. 50 may interfere with nervous function over a long period of time and create a clinical picture similar to, if not identical with, that of dementia.

Bedside Classification of Dementing Diseases of the Brain

The conventional classification of dementing diseases of the brain is usually according to etiology, if known, or pathology. Another more practical approach, which follows logically from the method by which the whole subject has been presented in this book, is to subdivide the diseases into three categories on the basis of the associated clinical and laboratory signs of medical disease and the accompanying neurologic signs. Once the physician has determined that the patient suffers a dementing illness, he must then decide, from the medical, neurologic, and laboratory data, into which category the case fits. This classification may at first seem somewhat artificial. However, it is likely to be more useful to the student or physician not conversant with the many diseases that cause dementia than a classification based on pathology.

CLASSIFICATION

I. Diseases in which dementia is usually associated with other clinical and laboratory signs of medical disease
  A. Hypothyroidism
  B. Cushing's disease
  C. Nutritional deficiency states such as pellagra, Wernicke's disease and Korsakoff's syndrome, pernicious anemia, and subacute degeneration of spinal cord and brain
  D. Neurosyphilis: general paresis and meningovascular syphilis
  E. Hepatolenticular degeneration
  F. Cerebral arteriosclerosis
  G. Bromidism

II. Diseases in which dementia is associated with other neurologic signs but not with other obvious medical disease
  A. Invariably associated with other neurologic signs
    1. Huntington's chorea
    2. Schilder's disease and related demyelinative diseases
    3. Amaurotic family idiocy and other lipid-storage diseases
    4. Myoclonic epilepsy
    5. Jakob-Creutzfeldt disease
    6. Cerebrocerebellar degeneration
    7. Dementia with spastic paraplegia
  B. Often associated with other neurologic signs
    1. Cerebral arteriosclerosis
    2. Brain tumor
    3. Brain trauma, such as cerebral contusion, midbrain hemorrhage, chronic subdural hematoma

III. Diseases in which dementia is usually the only evidence of neurologic or medical disease
  A. Alzheimer's disease and senile dementia
  B. Pick's disease
  C. Marchiafava-Bignami disease (sometimes with frontal lobe signs)
  D. Some cases of brain tumor of frontal lobes and corpus callosum

Many of these diseases are discussed more fully in other sections of this book. The special features of the dementia that accompanies arteriosclerotic, senile, syphilitic, traumatic, nutritional, and degenerative diseases are discussed in the appropriate chapters.

Differential Diagnosis

The first difficulty in dealing with this class of patients is to make sure of deterioration of intellect and personality change. It may be necessary to examine the patient several times before one is confident of the clinical findings.

There is always a tendency to assume that mental function is normal if patients complain only of nervousness, fatigue, insomnia, or vague somatic symptoms and to label the patients psychoneurotic. *This will be avoided if one keeps in mind that psychoneuroses rarely begin in middle or late adult life.* A practical rule is to assume that all mental illnesses beginning during this period are due either to structural disease of the brain or to depressive psychosis.

A mild dysphasia must not be mistaken for dementia. The aphasic patient appears uncertain of himself, and his speech may be incoherent. Furthermore, he may be anxious and depressed over his ineptitude. Careful attention to the patient's language performance will lead to the correct diagnosis in most instances. Further observation will disclose the fact that the patient's behavior, except for speech, is within normal limits.

The depressed patient presents another type of problem. He may remark that his mental function is poor or that he is forgetful and cannot concentrate. Scrutiny of his remarks will show, however, that he actually remembers all the details of his illness and that no qualitative change in mental ability has taken place. His difficulty is either lack of energy and interest or anxiety that prevents the focusing of attention on anything except his own problems. Even during mental tests his performance may be impaired by his emotions, in much the same way as that of the worried student during his examinations. This condition of emotional blocking is called *experimental confusion*. When the patient is calmed by reassurance, his mental function is normal, a proof that intellectual deterioration has not occurred. The hypomanic patient fails in tests of intellectual function because of his restlessness and distractibility. It is helpful to remember that the demented patient rarely has sufficient insight to complain of mental deterioration; and if he admits to poor memory, he seldom realizes the degree of his disability. The physician must never rely on the patient's statements as to the efficiency of mental function and must always evaluate a poor performance on tests in the light of the emotional state and the motivation at the time the test is given.

The neurologic syndrome associated with metabolic or endocrine disorders, i.e., ACTH therapy, hyperthyroidism, Cushing's disease, Addison's disease, or the post-partum state, may be difficult to diagnose because of the wide variety of clinical pictures that may be shown. As will be stated in Chap. 216, some patients appear to be suffering from a dementia, others from an acute confusional psychosis; or if mood change or negativism predominates, a manic-depressive psychosis or schizophrenia is suggested. In these conditions some degree of clouding of sensorium and impairment of intellectual function can usually be recognized, and these findings alone should be enough to exclude schizophrenia and manic-depressive psychosis. It is well to remember that acute onset of mental symptoms always suggests confusional psychosis or delirium. Inasmuch as many of these conditions are completely reversible, they must be distinguished from dementia.

Once it is decided that the patient suffers from a dementing disease, the next step is to determine by careful physical examination whether there are signs of a medical or focal neurologic disease. This enables the physician to place the case in one of the three categories in the bedside classification. X-rays of skull, electroencephalogram, and lumbar puncture should be carried out in most cases. Usually these procedures necessitate admission to a hospital. The final step is to determine by the total clinical picture which disease within any one category the patient has. Table 216-2 (p. 1291) shows the major points in differential diagnosis.

SPECIAL SYNDROMES CAUSED BY DISEASES OF PARTS OF THE CEREBRUM

Symptoms and signs of disease of one part of the cerebrum may occur singly or in combination with dementia, and they provide important information about the location of a disease process and at times about its nature. This is an appropriate place, therefore, to review briefly the known effects of disease of different parts of the cerebrum. Agnosia, apraxia, and aphasia will be only mentioned, since they are treated more extensively in Chaps. 49 and 52.

FRONTAL LOBES. In Fig. 54-1, it may be seen that the frontal lobes lie anterior to the central, or Rolandic, sulcus and superior to the Sylvian fissure. They consist of several functionally different parts, which are conventionally designated in the neurologic literature by numbers (according to a scheme devised by Brodmann) and by letters (in the scheme of von Economo and Koskinas).

The posterior parts, areas 4 and 6 of Brodmann, are specifically related to motor function. Voluntary movement in man depends on the integrity of these areas, and lesions in them produce spastic paralysis of the contralateral face, arm, and leg. This is discussed in Chap. 45, Motor Paralysis. Lesions limited more or less to the premotor areas (area 6) are accompanied by prominent grasp and sucking reflexes. Lesions in areas 8 and 24 of Brodmann interfere with the mechanism concerned with turning the head and eyes contralaterally. Lesions in areas 44 and 45 abolish or reduce vocalization, deglutition, and chewing. Lesions in area 44 of the dominant cerebral hemisphere, usually the left one, have often resulted in loss of verbal expression, the aphasia of Broca. Lesions in the medial limbic or piriform cortex (areas 23 and 24), wherein lie the mechanisms controlling respiration, circulation, and micturition have relatively unclear clinical effects.

The remainder of the frontal lobes (areas 9, 10, 11, 12, and 13 of Brodmann), sometimes called the *prefrontal areas*, have less specific and measurable functions. The following groups of symptoms have been observed in patients with diseases limited to one or both frontal lobes or to the central white matter and anterior part of the corpus callosum by which they are joined.

1. Change of personality, usually expressed as lack of concern over the consequences of any action, which may take the form of a childish excitement (moria of Jastrowitz), an inappropriate joking and punning (*witzelsucht* of Oppenheim), or an instability and superficiality of emotion, or irritability.

2. Slight impairment of intelligence, usually described as lack of concentration, vacillation of attention, inability to carry out planned activity, difficulty in changing from one activity to another, loss of recent memory, or lack of initiative and spontaneity.

3. Motor abnormalities such as decomposition of gait and upright stance, trunk ataxia of Bruns, abnormal postures, reflex grasping or sucking, incontinence of sphincters, and akinetic mutism.

The most pronounced changes have been observed in cases with bilateral disease of frontal lobes, and there has been much doubt as to the effect of a lesion involving only one frontal lobe. Nevertheless, the most careful psychologic tests on patients with lesions of either frontal lobe demonstrate a slight elevation of mood with increased talkativeness and tendency to joke, a lack of tact, inability to adapt to a new situation, and loss of initiative.

Several careful studies of lobotomized patients have now been published. Of course, very few of these patients were normal before the operation, so that base-line measurements of mental ability were not always obtainable. However, some patients of normal intellect have received this treatment for severe neurosis or intractable pain. They are said to have shown little or no loss of ability in their performance on intelligence tests, depending on the extent of the procedure; and if worry, fears, compulsions, and suffering from pain were incapacitating, the loss of these traits resulted in test scores actually higher than before the operation. However, careful examination usually will disclose a slight lowering of general intelligence, a decrease in drive or energy, a definite change of personality in the form of shallow emotional life, a lack of tact, and inability to direct and sustain activity toward future goals. Also there is a diminution of traits related to neuroticism, such as suggestibility, rigidity of character, self-criticism, and introversion.

The function of the frontal lobes cannot be determined simply by the study of human beings who have suffered injury or disease of this part of the brain. Symptoms from lesions of a part of the nervous system are not identical with the functions of that part. The symptoms of frontal lobe deficit must depend both on a loss of certain parts of the cerebrum and on the functional activity of the remaining portions of the nervous system. There is no doubt that the human mind is changed by disease of the frontal lobes, but it is difficult to say in what way it is changed. Intelligence, emotional feeling and expression, memory, visual fixation, postural control, regulation of respiration and blood pressure—all are intact in animals and human beings without frontal lobes. Perhaps at present it is best to regard the frontal lobes as that part of the brain which orients the individual, with all his percepts and concepts formed from past life experiences, toward action that is projected into the future.

TEMPORAL LOBES. The boundaries of the temporal lobes may be seen in Fig. 54-1. The Sylvian fissure separates the superior surface of each temporal lobe from the frontal and anterior parts of the parietal lobes. There is no definite anatomic boundary between the temporal and occipital lobes either inferiorly or laterally or between temporal and parietal lobes. The temporal lobe includes the superior, middle, and inferior temporal, fusiform, and hippocampal convolutions and the transverse convolutions of Heschl, which is the auditory receptive area present on the superior surface within the Sylvian fissure. The hippocampal convolution was once believed to be related indirectly to the olfactory bulb, but now it is known that lesions here do not cause anosmia. The fibers from the homolateral lower quadrant of each retina course through the central white matter en route to the occipital lobes, and lesions that interrupt them characteristically produce a contralateral homonymous upper quadrant defect of visual fields. Hearing and labyrinthine function, also localized in the temporal lobes, are bilaterally represented, which accounts for the fact that unless both temporal lobes are affected, there is no demonstrable loss of hearing. Loss of equilibrium has not been observed with temporal lobe lesions. Extensive disease in the superior and middle convolutions of the left temporal lobe in right-handed individuals results in Wernicke's aphasia. This syndrome, discussed in Chap. 53, Affections of Speech, consists of jargon aphasia and inability to read, to write, or to understand the meaning of spoken words. Probably the basic defect in all these is the loss of memory for words.

Between the auditory and olfactory projection areas there is a large expanse of temporal lobe which has no assignable function. This is the temporal association area. Patients with tumors and vascular lesions of this part of the brain have been examined on numerous occasions, but usually the full extent of the disease has not been determined, even by pneumoencephalography, arteriography, or isotopic scanning procedures. Cases of temporal lobectomy for tumor have provided more valuable material, but again it has seldom been possible to be certain that other parts of the brain were not involved. The most careful psychologic studies have shown a difference between cases involving loss of the dominant and the nondominant temporal lobe. With lesions of the dominant side there is impairment in learning verbal material presented aloud; with nondominant lesions there is a similar failure in tests with visually presented material. In addition about 20 per cent of such patients have shown a syndrome similar to that described for the prefrontal parts of the brain; but more significant is the fact that in the other cases little or no defect in personality was exhibited. The study of cases of uncinate epilepsy, with the characteristic dreamy state, olfactory or gustatory hallucinations, and masticatory movements, suggests that all these functions are organized through the temporal lobes. Similarly, stimulation of the posterior parts of the temporal lobes of epileptic patients during surgical procedures has brought to light the interesting fact that complex memories and visual and auditory images, some with strong emotional content, can be aroused in fully conscious human beings. Recent studies of the effect of stimulation of the amygdaloid nucleus, which is in the anterior and medial part of the temporal lobe, have shed additional light on this subject. There are remarkable autonomic effects. Blood pressure rises, pulse increases, respirations are increased in frequency and depth, and the patient looks frightened. Complex emotional experiences that have occurred previously may be revived. These effects have been discussed in Chap. 52, Recurrent Convulsions. Ablation of the hippocampal and adjacent convolutions bilaterally has been carried out recently, with a disastrous loss of ability to learn new experiences or to establish new memories (Korsakoff's psychosis). All this suggests the important role of the temporal lobes in auditory and visual perception and imagery, in learning and memory, and in the emotional life of the individual.

Bilateral ablation of temporal lobes, so far studied only in monkeys, produces an animal that displays a curious tendency to react to every visual stimulus without seeming to recognize it (psychic blindness) and to examine every object in its environment by oral and manual contact. Placidity, with lack of the usual emotional response to stimuli, was another prominent feature.

To summarize, in man the temporal lobe syndromes include the following:

I. Effects of unilateral disease of the dominant temporal lobe
   A. Quadrantic homonymous anopia
   B. Wernicke's aphasia
   C. Impairment in verbal tests of material presented through the auditory sense
II. Effects of unilateral disease of nondominant temporal lobe
   A. Quadrantic homonymous anopia
   B. Impairment of mental function with inability to judge spatial relationship in some cases
   C. Impairment in nonverbal tests of visually presented material

PARIETAL LOBES. This part of the human nervous system is the subject of one of the most interesting discussions of cerebral function that has occurred in this century: its role in the formation of the body image or body schema.

It has long been known that the postcentral convolution is the terminus of somatic sensory pathways from the opposite half of the body. It has also been learned that destructive lesions here do not abolish cutaneous sensation but instead cause mainly a defect in sensory discrimination with variable impairment of sensation. In other words, pain, touch, and thermal and vibratory sensation are largely retained, whereas stereognosis, sense of position, distinction between single and double contacts (two-point threshold), and the localization of sensory stimuli are lost. There is also the phenomenon of extinction, viz., if both sides of the body are touched simultaneously, only the stimulus on the normal side is perceived. This type of sensory disturbance, sometimes called *cortical sensory defect*, is discussed in Chap. 49, Disorders of Sensation. Later it was noted that extensive lesions deep in the white matter of the parietal lobes produce a contralateral homonymous hemianopia, and lesions in the angular gyrus of the dominant hemisphere result in an inability to read.

More recent investigations have centered about the function of the parietal lobes in perception of position in space and of the relationship of the various parts of the body to one another. Since the time of Babinski it has been known that patients with a large lesion of the minor parietal lobe are often unaware of their hemiplegia and hemianesthesia. Babinski called this condition *anosognosia*. Related psychologic disorders are lack of recognition of the left arm and leg when seen or felt by the other hand, neglect of the left side of the body in dressing, an imperception of external space on the left side, and constructional apraxia, an inability to perform the movements of constructing simple figures. *Agnosia* and *apraxia* are discussed in Chaps. 45 and 49.

Another frequent constellation of symptoms, usually referred to as *Gerstmann's syndrome*, occurs with lesions of the dominant parietal lobe. This consists of inability to write (agraphia), inability to calculate (acalculia), failure to distinguish right from left, and loss of recognition of various parts of the body. An ideomotor apraxia may or may not be conjoined.

The effects of disease of the parietal lobes differ according to whether the dominant (left hemisphere in a right-handed person) or nondominant lobe is involved. These may be tabulated as follows:

I. Effects of unilateral disease of parietal lobe, right or left
   A. Cortical sensory syndrome and sensory extinction (or total hemian esthesia with large acute lesions of white matter)
   B. Mild hemiparesis, unilateral muscular atrophy in children
   C. Homonymous hemianopia or visual inattention, and sometimes neglect of one-half of external space
   D. Abolition of opticokinetic nystagmus to one side
II. Effects of unilateral disease of dominant parietal lobe (left hemisphere in right-handed patients), additional phenomena
   A. Disorders of language (especially alexia)
   B. Gerstmann's syndrome
   C. Bimanual astereognosis (tactile agnosia)
   D. Bilateral apraxia of ideomotor type
III. Effects of unilateral disease of minor parietal lobe (right hemisphere in right-handed patients), additional phenomena
   A. Anosognosia
   B. Neglect of left side of body
   C. Neglect of visual space to the left of the midline

In all these lesions, if the disease is sufficiently extensive, there may be a reduction in the capacity to think clearly, inattentiveness, and impairment of memory.

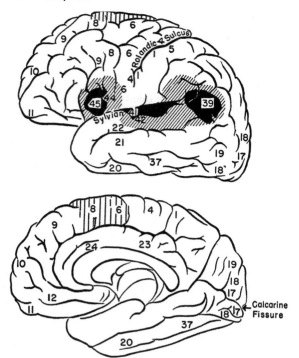

Fig. 54-1. Diagram to show cortical areas, numbered according to the scheme of Brodmann. The speech areas are in black, the three main ones being 39, 41, and 45. The zone marked by vertical stripes in the superior frontal convolution is the secondary motor area which, like Broca's area 45, if stimulated causes vocal arrest. (*Redrawn from "Handbuch der Inneren Medizin," Berlin, Springer-Verlag, 1939.*)

It is impossible at present to enunciate a formula of parietal lobe function in general. It does seem reasonably certain that the parietal and occipital lobes both participitate in sensory functions, especially in those which provide consciousness of one's surroundings, of the relationship of objects in the environment to one another, and of the position of the body in space. In this respect, as C. M. Fisher has recently suggested, the parietal lobe may be regarded as a suprasensory mechanism.

OCCIPITAL LOBES. The occipital lobes are the terminus of the visual pathways and are essential for visual sensation and perception. Lesions in one occipital lobe result in homonymous defects in the contralateral visual fields. Bilateral lesions cause cortical blindness, a state of blindness without change in optic fundi or pupillary reflexes. If areas 18 and 19 of Brodmann are affected (Fig. 54-1), there is loss of visual recognition, with retention of some degree of visual acuity, a state termed *visual agnosia* or *mind blindness*. In the classic form of this blindness an individual with intact mental powers is unable to recognize objects even though by tests of visual acuity and perimetry he appears to see sufficiently well to do so. Psychologists have demonstrated several special types of visual agnosia. In the simultagnosia of Wolpert, the patient, though able to see the individual parts of a picture, is unable to gather the

meaning of the whole. Similarly, in prosopagnosia the patient is unable to recognize a human face even though he sees all the individual details of it. Alexia, or inability to read, and visual spatial agnosia, or inability to recognize actual or abstract space, with resulting disorientation, are other special types of agnosia. Often the patient with bilateral lesions of the occipital lobes (cerebral cortical blindness) is unaware of his visual difficulty, i.e., has an agnosia for it. This state is known as *Anton's syndrome*. In *Holmes' syndrome* visual disorientation may be combined with a homonymous hemianopia.

This whole problem of both visual and tactile agnosia has recently been reexamined. In most of the reported cases tests of primary visual sensation or visual acuity have been inadequate. By controlling the time factor in visual perception and the adaptation time, and by testing the simultaneous perception of multiple points in the visual field, it is possible to show that the visual function is more often impaired than was at first suspected. The division of the visual process into sensation and perception becomes highly artificial.

Visual function is discussed further in Chap. 48.

DIAGNOSIS OF FOCAL CEREBRAL DISEASE. In summarizing the special effects of disease of different parts of the cerebral hemispheres, several points should be made. Extensive lesions in one or both frontal lobes often encroach on motor areas and, in doing so, cause a weakness of muscle groups on the opposite side of the body. This is especially noticeable in the face and is sometimes more pronounced during emotional expression than on voluntary movement. It may affect the arm and leg as well. In some instances the weakness may be rather slight, and a slowness and stiffness of movement with grasp reflex, slightly increased tendon reflexes, and Babinski's sign on the contralateral side are observed. A rather "absent-minded" type of urinary and fecal incontinence is also frequent. Expressive aphasia—an inability to speak—indicates involvement of the inferior frontal convolution of the dominant frontal lobe. Anosmia and blindness are neighborhood symptoms, resulting from extension of a lesion on the orbital surfaces of the frontal lobes to the olfactory bulbs and optic nerves.

An upper quadrantic homonymous anopia is the most reliable sign of disease of either the right or left temporal lobes; this localization should always be considered if dementia and this visual disturbance are conjoined. Uncinate or psychic seizures also establish a temporal lobe lesion but do not indicate the laterality. Bizarre disturbances of thinking and affect, often indistinguishable from schizophrenia, may follow temporal lobe seizures. In lesions of the dominant temporal lobe, Wernicke's aphasia is the most characteristic feature.

Cortical sensory deficit is the common neurologic abnormality in disease of either parietal lobe and is often combined with hemiplegia. With left-sided lesions in the inferior parietal lobule there is alexia and a contralateral homonymous hemianopia. Gerst-mann's syndrome localizes a lesion in the more posterior parts of the parietal and the lateral occipital lobes of the dominant hemisphere. The curious disturbances of body awareness or body scheme and of the midline are usually found with lesions of the non-dominant parietal lobe. Focal seizures arising in the parietal lobe usually consist of a focal or Jacksonian sensory disturbance.

Occipital lesions are distinguished by the almost exclusive affection of visual functions, a circumstance that rarely occurs in pure form with temporal or parietal lesions. The affection may take the form of homonymous hemianopia or of one of the more complex disorders of visual recognition.

Obviously, deterioration of intellect cannot at present be assigned to lesions in any one territory of the brain, and certainly not to any conventional division of the cerebrum. Stated in another way, the effects of disease of any of the known anatomic structures are not equivalent to dementia. Nevertheless, a disorder of personality and in thinking and memory does occur with a large lesion of any part of the cerebrum, particularly the frontal and temporal association areas.

THE APPROACH TO THE CLINICAL PROBLEM OF CONFUSION AND DEMENTIA

The physician presented with a patient suffering from a diffuse or focal cerebral disease must adopt an examination technique designed to expose fully the intellectual defect. Abnormalities of posture, movement, sensation, and reflexes cannot be relied upon for the full demonstration of the neurologic deficit, for it must be remembered that the association areas of the brain may be severely damaged without demonstrable neurologic signs of this type.

Three categories of data are required for the recognition and differential diagnosis of dementing brain disease:

1. A reliable history of illness
2. Findings on mental examination, i.e., so-called "mental status," as well as on the rest of the neurologic examination
3. Special laboratory precedures, lumbar puncture, x-rays of the skull, electroencephalogram, and sometimes pneumoencephalogram

The history should always be supplemented by information obtained from a person other than the patient, because through lack of insight he is often unaware of his illness; indeed, he may be ignorant even of his chief complaint. Special inquiry should be made about the patient's general behavior, capacity for work, personal habits, and such faculties as memory and judgment.

This performance of an examination of the mental status must be systematic. At a minimum it should include the following:

I. Insight (patient's replies to questions about his chief symptoms): What is your difficulty? Are you ill? When did your illness begin?

II. Orientation (knowledge of personal identity and present situation):

Person: What is your name? What is your occupation? Where do you live? Are you married?

Place: What is the name of the place where you are now? How did you get there? What floor is it on? Where is the bathroom? What are you doing now?

Time: What is the date today? What time of day is it? What meals have you had? When was the last holiday?

III. Memory:

Remote: Tell me the names of your children and their birth dates. When were you married? What was your mother's maiden name? What was the name of your first school-teacher?

Recent past: Tell me about your recent illness (compare with previous statements). What did you have for breakfast today? What is my name or the nurse's name? When did you see me for the first time? What were the headlines in the newspaper today?

Retention: Repeat these numbers after me (give series of 3, 4, 5, 6, 7, 8, digits at speed of 1 per second). Now when I give a series of numbers, repeat them in reverse order.

Visual span: Show the patient a picture of several objects and then ask him to name what he has seen and to note any anomalies.

IV. General information: Ask about names of presidents, well-known historic dates, the names of large rivers, of large cities, etc.

V. Capacity for sustained mental activity:

Calculation: Test ability to add, subtract, multiply, and divide. Subtraction of serial 7s from 100 is a good test of calculation as well as of attention.

Abstract thinking: See if the patient can detect similarities and differences between classes of objects, or explain a proverb or a fable.

VI. General behavior: Attitudes, general bearing, stream of thought, attentiveness, mood, manner of dress, etc.

In order to enlist the patient's full cooperation, the physician must prepare him for questions of this type. Otherwise, the first reaction will be one of embarrassment or anger because of the implication that his mind is not sound. It should be pointed out to the patient that some individuals are rather forgetful and that it is necessary to ask specific questions in order to form some impression about their degree of nervousness when being examined. Reassurance that these are not tests of intelligence or of sanity is helpful.

A more formal and reliable method of examining the mental capacity of adults is the Wechsler-Bellevue test. This can be given by a psychologist or by the physician if he has carefully read the instructions for administering and scoring the test. The *Mental Examiners' Handbook,* by F. L. Wells and J. Ruesch, published by the Psychological Corporation, is helpful to those not familiar with this type of examination. Tests of retention of verbal material and the recall of a series of learned digits or of visually presented objects are of value in estimating the degree of deterioration. In the Wechsler-Bellevue test the discrepancy between the vocabulary, picture completion, information, and object assembly tests as a group (these correlate well with premorbid intelligence and are relatively insensitive to dementing brain disease) and arithmetic, block design, digit span, and digit-symbol tests provide an index of deterioration.

Although the form of confusion or dementia does not indicate a particular disease, certain combinations of symptoms and neurologic signs are more or less characteristic and may aid in diagnosis. The mode of onset, the clinical course, the associated neurologic signs, and the accessory laboratory data constitute the basis of differential diagnosis. It must be admitted, however, that some of the rarer types of "degenerative" brain disease are at present recognized only by pathologic examination. The correct diagnosis of treatable forms of senile (over sixty years of age) or presenile (forty to sixty years) dementias, such as general paresis, subdural hematoma, brain tumor, bromide or other chronic drug intoxication, normal pressure hydrocephalus, pellagra and related deficiency states, and hypothyroidism, is of greater practical importance than the diagnosis of the untreatable ones.

Finally, with reference to the acute confusional states, one must also have a secure approach because such illnesses are observed almost daily on the medical and surgical wards of a general hospital. Occurring as they do during an infective fever, in the course of another illness such as cardiac failure, or following an injury, operation, or the excessive use of alcohol, they never fail to create grave problems for the physician, the nursing personnel, and the family. The physician often has to diagnose without the advantage of a lucid history, and his program of treatment may constantly be threatened by the agitation, sleeplessness, and uncooperative attitude of the patient. The nursing personnel are often sorely taxed by the necessity of providing a satisfactory environment for the convalescence of the patient and, at the same time, maintaining a tranquil atmosphere for the other patients on the ward. And the family is appalled by the sudden specter of insanity and all it entails.

Under such circumstances, it is a great temptation to rid oneself of the clinical problem by transferring the patient to a psychiatric hospital. This, in the author's opinion, is an unwise action for it may result in the inexpert management of the underlying medical disease and may even jeopardize the patient's life. It is far better for the physician to assume full responsibility for the care of such patients and to familiarize himself with this group of nervous disorders.

The first step in diagnosis is to recognize that the patient is confused. This is obvious in most cases; but, as pointed out above, the mildest form of confusion, particularly when some other acute alteration of personality is prominent, may be overlooked. In these mild forms a careful analysis of the patient's thinking as he gives the history of his illness and the details of his personal life will usually reveal an incoherence. The serial subtraction of 7s from 100 is a useful bedside test of the patient's capacity for sustained mental activity. Memory of recent events is one of the most delicate tests of adequate mental function and may be accomplished by having the patient relate all the details of his entry to the hospital, laboratory tests, etc.

Once it is established that the patient is confused, the differential diagnosis must be made between delirium, simple or primary mental confusion, a beclouded dementia, and Korsakoff's psychosis. This can be done usually by careful attention to the patient's degree of alertness and wakefulness, his capacity to solve new problems, his memory, accuracy of perception, and hallucinations. The presence of Korsakoff's psychosis may not become evident until the patient's general state improves. The distinction between confusional states and dementia is also difficult at times. It has been said that the patient with the acute confusional psychosis has a clouded sensorium, i.e., he is inattentive, and inclined to inaccurate perceptions and hallucinations, whereas the patient with dementia has a clear sensorium. However, it is the author's impression that many severely demented patients are as beclouded as those with confusional psychoses and that the two conditions are at times indistinguishable, except for their different time courses. All this suggests that the parts of the nervous system affected may be the same in both conditions. When the physician is faced with this problem, the history of the mode of onset becomes of great value. The confusional psychosis has an acute or subacute onset and is usually reversible, whereas dementia is always chronic and tends to be more or less irreversible.

Once a case has been classified as delirium, primary mental confusion, or Korsakoff's psychosis, it is important to determine its clinical associations. A thorough medical and neurologic examination and often a lumbar puncture should be done. The other medical and neurologic findings are of great value in indicating the underlying disease to be treated, and they also give information concerning prognosis. In the neurologic examination particular attention should be given to language functions, visual fields and visual-spatial discriminations, cortical sensory functions, and calculation and other test performances that require normal functioning of the temporal, parietal, and occipital lobes. Confusional states are frequent with diseases of these parts of the brain. Moreover, some of the signs of disease of these parts of the brain are often mistaken for a confusional psychosis.

Schizophrenia and manic-depressive psychosis can usually be separated from the confusional states by the presence of a clear sensorium and good memory.

The treatment is directed to the underlying disease process.

Care of the Delirious, Confused, and Demented Patient

There is an advantage to treating the delirious patient in a general hospital; he often suffers from a medical disease that can be dealt with more adequately there than in a psychiatric hospital. Furthermore, delirium seldom lasts more than a few days, and if the patient can be kept on a medical ward, the social stigma that attaches to incarceration in a mental institution is avoided. In the author's experience only a few delirious patients are so agitated and noisy as to annoy others; and should this happen, many general hospitals now have some facilities for isolating the mentally disturbed patient. Delirium of this severity is rare in infectious diseases but is, of course, not infrequent in alcoholism (delirium tremens), drug intoxication, and other medical diseases.

The first objectives are to quiet the patient and protect him against injury. A private nurse, an attendant, or a member of the family should be with the patient at all times, if this can be arranged. Depending on how active and vigorous he is, a locked room, screened windows that cannot be opened by the patient, and a low bed or mattress on the floor should be arranged. It is often better to let the patient walk about the room than to tie him into bed, which may excite or frighten him so that he struggles to the point of complete exhaustion and collapse. If he is less active, the patient can usually be kept in bed by leather wrist restraints, a restraining sheet, or a net thrown over the bed. Unless contraindicated by the primary disease, the patient should be permitted to sit up or walk about the room part of the day.

All drugs that could possibly be responsible for delirium—particularly opiates, barbiturates, bromides, atropine, hyoscine, cortisone, adrenocorticotropic hormone (ACTH), and salicylates in large doses—should be discontinued (unless withdrawal effects are believed to underlie the illness). Paraldehyde and chloral hydrate are the only sedatives that can be trusted under these circumstances. Paraldehyde, which is preferred, may be given orally or rectally in doses of 10 to 12 ml. For oral administration, mixing it with fruit juices makes it more palatable, though alcoholic

patients will take it in any form and seem to enjoy it. One must be cautious in attempting to suppress agitation completely. To accomplish this may require very large doses of drugs, and vital functions may be dangerously impaired. The purpose of sedation is to assure rest and sleep so that the patient does not exhaust himself. Continuous warm baths or warm packs are also effective in quieting the delirious patient, but very few general hospitals have proper facilities for this valuable method of treatment.

A fluid intake and output chart should be kept, and any fluid and electrolyte deficit should be corrected according to the methods outlined in Chap. 60. The pulse and blood pressure should be recorded at intervals of 2 hr in anticipation of circulatory collapse. Transfusions of whole blood and vasopressor drugs may be lifesaving.

Finally, the physician should be aware of many small therapeutic measures that may allay fear and suspicion and reduce the tendency to hallucinations. The room should be kept well lighted, and if possible, the patient should not be moved from one room to another. Every procedure should be explained in detail, even such simple ones as the taking of blood pressure or temperature. The presence of a member of the family may enable the patient to maintain contact with reality.

It may be some consolation and also a source of professional satisfaction to remember that most delirious patients tend to recover if they are placed in good hygienic surroundings and competently nursed. The family should be reassured on this point. They must also understand that the abnormal behavior and irrational actions of the patient are not willful but rather are symptomatic of a brain disease.

Dementia is a clinical state of the most serious nature, and usually it is worthwhile to admit the patient to the hospital for a period of observation. The physician then has an opportunity to see the patient several times in a new and fairly constant hospital environment, and certain special procedures such as x-rays of the skull, lumbar puncture, analysis for blood bromides, basal metabolic rate, an electro-encephalogram and often a pneumoencephalogram can be carried out at this time. The management of the demented patient in the hospital may be relatively simple if he is quiet and cooperative. If the disorder of mental function is severe, a nurse, attendant, or member of the family must stay with the patient at all times. Provision must be made for adequate food and fluid intake and control of infection, using the same measures outlined for the delirious patient.

Once it is established that the patient has an untreatable dementing brain disease, a responsible member of the family should be apprised of the medical facts. The patient should be told that he has a nervous condition for which he is to be given rest and treatment. Nothing is accomplished by telling him more. The family should be given the prognosis, if the diagnosis is sufficiently certain for this to be possible. If the dementia is slight and circumstances are suitable, the patient may remain at home, continuing activities of which he is capable. He should be spared responsibility and guarded against injury that might result from imprudent action. If he is still at work, plans for occupational retirement should be carried out. In more advanced stages of the disease mental and physical enfeeblement become pronounced and institutional care should be advised. Seizures should be treated symptomatically. Nerve tonics, vitamins, and hormones are of no value in checking the course of the illness or in regenerating decayed tissue. They may, however, offer some support to the patient and family.

Part Three

Biologic Considerations

Section 1

Inheritance and Growth

55 INHERITANCE OF HUMAN DISEASE

Victor A. McKusick

Increasingly in recent years the importance of genetics to medicine has come to be appreciated. The relative importance of those conditions in which genetic factors play a leading role has increased as some other etiologic categories of disease, e.g., infectious and nutritional, have become better understood and better treated.

The mutant gene should be considered an etiologic agent. The variability, yet predictability, of the clinical picture in a genetic disorder in which the etiologic agent, a gene, operates from within is very similar to that of an infectious disease in which the etiologic agent invades from the environment. In studying progressive muscular dystrophy of the pseudohypertrophic type, one is not searching for its cause. The cause, a sex-linked recessive gene, is known. It is the mechanism by which the mutant gene produces the clinical manifestations, and methods for interrupting that mechanism, or compensating for it, that are sought by research in muscular dystrophy.

In addition to those conditions for which a single mutant gene in single or double dose is quite directly responsible, and in addition to those disorders which result from chromosomal aberrations, there are many disorders, including some of the commonest affections of man, e.g., atherosclerosis, hypertension, and rheumatoid arthritis, in which genetic factors and environmental factors collaborate in a complex manner. For a majority of the diseases of man, causation must not be viewed in the rigid sense of a single etiologic agent —a pattern of thinking engendered by the bacteriologic era of medicine—but rather as a nexus, a network of multiple interacting factors among which the genetic factor or factors are always likely to be important. In coronary artery disease, for example, one cannot say that heredity, high-fat diet, cigarette smoking, particular forms of stress, or any other of many postulated factors is *the* cause. The controversy between genetics and environment, nature and nurture, of an early day has now subsided since it is appreciated that both types of factors are important.

The collaboration of heredity and environment is well illustrated by primaquine sensitivity (glucose 6-phosphate dehydrogenase deficiency) in which hemolytic anemia usually occurs only if the genetically predisposed person is exposed to a chemical of a particular type (p. 633); and by suxamethonium (succinylcholine) sensitivity (pseudocholinesterase deficiency) in which the genetically predisposed person suffers no obvious ill effects of his defect unless given the agent mentioned as a muscle relaxant in anesthesia.

An important principle of medical genetics is *heterogeneity.* Many genetic disorders which at first were thought to represent single entities have, on close study, been found to consist of two or more fundamentally distinct entities. There are known, for example, to be two types of X-linked hemophilia (A and B), and the genes for these are at loci rather far apart on the X chromosome. Four or five distinct varieties of hereditary intestinal polyposis can be distinguished on clinical grounds. Several recessively inherited varieties of familial goiter are found to have separate and distinct biochemical defects.

DEFINITIONS. *Congenital* means "present at birth" and is not synonymous with genetic. Genetic factors may or may not be of importance in the cause of individual congenital malformations. On the other hand, hereditary conditions are not necessarily congenital; at least, clinical manifestations may not appear until much later in life. *Hereditary, genetic,* and *heritable* are roughly synonymous. *Familial* and *heredofamilial* were used previously to designate conditions inherited as recessives, i.e., conditions which often occur in multiple siblings with both parents normal. Since a recessive disorder is as genuinely inherited as a dominant one, these terms have little justification. Possibly the only use for the term *familial* is in connection with disorders with a familial aggregation not yet proved to be genetic in basis.

The word *genotype* refers to the genetic constitution of the individual; *phenotype* refers to the outward

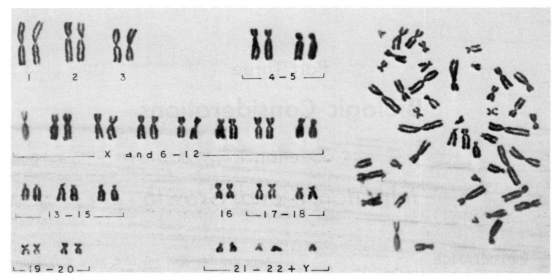

Fig. 55-1. The chromosomes of a normal male. On the right are shown the chromosomes of a single somatic cell in the metaphase stage of cell division. The photographic images of the chromosomes have been cut out and arranged, according to descending length and varying arm ratio, to form the karyotype shown on the left. The sex chromosomes in this normal male are an X, shown with the 6–12 chromosomes, which it resembles, and a Y, shown near chromosomes 21–22, which it resembles.

expression. The phenotype is, of course, what the physician observes, from which he makes deductions about the genotype. The difference is comparable to that between character and reputation—"genotype" and "character" refer to the true nature of the individual, "phenotype" and "reputation" to the apparent nature. *Karyotype* refers to the chromosomal complement of cells.

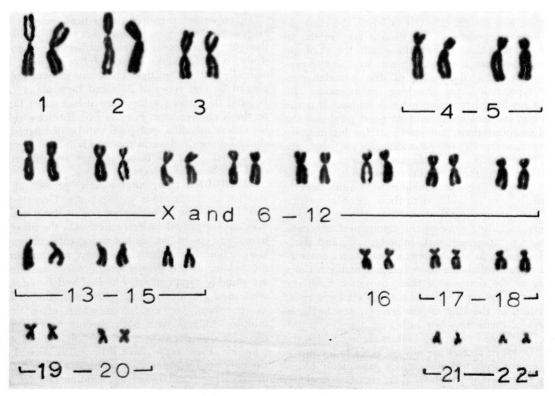

Fig. 55-2. The chromosomes of a normal female. No Y chromosome is present, and two X chromosomes are present with the 6–12 group.

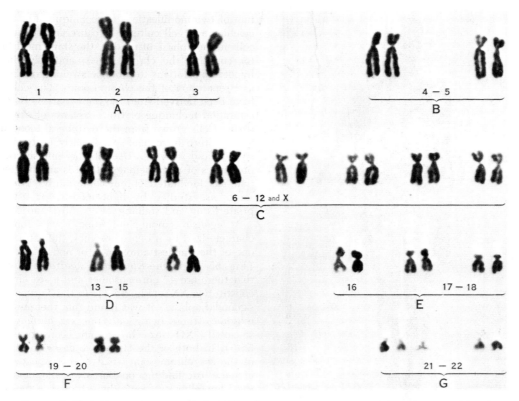

Fig. 55-3. The chromosomes in mongolism. The chromosoma constitution is that of a normal female except for the presence of an extra chromosome in the set numbered 21

Abiotrophy is a term introduced by Gowers (1902) to describe the behavior of genetic disorders, such as Huntington's chorea and the spinocerebellar ataxias, in which a system functions normally and may be histologically normal up to a stage more or less late in life. The term refers to an inborn defect which leads to premature deterioration of a particular tissue, organ, or system.

SYNDROMES. Many hereditary disorders have manifold manifestations, the combination of which is referred to as a *syndrome* ("running together"). (Of course, conditions predominantly nongenetic may also occur as syndromes.) Hereditary syndromes, excluding those like mongoloid idiocy which are due to a chromosomal aberration, appear to be produced by a single mutant gene which has multiple expressions in the phenotype because the protein, enzymatic, or other character, which is specified by the gene, has wide implications, at least multiple implications, in the economy of the organism. Genetic linkage—the location on the same chromosome of separate genes for each aspect of the syndrome—cannot account for the syndromal relationships observed in clinical medicine.

The investigation of members of a family with regard to a particular disease trait usually begins from a *proband,* or *propositus* (*-a*). The proband is the affected person through whom the family is ascertained. The proband is comparable to the *index* case of epidemiologic studies. Often in family studies it is

desirable to compare the frequency of a discontinuous trait or the mean level of a biometric trait in the relatives of probands and in the relatives of controls. Data are almost meaningless unless the degree of relationship of the relatives studied is indicated. It means little, for example, to state that 5 per cent of the relatives of patients with rheumatoid arthritis have rheumatoid arthritis, but more significance can be attached to the statement that 5 per cent of first degree relatives have rheumatoid arthritis. *First degree relatives* are parents, siblings, and offspring; on the average their genetic resemblance to the proband is 0.50, if genetic identity (as in monozygotic twins) is 1.0. *Second degree relatives* are grandparents, aunts and uncles, and grandchildren of the proband; on the average their genetic resemblance to the proband is 0.25.

The aspects of genetics of particular significance to clinical medicine are at least four: (1) cytogenetics, i.e., the study of chromosomes in relation to the phenotype; (2) pedigree patterns, i.e., the behavior in families of single-gene disorders; (3) biochemical genetics, i.e., the biochemical basis of inherited disease; and (4) the genetics of common disorders.

CYTOGENICS IN MAN

It was not until 1956 that the correct chromosome number in man (46) was known and not until 1959 that a microscopically identifiable chromosomal aber-

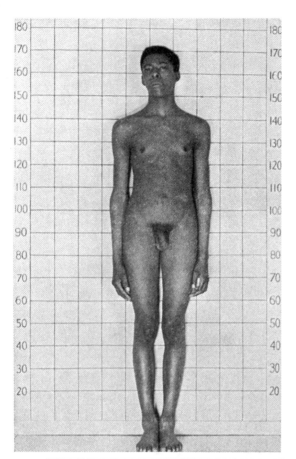

ration was reported to be the cause of disease in man. These advances were made possible by the introduction of two modifications of technique: (1) the use of colchicine in cell cultures to cause an accumulation of cells in metaphase of mitosis, the stage most favorable for counting the chromosomes; and (2) the use of hypotonic solutions to produce swelling of the nucleus and separation of the chromosomes. The cells studied have been derived from the bone marrow by the usual aspiration technique or from explants of skin or other tissue. Cells grown from the peripheral blood in short-term culture have been particularly useful for family studies and surveys. Use of the mitosis-stimulating properties of phytohemagglutinin is another technique that has facilitated chromosome study. The chromosomes are studied by light microscopy after appropriate fixing and staining (Figs. 55-1 and 55-2).

Mongolism (mongoloid idiocy) was found to be characterized by 47 chromosomes, the extra one being one of the smallest autosomes, or nonsex chromosomes (Fig. 55-3). In the *Klinefelter syndrome* it was found that there are 47 chromosomes and a sex chromosome constitution XXY (Fig. 55-4). In the *Turner syndrome* (gonodal aplasia) it was found that there are 45 chromosomes, there being only one sex chromosome, the so-called "XO sex chromosome constitution" (Fig. 55-5). In both of the latter two cases an abnormality of the sex chromosomes had been suspected because of paradoxic findings on Barr's test of nuclear sex. In the Klinefelter syndrome the subject is ostensibly male but shows the "chromatin-positive" pattern of the nor-

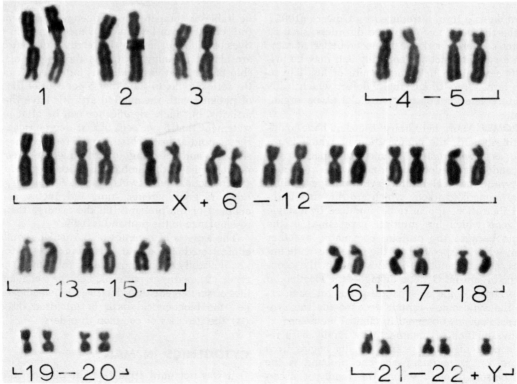

Fig. 55-4. *Upper*, a patient with the Klinefelter syndrome. Note the long legs, gynecomastia, and sparse body hair. *Lower*, the chromosomes in the Klinefelter syndrome. The karyotype is abnormal in the presence of three sex chromosomes (XXY).

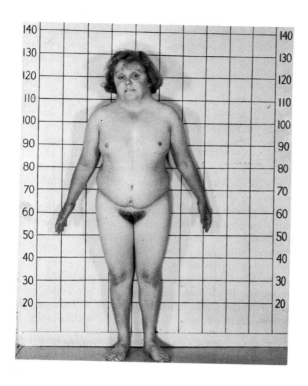

mal female; in the Turner syndrome the phenotypic female shows in a majority of cases the "chromatin-negative" pattern of the normal male (Fig. 55-6).

The three conditions above appear to arise through the accident of nondisjunction occurring either during meiosis in one parent (that is, in spermatogenesis or oogenesis) or in the first mitotic cleavage of the zygote. In meiotic nondisjunction both chromosomes of a given pair pass into one cell product rather than separating. Abnormal cells of two types are produced: one with one chromosome too many and one with one chromosome too few. In mongolism the strikingly higher frequency in the offspring of older mothers appears to be due to a higher risk of nondisjunction in older females.

Many other chromosomal aberrations have been discovered. Those which affect the sex chromosomes include XXX, XXXY, XXXXY, XXYY, and XXXX constitutions. Trisomic states (conditions in which, as in mongolism, three chromosomes rather than two of a particular set are present) have been described in which the chromosomes involved are different ones than in mongolism. Deletions and translocations have also been discovered and correlated with phenotypic changes.

The relationship of demonstrable changes in the chromosomes to neoplastic disease is under active investigation. In many cases of chronic myeloid leukemia

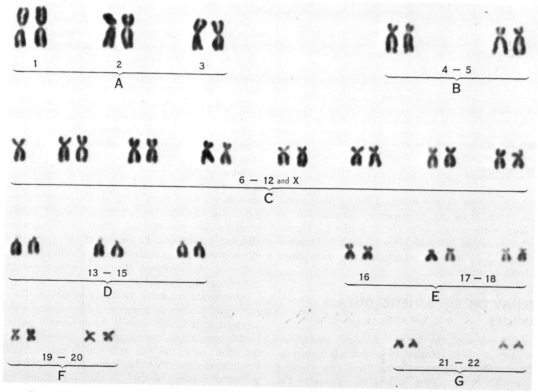

Fig. 55-5. *Upper,* a patient with the Turner syndrome. Note the short stature, broad shieldlike chest with wide intermammary distance, hypoplastic mandible, low-set ears, and webbed neck. Note the scar of the operation for resection of coarctation of the aorta. *Lower,* the chromosomes in the Turner syndrome. Only one sex chromosome, an X, is present.

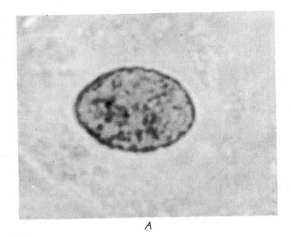

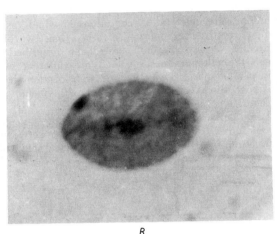

Fig. 55-6. *A.* Cell in buccal smear from normal male. No sex chromatin mass is seen in this "chromatin-negative" pattern, which is shown also by most patients with the Turner syndrome. *B.* Cell in buccal smear from normal female, showing a sex chromatin mass adjacent to the nuclear membrane. This "chromatin-positive" pattern is also shown by patients with the Klinefelter syndrome.

a consistent change in one of the four smallest autosomes has been observed. It appears that deletion, or loss, of part of the long arm of chromosome 21, resulting in the so-called "Philadelphia (or Ph¹) chromosome" (Fig. 55-7) may be responsible for most cases of this form of leukemia.

THE BEHAVIOR OF GENETIC DISEASE IN FAMILIES

In accordance with the laws of Mendel, many diseases in man occur in families in a characteristic pattern. The specific pedigree pattern depends on whether the responsible mutant gene is located on one of the autosomal chromosomes or on an X chromosome. It also depends on whether the effects of the gene are evident in single dose, that is, in the heterozygous state, or whether the gene requires double dosage, or

the homozygous state, for its expression. According to the type of chromosome bearing the gene in question, a trait is said to be either *autosomal* or *sex-linked*. Depending on whether expression of the gene occurs in the heterozygous state or only in the homozygous state, a trait is said to be either *dominant* or *recessive*, respectively.

Figure 55-8 presents an idealized pedigree pattern of an *autosomal dominant trait*. Within the limits of chance, half the sons and half the daughters of an affected person are affected. This follows directly from the fact that the mutant gene is carried by one of a pair of autosomes and that there is a 50 per cent chance of the affected parent contributing that chromosome to any given offspring.

As a generalization, dominant traits are less severe than recessive traits. In part an evolutionary or selective reason for this observation can be offered. A dominant mutation which determines a grave disorder that makes reproduction impossible will promptly disappear. On the other hand, even though in the homozygous condition a recessive mutation precludes reproduction, it can gain wide dissemination in heterozygous carriers, if it endows these carriers with a selective advantage.

A biochemical explanation is also possible for the greater severity of recessive traits. One might anticipate a greater derangement when both genes specifying a particular protein, let us say an enzyme, are of mutant type than if only one is mutant.

Another characteristic of dominant characters is wide variability in severity. The degree of severity is referred to as the *expressivity*. Sometimes the expressivity is so much reduced that the presence of the gene cannot be recognized at all, at least by the methods at one's disposal. When this is the case, the trait is said to be *nonpenetrant*. Sometimes in pedigrees of families with a dominant trait, so-called "skipped" generations occur. In the skipped individual, expressivity is so low that the presence of the gene is not recognizable, i.e., the trait is nonpenetrant in that person. The variability results from differences in the environment and in the rest of the genetic make-up, the *genome*. At least in part the variability of dominant traits may be the result of differences in the "normal" allele which accompanies the mutant allele in the heterozygous affected individual. Evidence of the last is provided when one can demonstrate that sib-sib correlations for behavior of the given disease are stronger than the parent-sibling correlations.

Autosomal recessive traits (Fig. 55-9) likewise occur equally often in males and females, as a rule. The affected individuals usually have normal parents, but both parents are heterozygous carriers of the gene in question. Since related individuals are more likely to be heterozygous for the same mutant gene, consanguineous mating, of first cousins, for example, is more likely to result in offspring affected by a recessive trait. Viewed in another way, a greater proportion of the parental matings in families affected by recessive traits are likely to be consanguineous than is true generally.

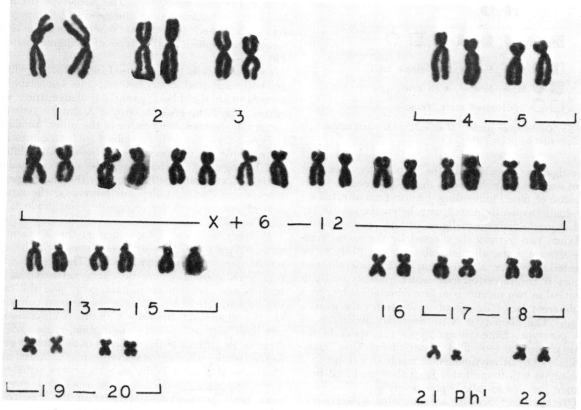

Fig. 55-7. The chromosomes of bone marrow from a female with chronic myelocytic leukemia. One chromosome 21, marked Ph¹ for Philadelphia chromosome, is missing part of its long arm.

The rarer the recessive trait, the higher is the proportion of consanguineous parental matings.

On the average, among the offspring of two heterozygous parents one-fourth of males and females are expected to be homozygous-affected. One-half will be heterozygous carriers for the trait, and one-fourth will be homozygous for the normal allele.

Affected sibships can usually be ascertained only through the appearance of one or more affected members. Since there is no way to recognize those matings of two appropriately heterozygous parents who are so fortunate as to have no affected children, a collection of sibships containing at least one affected child is a biased sample. More than the expected one-fourth

will be affected. Methods for correcting for the so-called "bias of ascertainment" are available.

If an individual affected by a recessive trait marries a homozygous normal person, none of the children will be affected, but all will be heterozygous carriers. If an individual affected by a recessive trait marries a heterozygous carrier, one-half of the offspring are likely to be affected. A pedigree pattern superficially resembling that of a dominant trait can result. It was previously thought that two genetic forms of alkaptonuria (p. 540) exist—one inherited as an autosomal recessive and one as an autosomal dominant. Closer

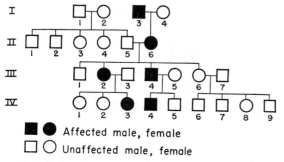

Fig. 55-8. Pedigree pattern of an autosomal dominant trait.

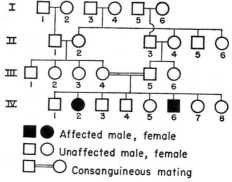

Fig. 55-9. Pedigree pattern of an autosomal recessive trait.

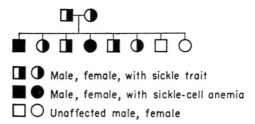

☐ ◑ Male, female, with sickle trait

■ ● Male, female, with sickle-cell anemia

☐ ○ Unaffected male, female

Fig. 55-10. Pedigree pattern of an autosomal intermediate trait as illustrated by sickle state.

investigation reveals that the apparently dominant form was the same disease as the clearly recessive one. Because of much inbreeding, homozygous affected individuals frequently mated with heterozygous carriers and a quasi-dominant pedigree pattern resulted.

When two individuals affected by the same recessive disease mate, all their offspring are likely to be affected. However, an exception to this generalization occurs if the recessive trait which phenotypically is identical in two parents is in fact determined by genes at different loci. The exception illustrates the genetic axiom: The phenotype is no necessary indication of the genotype. Different genotypes can result in the same phenotype (so-called "genetic mimics" or "genocopies"). Or an environmental insult can result in a phenotype indistinguishable from that produced by a mutant gene (a so-called "phenocopy").

Dominant and *recessive* are somewhat arbitrary concepts. When our methods are sufficiently acute, the effect of a recessive gene in heterozygous state can be recognized. Furthermore, a gene which has obvious expression in the heterozygous individual and is therefore considered dominant may have a different effect, quantitatively and even qualitatively, in the homozygous state. The gene for sickle hemoglobin and the states referred to as sickle-cell anemia and sickle-cell trait illustrate the arbitrary nature of the distinction. If sickle-cell anemia is considered as the phenotype, then the condition is recessive, since a homozygous

state of the gene is required. The phenotype sickling, however, is dominant since the gene in heterozygous state is expressed. *Intermediate inheritance* is the term sometimes applied to this type of pedigree pattern (Fig. 55-10).

Codominance is the term used for characters which are both expressed in the heterozygote. For example, persons with the blood group AB demonstrate the effects of both the gene for antigen A and the gene for antigen B. Neither is recessive to the other. Similarly the genes for different hemoglobins are both expressed, for example, in the person with both hemoglobin S and hemoglobin C. These examples of codominance again indicate that whether we view the phenotype as recessive or dominant depends largely on the acuteness of our methods for recognizing the products of gene action.

In traits determined by genes on the X chromosome, either dominance or recessiveness may be observed, just as in autosomal traits. The female with two X chromosomes may be either heterozygous or homozygous for a given mutant gene, and the trait can demonstrate either recessive or dominant behavior. On the other hand, the male with one X chromosome can have only one genetic constitution, namely, *hemizygous*. Regardless of the behavior of the mutant gene in the female, whether recessive or dominant, the mutant gene, if present in the male, is always expressed.

An important characteristic of sex-linked inheritance, both dominant and recessive, is the absence of male-to-male (that is, father-to-son) transmission of the disease. This is a necessary result of the fact that the male contributes his X chromosome to all his daughters but to none of his sons.

Sex-linked (X-linked) recessive inheritance (Fig. 55-11) is illustrated in a classic manner by hemophilia. The pedigree pattern of an autosomal dominant trait is a horizontal one, with affected persons in successive generations. The pedigree pattern of an autosomal recessive trait tends to be a vertical one, with affected persons confined to a single generation. The pedigree

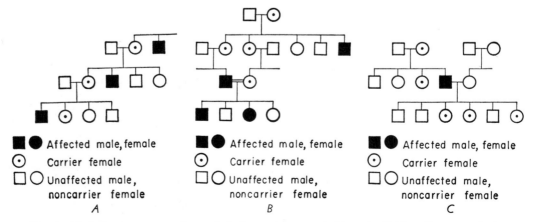

■ ● Affected male, female

⊙ Carrier female

☐ ○ Unaffected male, noncarrier female

A

■ ● Affected male, female

⊙ Carrier female

☐ ○ Unaffected male, noncarrier female

B

■ ● Affected male, female

⊙ Carrier female

☐ ○ Unaffected male, noncarrier female

C

Fig. 55-11. Pedigree patterns of a sex-linked recessive trait. A. Note the "oblique" pattern. B. An affected female can result from the mating of an affected male and a carrier female, as in the case of a consanguineous marriage shown here. C. An affected male mating with a normal, noncarrier female has all normal sons and all carrier daughters.

pattern of a sex-linked recessive character tends to be an oblique one because of transmission to the sons of normal carrier sisters of affected males. Bateson compared this pattern to the knight's move in chess. Tracing sex-linked recessive characters through many generations is often difficult because the patronymic of affected persons tends to change with each generation.

To have hemophilia a female must be homozygous for this recessive gene. She must have received a gene for hemophilia from each parent. Such can occur, and has been observed, when a hemophiliac male marries a carrier female (Fig. 55-11B). As with other recessive traits this homozygous state is more likely to result from consanguineous matings. A hemophiliac female may also occur if a carrier mother is impregnated by a mutant sperm from a normal father, or if the phenotypic female has in fact an XO sex chromosome constitution (the Turner syndrome) or an XY constitution (the syndrome of testicular feminization). (In these comments reference is, of course, made to sex-linked recessive hemophilia A and B and not to other hemophilioid states which occur equally frequently in males and females.)

A hemophiliac male can have gotten the hemophilia gene *only* from his mother and can transmit it only to his daughters but to none of his sons. *All* daughters of a hemophiliac male are carriers (Fig. 55-11C).

In man one can enumerate fifty or more other diseases inherited as sex-linked recessives, including such significant entities as primaquine sensitivity (p. 633), the Duchenne type of progressive muscular dystrophy (p. 1318), and agammaglobulinemia (p. 695). In some, for example, primaquine sensitivity and nephrogenic diabetes insipidus, a partial defect can be demonstrated in the heterozygous female carrier, and one might prefer to call the inheritance sex-linked intermediate. In another condition, choroideremia, hemizygous males, but only the males, have severe impairment of vision, and from this point of view the disease is a sex-linked recessive; but the heterozygous female carriers show striking changes in the fundus oculi on ophthalmoscopy, even though vision is unaffected.

At least one common trait, colorblindness, is inherited as a sex-linked recessive. It is sufficiently frequent (about 8 per cent of white males are colorblind) that the occurrence of homozygous colorblind females is no great rarity—0.08^2, or 0.6 per cent.

In sex-linked (X-linked) dominant inheritance both females and males are affected and both males and females transmit the disorder to their offspring, just as in autosomal dominant inheritance. Superficially the pedigree patterns in the two types of inheritance are similar, but there is a critical difference (Fig. 55-12). In sex-linked dominant inheritance, although the affected female transmits the trait to half her sons and half her daughters, the affected male transmits it to *none* of his sons and to *all* his daughters. Furthermore, in a series of cases females are expected to occur twice as often as males. One of the best studied sex-linked dominant traits is vitamin D–resistant rickets, or hypophosphatemic rickets (p. 388). In this condi-

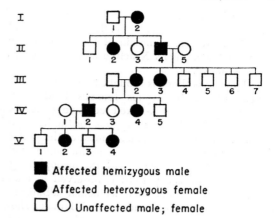

■ Affected hemizygous male
● Affected heterozygous female
□ ○ Unaffected male; female

Fig. 55-12. Pedigree pattern of a sex-linked dominant trait.

tion the hemizygous affected male tends to have more severe clinical involvement than does the heterozygous affected female.

One common trait is inherited as an X-linked dominant: the Xg(a+) blood group. In due course, antisera that directly identify the Xg(a−) blood group will probably be found. These will then be considered codominant traits.

Understanding of the behavior of X-linked traits and interpretation of findings in (1) females heterozygous for X-linked genes and (2) persons with an abnormal complement of X chromosomes have been greatly advanced by the *Lyon hypothesis.* There is now good evidence that at an early stage in development one X chromosome of the female becomes relatively inactive genetically (Fig. 55-13). The inactive X chromosome forms the *Barr body.* In each cell it is a random matter whether the X chromosome derived from the mother or that derived from the father is the one that becomes inactive. Once the "decision" is made in a

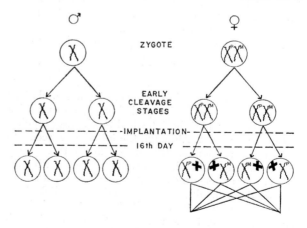

MOSAIC OF ADULT FEMALE

Fig. 55-13. Schematic representation of the phenomenon underlying the Lyon hypothesis. In the normal female, early in embryogenesis, probably soon after implantation, one X chromosome in each cell becomes inactive. Once it has been "decided" whether the maternal or paternal X chromosome will be the inactive one, all descendants of that cell "abide by the decision."

given cell, however, the same X chromosome remains inactive in all descendants of that cell. The adult female is, therefore, a mosaic of two types of cells, those with the mother's X active and those with the father's X active.

The Lyon hypothesis is thought to account for these findings: (1) Heterozygous females tend to vary widely in expression of X-linked recessive genes. As an extreme case, females heterozygous for the hemophilia gene have clinical hemophilia, if most of the pertinent anlage cells destined to produce antihemophilic globulin have the X chromosome with the hemophilia gene active. (2) A mosaic pattern is observed in females heterozygous for traits such as ocular albinism, an X-linked recessive. The fundi in such females show a mosaic of pigmented and unpigmented areas. (3) Persons with multiple X chromosomes, e.g., the XXX female, have two Barr bodies. All X chromosomes in excess of 1 are inactivated. These persons have much less drastic abnormalities than would be expected with such excess chromosomal material, if relative inactivation did not occur.

Occurrence of the following types of inheritance in man is uncertain: (1) *holandric (all-male) inheritance,* resulting from the possible location of a gene on the Y chromosome, and (2) *partial sex-linkage,* resulting from the location of a gene on possibly homologous parts of the X and Y chromosomes between which crossing over might occur.

Before leaving sex-linked inheritance, one should note the distribution between sex-linked inheritance and sex-influenced (or sex-limited) autosomal inheritance. Baldness appears to be such a sex-influenced autosomal trait. In man baldness is inherited as an autosomal dominant, but in women for baldness to occur the gene must be in homozygous state, that is, in women baldness behaves like a recessive. In women who develop masculinizing tumors of the ovary, baldness can occur if the genotype is proper. As another example, one can imagine a mutant gene whose sole effect was that of preventing lactation in the female. Even though it were located on an autosomal chromosome, it would not have expression in the male. Idiopathic hemochromatosis (p. 555) results from the pathologic effects of excessive accumulations of iron within the body, probably as a result of a hereditary defect in the intestinal mechanism regulating iron absorption. Although the inheritance seems to be autosomal dominant, females are rather rarely affected because they have a safety valve on excessive iron accumulation—menstruation and pregnancy.

Note the difficulties in distinguishing sex-linked recessive inheritance from sex-limited autosomal dominant inheritance, if the nature of the disease is such that reproduction of affected males does not occur. The syndrome of testicular feminization (p. 513) is an example. The affected individuals are genetic males but, because of the production of female hormones by the testis, female external genitalia and all the secondary sex characters of the female develop. The affected male does not reproduce and normal females are carriers. The pedigree pattern is precisely that of a sex-linked recessive trait. However, the inheritance can equally well be sex-linked autosomal dominant. In diseases too severe to permit reproduction of affected males—the Pelizaeus-Merzbacher disease (a form of cerebral degeneration), the Duchenne variety of muscular dystrophy (p. 1318), one variety of gargoylism (p. 1383)—there is on the basis of pedigree patterns no way to distinguish sex-linked and sex-limited inheritance.

GENETIC COUNSELING. Familiarity with the patterns of disease is useful in diagnosis; if the pedigree pattern is consistent with the mode of inheritance usual for a suspected entity, the diagnosis of that entity is thereby strengthened. Knowing what individuals in a kindred are at risk, one can watch for the earliest signs of hereditary disease.

Furthermore, familiarity with pedigree patterns is essential to genetic counseling. The risk of having an affected child can be stated as 1 in 2 for a person affected by a dominant trait and as 1 in 4 for a couple which has already had a child affected by a recessive disease. For the sister of a male affected by a sex-linked recessive trait the risk of being a carrier is (unless the affected brother represents a new mutation) 1 in 2, of having an affected son one-half of that, or 1 in 4, and the risk of any affected child (considering both sexes) one-half of that, or 1 in 8.

Other genetic considerations such as the severity of the disease in question, including its severity in the specific family, must be included in the evaluation. Only the risks should be stated to the persons seeking counsel. The decision as to what action they should follow must be theirs and must take account of factors such as economic status and emotional fortitude. Socially valuable traits partially determined by genetic constitution may be present in the family and outweigh the disadvantage of a mutant gene. Counseling will be strengthened when methods for detecting heterozygous carriers, for example, the female carrier of sex-linked recessive traits, are available.

Often the statement of risks is a relief to the persons involved and is not disturbing. For example, a young man with pseudoxanthoma elasticum (p. 1382), an autosomal recessive trait, was relieved to learn that the likelihood that his children by an unrelated wife would be affected by the severe eye involvement and tendency to hemorrhage is essentially nil. In families affected by a clear-cut, nearly fully penetrant autosomal dominant trait normal persons are sometimes surprised to learn, and considerably relieved, that there is virtually no risk of their offspring being affected.

Genetic counseling in common disorders of multifactor causation presents special problems, which are discussed later.

PRINCIPLES OF BIOCHEMICAL GENETICS IN MAN

Biochemical genetics had its origin in the early part of this century, with a physician, Archibald Garrod, and his "inborn errors of metabolism." The disorders he considered were defects in intermediary metabolism resulting from an inherited abnormality of particular enzymes. In its broader implications, biochemical genetics is concerned with the chemical nature of the genetic code and with all the biochemical steps by which that code is translated into an observed characteristic, for example, an inherited disease.

The genetic information passed from generation to generation is coded in some manner in the sequence of purine and pyrimidine bases in the deoxyribonucleic acid (DNA) of the chromosomes. The primary action of the so-called "structural genes" is to specify the amino acid sequence of a particular protein or of one polypeptide component of a protein. There is some rather direct relationship between the base sequence of DNA and the amino acid sequence of the protein specified. Ribonucleic acid (RNA) appears to be involved in transferring the code from its place of storage in the nucleus to the site of primary gene action, that is, protein formation, in the ribosomes of the cytoplasm.

In accordance with the current views, all properties of a protein are a consequence of its amino acid sequence. Probably the proteins specified by genes are not only enzyme proteins but also may be structural proteins, e.g., collagen, or proteins with other functions and properties, such as hemoglobin. The useful concept of "one gene, one enzyme" requires modification to "one gene, one polypeptide," or (see below) "one cistron, one polypeptide."

In the schema outlined above mutation represents a change in the code, that is, a change in the base sequence of DNA. Mutations may be of two types. In "mis-sense" mutations a different amino acid is substituted at a given site in the particular protein, for example, valine for glutamic acid, changing "normal" hemoglobin to sickle hemoglobin. In "non-sense" mutations the change in the base sequence of DNA is such that there is no corresponding amino acid and none of a given protein, e.g., an enzyme, may be found.

The limits of the gene have become clearer. As a functional unit, called by Benzer the *cistron*, the gene is that portion of DNA responsible for specification of a single polypeptide and a *locus* is physically that portion of the linearly arranged genetic material (DNA) occupied by the cistron or gene. The alternative forms of the gene which occur at the same locus are called *alleles*. For example, the genes for A, B, and O blood types are multiple alleles at one locus. Within a locus there are many mutable sites. Obviously if the gene at a locus is responsible for specifying all the many amino acids in a complex protein, many base pairs are vulnerable to mutation. This much smaller unit is called by Benzer the *muton*. In the third place the genetic unit as revealed by recombination is referred to as the *recon*.

As stated above, the mutant gene can result in the formation of a different protein or of no protein at all of a given type. If the protein in question is an enzyme, none at all may be formed or an enzyme may be formed which is so impaired in its function that the net effect is the same. In intermediary metabolism such a change can have pathogenetic consequences through any of several mechanisms or through some combination of these. We can represent a hypothetical metabolic process as follows:

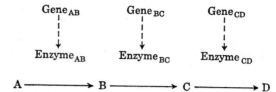

If a mutant form of $gene_{CD}$ results in no formation of $enzyme_{CD}$ or in the formation of functionally defective enzyme, then the effects may be of several types:

1. The disease characteristic may reflect the deficiency of product D:

$$A \longrightarrow B \longrightarrow C \longrightarrow\!\!\!/\!\!\!\longrightarrow (D)$$

Albinism (p. 544) might be cited as an example; melanin is not formed because of a block in tyrosine metabolism. In several forms of genetic cretinism (p. 427), thyroid hormone is not formed because of blocks of this type; in the adrenogenital syndrome (p. 523), hydrocortisone is not found.

2. A metabolite just proximal to the block may accumulate in toxic amounts.

$$A \longrightarrow B \longrightarrow \begin{matrix}C\\C\\C\end{matrix} \longrightarrow\!\!\!/\!\!\!\longrightarrow (D)$$

An example is alkaptonuria. Homogentisic acid is not metabolized normally. It is excreted in the urine in large amounts. Furthermore its increase in the body in some way leads to a form of degenerative arthritis.

3. If the reactions in question are reversible, there may be an accumulation of precursors farther back from the site of block.

$$\begin{matrix}A\\A\\A\end{matrix} \rightleftharpoons \begin{matrix}B\\B\end{matrix} \rightleftharpoons C \longrightarrow (D)$$

An example is the accumulation of glycogen in the form of glycogen storage disease (von Gierke's disease) in which the primary defect involves glucose 6-phosphatase (p. 571).

Glycogen $\rightleftharpoons$ glucose 1-phosphate $\rightleftharpoons$ glucose 6-phosphate

glucose 6-phosphatase

4. There may be production of products through an accessory pathway which is normally of minor significance.

$$A \longrightarrow B \longrightarrow C \longrightarrow\!\!\!/\!\!\!\longrightarrow (D)$$
$$\downarrow$$
$$X \longrightarrow Y \longrightarrow Z$$

In phenylketonuria, phenylketone products are produced in unusual amounts from phenylalanine, which is not properly metabolized. In hyperoxaluria, an excess production of oxalate may be the result of a defect in the normal metabolism of glyoxylate:

$$Glycine \rightleftarrows glyoxylate \longrightarrow formic\ acid + CO_2$$
$$\searrow$$
$$oxalic\ acid$$

Undoubtedly these do not exhaust the possible mechanisms of a pathogenetic effect from a mutation in a gene controlling an enzyme.

Metabolic processes are in most instances chains, indeed often networks. A mutation in the genes controlling any of several metabolic steps may lead to the same phenotypic result. Thus, the phenotype is not an indication of the specific genotype. Identical diseases may be produced by mutation of different genes; "genetic mimics," they are called.

Another type of process, not strictly enzymatic, by which mutations have pathogenetic effects involves changes in active transport mechanisms in the kidney and elsewhere. Cystinuria (p. 541) is an example. Other active transport systems can be cited, such as those involved in the movement of substances such as amino acids across the intestinal mucosa, of substances like bilirubin into and out of the liver cell, and of electrolytes across the muscle cell membrane. All these mechanisms are vulnerable to the effects of mutation in the determinant genes, and diseases for which such mutation is probably responsible can be cited.

Structural genes, i.e., those specifying the amino acid sequence of proteins, were briefly discussed above. "A pile of bricks is not a house," however. Other genes have a controlling role, ensuring an orderly interplay of the structural genes in development and in the adult organism. Mutation can occur also in these controlling genes with resultant disease. The evidence is coming mainly from the study of microorganisms; although a number of disorders of man are suspected to result from mutation in controlling genes, critical evidence is not easily assembled.

The complex machinery of protein synthesis, of which the framework is DNA-RNA-ribosomes, has become more clearly understood in recent years. Of potential therapeutic importance is the demonstration that intermediate steps in protein synthesis can be modified by various measures. It is possible, for example, that although a warped and enzymatically weak protein is formed in a given disorder, the amount synthesized can be increased by some means and the disease abolished or ameliorated.

The Genetics of Common Disorders

All disease is in some degree genetic and in some degree environmental in etiology and pathogenesis. As to the relative importance of endogenous and exogenous factors, disease can be thought of as falling on a spectrum (Fig. 55-14). Near the genetic end (G) are simply inherited disorders such as phenylketonuria and galactosemia, but these are not at the extreme end because exogenous factors, diet in these specific examples, can importantly modify the phenotype. Near the environmental end (E) are infectious diseases but again not at the extreme end because twin and other studies indicate a significant role of genotype in susceptibility.

In the analysis of disorders affecting all systems, two classes of disorders, with regard to the role of genetic factors, are evident: (1) rare, simply inherited disorders (near the G end of the spectrum); (2) common disorders in which genetic factors play some role. Examples in the gastrointestinal system are familial polyposis of the colon and peptic ulcer; in the cardiovascular system, hereditary hemorrhagic telangiectasia and coronary artery disease; in the connective tissue system, Marfan's syndrome and rheumatoid arthritis; in the eye, retinitis pigmentosa and glaucoma.

The common disorders are, for the most part, multifactorial in causation. The etiology is a nexus in which environmental and genetic factors collaborate in a complex way in determining the disease.

Questions asked in connection with common disease are mainly two: How significant are genetic factors in etiology? By what mechanism does the mutant gene contribute to the pathogenesis?

Methods for evaluating the role of genetic factors in common diseases are mainly six:

1. *Family studies.* If genetic factors are important, a familial aggregation for the disorder should be demonstrable. Familial aggregation can have other than a genetic basis; thus, evidence from family studies is per se not critical.

2. *Twin studies.* Monozygotic twins, because of genetic identity, should show a higher concordance rate (i.e., "both affected") than dizygotic twins show, if genetic factors are significantly involved.

3. *Interracial comparisons.* Races have different frequencies of many genes. If genetic factors are important in etiology, the frequency of common diseases may vary from race to race. A difficulty in interpretation of racial data is the uncertainty of environmental comparability. Races are social as well as biologic entities.

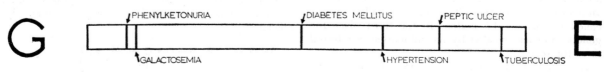

Fig. 55-14. Schematic representation of the spectrum of disease in regard to the relative importance of genetic (G) and exogenous (E) factors in etiology and pathogenesis.

4. *Component analysis.* Whenever a factor is shown to be an important element of the etiologic nexus, its genetics can be studied by family studies, twin studies, racial comparisons, and animal homologies. Lipid metabolism in atherosclerosis is an example.

5. *Blood group and disease association.* A simply inherited trait such as a specific blood group can, in some instances, be shown to occur more frequently with a given common disease than would be expected by chance. Some physiologic peculiarity of the person with that blood group seems to predispose him slightly but definitely to the disorder. The best example is the association between blood group O and peptic ulcer (p. 295). Demonstration of association is evidence of a genetic factor in the disorder. Failure to demonstrate association does not exclude the importance of genetic factors.

6. *Animal homologies.* If one has available in animals a disorder seemingly identical to a common disease of man, then one may be able to do breeding experiments and extensive biochemical and physiologic investigations that will throw light on the two questions stated above.

REFERENCES

Ferguson-Smith M. A.: Cytogenetics in Man, A.M.A. Arch. Int. Med., 105:627, 1960.
——: Chromosomes and Human Disease, in "Progress in Medical Genetics," vol. 1, A. G. Steinberg (Ed.), New York, Grune & Stratton, Inc., 1961.
Fraser-Roberts, J. A.: "Introduction to Medical Genetics," 3d ed., London, Oxford University Press, 1963.
McKusick, V. A.: "Human Genetics," Englewood Cliffs, N.J., Prentice-Hall, Inc., 1964.
——: "On the X Chromosome of Man," Washington, D.C., American Institute of Biological Sciences, 1964.
Stanbury, J. B., J. B. Wyngaarden, and D. S. Frederickson (Eds.): "The Metabolic Basis of Inherited Disease," 2d ed., New York, McGraw-Hill Book Company, Inc., 1965.

56 BLOOD GROUPS
M. M. Wintrobe

VARIETY OF BLOOD GROUP SYSTEMS AND FACTORS

In 1900 Karl Landsteiner studied the clumping which occurs when blood from one person is mixed with that of certain others and showed that this is due to completely normal properties in the cells and serum of the blood. These observations not only laid the ground for practical transfusion therapy but opened a field of knowledge which has not yet been exhausted. In addition to the A-B-O system with which Landsteiner first became engrossed, at least ten other "systems" of blood factors have been discovered (Table 56-1). The ramifications of these discoveries are of the utmost importance in human genetics and anthropology as well as in relation to disease and in the medicolegal field.

The number of different known blood factors is continuously enlarging. Thus it was found that there are qualitative differences in agglutinogen A. There are two main varieties, A_1 and A_2, thereby making two subgroups of A and two of AB (A_1B, A_2B). Still other variants of agglutinogen A exist, for example, A_x and A_m. It appears, furthermore, that group O is not the negative character (i.e., no A, no B) which was once assumed. Anti-O serums have been found to be of two kinds, namely, one which is inhibited by the addition of saliva of secretors of any group ("anti-H") and one which is not ("anti-O"). The H substance is found in almost all human red cells and is regarded as the basic substance from which the A and B substances are made under the influence of the A and B genes. Group O red cells contain the most H substance, since the O gene does not compete for this basic substance.

The discovery of a blood factor S related to the long-known M-N system, and the finding of still another blood factor, s, reciprocal to S, made it possible to distinguish nine M-N-S-s types. This, however, does not appear to be the end. There is evidence for a third allele at the Ss locus, Ss or S^u. There appear to be three alleles, M_1, M_2, and N, and perhaps still another, M^g. On the same chromosome but not allelic are Hu, He, Mi^a, Vw (Gr), and Vr. The P system, discovered at the same time as M and N and thought at first to be of little clinical or medicolegal significance, may prove to be of more importance than was thought at first.

As is well known, the Rh system, which came next in the expanding catalog of blood groups, has proved to be of major importance and also of great complexity. The discovery of anti-f made it necessary to postulate a fourth series of allelic antigens in the Rh system, f and a still hypothetical F, supplementing Dd, Cc, and Ee. However, f is now thought to be a "joint product" of ce. The Rh antibody anti-V now appears actually to be anti-ce^s, e^s and G may be another joint product. In addition, a number of alleles of these Rh antigens have been discovered, such as C^w, C^x, c^v, C^u, D^u, E^u, and E^w. The differences between the Fisher-Race and the Wiener systems of terminology and the genetic theories on which they are based cannot be considered here, but it should be mentioned that Wiener makes a distinction between an agglutinogen, a substance present on the surface of red blood cells that is identified by certain agglutination reactions with diagnostic reagents, and blood *factors*, which are attributes of the agglutinogen molecule that enable it to combine with antibodies. These have been named Rh^A, Rh^B, Rh^C, and Rh^D. Unfortunately, the inherent complexities of the subject are not being made easier by disagreement concerning nomenclature.

Other blood group systems listed in Table 56-1 include the reciprocal factors, Kell-Cellano (K, k) and several related alleles; antibodies for K have been

Table 56-1. BLOOD GROUP FACTORS

Name of system	Factors of clinical importance	Other identifiable factors
ABO.........	A, B	O, H
MNSs........	S, s, Ss, Miᵃ, Vw	M₁, M₂, N, Hu, He, Mᵍ
P..........	....	P₁, P₂, p, Pᵏ
Rh..........	{ D, Dᵘ { C, Cᵂ, Cˣ, cᵛ, Cᵘ, c { E, e, Eᵘ	Eᵂ
Kell.........	K	k, Kpᵃ, Kpᵇ, Kₒ
Duffy........	Fyᵃ	Fyᵇ
Kidd........	Jkᵃ	Jkᵇ, Jk
Lewis........	Leᵃ	Leᵇ
Lutheran.....	....	Luᵃ, Luᵇ
Diego........	....	Diᵃ
Sutter........	....	Jsᵃ, Jsᵇ

found in occasional serums from mothers of erythroblastotic babies and not infrequently in serums from persons who have had hemolytic transfusion reactions; Duffy (Fyᵃ, Fyᵇ), which has been responsible for a number of serious intragroup hemolytic transfusion reactions; and Kidd (Jkᵃ). The Lewis (Leᵃ, Leᵇ) and Lutheran (Luᵃ, Luᵇ) systems have not been thought to be of much importance antigenically in man, but anti-Leᵃ has been encountered in a few instances in which there was a history of transfusion. The Lewis system may be primarily an antigen system of the saliva and serum and only secondarily an antigen system of the red cells.

There is increasing evidence that the antigen *Diego* defines another locus controlling antigens of the red cells and saliva. This antigen is generally presumed to be a Mongolian character. It has been found in the blood of South American Indians, Japanese, and Chinese and only as an extreme rarity in the blood of Europeans and West Africans.

Still another well-established blood group system is Sutter and, besides this, a number of *"private" blood groups* have been discovered (Beᵃ, By, Swᵃ, Levay, and others) which are of such infrequent occurrence that they appear to be almost the private property of particular families. *"Public" antigens,* that is, those possessed by the vast majority of people, include Vel, Ytᵃ, and I.

MEDICOLEGAL AND ANTHROPOLOGIC IMPORTANCE

The three genes, A, B, and O, can occupy the same locus on a certain chromosome; that is, they are allelic. Each person inherits one of these genes from each of his parents. As a result six different combinations are possible, AA, BB, OO, AO, BO, AB. However, the factor O seems to be recessive to both A and B. Consequently the heterozygotes AO and BO cannot be differentiated by the usual typing techniques from the homozygotes AA and BB, respectively. For this

reason only four blood groups are distinguishable out of the six possible combinations.

The genes for the other blood group systems are thought to be present on different chromosome pairs, and there is no evidence that any of the groups are inherited together, or linked. Consequently the usefulness of serologic examinations in medicolegal and anthropologic work becomes apparent. It has been calculated that, with the ABO system and the two subgroups of A, the MNSs blood groups, P, the Rh system, Lutheran, Lewis, and Kell, the total number of possible different combinations of serologic recognizable phenotypes is 23,616 and the number of genotypes is 972,000. Because of technical and other difficulties, the P, Lewis, Kell, Duffy, and Kidd systems are not recommended for use in problems of parentage or identity, but even without them, when blood of the mother, the child, and the alleged father is available, it is possible to exonerate 51 per cent of all men wrongfully accused of paternity.

Of additional medicolegal importance is the fact that the antigens A, B, and H are present in saliva. The ability to secrete them is inherited as a mendelian dominant character not linked to the ABO genes. Persons whose red cells are Leᵃ positive are salivary nonsecretors of A, B, or H substance, whereas those who are Leᵇ are secretors. There are two distinct forms of the antigens: (1) a water-soluble form not present in the red cells or serum but present in most of the body fluids and organs of a secretor; and (2) an alcohol-soluble form, not influenced by the secretor gene, which is present in all tissues (except the brain) and in the red cells, but not present in the secretions. In secretors, blood group substances can be extracted with aqueous solutions from tissues and organs, especially salivary glands and gastric mucosa, and can be found in high concentration in secretions such as saliva, gastric juice, and semen. As a consequence it is possible to apply blood grouping to the examination of dried stains of saliva or semen and to saline extracts of muscle tissue.

In human genetics and anthropology the blood groups are of the utmost value for a number of reasons. The first is that they are sharply distinguishable "all-or-none" characteristics which do not grade into each other. Then again, they are simple, genetically speaking, and are inherited in a known way according to mendelian principles. Furthermore, they owe nothing to environment in their inheritance, nor are they subject to variations because of natural selection as is the case, for example, with skin color. Hence the blood groups are especially fitted to throw light on the moderately remote as well as the recent origins of mankind. Wide differences in frequency in different races have been observed. Consequently the blood groups provide valuable anthropometric measurements.

Considerable and interesting data are being accumulated concerning the ethnologic distribution of the blood groups. Thus the incidence of B has been found highest in certain parts of Asia and declines in

Table 56-2. DISTRIBUTION OF A-B-O, M-N, AND RH SYSTEMS

	A-B-O				M-N			Rh-Hr						
	O	A	B	AB	M	MN	N	cde	CDe	cDE	CDe/cDE	cDe	Cde	cdE
American Indians (Utah)....	97.4	2.6	0	0	58.7	34.6	6.7	0	33.7	28.8	37.5	0	0	0
Australian aborigines.......	48.1	51.9	0	0	2.4	30.4	67.2	0	58.2	8.5	30.4	1.3	1.7	0
Basques...................	57.2	41.7	1.1	0	23.1	51.6	25.3	28.8	55.1	7.8	6.0	0.6	1.8	
English..................	47.9	42.4	8.3	1.4	28.7	47.4	23.9	15.3	54.8	14.7	11.6	2.3	0.6	0.7
Negroes (U.S.A.)..........	51.5	29.5	15.5	3.5	23.0	51.5	25.5	8.1	20.2	22.4	5.4	41.2	2.7	0.5
White (U.S.A.)..........	42.2	39.2	13.5	5.1	29.9	50.2	19.9	13.5	33.5	13.0	13.8	2.5	0.5	0.5
Chinese..................	30.7	25.1	34.2	10.0	33.2	48.6	18.2	1.5	60.6	3.0	34.1	0.9	0	0
Asiatic Indians............	32.5	20.0	39.4	8.1	...	...	...	7.1	70.5	5.1	12.8	1.9	2.6	0

Italic figures—highest value in column; ... —no information.

all directions from central Asia except for a subsidiary high center in Africa. In the Old World the lowest figures have been found in the Scandinavian countries, and in Australia the gene seems to have been absent until very recent times. A similar complete absence has been found in the living aborigines of North America as well as in the Basques. Group O reaches levels of practically 100 per cent among certain Indian tribes in the United States. In the aborigines of America the gene for N is relatively rare, while in those of Australia it is very common. The factor P is much commoner in the blood of American Negroes than in that of American whites. The Rh-negative gene (cde) has been found in 13 to 17 per cent of modern inhabitants of Europe and in white inhabitants of America. In the Basques it reaches very high levels (28.8 per cent); in contrast, in a study of Eskimos only 1 out of 2,522 was found to be Rh-negative. Some representative figures are given in Table 56-2.

CLINICAL IMPORTANCE

Before discussing the relation of blood groups and blood transfusion, several other aspects may be considered briefly. It is well established that blood group incompatibility is responsible for at least one disease, hemolytic disease of the newborn (p. 635). From the standpoint of the pathogenesis of other acquired hemolytic anemias, the finding of anti-e in a patient with acquired hemolytic anemia whose red cells were of a genotype containing ee and other similar observations bring up the possibility that autosensitization may occur under special circumstances (p. 636).

It is possible that blood groups may be of clinical importance in other ways. It has been postulated that blood groups are examples of balanced polymorphism and that different combinations of genotypes may have different survival values. Unfortunately, information on this topic is as yet inadequate. Reports concerning an association between ABO blood groups and fertility are conflicting and difficult to interpret. It is also hard to evaluate the significance of reports concerning the relationship of these blood groups and prematurity and stillbirth or blood group "conflicts" and aberrant salivary secretion in spontaneous abortion.

It has been shown that there is a close association between blood group A and gastric cancer and with pernicious anemia. There is even a closer association between group 0 and duodenal ulceration, especially in nonsecretors. The association of ABO blood groups with diseases of the upper gastrointestinal tract suggests the possibility of some direct effect of the blood group mucoids since they are present not only in the saliva but also in the gastric and duodenal mucosa. Similar studies have been carried out with reference to many other conditions, but less strong support has been uncovered concerning the association of blood groups and these diseases.

As indicated in Table 117-1, blood transfusion reactions are of great variety. Those related to the blood groups are among the most serious and, unfortunately, though preventable, are all too frequent. The blood groups A and B or D (Rh) are involved in by far the great majority, perhaps 95 per cent of cases. This is because anti-A and anti-B antibodies occur naturally, and D is, like A and B, a strong antigen to which antibodies are produced readily. The first exposure to A or B of a person who does not possess the factor results in a hemolytic reaction if such blood is introduced. The transfusion of D blood to a person who is Rh-negative usually only sensitizes him; a second such transfusion may result in a hemolytic reaction. The Kell system (Kk) is also important because many K-negative persons can be sensitized to K by transfusion. The same holds true for E and c, but the danger is smaller. The remaining blood group factors are of still less importance. Nevertheless, it has been estimated that over 80 per cent of all transfusions given are possibly sensitizing ones. Scarcity of serums and the labor involved make it impractical to type routinely for all the known factors. The use of a sensitive cross-match test together with the Coombs test for "incomplete" antibodies is a helpful safeguard.

REFERENCES

Boyd, W. C.: "Genetics and the Races of Man," Boston, Little, Brown & Company, 1950.

Clarke, C. A., D. A. P. Evans, R. B. McConnell, and P. M. Sheppard: Secretion of Blood Group Antigens and Peptic Ulcer, Brit. Med. J., 1:603, 1959.

Owen, R. D., C. Stormont, I. B. Wexler, and A. S. Wiener: Medicolegal Applications of Blood Grouping Tests, J.A.M.A., 164:2036, 1957.

Plotkin, S. A.: The A-B-O Blood Groups in Relation to Prematurity and Stillbirth, J. Pediat., 52:42, 1958.

Race, R. R., and Ruth Sanger: "Blood Groups in Man," 3d ed., Oxford, Blackwell Scientific Publications, 1958.

Sussman, L. N.: Pitfalls of Paternity Blood Grouping Tests, Am. J. Clin. Pathol., 33:406, 1960.

Wintrobe, M. M.: "Clinical Hematology," 5th ed., Philadelphia, Lea & Febiger, 1961.

57 GROWTH AND DEVELOPMENT
Robert E. Cooke

The phrase "growth and development" has acquired a variety of vague meanings, ranging from changes in height to changes in emotional capacity. In this chapter, growth is defined as an increase in size with time, with particular emphasis on accretion of new protoplasm (largely protein and water) as opposed to changes in volume or weight such as might occur with edema. Development is defined as an increase with time in numbers of functions or in complexity of function, with biologic or behavioral aspects, or both, implied in that function.

Growth, as defined here, has two components— increase in cell number and increase in cell size. At various periods in life after conception, particularly early in gestation, increase in cell number may be primarily responsible for growth. During fetal life between 40 and 50 successive divisions take place, with an increase from one cell to 12×10^{12} cells at the time of birth. From birth to adulthood another four divisions occur. Early growth thereby occurs in a geometric progression. Subsequently there is a greater tendency for arithmetic accretion of protein. Numerous attempts have been made to develop equations describing growth. In general an S-shaped curve best fits the data.

In recent years more precise measurement of cell size has been possible by chemical analysis rather than by microscopic observations, including counts of mitotic activity. It has been determined that 6.2 to 7 $\mu\mu$g of DNA characterize most diploid cells. In the absence of polyploidy, measurement of total DNA content of one or more tissues establishes cell number. Protein and DNA analyses on similar samples make possible the calculation of cell size, since the water and protein contents of the body bear a straight-line relationship.

Liver nuclei demonstrate polyploidy under a variety of conditions, and the number and size of these cells cannot be determined readily by these simple analyses; actual counts of nuclei and chromosomes are necessary. Available data indicate that one tissue may differ markedly from another in respect to cell multiplication at various stages of growth. Muscle tends to approximate overall growth changes because it represents at least 40 per cent of the total lean body mass. Furthermore, cell multiplication may occur in spurts rather than as a continuous process. Likewise, growth as determined by changes in cell size varies markedly from one tissue to another and from one period of life to another.

The assessment of the growth rate of one tissue or another, or of the whole individual, must be related to the particular biologic age of the individual—i.e., the extent of maturation. In the human being, there is great variation in the onset of adolescence. The peak growth rate in height, for example, may occur anywhere over a 5-year period in chronologic age.

Development, as defined in this chapter, though far more difficult to quantify, also proceeds sporadically and in a nonlinear fashion. The appearance of marked increases in activity of certain enzymes—e.g., tyrosine hydroxylase—corresponds to certain biologic stages but may also exhibit considerable variability in time of peak activity. Likewise, the development of behavioral characteristics, when expressed in terms of norms, proceeds along a fairly smooth curve. However, the individual infant or child exhibits marked variability in rate of progress from one month or year to the next. For example, most infants show a fairly regular sequence of developmental milestones, but it is not unusual to see delays, then spurts; e.g., creeping may be delayed but walking accelerated.

CONTROL OF GROWTH AND DEVELOPMENT

Both phenomena obviously represent the interplay of genetic and environmental factors. Growth rates within a family show much less variability than when compared with those of the general population. Tall parents in general have tall children. However, in a process as complex as growth, many genes are involved, with rates of synthesis of many proteins being controlled by independently segregating genetic loci. It is not surprising, then, that physical size of a population has a normal Gaussian distribution. Environmental factors modify genetic expression considerably, however. Occasional monozygotic twins may differ markedly in size at birth, probably because of circulatory abnormalities. Geneticists some years ago predicted that the average height of the population would decrease because short persons were reproducing at a more rapid rate than the tall. Yet average height may actually be increasing because of environmental factors (possibly nutritional). At least greater growth rates are seen in the first 20 years of life now than in the previous generation.

A clearer understanding of the genetic control of development has come from the demonstration of various molecular forms of cell enzymes. Lactic dehydrogenase (LDH), for example, has been shown to be a variety rather than a single molecular species, with differing electrophoretic mobilities, amino acid sequences, and polypeptide groupings. The distribution of particular isozymes differs from one organ or tissue to another. Particular isozymes are present in varying amounts from one period in life to another. A variety of LDH appears in the testis in the human being and in several animal species only at sexual maturation. The mechanisms for turning genetic action on and off at a particular stage in the development of the individual remain unknown.

Exactly the same principles that apply to control of physical growth and maturation apply to behavioral development. The past tendency to attribute intelligence solely to genetic factors and the present tendency to disregard genetic factors in establishing relative limits for intellectual development are both contrary to the facts.

Gesell and others believed that behavior unfolded in an immutable manner, uninfluenced by experience and determined entirely by the innate potential of the individual. This hypothesis was supported by the fact that normative data collected on large numbers of infants and children indicated a fairly regular pattern for the appearance of a large number of items of behavior indicating cognitive and affective maturation.

Early experience, however, has been shown to alter behavioral development substantially. It has been shown that the longer the exposure to an underprivileged home the greater the fall in intellectual quotient. Children with inferior family and environmental histories, when placed in adoptive homes before the age of two years, despite obviously low IQ scores in the true parents and average but not superior IQ scores in the foster parents, had normal intelligence levels at five years, seven years, and thirteen years of age.

Studies of the intellectual development of twins reared in somewhat different environments show a greater correspondence in comparison with other children in the population but less than twins reared together.

The recent work of Hebb, Harlow, Riesen, and Piaget has reemphasized the influence of learning experiences on subsequent learning ability. Intelligent behavior results from the acquisition of and exploitation of many programs or schemata for solving problems. The initiative for searching for such programs is dependent on motivation—the genesis of which seems obscure but related in part to previous success or failure.

OPTIMAL GROWTH AND DEVELOPMENT

The possible relationship of longevity to rate of growth raises the issue that the maximal rate of growth may not necessarily be optimal. Much of the experimental data indicate that rate of growth in experimental animals and to an extent in human beings may be influenced by diet. Restriction of intake during gestation and prior to weaning may permanently slow growth despite free access to food thereafter. Increased longevity seemed to be associated with the limited food intake. Only one experiment has been designed to show that aging is probably associated with dietary factors rather than being directly related to accelerated rate of growth. The administration of growth hormone to animals previously subjected to dietary restriction restored growth rate to normal without shortening longevity. Diet, likewise, alters rate of maturation of certain tissues in a manner similar to the aging process. Concentrations of alkaline phosphatase, ATPase, and catalase and histidase increase with age in the rat liver.

The manipulation of diet can produce enzyme patterns in the younger rat comparable to those of a much older animal. Although changes in cell structure, water content, and the like may be responsible for some of these effects, the fact that changes in enzyme activity are in opposite directions lends significance to the findings.

Maximum behavioral development may or may not be optimal, just as with physical growth. Most of the evidence, however, indicates that superior intellectual performance is correlated with good emotional adjustment. Studies of the social success and accomplishments of gifted children negate the lay impression that "genius is tainted with madness." The more favorable environments of such children may be in part responsible for such adjustments. The fact that man has the longest ontogenetic preparatory period permitting opportunities for social training makes it possible for significant improvement of behavioral development providing the necessary condition for each child can be determined.

MEASUREMENT

The recording of changes in physical size and shape with age is important and a fairly reliable indicator of health. Many systems have been developed to facilitate comparisons with normal children of the same age, body build, weight, and height. The determination of prenatal growth and of premature birth in the past has been assessed primarily in terms of weight; gestational age, although necessarily inaccurate, is being utilized more frequently because of the relatively frequent occurrence of intrauterine growth disturbances. A combination of the two would seem desirable.

The prediction of adult size from measurements during childhood is reasonably accurate, paticularly if height and bone age are measured and if parental size is also appreciated. Height at three years shows a better correlation with height at maturity than at any other age. The correlation of childhood measurements with adult height were: birth, 0.77; one year, 0.67; two years, 0.75; and at five years, 0.79. One formula for prediction is that of Weech:

$$H_m = 0.545\,H_2 + 0.544\,A + 14.84 \text{ in.} \quad \text{(boys)}$$
$$H_m = 0.545\,H_2 + 0.544\,A + 10.09 \text{ in.} \quad \text{(girls)}$$

where H_m = height at maturity
　　　H_2 = height at two years
　　　A = average of parents' height

The standard deviation of difference in actual over predicted height is about 1 in.

The assessment of physical development is rapidly being improved. Such determinations as bone age, EEG, enzyme levels, and steroid excretion patterns indicate changes in function and serve to establish biologic age, particularly in the newborn period and at adolescence, when profound functional changes occur.

The measurement of intellectual development is now being criticized excessively—by modern psychologists especially. The evidence is irrefutable that there is a high correlation between test scores at ages four years and fourteen and school performance, although exceptions occur. Developmental quotients at one year correlate poorly with intelligence quotients in later childhood. However, low developmental scores at six, nine, and twelve months predict serious abnormality in later life with remarkable accuracy.

The major criticism of IQ predictions arises from the attempts of some investigators to attribute intelligence solely to genetic factors. The Gaussian distribution of intelligence test scores has been used as an argument for the genetic basis of intelligence. Unquestionably, there are multiple genetic factors with phenotypic manifestations far removed from primary gene action and, therefore, subject to great environmental alteration. The environmental factors probably have their greatest impact in the first 4 years of life, but, unfortunately, they have not been well characterized. Terms such as "cultural deprivation" and "inadequate stimulation" are used to describe the early environments of many children who later do poorly in school and in employment. The details of such experience that hinder or promote intellectual development in the human infant and child require much elaboration.

ABERRATIONS IN GROWTH AND DEVELOPMENT

Specific disturbances in physical growth and biologic development as well as behavioral development are discussed in other sections of this text. Retarded growth and slow intellectual development far exceed acceleration in frequency. The causes are multiple, and in no way can the terms "growth retardation" or "mental retardation" be considered as an adequate diagnosis. The etiology or pathophysiology leading to retardation must be searched for, even though at present the majority of cases cannot adequately be explained.

If the pathogenetic factor in growth can be ascertained and corrected, remarkable acceleration or "catch-up" growth may occur. In some cases of congenital heart disease, for example, surgical correction of the defect may lead to an increase in height age of several years occurring in several months. If excessive delay in correction occurs, eventual stature may be stunted.

Experience with correction of defects causing mental retardation is exceedingly limited. However, there are a few examples of young children reared in bizarre circumstances who seemed to have exhibited "catch-up" development when the biologic and behavioral environment was improved.

REFERENCES

Bloom, B. S.: "Stability and Change in Human Characteristics," New York, John Wiley & Sons, Inc., 1964.

Cheek, D. B., and R. E. Cooke: Growth and Growth Retardation: A Note on Normal Growth, Ann. Rev. Med., 15:357, 1964.

Riesen, A. H.: Effects of Early Deprivation of Photic Stimulation, in S. F. Osler and R. E. Cooke, "The Biosocial Basis of Mental Retardation," Baltimore, The Johns Hopkins Press, 1965, pp. 61–85.

Zinkham, W. H., A. Blanco, and L. J. Clowry, Jr.: An An Unusual Isozyme of Lactate Dehydrogenase in Mature Testes: Localization, Ontogeny, and Kinetic Properties, Ann. N.Y. Acad. Sci., 121:571–588, 1964.

58 AGING AND INVOLUTION
William Dock

DEFINITION AND GENERAL CONSIDERATIONS

Aging includes the acquired changes which need time for their development and also involutional changes which are as much a part of mammalian life as the autumnal involution of the leaves of deciduous trees. Accumulations of fat, of cholesterol in the arteries or gallbladder, of chalk in the cartilages, all require time; hence, they are more advanced in the aged than in the young. Changes in the subdeltoid tendon sheath or about the vertebral bodies occur from stress—the oftener the stress is repeated, the more marked the changes. Hence old persons show more change than younger ones. Involution probably also plays a part in altering the composition of the tissue in all these cases, but age and repeated exposure to a noxious influence are also necessary to evoke clinical evidence of impaired function.

Aging, then, may be defined as the sum of the losses of function and structure and of the callosities, scars, and nodular hyperplasias due to "wear and tear" and to involution. Wear and tear includes trauma; infection; overstimulation by emotional, dietary, or other abuses; dietary inadequacies; exposure to inclement weather; or exhausting exertion.

Involution may be defined as the physiologic changes in cellular activity leading to the altered structure and functional capacity characteristic of all senescent members of any species. The age at which, in any tissue, involution becomes manifest may show racial and often shows familial patterns, varying by years or even decades.

When degeneration is apparent at or soon after birth, or when it affects a minority of families, it sometimes is referred to as *abiotrophy*, but the boundary between classification as involutional or abiotrophic is arbitrary. If *involutional* designates "the usual or expected change occurring with age" and *abiotrophic* "the exceptional progressive anatomic and functional loss which may occur at any time during development or senescence," then gout and diabetes, idiopathic Parkinson's disease, and pernicious anemia are all abiotrophies, along with, perhaps, amyotrophic lateral sclerosis, Alzheimer's psychosis, and progressive muscular atrophy. In the future we may expect to learn more about the genetics and the external factors which control these disorders. Then we may include in aging many cases of Paget's disease, Graves's disease, myxedema, etc., which are now called idiopathic, or we may narrow aging to those disorders inevitably present in all men or women who reach the age of seventy, or ninety. Thus baldness and even graying of hair would be classified as abiotrophies, because they do not invariably manifest themselves before ninety.

Involutional changes cannot be distinguished from those due to mutagenic agents, such as cosmic radiation and that from radioisotopes, natural or from fallout, since these act uniformly on the population of large regions. There are data showing that irradiated animals and men with occupational exposure to high levels of gamma radiation age faster than do controls.

Abiotrophies cannot be distinguished from disorders which run in families, appear after adolescence, and are associated with autoantibodies. Classic examples are pernicious anemia and myxedema, with antibodies to human gastric mucosa and to the thyroid. Whether these antibodies result from age-dependent involution of such cells or are causative of the disease and result from involution of the thymolymphatic system has not been determined.

Under optimal conditions involutional tendency may remain subclinical. Thus gout, diabetes, or pernicious anemia, latent in a family, may not develop on a diet low in calories (for gout or diabetes) or rich in rare meat and liver (for pernicious anemia). The disorder might be blamed on dietary defect, although fundamentally it is due to innate metabolic fault.

AGING AND THE VASCULAR SYSTEM

Even in the aged, the vascular bed is able to grow and to adapt itself to circulatory needs. Tumors in the aged become well vascularized, and arteries leading to them enlarge strikingly. Only when the arterial lumen is severely encroached on by clots or atheromas does the vascular supply fail in the organs and brain of the aged. Inflammatory disease also may lead to vascular inadequacy at any age; and in the coronary arteries of the heart, atheromas may cause trouble soon after puberty in patients with very high blood cholesterol levels. The vessels of the legs also may suffer soon after maturity in such patients, and in severe hypertension, bilaterally symmetric and diffuse lesions of small arteries may become evident in the brain, retina, and kidneys, even before maturity. In the absence of initial unilateral lesions in the normotensive person, and in the absence of retinal lesions in the hypertensive one, it is never wise to ascribe changes in memory, judgment, and originality to cerebral arteriosclerosis. In the absence of angina or evidence of a myocardial infarct, it is equally unwise to ascribe cardiac failure to arteriosclerosis. In the heart there is only coronary atheromatosis involving the large epicardial branches; even in hypertension the arterioles in the myocardium usually remain unaltered.

The most vigorous objection must be registered to the notion that men are "as old as their arteries." Men may die of coronary atherosclerosis before they are old enough to vote; these arteries are diseased and not "old." Temporal arteries may stand out as large, tortuous vessels in men under thirty, yet at ninety the same men may be alert and in good health. This is due to fibrosis with ectasia, a clinically unimportant vascular involution. Men are as old as their skins, their scalps, their cerebral cortices, and all their other tissues. Since aging shows up most strikingly in the skin and brain, even when these have excellent vasculature, a man might be said to be no older than his ectoderm. He is vulnerable to death from a congenital weakness in 5 mm of his circle of Willis, or from an atheroma in 1 cm of one coronary artery.

MANIFESTATIONS OF INVOLUTION

The tissues of the body undergo aging at very different rates in different organs, species, and individuals. To some degree the rates are influenced by environment, nutrition, infection, trauma, or abuse, but even these influences are minimal—great variations in aging of specific tissues are obvious in individuals and in families as well as in species. Grizzly bears and gorillas have graying of the hair on reaching maturity; other bears and primates have none at advanced ages; some families turn white in the thirties, others not until after seventy. Wrinkling of the face and neck may occur early in members of families who become neither bald nor gray until old age. Pulmonary elastic fibers may age and emphysema become troublesome in men whose elastica ages slowly in the skin or the arteries.

The pattern of graying, baldness, and coarsening of the hair of the face, nostrils, and ears shows clearly how atrophy may proceed in one area while hypertrophy is occurring in another. Focal hyperplasia in the presence of atrophy is a commonplace of aging of the skin, breast, prostate, and thyroid, and in the gastric mucosa. Symmetric degeneration of neurones may occur in certain parts of the cerebral cortex, or the cerebellum, or the substantia nigra, while preservation of neurones in adjacent regions is still excellent. This is often incorrectly ascribed to vascular disease; in the scalp no loss of vascularity is necessary to cause baldness or graying, and in the brain no local ischemia precedes the symmetric loss of neurones. In many organs, involutional atrophy of the parenchyma precedes disuse atrophy of the vascular bed, which then undergoes secondary degenerative changes.

Physiologic involution, such as that in the lens and uveal tract which causes loss of near vision (presbyopia, or the "elder's eye"), may be associated with minimal histologic change. Anatomic involution, such as disseminated cortical atrophy of the frontoparietal regions, may be grossly striking, with almost no functional loss. In the former type, chemical systems age and wear out, but cell structure is little altered; in the latter, cells disappear but the effect is minimal because vital activity is carried on in adequate fashion by the remaining tissue. The aging heart recovers less rapidly during diastole than does the young heart; consequently, heart failure occurs under conditions which a few decades earlier did not even cause transient dilatation. In all such cases, the diagnosis of involution is made from two sets of facts. The mature patient may become senile in certain tissues at almost any age, and, therefore, maturity is one essential datum. The other is the demonstrated absence of infections or metabolic or vascular disorders capable of accounting for the phenomenon in question. Thus pellagra may simulate involution of the brain, beriberi simulate involution of the heart, and syphilitic aortitis simulate senile dilatation and elongation of the aorta. Much the most convincing evidence for involutional causation is a familial similarity in age of onset and distribution, and the widespread occurrence of similar disorders in aging mammals of various species.

Fortunately, many involutional losses are readily corrected—the hair can be dyed, the long hairs in the ears and nostrils clipped, the bald scalp can be wigged with a toupee. Others are turned to assets: the faulty memory of the aged and their deafness excuse much and spare effort and annoyance. Finally, some chemical involutions can be corrected. Those which cause pernicious anemia and combined cord lesions are effectively treated with vitamin B_{12}; senile heart failure is usually responsive to digitalis; presbyopia is easily corrected by eyeglasses, etc. Some physicians hesitate to diagnose disease as due to involution until after threescore years and ten, or avoid this diagnosis altogether because it suggests an incurable disorder. Both these reasons are incorrect. Many involutions, like presbyopia, can be demonstrated in larval stages in the twenties in nearly everyone; others, like baldness and the disorders of urate metabolism called gout, are manifest before forty in

a very appreciable percentage of all those finally recognized; and many involutions, after rapid progress for a few years, become arrested and often compensated.

The involution of greatest importance to society and to the physician is that of the central nervous system. Anatomically, this is characterized by loss of neurones, which is demonstrable in the spinal cords and brains of mice, rats, and men. Loss of motor neurones decreases the fiber count of the spinal nerves and probably contributes to the loss of agility and athletic prowess, with sustained capacity for prolonged heavy loads of work, which is typical of middle and old age. Loss of neurones in the basal ganglions accounts for tremor, rigidity, and even full-blown clinical disorders such as idiopathic parkinsonism.

But most important of all is the loss of cortical neurones which diminishes the acuteness of observation and, when severe, leads to the apathy, irritability, stolidity and garrulousness, overly great concern for minutiae, and loss of concern about essentials which are characteristics of senile psychoses and of many older people merely regarded as eccentric or bureaucratic. Older patients' histories are notoriously undependable. For every man or woman in whom "old experience do attain to something like prophetic strain," there are half a dozen in the asylums and several score who "ain't what they used to be." It is the physician's function to detect the remediable disorders, such as brain tumor, pellagra, pernicious anemia, or myxedema, which masquerade as senile behavior, and to do what is possible to secure maximum comfort and effectiveness from the waning powers of aging men and women. Nothing is gained by refusal to recognize the fact that all men age and die and that involution of many tissues sets in with maturity, not with old age.

One of the great tragedies of urban civilization is the treatment of elderly people slipping into second childhood or second infancy (with loss of concern for cleanliness, bowel or bladder function) as if they were insane. In rural or primitive cultures, such people are cared for by their relatives in the familiar environment of their homes. This can become impossible in small apartments, and there should be orphan asylums and foundling homes to provide for unwanted people in second childhood and infancy. They are not helped by psychiatric treatment, are upset by the strange environment of hospital or asylum, and deteriorate rapidly under sedative therapy.

This problem will grow as science brings arterial disease and neoplasia under control. These disorders, by removing aging people, serve an important biologic purpose, creating opportunity and removing burdens from those in the child-rearing age. During the nineteenth century when pneumonia killed more people, Sir William Osler called it "the old man's friend" for, like Ecclesiasticus, he considered death kind to the old and feeble. Inheritance of resistance to involution, arterial disease, and cancer is evident in many families, but this biologic blessing is often paid for by the necessity to live with or support aged relatives. In an urban society, such obligations favor late marriage and few or no children. Success in eradicating arteriosclerosis, cancer, and rapid aging will tend to be frustrated by natural selection, and the survival of more grandchildren in families with few living grandparents. Atherosclerosis and neoplasia are now the chief factors in determining that we do not decline into second childhood, do not overstay our biologically allotted span of life too long.

REFERENCES

Birren, J. E.: Human Aging, a Biological and Behavioral Study, U.S.P.H.S. Publication 986, 1963.

Bourne, G. H., et al.: "Structural Aspects of Aging," New York, Hafner Publishing Company, 1961.

Burch P. R. J..: Mutation, Autoimmunity, and Aging, Lancet, 2:299, 1963.

Corsallis, J. A. N.: "Mental Illness and the Aging Brain: The Distribution of Pathological Change in a Mental Hospital Population," London, Oxford University Press, 1962.

Korenchevsky, V., and G. H. Bourne: Physiological and Pathological Aging, New York, Hafner Publishing Company, 1961.

59 PRINCIPLES OF NEOPLASIA

Sumner Wood, Jr., and Ivan L. Bennett, Jr.

DEFINITIONS

A *neoplasm* is a proliferation of new cells that may progress, become quiescent, or regress. Although *tumor* literally signifies swelling from any cause, the terms neoplasm and tumor are often used synonymously in clinical parlance. Although the initiating factor in human tumors is usually unknown, it is clear that progressive, uncontrolled, and autonomous growth may continue after cessation of the provocative stimulus, indicating a heritable disorder of cellular multiplication.

A *benign* neoplasm is composed of normal or nearly normal cells whose growth is local, demarcated, or encapsulated. *Malignant* tumors, or *cancers*, are characterized by uncoordinated growth, usually without sharp delimitation of borders; as cellular multiplication progresses and becomes autonomous, morphologic characteristics frequently become atypical or undifferentiated ("anaplastic"), infiltration and invasion of adjacent tissues follow, and dissemination to remote sites may result in secondary growths, or metastases.

It is important to recognize that the word *cancer* designates disorders of many etiologies; biologically, physically, and chemically, the term is no more specific than *inflammation, degeneration,* or *infection*. Consequently, it is extremely difficult to generalize about many aspects of neoplastic disease; for detailed discussions, the reader should refer to the monographs listed at the end of the chapter.

Biochemical differences between neoplastic and normal tissues have been investigated extensively, but no universal specific or distinctive alteration has been found.

Even a consistent morphologic classification of tumors is lacking. Although malignant tumors usually show malignant aberrations in growth pattern and cytologic features, the histology of a malignant, metastasizing tumor, such as follicular carcinoma of the thyroid gland, may be indistinguishable from that of the normal tissue from which it arises. The recognition that many neoplasms are malignant has come only from careful correlation of the histologic patterns observed by the pathologist with the biologic behavior and clinical course of the tumors in man. It is obvious that the distinction between benign and malignant neoplastic disease is of fundamental importance in therapy and prognosis.

A malignant tumor derived from ectodermal or entodermal structures is a *carcinoma*, and one derived from mesoderm is a *sarcoma*. This basic distinction is not always clear-cut, an example being the melanoma or melanosarcoma, whose cellular origin is uncertain although its morphologic characteristics and clinical behavior are well established. Tumors of the central nervous system (see Chap. 206) are classified separately, and tumors arising from lymph nodes or related structures are often referred to as *lymphomas*.

A *teratoma* is a neoplasm arising from both mesodermal and ectodermal (or entodermal) tissues. Most teratomas are benign, but one or more components may be malignant; the recognition of the malignancy of a teratoma sometimes poses great difficulty for the pathologist.

A *hamartoma* is a focal proliferation of cells normally present in an organ and is probably best regarded as a congenital malformation rather than a true neoplasm.

ETIOLOGY

No precise causes are known for the majority of human tumors. It can only be hoped that accumulating knowledge of agents that will elicit cancer in experimental animals and of the many factors such as heredity, diet, and occupational exposure that seem to influence the incidence of neoplastic diseases in different ethnic groups and geographic areas will eventually clarify the situation.

GENETIC FACTORS. Experimentally, the role of heredity is easily demonstrable by inbreeding animals to produce strains which show a very low or very high incidence of spontaneous tumors. Isolated examples of human families in which tumors of several types have occurred with extraordinary frequency in as many as four generations are also well documented. Among the neoplastic diseases of man with known familial occurrence are von Recklinghausen's neurofibromatosis, polyposis coli, retinoblastoma, osteochondroma, and pheochromocytoma. Other new growths such as nevi, hemangiomas, chondromas, neurofibromas, teratomas, neuroblastomas, and Wilms's tumors of the kidney are often congenital, being present at birth. The high incidence of leukemia in patients with mongolism, now established as a chromosomal disorder, implies an association between chromosomal aberrations and neoplasms that is further suggested by the occurrence of the so-called "Philadelphia chromosome" in chronic myeloid leukemia.

VIRUSES. Viral etiology has been established for tumors in many experimental animals, including the chicken, frog, rabbit, mouse, and hamster. In man, present evidence indicates that a virus causes warts. However, it must be emphasized that the absolute identification of a virus as the causative agent of a human cancer would not be an indication for reclassifying the tumor. The lesion would still be a neoplasm —a neoplasm of known causation, similar to malignant growths induced by chemicals or ionizing radiation.

PHYSICAL AGENTS. The major physical agent known to produce both animal and human neoplasms is *ionizing radiation*. Examples in man include osteogenic sarcoma ("phossy jaw") after occupational exposure to radium, cutaneous carcinomas after x-ray exposure, and the high incidence of leukemia among those who were survivors of the atomic blast at Hiroshima. Thymic or pharyngeal irradiation during infancy has been associated with an increased frequency of thyroid carcinoma in young individuals, and therapeutic irradiation of benign giant-cell tumors of bone has resulted in osteogenic sarcoma. The so-called "Schneeberg carcinomas" of the lung in cobalt miners in Saxony are the result of the inhalation of radon. There is an increase in cutaneous cancer among individuals exposed chronically to actinic (sun) rays, noted especially in sailors, farmers, and fair-skinned races. Carcinoma of the skin is forty-five times as frequent in Caucasians living in Hawaii as it is among Orientals and Hawaiians. The congenital disorder *xeroderma pigmentosum*, characterized by unusual sensitivity to sunlight, is well known to predispose to cutaneous carcinoma at an early age.

Mechanical trauma is virtually never a primary or contributory cause of cancer.

CHEMICAL AGENTS. More than 500 different compounds of diverse chemical structure will produce experimental neoplasms. In man, the scrotal carcinoma of chimney sweepers was the first-recognized "occupational tumor." Others include cancer of the lip in Scottish fishermen who customarily held the tarred twine used in mending nets between the teeth, carcinoma of the lung in chromate workers (and possibly in nickel workers), malignant mesotheliomas of the pleura or peritoneum in asbestos workers, and carcinoma of the bladder among aniline-dye workers exposed to *beta-naphthylamine*. There is a strong statistic correlation between cigarette smoking and lung cancer; the controversy over the

etiologic significance of this will continue for a long time. Two examples of the role of chemical (or thermal) irritation in human tumorigenesis are observed in South Asia: the so-called "Andhra carcinoma" of the hard palate in South Indian women who smoke *chottas*, native cigars, "hotside in," and the well-documented increase in oral cancer among chewers of betel (areca) nut.

HORMONES. A variety of hormones, especially the sex steroids, is capable of inducing malignant tumors in animals. Although no direct causal relationship is known between hormones and tumors in man, striking alterations in the course of prostatic or breast cancer have been produced by giving sex hormones, by castration, by hypophysectomy, or by adrenalectomy. That these substances sometimes play a contributory or permissive role in human neoplasms seems beyond doubt.

MISCELLANEOUS FACTORS. A variety of studies illustrates the multiplicity of potential carcinogens or cocarcinogens. Laryngeal and esophageal cancer are more frequent in alcoholics. Hepatic cancer is associated with nutritional imbalance or dietary factors (e.g., aflotoxin) in Bantus; in the United States, more than 50 per cent of hepatomas occur in adults with cirrhosis of the liver. Studies among different ethnic groups in Hawaii have shown that gastric cancer is two and one-half times as common in Japanese males as in Caucasian men, that prostatic cancer is nine times as common in Caucasians as in Japanese, that the incidence of mammary carcinoma in Japanese women is less than one-fourth of that in Caucasian women, and that although Chinese compose only 6 per cent of the population, 76 per cent of nasopharyngeal carcinomas occur in Chinese patients.

The presence of neoplastic disease predisposes to further cancer, as evidenced by the observation that a patient with one malignant tumor is two to six times more likely than others to develop a second primary cancer.

There are, obviously, many "statistically significant" differences in the incidence of neoplasms among ethnic and racial groups, but the interpretation of these data is complicated by many differences in diet, climate, occupation, and coexisting endemic diseases. Presently, the usefulness of epidemiologic studies of human cancer is sharply limited by the problem of multiple factors that cannot yet be isolated from one another. Although findings in surveys often suggest excellent subjects for experimental testing, they rarely suffice for any new etiologic conclusions.

INCIDENCE

With increase in life expectancy and lowering of the number of deaths from infectious agents, incidence of and mortality from cancer have risen. As a cause of death in the United States, cancer is second only to circulatory disease in adults and to accidental trauma in children. About half the childhood deaths from malignant disease are caused by leukemia.

In the United States, the most frequent cancer in males is cutaneous, and mammary carcinoma is the commonest in women. The pattern varies enormously in other countries and geographic areas, and generalizations cannot be made.

PROPERTIES OF MALIGNANT NEOPLASMS

There are endless variations in the growth rate of different tumors, in their local invasiveness, and in their routes and sites of metastasis. Although multiplication of neoplastic cells may proceed more rapidly than that of many normal cells, this property alone does not imply malignancy of a tissue; indeed, the generation time of cells during embryogenesis, regeneration of liver, or the normal replacement of intestinal mucosa is shorter than that of most tumors.

Basal cell carcinoma of the skin is locally invasive, but metastasis is exceedingly rare. Epidermoid carcinoma of the skin frequently metastasizes by way of lymphatics, but melanomas can spread to regional nodes and also disseminate widely by the bloodstream while the primary lesion is still minute and inconspicuous.

Progressive growth, ulceration with bleeding, or pressure upon adjacent structures resulting in pain or obstructive phenomena may call attention to the primary tumor. Generally, cancer cells are less cohesive than normal cells, a property which may be of great importance in their detachment from the main growth, making possible their detection by the methods of exfoliative cytology.

PRECANCEROUS LESIONS, *IN SITU* CARCINOMA, AND MALIGNANT TRANSFORMATION. It is very rare for a benign tumor to become a cancer. However, on a purely empirical basis, it has come to be recognized that certain lesions are associated with later development of cancer frequently enough that excision or other active treatment is indicated. Leukoplakia of the oral cavity or female genitalia, senile keratosis of the skin, arsenical keratosis (Chap. 251), intestinal polyps, and cutaneous nevi showing "junctional activity" (Chap. 108) fall into this group. Other lesions that may be complicated by cancer are cirrhosis of the liver, thermal burn scars, and the atrophic gastritis of pernicious anemia (Chap. 112). Benign chondromas are often difficult to excise completely, and serial recurrences and removals for many years may lead to the development of chondrosarcoma at the local site. Whether this is the natural course of the tumor or malignant transformation resulting from repeated surgical trauma is not known. However, in the absence of repeated specimens indicating that a tumor was benign, the criticism can always be raised that it was malignant from the first and that no transformation was involved.

The terms *intraepithelial carcinoma* and *carcinoma in situ* are used interchangeably to describe foci of cytologically abnormal cells in which there is disruption of normal arrangement or sequence of cell types without invasion of adjacent tissue. They are used most often in connection with lesions of the uterine cervix and breast but are also applied to skin, stomach, bladder, bronchus, etc. The very names imply the malignant potential of the lesion, and it is customary to manage such foci as though they were indeed malignant. However, the true incidence of invasive carcinomas that arise in such lesions if they are undisturbed is not known. Indeed, to determine their existence requires excision and, consequently, those who prefer to believe that the lesion is premalignant can account for failure of cancer to appear in a patient with *carcinoma in situ* by claiming that the original biopsy also constituted surgical excision. Valuable as the definitive information would be, it seems unlikely that long-term studies in untreated patients will ever now be completed under conditions that will yield reliable answers.

METASTASIS. The occurrence of metastasis is the most decisive factor determining the choice of treatment and the success of therapy. Wound contamination by tumor cells can result in local *implant metastases*, largely preventable by meticulous surgical technique.

Invasion of lymphatics and spread to regional nodes are usually managed by excision of the primary with dissection and removal of the nodes or postoperative irradiation of them.

The occurrence of direct venous invasion and hematogenous transport of tumor cells is being recognized with increasing frequency. Venous invasion is demonstrable in about 40 per cent of resected carcinomas of the rectosigmoid, 70 per cent of lung cancers, and 80 per cent of gastric cancers. Manipulation or operative trauma may increase the number of cells released from the primary lesion into lymphatics and blood vessels. The prognostic significance of finding tumor cells in the blood has not as yet been established. *Tumor cell embolism does not necessarily mean metastasis.* Patients with venous invasion and circulating tumor cells have survived for many years after surgical excision of the primary growth. Experimental studies have revealed that an enormous number of cells must be injected into the bloodstream to produce a single metastasis.

The mechanisms responsible for the *organ selectivity* and latency (dormancy) of metastasis are unknown.

GRADING AND STAGING. For uniform evaluation of the natural behavior and response to therapy, methods of grading and staging have been proposed for specific tumors. *Grading* refers to the degree of histologic differentiation. Low-grade neoplasms (grade I) consist of well-differentiated, nearly normal-appearing cells; grade III and IV neoplasms are less differentiated or pleomorphic. *Staging* refers to extent; in the colon, stages include involvement of mucosa, or muscularis, of local lymph nodes, or distant sites.

SYSTEMIC EFFECTS

NUTRITIONAL. Weight loss and eventual inanition are frequent in extensive malignant neoplastic disease. This is usually attributable to a combination of anorexia, blood loss, diarrhea, fever, etc., rather than to any specific property of the tumor.

SPECIFIC METABOLIC CHANGES. The tissue concentrations of enzymes such as catalase and lactic acid dehydrogenase are nonspecifically lowered. Serum acid phosphatase level is elevated in disseminated prostatic cancer, and serum alkaline phosphatase level often rises when the liver or bones contain metastatic tumor. Peculiar neuropathy or myopathy and clubbing of the fingers may be reversed by removal of a small bronchogenic carcinoma. The systemic effects of serotonin elaborated by malignant carcinoid (Chap. 98), intractable peptic ulceration (Zollinger-Ellison syndrome, Chap. 180) accompanying tumors of the pancreatic islets or duodenum, and the hormonal effects of gonadal (Chap. 90), hypophyseal (Chap. 80), adrenal (Chap. 84), or pancreatic islet (Chap. 198) neoplasms are other systemic effects. *Thrombophlebitis* sometimes precedes other symptoms of pancreatic, bronchogenic, or gastric tumor by months, and intractable *pruritus* is the first manifestation of Hodgkin's disease in some patients. Elevation of blood uric acid level or of basal metabolic rate is seen in Hodgkin's disease and leukemia.

Many tumors of nonendocrine origin are now known to elaborate humoral substances which simulate hormonal action. Their systemic effects include hypercalcemia, hypoglycemia, polycythemia, Cushing's syndrome, inappropriate antidiuresis, thyrotoxicosis, and others which are reviewed in the article by Lipsett listed at the end of this chapter.

Fever, the mechanism of which is not understood, accompanies many tumors, especially lymphoma, renal carcinoma, and hepatic metastases.

PSYCHOLOGIC EFFECTS. No disease is more dreaded by the patient than cancer. Whether the patient should be told that he has this disease has been debated for years. As more and more patients are seen at the early stages of the disease when a cure may be expected and knowledge of the cure rate becomes known to the general public, the old fear may diminish, as it has for tuberculosis.

In the advancing stages of cancer an air of hope and optimism should be maintained not only for the patient but also for the relatives. Often the patient will suspect that he has cancer but will not ask, but a responsible member of the family should be informed of the diagnosis.

A combination of professional skill, common sense, and compassion will indicate the necessary management.

CANCER AND OTHER DISORDERS

The clinical association between benign or malignant tumors and other diseases is poorly understood in most instances. A partial list of tumors and diseases with which they seem to be clinically associated includes pernicious anemia (gastric carcinoma), cirrhosis or hemochromatosis (hepatoma), congenital cystic disease (bronchogenic carcinoma), polyposis coli (colonic carcinoma), chronic ulcerative colitis (colonic carcinoma), Paget's disease of the nipple (mammary duct carcinoma), Paget's disease of bone (osteogenic sarcoma), myasthenia gravis (thymoma), mongolism (leukemia), xeroderma pigmentosum (skin cancer), Peutz-Jeghers syndrome (colonic carcinoma), acanthosis nigricans (visceral carcinoma), and dermatomyositis (several types).

DIAGNOSIS

Other sections of this book describe the clinical manifestations of specific tumors and the use of laboratory tests, endoscopy, and x-ray studies in diagnosis. The discussion that follows is confined to the problem of the definitive diagnosis of tumors by microscopic examination of biopsy specimens or of smears of exfoliated cells.

In the examination of excised tissue, accurate diagnosis depends on the skill and experience of the pathologist. The clinician should remember that the interpretation of histologic findings in terms of the individual patient is not an "objective" exercise in exact morphology but may vary importantly with the patient's age, sex, medication, and x-ray findings (especially in bone tumors). All pertinent data should be made available to the pathologist, tissue specimens should be adequate in size, and the occasional need for additional biopsies should be recognized. It is not unusual, for instance, to find nonspecific and nondiagnostic changes in the structure of one or two excised lymph nodes, only to discover the characteristic lesion of Hodgkin's disease in a third specimen from the same patient.

The common practice of having histologic sections and x-rays reviewed and reinterpreted by another pathologist and radiologist when a patient comes under the care of another clinician illustrates the importance of individual skill and experience. This practice does not signify any innate unreliability of the methods employed or a distrust of the professional opinions of others; it is no more difficult to understand than is the insistence of a clinician on taking his own history and performing his own physical examination on a patient, no matter how frequently others may have carried out the same procedures.

Clinically benign lesions that may be mistakenly identified as histologically malignant include pseudoepitheliomatous hyperplasia secondary to insect bites or to a benign tumor called granular cell myoblastoma, juvenile fibromatosis, fibroxanthomas, intraductal hyperplasia or papillomas of the breast, chronic pancreatitis, oral lichen planus, myositis ossificans, and a poorly understood entity known as pseudosarcomatous fasciitis.

Lesions that may be histologically benign in appearance but can behave as malignant tumors include smooth-muscle neoplasms of the stomach, villous polyps of the colon, mixed salivary gland tumors, follicular thyroid tumors, and cartilaginous tumors. These can pose serious problems in clinical management because of the difficulty of accurate histologic distinction between malignant and benign forms.

EXFOLIATIVE CYTOLOGY. The examination of exfoliated cells in vaginal secretions by the method of Papanicolaou is accurate in detecting early carcinoma of the uterine cervix. The so-called "Pap smear" for this tumor is the only screening technique that is simple and sensitive enough to be applied in a practical way to mass examination of the population.

Accurate cytologic diagnosis is also possible for carcinoma of the larynx (sputum), lung (sputum, bronchial washings), kidney and bladder (urine), gastrointestinal tract (saline washings), biliary tract (duodenal washings), and breast (nipple secretions). Furthermore, the certain identification of cancer cells in cerebrospinal fluid, peripheral blood, and effusions into pleural, pericardial, peritoneal, or synovial cavities is feasible. However, for all these other tumors, the preparation of the patient, the collection and processing of specimens before cells degenerate, and the thorough examination of numerous smears require meticulous technique and many hours of the time of professional personnel. Simplification of tedious methodology, without sacrificing sensitivity and accuracy, is greatly needed.

The use of exfoliative cytology for the detection of cervical cancer in totally asymptomatic women is well established, and the Pap smear is becoming almost as routine as the blood count in physical checkups. However, no comparable test of the accuracy of cytologic methods for detecting *unsuspected* and *asymptomatic* tumors of other types has yet been possible. Most experience has been limited to patients with symptoms or signs of disease in a specific organ system, and it is probable that methods will never be simplified to an extent that will permit general "screening" of the population for malignant disease.

Presently, exfoliative cytology is a valuable diagnostic method in selected cases and supplements other diagnostic methods without eliminating the need for them.

THERAPY AND THE EVALUATION OF THERAPEUTIC RESULTS

The major avenues of attack on the neoplastic process are surgery, irradiation, and chemotherapy.

Total excision of tumors is desirable whenever possible. Advances in anesthesiology, general supportive care, and plastic surgery have made possible many radical and superradical operations. Surgical procedures have been extended to their anatomic limits. Further advances will be dependent on earlier diagnosis or the use of adjuvants to surgical treatment. Evaluation of the results in terms of cure and palliation balanced against immediate operative mortality and patient disability remains to be completed for many of these procedures. It is not surprising that there is considerable controversy over specific surgical techniques among different clinics and that the relative merits of surgery and irradiation are still unclear. The initial enthusiasm for radical operations has not yet been supported by a significant increase in survival rates.

Irradiation, including supervoltage therapy, is curative for some tumors. It is also occasionally of benefit in the management of disseminated diseases, e.g., treatment of skeletal metastases in cancer of the breast. Radioactive isotopes are effective with certain carcinomas of the thyroid (Chap. 82). The evaluation of results of treatment of "deep" tumors (lung, esophagus) using high-voltage beams awaits careful follow-up studies. Ionizing radiation should be avoided for benign or banal lesions except under very rare circumstances. A combination of radiation and surgery or radiation and chemotherapy sometimes gives better results than those achieved with the use of one modality. The judicious application of the available methods in the individual patient can prolong survival with many incurable tumors and enable a patient to continue an active, pain-free, and useful life for months or years.

With rare exceptions, chemotherapy is palliative or suppressive rather than curative. Since a unique metabolic system has not been found in the cancer cell, present chemotherapeutic agents are effective against any cell system with a high rate of synthesis of nucleoproteins. The gastrointestinal tract, hematopoietic system, and germinal cells are therefore as susceptible as most tumors. There are two general classes of antitumor drugs in wide use, the antimetabolites and the alkylating (sometimes called radiomimetic) drugs. Their use is usually limited by their effect on sensitive normal cells. This limits sharply their dosage and raises many problems because of undesirable, uncomfortable, and dangerous side reactions. Furthermore, the wide differences in tumors themselves make it just as unlikely that any single universal "cure" of cancer will be discovered as it is that any antibiotic will be found that can cure all bacterial, rickettsial, and viral infections.

The use of hormones and castration can produce striking remissions in prostatic or mammary carcinoma, and adrenal steroids often ameliorate symptoms of neoplastic disease without modifying its course. In certain cases of leukemia and lymphoma, corticosteroids may also exert some direct, though transient action upon the tumor itself.

Many other agents such as bacterial toxins, venoms, anticoagulants, protamine, dextran, fibrinolytic agents, and viruses have their advocates and are under continuing investigation. The therapy of cancer should be considered not only as the direct eradication of the tumor, but also antistromal therapy and augmentation of natural defense mechanisms of the host.

Intraarterial infusion or isolated perfusion of a diseased organ to allow delivery of larger doses of a drug to the tumor without systemic toxicity may be useful in special cases such as malignant melanomas involving the lower extremities, parotid tumors, and hepatomas.

An enormous program for discovery of new chemotherapeutic agents and generous support of cooperative clinical trails of their effectiveness and toxicity is sponsored on a continuing basis by the United States Public Health Service; eventually, improved agents may become available.

For many types of cancer, knowledge of the natural history of the disease and of the variations that may occur in the absence of treatment is incomplete, a fact which obviously makes the evaluation of therapeutic regimens difficult. For most tumors, the results of therapy may also be expected to depend on the extent of the lesion at the time treatment is initiated. It is in the attempt to standardize this variable that techniques of staging and grading have been developed for several common cancers. Controversy as to the optimal means of therapy can be resolved only by controlled, randomized series of cases, treated by the various modalities in question and followed for long periods of time after treatment.

The management of recurrent cancer presents an even greater challenge than the primary tumor. Aggressive treatment directed at the recurrence is usually not indicated, although notable exceptions with long-term survival warrant caution, care, and optimism. As in other chronic, disabling illnesses, attention to nutrition, judicious use of blood replacement, relief of pain, and maintenance of morale are of the utmost importance.

The results of therapy are often recorded as 5- and 10-year disease-free survival rates. For cervical, pulmonary, and gastric carcinomas, patients who live for 5 years without residual or recurrent disease can generally look forward to many more years of survival. However, recurrence or metastasis of carcinoma of the breast or thyroid is a threat for so many years after initial recognition and treatment of a tumor that the relative merits of therapeutic regimens are difficult to assess with certainty.

In most clinics, operative mortality rates are higher and 5-year survival rates lower for charity than for private patients. Survival figures are generally better for asymptomatic than for symptomatic tumors, regardless of grade or stage. The 5-year survival rates tend to be higher for females than for males treated in the same fashion for carcinoma of the lung, stomach, thyroid, esophagus, salivary glands, and tongue, and for melanoma and Hodgkin's disease.

REFERENCES

Ackerman, L. V., and J. A. Regato: "Cancer: Diagnosis, Treatment and Prognosis," 3d ed., St. Louis, The C. V. Mosby Company, 1962.

Cole, W. H., H. W. Southwick, S. Roberts, and G. O. McDonald: "Dissemination of Cancer: Prevention and Therapy," New York, Appleton-Century-Crofts, Inc., 1961.

Everson, T. C.: Spontaneous Regression of Cancer, Ann. N.Y. Acad. Sci., 114:721, 1964.

Greenstein, J. P.: "Biochemistry of Cancer," 2d ed., New York, Academic Press, Inc., 1954.

Koprowski, H.: Virus-induced Tumors and Leukemias, Am. J. Med., 38:716, 1965.

Kraybill, H. F., and M. B. Shimkin: Carcinogenesis Related to Foods Contaminated by Processing and Fungal Metabolites, Advan. Cancer Res., 8:191, 1964.

Lipsett, M. B., et al: Humoral Syndromes Associated with Nonendocrine Tumors, Ann. Internal Med., 61:733, 1964.

McGrady, P.: "The Savage Cell. The Fight Against Cancer," New York, Basic Books, Inc., 1964.

Quisenberry, W. B.: Sociocultural Factors in Cancer in Hawaii, Ann. N.Y. Acad. Sci., 84:795, 1960.

Shimkin, M. B.: "Science and Cancer," Washington, Public Health Service Publication 1162, 1964.

"Unusual Forms and Aspects of Cancer in Man," Ann. N.Y. Acad. Sci., 114:717, 1964.

Warren, S.: Criteria for Traumatic or Occupational Causation of Cancer, Ann. Surg., 117:585, 1943.

Wood, S., Jr., E. D. Holyoke, and J. H. Yardley: Mechanisms of Metastasis Production by Blood-borne Cancer Cells, Canadian Cancer Conference, 4:167, 1961.

Section 2

Biochemical and Immunologic Considerations

60 DISORDERS OF FLUIDS AND ELECTROLYTES

Louis G. Welt and Charles H. Burnett

PHYSIOLOGIC CONSIDERATIONS

Volumes of Body Fluid

The total volume of body fluid is equivalent to 50 to 70 per cent of the body weight. Since adipose tissue is relatively free of water, the figure is closer to 50 per cent in the obese and approximates 70 per cent in lean individuals. This fluid is compartmented into two major phases, the *intracellular* and the *extracellular,* and several subdivisions thereof. Approximately two-thirds of the total water is within the cells. The extracellular fluid (one-third of the total, approximately equivalent to 16 to 20 per cent of the body weight) is further partitioned between the plasma and interstitial fluid. The smallest component represents about 2.5 per cent of the total volume of water and is referred to as *transcellular*. It includes the fluid within the gastrointestinal tract, the tracheobronchial tree, the excretory system of the kidneys and glands, the cerebrospinal fluid, and the aqueous humor of the eye.

The volume of several of these major compartments can be estimated. The technique entails administration of some material whose distribution is considered to be uniform throughout the compartment in question. If a known amount of the test material is administered, and if the amount lost from the body during the time necessary for complete mixing can be determined and the concentration per liter at the time of equilibration can be estimated, the volume of distribution of the test substance can be calculated. The volume of total body water can be estimated by using water labeled with deuterium or tritium. A variety of substances, such as inulin, sucrose, and sulfate, have been used to define the volume of the extracellular fluid. The volume of the intracellular fluid cannot be estimated directly but may be inferred from the difference between the total volume of body water and the volume of the extracellular fluid. Plasma volume (approximately 4 per cent of the body weight) has been calculated from the volume of distribution of protein-bound dyes, such as T-1824, and of albumin tagged with I^{131}. However, since the proteins, particularly albumin, are not wholly confined to the vascular compartment and gain access to the interstitial spaces and the lymph, the volume of distribution of tagged albumin is likely to be in excess of the plasma volume itself. This extravascular distribution of labeled albumin may be exaggerated in many states of edema, and its use in these circumstances is thought by many to provide spuriously high values for the plasma volume. The volume of the red cell mass is considered to be more reliable and may be estimated utilizing erythrocytes tagged with an isotope of iron, phosphorus, or chromium. From the red cell mass and the hematocrit one can readily calculate the plasma volume.

Each of these measurements has been of value in investigating both normal and pathologic exchanges of water and electrolytes. There is no doubt that such measurements would provide considerable aid in managing patients whose illness is complicated by a disorder of hydration and of electrolyte imbalance.

Composition of Body Fluids

There are major differences in the composition of the intra- and extracellular fluids, and minor differences among the several components of the latter. The composition of the extracellular fluid is better understood and more precisely defined, both because it is a simpler fluid and because it is available for analysis in the form of serum and transudates into the serous cavities. The only cells that can be obtained in relatively pure form in any bulk are the erythrocytes. Generalizations from the characteristics of this unique and highly specialized cell to all cells would, of course, be most hazardous.

The *interstitial fluid* of the extracellular compartment is an ultrafiltrate of serum and differs from the latter in that it contains very low concentrations of large molecular species such as proteins and lipids. The usually accepted normal range of values for the concentrations of electrolytes in serum is as follows:

Cations, mEq/L

Sodium	132–142
Potassium	3.5–5.0
Calcium	4.5–5.5
Magnesium	1.5–2.0

Anions, mEq/L

Chloride	98–106
Total CO_2	26–30 (mM/L)
Phosphate and sulfate	2–5
Organic anions	3–6
Proteins	15–25

The average total cation concentration approximates 150 mEq/liter, and this is considered to be identical with the total anion concentration. Although these concentrations are conventionally expressed in relation to a unit volume of serum, it is understood that these ions are for all intents and purposes distributed in the aqueous phase of the serum. The average water content of serum is about 93 per cent, and hence to express these concentrations in terms of serum water, they should each be divided by 0.93. The concentrations in the water of serum can then be translated to the concentrations in the interstitial fluid by applying a correction factor to account for the asymmetric distribution of ions across the capillary membrane. This latter is related to the presence in the serum of nondiffusible ions, the proteins. The Donnan ratio that describes the relative concentrations between serum and an ultrafiltrate thereof is approximately 1.05 for the univalent cations and 0.95 for the univalent anions. For example, the calculations of the concentrations of sodium or chloride in the interstitial fluid are performed as follows:

$$Na_{IF} = \frac{Na_s}{SW} \times 1.05$$

and

$$Cl_{IF} = \frac{Cl_s}{SW} \times 0.95$$

where IF = interstitial fluid, SW = fraction of serum that is water.

The compositions of joint fluid, aqueous humor of the eye, and cerebrospinal fluid are all similar to an ultrafiltrate of serum, but there are enough differences in the aqueous humor and spinal fluid to suggest that these are not pure dialysates but are, in part at least, formed by active transport processes.

The composition of the intracellular fluids cannot be examined directly, and hence the characteristics of cell fluid are inferred from analyses of whole tissue and the use of certain "reasonable" calculations. The total tissue water can be readily estimated from the difference in weight between the fresh wet tissue and the weight after it has been dried. The volume of this water that is to be ascribed to the extracellular phase is calculated from knowledge of the concentration of some substance in the tissue and serum, with the assumption that that particular substance is confined to an extracellular position. In the past, most of these calculations were made on the assumption that chloride was confined to the extracellular phase. This is obviously not true, and for more precise data one must employ other agents such as inulin. The values for the volume of the extracellular fluid and the concentrations of sodium and potassium in this fluid (as derived from their values in serum) are

used to calculate the quantity of these two ions in the noncellular phase. The difference between the total tissue sodium and potassium and the quantity in the extracellular phase represents the amount in cells. The difference between the total water and the extracellular volume is the intracellular water. The concentration of sodium and potassium in the intracellular fluid can then be calculated. These details have been recited to emphasize the indirectness with which cell composition is defined.

The average data, derived largely from muscle analyses, obtained in this inferential manner are as follows:

Cations, mEq/L

Sodium	10
Potassium	150
Magnesium	40

Anions, mEq/L

Bicarbonate	10 (mM/L)
Phosphate and sulfate	150
Proteins	40

Granting the calculations are valid, much is still unknown about the physicochemical state of these materials. For example, the characteristics of the phosphate, sulfate, and proteins in terms of valence are unknown. It is not certain that all the potassium and magnesium is in a free and ionized state. Furthermore, it is probably unrealistic to speak of intracellular fluid as an entity, since diverse tissue cells have major differences in composition. Lastly, the intracellular fluid of a single cell type is probably not an entity, since it, in turn, is compartmented into extra- and intramitochondrial fluid, nuclear fluid, etc.

Another important technique to evaluate the composition of body tissues employs radioactive isotopes. These are used to calculate a value that is referred to as the *total exchangeable quantity* of a given ion. This method involves administration of a known quantity of the particular radioactive material. After a sufficient period of time, allowing the isotope to equilibrate with as much of the stable element as it will readily exchange with (approximately 24 hr), one then determines the specific activity in serum; with this datum plus knowledge of the quantity that has been lost by decay as well as that which has been excreted in the urine, one can calculate the total quantity of the ion that is readily exchangeable. This figure is usually expressed as a unit of body mass. The data collected by Moore and his colleagues provide the following average figures:

	mEq/kg body weight	
	Male	*Female*
Sodium	39.5	38.3
Potassium	48	39.4
Chloride	29.3	28.6

It must be cautioned that these figures do not represent the *total* quantity of these ions in the body, since the total is not readily exchangeable. For example, approximately 75 per cent of the total body sodium and 85 per cent of the total body potassium are exchangeable.

The most complicated characteristics of cell composition and the marked differences between it and the environment of the cells serve to emphasize the highly specialized functions of cells, the complex mechanisms that must be available to maintain these compositional differences, and the possibilities for alterations in metabolic pathways that may result from even subtle alterations in composition.

In contrast to the marked differences in the composition of these two major phases, it is believed that the total solute concentration in these fluids is identical. This, in turn, is due to the presumed free permeability of most of the cell membranes to water. This concept has been challenged in recent years. Although a categorical statement is not appropriate, the preponderance of evidence continues to support the concept that the cellular fluids are, in fact, isotonic with respect to their environmental fluid. This may not apply for those cells which secrete a hypotonic fluid, such as the sweat and salivary glands, and for the renal tubular cells that tolerate fluids of markedly different osmolalities on each surface.

Internal Exchanges of Water

When two aqueous solutions are separated by a membrane that is freely permeable to water, molecules of water will move from one compartment to the other. There will be an equilibrium with respect to water when the same number of water molecules pass in each direction per unit of time. At such a time there is no *net* alteration in volume in either of the compartments separated by the membrane. The tendency for the molecules of water to pass from one compartment to the other is spoken of as an "escaping tendency" and is referred to as the *chemical potential* of the water. Whenever the chemical potentials of the water of two contiguous solutions differ, there will be a net movement of water from the phase with the higher chemical potential to that with the lower, until equilibrium is reached. The chemical potential of water is reduced when solutes are added, and the reduction is proportional to the concentration of solutes. In contrast, the chemical potential of water molecules is enhanced by increases in hydrostatic pressure and temperature.

Thus, the addition of a solute that can traverse a membrane with freedom will result in its uniform distribution throughout the volumes of fluid separated by that membrane. The addition of this solute will diminish the chemical potential of the water molecules, but since the water in both compartments is influenced to the same degree, there is no *net* change in the volume of water on either side of the membrane. The only effect is that fewer molecules of water, but an equal number of them, move in each direction per unit of time. In contrast, if the added solute were unable to permeate the membrane in question, it would be confined to the side to which it was added and would diminish the chemical potential of the molecules of water on that side alone. Under this circumstance molecules of water would continue to *enter* this phase at the rate which obtained prior to the addition of the solute, but water molecules would *escape from* this compartment at a slower rate and there would be a net change in volume, such that water would accumulate in the compartment to which the solute had been added. The redistribution of water would continue until a new state of equilibrium was established.

This problem may be looked at a little more carefully in terms of the pore theory of membranes. In the context of the discussion just presented, imagine a membrane separating two aqueous solutions and visualize a pore that permeates the membrane. Assume that the solutions in the two phases are pure water and that exchange (with no *net* movement) occurs owing to the random movement of molecules of water. Now if one adds to Side I a solute that cannot permeate the membrane, it is clear that more molecules of water will move from the pore at its interface with Solution I than will move from Solution I into the pore. This loss of water molecules at the interface must promote a pressure drop across the pore and be responsible for the net movement of water into Solution I. This is emphasized by pointing out that there is only pure water within the pore and, hence, no tendency for the molecules of water to move more in one direction than another. The situation that conditions the movement must, in fact, be the pressure gradient across the pore. Ordinarily these problems are discussed in terms of osmotic pressure. In this context, the addition of a solute that can permeate membranes freely, such as urea, contributes to the total osmotic pressure, but it is not effective in promoting a redistribution of water. Glucose, which is not free to enter cells by passive diffusion, not only contributes to the total osmotic pressure of a solution to which it is added, but it contributes what is referred to as an *effective osmotic pressure* (as opposed to *total* osmotic pressure) and does condition a redistribution of water.

With respect to biologic fluids and membranes, it may be said that an increase in the concentration of those solutes that permeate membranes freely augments the total osmotic pressure (decreases the chemical potential of the water molecules) in all compartments of the body fluids. However, an increase in the concentration of a solute that cannot penetrate a membrane freely will increase the *effective* osmotic pressure as well as the total (diminish the chemical potential of the molecules of water) in the fluid in which the concentration has been altered. If this fluid is separated by a membrane freely permeable to water, there will be a net alteration in volume in favor of the compartment to which the solute has been added. Despite long usage and familiarity, the terms *total* and *effective osmotic pressure* will be replaced in the rest of this discussion with the terms *total* and *effective osmolality*. This should serve to recall that it is the activity of the molecules of water that is under discussion, and not the technique (utilizing hydrostatic pressure) used to estimate these activities. However, since hydrostatic pressure increases the chemical potential of molecules of water, a change in hydrostatic pressure may counterbalance the influence of solutes so that a *difference* in total solute concentration across a membrane may be unassociated with net transfers of water.

Sodium salts represent almost all the solutes that usually contribute to the effective osmolality of the extracellular fluid. Hence, in most instances an increase or a decrease in the concentration of sodium in the serum may be equated with an increase or decrease in the effective osmolality of the extracellular fluid and, in turn, will promote movement of water from or into the cellular compartment.

There are two circumstances when depressed concentration of sodium in serum may not necessarily represent diminished effective osmolality of the serum water. It will be recalled that it would be more precise to speak of the concentration of an ion such as sodium in terms of its concentration in the water of serum. Since the determination is actually performed on a diluted aliquot of serum, and since the percentage of serum that is water is so commonly between 90 and 93 per cent, the convention is to refer the concentration to a unit (usually a liter) of serum. In circumstances characterized by hyperlipemia, the lipids may occupy a significant volume of the serum, and the percentage of serum that is water may be drastically reduced, to as low as 70 to 80 per cent. An average concentration of sodium of 138 mEq/liter in a serum of which the water content was 93 per cent would represent a concentration of 148.3 mEq/*liter* of serum *water* (138/0.93). If this same concentration obtained in the water of a *lipemic serum* where the water content was only 75 per cent, the concentration per liter of *serum* would be 111.2 mEq (148.3 × 0.75). Thus, a striking hyponatremia in this instance would not mean a diminished effective osmolality of the water of the serum. This may also obtain with unusual hyperproteinemias.

Although glucose contributes to the effective osmolality of the extracellular fluid, the magnitude is usually small. At a concentration of 100 mg/100 ml (1,000 mg/liter) this would amount to 5.5 mOsm/liter. However, if hyperglycemia supervenes, the corresponding increase in the effective osmolality will promote a movement of water from the cells. This will dilute the concentration of sodium and may depress the level to the point of frank hyponatremia. In this instance the interpretation that the hyponatremia signifies a decrease in effective osmolality would be in error. For these reasons the concentration of sodium in a patient with diabetes mellitus should be interpreted with knowledge of the simultaneous concentration of glucose in the serum.

SIGNIFICANCE OF HYPONATREMIA. Hyponatremia is observed frequently in hospital practice. Not all instances of hyponatremia have the same pathogenesis; many are poorly understood, and a decision about management may be difficult. This discussion excludes those instances in which hyponatremia is not equivalent to a decrease in the effective osmolality of the body fluid, such as those cited in relation to hyperlipemia and hyperglycemia.

The commonest situations in which hyponatremia is observed are those cases of dehydration or edema in which salt has been lost in excess of water or water has been retained in excess of salt. A modest deficit of sodium is frequently accompanied by an equivalent loss of water. The sequence of events may be something as follows: (1) the loss of sodium induces a mild reduction of the concentration of this cation in the extracellular fluids; (2) this, in turn, suppresses the secretion of the antidiuretic hormone (ADH) (and furthermore the loss of salt impairs the ability to elaborate an appropriately concentrated urine); (3) the excretion of water is increased until the concentration of sodium has been restored. This is frequently referred to as a "sacrifice of volume in the interests of tonicity of the body fluids." However, as the volume deficit assumes more significant proportions, equivalent losses of water no longer follow further deficits of sodium salts and hyponatremia is established. It may be that the deficit in volume, or some expression thereof, is a stimulus for the secretion of ADH despite hyponatremia, and the volume deficit may influence renal function, in some fashion independent of ADH, to conserve water. It is clear from this sequence that one very important implication of a state of dehydration accompanied by hyponatremia is that the intensity of the dehydration is probably severe. In addition, the decrease in effective osmolality of the extracellular water will have promoted movement of water into the cellular compartment. Thus, the deficit in volume of the extracellular phase is greater than the total external loss. Lastly, the dilution of the intracellular fluid may be expected to have untoward consequences with respect to cell functions. These latter are most clearly expressed on a clinical level by a clouded sensorium, which may progress to frank coma and may be accompanied by seizures. In addition, there are data that hyponatremia (with or without cellular dilution) promotes an increased rate of production of urea nitrogen and induces a rise in the serum level of potassium.

Hyponatremia may occur in the absence of dehydration. In fact, there are some indications that it may develop in patients with no apparent alteration in the volume or disposition of body water; and it may certainly occur in patients with edema. There is some value in a tentative effort to characterize the several pathogeneses of hyponatremia other than that already discussed with regard to dehydration.

ESSENTIAL HYPONATREMIA. There is a group of patients who have hyponatremia but no other obvious disturbances in body fluid physiology. These are patients with advanced and debilitating diseases and are frequently in preterminal status. These patients excrete in the urine the approximate quantity of salt ingested. They are able to conserve sodium when this ion is removed from their regimen, and they are able to excrete an appropriately dilute urine when a water load is administered. No aspect of their symptom complex is apparently favorably modified by attempts to restore the concentration of sodium in serum to the normal range. If this is attempted, the patient becomes thirsty, ingests water, and then excretes salt and water until the volume and tonicity of the body fluids have been restored to the level from which they began.

It is clear that the basic defect of this syndrome is mysterious, but it may be suggested that a generalized cellular disorder promotes a new "setting" of the osmolality of the body fluids. Some have referred to this as the "sick cell syndrome." It is not difficult to discriminate between this syndrome and patients with hyponatremia and dehydration or patients who are deteriorating as a consequence of adrenal cortical insufficiency. The physical examination and collateral laboratory data such as a normal level of serum urea nitrogen and potassium are important clues. The disorder from which it must be differentiated is inappropriate secretion of antidiuretic hormone.

INAPPROPRIATE SECRETION OF ADH. More and more examples of this condition are noted continuously. These patients most commonly have intrathoracic lesions, both benign and malignant, or intracranial lesions of one sort or another. However, it is also noted in an odd variety of circumstances that make it difficult to provide reasonable explanations for the pathogenesis in each instance.

The problem is that the patient is secreting antidiuretic hormone (or an antidiuretic substance of other origin) under inappropriate circumstances. This implies that ADH is secreted in abundance in the absence of an osmometric or volumetric stimulus. The consequence is that the continued ingestion of water is not followed by its excretion and the patient develops a positive balance of water and dilutional hyponatremia. This hypotonic expansion of the body fluids usually promotes an increased glomerular filtration rate and an augmented excretion of salt. At this point, the urine osmolality may not be as high as it was initially, owing to the solute diuresis and perhaps in part to some suppressive influence on the secretion of ADH by the severe hypoosmolality of the body fluids. In any event, the urine osmolality is still inappropriately high for the degree of dilution consequent to the positive balance of water.

Since there is frequently an increased rate of glomerular filtration, it is not uncommon to find that these patients show serum urea nitrogen at the lowest levels of normal. Although these patients have an expanded volume of total body water, it is distributed throughout both the cellular and the extracellular compartments, and one usually finds only the most subtle signs of edema.

The disordered mechanisms that may be responsible for this concatenation of events are not altogether clear. However, it has been found that the pulmonary tumor of at least one such patient contained an antidiuretic substance. It is also known that there are receptors within the thorax such that when some component(s) of the intrathoracic cavity is filled with blood, stimuli are transmitted along the vagi which suppress the secretion of ADH. It is possible that a variety of intrathoracic lesions could disrupt and subvert this feedback mechanism. In those instances where there are intracranial tumors, it is not difficult to imagine their location as favoring an irritating stimulus to the secretion of ADH.

The treatment of these patients is clearly aimed at dissipating the positive balance of water. This is usually accomplished by drastic restriction in the volume of water ingested until a normal concentration of sodium in serum has been achieved. Then one must find, in an empirical fashion, what food and fluid regimen will be comfortable for the patient and yet not permit a positive balance of water to be achieved once again.

There are occasional circumstances when the level of hyponatremia is so extreme as to produce clouding of consciousness, coma, or seizures. These instances demand more rapid correction, and there are two courses available. One can administer solutions of mannitol, hypertonic glucose, or urea to induce a solute diuresis that will dissipate part of the positive balance of water via the urine and restore the concentration of sodium in serum to a more nearly normal level quickly. Alternatively, one can administer a volume of hypertonic saline solution sufficient to increase the concentration of sodium to a level where the hazards attendant on hyponatremia no longer obtain. This should be employed as the last resort, since, in fact, the patient already has an expanded body fluid volume.

It is almost certain that what was formerly referred to as "cerebral salt wasting" was, in fact, misinterpreted and represented instances of inappropriate secretion of ADH.

HYPONATREMIA WITH EDEMA. There are many instances of patients who have hyponatremia associated with lesser or massive degrees of edema. These patients are usually classified in two general categories: *chronic dilutional* and *acute dilutional hyponatremia.*

Chronic Dilutional Hyponatremia. (1) It seems reasonable that some of these patients may well represent examples of what is called *essential hyponatremia.* In that circumstance there would obviously be no value to restoring the concentration of sodium in serum to "normal." In fact, the patient would then have the discomfort of thirst added to his other problems. (2) Some of these patients may well represent instances of *inappropriate secretion of ADH*. The best management is to dissipate the relative positive balance of water by restricting intake. As in the instances of this syndrome without edema, there might be occasions when more aggressive measures were required, such as administration of a solution to provoke a solute diuresis. There may be *rare* occasions when the administration of small volumes of hypertonic saline solution is justified if the hyponatremia per se is truly hazardous. However, since these patients are already markedly expanded with fluids and may already have congestive heart failure, it is obvious that the treatment itself is dangerous and should be employed only under the most dire circumstances. (3) Lastly, it is quite probable that in many states of edema the rate of glomerular filtration is markedly reduced. Under these circumstances the quantity of water that escapes reabsorption in the more proximal portions of the nephron may be so small that very little gains access to the more distal segments where it might escape into the bladder. Why patients in such circumstances do not lose their thirst and thereby automatically prohibit a positive balance of water is certainly not clear. Nevertheless, drinking and eating patterns in man are such that a positive balance of water can be readily achieved under these circumstances. Once again, the treatment is dissipation of the positive balance of water.

Acute Dilutional Hyponatremia. (1) One example of this disorder is simply the consequence of administering water or urging a patient with edema to ingest quantities of water in excess of his ability to excrete the load. This is possible in any circumstance including health but is much more easily achieved in patients with edema who have altered renal hemodynamic and other parameters. In any event, the first point to emphasize is that this is preventable. Secondly, should it occur, the treatment again demands restriction of water to rid the body of this relative excess. Lastly, under duress the use of hypertonic solutions may be employed to encourage a solute diuresis. (2) A second example is observed in patients who develop considerable thirst after a successful therapeutic measure aimed at ridding the edematous patient of a volume of fluid. This may be noted after a brisk diuretic response and more commonly after a large abdominal paracentesis. The reasons for the intense thirst are not clear but may relate to a sudden loss of volume in some crucial segment of the vascular system. These complications are preventable. Patients should be warned that they may develop thirst, and their ingestion of water should be limited by themselves and carefully monitored and restricted when indicated by those responsible for their care.

The point of emphasis in managing patients with hyponatremia and edema is that if the concentration of sodium in serum is to be restored, it should be accomplished by dissipating the relative positive balance of water by restricting intake or by hastening

excretion through the use of an osmotic load. Some patients may, in fact, be more comfortable with hyponatremia than with "normal" concentrations of sodium in serum, and these may reflect a state referred to as essential hyponatremia. The indications for administration of hypertonic saline solutions are *exceedingly rare*, and the measure is only to control what are considered hazardous symptoms from the hyponatremia per se. Even under these circumstances saline solution should be administered in a small quantity sufficient only to restore the sodium concentration to levels that no longer represent a hazardous state.

Another way that hyponatremia might develop is by movement of sodium from the extracellular compartment to cells or to bone. There is some evidence that such an intercompartmental shift of sodium may occur in adrenal cortical insufficiency. Sodium may accumulate in cells deficient in potassium, and some investigators have considered that certain instances of hyponatremia are related to this transfer from the extracellular compartment.

An assessment of the pathogenesis of hyponatremia can usually be made on the basis of the above discussion, and hence the therapeutic implications can usually be arrived at according to the above criteria. It must be conceded, however, that the best opinion on this subject is confused.

SIGNIFICANCE OF HYPERNATREMIA. In contrast to hyponatremia, an increase in the concentration of sodium in the serum reflects loss of water in excess of salt or administration (or ingestion) of salt in excess of water. The hypernatremia, which is the chemical expression of a water deficit, in turn, incites the following responses, which result in the acquisition of more water, the most efficient conservation of same, and the most desirable distribution of the available water:

1. Thirst
2. Secretion of ADH, which promotes excretion of a concentrated urine
3. Movement of water from the cells to the extracellular space, thus mitigating the deficit of volume in this latter compartment
4. Diminution in the loss of insensible perspiration
5. Decrease in the rate of secretion of sweat

At least one report leaves little doubt that there may well be circumstances where there is hypernatremia with no other disorder in body fluid physiology and the patients appear to operate with a new "setting" of body fluid osmolality. This may be the counterpart of essential hyponatremia and perhaps should be referred to as *essential hypernatremia*.

COMMENTS ON CORRECTION OF HYPO- AND HYPERNATREMIA. One other implication of the free permeability of cell membranes to water and a uniform osmolality throughout the body fluids concerns the manner in which the concentration of sodium in the serum is restored to normal from both hypo- and hypernatremic levels.

If hyponatremia complicates an illness and it is

considered advisable to correct this abnormality by administering a hypertonic solution of sodium salts, the amount of sodium required is equivalent to the deficit in concentration per liter multiplied by the estimated number of liters of *total body water*. If there is to be osmotic equality throughout the body fluids, it is implicit that the concentration of sodium in the extracellular phase cannot be increased without an equivalent increase in solute concentration in the cellular fluid. The administered sodium will increase the osmotic activity of intracellular fluid, not by entering the cells, but by promoting movement of water from the cells to the extracellular compartment as the osmolality of the latter is increased. If it is desired to restore the concentration of sodium reasonably promptly, or if it is to be accomplished with a small volume of fluid, the sodium salts must be administered in hypertonic solution. The amount of sodium that must be administered to restore the concentration to normal is equal to the normal concentration of Na_s (138 mEq/liter) minus the current concentration of Na_s multiplied by the total volume of body water. For example, in a 70-kg adult with an assumed body water content of 60 per cent (42 liters) and a concentration of sodium in the serum of 128 mEq/liter,

$$(138 - 128) \times 42 = 420 \text{ mM deficit of sodium chloride}$$

Since there are 17.1 mM/Gm NaCl, 420/17.1, or 24.56 Gm NaCl would be necessary to restore the sodium to 138 mEq/liter. This could be supplied in 500 ml 5 per cent NaCl solution.

The same principles apply to estimating the volume of water that may be necessary to reduce the concentration of sodium in the serum from hypernatremic to normal levels. Since the intensity of the hypernatremia (due to the loss of water in excess of or without salt) is proportional to the deficit of total body water, the following relationship obtains:

$$\frac{\text{Normal concentration } Na_s}{\text{Elevated concentration } Na_s}$$

$$= \frac{\text{current vol total body } H_2O}{\text{assumed normal vol total body } H_2O}$$

The value for the current volume of total body water can be calculated, and the difference between it and the assumed normal volume for total body water represents the deficit of water. For example, in the same adult mentioned above but with a concentration of sodium in the serum of 160 mEq/liter:

$$\text{Current vol total body } H_2O = \frac{138}{160} \times 42 = 36.2 \text{ liters}$$

The deficit would be $42 - 36.2 = 5.8$ liters of water.

EXCHANGES BETWEEN PLASMA AND INTERSTITIAL FLUID. The net exchange of fluid between the plasma and interstitial space is conditioned by a series of forces. Some of these forces favor transudation from the vascular system, such as the hydrostatic pressure within the vessels and the colloid osmotic pressure of the tissue fluids. The tissue tension and the colloid osmotic pressure of the plasma favor the reabsorption of fluid from the interstitium (see Chap. 16). It should be emphasized that, unlike the cell membranes, the capillary endothelial membrane is freely permeable not only to water but to all the solutes of the plasma except the large molecular species such as the proteins and the lipids. Thus, the concentration of sodium and its salts does not influence the distribution of water between these two major components of the extracellular compartment. Although the proteins do not contribute a large osmolality, they alone contribute to the effective osmolality since they are unable to permeate the endothelial membrane except in very small quantity. Thus, hypoalbuminemia may promote expansion of the interstitial fluid, with diminution in plasma volume and hemoconcentration, with normal values for the concentration of sodium.

A change in the forces governing the net exchange between the plasma and the interstitial fluid need not necessarily condition a redistribution of volume between these two compartments. A net increase in transudation could be largely compensated by the return of this increment of fluid to the vascular system by way of the lymphatics. Lymphatic flow is frequently increased when the interstitial fluid volume is expanded, and this influence must be carefully considered when analyzing the forces that govern the disposition of fluid within the extracellular compartment.

Internal Exchanges of Electrolytes

Although it is apparent that ions such as sodium, potassium, and magnesium move in and out of cells, it is equally apparent that their net movements are not a consequence of free passive diffusion. The measurements of the electric potential differences across the membranes as well as the determination of the concentration gradients make it clear that these ions are not in a state of equilibrium but exist in what is referred to as a *steady state away from equilibrium*. This demands a series of operations dependent on sources of energy and referred to in general terms as *active transport*. The special permeability or "leakiness" characteristics of the plasma membranes of cells with regard to the several ionic species as well as the specific active transport mechanisms and the factors that regulate their rates are ultimately the determinants of the steady state composition of the several cell types. Any change in the permeability characteristics or rates of transport could readily influence the cell composition. It is presumed that metabolic reactions are necessary to maintain cell membrane structure, which, in turn, establishes the permeabilities to passive diffusion as well as the mechanisms involved in the active phases of transport. There are data which establish adenosinetriphosphate (ATP) as the ultimate source of energy for active transport, and, lastly, there is an enzyme within the membrane structure itself, ATPase, which may play an important role in making the energy available for the work of transport.

In some instances there appear to be elements of

active transport in which the movement of two ionic species in opposite directions may be linked. Although hypothetical, an illustration of the manner in which muscle cells become laden with sodium in the face of potassium deficits can be offered. For example, assume that the level of potassium outside the cell is one of the factors which regulates the rate at which sodium is actively extruded from within the cell. Assume, further, that the rate of extrusion of sodium from the cells controls the inward movement of potassium from the extracellular fluid to the intracellular space. When potassium is lost from the extracellular fluid owing to augmented urinary excretion, or losses from the gastrointestinal tract, etc., the level in the extracellular fluid tends to diminish. This creates initially a larger gradient for potassium from inside to outside the cell, and perhaps more potassium leaks out by passive diffusion. However, this is still inadequate to raise the extracellular fluid concentration of potassium to normal levels. At the same time sodium is constantly diffusing into the cells only to be actively extruded. However, if the diminished level of potassium in the extracellular fluid imposes a rate-limiting influence on the extrusion of sodium from the cells, the latter should accumulate within the cells. The advantage of this is that with the higher intracellular concentration of sodium more of this ion can now be extruded (despite the lower external concentration of potassium), and restoration toward normal of the rate of sodium extrusion at the expense of the higher intracellular concentration of this ion promotes the ability to implement the movement of potassium back into the cell. All these alterations induce a net change characterized by a loss of cell potassium, an increase of cell sodium, and the achievement of new steady state away from equilibrium. This may very well be fanciful in detail, but it provides an overall context in which one can view some of the problems.

The most prominent hypothesis relating to a mechanism of active transport is referred to as the *carrier hypothesis*. In an oversimplified fashion this may be described as suggesting that a compound resides at one side of the cell membrane and has a particular affinity for the sodium ion. Because of this characteristic it becomes linked with this ion; it is now a new species of compound with a higher concentration at one side of the membrane than the other. As a result, it diffuses passively to the other side of the membrane, where a reaction splits the sodium ion from the carrier. This reaction again modifies the compound, and it can be postulated that it now has an affinity for potassium. The latter ion articulates with the carrier and, again, owing to the establishment of a diffusion gradient in this fashion, it moves back to the original side of the membrane, where the potassium ion is split off and the carrier is returned to its original state with a great affinity for sodium, and the process is repeated over and over again.

This discussion of active transport has been too simple and succinct to provide more than a vague conceptual framework. The interested reader is referred to Ussing and other sources for detailed discussions of this fascinating and fundamental property. It should be emphasized that the active transport of ions is responsible at the least for the maintenance of cell volume and tissue excitability as well as what must be a vast array of phenomena that are dependent on the details of intra- and extracellular fluid composition.

Bone as a reservoir of ions other than calcium has attracted increased attention. Approximately one-third of the total body sodium is in bone, and only 15 per cent of this can be ascribed to the extracellular phase. About one-half of the total body content of magnesium is in bone. Potassium is present in much smaller amounts. Deficits of sodium, potassium, and magnesium are shared by bone, and this tissue participates in exchanges that articulate with alterations in acid-base relationships. (See also Chap. 61, Acidosis and Alkalosis.)

External Exchanges of Electrolytes and Water

THIRST. In considering the net exchange of water between the individual and his environment, it seems reasonable to begin with thirst. This is the sensory impression that motivates the ingestion of water. Several stimuli may give rise to the sensation of thirst, and the most important of these is an increase in the effective osmolality of the body fluids. This appears to hold true whether the hypertonicity is promoted by loss of water in excess of salt or by administration of salt in excess of water. These two circumstances differ in that in the first instance the volume of the extracellular fluid is decreased, and in the second this volume is expanded. However, in each circumstance the volume of the cells is diminished by virtue of a shift of water to the extracellular phase. A secondary stimulus is related somehow to a deficit of volume (or some expression of such a deficit) in some key portion of the extracellular space. Other factors that condition and modify the sensation of thirst include exposure of the oropharyngeal and esophageal tissues to water, the fullness of the stomach, and emotional as well as social factors. The central nervous system is responsible for the appreciation of and the response to thirst in both a specific and a nonspecific manner. There is now abundant evidence that lesions in key portions of the central nervous system—predominantly in the hypothalamus—may induce hypodipsia or polydipsia. The latter need not be accompanied by diabetes insipidus. The polydipsic center can be stimulated by exposing it to tiny volumes of hypertonic, but not isotonic, saline solutions. It can also be aroused by electrical stimulation.

In a less specific sense the central nervous system conditions the reception and response to stimuli provoking thirst in relation to the level of the state of consciousness. The frequency with which patients with a clouded sensorium or coma are allowed to develop significant deficits of water is sufficient justification for emphasizing the obvious fact that such patients can neither appreciate nor respond to their own thirst mechanism.

Potassium depletion may be accompanied by thirst and polydipsia. This may reflect, in part, the inability of the kidneys to conserve water appropriately in this condition. However, it is also possible that there may be a primary influence on some aspect of the stimulus-response pathways concerned with thirst.

INSENSIBLE PERSPIRATION. Water is continuously lost from the body in the expired air and from the skin. The sum of these losses is spoken of as "insensible loss" of water and is equivalent to about 600 to 1,000 ml per day in the average adult. This loss is augmented with increase in metabolic activity (fever, exercise, hyperthyroidism) and respiratory exchange. The catabolism of tissues produces 200 to 300 ml water per day; hence, the *net* loss of insensible water may be considered as 400 to 700 ml per day. Since this loss is water without solutes, it should be replaced as water without salt (e.g., 5 per cent glucose in water when fluid balance is being maintained by parenteral techniques).

SWEAT. The production of sweat is primarily responsive to heat. The latter presumably excites afferent impulses to centers that regulate motor activities promoting the loss of heat. The important centers in the central nervous system are in the anterolateral portions of the hypothalamus. Sweat is not a simple fluid, and the details of its secretion are not well understood. It is always a hypotonic solution except in adrenal cortical insufficiency and in patients with fibrocystic disease (mucoviscidosis) of the pancreas. Among other influences, the rate of sweating is diminished by an increase in the effective osmolality of the body fluids. An average composition for sweat, in millimoles per liter, is as follows: sodium 48.0, potassium 5.9, chloride 40.0, ammonia 3.5, and urea 8.6. The characteristics of this fluid dictate the replacement of losses incurred as sweat by a solution that is one-third to one-half isotonic saline. This is readily satisfied for intravenous administration with 1 part isotonic saline to 1 or 2 parts of 5 per cent glucose in water.

GASTROINTESTINAL TRACT. The exchange of water and solutes between the body fluids and the lumen of the gastrointestinal tract is large. It is contributed to by saliva and the secretions of the stomach, liver, pancreas, and intestinal mucosa. The volume of these secretions may exceed 8 liters per day under ordinary circumstances, but the net loss from the body is negligible. However, when there are losses through vomitus, diarrhea, or drainage from enterostomies, colostomies, or fistulas, the deficits of water and electrolytes may be prodigious. Loss of fluid through these routes probably represents the commonest pathogenesis of significant dehydration in clinical practice.

Aside from saliva, which is a hypotonic solution, the secretions mentioned are close to isotonicity with the extracellular fluids. However, they differ from the latter in composition. For example, the gastric secretion, if it contains free HCl, has a much lower pH, less sodium and bicarbonate, and more chloride than the extracellular fluid. In contrast, the pancreatic secretion has a higher pH and more bicarbonate. Most gastrointestinal secretions have more potassium than the extracellular fluid. Thus, although losses of gastrointestinal secretions per se represent isotonic deficits, the derangements that accompany the dehydration will be conditioned by the particular portion of the gastrointestinal tract from which the lost fluid derived. In many instances, however, these losses can be successfully replaced by equal volumes of isotonic saline solution. The potassium lost with these secretions and the consequences thereof must also be adequately managed.

RENAL EXCHANGES OF ELECTROLYTES AND WATER. The kidneys represent the major organs of conservation as well as of excretion in the net balance of water and electrolytes. The kidneys can excrete large volumes of excess water and large quantities of unwanted ions and other solutes. In addition, they respond to the need to conserve water by excreting small volumes of highly concentrated urine. Their response to a sodium deficit is to excrete a urine virtually free of salt. The conservation of magnesium is also good, and subjects subsisting on a diet deficient in magnesium may excrete as little as 1 mEq of this ion per day. Although the excretion of potassium is very much diminished when there is a deficit of this cation, the efficiency with which the kidneys conserve potassium is not quite so great as it is with sodium, chloride, or magnesium.

The excretion of sodium is markedly reduced when there is primarily a deficit of water, despite the fact that this is accompanied by hypernatremia. This has the advantage of eliminating a major solute from the urine and, by reducing urine flow, furthers the conservation of water.

The kidneys display other exquisitely sensitive responses to most of the alterations in the composition, volume, tonicity, and pH of the body fluids. Details of these responses and the mechanisms involved therein are discussed in Chap. 19.

CLINICAL CONSIDERATIONS

An understanding of the pathogenesis and management of disorders of fluid and electrolyte balance depends on an appreciation of the approximate net exchanges of water and the several ions that have occurred during the course of a patient's illness. In essence, many of the problems concerning clinical disorders of hydration are resolved by the simple expediency of setting up a balance sheet in which the total estimated losses are accumulated, the total intake is summated, and the net differences are calculated. Although not quantitatively precise, this practice usually defines the qualitative nature of the alterations and provides an approximation of the quantitative characteristics. Many of these data can be obtained from the carefully taken history or the well-documented hospital chart. In addition, the physical examination, the chemical analyses of serum and urine, and other laboratory data provide additional insights. The management of the problem then becomes largely one of providing those materials which will restore the normal state of hydration. It is not an oversimplification to state that the majority of these problems are easily resolved with simple arithmetic.

In many instances a disordered state of hydration could have been avoided by provision of adequate replacement of certain predictable and mandatory losses. It is desirable, therefore, to define the characteristics of the basal requirements for water and electrolytes, and to describe how these are modified by a variety of conditioning circumstances.

Basal Requirements

For the purposes of this discussion it will be assumed that the patient must receive the necessary water, electrolytes, and other materials by parenteral routes, that he has accumulated no antecedent deficits, that he is not sustaining any unusual losses, and that he has normal renal function. One other qualification is that the problem is one of short duration and that the need for calories and protein is not a major consideration. The task then is to prescribe a regimen which will maintain a normal state of hydration, avoid depletion of the major essential minerals, and minimize the most immediate threats of starvation.

The volume of water recommended per day is the sum of (1) the probable net insensible loss, 400 ml; (2) a reasonable volume for urine, 1,000 ml; and (3) perhaps a small additional volume, 400 ml, which is provided to anticipate other losses such as sweat but which, if not lost by extrarenal routes, can be readily excreted in the urine. These total 1,800 ml.

If a patient has been previously ingesting an average diet, he has probably been receiving about 8 to 10 Gm (135 to 170 mM) NaCl per day. If the intake of salt is suddenly eliminated, the patient will probably be able to excrete a urine essentially free of sodium in about 5 days. During this interval of 5 days a negative balance of sodium is allowed to develop. This is likely to be accompanied by an equivalent loss of water in the interests of maintaining a normal concentration of sodium in the extracellular fluid. This deficit in volume is probably not harmful in itself, but it prejudices the patient's ability to withstand subsequent losses. Therefore, unless there is some specific contraindication, it is recommended that the patient receive 4 to 5 Gm (70 to 85 mM) NaCl each day.

As noted earlier, the conservation of potassium is not quite so efficient as that of salt, and unless the urinary excretion of this cation is replaced, a deficit of potassium will be ultimately achieved. From 40 to 60 mM potassium per day should be adequate to avoid a negative balance of this cation.

Although the mechanisms of conservation for magnesium are quite good, one of the settings in which depletion of this cation is observed is prolonged parenteral fluid management. The administration of as little as 2.0 to 4.0 mM magnesium per day ought to suffice under most circumstances.

It has been stated that approximately 100 Gm carbohydrate is necessary for the operation of the Krebs cycle. Unless this is made available from preformed endogenous or exogenous carbohydrate, the catabolism of protein and fat will be accelerated and 4-carbon ketones will be formed faster than they can be utilized. The acid products of protein catabolism and the excess ketones must be excreted to avoid a metabolic acidosis; they are excreted in part as sodium salts, which adds another drain to the body's store of sodium. Each of these complications can be avoided by the provision of an adequate quantity, 150 to 200 Gm, of glucose per day.

The total basal requirements are the following:

Water . . . . 1,800 ml
NaCl . . . . 70–85 mM (4–5 Gm)
KCl . . . . 40–60 mM (3–4.5 Gm)
MgSO$_4$ . . . . 2.0–4.0 mM (1–2 ml 50% MgSO$_4$·7H$_2$O)
Glucose . . . . 150–200 Gm

An appropriate fluid prescription to meet these requirements is the following:

1,300 ml 10% glucose in water
500 ml 5% glucose in isotonic saline solution
4 Gm KCl (added to the total water to be administered)
2 ml 50% MgSO$_4$·7H$_2$O (added to the total water to be administered)

It should be reemphasized that this prescription is appropriate for the patient with qualifications set forth in the initial paragraph of this discussion on Basal Requirements.

ADDITIONAL REQUIREMENTS. There are many circumstances which would require revision of the above prescription. Fever, restlessness, and increased respiratory activity will augment the loss of water as insensible perspiration. A hot environment and fever will promote sweating. Water loss in urine will be accelerated during an osmotic diuresis due to glycosuria or unusual amounts of urea. The latter situation is observed when unnecessarily large amounts of protein are administered to patients who are experiencing a reaction to injury and hence are limited in the ability to store nitrogen. Additional amounts of salt may be lost with glycosuria. Impaired renal function will demand an increased volume of urine, and the conservation of sodium may be less efficient than in patients with normal kidneys.

FLUIDS AVAILABLE FOR PARENTERAL ADMINISTRATION. There are available a number of specially prepared solutions, such as "gastric replacement fluid" and "intestinal replacement fluid," aimed at meeting the requirements of particular types of loss. Their use should be discouraged. The basic tenet of the individualization of therapy applies here, as it does elsewhere in clinical practice. The proper management of disorders in fluid and electrolyte balance demands an analysis of the specific characteristics of the distortion in the particular patient at hand. The routine use of a special solution tends to diminish the diligence with which this analysis is made through the false sense of security provided by the claims of the value of the particular solution. This is not to imply that solutions other than glucose in water and isotonic saline are not frequently needed. However, when the need arises, the appropriate fluid should be designed for the particular patient and his problem. A great variety of special problems can be met by preparation of a special solution from the following list of raw materials:

5%, 10%, 50% glucose in water
0.9% NaCl (154 mM/liter)
5.0% NaCl (855 mM/liter)
7.5% NaHCO$_3$ (900 mM/liter)
14.9% KCl[1] (2,000 mM/liter or 2 mM/ml)
50%[1] MgSO$_4$·7H$_2$O (2mM/ml)

Lastly, it should be emphasized that the most appropriate replacement fluid for lost blood is whole blood; and where the particular need is to expand plasma volume, the use of whole blood, plasma, or a plasma expander is recommended.

Techniques of Administration of Fluids

Fluids may be given by vein, by hypodermoclysis, or by gavage into the stomach. The latter method has many advantages, especially where the problem is likely to last for some time and where the considerations of calories, proteins, and other essential foodstuffs merit attention. The intravenous route is convenient, and the use of plastic tubing threaded into larger veins has eliminated some of the technical problems. The rate of administration of fluid deserves some attention, and in patients with cardiovascular disease the patient should be observed carefully and frequently to ensure the earliest recognition of an untoward response. The potential hazard of cardiovascular complication may serve to modify the fluid prescription and the speed with which the fluids are administered. However, it should certainly not interfere with the proper management of dehydration.

The subcutaneous route may have some advantages in patients with heart disease. The access of fluid from the subcutaneous tissue to the blood stream is obviously slower than when fluid is introduced directly into the vein, but, in addition, its absorption may be even further delayed if there is a rise in venous pressure. In this fashion there is an added factor of safety. If fluids are administered by hypodermoclysis, two precautions must be borne in mind:

1. The fluid should be isotonic with the plasma. If it is hypertonic, there will be a tendency initially for water to leave the plasma and enter the clysis pool. This will cause an initial decrease in plasma volume, which is undesirable, especially if the patient is already dehydrated. Moreover, a hypertonic solution may be quite irritating to the subcutaneous tissue and result in a bad slough of tissue.

[1] These solutions are highly concentrated and should never be administered unless they are diluted.

2. A solution of 5 per cent glucose in water should not be administered by clysis if the patient is dehydrated. When glucose is administered in this fashion, concentration gradients are established for the diffusion of glucose from clysis pool to plasma and for diffusion of sodium from plasma to clysis pool. Sodium diffuses more rapidly than glucose, the fluid in the pool, therefore, becomes hypertonic, and this, in turn, promotes movement of water from the plasma. This reduction in plasma volume superimposed on the antecedent deficit may be sufficient to induce a state of peripheral vascular collapse.

Dehydration

The term *dehydration* continues to mislead, since it implies to many physicians the loss of water alone. Clinical dehydration is rarely a pure deficit of water. Dehydration is usually associated with losses of both salt and water (in proportionate or disproportionate quantities), with deficits of other ions such as potassium, and with the frequent complication of a disturbance in acid-base equilibrium. All these factors must be considered in planning appropriate management. For purposes of orientation and discussion, clinical dehydration may be classified into three major groups as follows:

1. Loss of water in excess of sodium
2. Loss of sodium in excess of water
3. Isotonic losses of sodium and water

LOSS OF WATER IN EXCESS OF SODIUM. The failure to drink is the commonest cause of a water deficit. This is observed most frequently in severely debilitated patients with clouding of consciousness or coma. Not only are these patients too weak and ill to respond to thirst, but they are even unable to communicate the fact that they are thirsty to their families or to their physicians. The size of the water deficit, though it may increase each day, may be small and hence easily overlooked. However, this deficit can achieve significant proportions and contribute greatly to the severity of the patient's illness.

Solute diureses due to glycosuria are usually characterized by a loss of water in excess of salt. This is the situation, for example, in almost all patients with significant degrees of diabetic acidosis.

Another type of solute diuresis may be responsible for a deficit of water. Many physicians have become impressed with the therapeutic value of feeding large quantities of protein. There are many situations in which this is desirable. However, in the early stages of reaction to injury, the ability to store nitrogen may be very seriously impaired, and large amounts of protein (usually administered by gavage) will find their way to urea, demanding excretion in the urine. If the patient is able, he may complain of thirst if the urine flow is large enough to induce a deficit of water. The unconscious patient cannot provide this help. Delay in recognition is due, in great measure, to misinterpretation of the significance of a large flow of urine, especially when the latter is not concentrated.

This is equated with an appropriate state of hydration, whereas, in fact, the large volume of unconcentrated urine may be causing the deficit of water (see Chap. 81).

Diabetes insipidus may be responsible for large deficits of water. Unfortunately, acute diabetes insipidus is commonly associated with trauma or infection in the central nervous system, and hence a clouded or comatose state is not unusual. Major deficits of water may occur in a matter of hours. A large volume of very dilute urine should alert the clinician to this possibility. The defect in the tubular reabsorption of water is easily corrected by the administration of pitressin (see Chap. 81).

The loss of sweat contributes to a deficit of water in excess of salt loss. To the extent that water alone is ingested and retained to replace the volume of lost sweat, a dehydration characterized by a loss of water in excess of salt loss is readily converted to one characterized by a loss of salt in excess of water loss. This serves to emphasize the point that the characteristics of the net deficit are conditioned not only by the quantity and quality of the fluid lost but also by the characteristics of the replacement fluid.

The hallmark of dehydration characterized by a loss of water in excess of salt loss is an increase in the effective osmolality of the extracellular fluids. In most instances this is reflected in an increase in the concentration of sodium in the serum, and the intensity of the hypernatremia may be used as a gauge to calculate the relative deficit of water (see above).

DEFICIT OF SALT IN EXCESS OF WATER DEFICIT. *Adrenal cortical insufficiency* is probably the classic example of this type of dehydration. Although the loss of sodium may be the primary event in the pathogenesis of the dehydration in this disorder, it does not necessarily follow that the concentration of sodium will be depressed in the early phase (see Significance of Hyponatremia). However, as the contraction of volume becomes more significant, further deficits of sodium salts are not accompanied by equivalent deficits of water and hyponatremia supervenes. The dehydration is severe, the cells are overhydrated, and the contracted volume of the plasma may compromise the renal blood flow and glomerular filtration rate, leading to azotemia and some degree of acidosis. The excretion of potassium is diminished. This is owing to the failure to reabsorb sodium at a site in the renal tubule where potassium secretion is coupled with sodium reabsorption. Hyperkalemia out of proportion to the azotemia and hyponatremia is characteristic of this disorder. Peripheral vascular collapse is common, as are hypoglycemia, restlessness, and an altered sensorium.

Patients with chronic renal insufficiency may exhibit an inability to conserve salt properly. This may be of striking proportions and has been known to mimic and be misdiagnosed as adrenal cortical insufficiency. More commonly, the defect is much less intense and may be unmasked only when such patients are advised to restrict the use of dietary salt. The loss of salt each day may not be great, but in the course of time a significant deficit may develop, accompanied by hyponatremia. The dehydration is associated with alterations in renal hemodynamics, and further reduction of an already deficient renal function is a common and dangerous complication. The hazard of a salt-poor regimen in patients with chronic renal disease should be recognized, and it is the responsibility of the physician to make certain that the patient can tolerate the treatment. Careful evaluation of daily weights, observations with respect to changes in concentration of blood urea nitrogen and the concentration of sodium in serum, and an estimation of the total 24-hr excretion of salt in the urine are helpful in evaluating the response.

Some patients with lesions in the central nervous system may excrete large quantities of salt in the urine. As alluded to earlier, these are almost certainly instances of inappropriate secretion of antidiuretic hormone.

ISOTONIC DEFICITS OF SALT AND WATER. In general, these deficits are primarily incurred by losses of fluid from the gastrointestinal tract. The ultimate character of the net deficit will be determined in part by the quality and quantity of fluids that the patient may receive. If the patient refrains from taking fluid and none has been administered by a parenteral route, the continued loss of insensible perspiration, sweat, and urine will determine a net deficit characterized by the loss of water in excess of salt loss. If the patient drinks water and vomits, the net deficit will be a loss of salt in excess of water loss.

ANALYSIS OF THE CHARACTERISTICS OF DEHYDRATION. The discussion presented above concerns the pathogenesis of dehydration in rather isolated terms, and in the hope of achieving clarity the price of oversimplification has been paid. Most patients have experienced a variety of insults of different magnitudes and for shorter or longer periods of time. The essence of the analysis of the characteristics of the dehydration is an assessment of all the data, in both quantitative and qualitative terms. These data are derived from the history, the physical examination, and the laboratory.

History. A careful review of the sequence of events during the course of the illness provides most important information concerning the quality and magnitude of the deficits of electrolytes and water. These data should actually be tabulated, and it is most desirable to develop the habit of preparing a balance sheet to use in the analysis. A sheet with the simple headings indicated below will usually suffice:

Intake:	Output:
Date/time	Diarrhea
Weight	Vomitus
Character of fluid	Urine
Volume	Insensible loss
	Sweat
	Blood

The systematic analysis of these data should provide a fair estimate of deficits in terms of volume, salt, potassium balance, and acid-base equilibrium. In an illness of short duration, information relating to the patient's usual and current weight may be helpful in estimating the volume of fluid that has been lost. The presence or absence of fever and sweating is relevant, as are data concerning the possibility of renal insufficiency or diabetes mellitus. Information concerning the usual level of blood pressure is helpful, since a "normal" blood pressure may be hypotensive for a patient whose blood pressure is usually in the hypertensive range. The symptom of thirst is most significant and can be most helpful in calling the physician's attention to a disorder of hydration which might otherwise be neglected. Thirst is most often due to a primary deficit of water, although it may also reflect a contracted volume, even when salt has been lost in excess of water.

A disorder of hydration may develop during the course of hospitalization. The data referred to above should certainly be available in a precise fashion in the hospital chart. The administration of parenteral fluids should be recorded with as much attention to detail as the record of drug therapy.

Physical Examination. The physical signs may provide important information for the analysis of the deficits of electrolytes and water. The appearance of the skin, its elasticity, texture, temperature, and color, the appearance of the mucous membranes, the tension of the eyeballs, the blood pressure, and the pulse rate all contribute to an estimation of the magnitude of the deficit. The state of consciousness may be related to the magnitude of the deficit. Muscle weakness and diminished-to-absent deep tendon reflexes may suggest potassium depletion.

The character of respiratory activity may suggest a disequilibrium in acid-base relationships. The respirations in metabolic acidosis, with dehydration as an almost invariable concomitant feature, are deep and eventually accelerated, and one can usually detect an effort toward the end of expiration. A systemic alkalosis is suggested by a positive Chvostek reflex; this may also be present if the patient has hypocalcemia despite a concurrent acidosis. Clinically detectable changes in respiration in alkalosis can rarely if ever be appreciated. The odor of acetone on the breath implies a ketonemia.

Laboratory Data. The value of the *packed cell volume* (hematocrit), the concentration of *hemoglobin*, and the concentrations of *total proteins* in the serum can help in evaluating the degree of contraction (or expansion) of the plasma volume. Since this inference is dependent on *changes* in the concentrations, these data are of help primarily in evaluating those disorders that develop while the patient is under observation and in following the progress of a patient whose dehydration is undergoing correction.

It is worthwhile to reemphasize that the concentration of sodium per se cannot possibly be equated with the presence or absence of a state of dehydration. The *concentration* of sodium is merely a statement of the amount of sodium in a liter (or any other unit of volume) of extracellular fluid. The patient with a normal concentration of sodium in the serum may have no disorder of hydration, he may have gained many liters of fluid, or lost a large volume of fluid.

The excretion of urea is related to the amount filtered less the amount reabsorbed through the renal tubules. This latter process is considered to be primarily passive. There are new data suggesting that some component of urea reabsorption may be active. However, to the extent that it is passive it is favored by high concentration gradients between renal tubular and interstitial fluid. Therefore, it is clear that a diminished rate of filtration at the glomerulus, or a highly concentrated urine, or both will favor a diminished rate of excretion and an increase in urea concentration in the body fluids. To the extent that dehydration is responsible for these alterations in renal function, the concentration of urea in blood may serve as a gross index of the severity of the dehydration.

The urinalysis contributes considerable information. In the first place it provides information concerning the probability of renal disease. A urine of high specific gravity, in the absence of glucose or protein, suggests good renal function and an antidiuretic response. This, in turn, carries certain implications with respect to alterations in the internal environment. The excretion of salt despite hyponatremia may indicate one of the salt-wasting disorders.

The concentrations of potassium and total CO_2 content of the serum may be altered, and these deviations are frequently accompanied by disturbances in acid-base equilibrium. These matters are discussed in more detail in Chap. 61. Hypo- or hypermagnesemia may be present. The former is not uncommon in the same situations that are characterized by deficits of potassium such as diabetic acidosis, gastrointestinal disturbances including the malabsorption syndrome, and the postoperative period.

Deficit of Magnesium

There are approximately 2,000 mEq magnesium in the average 70-kg adult, and of this approximately one-half resides in bone. The concentration in serum is between 1.5 and 2.0 mEq/liter and is remarkably constant; approximately one-third of this is bound to protein. The residual magnesium is in the skeletal muscles and parenchymatous tissues.

Much more is known about experimental magnesium deficiency, and most of these data have been obtained in rodents. Nevertheless, a brief review of this information may provide the clues necessary to make new observations at the bedside.

Growing animals made deficient in magnesium with a diet free of this mineral develop hyperemia of the skin, appear ill, lose their appetite, and, finally, startle easily and may have generalized seizures. The common chemical findings in serum include hypomagnesemia, hypercalcemia, hypophosphatemia, mild azotemia, and, significantly, normal levels of potassium and total CO_2 content. The muscle analyses reveal depressed levels of magnesium, and a mild but consistent and significant deficit of potassium despite the fact that the animals received more than what is usually considered adequate quantities of potassium in the dietary regimen. This alteration, in addition to evidence that there is a higher concentration of sodium in the erythrocytes of magnesium-deficient animals, suggests that this deficient state promotes one or more defects in the mechanisms of transport across cell membranes which are crucial to the steady state composition of cell fluid.

The hypercalcemia and hypophosphatemia are accompanied by hyperphosphaturia. The first two observations are not present when control and magnesium-deficient animals which have been parathyroidectomized are compared, but the magnesium-deficient animals still excrete more phosphorus. Thus, some but not all of these alterations reminiscent of hyperparathyroidism are dependent on increased parathyroid activity.

The pathology of this deficient state includes alterations in skeletal and cardiac muscle with myocytolysis and necrosis; and in the kidneys there is a striking nephrocalcinosis. This is unique in that it is confined to the broad ascending limb of the loop of Henle and consists primarily in the formation of microliths within the lumen, with only secondary damage to the cells as the lamellated stone expands in size.

It is, of course, not surprising that deficits of this cation should be accompanied by architectural and functional changes. This ion is known to be an important activator of many enzyme systems. In particular, attention is drawn to alkali-metal-sensitive ATPase, which demands magnesium and which may be important in the mechanisms of active transport.

The clinical circumstances in which magnesium deficiency is likely to be observed include the malabsorption syndromes, chronic alcoholism, prolonged and severe losses of body fluids, diabetic acidosis, cirrhosis of the liver, and primary aldosteronism. It is also noted following removal of a parathyroid adenoma, and this is more likely when there is evidence of bone demineralization. Lastly, patients who must be treated for long periods of time by the parenteral route may develop some deficit of magnesium when this ion is not added to the maintenance fluids.

The symptoms consist primarily of neuromuscular disorders and others related to the central nervous system. In the former area the prominent features include weakness, muscle fasciculation, tremors and occasionally a positive Chvostek's sign, and tetany. With reference to the central nervous system there may be personality changes, agitation, delirium, frank psychoses, and coma. Choreiform and athetoid movements have been noted.

It is important to emphasize that it is difficult to evaluate the specific characteristics of the response to magnesium therapy. This is because magnesium in pharmacologic doses may readily improve some of the signs and symptoms noted above when their origins are not necessarily ascribable to magnesium deficit.

Nevertheless, in the presence of these symptoms with evidence of magnesium deficiency, these patients should be treated with appropriate amounts of magnesium.

Since one cannot define antecedently the quantitative nature of the deficit, the repletion program must be empirical. The use of the intramuscular route for the injection of magnesium sulfate is appropriate, and if modest doses, such as 10 mEq magnesium (2.5 ml 50 per cent $MgSO_4 \cdot 7H_2O$), are given at intervals and the serum levels checked, it is unlikely that one will promote hazardous hypermagnesemia. In general, levels as high as 3 to 4 mEq/liter in the serum are unassociated with untoward effects.

Principles of Management of Dehydration

The initial goals of the management of a state of dehydration are simple and include the restoration of the body fluids to normal volume, effective osmolality, composition, and acid-base relations. The quality and quantity of fluids required to satisfy these goals depend on the analysis of the characteristics of the dehydration. On the basis of this analysis it should be possible to outline a course of action. Since the analysis cannot be expected to be precise, it is wise to include in the outline a plan to interrupt therapy at an appropriate point to allow a reevaluation of the status of the patient. This reevaluation should employ all the available clinical and laboratory data relevant to the problem. The initial plan of management may then be modified in accord with this second analysis. Like the management of many other clinical problems, management of dehydration requires a combination of information, logic, and empiricism. In many instances the restoration of normal volume and tonicity of the body fluids, and the repair of a deficit of potassium, if present, will be accompanied by the coincidental correction of a complicating disturbance in acid-base balance. The administration of insulin and, at an appropriate time, of glucose and potassium is obviously necessary in a patient with diabetic acidosis. Since the alleviation of the acid-base disturbance is dependent on normal renal and respiratory function, these problems are more complex in patients with renal and pulmonary disease (see Chap. 61). The basic principles of the management of adrenal cortical insufficiency do not differ from those presented above; however, cortisone or hydrocortisone and 9-α-fluorohydrocortisone are added to the regimen. The management of the water deficit in diabetes insipidus differs from that of other deficits of water only insofar as the patient with diabetes insipidus should be given a preparation of the posterior pituitary gland to replace the deficiency of the ADH.

When these first goals have been realized, plans must be made to maintain the normal state of hydration. The fluid prescription must be developed in relation to the usual basal requirements and their possible alterations in this particular patient and to the need to replace losses other than those included in the former category.

REFERENCES

Elkinton, J. R., and T. S. Danowski: "The Body Fluids, Basic Physiology and Practical Therapeutics," Baltimore, The Williams & Wilkins Company, 1955.

Moore, F. D., H. Olesen, D. McMurrey, H. V. Parker, M. R. Ball, and C. M. Boyden: "The Body Cell Mass," Philadelphia, W. B. Saunders Company, 1963.

Ussing, H. H., P. Kruhøffer, J. H. Thaysen, and N. A. Thorn: The Alkali Metal Ions in Biology, in "Handbuch der Experimentellen Pharmakologie," O. Eichler and A. Farah (Eds.), Berlin, Springer-Verlag, 1960.

Welt, Louis G.: Water Balance in Health and Disease, p. 449, in "Diseases of Metabolism," 5th ed., G. G. Duncan (Ed.), Philadelphia, W. B. Saunders Company, 1964.

61 ACIDOSIS AND ALKALOSIS

Louis G. Welt and Charles H. Burnett

PHYSIOLOGIC CONSIDERATIONS

An understanding of the physiologic regulation and the clinical disorders of acid-base balance is often needlessly difficult because of the multiple uses and misuses of the terms *acid* and *base*. In the past these terms have been applied to anions and cations. This is not now acceptable, although the respectability of long usage has tended to perpetuate the error. Moreover, this is not a semantic quibble, since the use of these inadequate and misleading definitions creates a major handicap in the efforts to appreciate the very nature of the problem. In this discussion the term *acid* refers to any substance that can donate a hydrogen ion (H^+), and *base* means any substance that can accept a hydrogen ion. This statement may be rewritten as follows:

$$Acid \rightleftharpoons base + H^+$$

Some substances may serve as an acid *or* a base. For example, $H_2PO_4^-$ can dissociate to H^+ and HPO_4^{--}, or it can accept a hydrogen ion to form H_3PO_4. In the first instance it serves as an acid, and in the second as a base. These definitions serve to focus attention on the hydrogen ion as the significant item in acid-base balance. The manner in which the concentration of hydrogen ions may be expressed and the inferences drawn from this expression therefore become highly relevant.

The dissociation of an acid, HA, may be expressed in the following manner:

$$HA \rightleftharpoons H^+ + A^- \qquad (1)$$

The rate at which this reaction proceeds to the right is proportional to the molar concentration of the acid and may be said to be equivalent to $k_1[HA]$. Like-

wise, the rate at which the reaction proceeds to the left is proportional to the product of the molar concentrations of H^+ and A^- and may be described as equivalent to $k_2[H^+][A^-]$. At equilibrium the two rates are equal, and therefore

$$k_1[HA] = k_2[H^+][A^-] \qquad (2)$$

This equation can be rearranged to

$$\frac{k_1}{k_2} = \frac{[H^+][A^-]}{[HA]} \qquad (3)$$

The ratio of the two constants can be included in one new constant, K, and the statement can be rearranged to function as an expression of the concentration of hydrogen ions:

$$[H^+] = K \frac{[HA]}{[A^-]} \qquad (4)$$

Sorenson introduced the alternative method of expressing the concentration of hydrogen ions as the negative logarithm. The latter is denoted as pH, and the following statement emerges:

$$pH = pK + \log \frac{[A^-]}{[HA]} \qquad (5)$$

This may be stated in the more general form:

$$pH = pK + \log \frac{[base]}{[acid]} \qquad (6)$$

which is referred to as the *Henderson-Hasselbalch equation*. The logarithm of 1.0 is zero, and therefore when the concentrations of the base (the hydrogen ion acceptor) and the acid (the hydrogen ion donor) are equal to each other, the pH is equal to pK.

Buffers

A buffered solution is able to minimize the deviation of pH by adding to that solution a strong acid or a strong base. A buffer pair is composed of a weakly dissociated acid or base and a highly dissociated salt. Such a pair might be designated as HA and NaA. The addition of a strong acid, such as HCl, to this solution would promote the following reaction:

$$HA + NaA + HCl \rightarrow 2HA + NaCl$$

In this fashion a weak acid is substituted for the strong acid. The concentration of hydrogen ions will be increased to the extent that the increment of weak acid dissociates. This increase is clearly considerably less than that which would have occurred had the HCl been added to pure water.

The pH of a buffered solution will be defined by the ratio of the molar concentrations of the members of the buffer pair:

$$pH = pK + \log \frac{[NaA]}{[HA]}$$

Several characteristics of buffer activity are implicit in this equation. The deviation in pH consequent to the addition of an acid stronger than HA will be equated with a decrease in the concentration of A$^-$ (represented by the numerator of the ratio) and an increase in the concentration of HA. This implies that, for a given increment of acid, the least change in pH will occur when the buffer ratio has a value of 1. Another implication is that, at *any* specific ratio of the concentrations of the pair, the addition of a given quantity of acid will alter the ratio less if the concentrations of the members of the pair are high rather than low. Finally, it is apparent that the capacity to buffer is lost when there is no hydrogen ion acceptor (base) left.

A solution may contain several buffers. The ratio of the concentrations of the components of each buffer pair is determined by the pH and, in turn, determines the pH. The ratios of each pair will be different at a specific pH in accordance with the individual dissociation constant for the system. Therefore, in a solution with several buffers a change in one component of any pair will dictate a change in the ratio for every other pair.

As mentioned in the preceding chapter, the body fluid most accessible for analysis is the plasma, and the pH of the extracellular fluid can be defined by the relationship between NaHCO$_3$ and H$_2$CO$_3$, or, more precisely, the tension of CO$_2$(P_{CO_2}).[1] This is expressed by the equation

$$pH = 6.1 + \log \frac{NaHCO_3}{\underset{\underset{CO_2 + H_2O}{\Updownarrow}}{H_2CO_3 + \text{dissolved } CO_2}}$$

The ratio of the concentrations of sodium bicarbonate and the carbonic acid plus dissolved CO$_2$ is 20:1 at the pH of serum 7.40. This is far removed from the more efficient ratio of 1:1, and in a closed system this would be a poor buffer pair at that pH. However, the buffer is unique in that its acid component is a gas whose excretion can be rapidly accelerated or diminished by variations in respiratory exchange, and it is ubiquitous in that it is constantly being formed as a metabolic end product.

Although much of the buffer activity within the body is reflected and mirrored in the bicarbonate–carbonic acid system, this is by no means the only important buffer system in the body's fluids. The proteins of the plasma, the hemoglobin of the red blood cells, and the bicarbonate, phosphate, and proteins of the intracellular fluids all play a significant role in buffer activity. The sum total of the anions of the buffer salts capable of accepting hydrogen ions (i.e., the sum total of *base*) represents the first line of defense in absorbing the insult of the accession of an acid load in the body. The total of all body buffers (including those contributed by cations from cells and bones) cannot be estimated readily; some indication of their magnitude and a reflection of changes

[1] The term P_{CO_2} refers to the partial pressure of carbon dioxide and is usually close to 40 mm Hg.

therein may be obtained from a consideration, as developed by Singer and Hastings, of the buffers present in whole blood alone.

The buffers in whole blood include the bicarbonate, proteins, and phosphate of the plasma and the hemoglobin, bicarbonate, and phosphate salts in the red blood cells. In addition, since the anionic properties of hemoglobin vary between the reduced and oxygenated state, the degree of saturation of hemoglobin with oxygen must be stipulated. The sum of these buffers has been referred to as *buffer base*. Initially this term was used to mean the cation equivalents of the buffer anion. It is now more proper to use the term interchangeably with *buffer anion* itself. The range of normal values for the sum of the buffer base is 46 to 52 mM/liter. The values for buffer base and P_{CO_2} can be read from a nomogram prepared by Singer and Hastings if the pH of the blood, the hematocrit, and the total CO$_2$ content of whole blood or plasma are known. Since the anionic properties of the proteins vary directly with pH, the primary retention or loss of carbon dioxide and bicarbonate, as in respiratory disturbances, is accompanied by reciprocal changes in the buffer base value for the proteins. Hence, the characteristic of respiratory acidosis and alkalosis will be the lack of deviation from normal in the value for buffer base. In contrast, the value for buffer base will be diminished in metabolic acidosis and increased in metabolic alkalosis.

Astrup and Siggaard-Andersen have emphasized the concept of *standard bicarbonate,* from which one can calculate a base excess or a base deficit. In a sense this represents a somewhat more refined and sophisticated method of determining what was alluded to above as the buffer base of Singer and Hastings. The essence of the concept is to remove from consideration the contribution made by the respiratory regulatory defenses. In this technique the pH of the blood is determined as drawn. Following this the pH is again measured at two different levels of P_{CO_2}, and the hemoglobin is rendered fully oxygenated. From a nomogram one can then determine the standard bicarbonate. The normal values range between 21 and 25 mEq/liter. If the determined value is greater, there is a base excess and, if lower, a base deficit. Thus, if the pH of the blood as originally drawn is depressed or elevated and there is neither a base excess nor deficit, the disturbance is respiratory in origin. Those who champion this system consider an additional advantage to be the quantitative nature of the determination and stress its usefulness in management of the clinical problem. In contrast, others have indicated that this technique offers little that is not readily available through less elaborate methods; and they point out in addition that the specific datum of base excess or deficit can be misleading.

ACIDOSIS AND ALKALOSIS

It should be clear from the above that the status of the acid-base relationship cannot be evaluated solely from knowledge of the total CO_2 content of the serum. This latter represents the sum of the members of the buffer pair and includes bicarbonate as well as carbonic acid and CO_2 gas. The total provides no information with respect to the relative proportions of the components of the buffer pair. In fact, a high or low concentration of total CO_2 is compatible with either acidosis or alkalosis. The pH of arterial blood (or blood obtained from a limb vein after warming the part at 45°C for about 10 min) is ultimately necessary to define the acid-base relationship. The pH, however, may be found to be disturbed more or less than the deviation in total CO_2 content of the serum. This depends, in part, on the sequence of events, the speed with which the distortion has supervened, and the success or failure of the compensatory mechanisms. Furthermore, in more complicated circumstances, the estimation of both P_{CO_2} and whole blood buffer base may be necessary to unravel the nature of the disturbance in acid-base relationships.

CALCULATION OF P_{CO_2} AND PARTITION OF TOTAL CO_2 CONTENT

The quantity of carbon dioxide dissolved in a liquid is proportional to the P_{CO_2} and can be expressed in millimoles per liter as equal to alpha P_{CO_2}. The term *alpha* is equal to 0.0301 (mM/liter/mm Hg) for plasma at a temperature of 38°C. At different body temperatures an appropriate correction must be made. In turn, dissolved CO_2 is in equilibrium with H_2CO_3, and therefore the sum of dissolved CO_2 and carbonic acid can be said to be proportional to P_{CO_2}. Since the quantity of dissolved CO_2 is so much greater than the concentration of carbonic acid, this value will be used as the denominator in the Henderson-Hasselbalch equation.

In the sample calculation to follow, it will be assumed that the pH is 7.40, the total CO_2 content is 26 mM/liter, and the pK for the bicarbonate–CO_2 system is 6.10. The Henderson-Hasselbalch equation may be written as follows:

$$pH = 6.10 + \log \frac{(HCO_3^-)}{(\alpha P_{CO_2})}$$

Since the concentration of bicarbonate in plasma is equal to the difference between the total CO_2 content and P_{CO_2}, the equation may be rewritten:

$$pH = 6.10 + \log \frac{(\text{total } CO_2) - (\alpha P_{CO_2})}{(\alpha P_{CO_2})}$$

$$7.40 = 6.10 + \log \frac{(26) - (0.0301\, P_{CO_2})}{(0.0301\, P_{CO_2})}$$

$$7.40 - 6.10 = 1.3 = \log \frac{(26) - (0.0301\, P_{CO_2})}{(0.0301\, P_{CO_2})}$$

$$\text{Antilog } 1.3 = \frac{(26) - (0.0301\, P_{CO_2})}{(0.0301\, P_{CO_2})}$$

$$\text{Antilog } 1.3 = 19.95$$

therefore,

$$19.95\,(0.0301\, P_{CO_2}) = (26) - (0.0301\, P_{CO_2})$$
$$19.95\,(0.0301\, P_{CO_2})$$
$$+\ (0.0301\, P_{CO_2}) = 26$$
$$0.6306\, P_{CO_2} = 26$$
$$P_{CO_2} = \frac{26}{0.6306}$$
$$P_{CO_2} = 41.2 \text{ mm Hg}$$

The sum of the concentrations of dissolved CO_2 and H_2CO_3 is equal to

$$0.0301\, P_{CO_2} = 0.0301 \times 41.2 = 1.24 \text{ mM/L}$$

Since the concentration of bicarbonate ion is the difference between total CO_2 content and the value for dissolved CO_2 and H_2CO_3,

$$(HCO_3^-) = 26 - 1.24 = 24.76 \text{ mM/L}$$

REGULATION OF ACID–BASE EQUILIBRIUM

In general, the problem of regulating acid-base balance in health is to protect the pH from alterations induced by the continuous formation of acid end products of metabolism. In health the pH of the extracellular fluids is maintained at a level between 7.35 and 7.45. This is accomplished by buffer activity (discussed earlier), by exchange of ions between the two major fluid compartments, and by adaptations of respiratory and renal function.

REGULATION BY ION EXCHANGE. The exchange of *anions* across membranes appears to be restricted to the red cells and, probably, the renal tubular cells. Chloride and bicarbonate ions can diffuse across the erythrocyte membrane, and their distribution between the red cell and plasma water is responsive to changes in their concentrations and pH. For example, an increase in the P_{CO_2} of the plasma due to the addition of carbon dioxide is followed by diffusion of the gas into the red cell, where part of it is hydrated to H_2CO_3. The dissociation of this acid increases the concentration of bicarbonate ions, and these diffuse from the cell. This, in turn, is accompanied by a movement of chloride into the red cells. The net effect of this redistribution of anions in terms of the acid-base relationships of the extracellular fluid is to increase the concentration of bicarbonate in this compartment. This increase in the concentration of HCO_3^- tends to offset the effect of the initial increase in P_{CO_2} on the buffer ratio of the Henderson-Hasselbalch equation.

The exchange of *cations* such as sodium, potassium, and perhaps calcium as well from muscle cells and bone for hydrogen ions in the extracellular fluid (and vice versa) plays a significant role in modifying the alterations in pH of the extracellular fluids. It has been estimated, for example, that approximately 50 per cent of an acid load administered to dogs was neutralized by such an exchange of sodium and potassium for hydrogen ions. In another study it was suggested that 25 per cent of the "neutralization" of an infusion of $NaHCO_3$ had been achieved by the exchange of extracellular sodium for intracellular hydrogen ions. Similar exchanges are reported in studies of both respiratory acidosis and respiratory alkalosis.

RESPIRATORY REGULATION. The lungs play a major role in the excretion of acid as carbon dioxide. Moreover, the centers that regulate the rate and depth of ventilation are exquisitely sensitive to subtle changes in the composition of the blood and extravascular fluids. The central chemoreceptors located in the medullary respiratory centers are responsive to the P_{CO_2} and pH of their environment in such a way that an increase in P_{CO_2} or hydrogen ion concentration promotes an increase in pulmonary ventilation. In contrast, a decrease in CO_2 tension or increase in pH tends to inhibit ventilation. In either case it is clear that the alteration in respiratory activity tends to correct the primary deviation in P_{CO_2} or pH. The P_{CO_2} appears to be the more potent stimulus of the two. In addition, there are peripheral chemoreceptors located in the carotid and aortic bodies. These are relatively insensitive to pH and P_{CO_2} but are responsive to the arterial oxygen tension (P_{O_2}).

An interesting aspect of the chemoregulation of pulmonary ventilation concerns the phenomenon of a change in the "sensitivity" of the central respiratory centers to a specific P_{CO_2}. It appears as though a period of hypercapnia diminishes "sensitivity," and hypocapnia enhances the intensity of the response to a given tension of CO_2. The precise nature of this altered response is not clear. An appreciation of this adaptation is helpful in understanding certain complications of acid-base disorders, which will be discussed in more detail later (see Chap. 15 for a more complete discussion of respiratory regulation).

RENAL REGULATION. The kidneys contribute to the regulation of acid-base balance by varying the net rate of excretion of hydrogen ions and by processes of selective reabsorption and rejection of cations and anions. These two processes are interdependent to the extent that the reabsorption of sodium is closely related to the secretion of hydrogen ions and potassium. The total rate of *secretion* of hydrogen ions by the tubular cells may be calculated from the sum of the titratable acid, ammonium ion, and a fraction equivalent to the difference between the filtered and excreted bicarbonate. The part each of the above phenomena plays in the urinary *excretion* of acid or alkaline loads is discussed below.

The titratable acid is equivalent to the quantity of NaOH that must be added to the urine to change its pH to that of the plasma. It represents the hydrogen ions present in free acid compounds and incorporated in the buffer components of the urine. Caution must be exercised to avoid the error of necessarily equating a low urinary pH with a high rate of excretion of acid. A small quantity of dissociated acid in a poorly buffered urine will lower the pH considerably. This same quantity of titratable acid in a

buffered solution might be accommodated with very little depression of pH.

Pitts and his collaborators demonstrated that the urinary excretion of acid may be in excess of what can be accounted for by filtration and preferential reabsorption. They developed the hypothesis that hydrogen ions are secreted into the tubular fluid in exchange for sodium. The source of the hydrogen ions for this secretory process is not known for certain, although it is usually represented as having been derived from carbonic acid. The latter, in turn, is believed to be formed from the hydration of carbon dioxide:

$$H_2O + CO_2 \atop \updownarrow \atop H_2CO_3 \atop \updownarrow \atop H^+ + HCO_3^-$$
This reaction accelerated by the enzyme carbonic anhydrase

The rate of tubular *secretion* of hydrogen ions is probably conditioned by many factors, some of which include the pH of the renal tubular cell fluid, the P_{CO_2} (rather than the pH) of the extracellular fluid, the availability of buffers in the tubular fluid, the intensity of the stimuli primarily responsible for the reabsorption of sodium, and the status of the stores of potassium in the tubular cells. A decreased pH in the cell fluid, hypercapnia, and a diminished content of potassium in the renal tubular cells tend to favor the secretion of hydrogen ions. These ions cannot be secreted against a concentration gradient in excess of approximately 800:1. A diminished tubular content of buffer will therefore impose a restriction on the rate of secretion of hydrogen ions by failing to resist the decrease in pH consequent to this secretion.

In essence one can view the major role of the kidney in combating acidosis as reabsorbing all the filtered bicarbonate and, in addition, regenerating the bicarbonate that is continuously dissipated by the buffer action of strong acids with the bicarbonate–carbonic acid system. These operations can be portrayed in the following fashion:

1. The reabsorption of filtered bicarbonate

It will be noted that the reabsorption of the filtered bicarbonate is somewhat indirect. The sodium which is reabsorbed by exchange with hydrogen ion is then transported from the cell to the interstitial fluid of the kidney along with the bicarbonate remnant of the carbonic acid that donated the hydrogen ion. The carbonic acid left behind in the tubular fluid is then dehydrated to CO_2 and H_2O, and the carbon dioxide diffuses back to the body fluids.

2. The reabsorption of bicarbonate that is *not* filtered

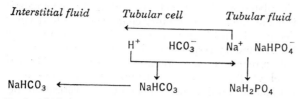

In this fashion sodium of a salt other than bicarbonate is reabsorbed in exchange for a hydrogen ion that becomes incorporated in a buffer. In a somewhat similar fashion the following reaction may obtain when the anion accompanying sodium is relatively unable to permeate the tubular cell membrane:

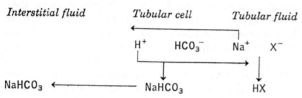

In addition to excretion as titratable acid, as illustrated above, hydrogen ions are excreted as ammonium, NH_4^+, as well. The sequence of events leading to enhanced excretion of ammonium depends in part on the reaction just described. The active transport of sodium produces a potential difference across the tubular membranes such that the lumen is negative. This creates a driving force which can be accommodated either by reabsorption of an anion with a negative charge along the established electrochemical gradient or by secretion of a positively charged cation. If the anion cannot permeate, the second alternative must obtain. Hydrogen ions can be secreted until the luminal fluid pH falls to a level against which no more hydrogen ions can be transported. Ammonia is considered to be in diffusion equilibrium between tubular cells and lumen and can move freely in either direction, but NH_4^+ cannot. Thus, if hydrogen ions are secreted and all filtered buffers are exhausted, the NH_3 in the luminal fluid can buffer the hydrogen ion. The NH_4^+ which is formed cannot diffuse back and hence is excreted into the urine. This sets the direction of the reaction pathway for ammonia, the hydrogen ion gradient is reduced, and now more hydrogen ions can be secreted. This may be illustrated in the following fashion:

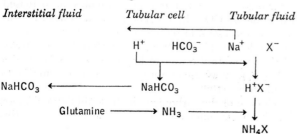

The rate of excretion of ammonia does not change as acutely as is the case with titratable acid, but in appropriate circumstances it may make a greater contribution in quantitative terms. Ammonia is formed in the tubular cells, and the largest fraction is derived from glutamine. The deamidation of glutamine is accelerated by the enzyme glutaminase, which is present in the kidneys.

Thus, in these several ways the renal tubules regenerate the bicarbonate that is dissipated (and excreted as CO_2) by the buffer activity consequent to the accession of an acid load in the body fluids.

The reabsorption of sodium may be associated with an exchange for potassium in lieu of hydrogen ion. These alternatives are frequently pictured as competing one with the other. These interrelationships may explain, in part, the aciduria which may accompany potassium depletion despite an extracellular alkalosis; and this may also explain why the administration of $NaHCO_3$ is accompanied by an augmented excretion of potassium.

The administration of a carbonic anhydrase inhibitor suppresses all these reactions that depend on a readily available source of hydrogen ions. Such an agent promotes increased excretion of sodium, bicarbonate, and potassium and decreases the rate of excretion of titratable acid and ammonia. Some of these alterations are observed in patients with renal disease characterized by tubular dysfunction. The defect in some instances is due to inability to transport hydrogen ions against a concentration gradient.

The role of the kidneys in acid-base regulation will be discussed further later in this chapter. The nature of the specific responses in each type of acid-base disturbance will serve to illustrate the particular contributions of the kidneys.

A comment is in order concerning the significance of *compensation*. The responses just described are initiated by a distortion of one or more of the physicochemical characteristics of the body fluids. If the response were such as to efface the distortion, the stimulus for the response would be removed and the distortion would reappear. Thus, it is unlikely that compensation can ever be perfect since it would automatically be self-destructive so long as the initial basis for the disturbance persisted. Hence, if a patient with an obvious acid-base disturbance has a normal value for pH, or P_{CO_2}, or total CO_2 content, the implication is that this is almost certainly an instance of a *mixed* acid-base disturbance.

CLINICAL CONSIDERATIONS

There are four major disturbances in acid-base equilibrium, and it is convenient to discuss them individually and as separate entities. Nevertheless it should be remembered that mixed disturbances occur fairly frequently. In this discussion the aim is to analyze each disorder in terms of the primary alteration, the impact of this insult and the compensatory respiratory and renal responses on the Henderson-Hasselbalch equation, the nature of the compositional changes, and the approach to the management of the disorder. The Henderson-Hasselbalch equation is re-presented here with respect to the bicarbonate–carbonic acid buffer system. Reference to this equation, which defines the pH, is most helpful in visualizing the sequence and consequence of primary and secondary events in the pathogenesis of acidosis and alkalosis:

$$pH = 6.1 + \log \frac{NaHCO_3}{\underset{\underset{CO_2 + H_2O}{\Updownarrow}}{H_2CO_3 + \text{dissolved } CO_2}}$$

The ratio of the concentrations of the buffer pair is 20:1.

Respiratory Acidosis

Respiratory acidosis is due to inadequate elimination of CO_2 by the lungs because of hypoventilation or because of uneven ventilation in relation to blood flow. It is unlikely to be associated solely with impaired diffusion across the alveolar capillary membranes, since the diffusion of CO_2 is so rapid. Respiratory acidosis is found commonly in patients with conditions such as emphysema, pulmonary fibrosis, and cardiopulmonary disease.

The retention of CO_2 will increase the P_{CO_2} and the concentration of carbonic acid. The increase in the value for the denominator of the buffer ratio will change this to something less than 20:1 and will define a decrease in the pH. The CO_2 can penetrate cell membranes freely, and in this fashion a considerable quantity of acid can be buffered in the intracellular fluids. In addition, there is evidence that hydrogen ions from the extracellular fluids exchange for potassium and sodium from cells and bone.

The increase in P_{CO_2} and the decrease in pH both serve to stimulate ventilation, and further accumulation of CO_2 may be prevented or at least retarded thereby. The renal response is characterized by increased excretion of titratable acid, ammonium, and chloride and diminished excretion of bicarbonate. The above-mentioned response clearly implies a net increase in the total rate of *secretion* of hydrogen ions by the renal tubule, which is not necessarily the case in metabolic acidosis (see below). In this manner the kidneys help eliminate acid, but, in addition, they alter electrolyte composition so that the concentration of bicarbonate in the extracellular fluid increases at the expense of chloride. To the extent that this increase in the concentration of bicarbonate restores the buffer ratio toward 20:1, the deviation of the pH is minimized. The ability to tolerate a high P_{CO_2} has an additional advantage in that a greater quantity of CO_2 is excreted per unit of ventilation. This increment may be sufficiently large to allow the excretion of CO_2 to

equal its production. In this circumstance no further increase in P_{CO_2} will occur unless the primary disease worsens.

It was stated earlier that the increase in CO_2 tension stimulated respiratory activity, but as the hypercapnia is maintained the respiratory centers appear to develop decreased sensitivity to this stimulus. A diminution in the respiratory response to the next increment of P_{CO_2} will promote a more intense hypercapnia. This new level of P_{CO_2} serves to maintain some increase in ventilation until a new level of desensitization develops, and the vicious cycle is repeated. Ultimately the hypercapnia becomes extreme, and the increased P_{CO_2} no longer serves as an appropriate stimulus to increase ventilation. At this time the most important stimulus for respiratory activity is the accompanying hypoxia. It has been said that if patients with respiratory acidosis were left to their own devices, they would probably succumb to hypoxia rather than to hypercapnia or acidosis. The slower diffusion of oxygen would be expected to promote incapacitating hypoxia before the development of CO_2 narcosis or a pH incompatible with life. However, if such patients are treated by exposure to a breathing mixture with a high content of oxygen in an effort to relieve the hypoxemia, they may quickly become confused, lapse into coma, and die. The improvement in the hypoxia may remove the last effective stimulus for respiratory activity. As a result of the diminished ventilation, there is a further decline in the excretion of CO_2, leading to the grave consequences of extreme hypercapnia. This should not be interpreted to suggest that such patients should never be treated with oxygen; it emphasizes the need for close observation when oxygen therapy is used to detect the earliest evidences of this complication. If morphine is given these patients, it should be administered with caution, since this drug may affect the respiratory center in such a manner as to induce hypoventilation. This, in turn, will promote a sharp increase in the P_{CO_2}, the intensity of the acidosis, and the degree of hypoxia.

The management of these patients includes all those measures which may be expected to improve the basic disease condition responsible for pulmonary insufficiency, as discussed in Chap. 176. However, these measures may fail, and the extreme hypoxia and hypercapnia may require immediate attention. In this situation artificial respiration (by mechanical respirator) may offer a valuable therapeutic approach. The increase in ventilatory exchange induced by the respirator improves the hypoxia and promotes an increased excretion of CO_2. In the course of a few days this may be successful in reducing the P_{CO_2} to more nearly normal levels. This, in turn, may restore the sensitivity of the respiratory center to lower levels of CO_2, and a rising P_{CO_2} may again serve as a proper stimulus to respiratory activity.

The use of the carbonic anhydrase inhibitor Diamox has been recommended in the management of this problem. Although it has not been uniformly successful, some patients appear to have improved as a result of its use. Furthermore, the observed data are not sufficiently consistent to permit certainty as to the precise sequence of events by which it has been effective. A reasonable working hypothesis suggests that the first event is augmented excretion of bicarbonate in the urine, leading to decreased concentration of bicarbonate in the extracellular fluids. This change should dictate a decrease in pH. If this latter were successful in stimulating an increase in respiratory activity with an augmented excretion of CO_2, the pH would be restored toward normal and the P_{CO_2} would be diminished. The decrease in hypercapnia would be expected to restore the sensitivity of the respiratory centers to lower tensions of CO_2, and this would have the same beneficial effect as that described above with respect to artificial respiration. However, the data do not always support this hypothesis, and some suggest that Diamox has an effect on the respiratory center itself which may serve to improve ventilation. Another agent that may be useful is salicylate, which may be ingested as aspirin or administered intravenously as the sodium salt. This drug definitely increases the sensitivity of the respiratory center to carbon dioxide and may be helpful in patients with chronic hypercapnia. Progesterone has been reported to influence the sensitivity of the respiratory center to carbon dioxide. Vanillic acid diethylamide improves ventilation primarily by increasing the depth rather than the rate of respiration. It may be useful in the management of acute as well as chronic respiratory insufficiency. One other agent has been suggested to combat respiratory acidosis, namely, THAM (tris hydroxy methyl amino methane). This agent combines with CO_2 and in this fashion aids in restoring the pH toward normal. However, this by itself might have undesirable consequences by reducing ventilation and oxygenation. Hence, its use without mechanical assistance may be harmful, and if the latter is provided, the use of THAM would appear unnecessary.

The compositional changes in the serum have been mentioned; a fairly typical pattern of concentrations of electrolytes in a patient with respiratory acidosis is

Na.	137 mEq/L
K.	4.5 mEq/L
Total CO_2.	40 mM/L
Cl.	90 mEq/L
pH.	7.31
P_{CO_2}.	79 mm Hg

The pattern, neglecting pH and P_{CO_2}, would also be compatible with metabolic alkalosis. The gross characteristics of the underlying clinical problem will usually dictate the appropriate selection between these two alternatives. The normal concentration of potassium suggests that this is not metabolic alkalosis. The arterial pH clearly resolves the problem in the above instance.

Metabolic Acidosis

Metabolic acidosis is due to either an accumulation of acids or a primary loss of bicarbonate. An accumulation of acids is observed classically in diabetic acidosis and in renal insufficiency, and a primary loss of bicarbonate may be observed in renal disease as well. In diabetes the offenders are the 4-carbon ketones, and if these may be represented by the expression HK, the consequences of their accession to the extracellular fluid may be visualized as follows:

$$HK + NaHCO_3 \rightleftharpoons NaK + H_2CO_3$$

If this buffering of the ketone acid is related to the effect on the Henderson-Hasselbalch equation, it is readily observed that the reduction in bicarbonate and increase in carbonic acid will decrease the ratio to something less than 20:1 and will define a decrease in the pH. The latter as well as the presumed initial increase in P_{CO_2} both serve as stimuli to increase pulmonary ventilation, the excretion of CO_2 will be accelerated, P_{CO_2} will fall, the buffer ratio will be restored toward 20:1, and the deviation in pH is minimized. The violent respiratory response to acidosis characterized by an increase first in depth and later in frequency of respirations is referred to as *Kussmaul breathing*. If one observes the characteristics of this respiratory activity closely, it is usually noted that the effort appears to be on the expiratory phase in contrast to the inspiratory effort noted in patients with oxygen lack.

Since the P_{CO_2} is depressed along with the decrease in pH, the inference is either that the latter is now solely responsible for the increased respiratory activity or that the hypocapnia has induced a state of increased sensitivity of the respiratory centers to low tensions of CO_2. The latter appears quite likely, and it has been pointed out that during the recovery phase of several types of metabolic acidosis, the pH reaches normal values while the P_{CO_2} is still depressed. This would be an unlikely event unless the respiratory center was responsive to these lower levels of P_{CO_2}.

The renal response to this metabolic acidosis includes virtual total reabsorption of filtered bicarbonate and an increase in the net *urinary excretion* of acid as titratable acid and ammonia. The increase in net excretion of acid does not necessarily imply an increase in the net *secretion* of hydrogen ions. This will be apparent if it is recalled that the secretion of hydrogen ions to effect total reabsorption of a small filtered load of bicarbonate may be considerably less than that needed for incomplete reabsorption of bicarbonate when there is a much higher filtered load, as is the case normally or in respiratory acidosis. The net rates of excretion of acid may be similar in respiratory and metabolic acidosis, although presumably more hydrogen ion is secreted in the former to effect the larger bicarbonate reabsorption. Thus, although higher levels of P_{CO_2} favor the secretion of hydrogen ions, the renal response, in terms of the *net excretion* of acid, is not jeopardized by the hypocapnia of metabolic acidosis.

A fairly typical pattern of the concentrations of electrolytes in the serum in diabetic acidosis is

Na	125 mEq/L
K	3.5 mEq/L
Total CO_2	5 mM/L
Cl	90 mEq/L
Glucose	800 mg per 100 ml
pH	7.01
P_{CO_2}	19 mm Hg

It will be noted that the sum of the concentrations of CO_2 and chloride is 95 mEq/liter. The difference between this sum and the concentration of sodium is 30 mEq/liter, which is significantly higher than the usual difference of 5 to 10 mEq/liter and implies an unusual concentration of some anion other than bicarbonate and chloride. In diabetic acidosis this is likely to be almost all represented by ketones. (Although the concentration of sodium is depressed, the effective osmolality of the extracellular fluids will be found to be increased if one calculates the osmolar contribution of the elevated concentration of glucose.)[2]

The management of the acid-base disturbance in diabetic patients is not usually a primary concern. The administration of adequate amounts of insulin can be expected to promote the utilization of glucose and to decrease the production of ketones. Under these circumstances the ketonemia is soon dissipated by utilization and excretion, and as the ketonemia subsides, the concentration of bicarbonate increases and the pH is soon restored to more nearly normal levels.

Metabolic acidosis due to the loss of bicarbonate in the urine is not uncommon in chronic renal insufficiency. It is due, presumably, to inadequate reabsorption of bicarbonate by the renal tubular cells. This may, in turn, be due to one of several steps that must precede the actual secretion of hydrogen ions in the process of exchange with sodium. Since this is primarily a reflection of tubular dysfunction, it has been stated that it is seen more commonly in chronic pyelonephritis than in glomerulonephritis or other forms of chronic Bright's disease; it may occur, however, in all types of chronic renal failure. In one rather rare form of renal disease there is relatively little functional evidence of glomerular disease. In some of these disorders, the tubular defect may be congenital in origin. In this last instance the defect appears to be concerned not with the formation of hydrogen ions but with the inability to secrete these ions against the concentration gradient. The net effect of the defect is reduced concentration of bicarbonate in the extracellular fluids, accompanied by reciprocally increased concentration of chloride. The diminution in concentration of bicarbonate defines a decrease in the pH of the extracellular fluid. This latter serves as a stimu-

lus to respiratory activity, increased excretion of CO_2 promotes a decrease in P_{CO_2}, and pH approaches a normal value as the ratio of the buffer pair approaches a value of 20:1. Since the ability to secrete hydrogen ions is not totally defunct, the excretion of bicarbonate diminishes only to the point where the filtered load of bicarbonate reaches a value no longer in excess of the residual capacity to secrete hydrogen ions. This disorder may also be associated with increased excretion of calcium and potassium. The latter is not unexpected by virtue of the competitive relationship between hydrogen ions and potassium for exchange with sodium. The reason for the augmented excretion of calcium is less clear. It may be due, in part, to the effect of systemic acidosis in mobilizing calcium from bone. It may also represent some specific renal response of an adaptive nature.

A characteristic set of concentrations of electrolytes in the serum is

Na	134 mEq/L
K	3.5 mEq/L
Total CO_2	12 mM/L
Cl	115 mEq/L
PO_4	2 mEq/L
pH	7.25
P_{CO_2}	26 mm Hg

It should be noted that the sum of the concentrations of CO_2 and chloride, 127 mEq/liter, differs only by 7 mEq/liter from the concentration of sodium and that the phosphate concentration is normal. This makes it clear that the depression of CO_2 cannot be ascribed to the accumulation of anions other than chloride. This same pattern might be observed in a patient who had received large doses of NH_4Cl or Diamox or who had respiratory alkalosis. The determination of the pH readily resolves the directional deviation in this instance. In clinical situations the history alone should reveal whether this pattern resulted from a renal lesion or from the administration of ammonium chloride or a drug.

In instances of renal insufficiency accompanied by a significant decrease in filtration rate and renal mass, there is an inability to regenerate bicarbonate. This may be due in part to the filtration of lesser quantities of sodium salts, diminished buffer capacity in the tubules, and failure to excrete ammonia properly owing to the loss of the tissue responsible for this function. The diminished filtration rate is presumably responsible for the retention of phosphate, sulfate, and other anions of fixed acids as well. This constellation of defects is characterized by a diminution in the total CO_2 content as well as an increase in what is commonly referred to as the *undetermined anions*. Hence, the sum of the concentrations of total CO_2 and chloride subtracted from the concentration of sodium in the serum will usually equal a value in excess of 5 to 10 mEq/liter. This type of acidosis is the one most commonly encountered in chronic renal failure. A characteristic set of concentrations is

---

[2] 180 mg per 100 Gm glucose is approximately equivalent to 10 mOsm/liter.

$$
\begin{array}{ll}
\text{Na} \dots\dots\dots\dots & 130 \text{ mEq/L} \\
\text{K} \dots\dots\dots\dots & 5 \text{ mEq/L} \\
\text{Total CO}_2 \dots\dots & 12 \text{ mM/L} \\
\text{Cl} \dots\dots\dots\dots & 93 \text{ mEq/L} \\
\text{PO}_4 \dots\dots\dots & 7 \text{ mEq/L} \\
\text{pH} \dots\dots\dots & 7.25 \\
P_{\text{CO}_2} \dots\dots\dots & 26 \text{ mm Hg}
\end{array}
$$

Note that the total CO_2 plus chloride subtracted from the sodium equals 25 mEq/liter. The hyperphosphatemia accounts for part of this excess, and sulfates would, if measured, probably be equally increased. Note also the slight hyperkalemia.

Metabolic acidosis due to renal insufficiency can be corrected by administering sodium bicarbonate. In this fashion the concentration of bicarbonate can be increased and the buffer ratio restored to a normal value. Correction can be made effectively in many instances simply by prescribing the ingestion of sodium bicarbonate either in addition to or in lieu of table salt. The reduction in the intake of NaCl is particularly desirable where there is some reason to avoid an excessive intake of sodium or where the substitution of sodium bicarbonate for sodium chloride is indicated because acidosis is due to a primary loss of bicarbonate and the concentration of chloride is already high. The amount of sodium bicarbonate necessary as a daily supplement must be gauged in an empirical manner by correlating the dosage with the response. The use of 2 to 4 Gm $NaHCO_3$ per day is safe to start with. Two complications may mar the success of this treatment. Since the kidneys of these patients have lost the capacity to discriminate properly, it is possible to overcorrect the acidosis. The possibility of overcorrection may be increased by the maintenance of a low P_{CO_2} due to increased sensitivity of the respiratory center to CO_2 as a stimulus. The second complication deals with the possible development of tetany. Many of these patients have hyperphosphatemia and hypocalcemia. The acidosis may protect against tetany from hypocalcemia, and this protection may be lost as the pH is corrected with $NaHCO_3$. The ingestion of several grams of calcium gluconate or lactate may prevent this complication. The obvious advantages of the correction of the metabolic acidosis include elimination of the hyperpnea which may be a troublesome symptom, in most cases some relief from subjective discomfort, and maintenance of an internal environment better able to buffer sudden increments of acid. The increase in excretion of calcium and potassium that may accompany the acidosis may be diminished as well. However, it is unnecessary to raise the level of bicarbonate in excess of 20 mM/liter.

So far this discussion has concerned management in a noncritical chronic phase of the disease. When patients with renal insufficiency experience an episode of dehydration with further decompensation in renal function, they may develop acute and more intense disturbances in acid-base balance. However, it is frequently in these very circumstances that the physician may be most effective in correcting a disabling acidosis. The efficient correction of acidosis depends on increasing the concentration of bicarbonate in the extracellular fluid. This can be accomplished most dramatically when hyponatremia accompanies the disorder, since the concentration of sodium can be raised together with the bicarbonate by administering a hypertonic solution of $NaHCO_3$. The quantity of sodium to administer is calculated as discussed in Chap. 60. This should represent too much bicarbonate, but, in fact, it rarely does. The second most dramatic correction may be accomplished when the patient with acidosis has a normal concentration of sodium but is dehydrated. The administration of an isotonic solution of a sodium salt will expand the volume of the extracellular fluid and repair the dehydration. If the salt is the bicarbonate, the concentration of this anion will be increased.

The possibility of provoking hypocalcemic tetany must always be considered when sodium bicarbonate is administered in these circumstances. It is recommended that prior to the infusion of $NaHCO_3$ the patient should receive at least 10 ml 10 per cent solution of calcium gluconate intravenously. In addition, the presence of Chvostek's reflex should be checked during the administration of the bicarbonate and more calcium administered if the reflex is elicited. The solution of calcium should not be mixed with bicarbonate, since calcium carbonate will precipitate.

Respiratory Alkalosis

Respiratory alkalosis is due to hyperventilation and results from the excretion of carbon dioxide in excess of its production. This reduces the tension of CO_2, increases the value for the ratio of the buffer pair, and defines an increase in pH. This disorder may be observed in the early phases of pulmonary and cardiopulmonary disease when hyperventilation is induced by hypoxia. It is more commonly observed as a manifestation of anxiety and tension, and it may be due to a lesion in the area of the central nervous system responsible for respiratory regulation. This last is the least common variety, but it is the circumstance in which one may see the most significant deviations from normal.

The anxious and tense patient, usually a woman, who hyperventilates in response to emotional stimuli may develop acute, although transient, alkalosis accompanied by a variety of symptoms, which include giddiness and light-headedness, circumoral and peripheral paresthesias, muscle tremors, and frank carpopedal spasm. Since these episodes are shortlived, there is insufficient time for a significant renal response in the nature of a compensatory effort. For the same reasons the only compositional changes are the increase in pH and decrease in P_{CO_2}.

In those instances of relatively sustained hyperventilation, as with an irritative lesion in the reticular formation of the medulla, compensatory responses and compositional changes may be prominent. The renal responses are characterized by increased excretion of bicarbonate, decreased excretion of chloride, and augmented excretion of potassium and sodium. The diminution in renal tubular reabsorption of bicarbonate is due, presumably, to decreased secretion of hydrogen ions for the exchange with sodium. This may be due to hypocapnia. The lessened secretion of hydrogen ions may be responsible for an increase in the secretion and excretion of potassium. The most significant consequence of these renal responses is decreased concentration of bicarbonate in the extracellular fluids. This alteration tends to reduce the value for the ratio of the buffer pair toward 20:1 and hence minimizes the deviation in pH. The other alterations in composition include an increase in the concentration of chloride in the serum, along with a tendency to a lowered concentration of sodium and potassium.

These alterations in the electrolyte pattern may mimic those of metabolic acidosis. It is important to recognize respiratory alkalosis as distinct from metabolic acidosis, since the administration of bicarbonate, which may be desirable for acidosis, may be detrimental to the patient who is already alkalotic.

The management of patients with hyperventilation as a manifestation of anxiety and tension is primarily directed toward helping the patient to understand the pathogenesis of the disorder. It is frequently helpful to have the patient induce an episode by voluntary hyperventilation and then to demonstrate how this may be modified by rebreathing into a paper bag or by holding the nose and covering the mouth. This demonstration is usually quite convincing and helps to furnish the motivation for the patient to train herself to discontinue this habit. In those instances where hyperventilation has provoked carpopedal spasm, the immediate need is to use some technique to increase the P_{CO_2} of the body fluids. This is most easily accomplished by having the patient rebreathe into a paper bag.

Metabolic Alkalosis

Metabolic alkalosis is characterized by increased concentration of bicarbonate unattended by an equivalent increase in the P_{CO_2}, so that the ratio of the concentrations of the buffer pair is in excess of 20:1 and the pH is elevated. This condition may arise as a consequence of (1) the administration of sodium bicarbonate (or sodium salts of organic acids such as citrate or lactate); (2) the loss of chloride as HCl, as in vomiting or gastric suction; (3) the loss of chloride with sodium in a ratio in excess of that which characterizes their relative concentrations in the extracellular fluid; (4) excessive excretion of acid in the urine; (5) the movement of hydrogen ions from the extracellular fluid to the cells in consequence of a deficit of potassium. The interrelationships among these possible primary events are intimate, and each of them provokes responses of an interdependent character, so it is rare to find metabolic alkalosis that is not multicausal. The interplay of primary events and subsequent responses can be illustrated by examining the sequence that may follow each of the major initiating events.

Throughout the discussion it will be well to visualize the effects of compensatory mechanisms that tend to mitigate the deviation in pH as these may be surmised from the Henderson-Hasselbalch equation. These include an increase in the CO_2 tension, which may be induced by hypoventilation, and a reduction in the concentration of bicarbonate in the extracellular fluid. Hypoventilation would, presumably, be favored by the increase in pH. However, this path of compensation is not usually of great quantitative significance. There are limiting influences on hypoventilation, which include the development of hypoxia and hypercapnia. These are both stimuli to increased respiratory activity. Reduction in the high concentration of bicarbonate may be achieved to some extent by the accelerated excretion of $NaHCO_3$ in the urine. To the extent that an increase in P_{CO_2} tends to enhance the reabsorption of bicarbonate, it may be said that a more successful hypoventilatory response would impose serious limitations on the efficiency of the renal response. Other limitations imposed on the compensating mechanisms will be illustrated in the discussions to follow. Furthermore, there may be specific deleterious effects on renal function and anatomic integrity as a consequence of certain features of metabolic alkalosis. One of these effects is potassium depletion, and another may be the alkalosis per se, although there really are no good data to substantiate this.

ALKALOSIS INDUCED WITH SODIUM BICARBONATE. The administration of $NaHCO_3$ will induce metabolic alkalosis, which depends, in part, on the magnitude and rapidity with which a particular load of this salt is administered. However, the ability to accelerate the excretion of $NaHCO_3$ in the urine is so great that it is difficult to maintain any serious degree of alkalosis in this fashion in the absence of other conditioning influences. The ingestion or administration of $NaHCO_3$ is accompanied by an augmented excretion of potassium. If the ingestion or administration of potassium is inadequate to match the accelerated urinary loss, a deficit of potassium develops. The depletion of potassium has several consequences that tend to intensify rather than mitigate alkalosis:

1. A potassium deficit tends to diminish the secretion of potassium and enhance the exchange of hydrogen ions for sodium in the renal tubular reabsorptive mechanism. The augmented secretion of hydrogen ions promotes increased reabsorption of sodium as bicarbonate, which imposes a limit on the efficiency with which bicarbonate may be excreted.

2. A large experimental literature dealing with the production of potassium depletion utilizing diets essentially free of this cation and administering $NaHCO_3$ describes an increase in the quantity of sodium in tissue cells. However, in most instances the quantitative relationship is such as to suggest that some other

cation has gained access to the cell along with sodium. In some instances, at least, this appears to be hydrogen ion. To the extent that this transfer of hydrogen ions from the extracellular fluids to cells operates, the intensity of the extracellular alkalosis will be augmented.

As long as potassium depletion is avoided, large amounts of administered bicarbonate may fail to induce significant alkalosis.

METABOLIC ALKALOSIS DUE TO LOSS OF GASTRIC SECRETION BY VOMITING OR SUCTION. The primary cause of alkalosis in this instance is the loss of HCl with the consequent increase in the bicarbonate concentration and decrease in the chloride concentration in the extracellular fluids. The renal response to this alkalosis is similar to that just described and is characterized by accelerated excretion of sodium and potassium bicarbonate in the urine. The loss of potassium in the urine added to the loss of this ion in the gastric fluid represents an early potassium deficit. The nature of the primary event precludes retention of ingested food or fluid, and if potassium is not administered parenterally and the gastric losses continue, the intensity of the potassium depletion increases. Furthermore, the loss of sodium in the gastric fluid and in the urine, if unreplaced, induces a deficit of this ion as well. The deficits of potassium and sodium both impose limitations on the mechanisms that tend to compensate for alkalosis. Those related to potassium depletion have just been described. The limits imposed by sodium depletion may operate as follows: As the deficit of sodium develops, there is a loss of fluid. If no water is ingested or administered, the net deficit tends toward a loss of water in excess of sodium loss. If water is ingested and promptly vomited, or if water without salt (e.g., glucose in water) is administered by vein, the net deficit will be of sodium in excess of water. In either event, there will be a contraction of the extracellular volume. This, in turn, will promote a decreased rate of sodium excretion. To the extent that renal tubular reabsorption of sodium is increased, a serious limitation is imposed on the excretion of bicarbonate. Moreover, if sodium reabsorption is virtually complete and that fraction of sodium reabsorption which transpires by cation exchange is achieved with exchange for hydrogen and ammonium ions in lieu of potassium (because of deficit of the latter), the urine may no longer be alkaline but acid. This implies an increase in the *net* excretion of acid despite the extracellular alkalosis. These conditioning factors are, presumably, the genesis of the paradoxical aciduria that may be noted in clinical disorders associated with metabolic alkalosis. It is probable that aciduria is conditioned not only by the deficit of potassium but also by a condition which demands virtually total reabsorption of sodium.

These considerations have very important therapeutic implications and serve to emphasize the need for an overall evaluation of the problem in management. For example, administration of ammonium chloride to such a patient could correct the state of alkalosis but add the complications of metabolic acidosis; it would probably enhance the loss of potassium and sodium and serve very poorly to improve the patient's status. In contrast, the clearly indicated therapeutic measures include the following:

1. Dehydration should be corrected by administration of salt and water. The proportion in which they should be administered depends on the net character of the deficits. If there is hypernatremia, the patient needs more water than salt; if he is hyponatremic, the need is for more salt than water. If one is in doubt, isotonic saline solution will usually be adequate. The amount to administer must be judged by an evaluation of the quantity of the deficit, made on the basis of history, physical examination, laboratory data, and the observed response to therapy (see Chap. 60).

2. The deficit of potassium must be corrected. The manner in which this may safely be accomplished will be discussed below under Deficit of Potassium.

3. Sufficient carbohydrate should be administered to minimize protein catabolism and ketonemia.

Once the antecedent deficits are restored, care must be taken to ensure appropriate replacement of current losses so that a new state of depletion will not obtain.

ALTERED URINARY COMPOSITION DUE TO DIURETIC AND STEROID THERAPY. The administration of many diuretic agents promotes potassium loss and alkalosis. The precise manner in which this occurs is not clear. However, it is most probably a consequence of the delivery of greater quantities of sodium to sites where its reabsorption articulates with secretion of hydrogen ions or potassium. In the first instance this would tend to induce alkalosis with its attendant consequences; and in the second instance it induces a loss of potassium, which, in turn, tends to provoke a state of alkalosis.

The naturally existing adrenal cortical hormones tend to enhance the excretion of potassium. This appears to be a secondary rather than a primary event, since it does not occur when the dietary regimen is free of sodium. The suggestion is that the steroids enhance reabsorption of sodium and to the extent that this promotes the secretion of potassium, more of this latter ion is excreted in the urine. The synthetic steroids, employed for reasons other than replacement therapy, have a considerably diminished activity in this regard.

DEFICIT OF POTASSIUM. The manner in which a deficit of potassium interrelates with a state of metabolic alkalosis has already been described. There are many causes of a deficit of this ion, including prolonged periods of parenteral alimentation without addition of potassium, excessive losses in gastrointestinal fluid, diarrhea due to disease or induced with cathartics, excessive losses in the urine as with the use of organic mercurial diuretics, chlorothiazide, and steroid hormones, potassium-losing renal disease, Cushing's syndrome, and primary aldosteronism.

Potassium is the major intracellular cation, and depletion is accompanied by disorders of structure and function in various tissues. These tissues include skeletal muscle, smooth muscle of the gastrointestinal tract, myocardium, cartilage, kidneys, and gastric mucosa. Weakness of the muscles and hyporeflexia are common, alterations in the electrocardiogram are well-established, and abnormalities in the motor and secretory activity of the gastrointestinal tract are well-documented. Inability to concentrate the urine appropriately, decreased rate of filtration at the glomerulus, and defective transport of para-aminohippurate have all been reported.

Although a potassium deficit may have serious consequences, judgment must be exercised in the technique of repletion to avoid the complications of therapy. The most significant hazard is the possibility of administering a potassium salt in too great a quantity or too rapidly so that cardiotoxic levels are reached in the serum.

In the course of the development of a potassium deficit, the patient may become sufficiently dehydrated or acidotic that the depletion is not mirrored in hypokalemia. This is seen quite often, for example, in diabetic acidosis. It would appear to be safer under these circumstances to refrain from administering potassium until partial correction of the dehydration and utilization of the carbohydrate have induced a decrease in the concentration of potassium in the serum and there is clear evidence of satisfactory flows of urine. Potassium salts may be administered more safely by mouth than parenterally. There is sufficient delay in absorption from the gastrointestinal tract to provide some assurance that a sudden increase in the concentration of potassium in the serum will not obtain.

These precautionary comments should not be interpreted to mean that potassium salts cannot be safely administered intravenously. There are many circumstances where for obvious reasons the salt cannot be administered orally and potassium repletion is clearly indicated. However, some control should be exercised with respect to the rate of administration. It is reasonably safe to administer potassium at a rate of about 20 mEq/hr, but it would be desirable to limit the first replacement to 50 to 100 mEq. After this first phase of replacement has been completed, the level of potassium in the serum should be determined. A change in the pattern of the electrocardiogram can also be used as a guide. The change in concentration will provide some indication as to the safe dosage for the next phase of therapy. Unfortunately, there is no way to estimate the magnitude of the deficit with any precision from knowledge of the concentration of potassium in the serum. There is, of course, a gross correlation, but this is an inadequate premise on which to base a safe prediction.

Since the rate of infusion may vary with change of position of the needle, it is always possible that the plan of administration may fail. An additional safeguard is provided by limiting the concentration of potassium in the infusate to approximately 50 mEq/liter. Under this circumstance an accidental increase in the rate of administration of the infusion will have less effect on the rate of administration of potassium.

The particular salt of potassium that is used may be very important. If there is no source of chloride in the diet (as might well be the case with hypertensive or edematous patients who have become potassium-depleted), the potassium should be given as potassium chloride. Other salts of potassium such as acetate, bicarbonate, or citrate may make it difficult to retain potassium under these circumstances. The reasons for this relate to some of the earlier discussion of renal regulation of acid-base equilibrium. Chloride is quite able to permeate the renal tubular epithelium, so when sodium is reabsorbed and an electric gradient established, the reabsorption of sodium will usually be accompanied by chloride if it is present. However, when there is a deficit and no dietary source of chloride, more sodium may be reabsorbed at sites where chloride is no longer present. Since the other anions are less able to permeate, there will be a tendency for the reabsorption of sodium to articulate with the secretion of hydrogen ions or potassium. If it is the former, alkalosis will be established that promotes potassium excretion; if it is potassium, it is obvious that its excretion will be enhanced. In either event the retention of potassium is not as efficient. This has several important consequences. First, the ill effects of potassium depletion are not reversed appropriately. Secondly, if the patient has hypertension and is potassium-depleted and it appears difficult to effect repletion, the clinical state may be misinterpreted as primary aldosteronism.

Once again it must be emphasized that, although this discussion has presented the disturbances of acid-base equilibrium as four distinct and separate entities, mixed clinical pictures are common. However, these should not be too difficult to analyze if the principles described are recalled. In addition, it must be remembered that a disturbance in acid-base equilibrium may be only one aspect (and not necessarily the most important) of the patient's total disease picture. In fact, in some instances attention to the primary disorder may improve the disturbance in acid-base equilibrium so that no therapy for the disequilibrium per se is necessary. Moreover, there are circumstances in which a correction of abnormal chemical values may be undesirable in that it may destroy an adequate compensation.

REFERENCES

Davenport, H. W.: "The ABC of Acid-Base Chemistry," 4th ed., Chicago, The University of Chicago Press, 1958.

Pitts, R. F.: "Physiology of the Kidney and Body Fluids," Chicago, Year Book Medical Publishers, Inc., 1963.

Siggaard-Andersen, O.: "The Acid-Base Status of the Blood," 2d ed., Copenhagen, Munksgaard, 1964.

Singer, R. B., and A. B. Hastings: An Improved Clinical Method for the Estimation of Disturbances of the Acid-Base Balance of Human Blood, Medicine, 27: 223, 1948.

62 INTERMEDIARY METABOLISM OF PROTEIN, FAT, AND CARBOHYDRATE

Frederic L. Hoch and George F. Cahill, Jr.

Life may be defined as a system of matter having heritability and mutability; as such, it requires continued or intermittent capture of both energy and matter. The processes maintaining life in the cell may be divided accordingly: the transformation of captured energy into forms useful to and usable by cells, and the transformation of matter (molecules) to make more available their energy content or to use the matter to replace the machinery of the cell or to synthesize new machinery for growth or reproduction. Disturbances in transformation of energy or molecules may become manifest as disease processes, though our knowledge of the precise metabolic events in most cases is as yet fragmentary.

These functions of the cell are carried out in specialized subcellular compartments: maintenance and renewal of cell structure is governed by information contained in nuclear deoxyribonucleic acid (DNA); energy transformations are performed mainly by mitochondria; and synthetic and degradative processes are accomplished in microsomes and in the surrounding soluble fluid or cytoplasm.

ENZYMES. The functioning unit of the cell which catalyzes all the molecular changes is a protein molecule, an "enzyme." A biochemist's view has been summarized: "Except for those rare phenomena in biology which are purely physical, the 'aliveness' of cells is basically the summation of enzymatic catalysis and its regulation" (Anfinsen). Enzyme function is localized to a small portion of the usually large polypeptide sequence, the active site E. This site binds the substrate molecule S transiently during the act of catalysis to form the enzyme-substrate complex ES, which then dissociates to liberate free enzyme and product P. The process of catalysis by the enzyme can be formulated as a set of rates maintaining a chemical equilibrium:

$$E + S \underset{k_{-1}}{\overset{k_1}{\rightleftharpoons}} ES \overset{k_2}{\rightarrow} P + E \qquad (1)$$

The velocities are expressed by the constants k_1, k_{-1}, and k_2 and are properties of the enzyme molecule arising from its three-dimensional structure and from the arrangement of its active sites. The overall chemical equilibrium $S \rightleftharpoons P$, which in the absence of the catalytic enzyme might be reached only after a prolonged period of time, is accelerated by the enzyme, which, by forming complexes as in Eq. (1), imparts much higher velocities to some of the individual steps of the reaction. An interrelationship between these velocity constants can be expressed through a constant that depends on the features of the enzyme and the conditions of the reaction:

$$K_m = \frac{k_{-1} + k_2}{k_1} \qquad (2)$$

K_m is the Michaelis constant. When k_2 is small compared with k_{-1}, K_m is also the measure of the affinity of the active site for the substrate, the dissociation constant of the enzyme-substrate complex; K_m can also be thought of as the concentration of substrate that half-saturates the active enzyme sites. These concepts are of increasing importance in understanding normal and disease mechanisms, since controls can be exerted on enzymes which catalyze "rate-limiting" steps in a sequence of reactions or on enzymes at points in the pathways of intermediary metabolism (or of energy transfer) which are "switching stations," where more than one path is possible. The mechanism of control at these points may be a chemical reaction between the controlling agents and the effector molecule, and is governed by the properties of the enzyme and agent and their interactions, much the same way as the reactions shown in Eq. (1).

CONTROL MECHANISMS. The state of simple chemical equilibrium is probably seldom attained in reactions in the living cell. Since the product is usually being removed by another process, the reaction, although potentially bidirectional, usually carries substrate in only one direction. In certain cases, the nature of the reaction catalyzed by the enzyme is so heavily favored in one direction, because of loss of free energy in the reaction (exergonic), that the enzyme catalyzes a reaction which is essentially unidirectional. Wherever this occurs there appears to be an important site of overall metabolic control, as by a hormone or some other regulatory process, which by changing the activity or quantity of the enzyme is able to alter profoundly the rate of the reaction and therefore the flow of substrate over this and subsequent reactions.

Knowledge of enzymes has so far been of medical value in two areas: the empiric use of enzyme activity measurements as diagnostic aids and the recognition that certain genetically transmitted diseases or disease traits are the result of a single discrete biochemical lesion, due to a defect either in synthesis or in the action of an enzyme. The usefulness of diagnostic enzymology is being increased by observations that "isozymes," enzymes catalyzing the same reaction but possessing different structural or functional (e.g., K_m) properties, can be identified in body fluids as originating in a specific organ or tissue. The catalytic nature of enzymes (some enzymes handle the alteration of

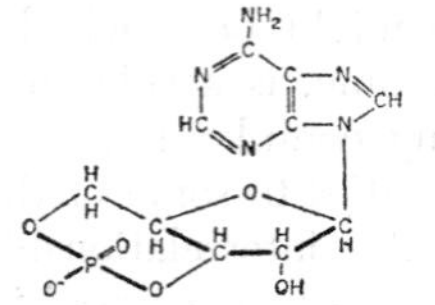

ADENOSINE-3',5'-MONOPHOSPHATE
(CYCLIC-3',5'- AMP)

Fig. 62-1. The structure of cyclic-3',5'-adenosinemonophosphate (cyclic-3',5'-AMP or cyclic adenylate). It is produced in the cell from adenosinetriphosphate (see Fig. 62-2).

more than 5 million substrate molecules per minute per molecule of enzyme) makes them key control points for the regulation of metabolic flux by hormones, vitamins, trace metals, pharmacologic agents and toxins, and specific metabolites which can bind to an enzyme and either alter the three-dimensional conformation of the enzyme (allosteric transitions) or compete with the substrate and cause inhibition.

Other control mechanisms include (1) changes in the state of polymerization of enzyme molecule structure; e.g., the transformation of inactive phosphorylase dimers into the active tetramer under the indirect influence of a unique molecule, cyclic-3',5'-adenosine-monophosphate (Fig. 62-1); (2) the availability of oxidized or reduced coenzymes; (3) actions on membrane permeability. There is also evidence that hormones act on membranes that enclose and partition the interiors of cells to control the transport of substrates or cofactors from one compartment to another. With the discovery that the membrane of the mitochondrion, for instance, contains oriented enzymes, this distinction may lose some of its sharpness. Nevertheless, the phenomena of diffusion, active membrane transport, and pinocytosis (an action engulfing external particles or molecules, in which part of the membrane forms a shell around the object of transport) have been shown to be affected by hormone action. (4) The amount of an enzyme present in the cell also controls the catalytic action exerted. Enzymes are made via the usual routes of synthesis of proteins, but there are more specific influences on enzyme synthesis than those governing the general production of proteins. In primitive unicellular organisms, where the supply of substrates can be controlled, production of an enzyme can be induced *de novo* by supplying a new substrate. The role of enzyme induction in mammals is not so clear, although some examples of adaptation of tissues to metabolize certain compounds more rapidly have been reported. When an enzyme contains a special organic or inorganic prosthetic group that is not synthesized via the ordinary metabolic routes, interference with the supply of the prosthetic group may decrease the amount of active enzyme synthesized; conditioned or dietary deficiencies of vitamins and inorganic elements may also cause such defects.

ENERGY TRANSFORMATION. The energy that allows living protoplasm in heterotrophic cells to maintain its structure and growth and therefore its function against the demands of the less-organized environment is derived from the potential energy inherent in the chemical bonds of large, moderately complex organic molecules—biologic fuels. This energy is transformed by various catalytic mechanisms partly into heat, which in homotherms maintains a constant body temperature higher than that of the environment, facilitating enzyme catalyses. In autotrophic cells, energy for useful work is derived not from organic molecules, but from sunlight, which is used to fix carbon dioxide from the air and to synthesize carbohydrate; this is the ultimate source of the substrates needed by heterotrophic cells to survive.

HIGH-ENERGY BONDS. The carrier molecule for the free energy derived from foodstuffs (or from sunlight) is adenosinetriphosphate (ATP) (Fig. 62-2). In the cells, the terminal phosphate groups are transferred to "activate" other molecules; the free energy of the ATP molecule is conserved in part in this transfer so that the activated acceptor molecule can thereafter participate in energy-requiring processes such as muscle contraction or syntheses. The high-energy bond of ATP is the pyrophosphate linkage of its terminal phosphate groups ($\sim$P), and the free energy content of each $\sim$P is about 8 kcal per mole. This may be thought of as the energy evolved when the phosphate ester linkage is simply hydrolyzed in solution. Ordinary "energy-poor" phosphate ester linkages have a free energy content of approximately 2 kcal per mole. The high energy is apparently imparted to the bond by the other resonant chemical bonds immediately adjacent to the phosphate group: it is as if these supplied negative charges like the negative poles of a magnet, kept together only by the phosphate bond; when hydrolysis or transfer occurs, this highly "stressed" bond releases or transfers its potential energy content.

High-energy bonds are not found solely in ATP, although it is probably the source for most of the others in the cell. In mammalian muscle, the main storage form of high energy is in the phosphoamide bond of creatine phosphate (in lower animals, in arginine phosphate). Other forms are the phosphoenols like phosphoenolpyruvate and acetyl phosphate; pyrophosphate and polypyrophosphate; thioesters like acetyl-coenzyme A; and sulfonium compounds like S-adenosylmethionine, which activate methyl groups for the

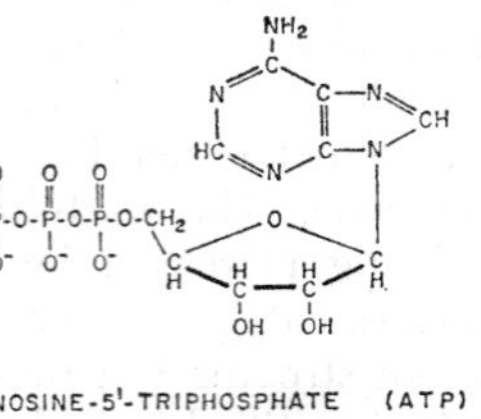

ADENOSINE-5'-TRIPHOSPHATE   (ATP)

Fig. 62-2. The structure of adenosinetriphosphate (ATP). Energy is stored in the two terminal high-energy phosphate bonds (denoted in the text as $\sim$P) and is released or transferred to support reactions requiring energy (endergonic).

synthesis of choline, creatine, N-methylnicotinamide (for coenzyme I or DPN+),[1] and norepinephrine.

There are two major pathways by which high-energy bonds in ATP are generated. (1) *Intramolecular* H transfer (hydrogen atom transfer), which is performed by single or complex soluble enzymes in the cytoplasm or in the free fluid inside mitochondria. (2) *Inter*molecular H transfer, which is performed by solid-state, insoluble complexes of oriented enzymes in mitochondrial membranes. Mitochondria transduce energy in heterotrophic cells, transforming substrate energy to ATP bonds through the use of over 90 per cent of the O_2 consumed by the cell.

In mitochondria, the enzymes, starting with that one specific for the substrate being utilized, transfer H atoms or electrons stepwise to each other [diphosphopyridine nucleotide (DPN+), flavins, cytochromes] in the membrane portion, and at the same time esterify inorganic phosphate to make an (as yet hypothetic) high-energy intermediate compound, $X \sim P$ (Fig. 62-3). In the presence of adenosinediphosphate (ADP) the high-energy phosphate is transferred from the intermediate compound on the mitochondrion to make ATP; three ATP molecules are produced for each atom of oxygen used in oxidizing most substrates. This process is *oxidative phosphorylation.* The mitochondrial apparatus, besides transforming energy, also contains its own control mechanism for respiration. When the high-energy intermediate remains *in situ,* i.e., when no ADP is present to accept the high-energy bond from $X \sim P$, oxidation proceeds at a relatively slow rate; when acceptor ADP is added, the oxidative rate increases up to tenfold or more as substrate is consumed. The demand for useful energy thus controls the generation of useful energy, a mechanism of *respiratory control.* Living cells, surprisingly perhaps, respire at the lower rate and so are in a state of controlled respiration. The oxygen consumption of man, measured as the BMR, is predominantly due to this basal mitochondrial oxygen utilization. The coupling between oxidation and phosphorylation in the normal cell may be compared to the clutch of a car, which engages and harnesses the consumption of fuel and oxygen to rotating the wheels; the phosphate-acceptor function of ADP is like releasing a set brake and advancing the throttle.

The transformation of energy by oxidative phosphorylation in mitochondria can be inhibited by chemical agents in vitro and in vivo. Dinitrophenol and salicylates act this way, reducing phosphorylation but allowing oxidation to continue. Indeed, when this "uncoupling" of phosphorylation occurs, the rate of oxidation increases severalfold, as if the clutch of the car had been disengaged while the throttle was still advanced, allowing the motor to run faster and overheat without doing useful work. This accounts for the toxic actions of dinitrophenol and salicylates, which raise the BMR and eventually the body temperature; toxic amounts of thyroid hormone induce a similar change.

INTERMEDIARY METABOLISM

MITOCHONDRIAL OXIDATION. Mitochondria can oxidize a number of substrates as fuel for generation of high-energy bonds, through the presence of enzymes specific for the substrate; the H atoms so obtained all traverse the common mitochondrial membrane pathway of electron transport and H transport to produce useful energy. The following metabolic fuels or molecules derived from them can be oxidized by mitochondria to serve as the important sources of energy (Fig. 62-3): (1) glucose, (2) amino acids, (3) ketone bodies, and (4) fatty acids. As detailed below, the proportion and amount of each of these utilized is under physiologic and biochemical control. Products of the metabolism of glucose and amino acids (after transamination) enter the Krebs cycle in the soluble matrix of the mitochondrion mainly as acetyl CoA, an activated thioester of acetate and coenzyme A, which contains the vitamin pantothenic acid. The esterification proceeds from energy derived from ATP. Fatty acids and ketone bodies are also oxidized by mitochondria as CoA esters. Studies suggest that the fatty acid molecules enter mitochondria combined with carnitine, a known growth factor. There is a complex mitochondrial fatty acid oxidation cycle, whereby fatty acids are activated using CoA and ATP. Dehydrogenation is accomplished by flavoproteins which contain the vitamin riboflavin and the metals Cu or Fe. The unsaturated fatty acid is then hydrated, dehydrogenated (using DPN+, containing the vitamin nicotinamide); and split by a molecule of CoA, liberating acetyl CoA to enter the Krebs cycle and generate ATP). From this process there remains a fatty acid two carbons shorter than the original, which in turn reenters the fatty acid cycle for another repeat of the above sequence. In the cycle, the reducing equivalents obtained from the two dehydrogenation steps may also enter the electron-transport chain to generate high-energy bonds.

GLUCOSE METABOLISM. Mitochondrial generation of ATP is not the only source of utilizable energy in the cell, though it accounts for more than 90 per cent. Anaerobic glycolysis in the cytoplasm also produces via intramolecular H-atom transfers two ATP molecules per molecule of glucose oxidized, as indicated in Fig. 62-3. The efficiency of energy transformation, the amount of useful energy obtained per unit of fuel burned, is much lower in glycolysis than in mitochondrial oxidative phosphorylation; in other words, glycolysis is a relatively inefficient means of supplying large amounts of energy.

In the utilization of glucose by a cell, it is first phosphorylated to glucose 6-phosphate by the enzyme

---

[1] Diphosphopyridine nucleotide (DPN+) and reduced diphosphopyridine nucleotide (DPNH) have recently been renamed nicotinamide adenine dinucleotide (NAD+ or NADH), and the respective triphosphopyridine nucleotide compounds TPN+ and TPNH, renamed nicotinamide adenine dinucleotide phosphate (NADP+ and NADPH).

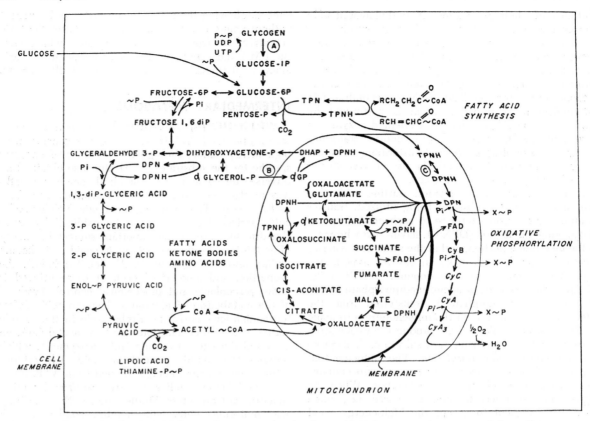

Fig. 62-3. A general scheme of energy and molecular transformations in compartments of the cell. Glucose is transported across the cell membrane, phosphorylated through use of a high-energy phosphate bond (∼P), and then transformed either to store its energy content (upward, glycogenesis) or to release its energy content (downward) via (1) breakdown of glycogen by phosphorylase (A); (2) oxidation through the glycolytic cycle to form acetyl CoA; (3) hydrogen transfer (B) to enter the mitochondrial apparatus; (4) oxidation through the pentose pathway. Energy is transformed into useful form via the consumption of O_2 in mitochondrial membranes, with concomitant esterification of inorganic phosphate (P_i) to form a (hypothetic) high-energy phosphate intermediate compound (X∼P) which can then be used to synthesize ATP (see Fig. 62-2); this mitochondrial process is oxidative phosphorylation. The mitochondrial matrix contains enzymes catalyzing the Krebs (tricarboxylic acid) cycle, transforming the energy released from acetyl CoA produced from glucose, amino acids, ketone bodies, or fatty acids. Further details are discussed in the text.

hexokinase. Adenosinetriphosphate is utilized in the process, yielding ADP and glucose 6-phosphate. Thus a high-energy phosphate bond is transferred to form a low-energy bond with loss of heat, which makes the reaction essentially unidirectional and therefore a potential site of metabolic control. Glucose 6-phosphate occupies a strategic position with reference to several biochemical pathways (see further on).

Glycolysis. This sequence of reactions is the most important route of glucose 6-phosphate metabolism. The first step is the conversion of glucose 6-phosphate to fructose 6-phosphate by phosphoglucose isomerase. Then another high-energy phosphate is added from ATP by phosphofructokinase to form fructose 1,6-diphosphate. This is another exergonic or unidirectional step, and it has been suggested that this step controls the entire glycolytic pathway. Phosphofructokinase action is opposed by another enzyme, fructose 1,6-di-

phosphatase, which converts fructose 1,6-diphosphate back to fructose 6-phosphate. This latter enzyme, as expected, is located in tissues which *produce* glucose, and therefore is found in liver; there its activity is increased by any one of a numerous group of metabolic stimuli which accelerate gluconeogenesis, e.g., glucocorticoids. Conversely, fructose 1,6-diphosphatase is essentially lacking in tissues such as muscle, adipose tissue, or brain, where the only route of glucose metabolism is via glycolysis to pyruvate and lactate and then via acetate and the Krebs cycle to CO_2, in the presence of oxygen.

After formation of fructose 1,6-diphosphate, the hexose unit is split into two interconvertible 3-carbon phosphorylated sugars. One of these, glyceraldehyde 3-phosphate, is dehydrogenated and phosphorylated to form DPNH (NADH)[1] and 1,3-diphosphoglyceric acid, which through a series of reactions yields pyruvate and two high-energy phosphate bonds. Thus the overall reaction is:

$$\text{Glucose} + 2 \sim P + 2\ Pi + 2\ DPN^+ \rightarrow 2\ \text{pyruvate}$$
$$+ 4 \sim P + 2\ DPNH + 2\ H^+$$

If oxygen is lacking and the DPNH cannot be oxidized to DPN^+, its hydrogen atom can be disposed of in the conversion of pyruvate to lactate, and thereby DPN^+ is replenished for further glycolysis. Thus the overall reaction is:

$$\text{Glucose} + 2 \sim P \rightarrow 2\ \text{lactate} + 4 \sim P$$
$$\text{or} \qquad \text{Glucose} \rightarrow 2\ \text{lactate} + 2 \sim P \qquad (3)$$

This sequence, termed *anaerobic glycolysis* since it can occur in the absence of oxygen, can provide a small but, in an emergency, significant and necessary amount of energy. *Anaerobic glycolysis is limited, however, by the accumulation of lactic acid which eventually lowers the pH to a degree not compatible with cellular function.*

Glycogenesis. Glucose 6-phosphate can alternatively be converted to glycogen by first being altered to glucose 1-phosphate by phosphoglucomutase. The glucose 1-phosphate is condensed with uridine triphosphate (UTP) to form uridine diphosphoglucose (UDPG) and pyrophosphate, which in turn is hydrolyzed to free inorganic phosphate. Thus two high-energy phosphate bonds are utilized, an exergonic reaction. As expected, the activity of this system is a site of metabolic control, being increased in muscle by insulin, and possibly also in liver. The UDP-glucose is then condensed with one of the many outer chains of an already existing glycogen molecule to form one more glucose unit attached by a 1,4 link. The glycogen chain can be modified by the "branching" enzyme to form another chain. In the opposite direction, glycogen is broken down to glucose 1-phosphate by another enzyme, phosphorylase (Fig. 62-3,A). This also is an exergonic process and essentially unidirectional. Phosphorylase activity is increased by different hormones in different tissues, e.g., epinephrine and glucagon in liver, epinephrine in muscle, norepinephrine and epinephrine in adipose tissue, and probably others. The precise activations of phosphorylase are different in various tissues, i.e., in muscle a condensation of two proteins takes place, in liver a phosphate is joined to the inactive enzyme. In all tissues, cyclic-3',5'-adenosinemonophosphate (Fig. 62-1) appears to be the intermediate effector molecule between the stimulator and the activation of phosphorylase. The end result is glycogenolysis and presentation of extra fuel for glycolysis in whatever tissue is activated. These reactions are discussed in further detail in Chap. 104.

Direct Oxidative Pathway. In several tissues (adipose, liver, adrenal, mammary) reduced TPN^+ (TPNH or NADPH) is required to provide the hydrogen and electrons for synthesis of lipid. Thus a certain proportion of glucose 6-phosphate and TPN^+ is oxidized by glucose 6-phosphate dehydrogenase to TPNH and 6-phosphogluconic acid, and the last in turn to a

compound which loses carbon-1 as CO_2 and produces another TPNH and a pentose phosphate, ribulose 5-phosphate. Through a complicated series of reactions, the pentose phosphates return to the main glycolytic sequence as fructose 6-phosphate or triose phosphate.

Glucose 6-Phosphatase. This enzyme comprises yet another pathway of glucose 6-phosphate metabolism and is located only in those tissues capable of producing glucose: liver and kidney, and also placenta. In the liver, it is the final common pathway for glucose production, and opposes the activity of the glucose-phosphorylating system. The activity of glucose 6-phosphatase in liver is increased in states associated with increased glucose production (diabetes, excess adrenal glucocorticoids) and is decreased in those associated with increased insulin or carbohydrate intake. Again there are two "unidirectional" enzymes at an important site of metabolic control, the production or uptake of glucose by liver. The role of the enzyme in kidney is apparently different and may be related to the process of reabsorption of metabolic intermediates which are converted to glucose 6-phosphate and then released into the bloodstream. It is clearly not related to the renal tubular reabsorption of glucose, since this process does not involve phosphorylation or dephosphorylation.

Glucuronic Acid Pathway. An alternative route of glucose 6-phosphate metabolism is the oxidation of carbon-6 of glucose, the glucose having been condensed with UTP to form uridinediphosphate glucose, similar to its route to glycogen. The glucuronic acid thus formed may become a moiety in many of the complex carbohydrates which serve as structural units (glycoproteins) or may be used to conjugate and detoxify endogenous and exogenous compounds prior to their elimination from the body. As part of this pathway, carbon-6 of UDPG can be cleaved to form CO_2 and a 5-carbon sugar which, through a series of reactions, enters the glycolytic pathway. One of the intermediates in this sequence, *l*-xylulose, may accumulate and be excreted in the urine in the benign disease of essential pentosuria, which is due to lack of the enzyme which catalyzes the subsequent step in the sequence (Chap. 87).

ACETATE AND PYRUVATE METABOLISM. Just as glucose 6-phosphate occupies a position at the crossroads of many metabolic reactions, so do acetate and its closely related products. Pyruvate, the terminus of the previously mentioned pathways, to be further metabolized, must be decarboxylated in the presence of DPN^+ and coenzyme A (thiamine or vitamin B_1 and lipoic acid are essential cofactors) to form CO_2 and acetyl CoA (see Chap. 73). Free acetate itself is of only minor importance in nonruminants as a metabolic fuel. It is the acetyl CoA, therefore, which can enter the subsequent metabolic routes.

In the process of fatty acid synthesis, the acetyl CoA accepts CO_2 to form malonyl CoA and through a series of reactions involving condensations and reductions [TPNH derived from glucose oxidation via the direct oxidative pathway or via transhydrogenation from DPNH (Fig. 62-3,C) is the reducing agent] a 16-carbon, saturated, long-chain fatty acid, palmitic acid, is formed; this can then be extended or unsaturated by other enzyme systems. This sequence takes place primarily in adipose tissue but also in liver and to a lesser extent in other tissues. Another route open to acetyl CoA is the formation of ketone bodies, a reaction which occurs exclusively in liver. There is some question as to whether ketones are formed by direct condensation of two acetyl CoA's or via an intermediate comprised of three acetyl CoA's, namely, β-hydroxy-β-methylglutaryl CoA. A third route for acetyl CoA metabolism, via β-hydroxy-β-methylglutaryl CoA, is in the formation of the steroid nucleus and the various compounds derived from it by further metabolic changes, such as cholesterol, steroid hormones, and bile salts. The fourth and perhaps most important route is the condensation of acetyl CoA with oxaloacetate to form citrate, the first step in the sequence of intramitochondrial reactions involving the Krebs or citric or tricarboxylic acid cycle, as previously described.

Another pathway of pyruvate metabolism is the direct condensation with CO_2 to form oxaloacetate. This sequence is unique in liver and is catalyzed by an enzyme, pyruvic carboxylase. In fasting, or in diabetes mellitus in which fat breakdown to acetyl CoA occurs at a rapid rate, the high level of acetyl CoA accelerates this reaction. Normally oxaloacetate would accept the acetyl CoA to form citrate for oxidation via the citric acid cycle, but this reaction is apparently blocked under fasting conditions or diabetes, and under these conditions the oxaloacetate is phosphorylated and decarboxylated to form phosphoenolpyruvate by another enzyme unique to liver, phosphoenolpyruvate carboxykinase. By this sequence, pyruvate is converted to phosphoenolpyruvate and then to glucose, a reaction which cannot proceed directly in this direction because of the energy differential.

HYDROGEN SHUTTLES. H atoms (reducing equivalents) can be shunted between different metabolic or structural compartments or pathways which eventually generate ATP. Thus, H atoms can be transferred from the low-efficiency glycolytic-cytoplasmic pathway to the high-efficiency mitochondrial apparatus, increasing the generation of ATP. Any metabolite that is reduced in the cytoplasm to a product which is a substrate for an intramitochondrial oxidation can act as an H carrier. One such system is the α-glycerophosphate-dihydroxyacetone shuttle:

$$\alpha\text{-Glycerophosphate} + DPN^+ \rightleftharpoons$$
$$\text{dihydroxyacetone phosphate} + DPNH + H^+ \quad (4)$$

A soluble cytoplasmic α-glycerophosphate dehydrogenase uses DPN^+ to oxidize α-glycerophosphate (αGP) to dihydroxyacetone phosphate (DHAP) (both produced by the glycolytic cycle) and DPNH. DPNH cannot apparently enter mitochondria to act as a

carrier of H equivalents from the cytoplasm, but α-glycerophosphate can (Fig. 62-3B). Then a distinctly different α-glycerophosphate dehydrogenase within mitochondria oxidizes αGP to DHAP, producing intramitochondrial DPNH, which in turn generates mitochondrial ATP. The DHAP then diffuses into cytoplasm to reenter the shuttle cycle. In rats, thyroid hormone rapidly produces a marked increase in the activity of only the mitochondrial dehydrogenase, making possible increased H-shuttle activity, which in turn increases metabolic ATP generation. A similar H shuttle exists between the fatty acid synthetic cycle and mitochondria, consisting of two β-hydroxybutyric acid dehydrogenases, DPN^+, β-hydroxybutyric acid, and acetoacetate.

A different sort of H shuttle can transfer H atoms between the two coenzymes for dehydrogenation, DPN^+ and TPN^+ (Fig. 62-3C). This is of importance in that H atoms carried into the mitochondrial electron-transport system by DPNH generate ATP; H atoms carried into extramitochondrial oxidizing systems by TPNH generate no high-energy phosphate bonds but are available for the reductive steps of fatty acid and other syntheses. These transhydrogenations between DPN^+ and TPN^+ are thus a switching point where reducing equivalents generate useful energy, are used in syntheses directly, or are dispelled as heat. A specific transhydrogenase enzyme is found in mitochondrial membranes, and there are probably many additional *de facto* transhydrogenases. Any enzyme that has a coenzyme specificity broad enough so that it can react with both DPN^+ and TPN^+, e.g., glutamic dehydrogenase in mitochondria or steroid dehydrogenase in microsomes, can act as a molecular H shuttle.

USES OF ATP. A detailed listing of specific reactions into which ATP enters may be found in standard biochemical texts. A selected few are of illustrative interest. Studies indicate that the mitochondrion, a self-sufficient apparatus in many ways while it transforms energy, also has a capacity to maintain high internal electrolyte concentrations when it is functioning in its energy-producing role. Mitochondria can accumulate K^+, Ca^{++}, Mg^{++}, Mn^{++}, and phosphate ions while oxidizing and phosphorylating, but not when phosphorylation is uncoupled. The purpose of the accumulation is as yet obscure, for Ca^{++} ions, for instance, are themselves uncoupling agents. However, demonstrations that parathyroid hormone is capable of affecting phosphate and Ca^{++} exchanges in mitochondria in vitro are of obvious importance in understanding the mechanism of action of the hormone. The contribution of the osmotic work done by mitochondria toward that of the whole cell is not yet clear.

A major role of ATP in the body is to serve as the ultimate energy source for muscle contraction. The detail of the molecular events concerned with this physical process is still a matter for investigation, but ATP is necessary for the relaxation phenomenon, whereby the contracted actomyosin fibrils resume their more elongated form, primed for the next contraction. Indeed, so definite is the association between the use of ATP and muscle contraction that the actomyosin molecule is called an "ATPase." The dependence of muscle contraction on ATP is reflected in the demands of the myocardium, for instance, for a continued supply of utilizable energy derived from oxidation. The myocardium is supplied with large intricate mitochondria, and interference with the supply of oxygen by a decrease in blood flow produces *noncontracting* myocardial areas with differences in electric potential (see Chap. 138). Such changes probably increase cellular permeability so that enzymes (e.g., lactic dehydrogenase and the transaminases from cytoplasm, and intramitochondrial enzymes such as malic dehydrogenase) leak into the circulation to provide biochemical diagnostic criteria of impaired myocardial function. Biochemical lesions of the myocardium that interfere with the generation of ATP occur in anemia, thyrotoxicosis, and beriberi, and result in a myocardial contractile defect which is not susceptible to the beneficial action of digitalis, ordinarily so effective when the contractile mechanism itself operates at a disadvantage but has an adequate energy supply. Defects in energy transformation in *skeletal* muscle appear to be present in at least two diseases, as demonstrated by functional and structural changes in muscle mitochondria in patients with thyrotoxicosis, and in a reported case of hypermetabolism in a euthyroid woman.

Another significant use of ATP is the generation of heat to maintain body temperature. In the synthesis of ATP by oxidative phosphorylation, for example, only 60 per cent of the energy liberated from oxidation of its substrates is transformed by the mitochondrion to phosphate bond energy. An appreciable portion of the liberated energy is evolved as heat, which assists in maintaining body temperature. When the external environment increases the need for heat production, the body responds with an increased rate of oxygen consumption. Fat depots may function actively in controlling body temperature, not only as an insulator but possibly by increased heat production. The free fatty acids liberated under hormonal control from adipose tissue are reesterified and reincorporated through a burst of O_2 consumption and ATP utilization, and heat is generated concomitantly. The major toxic symptom of agents that uncouple oxidative phosphorylation is hyperthermia, seen with salicylates and dinitrophenol, and in thyroid crisis.

The syntheses of the polymeric compounds that store energy in the body require ATP, e.g., the condensation of glucose 1-phosphate to form glycogen, of acetyl CoA to form fatty acids, of soluble RNA–amino acid complexes to form polypeptides and proteins, and of nucleosides to form nucleotides.

ENERGY TRANSFORMATION

To survive, a species must possess mechanisms whereby it can deposit and store fuel during periods of availability, and be able to mobilize this fuel at times of increased need, in addition to storing and mobilizing fuel for the necessary chemical reactions required to maintain the integrity of its structure.

The human body contains numerous organic compounds with energy potential: lipids, carbohydrates, proteins, and nucleic acids. The lipids are by far the most quantitatively important form of storage of fuel, in addition to providing other functions such as insulation of the body as a whole or as essential components in the structure of cell walls, myelin, and other membranes. Carbohydrates serve as a lesser form of fuel storage except for the nervous system. Protein serves as the structural basis for all enzymes, as well as for contracting elements such as muscle or supporting structures such as collagen, and as a fuel, as a precursor for carbohydrate in the process of gluconeogenesis. Nucleic acids form fundamental components in the hereditary and synthetic mechanisms and, fortunately, are not available as fuels. The body can be divided into four main metabolic compartments, adipose tissue, nervous tissue, muscle, and liver.

ADIPOSE TISSUE. Adipose tissue is composed of between 60 and 90 per cent triglyceride and thus contains 6 to 8 kcal per Gm tissue. A normal 70-kg male may have 10 kg adipose tissue and thereby a potential fuel reserve of approximately 75,000 kcal, which theoretically could support life for well over 2 months. In obesity, 100 kg of adipose tissue may be present—an entire year's supply!

Adipose tissue metabolism (Fig. 62-4) is controlled by many factors, which may be grouped into two general classes, anabolic and catabolic. A rise in blood glucose level following ingestion of carbohydrate

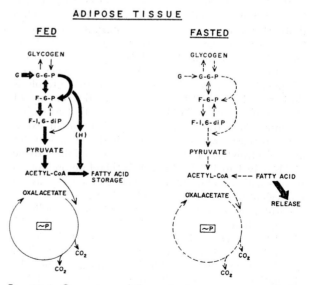

Fig. 62-4. Comparison of flow of substrate across metabolic pathways in adipose tissue in the fed and fasted state. In the former, glucose (G) is metabolized to acetyl CoA, which is then resynthesized to fat and stored. During fasting, glucose metabolism is limited and fatty acids are released for fuel for the remainder of the body.

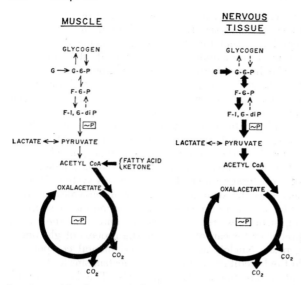

Fig. 62-5. Muscle tissue utilizes predominantly fatty acid or ketone as a source of fuel, but it is also able to derive limited amounts of energy ($\sim$P) from the conversion of glucose to lactate (anaerobic glycolysis). Nervous tissue is able to utilize only glucose as its metabolic fuel, and requires a constant supply of oxygen for total combustion of the glucose to CO_2 in order to derive energy for adequate function.

stimulates insulin production; insulin directly increases glucose uptake into adipose tissue, where, in the process of lipogenesis, it is metabolized via acetate into fatty acids, which are then esterified with glycerol to form triglycerides. Thus the individual has converted a less efficient fuel on a weight basis (carbohydrate) to a more efficient form of energy storage (lipid). Some of the ingested glucose may be converted to glycogen in liver, muscle, and adipose tissue. These carbohydrate stores serve two ancillary purposes (1) as a temporary storage site during ingestion of large amounts of carbohydrate until the lipogenetic process can store the energy as fat; (2) as an emergency store of quickly available glucose for anaerobic glycolysis during periods of stress. The increased economy of storage of energy as lipid far surpasses that as carbohydrate, since triglyceride is deposited in an extra-aqueous phase, whereas glycogen is stored with water and electrolytes; 1 Gm glycogen-containing tissue yields only 1 to 1½ kcal and it is therefore one-fourth to one-sixth as efficient for storage of energy as an equivalent unit of lipid-containing tissue.

Insulin appears to exert other effects on adipose tissue. Following a fatty meal, triglycerides enter the bloodstream as particulate aggregates—chylomicrons—via the thoracic duct. They may then enter the liver and be chemically remodified and released into the circulation or they may be directly incorporated into adipose tissue where they are hydrolyzed into free fatty acids and reesterified into triglyceride. These many rearrangements of the originally ingested fat may be the animal's mechanism to ensure that the fat which it stores in its adipose tissue contains the cor-

rect number and types of fatty acids. Insulin in the fed individual apparently plays an important role in the uptake of circulating triglycerides into adipose tissue, in addition to its role in promoting lipogenesis from glucose.

Fuel stored as adipose tissue triglyceride is released in only one form, free fatty acids. Adipose tissue free fatty acid concentration is in equilibrium with the fatty acid bound to albumin in the circulation; thus, a rise in adipose tissue free fatty acids induces a release of these into the circulation. The level of free acids in adipose tissue is controlled by several factors. Insulin decreases this level by providing increased glucose uptake, which supplies increased glycerol acceptor for esterification of fatty acids in the cell. Insulin also inhibits the breakdown of triglyceride into free fatty acid. Conversely, lack of insulin, as in fasting, increases adipose tissue free fatty acid by a reversal of these processes, and thereby augments fatty acid release. Among other substances which increase fatty acid production by adipose tissue are norepinephrine, epinephrine, and growth, thyroid, and adrenal hormones. The action of epinephrine on free fatty acid mobilization depends on the thyroid status, being increased in hyperthyroidism and decreased or absent in hypothyroidism.

NERVOUS TISSUE. Nervous tissues require glucose as fuel at all times (Fig. 62-5). This glucose utilization is independent of insulin, or of glucose concentration (as long as it is adequate), or of the state of nervous activity. Only in severe metabolic derangements producing coma is there a significant decrease in the use of glucose (except for a gradual slight decrease with age). In nervous tissue glucose is totally glycolyzed and then oxidized to CO_2 by the tricarboxylic acid cycle. Thus glucose and oxygen must always be available; if their supply is interrupted, brain function ceases immediately.

MUSCLE. Muscle tissue is versatile in that it can utilize several different fuels to support activity (Fig. 62-5). Glucose is readily removed by muscle from the circulating fluids under the stimulus of insulin, although increased muscular activity or anoxia can also increase glucose uptake. The glucose in muscle is readily glycolyzed to lactic acid, and, if there is adequate oxygen, to CO_2 and water. The glucose may also be stored to be used as emergency fuel for glycolysis when oxygen is unavailable or relatively inadequate.

Muscle mitochondria also readily utilize fat as fuel. The fat can come from several sources, from circulating particulate fat (triglyceride) derived from the diet or secondarily from the liver, from free fatty acids circulating in the blood, having been released from adipose tissue, or from a third source, fat stored directly in the muscle itself. Whatever the origin, the fatty acid is oxidized completely to CO_2 and water, and it is fat which serves as the major contributor of energy to muscle metabolism.

A third type of fuel for muscle is derived from the liver as product of the incomplete combustion of fatty acids, namely, acetoacetic and β-hydroxybutyric acids, which, with acetone, form the *ketone bodies*. These two acids are also completely metabolized to CO_2 and water in muscle and in certain circumstances can provide a major share of muscle fuel.

By mechanisms not yet clarified, muscle selectively metabolizes ketone bodies, then fatty acids, and, as a last resort, glucose. If ketones are unavailable and free fatty acid concentration is low, as after carbohydrate or insulin administration, muscle will then readily metabolize glucose. Conversely, if ketone or fatty acid concentrations are high, glucose metabolism is minimized, even in the presence of insulin and the glucose which is taken into the tissue is converted to and stored as glycogen.

One major role of muscle is to serve as a storehouse for amino acids. It is now accepted that a primary site of insulin action is to stimulate the incorporation of circulating amino acids into muscle protein. This action is biochemically distinct from the effect on glucose. If insulin is lacking, this process is decreased or even reversed, and amino acids are mobilized. Adrenocortical hormones oppose the insulin effect. In fasting, amino acids are mobilized from muscle, and during feeding, when insulin increases, amino acids are incorporated into muscle protein. Removal of both insulin and adrenal hormones achieves a new balance, but one without flexibility in either direction.

LIVER. Of the four groups of tissues playing a major role in body fuel economy, liver (Fig. 62-6) serves as the director of traffic and, as such, is more complicated than adipose, nervous, and muscle tissues. During fasting, it must provide glucose for those tissues requiring glucose for survival (mainly the brain), and during times of carbohydrate ingestion, it stops producing glucose and, instead, removes glucose and stores it as glycogen, transiently if the glycogen reserve were already adequate, or more permanently if the glycogen reserve had been previously depleted by prolonged fasting or other stress.

Unlike peripheral cells, the liver cell is freely permeable to glucose, and the concentration of glucose in the blood is approximated by the concentration in the liver cell, being slightly greater if glucose is being produced by the liver and slightly less if glucose is being removed. The net flow of glucose inside the liver cell into and out of the metabolically activated pool of glucose, glucose 6-phosphate, is a function of two enzymes unique to liver, glucokinase and glucose 6-phosphatase. The activity of the former of these is increased by insulin or carbohydrate feeding, and that of the latter by fasting, insulin insufficiency, or adrenal steroids. Thus the activities of these two opposing systems direct the net flow of glucose into and out of the liver, and are a control over the concentration of glucose in the circulating fluids.

Liver is also unique in possessing other enzymes which are located at metabolic control sites in the sequence of reactions between amino acids and glucose and which increase in activity during times of in-

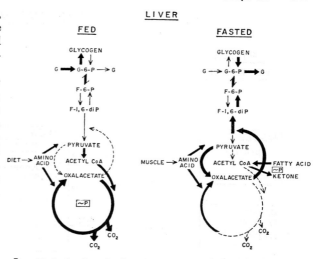

Fig. 62-6. As described in the text, the liver in the fed animal stores glucose as glycogen and derives its own energy from amino acid metabolism. During fasting, its energy ($\sim P$) is derived from the conversion of fatty acids to ketone, and amino acids are diverted into glucose synthesis.

creased gluconeogenesis, as associated with fasting, diabetes, or adrenal steroid administration, and are decreased by carbohydrate feeding or insulin administration.

During fasting, liver must provide glucose for fuel for those tissues requiring glucose, primarily brain, but also spinal cord, peripheral nerve, leukocytes, erythrocytes, renal medulla, and probably others. This it does by synthesizing new glucose (gluconeogenesis) from glycogenic amino acids released into the circulation from muscle, and, to a lesser extent, from lactate or pyruvate returning to the liver from peripheral tissues, as well as from glycerol arising from lipolysis in adipose tissue. Normally liver contains only 70 to 80 Gm glycogen, less than one-half a day's supply of carbohydrate, should gluconeogenesis not be stimulated to provide the glucose needed by the organism. The liver in a fasting normal man produces approximately 180 Gm glucose daily, of which approximately 144 Gm is oxidized to CO_2 and water and 36 Gm is returned as lactate and pyruvate. To accomplish this, about 75 Gm muscle protein is metabolized to amino acids and removed by the liver as precursors for the bulk of the glucose which has to be synthesized. Although net conversion of fat into carbohydrate has not been shown in mammalian tissues, 128 Gm glucose (glycerol from adipose tissue mobilization of triglyceride provides about 16 Gm) cannot be synthesized from 75 Gm protein; many explanations for this process have been offered, such as utilization of fat or ketones or utilization of a small amount of the stored glycogen for a brief period of time.

The liver in the normal fed individual uses as its source of fuel mainly amino acid. During fasting, the amino acid which is presented to the liver is diverted, for economical reasons, into glucose synthesis and the

FASTING MAN

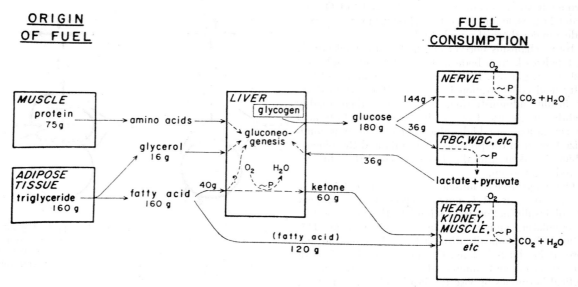

Fig. 62-7. Quantitative estimation of the flow of metabolic fuels required by a normal fasted man for a period of 24 hr, utilizing 1800 kcal.

FED MAN

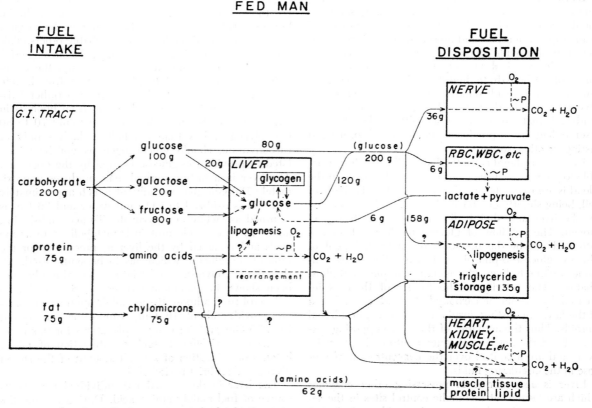

Fig. 62-8. Quantitative estimation of the flow of metabolic fuel of a man eating a theoretic meal containing 200 Gm carbohydrate (100 Gm as glucose, 20 Gm as galactose, and 80 Gm as fructose), 75 Gm protein and 75 Gm fat and disposing of the meal in peripheral depots in 4 hr.

liver now uses for its own energy needs the partial oxidation of fatty acids to ketone bodies, from which one-third of the total potential energy of the fatty acid is derived. Thus the process of gluconeogenesis, amino acid metabolism (and therefore urea production), and the production of ketone bodies are intimately related.

When the animal is fed, liver metabolism is grossly altered through a number of complicated mechanisms. Gluconeogenesis ceases, those amino acids which enter the liver are metabolized, providing the needed energy for the liver's own metabolic processes, and ketone production ceases. The level of free fatty acids in the circulation falls, since their release from adipose tissue is inhibited. The liver, however, continues to remove about one-fourth of the total turnover of free fatty acids, but now, since its own energy is adequately provided by amino acid oxidation via its citric acid cycle, esterifies these free fatty acids and returns them to the periphery instead of converting them to ketone bodies. In other words, during fasting, amino acid carbon is diverted into gluconeogenesis, the liver citric acid cycle is inoperative, and the liver's energy is derived from ketogenesis. During feeding, the citric acid cycle predominates, amino acids are deaminated, and their products are oxidized via the cycle, and ketone production essentially ceases.

TOTAL ORGANISM. Figures 62-7 and 62-8 summarize the two metabolic phases of fasting and feeding in a normal man at rest. The basal metabolic

expenditure, that amount of fuel as determined by the oxygen consumed to burn it, is a function of body surface, age, and sex, and is remarkably constant in a single person and, more important, between persons of similar age, size, and sex. The basal metabolic rate (BMR) is expressed as a percentage variation of the mean oxygen consumption obtained from a normal population of similar sex and surface area, or substituting for surface area, height, and weight, from which surface area is derived. The appetite mechanism in a normal individual appears to be exquisitely set so as to maintain the body at constant weight, and to be able to compensate for the increased fuel consumption during muscular work. Thus the weight normally varies little from year to year. For example, if an additional 100 kcal, i.e., one slice of bread, were to be stored daily as adipose tissue, at the end of the year there would have been over a 10-lb weight gain. The sensitivity of the appetite mechanism, and obviously, of the capacity to expend the calories beyond those required to maintain basal metabolism, and the equality between these two processes in the normal individual are overtly disturbed in states of abnormal energy storage such as anorexia nervosa, or its antithesis, obesity (discussed further in Chaps. 68 and 78).

DIABETES. The metabolic changes of the normal fasted man may be extrapolated into those of the subject with diabetes, who loses glucose in the urine be-

SEVERE DIABETES

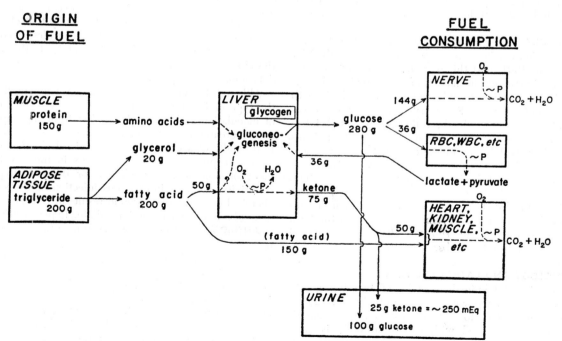

Fig. 62-9. Quantitative estimation of the flow of metabolic fuel for a period of 24 hr in a subject with diabetes mellitus; the subject was losing 25 Gm ketone and 100 Gm glucose in the urine. This glucose is *in addition* to that amount lost in the urine if the subject were eating and spilling the ingested carbohydrate. Thus a *net* negative carbohydrate balance of this degree is the causative factor which necessitates increased gluconeogenesis and the resultant ketosis. Net energy loss is 2400 kcal.

cause of hyperglycemia (Fig. 62-9). Thus, muscle protein is mobilized at a faster rate to supply precursors for the accelerated gluconeogenesis. Fatty acids are released more rapidly from adipose tissue, and concomitantly ketones are produced more rapidly by the liver, and these also are spilled in the urine; being relatively strong acids, their loss is associated with sodium and potassium loss, thereby producing a metabolic acidosis. The entire sequence progresses (as described in Chap. 86) until reversed by the administration of insulin.

REFERENCES

Anfinsen, C.: "The Molecular Basis of Evolution," New York, John Wiley & Sons, Inc., 1959.

Lehninger, A. L.: "The Mitochondrion," New York, W. A. Benjamin, Inc., 1964.

Stanbury, J. B., J. B. Wyngaarden, and D. C. Fredrickson: "The Metabolic Basis of Inherited Disease," 2d ed., McGraw-Hill Book Company, New York, 1965.

63 THE IMMUNE PROCESS IN DISEASE

Leighton E. Cluff and Philip S. Norman

DEFINITION. *Allergy* designates the adverse reactions and *immunity* designates the protective reactions observed upon exposure to a foreign substance (antigen) following an initial sensitizing or immunizing contact.

HISTORY. Acceleration of the local reaction to cowpox vaccination in immune persons was described by Jenner in 1801, and this was the first recognized immunologic reaction in man. Koch described the hypersensitivity reaction to tuberculin in individuals with tuberculosis in 1890. Severe systemic reactions, occasionally leading to death, following repeated intravenous inoculations of foreign protein into animals were described by Portier and Richet and by Theobald Smith in 1902. This phenomenon was called *anaphylaxis,* the antithesis of prophylaxis or protection. Rosenau and Anderson showed that anaphylaxis was elicited only by the specific *antigen* to which an animal had been sensitized. Von Pirquet coined the term *allergy* in 1907 to describe the altered reaction and clinical manifestations observed after exposure of human beings to foreign proteins.

ETIOLOGY AND PATHOGENESIS. Allergy in man and in experimental animals may be of two types: (1) reactions associated with serum antibody and (2) reactions unrelated to serum antibody. The allergic reaction unassociated with serum antibody is often referred to as *delayed hypersensitivity,* whereas the reaction related to serum antibody is referred to as *immediate hypersensitivity.*

Allergic reactions in man attributed to serum antibody primarily involve smooth muscle and blood ves-

sels, as illustrated by hay fever, asthma, anaphylaxis, urticaria, and periarteritis nodosa, resulting in increased vascular permeability, edema, vasculitis, granulocytic or eosinophilic inflammation, and probably smooth-muscle contraction. Anaphylaxis, serum sickness, arteritis, and glomerulonephritis can be induced in experimental animals by injection of foreign protein. These allergic reactions appear when antigen is in excess of serum antibody and soluble antigen-antibody complexes are present in the circulation, illustrating the important quantitative relationship between antigen and antibody in the production of disease.

Delayed hypersensitivity reactions not related to serum antibody may not be primarily associated with vascular lesions but are characterized by perivenous inflammation with mononuclear cells, and tissue injury results from effects other than vasculitis and smooth-muscle contraction. Allergic reactions to bacterial antigens following infection, such as the tuberculin reaction, contact dermatitis, and possibly others, are attributed to delayed hypersensitivity.

The relationship of immediate hypersensitivity reactions to serum antibody is illustrated by passive transfer of the allergic state with serum. Delayed hypersensitivity reactions, on the other hand, can be transferred only with mononuclear cells from the sensitized individual.

ANTIGENS. Most antigens of organic substances, including pollen, dust, and dander, which are common causes of allergy in man, are proteins. Other substances capable of inducing an immunologic response, however, may be polysaccharides, chemicals such as drugs, and possibly lipids. From the classic studies of Landsteiner, Chase, and others, it is likely that chemicals or drugs, and frequently polysaccharides, become antigenic only when complexed to protein. In this way the chemical or polysaccharide serves as an antigenic determinant, or *hapten.*

Although the character of an antigen may condition the type of immunologic response induced, the route of inoculation and the conjugated state of the hapten are of greater importance. For example, injection intradermally of a chemical such as picryl chloride into man or experimental animals results in the development of non-antibody-mediated, or delayed, hypersensitivity, whereas intravenous injection of the same chemical conjugated to protein results in development of antibody-mediated, or immediate, hypersensitivity.

ANTIBODIES. Serum antibodies in man fall into three main physicochemical and immunologic classes. The term *immunoglobulins* is employed to describe the diverse proteins associated with antibody activity. According to the WHO Meeting on Nomenclature of Immunoglobulins, the *first class* is referred to as γG or I_gG. These antibodies have a molecular weight of about 160,000, are gamma-globulins in electrophoretic mobility, and have a sedimentation constant of 7S. Other terms are $\gamma 2$, $7S\gamma$, or $6.6S\gamma$ globulins. The *second class* is known as γA or I_gA. These antibodies are beta-globulin in electrophoretic mobility. They sediment as 7S or intermediate proteins in the ultracentrifuge. Other terms are β_2A and γ_1A globulins. The *third class* is referred to as γM or I_gM. These have a molecular weight of about 1,000,000, are fast globulins in electrophoretic mobility, and have a sedimentation constant of 19S. Other terms are γ_1M, β_2M, $19S\gamma$, or macroglobulins.

REAGINS. Antibodies specifically associated with certain diseases such as hay fever, urticaria, and asthma frequently are referred to as *reagins*. Reagins are not detectable by the usual in vitro immunologic procedures (precipitation and complement fixation with antigen), they are less resistant to heat than other antibodies, and they are firmly fixed in the skin at the site of inoculation. The titer of a reagin in serum correlates with the wheal and erythema elicited by intracutaneous injection of antigen and bears a rough relationship to the presence or the severity of clinical allergic disease.

Reagins are usually γA immunoglobulins. The capacity to produce reagins is not confined to persons with atopic allergies, for a majority of individuals can be stimulated to produce reagins upon inoculation of antigens such as Ascaris extract. Furthermore, most allergic patients have γG and a few have γM immunoglobulins directed toward the antigens to which they are allergic. The relationship of these antibodies to the disease is unclear, but they may inhibit the hypersensitivity reaction that occurs upon exposure to the antigen. Proteins which have been immunologically identified as γA immunoglobulins are selectively secreted by exocrine glands and are found in colostrum, milk, saliva, tears, and respiratory mucus. In this way they may play a role in respiratory allergies.

Important quantitative relationships between antigen and antibody are required to elicit a hypersensitivity reaction. For example, an Arthus skin reaction, characterized by acute inflammation and hemorrhagic necrosis, regularly can be induced only when the intracutaneous dose of antigen is specifically related to the amount of antibody an animal possesses. Furthermore, as mentioned previously, anaphylaxis and serum sickness are most readily elicited only when antigen is in excess of the available specific antibody.

COMPLEMENT. Serum complement often is involved in the interaction of antigen and serum antibody, and it is probable that complement plays an essential role in some allergic reactions. Allergic reactions associated with serum antibody are commonly characterized by the elaboration of histamine, proteolytic enzyme activity, and changes in blood potassium, adenosine, serotonin, heparin, "slow-reacting substances," and other substances. None of these biochemical changes has led to a satisfactory understanding of the mechanisms of allergic disease in human beings, but the liberation of histamine probably accounts for the wheal and flare in reaginic skin reactions and may account for some of the effects of hay fever, as these reactions can be reproduced with histamine and are alleviated with histamine inhibitors.

ANTIBODY PRODUCTION. The ability to produce antibodies is probably genetically determined, although this has not been satisfactorily defined. In addition, selective animal breeding can evolve strains with varying immunologic responsiveness. Congenital agammaglobulinemia (Chap. 130), characterized by a defect in serum antibody synthesis, is a gross example of varying immunologic responsiveness in the human being. In addition, acquired diseases may significantly alter immunologic responsiveness; there is failure to develop delayed hypersensitivity in sarcoidosis and Hodgkin's disease. Furthermore, patients with lymphatic leukemia are often defective in the ability to produce serum antibody, as are patients with multiple myeloma. It has been shown that exposure to ionizing radiation and several cytotoxic drugs can impair immunologic responsiveness.

TISSUE TRANSPLANTATION. Antigenic differences exist between individuals, except identical twins. This accounts for the rejection of tissue or organ transplants from one person to another. Identification of genetically determined antigenic types of erythrocytes common to groups of human beings, however, has enabled the safe use of blood transfusions (Chap. 56). No such antigenic groups among other tissues, organs, or cells have been clearly defined. Skin and other organ transplants between individuals of the same species (homografts) survive usually for 7 to 12 days but then become necrotic and slough. Repeated transplantation of skin from the same donor to the same recipient results in acceleration of the graft rejection. Similar transplant rejection is observed with other tissues or organs. Cytotoxic drugs and x-irradiation which destroy immunologically competent cells such as plasma cells and lymphocytes can abort the reactions to transplants and prolong graft survival. Corticosteroids can also inhibit graft rejection, particularly when combined with immunosuppressive drugs. These techniques are being employed extensively in attempts to transplant kidneys and other organs.

ALLERGY. Allergy, itself, is not inherited, but the existence of a *familial predisposition* to its development seems firmly established. Familial allergic disease is commonly called *atopic*. About 50 per cent of patients with hay fever or asthma will have a family history of allergic disease, as opposed to only 15 per cent of the remaining population.

The characteristics of antigen, antibodies, and the immunologic mechanisms probably associated with certain allergic diseases of man are listed in Table 63-1.

HYPOSENSITIZATION (DESENSITIZATION). This has been the principal means of specific treatment in allergic disease of man. The immunologic mechanisms involved in specific reduction of hypersensitivity reactions have been extensively studied but still are poorly understood. In experimental animals and in the human being, desensitization can be accomplished by two principal methods of antigen administration: (1) by repeated and frequent injection of small but increasing doses of antigen over an extended period of time; (2) by injection of a large dose of antigen in one inoculation or several doses over a short period of

Table 63-1. IMMUNOLOGIC CHARACTERISTICS OF HUMAN DISEASE

	Antibody			"Delayed" hypersensitivity
	γG	γA	γM	
Clinical types				
Anaphylaxis (insect, drug, infection)		+		
Hay fever	+	+	±	
Asthma	±	+		
Urticaria		+		
Serum sickness	+?			
Contact dermatitis				+
Homograft rejection	+			+
Sympathetic ophthalmia				+
Isoimmune encephalomyelitis				+
Chronic (Hashimoto's) thyroiditis	+		+	+
Systemic lupus erythematosus	+			
Periarteritis nodosa	+?			
Cold agglutinin syndrome			+	
Paroxysmal cold hemoglobinuria	+			
Autoimmune hemolytic anemia	+		+	
Erythroblastosis fetalis	+			
Immunologic posttransfusion thrombopenia	+			
Immunologic neonatal thrombopenia	+			
Properties				
Mol. wt. (approx.)	160,000	160,000 or more	1,000,000	
Ultracentrifuge	7S	7–13S	19S	
Electrophoresis	mid	slow β	slow β or fast	
Cross placenta	+	0	?	
Skin fixation		+		
Quantity in normal serum, Gm/100 Gm	1.2	0.4	0.1	

time. The first method is the one commonly used to desensitize patients with allergic diseases such as hay fever and asthma, and the second is usually employed to desensitize patients to horse serum.

Injection of a large but sublethal dose of antigen into the sensitive individual is followed by decrease or disappearance of specific serum antibody, and the accompanying desensitization persists as long as the serum antibody is suppressed. When the serum antibody reappears, however, sensitivity to the antigen reappears.

Repeated and frequent injection of antigen into the sensitive individual may result in an increase rather than a decrease in serum antibody. One possible explanation suggested for desensitization accomplished in this way is a change in the quantitative relationships between level of antibody and dose of antigen required to elicit a hypersensitive reaction. In other words, as the antibody titer rises, larger amounts of antigen would be required to elicit a hypersensitivity reaction, and there is decreasing reactivity to doses of antigen that were previously harmful.

From the studies of Cooke and Loveless it seems clear that in atopic or reaginic disease there may be an alternative explanation for desensitization in man accomplished by repeated injections of small doses of antigen. Following *parenteral* injections of pollen antigens into the sensitive or normal person, *blocking antibody* may develop that can block the reaction of antigen with reagin. These antibodies are usually γG immunoglobulins. Reduction in sensitivity by repeated injection of small doses of antigens, whether attributable to increased levels of serum antibody or appearance of blocking antibody, may persist for a very limited period of time.

Nonspecific Desensitization. Suppression of allergic reactions can be accomplished with a variety of drugs and other substances. For example, adrenal cortical steroids can suppress the inflammation associated with cellular hypersensitivity but are less effective in suppressing most reactions mediated by serum antibody in experimental animals. In this respect, it is of interest that adrenal steroids have such a profound effect in suppressing the symptoms of hay fever, urticaria, and serum sickness, which are probably mediated by serum antibody. Antihistamines, bacterial endotoxin, and other substances also will reduce many experimental and clinical allergic reactions.

REFERENCES

Fahey, J. L.: Heterogeneity of Gammaglobulins, in "Advances in Immunology," vol. 2, New York, Academic Press, Inc., 1962.

Lawrence, H. S.: "Cellular and Humoral Mechanisms of the Hypersensitive States," New York, Paul B. Hoeber, Inc., Medical Department of Harper & Brothers, 1959.

Shaffer, J. H., G. A. LoGrippo, and M. W. Chase: "Mechanisms of Hypersensitivity," Boston, Little, Brown & Company, 1959.

Stanworth, D. R.: Reaginic Antibodies, in "Advances in Immunology," vol. 3, New York, Academic Press, Inc., 1963.

Part Four

Nutritional, Hormonal, and Metabolic Disorders

Section 1

Disorders of Nutrition

INTRODUCTION

Broadly speaking, nutrition is the science of food. More particularly, nutrition is concerned with types and amounts of foodstuffs with respect to their basic components (minerals, amino acids, lipids, carbohydrates, or vitamins) and how these nutrients are carried through the processes of digestion, absorption, transport, utilization, and excretion.

The term *nutrition* does not confine one necessarily to a consideration of dietary or exogenous materials. The title of this section, Disorders of Nutrition, is used in a broad sense and refers not only to disease resulting from a dietary lack of any of the 40-odd essential nutrients, but includes those situations whereby, even in the presence of adequate nutrients in the diet, a variety of causes may precipitate conditioned deficiency states for cells and tissues.

Persons concerned with international health matters speak of "developed" and "developing" nations. In the first category are those in which technology, education, law and order, social security, medical services, food, clothing, housing, and many other socioeconomic factors are highly developed. In the developing nations, these characteristics have not evolved so well.

The disorders of nutrition differ in developed and developing societies. In developed societies, food of all types is abundant, sometimes too plentiful. Disorders of nutrition are generally due to factors which interfere with assimilation or absorption of nutrients, produce excess loss, or cause excess elimination of an adequate intake. Psychic factors, such as those which play such an important role in anorexia nervosa or food fads, are also important considerations.

In contrast, in developing societies, reduced intake of calories and essential nutrients is likely to be the most important cause, the result of poverty, insufficient education, and a host of other socioeconomic factors. In order to understand the complex natural history of deficiency diseases such as kwashiorkor and pellagra, the physician needs the help of many other disciplines besides medicine: economics, sociology, anthropology, geology, agriculture, food technology, biochemistry—the list is virtually endless.

64 THE ESSENTIAL NUTRIENTS: REQUIREMENTS

Richard H. Follis, Jr.

A number of inorganic elements, amino acids, unsaturated fatty acids, and organic molecules called *vitamins* have been shown to be essential for normal function and structure of vertebrates. Not all these nutrients have been specifically demonstrated to be indispensable for man, though it is likely that they are. Perhaps the most fundamental approach to the definition of minimal requirements is to determine the basic minimal needs to effect balance in the normal individual. Such requirements will be affected by growth, pregnancy, lactation, muscular activity, and general metabolic rate. In addition, stresses induced by various disease states will affect requirements. Hence, the nutritional allowances recommended are usually higher than minimal requirements.

CALORIES. Before discussing the requirements of the essential nutrients, it will be advantageous to survey briefly certain aspects of energy metabolism and caloric requirements. If we take as an example an average individual not gaining or losing appreciable weight, of the total energy derived from food each day, approximately half is expended to meet basal metabolic needs. The remainder is utilized for muscular work, the specific dynamic effect, weight gain (if any), and as food energy lost in urine and feces. Energy diverted to the specific dynamic effect and excreta represents roughly 15 per cent of the total intake. Hence, about 35 per cent of the food energy is either used for muscular work or stored as fat. Energy may be derived from carbohydrates, fats, and proteins.

Caloric requirements for normal individuals are affected by variable factors: (1) physical activity, (2) body size and composition, (3) age, and (4) climatic environment. In childhood and adolescence, there are additional caloric needs for growth; so, too, during pregnancy and lactation more calories are necessary for growth of the fetus and placenta and certain maternal organs as well as for milk production after the baby is born. Caloric requirements are much affected by disease, particularly when it is accompanied by fever, leukocytosis, tissue regeneration, or neoplasia. As an example, consider the caloric allowance for a "reference" man, aged twenty-five years, weighing 70 kg (154 lb), living in the United States at an average environmental temperature of 20°C, presumed to be in health, and leading a moderately active life. The allowance for such a man has been set at 2900 Cal. This figure must be adjusted for other persons who may differ in physical activity, body size and composition, age, and climatic environment. Adjustment for temperature variations from 20°C must be made either up or down. Caloric requirements at high temperatures are probably less because of the natural inclination to reduce activity. Adjustments for differences in physical activity are important. Caloric allowances for growing infants, children, and adolescents, as well as for pregnant and lactating women, must be increased on a per-kilogram basis (Table 64-1).

INORGANIC ELEMENTS. Oxygen, hydrogen, and carbon are obviously indispensable. Nitrogen and sulfur are found in amino acids as well as in certain vitamins. The subject of nitrogen nutrition will be considered more fully below. This leaves for discussion the other elements which are nutritionally important.

CALCIUM. Approximately 99 per cent of all body calcium is found in the skeleton combined with phosphate to form hydroxyapatite. Calcium ions have other functional activities, such as in blood coagulation and neuromuscular activity. It has been estimated that the calcium content of adults weighing from 50 to 70 kg varies from 850 to 1,400 Gm. If an average adult is to contain 1,200 Gm calcium by age twenty, 165 mg must be retained each day during the 20-year period. How may this requirement be met? Before one can begin to assess requirements for calcium, certain fundamental principles must be understood. Under ordinary conditions dietary calcium is incompletely absorbed. Certain components of the diet affect absorption. Vitamin D appears to enhance calcium absorption directly. On the other hand, excessive amounts of certain anionic complexes, such as phosphate, phytate, oxalate, or fatty acids, may form poorly soluble compounds with calcium and thus decrease absorption. The intestinal mucosal cells of many individuals are able to adapt themselves to low levels of calcium intake by absorbing greater quantities of the element. Certain mandatory losses must be considered when determining calcium requirements. In adults urinary losses approximate 175 mg per day and an additional 125 mg of calcium is lost in the feces. In tropical or

Table 64-1. FOOD AND NUTRITION BOARD, NATIONAL ACADEMY OF SCIENCES–NATIONAL RESEARCH COUNCIL, RECOMMENDED DAILY DIETARY ALLOWANCES,[1] REVISED 1963

Designed for the maintenance of good nutrition of practically all healthy persons in the U.S.A.
(Allowances are intended for persons normally active in a temperate climate)

	Age,[2] yr	Weight		Height		Calories	Protein, Gm	Calcium, Gm	Iron, mg	Vitamin A value, IU	Thia-mine, mg	Ribo-flavin, mg	Nicotinic acid equiv.[3] mg	Ascorbic acid, mg	Vitamin D, IU
		Kg	Lb	Cm	In.										
Men........	18–35	70	154	175	69	2900	70	0.8	10	5,000[5]	1.2	1.7	19	70	
	35–55	70	154	175	69	2600	70	0.8	10	5,000	1.0	1.6	17	70	
	55–75	70	154	175	69	2200	70	0.8	10	5,000	0.9	1.3	15	70	
Women......	18–35	58	128	163	64	2100	58	0.8	15	5,000	0.8	1.3	14	70	
	35–55	58	128	163	64	1900	58	0.8	15	5,000	0.8	1.2	13	70	
	55–75	58	128	163	64	1600	58	0.8	10	5,000	0.8	1.2	13	70	
	Pregnant (2nd and 3rd trimester)					+200	+20	+0.5	+5	+1,000	+0.2	+0.3	+3	+30	400
	Lactating					+1000	+40	+0.5	+5	+3,000	+0.4	+0.6	+7	+30	400
Infants[4]......	0– 1	8	18			kg × 115 ±15	kg × 2.5 ±0.5	0.7	kg × 1.0	1,500	0.4	0.6	6	30	400
Children.....	1– 3	13	29	87	34	1300	32	0.8	8	2,000	0.5	0.8	9	40	400
	3– 6	18	40	107	42	1600	40	0.8	10	2,500	0.6	1.0	11	50	400
	6– 9	24	53	124	49	2100	52	0.8	12	3,500	0.8	1.3	14	60	400
Boys........	9–12	33	72	140	55	2400	60	1.1	15	4,500	1.0	1.4	16	70	400
	12–15	45	98	156	61	3000	75	1.4	15	5,000	1.2	1.8	20	80	400
	15–18	61	134	172	68	3400	85	1.4	15	5,000	1.4	2.0	22	80	400
Girls........	9–12	33	72	140	55	2200	55	1.1	15	4,500	0.9	1.3	15	80	400
	12–15	47	103	158	62	2500	62	1.3	15	5,000	1.0	1.5	17	80	400
	15–18	53	117	163	64	2300	58	1.3	15	5,000	0.9	1.3	15	70	400

[1] The allowance levels are intended to cover individual variations among most normal persons as they live in the United States under usual environmental stresses. The recommended allowances can be attained with a variety of common foods, providing other nutrients for which human requirements have been less well defined.

[2] Entries on lines for age range range 18–35 years represent the 25-year age. All other entries represent allowances for the midpoint of the specified age periods, i.e., line for children 1–3 is for age 2 years (24 months); 3–6 is for age 4½ years (54 months), etc.

[3] Nicotinic acid equivalents include dietary sources of the preformed vitamin and the precursor, tryptophan. 60 mg tryptophan represents 1 mg niacin.

[4] The calorie and protein allowances per kg for infants are considered to decrease progressively from birth. Allowances for calcium, thiamine, riboflavin, and nicotinic acid increase proportionately with calories to the maximum values shown.

[5] 1,000 IU from preformed vitamin A and 4,000 IU from β-carotene.

subtropical areas and under conditions of muscular activity in temperate regions, as much as 20 mg calcium per day may be lost in sweat. Thus, under normal conditions, approximately 320 mg calcium may be needed to replace these losses each day. If we assume that only 40 per cent of what is available is absorbed, the value of 320 mg must be raised to 800 mg; this has been recommended as the daily allowance for adults by the U.S. National Research Council. Many believe this value is too high, particularly in areas of the world where less calcium is available and where inhabitants may have adapted to low intakes by increased absorption. Requirements of 400 to 500 mg have been recommended by other agencies. In growing infants, children, and adolescents, as well as during pregnancy or lactation, intakes must necessarily be higher in proportion to body weight (see Table 64-1).

PHOSPHORUS. Phosphorus is present in bone and tooth mineral and occurs in organic combination in proteins, lipids, and energy-transfer systems. Available data indicate that the average adult maintenance requirement for phosphorus is 16.7 mg/kg/day. The maintenance phosphorus requirement for a 20-kg adult would therefore be 1.17 Gm per day. This value may be raised to 1.32 Gm to take care of individual variations and ordinary physiologic stresses.

MAGNESIUM. Because of its important role in enzyme reactions and in neuromuscular activity, magnesium is an indispensable element for man. From balance experiments, the human requirement for magnesium is estimated to lie between 200 and 300 mg per day.

SODIUM. Estimates of sodium intake per day for adults in the United States range from 3 to 7 Gm, the equivalent of about 7.5 to 18 Gm of table salt. In certain other countries much higher salt intakes may be encountered, up to 30 to 35 Gm per day, a good proportion of which may be present in various sauces. No dietary allowances have been established for sodium. Dietary deficiencies are not encountered under ordinary conditions. However, states associated with hyponatremia are well recognized (see Chap. 77).

POTASSIUM. The potassium content of food derived from plant and animal sources is high. Dietary allowances for potassium have not been established because of its ubiquity. Hypokalemic states are discussed elsewhere (see Chap. 77).

IRON. Iron requirements are discussed in Chap. 111 (see Table 64-1).

COPPER. The body of the human adult contains about 75 to 150 mg copper. An intake of 2 mg daily appears to maintain balance. Ordinary diets provide 2 to 5 mg copper per day.

COBALT. Cobalt is an integral constituent of vitamin B_{12}. As far as is known, man needs no source of cobalt other than vitamin B_{12}.

IODINE. The requirements for iodine are discussed in Chap. 71, Endemic Goiter.

FLUORINE. This element, found in varying quantities in foods and water, has not been unequivocally demonstrated to be indispensable for man or animals. However, its efficacy in the prevention of dental caries has been amply shown. The addition of fluoride to community water supplies in amounts which bring the final content to 1 part per million is a safe and economical way to reduce the prevalence of dental caries among groups whose flouride intake may be low. At this level of fluoridation, there is no risk of producing any evidence of excess, the commonest manifestation of which is mottling of the enamel.

TRACE ELEMENTS. The elements manganese, zinc, molybdenum, and selenium are indispensable for some vertebrates, and it is likely that they are also for man. All are present in ordinary foodstuffs. Hence, requirements have not been set, nor is it likely that deficiency states occur as a result of dietary insufficiency. Whether cells in human beings ever become deprived of these elements so as to give physiologic or morphologic evidence of disease remains to be proved. A syndrome characterized by dwarfism, hypogonadism, and anemia and in which abnormalities in the metabolism of zinc were noted has been described in young males in Iran and Egypt. The precise relationship of zinc to the pathogenesis of this syndrome is not yet clear.

UBIQUITOUS ELEMENTS. When tissues or their secretions are analyzed, a number of elements, in addition to those mentioned above, are found in various concentrations. The indispensability of some of these has been tested in lower animals with negative results. Others have not been evaluated. These ubiquitous elements include boron, chromium, aluminum, silicon, bromine, arsenic, rubidium, cesium, barium, vanadium, lead, bismuth, strontium, tin, and titanium.

NITROGEN. Nitrogen is continually being lost from the organism, principally in the urine and feces, and to a lesser extent in sweat, hair, and nails. It is possible to obtain an estimate of balance between nitrogen intake and loss by determining the quantitative excretion of nitrogen in urine and feces, neglecting loss from other sources. The quantity of protein required to produce nitrogen balance then provides some indication of the daily dietary protein requirement. However, the amount of protein needed to produce nitrogen balance may vary, depending on its composition. For instance, 30 Gm protein A may be necessary to produce balance in a particular individual, whereas 60 Gm protein B will be needed. Thus, the nutritive value, or quality, of proteins differs. This fact led to the concept of *biologic value* of a protein, which can be defined as the percentage of absorbed nitrogen retained in the body of a test animal. Biologic value is intimately related to amino acid composition, particularly with respect to the essential ones: lysine, leucine, isoleucine, valine, tryptophan, phenylalanine, threonine, and methionine. Extra histidine is necessary for human beings during active growth.

When the nutritive value of a foodstuff with respect to protein quantity and quality is being evaluated, the biologic value of the one or more proteins it may contain must be considered; also, the total content and digestibility of the protein must be known. Digestibility varies considerably, particularly among cereal products.

The nitrogen-containing components of the diet can thus be divided into two categories: one containing the indispensable amino acids, so-called "essential" nitrogen, and the other containing those amino acids which can be synthesized in vivo together with other nitrogenous materials such as urea and ammonium compounds, so-called "unessential" nitrogen. Nitrogen requirements are based on proper amounts of nitrogen contributed from both categories. An estimation of minimal nitrogen (or protein) requirements in children and adults may be obtained by determining the minimal amounts of nitrogen excreted after an individual has been placed for a certain number of days on a nitrogen-free diet. This minimal value, which is closely correlated with the basal metabolic rate, approaches 2 mg nitrogen per basal Calorie. Thus, the obligatory nitrogen excretion of an individual with a basal metabolic rate of 1500 Cal is 3.0 Gm per day. This value may be multiplied by 6.25 to give the minimal amount of protein per day, which in this case is 18.75 Gm. Further corrections are necessary to take into account the biologic value and digestibility of the protein ingested, together with the total amount of protein in the foodstuff. For a protein such as egg or milk, which has a biologic value of 100 and digestibility of practically 100 per cent, a minimal requirement of 18.75 Gm, plus another 2.5 Gm for obligatory excretory losses, will be adequate. In contrast, a protein of biologic value 70 and less digestibility will necessitate a higher minimal protein intake.

The recommended protein allowance for adults has been set at 1 Gm per kg body weight, or about 70 Gm for men and 58 Gm for women. These values must be increased during the growing period, pregnancy, and lactation (see Table 64-1). Dietary protein should furnish at least 10 per cent of the total caloric intake.

Short-term studies in human adults and infants have provided data on the requirements for the essential amino acids, which have led to the quantitative definition of ideal reference patterns of minimal or recommended allowances for these nutrients. The practicability of such data is open to some question. More attention should be given to assessing protein quality on the basis of ideal foods such as human milk or whole egg, not on absolute quantities of individual amino acids.

LIPIDS. Fats and oils are important nutrients, though, except for certain unsaturated fatty acids, the organism can get along without dietary lipid. The caloric value of lipids is high. In many areas of the world, 40 or more per cent of the daily caloric intake is derived from this source. The fatty acids considered essential for the organism are linoleic, linolenic, and arachidonic acids, which have, respectively, two, three,

and four double bonds. Of these, linoleic acid is the most important. It is estimated that 2 to 3 Gm dietary linoleic acid daily will more than meet the requirements for essential fatty acids.

CARBOHYDRATE. Approximately 45 per cent of the total caloric intake in the United States today is provided by carbohydrates. In developing countries, where cereal grains comprise a large portion of the diet, the proportion of carbohydrate calories may rise to 80 per cent.

VITAMINS. Vitamin A. For practical purposes, 2 International Units (IU) of β-carotene are equal to 1 IU of vitamin A. The IU for vitamin A is equal to 0.30 μg vitamin A alcohol. Levels of intake providing 20 IU vitamin A/kg/day meet minimal requirements for adults. The β-carotene content of the diet will affect the requirements of exogenous vitamin A itself. The average diet in the United States provides about two-thirds of its vitamin A activity as carotene and one-third as vitamin A. The recommended allowance for vitamin A is 5,000 IU (4,000 IU carotene and 1,000 IU preformed vitamin A). Further aspects of vitamin A nutrition will be found in Chap. 76.

Vitamin D. See Chap. 75, Rickets and Osteomalacia.

Vitamin E. The per-capita consumption of vitamin E (α-tocopherol) is estimated to be approximately 14 mg per day. The needs for adults vary between 10 and 30 mg tocopherol per day. Because other antioxidants, such as selenium, decrease tocopherol requirements, a precise value is difficult to set. No recommended allowance has been defined.

Vitamin K. The vitamin K content of edible vegetables and the synthetic activities of the intestinal flora furnish adequate amounts of vitamin K save in the newborn infant. A single parenteral dose of 0.5 to 1.0 μg, or oral dose of 1.0 to 2.0 mg, is considered adequate for prophylaxis. No recommended allowance has been defined.

Ascorbic Acid. The minimal daily requirement for ascorbic acid to prevent scurvy in adults is in the neighborhood of 10 mg. The estimated minimal requirement for infants is approximately 20 mg daily, which is supplied by milk from well-nourished mothers. The recommended daily allowances are much higher, 70 mg for adults and 30 mg for infants during the first year, increasing thereafter until adult life is reached. Further aspects of ascorbic acid nutrition will be found in Chap. 74.

Thiamine. The thiamine requirement is intimately related to caloric intake. The minimal requirement, derived from studies in adult human beings, approximates 200 μg per 1000 Cal. The recommended allowance has been set at twice this value, 400 μg per 1000 Cal. It is likely that these needs are increased during pregnancy. The recommended allowance for infants is the same as for adults. Further aspects of thiamine nutrition will be found in Chap. 73, Beriberi.

Riboflavin. The recommended allowance has been set at 600 μg per 1000 Cal, or about 1.74 mg per day for a caloric intake of 2900. During pregnancy

Table 64-2. FOOD CONSUMPTION PATTERNS IN DIFFERENT AREAS OF THE WORLD, GRAMS PER CAPITA PER DAY

	Thailand[1]	Japan (all)[2]	Uganda[3]	Guatemala[4]	Colombia[5]	United States[6]
Cereals...................	449	453	50	475	92	180
Fruits and Vegetables.......	147	435	1,400	176	268	357
Meats...................	50	96	...	27	10	238
Milk and Eggs.............	2	52	0	15	0	580
Fats and Oils.............	8	6	7	1	5	50
Sugars...................	1	12	56	30	132	140

[1] ICNND Nutrition Survey, 1960, Chieng Mai.
[2] Ministry of Health and Welfare, Japan, 1961.
[3] Courtesy Dr. R. F. A. Dean. In this area meat is available two or three times a week.
[4] Courtesy D. Bocobo, FAO.
[5] ICNND Nutrition Survey, 1960, Manizales.
[6] Urban area, USDA, Household Food Consumption Survey, 1955.

an additional 300 μg riboflavin per day is advised. The minimal riboflavin requirement of infants has been estimated to be 400 to 500 μg per day; the recommended allowance is set at 600 μg per 1000 Cal.

Nicotinic Acid. Tryptophan is a precursor of nicotinic acid, so the amount of this amino acid in the diet must be added to the nicotinic acid content. In human beings, 60 mg tryptophan will yield 1 mg nicotinic acid. The minimal requirement to prevent the development of dermatitis and certain other manifestations of pellagra in adults is approximately 4.5 mg nicotinic acid equivalents per 1000 Cal. The recommended daily allowance is set at 6.6 mg nicotinic acid or its equivalent per 1000 Cal. During the second and third trimesters of pregnancy an additional 3 mg is recommended. Minimal requirements for infants are about 5 mg nicotinic acid equivalents. The recommended allowance for infants and children is about 6.6 equivalents per 1000 Cal.

Vitamin B$_6$ Group. Vitamin B$_6$ is used as an inclusive term for three naturally occurring substances: pyridoxine, pyridoxal, and pyridoxamine, which are metabolically interconvertible. The average adult consuming 2900 Cal is estimated to require a minimum of 750 μg. The recommended allowance has been set at 2.0 mg. For infants the requirement, based on xanthurenic acid excretion, ranges from 200 to 500 μg per day. A reasonable allowance is 400 μg. Vitamin B$_6$ deficiency is discussed in Chap. 77.

Pantothenic Acid. Normal adults excrete from 1 to 7 mg pantothenic acid per day. Average diets consumed in the United States contain approximately 15 mg. It is estimated that 10 mg will satisfy human needs.

Folic Acid. The requirement is estimated from the amount necessary to induce therapeutic responses in patients with megaloblastic anemia, from serum folic acid values, and from experimental deficiency in man. The minimal requirement for the adult appears to be

Table 64-3. NUTRIENT CONSUMPTION PATTERNS IN VARIOUS AREAS OF THE WORLD, PER CAPITA PER DAY

	Thailand[1]	Japan (all)[2]	Uganda[3]	Guatemala[4]	Colombia[5]	United States[6]
Calories...................	1700	2096	2075	2182	1723	3200
Protein:						
Total, Gm...............	43	69	40	58	32	103
Animal, Gm.............	10	24				
Fat, Gm...................	15	22	...	27	13	155
Calcium, mg...............	351	395	138	1,000	180	1,150
Iron, mg...................	8	14	7.5	20	33	18
Vitamin A, IU.............	4,160	1,050	1,185	4,900	1,913	8,540
Ascorbic acid, mg..........	69	79	175	44	32	106
Thiamine, mg 1000 Cal......	0.4	0.5	0.6	1.0	0.25	0.5
Riboflavin, mg.............	0.45	0.7	0.65	0.7	0.75	2.3
Niacin, mg.................	11	...	20	10.2	7.1	19

[1] ICNND Nutrition Survey, 1960, Chieng Mai.
[2] Ministry of Health and Welfare, Japan, 1961.
[3] Courtesy Dr. R. F. A. Dean. In this area meat is available two or three times a week.
[4] Courtesy D. Bocobo, FAO.
[5] ICNND Nutrition Survey, 1960, Manizales.
[6] Urban area, USDA, Household Food Consumption Survey, 1955.

about 50 μg per day. An average diet, containing approximately 150 μg folic acid, should more than meet this requirement.

Vitamin B$_{12}$ (Cyanocobalamin). Requirements have been derived in large part from data obtained from therapeutic response in Addisonian anemia. As little as 0.1 μg vitamin B$_{12}$ administered parenterally may produce a response; regular remissions of pernicious anemia are obtained with 1 to 2 μg, but such amounts daily will not replenish liver stores; for this 5 to 6 μg is necessary. After repletion with vitamin B$_{12}$, 1.5 μg will generally meet requirements.

Biotin. A deficient state has been produced experimentally in man by feeding large amounts of egg white, which contains a biotin-binding material, avidin. Daily needs are in the range of 150 to 300 μg, a quantity present in average American diets.

FOODSTUFFS AND DIETARY PATTERNS. The kinds of food consumed in a given area are intimately related to ecologic factors. Tables 64-2 and 64-3 present data on food and nutrient consumption per capita per day for certain selected areas, which can be compared with one another and with the United States. The amounts consumed per capita per day of six food groups are shown in Table 64-2. In Thailand and Guatemala, the dependence on cereal grains is striking. However, the types of grain are different: rice in the former area, maize in the latter. In Uganda, cereal grain consumption is low and is compensated by large amounts of low-protein-containing starchy vegetables. In some countries no dairy products whatsoever are available, except an occasional egg. Differences in meat consumption found from area to area indicate the degree of sophistication of agricultural practices, as well as economic status of the area and the presence or absence of overcrowding.

Table 64-3 shows the intake of certain essential nutrients per capita per day in selected areas. Caloric values are strikingly different, though variations in caloric needs based on differences in body size and environmental conditions must be borne in mind. Calcium intakes vary as much as tenfold. The variations in iron intake are not so marked. The intakes of other nutrients should be compared with the recommended allowances already discussed.

COOKING PROCEDURES. Cooking is mentioned only to stress the importance of nutrient loss through poor cooking procedures. Such losses occur either from excess leaching of plant and animal foods by the cooking water or from destruction of some nutrients by excess heat. A good example of the first category is the losses that may occur during the cooking of rice. If the grain is washed and then boiled in an excess of water that is discarded, over one-half the vitamin content will be lost. Much has already been removed by the miller. Hence, the nutrient content of rice may be seriously impaired. Heat losses may be significant, particularly with respect to temperature-sensitive vitamins, such as thiamine and ascorbic acid.

REFERENCES

National Academy of Sciences–National Research Council, "Evaluation of Protein Nutrition," Pub. no. 711, Washington, 1959.

National Academy of Sciences–National Research Council, "Recommended Dietary Allowances," Pub. no. 1146, Washington, 1964.

65 THE PATHOGENESIS AND PREVALENCE OF NUTRITIONAL DISEASE

Richard H. Follis, Jr.

Except for the possibility that certain trace elements may yet join the list of indispensable factors, all the nutrients essential for vertebrates appear to have been identified. Certain disease states occur in man when his diet lacks one or more of the essential nutrients. A number of factors may operate to produce such an ecologic imbalance. In the first place, man's foodstuffs may be deficient through no fault of his own. For instance, soil and water may be so low in iodine concentration that, if outside sources are not available, goiter will develop. For economic and cultural reasons, man sometimes finds it necessary to subsist largely on a single foodstuff, such as plantain or maize; as a consequence, kwashiorkor or pellagra may develop. In earlier times, when food preservation was difficult on shipboard, the sailor's diet would lack fresh meats, fruits, and vegetables. Scurvy then appeared. Man has inadvertently brought certain deficiency states upon himself. With the coming of the Industrial Revolution, he congregated in cities, spent more time indoors, and built factories which filled the atmosphere with smoke. All this deprived him of the sun's ultraviolet radiations so necessary to form endogenous vitamin D in his skin; rickets in his children was the result. The Industrial Revolution increased the prevalence of beriberi in the Far East when power-driven rice milling machinery was introduced during the latter part of the nineteenth century. This, of course, did a better job of removing the outer nutritive layers than did hand-milling procedures. Man has brought nutritional disease upon himself by adopting certain unnatural dietary habits, religious or otherwise. Finally, man's food may be scanty as a result of lack of money or because of natural events over which he has little control: droughts, floods, or diseases of crops and animals.

During the early development of knowledge of nutritional deficiency disease, situations such as those mentioned above attracted the most attention. Soon, however, it came to be realized that evidences of deficiency disease might be present in the face of no apparent environmental dietary lack and that certain ancillary endogenous factors might interfere with the ingestion, absorption, utilization, storage, excretion, or requirements of essential nutrients. In the 1930s, the term *conditioned malnutrition* was introduced to include this group. This concept has greatly broadened the scope of nutrition. All the situations that may lead to conditioned deficiency states cannot be discussed here. The main categories will be delineated and examples provided in each.

INTERFERENCE WITH INGESTION. Here it is assumed that adequate food is available but for some reason it is not eaten. Anorexia may be present during the course of acute or chronic infectious diseases, during congestive heart failure, following surgical operation, following therapeutic irradiation, or in association with alcoholism. Diseases of the gastrointestinal tract often accompanied by pain, such as gastric or duodenal ulcers, obstructive lesions, acute gastroenteritis, pancreatitis, and cholecystitis, are important. In addition, neuropsychiatric disorders, food allergy, adentia, and pregnancy may interfere with the ingestion of adequate amounts of food.

INTERFERENCE WITH ABSORPTION. Although adequate amounts of one or more nutrients may be ingested, optimal quantities may not be absorbed for a variety of causes, most of which involve some abnormality in the gastrointestinal tract. Disease of the stomach accompanied by achlorhydria and a lack of biliary or pancreatic secretions are significant. So, too, are sprue, celiac disease, and other states of malabsorption. Finally, iatrogenic factors such as excessive use of cathartics, surgical procedures, or irradiation damage to the intestines must be considered.

INTERFERENCE WITH STORAGE OR UTILIZATION. Even when absorption is normal, foodstuffs may not be stored or utilized. For instance, hepatic disease may result in poor storage and therefore poor utilization of vitamin A. Therapeutic goitrogens interfere with the synthesis of thyroid hormone by blocking the metabolism of iodine.

INCREASED EXCRETION. Even though nutrients may be ingested and absorbed in adequate amounts, they may be excreted so rapidly that deficiency states result. Polyuria, due to a variety of causes including diuretics, may be associated with such losses. Functional or structural disturbances in the renal tubule may lead to loss of phosphate, glucose, and amino acids. Several forms of renal disease result in prodigious losses of nitrogen. Endocrine disease with resulting losses of sodium or potassium can have disastrous results. Parathyroid disease may lead to excess losses of phosphorus and calcium from the organism. Appreciable amounts of nitrogen, calcium, and other nutrients may be excreted in sweat. Lactation may deplete the maternal organism of one or more essentials.

EXCESS LOSS. In addition to the losses mentioned above, depletion may occur in certain disease states. Continuous loss of blood by any means may lead to iron deficiency. Acute nitrogen loss may occur as a result of burns. Chronic nitrogen depletion may occur in patients with continuously forming ascitic fluid that must be removed for therapeutic reasons.

INCREASED REQUIREMENTS. The normal needs for one or more nutrients may be exceeded for a variety of reasons. Some obvious examples are fever and the increased metabolic needs in hyperthyroidism. Normal growth processes, as well as pregnancy, require an increased intake of certain nutrients.

INHIBITION BY "ANTI" SUBSTANCES. Certain materials closely related in structure to vitamins and amino acids may block the action of these essential nutrients. Analogs of thiamine, nicotinic acid, riboflavin, pantothenic acid, vitamin B$_6$, and folic acid are all well known and have been used either therapeutically or experimentally.

These represent ways in which the nutrient content of the total organism may be reduced below its requirements. How does the cell suffer? Most nutritionists have adopted the hypothesis that physiologic and anatomic changes that result from lack of indispensable nutrients develop in a definite and orderly sequence: (1) decreased concentration in blood and intercellular fluids; (2) decreased intracellular concentration in one or more tissues; (3) biochemical alterations that lead first to evidences of physiologic abnormalities followed by structural changes, which are seen initially under the microscope and later may become grossly visible.

PREVALENCE. Few qualified observers will question the statement that hunger, whether due to lack of calories or of specific nutrients, is a problem in many developing nations of the world today. A precise assessment of the numbers involved is difficult. However, some generalizations can be made. When data for total food production are compared with those of population growth, it is obvious that in many areas the increase in persons has passed that of food production per capita. This trend is particularly prominent in many of the nations of Latin America, Africa, and the Far East. In contrast, in most countries of Western Europe, North America, Oceania, and the Near East, food production per capita continues to be maintained above the increase in population growth. It is generally conceded that the situation will continue to worsen in developing countries rather than improve. Annual data compiled by the Food and Agriculture Organization bear out this pessimistic prediction, the implications of which are obvious enough for physicians and health workers in these areas.

As for the prevalence of specific nutritional diseases, here one can only generalize; more specific data will be presented in the following chapters. Three disease entities of nutritional origin stand out by their high prevalence in developing countries. These are the nutritional anemias, protein malnutrition in children, and endemic goiter. Of the other classic deficiency states, some have definitely decreased in recent years. For instance, beriberi incidence appears to have declined. On the other hand, thiamine malnutrition, when viewed in the light of present-day requirements for this nutrient, is a problem in many parts of Southeast Asia. Riboflavin deficiency, as assessed by dietary and biochemical criteria, is widespread in developing countries; the public health significance of this is not clear. The prevalence of pellagra has certainly decreased; today only a few endemic foci remain. Scurvy and rickets are rare in developed countries. However, in the crowded cities of Latin America, Asia, and Africa, rickets is being encountered with increasing frequency. One may also wonder whether infantile scurvy will not appear in developing countries as it did in Europe and North America when artificial feeding supplanted the breast. Xerophthalmia is a serious cause of blindness in certain areas.

The problem posed by the expansion of the world's population is and will continue to be the most important one for some time to come. Control of the death rate in the absence of birth control is already disastrous and will become increasingly so in the years ahead. How a balance between food production and population growth is to be attained awaits solution.

66 EVALUATION OF NUTRITIONAL STATUS AND DIAGNOSIS OF MALNUTRITION

Richard H. Follis, Jr.

The diagnosis of nutritional disease is intimately related to the evaluation of the nutritional status of an individual patient or to samples of population groups. Certain principles relating to the dietary evaluation of nutritional status will be discussed first, followed by pertinent aspects of clinical and biochemical appraisals of nutriture.

DIETARY EVALUATION. Indirect or direct approaches may be used. The indirect method is applied to large population groups, frequently nationwide. From data pertaining to total food production, food imports, and food exports, the amounts of calories, protein, and other nutrients available to the population can be calculated on a per capita basis.

The direct method of evaluation of dietary intake may be applied to groups in institutions or the military forces, to families, or to individuals. The easiest procedure, though the least accurate, is dietary recall, which is usually accomplished by a questionnaire on which can be entered types and amounts of food bought and consumed for each meal during one or more days. The approximate intake of nutrients for each individual can then be calculated from standard food composition tables. A more accurate method requires that a dietitian be present for one or more days during the preparation and consumption of each meal. All dietary components are weighed, and after wastage is noted, accurate estimations of nutrient intake can be established from food composition tables. The most accurate method is to obtain composite samples of meals upon which chemical analyses may be performed.

The history assumes great importance in the dietary assessment of an individual. Dietary habits, food idiosyncrasies, income expended on food, mode of living, i.e., whether eating at home or in a restaurant, are some of the important particulars that should be determined.

STATISTICAL EVALUATION. Since malnutrition may affect morbidity and mortality rates in the one- to four-year age group, the mortality rate at this age is considered to be a useful index of the nutritional status of a country, even though it is difficult to separate the effects of malnutrition and of infection.

CLINICAL EVALUATION. Three important parameters of nutritional status are *skeletal development, weight,* and *body composition.* In considering these, the importance of the genetic constitution of the individual must always be borne in mind.

Skeletal Development. Increases in height are usually within normal ranges in any population during the first six to nine months, i.e., during the period of breast feeding. After this, particularly in developing countries, increments in height may tend to decline when compared with normal subjects for that country or with the picture in developed countries. This decline is generally ascribed to malnutrition.

Poor height increments can be further documented by roentgenologic examination of selected areas, such as the wrist where the presence and development of the centers of ossification of the epiphyses of the long bones, carpals, and bones of the hand may be compared with that of normal subjects at a given chronologic age. In malnourished children, the bone age may be far below the chronologic age. The measurement of the width of the cortex of a metacarpal may reveal decrease in comparison with normal.

The x-ray may reveal the presence of lines or zones of arrested bone growth. These are commonly seen when skeletal x-rays are made of children recovering from kwashiorkor and marasmus. These growth-arrest lines represent the deposition of a stratum of bone on the undersurface of an epiphyseal cartilage plate that has virtually ceased growing. When growth resumes as a result of improved nutrition, the cartilage cells begin to proliferate again and grow away from the stratum of bone. Hence, in time, a line or zone of bone appears below the epiphyseal area. Obviously, this line has not moved. The epiphysis has simply grown away from it.

Weight. Changes in weight are an even more sensitive index of nutritional status than are alterations in height, since weight changes are usually detectable before the slower and less pronounced changes in height become apparent.

Body Composition. The chemical composition of the whole body is pertinent to any evaluation of nutritional status. Various techniques yield important information on the composition of the body in healthy and diseased subjects. Methods for estimating total body water, lean body mass, body fat, and skeletal mass furnish important information. The concept of a "reference man" has been developed; his composition is as follows: water, 61 per cent; protein, 19 per cent; minerals, 6 per cent; and fat, 14 per cent.

Water and electrolytes (Na, K, Cl) may be estimated by isotopic dilution procedures using tritiated water, K^{42}, Na^{24}, and Br^{82} (for Cl). Nonradioactive materials, such as antipyrine and urea, furnish information on total body water. Extracellular fluid may be measured by determining the plasma dilution of substances that do not enter cells, such as sucrose, inorganic sulfate, and sodium thiocyanate. Whole body counters can be used to estimate total K^{40} content and are of value in studies dealing with iron and calcium metabolism.

The term *lean body mass* includes cells, extracellular water, and skeletal mass. The remainder of the body is fat. A value for lean body tissue may be estimated by determining the total body water and dividing by the factor 0.72. This figure, subtracted from the total body weight, yields an estimate of total body fat. The entire body may be weighed in water and then in air to determine its density. Since fat has a lower density than lean tissue, body fat can then be computed. The nearer the whole body's density comes to that of fat, which is 0.901, the fatter the subject. The density of the lean body is calculated to be approximately 1.097. Fat-soluble materials such as cyclopropane and radioactive krypton may be introduced to estimate the fat content of the body. Finally, the thickness of skin folds in selected areas may be measured with appropriate calipers to provide an estimate of subcutaneous fat.

SKIN. In the past, examination of the skin was very important in evaluating nutritional status. Today, however, with certain exceptions, less stress is placed on examination of the skin, because it is realized that certain changes previously ascribed to nutritional deficiency may be due to some other cause. For instance, factors such as sunlight, chronic infection, and poor hygiene clearly play significant roles in lesions previously ascribed to nutritional causes. Moreover, the specificity of certain lesions has been negated, for it has been established that deficiency of more than one nutrient may play a role in producing a given lesion.

Skin lesions may be prominent in kwashiorkor, pellagra, and scurvy and are described in the chapters dealing with these entities.

Hyperkeratotic lesions of hair follicles (follicular hyperkeratosis), which are unrelated to ascorbic acid deficiency, have been probably the most controversial subject in the clinical evaluation of nutritional status. Localized or diffuse areas of the skin in which the lumens of the follicles become plugged by keratinized material were described as a specific manifestation of vitamin A deficiency in the 1930s. Eye changes might or might not be present. A response to vitamin A administration was sometimes reported. The prevalence of such skin lesions did not necessarily correlate with low dietary intake of vitamin A or with reduced serum concentrations of carotene and vitamin A. The lesions ascribed to vitamin A deficiency are identical with those observed in the well-known skin disease keratosis pilaris. The role of animate agents in producing prominence of the follicles has been stressed. Follicular lesions may be associated with the secondary stage of syphilis and prominent follicles are seen in individuals with the fungus disease *taenia versicolor*. There is evidence to support the thesis that essential fatty acid deficiency, rather than lack of vitamin A, causes the lesions. Successful therapeutic response has been obtained by the administration of unsaturated fatty acids. Skin lesions of the follicular type are not so prominent in assessment of nutritive status as in the past, particularly as a specific manifestation of vitamin A deficiency.

Certain other skin changes that have been ascribed to nutritional deficiency are *xeroderma*, or dry skin, and *crazy pavement skin*, which has a crackled appearance. These are nonspecific alterations associated with excess sunlight and poor hygiene.

NASOLABIAL SEBORRHEA. An increased prominence of sebaceous glands, plugged with secretions, has been regarded as a manifestation of nutritional disease. Since this change is observed at puberty, its significance is questioned by many. A true erythematous seborrheic dermatitis, involving the nasolabial folds, has been observed in experimental vitamin B_6 deficiency in man.

SCROTAL DERMATITIS. Erythema and hyperkeratosis of the dorsum of the scrotum is one of the less common lesions encountered in pellagra. The dermatitis does not respond to nicotinic acid but heals after administration of riboflavin. Scrotal dermatitis has been one of the conspicuous abnormalities to develop in the course of experimentally induced ariboflavinosis in man. Currently, the lesion must be regarded as specific for riboflavin deficiency, since it has not been seen in other deficient states induced experimentally in human beings.

DERMAL PIGMENTARY CHANGES. Small or large areas of dyspigmentation are seen as one of the earliest skin changes in kwashiorkor. Hyperpigmented, hyperkeratinized plaques of skin occur in both kwashiorkor and pellagra; the underlying regenerating epithelium may be depigmented when these plaques are lost. In states of chronic malnutrition, a grayish skin color has been noted.

HAIR. In kwashiorkor the hair loses its crinkly structure, tends to fall out or can easily be plucked, and may exhibit decrease or loss of pigment. Examination of the hair is of little other help in clinical assessment of nutritional status.

EYES. The appearance of the conjunctiva and cornea may be affected in vitamin A deficiency (see Chap. 76).

Ingrowth of blood vessels into the cornea, or corneal vascularization, was once regarded as a significant sign of riboflavin deficiency. The nonspecificity of these lesions and lack of relation to nutritional status has tended to eliminate corneal vascularization from consideration.

LIPS. Changes at the corners of the lips which may extend to the entire labial margin have been recognized for many years in association with states of malnutrition. The terms *perlèche* and *cheilosis* have been applied to these abnormalities. The earliest and commonest change consists of whitened areas at the angles of the lips wherein the mucous membrane appears to be macerated. Then appear small ulcers with crusting. The area of ulceration may increase, but rarely is the mucous membrane of the mouth involved. If healing occurs, scars may result. From experimental studies of single deficiency states in man, it is clear that this alteration may result from a lack of one of several essential nutrients: iron, riboflavin, tryptophan–nicotinic acid, and pyridoxine. It is important to realize that angular lesions unrelated to malnutrition may be encountered, particularly in edentulous individuals.

TONGUE. Alterations in the tongue range from painful erythema to complete atrophy of the surface. The erythematous change usually begins at the margins and may extend to involve the entire surface. The buccal mucosa may also be involved. The tongue is usually beef-red and edematous. Sometimes the structure has a magenta tint. Color of the tongue will naturally be affected by anemia, if present. Associated with such evidences of inflammatory change are varying degrees of atrophy, ranging from loss of papillae at the margins to complete absence of these structures, so that the entire surface of the tongue is smooth. Tongue changes are nonspecific in character. This does not negate the value of careful examination of the tongue, which provides valuable information in the individual patient as well as in assessing nutritional status of population groups. Changes in the tongue may occur with naturally occurring or experimentally produced deficiencies of the following essential nutrients: iron, tryptophan-nicotinic acid, pyridoxine, folic acid, vitamin B_{12}, and biotin.

TEETH. If general growth is defective as in kwashiorkor and marasmus, the time of eruption and development of dental structures will be affected. In scurvy, the attachments of the teeth become defective, with loosening and loss of these structures. Enamel hypoplasia may be seen as a result of vitamin D deficiency. The precise relation of nutrition to dental caries is difficult to assess. The number of decayed, missing, or filled teeth, the *DMF index,* may be used to rate the degree of caries in individuals or in groups.

Caries prevalence is affected by fluoride intake. In areas where DMF indices are low, fluorosis may be present and is often severe enough to be detected clinically.

GUMS. Changes in the gums have always been part of the scurvy syndrome, yet studies of experimentally produced scurvy in man have not revealed particu-

larly conspicuous gum changes. The state of oral hygiene is an important factor in development of gum lesions in the presence of ascorbic acid deficiency. Periodontal disease is widespread in areas where dental hygiene is poor or entirely lacking. Periodontal disease is considered by dentists to be the most important single factor in the loss of teeth. Any relation of periodontal disease to nutritional status is not clear at this time.

PAROTID GLAND. Enlargement of the parotids, usually bilaterally, has been noted in malnourished individuals. This is a nonspecific sign of obscure pathogenesis.

THYROID GLAND. Thyroid enlargement (goiter) is often, though not always, a manifestation of iodine deficiency. Hence, examination of the neck by observation and palpation is important (see Chap. 71).

RESPIRATORY SYSTEM. In malnourished states, respiratory rate and vital capacity are decreased.

CARDIOVASCULAR SYSTEM. Decreased pulse rate and blood pressure are found in malnourished individuals. Usually patients complain of coldness. The circulation time and cardiac output are decreased. Electrocardiographic changes may be detected in the presence of hypocalcemia, hypokalemia, and thiamine malnutrition.

GASTROINTESTINAL TRACT. The history is important, since the story of previous or current malfunction or past surgical intervention may provide pertinent data. The number of stools and their appearance are important. Diarrhea is a common accompaniment of undernutrition, whether or not it is related to any animate agent of disease. The incidence of gastric ulcer increases during periods of malnutrition. Reduced gastric acidity is also prominent. Examination of the stool is extremely important, particularly with relation to the presence of parasites.

GENITOURINARY TRACT. Polyuria is virtually always present in malnourished states. Alterations in the urine as measured by routine urinalysis are not particularly significant, though biochemical assessment of urinary metabolites is important.

NERVOUS SYSTEM. Neurologic examination may reveal changes in motor function or sensation. A large number of subjective complaints may be elicited in states of malnutrition.

SKELETAL SYSTEM. Roentgenologic examination of the skeleton is useful in both children and adults but more particularly in the former. The diagnosis of scurvy and rickets by x-ray may frequently be made before other clinical manifestations become apparent.

BIOCHEMICAL ASSESSMENT. Any number of direct chemical determinations of essential nutrients or studies of reactions in which they participate may be applied to assess nutritional status. Some may be simple and within the competence of the routine laboratory; others are more complex and require special skills. Some more commonly employed procedures of well-established value are listed here.

Minerals. Determination of serum calcium and phosphorus are important in metabolic studies but of little use in nutritional assessment. Estimates of calcium excretion have received insufficient attention, although the assessment of calcium intake by studies of calcium-creatinine concentrations in the urine has been recommended. Serum sodium, potassium, and magnesium determinations have proved their usefulness in individual cases. Little attention has been given to the concentration of these three elements in the urine. Plasma iron, iron-binding capacity, and iron tissue levels are of use in assessing the nutriture of this element. The 24-hr urinary excretion of iodine or the iodine-creatinine content of casual urine specimens provide important information on the intake of this element. Urinary concentrations of fluoride are also important in assessing intake.

Nitrogen. Plasma protein concentrations, with particular emphasis on albumin, may provide important information. Creatinine excretion has been utilized to assess protein nutriture. Quantitative study of urinary nitrogen excretion has been recommended to assess protein intake patterns. Radioactive-labeled albumin may provide important information in specialized studies of protein metabolism. Hematocrit and hemoglobin determinations are of obvious importance in assessing anemia. A large number of studies of enzyme concentrations in serum and various secretions have been applied in attempts to assess protein nutriture.

Vitamins. For the fat-soluble group, the following are pertinent: Vitamin A, serum values of vitamin A and β-carotene; vitamin D, biologic assay of serum content and alkaline phosphatase activity; vitamin E, chemical estimation of α-tocopherol and red cell hemolysis with peroxide; vitamin K, prothrombin determinations.

For the water-soluble group, the following are pertinent: ascorbic acid, serum levels and load tests; thiamine, 24-hr excretion or concentration in urine related to creatinine content of specimen and transketolase activity of red cells; riboflavin, 24-hr excretion or concentration in urine in relation to creatinine content; nicotinic acid, 24-hr N-methyl nicotinamide concentration of urine or in relation to creatinine content in casual samples; vitamin B_6, xanthurenic content of urine following tryptophan load; pantothenic acid, microbiologic assay; folic acid, microbiologic assay of serum and FIGLU content of urine following histidine load; vitamin B_{12}, concentration in serum by microbiologic or *euglena* assay and absorption or clearance of radioactive cobalt–labeled vitamin B_{12}.

REFERENCES

Brozek, J., and A. Henschel (Eds.): "Techniques for Measuring Body Composition," National Academy of Sciences–National Research Council, Washington, 1961.

Interdepartmental Committee on Nutrition for National Development: "Manual for Nutrition Surveys," Washington, 1964.

67 STARVATION AND CALORIE-PROTEIN MALNUTRITION

Richard H. Follis, Jr.

HISTORY. The outward effects of severe malnutrition in man were well known before the beginnings of written history. More recent descriptions are vivid enough: "walking skeletons covered with skins of tanned leather," of the slave trade; "shadows and spectres, the impersonifications of disease," of the potato famine; "bodies, nothing but skin and bone," of mutinous sailors; or "crying children, begging in vain for bread, and falling dead like flies," during a famine in Europe.

By 1860, the changes in chemical structure which occur during undernutrition were shown to be principally loss of fat and protein, and some proportional gain of water. Subsequent observations on animals and man provided certain fundamental data on the day-to-day history of the starving organism. During the first days of complete starvation, glycogen stores are rapidly used up, after which the organism must depend in large part on depot fat with all possible economy of protein. The importance of studies of complete and partial starvation for clinical medicine was recognized at the turn of the century by von Noorden, who remarked that "changes in metabolism produced by sickness cannot be understood without a knowledge of the changes due to simple inanition."

Although increases in body water during states of malnutrition had attracted attention, not until famine edema became so prevalent in Central Europe during World War I was this problem studied in any detail. Lack of dietary protein was assumed to lead to a fall in serum protein concentration; this hypoproteinemia was considered to be the cause of the excessive accumulation of extracellular fluid. By 1920, edema had been produced in experimental animals fed diets deficient in protein. It remained, however, for studies during World War II to reveal how complicated the edema problem really is. Further understanding of malnutrition, particularly that of protein, came from studies on nitrogen metabolism in disease. During the latter part of the nineteenth century and early years of the twentieth, careful investigations revealed that nitrogen losses were markedly increased during acute and chronic infections such as erysipelas, typhoid fever, tuberculosis, and malaria. These studies led to the conclusion that increased protein catabolism in these infections is due not only to increased energy requirements associated with fever but also to tissue destruction. It was further demonstrated that traumatic episodes, such as fractures, lead to marked losses of nitrogen for some time during the healing stage. Studies such as these provide insight into a relatively new aspect of the science of nutrition, i.e., the nutrition of disease.

PREVALENCE. Famines resulting from natural causes or associated with war have been common throughout history. As many as 1,869 famines were recorded during a 2,000-year period in China. Currently famine is not so prevalent. The incidence of undernutrition is difficult to assess. The World Health Organization has estimated that between one-half and two-thirds of the world's population suffers from malnutrition, the result of a total insufficiency of food or inadequacy of protective foods necessary for health, or a combination of both. The problem is intimately related to the present race between population growth and food production. The seriousness of the situation can best be gauged by current statistics, which indicate that per capita food production is falling in many areas as populations increase.

CLINICAL FINDINGS. Malnutrition, exemplified primarily as loss of weight, is encountered in adults and children throughout the world as a direct effect of lack of food, brought on principally by socioeconomic factors. This form of malnutrition is seen in adults as wasting, with or without edema, which is observed in victims of famine or those suffering from less severe forms of calorie-protein malnutrition. It must be stressed that whenever sources of calories are deficient, protein supplies are also likely to be low. In infants, calorie-protein malnutrition is characterized by the syndromes of kwashiorkor and marasmus. Certain forms of conditioned calorie-protein malnutrition are important, including metabolic effects of trauma, infections, neoplastic disease, alcohol, and psychogenic malnutrition, as exemplified by anorexia nervosa.

Total Starvation. The clinical changes that result from the most severe form of malnutrition, i.e., total deprivation of water and food, are muscular fatigue, intestinal discomfort, nausea, headache, and dyspnea. Fortunately, consciousness appears to be lost for a considerable period before death. On the basis of observations in man and on theoretic grounds, 12 days is about the maximum limit of man's survival without water. The end result is affected by the rate at which water losses occur from the skin.

Chronic Malnutrition in Adults. The individual suffering from various degrees of chronic undernutrition but supplied with water complains of weakness, easy fatigability, increased sensitivity to cold, constant hunger, dizziness on sudden movement, polydypsia, polyuria, nocturia, swelling of the legs, depression, loss of ambition, amenorrhea, impotence, and a sensation of being old. Diarrhea is a conspicuous complaint. Evidence of weight loss is the most prominent alteration. In the adult, depending upon the degree of malnutrition, body weight begins to fall rapidly. Death may occur after one-third to one-half of the initial body weight is lost. Survival time will naturally depend on the initial state of nutrition. Histories of individuals who have subsisted for 30 to 60 days with water but without food are well-documented. Loss of weight gives rise to certain characteristic changes in physique. The face has a gaunt, emaciated appearance, resulting from atrophy of the musculature. The neck is thin and appears increased in length. The outlines of the clavicles are sharp. The width of the shoulders is decreased. The ribs are prominent; the scapulas appear as wings. Breasts are atrophic. The vertebral column stands out prominently. The iliac crests project. The buttocks become flat; the arms and legs appear spindly.

On examination the skin is dry, scaly, and inelastic. In severely malnourished individuals, the color is a dirty gray. Areas of brownish pigmentation are sometimes present. The hair is dry and may be plucked more easily than normal. Skin fold thickness in various areas is decreased. On palpation muscle mass is diminished. The eyes are glazed and lusterless due to decreased formation of tears. Conjunctivas are pale. Certain nonspecific changes about the lips and tongue, mentioned in Chap. 66, may be present. Secretion of saliva is diminished. Body temperature may be decreased. The heart rate and blood pressure are reduced. The position of the heart is changed; the major axis tends to be more vertical. Heart sounds are distant. Syncope is common. Respiratory rate and pulmonary ventilation are decreased. Neurologic alterations resulting from chronic calorie-protein malnutrition are uncommon.

In times of famine, edema is likely to appear. In addition to reduced serum protein concentration, other factors must be considered in its pathogenesis. These are an overall increase in body water which replaces lipid and cytoplasm lost during malnutrition, salt intake, posture, tissue tension, cardiovascular factors, renal function, and hormonal effects. The pathogenesis of edema is discussed in Chap. 16.

Kwashiorkor and Marasmus. In the middle 1930s, a disease characterized by edema, wasting, diarrhea, irritability, and skin lesions was described in poorly nourished children, aged one to four years, in Africa. It was given the name *kwashiorkor*, a term used in that area to designate the condition that develops in a child who is weaned because another is expected; in other words, it is the disease of the deposed baby. Kwashiorkor and general malnutrition in children have come to be regarded by public health authorities and pediatricians in many developing countries as the most important nutritional disturbances in children.

The disease occurs predominantly in children twelve to thirty-six months of age. The commonest clinical signs are growth failure, edema, atrophy of the muscles, misery and loss of activity, changes in the pigmentation of the hair, and pallor of the skin. A history of poor appetite, diarrhea, and some preceding infectious disease may usually be elicited. Other signs, which may or may not be present, are pellagralike skin lesions, enlargement of the liver, anemia, and other evidences of nutritional deficiencies, such as angular stomatitis, glossitis, and xerophthalmia. Furthermore, a whole spectrum of changes may be encountered beginning with those just enumerated, which denote classic kwashiorkor, over to a stage of virtually complete starvation, or nutritional marasmus of the skin-and-bones variety. In such cases subcutaneous fat is absent and the musculature is severely wasted. Changes in the skin and hair are absent. Edema and liver enlargement are not present.

Socioeconomic factors are important in the pathogenesis of the disease. As a result of poverty, ignorance, poor sanitation, urbanization, custom-directed dietaries, and many other factors, protein malnutrition is likely to occur at weaning. Cow's milk and other sources of animal protein are practically nonexistent in most underdeveloped countries. The child is weaned to a diet that consists predominantly of maize in Mexico, Central America, and South Africa, or low-protein-containing staples such as cassava, plantain, and sweet potatoes in Central Africa. Thus, at a time when growth should be proceeding rapidly, the infant is deprived of protein, minerals, fat, certain vitamins, and sometimes even calories. That protein deficiency, accompanied by varying degrees of caloric restriction, is primarily responsible for the disease is clear, both from an evaluation of the diets consumed as well as from the prompt response to feeding with protein and calories. Equally important in precipitating the disease is infection of one type or another. Some authorities would go so far as to say that, although clinical kwashiorkor may develop on the basis of dietary deficiency alone, virtually all cases result from the synergism between malnutrition and some infectious process, such as measles or pneumonia, particularly when diarrhea is present. Depending on the geographic area in which the disease occurs, evidences of other nutritional deficiencies may be present. Angular lesions, which may denote riboflavin deficiency; xerophthalmia, the result of vitamin A deficiency; and rickets or scurvy may be present.

LABORATORY FINDINGS. During states of total water and food deprivation, plasma concentrations of sodium, chloride, potassium, nonprotein nitrogen, and protein increase. Blood volume decreases, as the hematocrit increases. The volume of urine is much reduced. Excretion of sodium and chloride is negligible. Potassium concentrations in urine rise as volume decreases.

In the various states of calorie and protein undernutrition, prominent alterations occur in the body fluids depending on the degree and duration of the deficient period. If all food is withheld, serum glucose concentrations fall and remain low, sometimes reaching values comparable to those observed in insulin shock. The concentrations of total fatty acids in the serum become elevated and generally remain so during the starvation period. Serum ketone bodies rise. The nonprotein nitrogen content of serum is elevated during the first few days of starvation. Uric acid concentrations are also increased. Changes in electrolytes are not prominent unless trauma or diarrhea are present. The above alterations are less marked in states of partial, more chronic calorie-protein malnutrition. Ketosis, increase in fatty acid concentrations of the serum, and depression in cholesterol and phospholipid concentration are present. Initially, serum protein concentrations remain in the normal range. With decreasing sources of essential and unessential nitrogen, albumin concentrations begin to fall. In addition, certain other plasma protein fractions, such as beta-globulin C and haptoglobins, are depressed. Plasma concentrations of many enzymes may be decreased. Plasma amino nitrogen content of serum tends to fall. Patterns of amino acid concentration in the serum vary; in general, the unessential amino acids tend to rise, while the essential ones decrease. Anemia may be present. Loss of tissue is evidenced by increased concentrations of nitrogen, sodium, potassium, chloride, sulfur, phosphorus, calcium, and magnesium in the urine. Ketonuria is present.

Marked changes in total body composition occur in various stages of malnutrition. These may be demonstrated by the isotope dilution techniques mentioned in Chap. 66. As body weight falls, body fat decreases, yielding a gradual increase in relative body water. If this water is not excreted, an absolute increase in body water ensues. A loss of lean tissue (muscle mass) can be demonstrated by loss of exchangeable potassium and by negative nitrogen balance. Total extracellular volume and exchangeable sodium tend to remain as they were in the normal state. Relatively, however, as weight falls, these increase. Plasma volume maintains its normal value. Erythrocyte volumes tend to fall. During starvation a tendency toward antidiuresis and salt retention is usually present. Hence, there is disproportionate water retention.

PATHOLOGY. The principal findings at autopsy in all these states are widespread loss of adipose tissue and atrophy of most organs. The latter include heart, liver, spleen, pancreas, kidneys, testes, uterus, ovaries, thyroid, and pituitary. The adrenals may or may not be decreased in size and sometimes are enlarged. The amounts of lymphoid tissue and marrow elements, as well as the size of the spleen, are all greatly reduced. Some degree of osteoporosis is usually present. No change is found in brain weight.

In infants and children, the loss of weight of various organs varies with respect to the age at which the state of malnutrition begins and is related to the stage of functional and anatomic maturity of the organ concerned, together with its growth activity at that particular period of development. Hence, growth of some organs may have continued, though at reduced rates, while that of others may have stopped or even regressed as far as their relation to total body size is concerned. The heart, liver, and kidneys undergo most of their development during fetal life; hence, these change least in size. Skeletal muscle has its principal growth period after birth and will be more markedly affected. As far as the skeleton is concerned, cartilage growth is severely retarded; hence, bone growth in length virtually ceases. The activity of cells in the periosteum and endosteum may continue. Cellular proliferation in lymphoid tissue, spleen, and bone marrow is severely diminished.

Under the microscope, adipose tissue is a meshwork of fibroblasts traversed by capillaries. Cells of most organs are atrophic as a result of loss of cytoplasmic mass. Size of nuclei change little. In states of severe malnutrition cells may die, particularly in those tissues in which cells renew themselves under normal circumstances. Liver cells may contain an excess amount of neutral fat. Frequently present are evidences of some infectious disease, which is usually the cause of death.

PATHOGENESIS. When all food and water are withheld, the course is short. Dehydration is the most prominent manifestation. When all food is withheld in the presence of adequate water, the organism is forced to live upon itself. Glycogen stores in the liver are rapidly consumed. From then on energy is largely derived from depot lipid. Mobilization of fatty acids from the fat depots is represented by increase in free fatty acid concentration of serum. Fat accumulates in the liver. As the metabolism of fatty acids proceeds at an increased rate, the increased acetyl CoA produced cannot be resynthesized into fatty acids because of the reduced energy supply from glycolysis due to carbohydrate lack. The excess acetyl CoA results in an increased formation of acetoacetate and its derivatives, acetone and beta-hydroxybutyrate. Ketosis is accompanied by acidosis, with fall in serum chloride and bicarbonate and some reduction in serum sodium concentrations. Blood sugar values fall during the first 48 hr of total food deprivation and subsequently remain low.

The amount of depot lipid at the time food is withheld will determine the degree of nitrogen depletion of the organism. If protein must be utilized as a source of energy relatively early, nitrogen excretion will be high initially. Otherwise, the protein in tissues, particularly muscle, will only be called upon to replace the constant nitrogen drain in urine and feces. Serum protein concentrations are normal initially. These may fall. Some of the change is due to increased hydration, though later in the course of starvation, serum albumin values may be absolutely reduced. Such decreases may account for the slight fall in total serum calcium concentrations that may be observed.

THE METABOLIC REACTION TO INJURY. When the organism sustains injury, whether by any one of the many animate agents of disease, from physical trauma or heat, or as a result of neoplasia, a number of biochemical changes occur, involving the metabolism of all essential nutrients. The alterations are fairly stereotyped, regardless of the type of injurious process. They resemble the metabolic responses to starvation or calorie-protein malnutrition just described.

Following traumatic injury or some infection, as much as 40 Gm nitrogen (250 Gm protein) may be lost in the urine each day, even when protein intake is about 1 Gm per kilogram. The increased nitrogen excretion begins soon after onset of the disease, reaches its peak in a few days, continues for the duration of the acute phase of the illness, and in many cases is present well into the convalescent period. Loss of nitrogen is accentuated in individuals whose disease is complicated by loss of whole blood or exudation, such as occurs in burns. The nonprotein nitrogen concentration of the serum may rise, particularly if renal function has decreased.

In addition to nitrogen losses, deficits in phosphorus, potassium, sulfur, calcium, and magnesium will occur. How may these losses be explained? In the individual with a serious infectious disease, or after trauma, food intake will have decreased or even stopped entirely. Some loss of tissue will accompany the inactivity of bed rest. The principal losses result, however, from the destruction of tissue itself, as well as from the increased needs associated with fever, leukocytosis, and reparative processes. The extent of loss of body constituents is clearly dependent on the previous state of nutrition of the individual. Endocrine effects also play a role, particularly in the acute stage following trauma. Changes in sodium and potassium metabolism as a result of excessive stimulation by aldosterone and the metabolic effects associated with the liberation of 17-hydroxy adrenal corticoids are prominent. The presence of increased amounts of epinephrine and norepinephrine in serum and urine help to explain cardiovascular abnormalities that accompany trauma.

ALCOHOL AND NUTRITION. On superficial examination an alcoholic may appear to be well-nourished; such an impression is commonly erroneous. The alcoholic's dietary, whether he is living in a well-developed country such as the United States or a less developed area such as South Africa, is notoriously poor. This is brought out by the prevalence of polyneuropathy, Wernicke's disease, and pellagralike syndromes so commonly seen in alcoholics. Even more important in areas where alcohol consumption is high is the relation of alcohol to liver disease. Two viewpoints have been vigorously argued for some time: (1) that alcohol has a toxic effect, particularly on the liver, and (2) that the poor dietary of the alcoholic predisposes to liver disease. There appears to be truth in each of these views; the first is probably the more important. In the presence of an adequate diet, large amounts of alcohol have definite effects on lipid, carbohydrate, and protein metabolism. Structurally, the liver appears to suffer more than any other tissue. Space does not permit a discussion of the metabolic derangements alcohol induces in the liver. Increased accumulation of lipid probably results from increased mobilization of free fatty acids from adipose tissue. Once in the liver the free fatty acids are esterified and remain. States of hypoglycemia are well-recognized in alcoholics. Alcohol appears to interfere with protein synthesis and uric acid metabolism.

The term *nutritional liver disease* is commonly used. The fatty liver of kwashiorkor and calorie-protein malnutrition in adults is real enough. That such a fatty liver can progress to cirrhosis in man without the effects of alcohol, another toxic material, or an animate agent appears unlikely.

DIAGNOSIS. The principal manifestation of calorie-protein malnutrition in both adults and children is loss of weight. Naturally, the most important aspect is determination of the cause, whether economic or some disease process. The general approach to the diagnosis of malnutrition has been discussed in Chap. 66.

TREATMENT. In states of severe calorie-protein malnutrition, treatment centers on three items: correction of fluid and electrolyte deficits, administration of an appropriate diet, and treatment of infection. Many malnourished individuals have diarrhea; hence, dehydration and electrolyte deficits are usually present. These should be corrected by oral or parenteral administration of solutions containing glucose and electrolyte. Frequent small feedings should be initiated. Finally, since infections of one type or another are so common in malnourished individuals, appropriate antibiotic therapy is usually indicated after the infectious agent has been identified.

REFERENCES

Isselbacher, K. J., and N. J. Greenberger: Metabolic effects of alcohol on the liver, New England J. Med., 270: 351, 402, 1963.

Jeliffe, R. B., and R. F. A. Dean: Protein-calorie malnutrition in early childhood (practical notes), J. Trop. Ped., 5:196, 1959.

Keys, A., J. Brozek, A. Henschel, O. Mickelsen, and H. L. Taylor: "The Biology of Human Starvation," Minneapolis, University of Minnesota Press, 1950.

Levinson, S. M., and D. M. Watkin: Protein requirements in injury and certain acute and chronic diseases, Fed. Proc., 18:1155, 1959.

Medical Research Council: "Studies of Undernutrition, Wuppertal, 1946–9," London, 1951.

Monro, H. N., and J. B. Allison (Eds.): "Mammalian Protein Metabolism," vols. I and II, New York, Academic Press, 1964.

Moore, F. D.: "Metabolic Care of the Surgical Patient," Philadelphia, W. B. Saunders Company, 1959.

68 ANOREXIA NERVOSA
George W. Thorn and Henry M. Fox

Anorexia nervosa is a psychosomatic disorder with complex interrelations between psychologic and somatic factors. Although the condition may and sometimes does lead to death, there is no apparent somatic pathology. However, the patient adamantly refuses to eat. Richard Morton (1689) has generally been credited with publication of the first medical account. Sir William Gull gave a detailed description of the condition in 1873 and termed it *anorexia nervosa*. In the same year, Lasegue published an article (*De l'anorexie hysterique*) which conveyed a vivid description of the disturbed relationships and intrapsychic turmoil of the patients.

ETIOLOGY. The disorder occurs predominantly (85 to 90 per cent) in young women. Although patients with anorexia nervosa manifest features ranging from those of psychoneurosis to those of schizophrenia, the underlying conflict is most often a primitive struggle for control between the patient and the mother and the severity of the regression varies from one patient to another. This struggle is always pervaded by an exceptionally intense negativism related to the earliest forms of self-assertion in the developing infant, when breath holding, rejecting food, retaining feces, and refusing to smile or speak are the only means of resisting the mother's attempts to control bodily functions. This intense negativism is sometimes initially passive and indirect in a patient who has always been obedient outwardly, but as the illness progresses, the primitive nature of the process often becomes more painfully direct and undisguised.

In some patients the precipitating factor is initiation of a reducing diet because the patient thinks she is too "fat." This may have resulted from self-appraisal or from a remark by someone else about her appearance. In other patients the condition begins with loss of an important relationship by death, illness, or separation. In some the disturbance may have begun in the setting of an urge to leave the shelter of the family in the course of adolescent development.

All these patients place a disproportionate emphasis on food and eating, and there is often a history of preexisting obesity. Fantasies about pregnancy and sexual attractiveness as well as reactivation of early conflicts with the mother can usually be demonstrated. A typical finding in the vast majority of cases is complete cessation of menses. In a goodly proportion the amenorrhea begins before or simultaneously with the disturbances in eating. Although failure to eat is the obvious and striking phenomenon, almost all the patients are found to have a variety of other symptoms referable to the gastrointestinal tract, including vomiting, which may be spontaneous or self-induced. In some patients excessive use of cathartics may be a noticeable aspect of their behavior.

CLINICAL PICTURE. Weight loss may be extreme, down to as little as 40 to 50 per cent of the normal weight (Fig. 68-1). However, in contrast to famine victims, patients usually maintain their strength and activity at near normal levels, or at least strength is disproportionate to the degree of emaciation. Many patients are able to carry out their usual activities to a remarkable degree. They appear characteristically unconcerned with their undernourished state and lack the constant hunger of the famine victim.

The blood pressure may be low; there is no change in pigmentation, no loss of axillary or pubic hair, and the breasts are relatively well preserved in contrast to the atrophy so commonly seen in other forms of undernutrition. Other manifestations of severe undernutrition are present, i.e., lowered basal metabolic rate, anemia, reduced serum cholesterol, urinary gonadotropin levels, and 17-ketosteroid values. The serum protein-bound iodine is normal, as are most other laboratory tests. Hypoproteinemia may or may not be present, but edema is conspicuous by its absence.

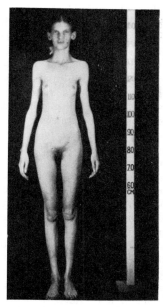

Fig. 68-1. A patient showing signs of marked undernutrition due to anorexia nervosa.

DIAGNOSIS. The usual causes of emaciation must be considered in differential diagnosis, but such diseases as disseminated cancer, diabetes, or intestinal malabsorption syndromes are usually easily excluded because of the patient's subjective feeling of good health. Much has been said in the past about differentiating anorexia nervosa from hypopituitarism. Actually, the only similarity between these diseases is that menstruation ceases in both. Otherwise, the persistence of normal body hair, normal breast tissue, normal thyroid and adrenal function, and good subjective strength and health serve to eliminate pituitary dysfunction from consideration. However, *very late* in the disorder with *long-continued, severe undernutrition* secondary pituitary deficiency may develop.

TREATMENT. Since the emotional disorder associated with this disease is usually severe and potentially self-destructive, these patients should be treated with the full cooperation of a psychiatrist. Although the physician is necessarily preoccupied with increasing the patient's caloric intake, it is important to establish a relationship with the patient that does not duplicate the struggle with the mother. Exhortations about the importance of eating should be avoided. The patient should be fed a high-vitamin diet in small feedings if she complains that larger quantities of food result in discomfort. If the patient begins to eat adequately, it is important not to restrict her activities by keeping her in bed, as this activates conflicts concerning dependency and helplessness. Even without treatment subsequent to their initial hospitalization some patients make a good recovery, marry, raise families, and do not have relapses. Many patients, however, remain maladjusted, and a considerable number die despite all attempts to maintain improved nutrition. Tube feedings may be necessary to prevent the patient from starving to death. Numerous appetite stimulants have been suggested, including vitamins, "tonics," wine, and even cortisone. Any of these items may on occasion help, but they do not relieve the basic disorder and should therefore be used only as adjuncts to treatment rather than as substitutes for more fundamental psychotherapeutic approaches.

REFERENCES

Nemiah, John C.: Anorexia Nervosa: Fact and Theory, Am. J. Digest. Dis., 3:249, 1958.

Bliss, Eugene L., and C. H. Hardin Branch: "Anorexia Nervosa—Its History, Psychology, and Biology," New York, Paul B. Hoeber, Inc., Medical Department of Harper & Brothers, 1960.

69 MALABSORPTION SYNDROMES AND SPRUE

Frank H. Gardner

DEFINITION. "The malabsorption syndrome is the consequence of impaired absorption of foods, minerals and water by the small bowel. The majority of the clinical symptoms of the syndrome are manifestations of the nutritional deficiencies which result from impaired absorption or from altered intestinal activity."

CLASSIFICATION. Recurrent diarrhea among Europeans living in the Far East initiated interest in malabsorption by the small bowel. This disorder was called *tropical sprue,* and clinicians assumed that it was limited to hot humid tropical climates. In 1932 Thaysen reported that a similar malabsorption syndrome occurs in the temperate zones, and the term *nontropical sprue* was introduced. Clinical observations in the past decade have emphasized the marked similarity of celiac disease in children and the gastrointestinal dysfunction of nontropical sprue. Numerous adult patients probably have nontropical sprue as the continuing manifestation of childhood celiac disease. Hence, nontropical sprue should be called *adult celiac disease.*

Malabsorption disorders have been classified for convenience as primary and secondary; in primary disorders a defect of intestinal epithelium predominates. Primary types include acute and chronic forms (Table 69-1). Acute types are usually self-limited and may be associated with a variety of infections that irritate the epithelial surface. Malabsorption from viral infection (hepatitis) or bacterial invasion (cholera) is self-limited. In the chronic form of primary malabsorption, adult celiac disease, β-lipoprotein and certain primary disaccharidase deficiencies can be considered as hereditary in nature. Most patients with a chronic form of primary malabsorption usually are first recognized many years after the onset of symptoms.

Table 69-1. CLASSIFICATION OF MALABSORPTION

I. Primary (epithelial disease)
   A. Acute (self-limited)
      1. Infections (cholera, salmonella, infectious hepatitis, giardiasis, hookworm infection, rhinoenteric viruses)
      2. Drug (neomycin)
      3. Radiation injury
   B. Chronic
      1. Tropical sprue
      2. Adult celiac disease (nontropical sprue, gluten enteropathy)
      3. Idiopathic protein-losing enteropathy
      4. β-Lipoprotein deficiency
      5. Hypogammaglobulinemia
      6. Disaccharidase deficiency
II. Secondary
   A. Intrinsic bowel wall alterations
      1. Intestinal tuberculosis
      2. Regional enteritis
      3. Amyloid disease
      4. Lymphoma
      5. Mesenteric artery insufficiency
      6. Vasculitis (collagen disease)
   B. Obstruction of intestinal lymphatics
      1. Intestinal lipodystrophy (Whipple's disease)
      2. Lymphoma
      3. Intestinal lymphangiectasia
      4. Heart failure
   C. Anatomic alterations
      1. Postgastrectomy syndrome
      2. Diverticula of small bowel
      3. Enteric fistula and blind loops (enteroenterostomy)
      4. Vagotomy
      5. Bowel resection
   D. Hormonal
      1. Addison's disease
      2. Diabetes mellitus
      3. Hypoparathyroidism
      4. Pancreatic adenoma (multiple endocrine adenomas)
   E. Maldigestion
      1. Pancreatic insufficiency

The secondary forms of malabsorption listed in Table 69-1 represent a wide range of malabsorption states. For the most part, all these disorders are quite rare except for malabsorption associated with anatomic alterations, especially the postgastrectomy syndrome and regional enteritis.

ETIOLOGY

PRIMARY MALABSORPTION. The acute self-limited disorders improve with control of the infection or cessation of drug administration. Rarely bowel dysfunction continues for months after control of the enteric bacterial infection. The cause of tropical sprue is not known. Efforts have been made to associate the disorder with vitamin deficiencies or an imbalance of the bacterial flora of the small bowel. Despite un-

successful efforts to isolate a particular infectious agent, tropical sprue has responded well to sulfonamides and antibiotic therapy. Severe anemia and nutritional depletion will improve if antibiotics are administered for months. Folic acid has been cited as a specific nutritional defect in tropical sprue but, by the methodology available, a systemic dietary folic acid depletion has not been demonstrated. Hence it is difficult to explain the infrequency of tropical sprue in the geographic areas where nutritional deficits are widespread. It is noteworthy that the symptoms of sprue may develop after 1 or 2 months' residence in tropical areas where the disease is endemic, or they may appear years later after return to nontropical areas. Such observations should encourage further search for infectious agents. The infrequency of sprue in Africa compared to the incidence in the Far East may reflect racial, dietary, and constitutional factors.

ADULT CELIAC DISEASE. Studies in Holland and England have demonstrated that most children with celiac disease respond dramatically when wheat, barley, and rye flour are excluded from the diet. Similar results have been observed in the majority of adult patients with nontropical sprue, especially if dietary control is rigid and is followed for at least 6 months. More specifically, the offending agent appears to reside in the protein fraction of the flour (gluten). Gluten is the water-insoluble portion of flour. The gliadin fraction of gluten is most active in initiating symptoms. Although gliadin has a high glutamine content, it must be emphasized that glutamine has no ill effect in celiac disease. The exact mechanism for interference with absorption by gluten is not known. Two widely held views are (1) that an antibody immune response is involved, or (2) that an enzymatic defect in the epithelium is responsible. The possibility cannot be excluded that other food substances may act in a fashion similar to gluten, since some patients do not respond to a gluten-free diet. Recently adults with disaccharidase deficiency have been aided by the dietary elimination of the specific disaccharide.

SECONDARY MALABSORPTION. The invasion of the bowel epithelium or submucosal area by tumor (lymphoma) or the development of lymphatic obstruction (Whipple's disease) impairs absorption or transport of foodstuffs. Diverticula or blind loops allow stagnation of chyme, with a resultant profuse bacterial overgrowth. It has been suggested that the competitive demands of such bacterial flora consume or bind vitamins and nutrients or that the metabolic products of the bacteria may irritate the bowel mucosa (jejunitis). Normally, there is no resident bacterial population in the small bowel as far down as the terminal ileum.

Alterations in motility of the small bowel produced by the absence of the pylorus (subtotal gastrectomy) or the ileocecal valve (ileocolostomy) decrease transit time and reduce absorption. Following massive small-bowel resection (usually for vascular lesions), the remaining bowel is an inadequate absorptive area for proper nutrition. Inadequate mixing of stomach contents with pancreatic enzymes probably is the most important defect to account for malabsorption after subtotal gastrectomy. In some patients excessive bacterial overgrowth in a proximal redundant afferent loop following subtotal gastrectomy has been the primary mechanism of malabsorption (jejunitis).

PATHOLOGY

In the small bowel changes are found in association with acute bacterial, protozoan, and viral infection. Cellular infiltration of the lamina propria is associated with blunting of the villi and increased depth of the crypts. Some of these changes may persist for months during recovery from the infectious process. Similar changes may be noted in tropical sprue, often within a month of arrival in tropical climates. Such observations add further support to the hypothesis that tropical sprue is infectious in origin. In celiac disease, in contrast, extensive histologic alterations are found, more severe in the jejunum than in the ileum. As in tropical sprue, jejunal biopsy specimens show short blunted villi and increased depth of the crypts of Lieberkühn, but, in addition, the columnar cells of the epithelium are distorted; increased mitotic figures are observed as well as plasma cell infiltration of the lamina propria. Histochemical and biochemical studies emphasize the deficient enzymatic function of the epithelium. The microvilli (brush border) are sparse, blunted, and fused. The mitochondria are abnormally enlarged and vacuolated. The shortened villi and sparse microvilli reflect a loss in the absorption surface of the bowel in both tropical and nontropical sprue (Fig. 69-1). Installation of wheat flour into the ileum of patients with adult celiac disease, where the epithelial changes are minimal, will cause mucosal alterations of the villi within hours and is associated with lassitude and onset of diarrhea. To gross inspection the small and the large bowel are dilated and may be transparent through areas of the blunted villi.

There are no specific epithelial alterations in the other chronic types of primary malabsorption except for β-lipoprotein deficiency. In this disorder the epithelial cells are engorged with lipid since the cells can absorb triglycerides but are unable to discharge the lipid into the lacteals. The fatty cellular infiltration has a characteristic histologic appearance. Malabsorption associated with acquired hypogammaglobulinemia in the adult is accompanied by normal epithelial patterns, and plasma cells may or may not be observed in the lamina propria. Malabsorption is not characteristic of congenital agammaglobulinemia.

Treatment of tropical sprue with folic acid and vitamin B_{12} will allow the villi to return to a normal state in half the patients. In a limited number of patients, prolonged antibiotic therapy has reversed the abnormalities. After prolonged use of the gluten-free diet, the adult celiac patient shows a reversal

toward normal of the severely blunted villi and disordered epithelium. In neither type of malabsorption can clinical improvement be correlated with the morphology; many patients may be asymptomatic in spite of an abnormal villus histology.

Secondary malabsorption disorders usually do not involve the epithelium. In instances of diverticula or fistula, the bacteria may cause an inflammatory reaction (jejunitis) with cellular infiltration of the lamina propria. Such changes are reversible when the bacterial contamination is eliminated. However, the malabsorption that may follow acute enteric infections is not associated with chronic persistence of the organism. Giardiasis and hookworm disease can cause malabsorption from a reactive enteritis. In Whipple's disease mild blunting of the villi and a diffuse macrophage infiltration of the lamina propria are observed. These are associated with lacteal dilatation and lymphatic obstruction. Intracellular bacilluslike organisms have been seen in these macrophages by electron microscopy, thus suggesting a bacterial etiology for this disease, especially since these organisms and symptoms disappear with antibiotic therapy.

In intestinal lymphangiectasia there is a congenital dilatation of the lacteals with leakage of protein into the bowel lumen and an associated protein depletion. Intestinal protein loss may be associated with chronic inflammatory disease, ulcerating tumors, and prolonged heart failure (constrictive pericarditis). The steatorrhea that may be seen with severe heart failure has been attributed to the lymphatic congestion and impaired pancreatic function.

The ischemia of the bowel wall from the vascular insufficiency of arteriosclerosis or from vasculitis associated with collagen disorders results in a generalized atrophy of all tissues. It is presumed that a combination of inadequate villi and impaired circulation explains the malabsorption in these rare patients. Chronic skin disorders (psoriasis, rosacea, exfoliative dermatitis) are associated with steatorrhea and flattened small bowel villi, such as are seen in adult celiac disease. Altered blood flow with ischemia of the mucosa has been suggested as a mechanism for these changes. There are no pathologic alterations associated with hormonal types of secondary malabsorption.

Small-bowel biopsy specimens obtained by means of various intraluminal instruments passed into the bowel by mouth allow a more definitive diagnosis of the bowel lesion. For complete understanding of these disorders, microscopic study of the mucosa should always be done to facilitate classification and therapy.

With prolonged folic acid and vitamin B_{12} depletion, megaloblastic erythroid hyperplasia of the bone marrow develops. Similar enlargement of the cells occurs in the proliferating crypt cells of the bowel. Such changes may contribute to the altered villus height as well as to the malfunction of intracellular enzymes. Young children with severe iron deficiency have blunted and fused villi with an associated mal-

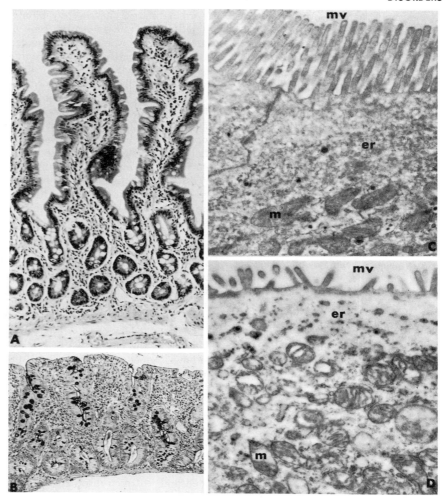

Fig. 69-1. *A.* Biopsy specimen of normal jejunum. The villi are prominent, slender, and erect, and the columnar cells are arranged in an orderly palisade (H and E approximately × 100).

B. Biopsy of specimen of jejunum in adult celiac disease (nontropical sprue). Villi are virtually absent; when present, they are severely blunted. The epithelial surface is diminished considerably, whereas, proportionately, the depth of the crypts of Lieberkühn appears to be increased (PAS and H approximately × 100).

C. Electronmicrograph of a portion of a normal jejunal columnar villous cell. A distinct border of microvilli (*mv*) faces the intestinal lumen. Under this border is a region of fine cytoplasmic tubules of the endoplasmic reticulum (*er*), beneath which are an abundance of normal-appearing mitochondria (*m*) (approximately × 20,000).

D. Electronmicrograph of a portion of an absorptive columnar cell of jejunum in adult celiac disease (nontropical sprue). The microvilli (*mv*) are shorter, fewer, and relatively irregular. The cytoplasmic tubules of the endoplasmic reticulum (*er*) appear to be reduced in number and compactness. Mitochondria (*m*) exhibit abnormalities of form and internal structure. Histochemically, these mitochondria show a deficiency in succinic dehydrogenase (approximately × 20,000). (*Prepared by Dr. A J. Ladman.*)

absorption. These abnormalities disappear with iron therapy. There are no conclusive data to imply that iron deficiency can alter the small-bowel mucosa in the adult.

PHYSIOLOGY

The term *idiopathic steatorrhea* was used by clinicians because the impaired absorption of fat alters the character of the feces in a striking fashion. The morphologic changes of the mucosa in reality impair the absorption of all foodstuffs in varying degrees. In adult celiac disease and tropical sprue, fat intolerance is the most sensitive dietary component and develops early. More extensive deficiencies of vitamin absorption appear later. The impaired absorption results from the immense loss of bowel-wall epithelial area caused by blunted villi and the impaired propulsion of the emulsified chyme. Secondly, there is a large secretion of protein into the lumen, associated with gastric and bowel enzymes that participate in digestion. These proteins are prepared for reutilization by autodigestion. With epithelial damage these materials in the succus entericus are reabsorbed poorly and contribute to the azotorrhea. Alterations in mucoprotein secretion and increased viscosity of the succus entericus have been demonstrated in adult celiac disease and tropical sprue. These viscous secretions also may interfere with absorption. Finally, histochemical and biochemical depletion of enzymes in the epithelium has been noted. Damage to the epithelium impairs absorption of all disaccharides. Impairment of lactase secretion is observed early by tissue biopsy assay, and this may persist even after other absorptive measurements return to normal. Disacchariduria is associated with the depletion of epithelial disaccharidase in tropical sprue and adult celiac disease. Further elucidation of other enzyme defects can be expected. In β-lipoprotein deficiency the impaired transport of fat from the columnar cells represents an effective block to epithelial cell function.

Analysis of the duodenal secretions in primary malabsorption reveals normal values for pancreatic enzymes and bile salts. In the jejunum there is adequate emulsification of fats and digestion of proteins. In pancreatic disorders steatorrhea often occurs from lack of lipase. Hence one notes inadequate lipolysis in congenital cystic fibrosis (mucoviscidosis), chronic pancreatitis, and carcinoma of the pancreas. In these diseases the bowel epithelium is normal, but the fat is not prepared for absorption. Carbohydrates are absorbed normally, and diabetic blood sugar curves are not uncommon. This selective fat malabsorption with normal carbohydrate absorption helps to differentiate pancreatic insufficiency.

Ulcerogenic tumors of the pancreas (Zollinger-Ellison syndrome) may be associated with pancreatic steatorrhea because the excess of stomach acid inactivates the pancreatic enzymes in the duodenal juice. In the malabsorption associated with hormonal disorders listed in Table 69-1 steatorrhea is the predominant abnormality. The defect is usually mild and often overlooked. Impaired motility of the small bowel has been the mechanism ascribed to hypoparathyroidism. Electrolyte imbalance with impaired epithelial metabolism has been proposed as the explanation in adrenal insufficiency. The steatorrhea of diabetes mellitus may improve with tetracycline therapy. Therefore an altered bacterial flora with epithelial irritation has been proposed for this disease. Alternatively, motility defects from neuropathy have also been suggested to explain malabsorption in diabetes.

Decreased absorption of simple molecular substances (D_2O, KI^{131}, Fe^{59}, $S^{35}O_4$, and $Na^{29}Cl$) may be detected with isotope-labeling procedures. The absorption of more complex foodstuffs such as fats, amino acids, sugars, and vitamins can be measured by dietary balance studies. Not all substances are associated with the same degree of impaired transfer across the mucosa. The presence of an abnormal bacterial flora in diverticula and blind loops is especially prone to impair absorption of vitamin B_{12}. This defect is noted when there is ileal involvement (regional enteritis) since, in human beings, most of the vitamin B_{12} is absorbed from this area of the bowel. Folic acid is absorbed preferentially in the jejunum. In tropical sprue and adult celiac disease folic acid absorption decreases since the jejunum is the area of marked mucosal damage. The abnormal mucosa also impairs the reabsorption of the vitamin B_{12}, folic acid, and cholesterol excreted in the bile. Disaccharides may be poorly absorbed because of rapid transit time following gastric surgery. Other patients may have lactosuria related to this disaccharide enzyme depletion. The impaired absorption of carbohydrates can be associated with weight loss and steatorrhea from an osmotic and fermentative catharsis.

Impaired absorption of vitamin K often produces hypoprothrombinemia. Secondary physiologic alterations are associated with deficiency of electrolytes. Hypomotility of the small bowel may be enhanced by hypopotassemia. Hypocalcemia and demineralization of the skeleton are observed to occur with a negative calcium balance most frequently in adult celiac disease. There is an impaired absorption of water, which has been attributed to the decreased motility of the small bowel. As a consequence many patients have a recurrent nocturnal diuresis resulting from delayed fluid absorption during the daylight hours.

CLINICAL PICTURE

The malabsorption syndromes are characterized in most instances by an insidious onset. Often patients are treated for prolonged intervals symptomatically before the diagnosis is made. A history of intermittent diarrhea for months or years may be elicited. In 40 per cent of adult patients with celiac disease one obtains a history of stunted growth and intestinal disorders in early childhood. During the episodes of diarrhea, the stools may be mushy, light-colored, frothy, foul-smelling, and associated with explosive flatus. At onset, the diarrhea may be limited to two or three bulky stools in the morning without additional stools during the day. Intermittent constipation often is present between bouts of diarrhea. Severe lassitude and fatigue are associated with the diarrhea, possibly because of excessive loss of electrolytes in the feces. Moderate to severe weight loss is noted in all patients, depending on the duration and severity of the disorder. Often patients become accustomed to an altered bowel habit and do not seek medical advice until secondary deficiencies become prominent. Severe emotional or physical stress may convert intermittent diarrhea to a constant condition, which in turn is associated with more generalized clinical manifestations of nutritional deficiencies. When there is more active diarrhea, nausea and vomiting may be noted as well as bloating and abdominal pain. In rare instances, the abdominal distress may simulate intestinal obstruction or volvulus. Progressive abdominal distension during the day, which disappears at night, is a frequent observation. Nocturnal diuresis often is observed in the patient with adult celiac disease, and such a symptom may be helpful in orienting the physician to the correct diagnosis. Patients with pancreatic insufficiency have a selective steatorrhea and do not have anemia or electrolyte depletion.

As malabsorption becomes chronic, clinical signs and symptoms of nutritional deficiencies develop. Muscle cramps occur at some time in all patients, and a few may have tetany. Hypoprothrombinemia is associated with widespread hemorrhagic lesions. Glossitis is seen at some time in all patients with chronic malabsorption. The lesions may be limited to mild atrophic changes at the tip of the tongue or associated with widespread denudation of the papillary surface, and numerous small aphthous lesions. Tongue changes may appear within a few days but cannot be distinguished from those of other states of nutritional deficiency. With severe glossitis dysphagia contributes to further weight loss. Progression of secondary deficiencies results in inadequate reserves of iron, folic acid, and vitamin B_{12}. All the symptoms of anemia may therefore be present. Clubbing of the fingers and toes may be seen rarely. Edema and ascites may result from hypoproteinemia. Fractures, especially of the long bones, are associated with osteomalacia. Hypocalcemia with tetany is seen in adult celiac disease but is rare in tropical sprue, possibly because of the greater exposure to sunlight in the tropics.

LABORATORY FINDINGS

Stools are not consistently altered; in mild cases their appearance may be normal. In more severe disease the stools are light tan (almost acholic in appearance), frothy, greasy, and foul-smelling, and they tend to float on water. These changes are associated primarily with the content of fat and will not be detected if the patient has avoided fat. Neutral fat particles and fatty acid crystals may be detected by microscopic examination of the stool.

EXAMINATION FOR FAT. A small, 5-mm sample of stool is emulsified with a few drops of water, and an aliquot is placed on two glass slides. To the first slide is added 2 drops of 95 per cent ethanol, followed by 3 drops of a saturated 95 per cent ethanol solution of Sudan III. The stool aliquot must be mixed with the Sudan III with an applicator stick for 5 min. A cover slip is then applied, and after another 5 minutes the preparation is examined microscopically for yellow, pale orange refractile globules of fat with a low and a high dry lens ($430\times$). The edge of the cover slip should be examined especially carefully. These globules represent neutral fat and may also be seen following the ingestion of oily laxatives. Fat droplets are not seen in most patients because bacterial activity converts fat to soaps.

EXAMINATION FOR FATTY ACIDS. On the second prepared slide, the aliquot of stool is mixed with 3 drops of 36 per cent acetic acid, followed by 3 drops of a saturated solution of Sudan III. A cover slip is applied after mixing, as described above, and the slide is heated gently over a low flame until bubbling is noted under the cover slip. The heating allows hydrolysis of the soaps with the release of fatty acids in the presence of acetic acid. After cooling, the slide is examined as described above. With cooling, the fatty acids may crystallize as colorless, needlelike sheaves.

The normal stool usually contains as many as 100 globules of fatty acid per high dry field, usually less than 4 μ in diameter. With increased fatty acids the globules are larger, ranging from 10 to 75 μ in diameter, and the relationship to fecal material in the background varies with the degree of steatorrhea. With profound steatorrhea only fatty globules may be observed. These fecal examinations are of no value without adequate fat intake in the diet (more than 60 Gm daily). The examiner must train himself by repeated examinations of normal stools.

The stool bulk is increased (normal, 100 to 200 Gm; malabsorption, 500 to 1,000 Gm) and reflects increased liquid volume. No consistent bacterial flora are observed, although the absolute number of bacteria is increased, probably reflecting the utilization of unabsorbed nutrients from the small bowel.

ABSORPTION AND OTHER LABORATORY STUDIES. Dietary balance studies reveal increased fecal loss of nitrogen and fats. Normal subjects excrete 5 Gm or less of fecal fat when consuming the average 50 to 100 Gm daily of dietary fats. Usually, in severe malabsorption 15 to 30 Gm or more of fat will be excreted daily. In most instances 3- to 6-day determinations are needed for careful evaluation, inasmuch as wide fluctuations in daily excretion occur. A variety of tests may be used, but there is no substitute for this intake-excretion evaluation of fat balance. It is the only reliable method for defining mild degrees of steatorrhea and quantitating fat loss. This procedure should be carried out, if possible, on all patients as a base line to evaluate the severity of malabsorption as well as to measure effects of treatment.

The chronic deficiency state is reflected in low fasting serum levels of neutral fats, cholesterol, phospholipids, vitamin A, carotene, vitamin B_{12}, folic acid, vitamin C, iron, copper, total proteins, calcium, potassium, and prothrombin. However, the various nutritional components are not depressed uniformly in all patients. The fasting serum *carotene* level has been the most useful screening laboratory measurement. Serum mucoprotein levels are elevated in all malabsorption states associated with inflammatory response of the lamina propria.

Many types of malabsorption are associated with increased amounts of urinary tryptophan metabolites. Usually these are measured as 5-hydroxyindoleacetic acid (5-HIAA). With correction of the malabsorption

5-HIAA excretion returns to normal. These changes demonstrate a metabolic defect of serotonin in the bowel wall but are not diagnostic, aside from indicating malabsorption.

Serologic factors (antibodies) to a fraction of gluten are present in childhood and adult celiac disease, but these measurements are not diagnostic. Some patients also have increased antibody titers to milk proteins; the significance is not known. Further improvement may occur when milk as well as gluten protein is eliminated from the diet. These observations may indicate an immune response to the systemic passive absorption of undigested substances through the damaged epithelium.

A variety of oral tolerance tests have been used to evaluate the impaired bowel function. Although glucose absorption has been popular, one-third of normal adults may have a "flat tolerance curve," and the procedure should be discarded. However, the test has been retained by some physicians because a diabetic type of oral glucose tolerance curve can indicate pancreatic insufficiency. Two screening procedures can be used with ease to estimate sugar and fat absorption.

ABSORPTION OF d-XYLOSE. The fasting patient ingests 25 Gm d-xylose with several glasses of water. The urine is collected for a 5-hr period thereafter, and the amount of the pentose excreted is determined (normal persons excrete 5 to 8 Gm; malabsorption patients excrete 3 Gm or less).

POSTPRANDIAL LIPEMIA. Lipemia curves can be standardized by semiquantitative measurements of changes in serum optical density (O.D.). The fasting patient receives a standard breakfast meal of 30 Gm butter, two slices of bread with jelly, 100 ml fruit juice, and sweetened tea or coffee. A fasting serum sample, as well as collections at 2, 3, 4, and 5 hr, are measured in a colorimeter at 540 mμ for optical density changes, with the fasting sample as a control. In the normal subject the peak of lipemia occurs in the second to fourth hour, with an optical density above 0.1. For reproducible results, the patients should be resting and refrain from smoking during the test. In the sprue patient values below 0.05 are found, and there is evidence of postprandial lipemia in this short interval. Radioactive iodinated triolein can be used instead of butter fat with similar results. However, the steatorrhea of pancreatic disease can be differentiated in part by comparing absorption (blood levels) of radioactive iodinated triolein and oleic acid, there being good absorption of the fatty acid in the absence of lipase. Other tolerance tests are more difficult to perform and add little diagnostic information.

HEMATOLOGY. About two-thirds of patients with primary sprue demonstrate mild to severe macrocytic anemia. Morphologic changes of the peripheral blood and bone marrow are indistinguishable from those of Addisonian pernicious anemia. Folic acid deficiency may be detected early by careful examination of the blood film for multilobed neutrophils; they may be found before anemia has developed. With impaired iron absorption, anemia may be normocytic or hypochromic. At that time a double red cell population may be present; such changes are referred to as dimorphic anemia. Urinary and fecal assays for folic acid, Fe^{59} salts, and Co^{60}-vitamin B_{12} have revealed impaired absorption of these erythropoietic agents. Diverticula and blind loops, especially, are associated with impaired absorption of vitamin B_{12}, possibly by competitive bacterial utilization of the vitamin or binding of intrinsic factor.

ROENTGENOLOGIC OBSERVATIONS. Ingestion of a barium sulfate suspension normally reveals a fine feathery pattern of the jejunal and ileal mucosa. In most types of malabsorption, segmentation and clumping of the barium meal and prominent haustral marking are found instead (Fig. 69-2). Such "puddling" of the barium meal may be absent earlier, but in chronic disease alterations of the bowel pattern are always observed. The flocculation of the barium suspension has been attributed to excess mucus or fluids in the small bowel, but aspiration studies have not demonstrated increased secretion. Transit time of the barium meal is delayed in the small bowel. With colloidal barium suspensions dilatation of small bowel loops and of the colon is noted. The dilatation of the bowel may explain the volvulus of the intestine, especially the sigmoid colon, that has been reported in many types of malabsorption syndrome. The observer should be aware that the well-known flocculation pattern is noted only with barium suspensions. If studies are done with colloidal preparations, these changes are not found and only dilatation of the bowel may be seen. Secondary malabsorption associated with intrinsic bowel wall alterations or obstruction of lymphatics may show a similar pattern with the barium suspension. Radiologic examination is the only method by which anatomic lesions (blind loops, enteritis, diverticula, fistulas) can be detected and differentiated from those of primary malabsorption. Calcifications in the pancreatic area may be observed during bowel studies and suggest chronic pancreatitis. Since the results of absorption tests may be similar, x-ray studies and biopsy specimens of the small bowel are necessary for adequate differentiation. With prolonged impaired calcium absorption, demineralization of the skeleton occurs. The growth of the long bones may be altered in the adult patient whose illness represents a recrudescence of a childhood celiac disease.

The general appearance of these patients, as well as their associated weight loss, anemia, and weakness, often suggest the diagnosis of postpubertal panhypopituitarism. However, the target glands are normal when measured by their response to pituitary hormones.

When malabsorption is suspected, the physician should examine the stool grossly for color, volume, and texture and study a sample for fatty acid crystals. Concurrently, fasting serum samples should be collected for carotene, cholesterol, and iron determinations. The tests for absorption of d-xylose and butter fat are performed. If these observations confirm the

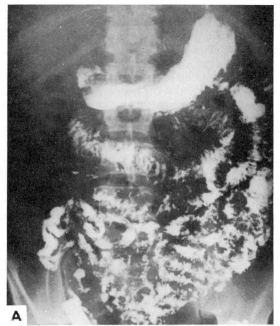

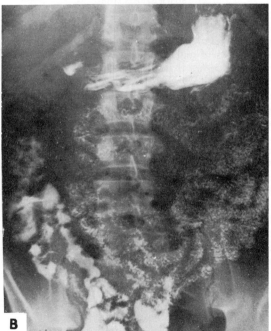

Fig. 69-2. A. Small bowel x-ray studies in tropical sprue. The barium suspension is segmented. (puddled) in the small bowel. B. Tropical sprue (same patient) during folic acid therapy. A normal feathery appearance is observed throughout the jejunum and upper ileum.

clinical diagnosis of malabsorption, the radiologic pattern of the small bowel should be studied and a mucosal biopsy performed. Before therapy is started, fecal fat balance for a minimum of 3 days should be determined.

In steatorrhea with pancreatic disease, usually

chronic pancreatitis, there is impaired fat absorption but absorption of d-xylose is normal. The small-bowel radiologic pattern and the mucosal biopsy are normal. To clarify a diagnosis of pancreatic insufficiency the physician must study duodenal secretions for lipase and trypsin. If possible a secretin stimulation test with measurements of duodenal content for volume, bicarbonate, and enzyme activity should be done.

TREATMENT

Acute malabsorption following enteric infections requires no therapy aside from the specific antimicrobial agent for the infection. Bland diets and vitamin replacement therapy may be tried. Tropical sprue in the early or chronic phase of the illness responds to oral folic acid therapy (5 mg daily). Physical and emotional rest in the acute phase hastens recovery. The diet should be bland (skim milk, bananas, liver soups, and puréed meats) and of low residue. This treatment relieves lassitude, diarrhea, and weight loss, even in the absence of anemia or clinical evidence of secondary nutritional deficiencies. Folic acid therapy should be given for 4 to 6 months. Then the drug may be withdrawn for evaluation. The vitamin may be needed indefinitely in the tropics or if symptoms recur. Good results with tetracycline therapy have been reported: 1.0 Gm daily for 2 to 3 months should be used. Possibly the success of various dietary programs is attributable to the alteration of bacterial flora associated with a high protein diet. Return to the temperate zone brings remission of the disorder. Tropical sprue does not respond to elimination of gluten from the diet.

The secondary nutritional deficiencies and megaloblastic anemias likewise respond to folic acid. Usually oral or parenteral iron salts are necessary for a complete hematologic remission. However, some patients continue to manifest some degree of impaired absorption of all foodstuffs. In such instances dietary limitation of fats and starches may be necessary to control intermittent diarrhea. Parenteral vitamin B_{12} likewise has been successful in amelioration of anemia, but the ease of oral folic acid administration for patient care has made it the treatment of choice.

Patients with adult celiac disease must be given a gluten-free diet. The patient may use any food that does not contain wheat, barley, or rye gluten. The absorption defect is altered slowly, and the dietary restriction must be continued for at least 6 months before the physician can conclude that it is not helpful. The physician and patient must evaluate the diet carefully, for wheat flour is used in many prepared foods as a binding agent or filler without designation on the package labels. These patients need folic acid, vitamin B_{12}, and other vitamins only if anemia and nutritional deficiencies are present. The use of vitamins and hematinics may correct anemia and initiate clinical improvement, but this is not comparable to the more spectacular responses noted in tropical sprue. Even in the absence of a childhood history of intestinal complaints, a gluten-free diet may be tried empirically. Instructions for careful dietary restriction of fats and starches should be given and a high protein diet provided. Elimination of milk products should be considered if the response to gluten-free diet is inconclusive. Chronic dermatitis associated with steatorrhea will disappear with corrective local therapy. Some patients also have benefited from a gluten-free diet. Folic acid should be prescribed in view of the nutritional requirements for increased dermal proliferation. In patients with malnutrition, therapy may be initiated with adrenocortical hormones (cortisone acetate or prednisone, 200 and 40 mg, respectively), but prolonged therapy is not advised. The results of hormonal therapy may be dramatic, with improved absorption and relief of diarrhea noted in 2 to 3 days. Some patients have been given corticosteroids when the gluten-free diet is started, with the expectation that the hormone therapy will be discontinued in 4 to 8 weeks. If the drug is used alone, most patients require 50 to 75 mg cortisone acetate or 10 to 15 mg prednisone daily to control bowel symptoms. Improved absorption of foodstuffs is noted within one week and is maintained for the duration of hormone therapy. Initially, corticosteroids often accentuate tetany (possibly by increased fecal calcium loss and decreased absorption of vitamin D), and calcium salts should be given orally. Prolonged administration of corticosteroids will accentuate osteoporosis. Tetany from hypocalcemia can be controlled rapidly with intravenous 10 per cent calcium gluconate. Special attention to electrolyte replacement, especially potassium salts, is of great importance in the relief of lassitude and weakness. Usually potassium chloride solution is given, 2 to 3 Gm daily. Hemorrhagic complications (hypoprothrombinemia) respond to intramuscular menadione (10 mg daily).

Secondary malabsorption associated with specific defects in the small bowel can be treated only after recognition of the cause. Diverticula, intestinal strictures, and blind loops may improve dramatically with antibacterial therapy. However, relapse follows when the bacterial flora grow again. Antibacterial therapy helps to prepare the patient for surgical correction of the anatomic defect. Jejunal biopsies are helpful to plan proper chemotherapy for lymphosarcoma and Hodgkin's disease. Intestinal lipodystrophy may respond to adrenocortical hormones, but most patients have had complete remissions with antibiotic (chloramphenicol, tetracycline) treatment. This response may be related to the elimination of the intracellular bacilluslike organisms in the lamina propria. Congenital β-lipoprotein deficiency may be aided by a diet of short-chain (less than 12) fatty acids, to allow direct transport through the portal venous circulation without esterification. Acquired hypogammaglobulinemia is improved with intramuscular injections of gamma-globulin. As an estimate, most adults require 10 ml weekly. Disaccharidase deficiency requires careful dietary carbohydrate selection.

The treatment of the postgastrectomy patient has been difficult. Weight gain has been associated with (1) frequent small feedings to assure adequate pancreatic secretions from the proximal loop of the anastomosis, addition of 5.0 Gm of powdered pancreatin with each meal, (3) antibiotics (tetracycline, 1.0 Gm daily) to alter bacterial flora in the proximal jejunal loop, and (4) an androgen, testosterone propionate, 100 mg parenterally twice weekly, for its anabolic effects. In many patients, the malabsorption defect lessens over a period of years. These patients absorb iron poorly, and an iron-deficiency anemia is observed frequently within 5 years after surgery. Symptoms of the "dumping syndrome" may be associated with hypoferremia and are relieved in part by parenteral iron therapy (iron dextran intramuscularly 250 mgm weekly for a total dosage of 2.0 Gm).

PROGNOSIS

Diagnostic procedures are now available to define the various types of malabsorption. With such information, therapy can be planned with the expectation of improved bowel function. Information is still sparse regarding the mechanisms of absorption across the bowel mucosa. The accumulated evidence relating nontropical sprue to a similar defect found in celiac disease has emphasized the long duration (lifetime) of these disorders and points to additional epithelial enzyme deficiencies. There is evidence to suggest an increased incidence of neoplasm in the small bowel of adult celiac patients. Although this is not proved, dietary therapy may protect the patient by eliminating the abnormal bowel epithelium.

REFERENCES

Benson, G. D., O. D. Kowlessar, and M. H. Sleisenger: Adult Celiac Disease with Emphasis upon Response to the Gluten-free Diet, Medicine, 43:1, 1964.

Gardner, F. H., and E. W. Strauss: Disorders Related to Disturbed Absorption of the Small Bowel, Advances Int. Med., 10:137, 1960.

Padykula, H. A., E. W. Strauss, A. J. Ladman, and F. H. Gardner: Morphological and Biochemical Analysis of Human Jejunal Epithelium in Non-tropical Sprue, Gastroenterology, 40:735, 1961.

Sheehy, T. W., and M. H. Flock: "The Small Intestine: Its Function and Diseases," New York, Harper & Row, 1964.

Thaysen, E. H.: "Non-Tropical Sprue: A Study in Idiopathic Steatorrhea," Copenhagen, Levin and Munksgaard, 1932.

Wilson, T. H.: "Intestinal Absorption," Philadelphia, W. B. Saunders Company, 1962.

Wiseman, G.: "Absorption from the Intestine," London, Academic Press, Inc., 1964.

70 NUTRITIONAL ANEMIAS
Richard H. Follis, Jr.

For those who may be concerned with worldwide problems of nutrition, nutritional anemia is perhaps the most important after calorie and protein deficiency states (Chap. 67). Detailed discussions of the anemias resulting from deficiencies of iron, folic acid, and vitamin B_{12} are presented in Chaps. 111 and 112. Herein, it is only desired to stress the importance of the place of nutritional anemias in any review of nutritional deficiency states, whether dietary or conditioned in origin.

The prevalence of nutritional anemia varies from area to area around the world, and socioeconomic factors loom large in any discussion. Of the two main groups, microcytic and macrocytic, the former, which is usually associated with iron deficiency, is the more common. In a developed country such as the United States, one can gain some impression of the prevalence of anemia in the population at large from data accumulated in blood bank programs, for a certain level of hemoglobin is necessary before a donor is bled. This is set at about 12.5 Gm hemoglobin. In the age group from eighteen to fifty-nine years, 0.8 per cent of men and 12.6 per cent of women may be disqualified because of low hemoglobin levels. Cases of iron-deficiency anemia comprise the largest portion. In selected populations in Europe, similar data have been reported. In infants, the prevalence of iron-deficiency anemia in developed countries is higher, reaching 25 to 30 per cent of various groups that have been studied. The prevalence of macrocytic anemias in the United States and countries of northern Europe is low. In this group, 90 per cent, or even more, is composed of cases of Addisonian pernicious anemia. Only occasional instances of macrocytic anemia, usually associated with gastrointestinal disease or peculiar dietary habits, are encountered.

In some areas of developing countries, 50 per cent or more of the entire population may have hemoglobin values below 12 Gm per 100 ml. Iron-deficiency anemia is the most common type. Hookworm infestation leading to chronic blood loss is important in the pathogenesis of hypochromic microcytic anemia. Precise data on prevalence are usually not available. The proportion of cases with macrocytic anemias is lower; the geographic distribution may be different. This group is associated with dietary deficiency of folic acid or vitamin B_{12}. Assessment of the prevalence of iron, folic acid, or vitamin B_{12} deficiency, rather than anemia, is naturally most important. Only a start has been made at collecting such data.

71 ENDEMIC GOITER
Richard H. Follis, Jr.

HISTORY. That groups of people living in certain regions had swelling of the neck was well known to ancient writers (Pliny, Juvenal, Vitruvius). Such swellings were further described during the Middle Ages and are pictured in illuminated manuscripts of the times. By 1850, goiter was recognized as a common entity in many areas of the world, particularly mountainous sections, such as the Pyrenees, Alps, Carpathians, Himalayas, Sierras of Mexico and Central America, and the Andes. Mentally retarded dwarfs, called *cretins*, were also observed in groups in whom thyroid enlargement was prevalent.

Shortly after the discovery of iodine in seaweed in 1811, the element was introduced in the treatment of goiter, though soon its use came to be discredited. The situation changed abruptly in 1895 when iodine was found to be a normal constituent of the thyroid gland.

In 1905 Marine began to correlate the histologic appearance of thyroid glands from human beings and animals with their iodine content. He soon formulated the hypothesis that the hyperplastic form of goiter is the response of the thyroid gland to iodine deficiency. In 1917 Marine tested this fundamental hypothesis by administering sodium iodide to a group of schoolgirls in Akron, Ohio, then an area in which goiter was endemic. One group, with or without goiter, received a total of 2 Gm sodium iodide in multiple doses spring and fall. An equal number of girls served as controls. During an observation period of 3 years, among the girls receiving iodine there was either a decrease in or a disappearance of goiters or no enlargement developed; among the control subjects either more enlargement occurred or goiters appeared. These observations were soon confirmed in other parts of the world.

PREVALENCE. In 1960 the World Health Organization estimated that approximately 200 million persons were affected. In some countries, such as the United States, Canada, Switzerland, and New Zealand, where goiter had been prevalent during the first part of this century, the disease has decreased appreciably. Endemic goiter is a problem in certain parts of all countries of Latin America and in many areas in Africa, Europe, and Asia.

CLINICAL FINDINGS. In areas where it is highly endemic, goiter may be noted at birth. It is more usual, however, to find an increase in the size of the thyroid at five to seven years of age, the swelling slowly increasing so that visible enlargement is present at puberty. When adult life is reached, goiters in endemic areas tend to continue to increase in size, particularly in child-bearing women. In addition, nodules may appear. Such nodules are palpable in children; during adult life they may become more numerous and grossly evident, and the entire gland may have a visibly nodular appearance.

For the clinical assessment of the severity of goiter, the World Health Organization has recommended the following classification: Group O, persons without goiter by palpation; Group I, persons with palpable goiter or goiter visible with the head thrown back and neck fully extended; Group II, persons with plainly visible goiters; Group III, persons with large goiters.

This classification is particularly helpful in goiter surveys of population groups. As a general rule, goiters in females tend to be larger than those in males.

In an endemic area in a developing country, little complaint may be made by an individual with goiter, for the enlargement of the neck may be so common that the condition ceases to be noticed. Sometimes medical assistance is sought for cosmetic reasons, but this is unusual. The principal complaints, which fortunately are not common, include difficulty in breathing or swallowing, which results from pressure on the trachea or esophagus either in the cervical region or substernally. Coughing and hoarseness may result from pressure on the recurrent laryngeal nerve. The neck veins may be engorged. A thrill or bruit may be felt or heard over the gland. Virtually all individuals with large goiters in endemic areas are euthyroid. Myxedema is rare. Toxic goiter is uncommon in endemic goiter areas. There is no convincing evidence to implicate endemic goiter in the pathogenesis of carcinoma of the thyroid.

As already noted, cretins have been and continue to be found in areas where goiter is highly endemic. The mothers of such individuals are usually goitrous. The appearance of the cretin is characteristic: the head is large with wide fontanels; body movements are sluggish; growth is impaired; walking is retarded; speech is limited; deafness may be present; the tongue is large and protruding. Goiter may or may not be present, more often not.

LABORATORY FINDINGS. The uptake of radioactive iodine (I^{131}) by the thyroid is increased. So, too, the clearance of I^{131}, that is, its removal from the plasma per minute, is greatly increased, sometimes to three or four times normal. The urinary excretion of iodine per 24 hr is greatly reduced. Values less than 10 μg per day have been reported. The concentration of plasma *inorganic iodine* is decreased. Protein-bound iodine (PBI) concentrations are usually not changed or at least do not fall much below the lower limits of normal. However, in certain areas where goiter is severely endemic, the PBI levels may be distinctly low. Except in such areas, the basal metabolic rate is unaffected, although it may be reduced in areas where goiter is only slightly less endemic. In endemic cretins the urinary excretion of iodine is low. The I^{131} uptake by the thyroid may be reduced below normal in cretinous individuals without goiter; serum PBI levels are reduced.

PATHOLOGY. The anatomic changes that occur in the thyroid depend on the age of the individual, as well as the severity and possibly the fluctuations in the thyroid-stimulating hormone (TSH) acting on the gland. In newborn infants coming to autopsy in endemic areas, glands weigh more than normal; the cells are increased in size and number; the follicles contain little colloid; and the blood vessels are prominent. Although these anatomic changes may persist, it is commoner to find that the follicles of the adolescent gland contain more colloid. Foci of hyperplasia may

also be present. With increasing age, nodules, sometimes cellular, i.e., parenchymatous, and sometimes colloid, appear. There may be hemorrhage into these nodules with repair by connective tissue proliferation. Large colloid cysts are frequently present. Sclerosis of the abundant blood vessels is prominent. The thyroid of the endemic cretin is frequently reduced in size, with excess connective tissue separating foci of hyperplastic tissue.

PATHOGENESIS. Stated in simplest form, endemic goiter represents the response of the thyroid gland of the host, man, to a deficient supply of iodine in the diet he obtains from his environment. Iodine is present in soils derived from igneous, sedimentary, and metamorphic rocks. Plants obtain much of their iodine from the soil and its water, a little from the atmosphere. Iodine is returned to the soil as plants die or is transferred to animals as they consume the vegetation. Man derives some of his dietary iodine from terrestrial plants and animals. Richer sources are marine plants and animals, for much iodine has been washed from the land into the sea and some sea-living plants and animals have developed an extraordinary ability to concentrate iodine. Seaweeds favored by the Japanese and the various species of salt-water fish eaten by coastal inhabitants augment daily dietary supplies of iodine. In developed countries dairy products may be a source of iodine if cows receive iodine-supplemented salt. Iodate is used in commercial baking procedures. Under normal circumstances, about 30 to 40 per cent of ingested iodine is taken up by the thyroid. The remainder will be excreted in 24 hr, most of which appears in the urine. Hence, measurements of the iodine content of 24-hr urine samples give a fair approximation of iodine intake. Further aspects of iodine metabolism are discussed in Chap. 82.

The reaction to a decreased supply of iodine is as follows. Plasma *inorganic iodine* concentrations fall, and the concentrations of circulating active principles produced by the gland are decreased. The pituitary then releases more TSH, which causes hypertrophy and hyperplasia of the thyroid cells, loss of colloid, and increased vascularity. If the iodine supply of the gland is restored, concentration of active principles is increased, which leads to a decrease in TSH production; the gland returns to as "normal" a state as it can, i.e., a colloid goiter. Any mechanism that inhibits thyroid hormone synthesis will result in excess TSH production and goiter. The chemical goitrogens are examples, and the well-known genetic disturbances in hormone synthesis (Chap. 55) further demonstrate this principle. As far as is known today, TSH is the only chemical compound that will directly stimulate thyroid cells to increase in size and number.

Following the discovery of chemical goitrogens in 1941, such agents were invoked by many to explain the pathogenesis of endemic goiter in certain areas. No conclusive evidence has ever been presented to incriminate any goitrogen in food or water as a cause of endemic goiter in man. Evidence pointing unequivocally to iodine deficiency has been even further strengthened. Colloid goiter has been readily produced in experimental animals. Further studies have confirmed the prophylactic effects of iodine. Finally, numerous reports from various parts of the world indicate that the urinary excretion of iodine is low in areas of endemic goiter and that the uptake of radioactive iodine is increased. The pathogenesis of the changes that occur in the thyroid gland of the endemic cretin is not clear. Reduced size resulting from loss of cells and scarring has been referred to as "exhaustion atrophy." Precisely how this comes about is obscure. That genetic factors may influence the response of the organism to iodine deficiency must be borne in mind, though no proof of this has been derived from studies of endemic goiter in man or experimental goiter in animals. The effects of environment, particularly temperature, which may influence metabolic rate, must also be taken into consideration in any discussion of the pathogenesis of endemic goiter. Physiologic alterations, such as those which occur during pregnancy, must also be kept in mind.

DIAGNOSIS. The diagnosis of endemic goiter is a simple matter in areas where large numbers of the population are affected. The World Health Organization has suggested that any area in which more than 10 per cent of the population has thyroid enlargement should be classed as a region of endemic goiter.

Much more important is the assessment of iodine nutriture. Studies from areas of endemic goiter throughout the world have shown that radioactive iodine accumulation by the thyroid is increased, sometimes to over 90 per cent in 24 hr.

The excretion of iodine in the urine provides a fairly satisfactory assessment of iodine intake. The ideal procedure is, of course, to collect 24-hr urine samples, but this is difficult under field conditions. The few studies of 24-hr excretion which have been performed in endemic goiter areas have revealed low values. Casual urine samples may be used instead; the concentration of stable iodine (I^{127}) is equated to the concentration of creatinine, which may be regarded as a fairly constant value for a given individual. The result is expressed in micrograms of stable iodine per Gram of creatinine. The normal range is above 100 μg iodine per Gm creatinine.

TREATMENT. The best treatment is prevention. An intake of 100 to 150 μg iodine per day is recommended for adults. Programs for goiter prophylaxis or prevention by use of some form of iodine administration are difficult to effect, particularly if laws must be passed. The United States took the lead in 1924 when salt manufacturers agreed to sell iodized salt for the same price as the ordinary product. Today in the United States, approximately half the salt bought for home consumption is iodized. It is obvious that more education is needed concerning the advisability of purchasing iodized salt. There is no law pertaining to salt iodization in the United States. In certain other countries, however, salt is iodized by law. In Canada,

Guatemala, Colombia, and Switzerland, salt iodization programs are in effect and appear to be working satisfactorily. Other methods, such as the addition of iodate to bread or administration of iodized oils, are being used.

Obviously, because of the large numbers of people involved, surgical intervention in endemic areas is virtually impossible unless obstruction is present. Although thyroid extract or thyroxin have been recommended in the therapy of sporadic goiter in nonendemic areas, such treatment has not been tried on a large scale in endemic regions.

PROGNOSIS. Once a goiter has developed, particularly after puberty, there is little that can be done, save to prevent the gland from growing any larger. If treatment begins before puberty, particularly if the gland is not too enlarged, a reduction in size may occur. Some of this decrease in swelling may be due to diminished vascularity as the hyperemic hyperplastic structure involutes to a less vascular colloid gland. Once nodules or cysts have appeared, there is no treatment other than surgical intervention.

REFERENCES

Follis, R. H., Jr.: The ecology of endemic goiter, Am. J. Trop. Med. Hyg., 13:137, 1964.
——: Recent studies of iodine malnutrition and endemic goiter, Med. Clin. N. America, 48:1219, 1964.
Marine, D.: Etiology and prevention of simple goiter, Medicine, 3:453, 1924.
Stanbury, J. B., G. L. Brownell, D. S. Riggs, H. Perinetti, J. Itoiz, and E. B. Del Castillo: "Endemic Goiter: The Adaptation of Man to Iodine Deficiency," Cambridge, Mass., Harvard University Press, 1954.
Wayne, E. J., D. A. Koutras, and W. D. Alexander: "Clinical Aspects of Iodine Metabolism," Philadelphia, F. A. Davis, 1964.
World Health Organization: "Endemic Goiter," WHO Monograph Series, no. 44, Geneva, 1960.

72 PELLAGRA
Richard H. Follis, Jr.

HISTORY. During the eighteenth century, a disease hitherto undescribed by physicians began to appear with increasing frequency in northern Spain and Italy. First called by Casal *mal de la rosa* (from the erythematous skin lesions), the malady soon came to be known as *pelle agro* (skin, rough), from which the present-day name, *pellagra*, is derived. Casal described the prominent features: "a horrible crust" involving the skin, particularly of the hands and neck; "painful burning of the mouth"; "perpetual shaking of the body"; and "mania." Casal mentioned the prominence of maize in the diet of the people whom he had studied. During the nineteenth century, the principal focus of the disease was northern Italy, where in some areas as many as 5 per cent of the population in a given area might be affected. A number of theories were advanced as to the cause: that maize acquired toxic properties as a result of infestation with molds or fungi; that a material present in the grain was transformed into a poisonous substance in the intestinal tract of man; that maize contained some chemical that sensitized the skin to the photodynamic action of sunlight; that some specific microorganism was present; or that a diet predominantly of maize was a poor source of nourishment.

Pellagra appeared with an epidemiclike prevalence in the southern part of the United States in the early 1900s. Joseph Goldberger, of the U.S. Public Health Service, soon showed that diet alone would cure or prevent as well as produce the disease. He demonstrated the importance of protein in the diet and for a short time favored the idea that lack of specific amino acids was the cause. His interest then shifted to the curative effects of yeast and to the identification of an antipellagra vitamin. In 1937, Elvehjem and his coworkers showed that nicotinic acid would cure black tongue, a pellagralike disease, in dogs. Shortly thereafter nicotinic acid proved effective in the therapy of clinical pellagra. The story was not complete, however, for soon the amino acid, tryptophan, was demonstrated to be a precursor of nicotinic acid. Today it is clear that pellagra results from a deficiency of dietary tryptophan and/or nicotinic acid; other nutrients, such as riboflavin, thiamin, folic acid, and vitamin B_{12} may also be involved.

PREVALENCE. From 1940 on, the prevalence of endemic pellagra diminished greatly in the United States. The disease is still being encountered in Yugoslavia, Rumania, Egypt, India, South Africa, and Yucatan. Cases of sporadic pellagra are observed, usually in large urban clinics, in the United States; these accompany many chronic disease states, particularly those affecting the gastrointestinal tract. In addition, pellagra occurs in individuals who consume large quantities of alcohol and whose diets are usually restricted with respect to a number of essential nutrients.

CLINICAL FINDINGS. Before pellagra becomes clinically manifest and the patient seeks the help of a physician, certain prodromal subjective symptoms may be present. These include loss of appetite leading to weight loss, indigestion, diarrhea or constipation, generalized weakness, lassitude, burning sensations in various areas, headache, and insomnia. These vague, nonspecific symptoms are usually followed after varying periods of time by the principal manifestations of full-blown endemic pellagra, which affect the skin, alimentary tract, nervous system, and, to a lesser extent, the blood.

The skin lesions may begin as an erythema that looks very much like sunburn. Burning or itching may be intense. The initial changes may be followed by the formation of vesicles or by peeling. In some cases the erythematous skin assumes a dirty-brown color and then becomes rough and scaly. This stage, which may not necessarily be preceded by erythema, may remain for prolonged periods. Characteristically, the skin lesions are symmetric and tend to be localized over exposed areas: backs of hands in adults and backs of feet in children, face, neck, elbows, and knees. In addition, the scrotum, vulva, and perianal region may be involved. Unilateral dermatitis is usually associated with local pressure, trauma, heat, or sunlight. The evolution of the lesions may differ; erythema of the hands may appear while hyperkeratosis of the legs is already present. Seborrhea about the nose with comedo formation may be conspicuous in some patients.

Sore mouth is a common complaint. Changes in the tongue are conspicuous, and glossitis is thought by some to be a more sensitive gauge of the disease than skin lesions. The tip and margins of the tongue become hyperemic, a change that may spread to involve the entire surface so that the structure acquires a beef-red appearance. Small ulcers sometimes appear. Inflammatory lesions may be found in the mucous membrane of the mouth. Secondary infection is common, particularly with fusospirochetal organisms. In advanced stages of the disease, the tongue may be pale with complete atrophy of the papillae. Angular lesions, i.e., gray macerated or ulcerated areas at the corners of the mouth, are frequently present. Pain on swallowing is common. Anorexia, accompanied by epigastric discomfort, is a frequent complaint. Diarrhea has always been a prominent part of the pellagra syndrome. Stools are small, frequent, and watery, quite different from those in sprue. The liver is ordinarily not enlarged.

Neurologic signs rarely appear at the beginning of the disease but are common when skin or alimentary manifestations are prominent. Subjectively, the patient may complain of vertigo, weakness, headache, paresthesia, anesthesia, and general aches. Severe pain of the hands and feet may be present. Objectively, tendon reflexes are abnormal, usually diminished. Coarse tremors of the tongue, head, or extremities may be noted on examination. Muscular spasms are sometimes prominent. Mental disturbances have always been a feature of endemic pellagra; they include general "nervousness," confusion, depression, insomnia, apathy, and delirium. The picture is a varied one.

Pellagra is seen in children, usually in the five to fifteen age group. Skin manifestations are the most prominent feature at this age. Involvement of the gastrointestinal tract and nervous system is not common. Pellagra and kwashiorkor may occur in the same area. The former disease tends to affect older children, who do not appear as ill as those with kwashiorkor. The distribution of the skin lesions in the two conditions is different.

LABORATORY FINDINGS. Chemical examinations of the blood reveal very little in pellagra. Occasionally hypoproteinemia, with low serum albumin values, is found. Gastric analysis reveals achlorhydria in about one-half the cases. On examination, the stools may show the presence of hookworm ova or other parasites in areas where infestations are prevalent. The N-methyl nicotinamide content of the urine is helpful in assessing tryptophan–nicotinic acid nutriture in population groups, but this determination is of little help in the individual case. The urinary excretion of riboflavin may be decreased in pellagra.

Anemia may be present in approximately one-half the cases of pellagra, but in only about one-quarter is it of any consequence. The anemia is not particularly specific; it may be normocytic hypochromic, microcytic, or macrocytic in character, according to the presence of associated iron, folic acid, or vitamin B_{12} deficiencies. There is usually no alteration in the white blood cell count unless infection is present.

PATHOLOGY. Under the microscope the earliest skin lesions show dilatation of the superficial blood vessels and proliferation on their endothelial cells. The superficial connective tissue elements of the corium assume a spongy appearance. The epidermis, which may already show hyperkeratosis, separates from the corium with the formation of a vesicle. There may be increased pigmentation of the superficial hyperkeratotic layer with decrease in pigment cells in the basal region. Chronic lesions merely show hyperkeratosis. The epithelium of the tongue is atrophic, with loss of papillae; a subacute inflammatory reaction may be present. The esophagus is commonly the site of acute inflammation with loss of epithelium. Alterations in the remainder of the intestinal tract are not particularly noteworthy, save in the colon. Here small ulcers may be present with abscess formation in the submucosa. Cystic dilatations of the mucous glands are prominent. The liver may contain excessive fat, which is usually periportal in distribution. The lining of the vagina is frequently acutely inflamed with superficial ulceration. The neurologic changes are variable and consist of atrophy of cerebral neurones, degeneration of peripheral nerves, nerve roots, and tracts in the spinal cord. Bone marrow, if abnormal, may show a megaloblastic response or erythroblastic hyperplasia.

PATHOGENESIS. When man subsists on a diet of which the main staple is maize and in which there is little other protein, pellagra is likely to ensue. Pellagra has always been an affliction of the poor man and his family, sometimes even the canine members. Fluctuations in the prevalence of endemic pellagra can usually be correlated with "good times" and "hard times." In the southern United States the increased prevalence of pellagra was associated with a decrease in general prosperity and, in particular, with regional changes in income, caused by rise or fall in the price of cotton.

What is there about maize, when this grain comprises a large part of the diet of man, which leads to the appearance of pellagra? Whole ground maize is nutritionally inferior in a number of ways, particularly when modern milling procedures are employed. First and foremost, its protein is low in *quantity* and, even more important, in *quality*. Maize protein is deficient in two amino acids, since it contains only a trace of tryptophan and insufficient lysine. Although maize contains appreciable quantities of nicotinic acid when assayed chemically, much of this vitamin is unavailable since it cannot be broken down in the intestinal tract. Nicotinic acid is found in high concentrations in liver, yeast, red muscle meats, fish, and wheat germ. Vegetables and cereals contain much less.

Maize is deficient in calcium, magnesium, sodium, chlorine, and iodine. The phosphorus content is high, but a large proportion is in the form of phytate, much of which is unavailable. Maize is low in thiamine and riboflavin content, particularly if highly milled. The concentration of pantothenic acid and pyridoxine is usually considered adequate. Maize contains no vitamin B_{12}, and its folic acid content is relatively low. Vitamin A and carotene are absent in white maize but high in yellow cornmeal.

Meat protein, dairy products, and eggs are generally either present in small amounts or entirely lacking in the pellagrin's diet. Diets that have been associated with pellagra are deficient in protein, with respect to both quantity and quality, and deficient in available nicotinic acid, riboflavin, thiamine, and vitamin B_{12}. Coffee is a source of nicotinic acid.

Although maize is most often the source of poor-quality protein in the pellagrin's diet, this is not invariable. In India, for instance, pellagra is associated with the use of a millet, sorghum (*jowar*), in the diet.

The multiple deficiency aspects of pellagra have been recognized for some time, and they cause one to ask: What is the definition of pellagra? Some workers would be restrictive and define the disease as pure tryptophan–nicotinic acid deficiency. The argument is that since the cardinal symptoms respond to nicotinic acid, pellagra should be regarded as a deficiency of this vitamin. Since, however, some of the classic symptoms and signs are alleviated not by nicotinic acid therapy but by other nutrients, it may be preferable to define pellagra as a multiple deficiency syndrome produced principally by deficiencies of tryptophan–nicotinic acid, riboflavin, and thiamine, and occasionally by folic acid, vitamin B_{12}, and possibly pyridoxine.

It is generally agreed that exposure of the skin to ultraviolet radiation may precipitate the appearance of dermal lesions or may increase the severity of those already present. In addition, the exposure of pellagrous subjects to sunlight may lead to effects in areas other than the skin; for instance, glossitis may be induced, nausea and vomiting may occur, or diarrhea may appear. The effect of sunlight helps to explain the seasonal variations in the prevalence of pellagra in the north temperate zones.

Individuals of different age groups are not equally affected by the disease. The greatest prevalence is in females, aged twenty to forty-five, i.e., the childbearing, lactating group. The next most common prevalence is usually found in children aged nine to fifteen years, though these data come from Goldberger's studies in the southern United States at a time when child labor was extensive.

Mention has been made that, in addition to classic endemic pellagra generally associated with a maize diet, sporadic cases occur. These are important, for today they comprise in most urban clinical centers the commonest groups of pellagrins. Several types of "secondary" or conditioned pellagra have been designated. A large group comprises cases of pellagra developing in persons who have some other disease. In general, disturbances of the gastrointestinal tract are the most numerous; gastric ulcer or carcinoma and various disturbances of the large and small intestine, particularly those which lead to diarrhea. The diet of such individuals may or may not be adequate. The second most important group is chronic alcoholics. Although the inveterate drinker may consume 3000 to 4000 Cal per day in the form of alcohol, his intake of other essential nutrients may be virtually *nil*. It is more usual for the chronic alcoholic to develop symptoms of thiamine deficiency rather than those due to lack of nicotinic acid and other essentials. However, polyneuritis, as well as the skin and other characteristics of pellagra, may be observed in the same individual.

DIAGNOSIS. Symptoms and signs in endemic pellagra are specific enough. Dietary history is also significant. More difficult is the diagnosis of incipient pellagra or cases without skin manifestations, which have been termed *pellagra sine pellagra*. Here is may be necessary to evaluate the response to therapy with nicotinic acid and other nutrients. The estimation of N-methyl nicotinamide concentration in the urine may be of help in this respect also. The possibility of overt or subclinical pellagra should be considered in every person who suffers from gastrointestinal disease, particularly those conditions which lead to the malabsorption syndrome. So, too, with any chronic alcoholic, the question of adequate nutrition with respect to nicotinic acid and other vitamins must always be in the forefront.

In the differential diagnosis of pellagra, certain other disease states need to be considered. Such are sprue, chronic pancreatitis with steatorrhea, pernicious anemia, and tuberculosis or other forms of chronic enteritis. In sprue, skin lesions are usually absent, although alterations in the tongue may be present. The large, bulky stools are characteristic. Mental changes are not present. The clinical picture of chronic pancreatitis is similar. Pernicious anemia may sometimes closely resemble the clinical picture of pellagra with stomatitis, glossitis, anemia, and gastrointestinal disturbances. The differential diagnosis of pellagra should not be difficult in cases exhibiting chronic gastrointestinal disease since skin and neurologic changes are absent.

Three forms of pellagralike skin lesions, though uncommon, are worthy of mention. The first is an hereditary affliction, initially reported over 10 years ago in a patient named Hartnup, and hence called *Hartnup's disease*. This syndrome consists of a pellagralike skin rash following exposure to sunlight, intermittent cerebellar ataxia, renal amino aciduria, and the excretion of large amounts of indole-3-acetic acid and indican in the urine. Increased quantities of protoporphyrin are found in the stool. The skin lesions are the only pellagralike changes that have been described. No glossitis, stomatitis, or gastrointestinal symptoms are present. The skin lesions respond to nicotinic acid therapy.

A second form of a pellagralike disease has been reported in patients receiving isoniazid, a vitamin B_6 antagonist. In such patients peripheral neuritis and pellagralike skin lesions appear and may not even regress when the drug is discontinued. Treatment with nicotinic acid is efficacious in curing skin lesions. Pyridoxine or B-complex preparations will usually improve the neurologic manifestations.

The third disturbance in which pellagralike skin lesions have been observed is associated with malignant carcinoid tumors (*malignant argentaffinomas*). In individuals with such tumors large amounts of 5-hydroxytryptamine (serotonin) are produced so that a conditioned form of tryptophan deficiency results. In addition to skin lesions, patients may exhibit other characteristics of pellagra: mental confusion, diarrhea, and glossitis.

TREATMENT. Severely ill patients, particularly those with diarrhea and dementia, should be treated as emergencies. Water and electrolyte deficits must be corrected immediately. Intravenous administration of nicotinic acid or nicotinamide in doses of 100 mg two or three times a day is recommended. These amounts can be added to physiologic salt solution containing 5 per cent glucose. The administration of 100 mg nicotinic acid divided into two daily doses should be adequate for most patients. Nicotinamide in the same dosage is equally effective and is free from the unpleasant vasomotor effects of nicotinic acid. Naturally, other nutrients, particularly riboflavin, are usually also necessary. The most practical form of therapy is the administration of $\frac{1}{2}$ to 1 oz debittered brewer's yeast in tomato juice three times a day. Naturally, a high calorie (3000 to 4000), high protein diet is desirable. Frequent feedings are advocated at first. Stomatitis, diarrhea or constipation, and oozing or ulcerated lesions of the skin will necessitate symptomatic medication.

PROGNOSIS. Until the advent of yeast and vitamin therapy, the prognosis of pellagra was grave. Today the prognosis is excellent. The glossitis begins to decrease in 24 hr; the papillae of the tongue will begin to regenerate by the end of the first week. Lesions of the lips begin to heal in 2 to 3 days. Gastrointestinal symptoms improve in 24 to 48 hr, and diarrhea will usually have ceased by the end of the first week. Demented patients usually become rational after 3 or 4 days, unless, of course, damage to the brain has been irreversible. Polyneuritis, if present, may take some time to improve.

REFERENCES

Bean, W. B., T. D. Spies, and M. A. Blankenhorn: Secondary Pellagra, Medicine, 23:1, 1944.

FAO Nutritional Studies, "Maize and Maize Diets," no. 9, Rome, 1953.

Gillman, J., and T. Gillman: "Perspectives in Human Malnutrition: A Contribution to the Biology of Disease from a Clinical and Pathological Study of Chronic Malnutrition and Pellagra in the African," New York, Grune and Stratton, Inc., 1951.

Goldsmith, G. A., H. P. Sarett, V. D. Register, and J. Gibbens: Studies of Niacin Requirement in Man: I. Experimental Pellagra in Subjects on Corn Diets Low in Niacin and Tryptophan, J. Clin. Invest., 31:533, 1952.

Sydenstricker, V. P.: The History of Pellagra, Its Recognition As a Disorder of Nutrition and Its Conquest, Am. J. Clin. Nutrition, 6:409, 1958.

Terris, M. (Ed.): "Goldberger on Pellagra," Baton Rouge, La., Louisiana State University Press, 1964.

73   BERIBERI

Richard H. Follis, Jr.

HISTORY. During the seventeenth, eighteenth, and nineteenth centuries, as a result of the increasing contacts of European physicians with the Far East, a disease peculiar to that area was added to Western medical knowledge. The principal characteristics of this disease, oriental beriberi, as described by a nineteenth-century physician, were "a feeling of numbness, sense of weight and weakness" in the legs, "edema of the feet," "unsteady and tottering walk" with "almost total palsy," "rigidity and various affections of the nerves," "oppression and weight in the precordium," and, occasionally, "sudden death." The disease was endemic throughout South China, Southeast Asia, the Philippines, the East Indies, and parts of India.

When studies on the cause and prevention of beriberi were begun, the close relationship of rice to the disease was soon recognized. Beriberi was eradicated from the Japanese Navy by Takaki, who recommended adding meat, vegetables, and condensed milk to the rice diet of the common sailor. In Batavia (now Djakarta), Eijkman observed a beriberilike disease in fowl fed polished rice; the birds could be cured with unpolished grain. In Malaya, differences were noted in the prevalence of beriberi among persons who consumed parboiled rice and those who were accustomed to eat a highly polished grain. By 1912, the therapeutic effectiveness of rice polishings had been demonstrated, particularly in patients with acute cardiac manifestations of beriberi. This led E. B. Vedder, a young U.S. Army physician, to recommend

to R. R. Williams, a chemist then working in Manila, that the protective substance be isolated. Twenty years later Williams and his coworkers announced the chemical structure and synthesis of the active principle, thiamine. The metabolic role of thiamine was demonstrated at once.

PREVALENCE. Today the prevalence of clinical beriberi in the Far East is much reduced. One may encounter occasional cases of the disease, particularly in infants and pregnant or lactating women. Of particular importance, though difficult of interpretation, is the occurrence of thiamine malnutrition in countries, particularly in Southeast Asia, where polished rice comprises a large portion of the diet and where recent studies in some areas indicate low values of urinary thiamine excretion.

CLINICAL FINDINGS. For years clinical beriberi in the Orient has been classified into three main types: a chronic form in which neurologic involvement is prominent, an acute form with heart failure, and a less acute state in which edema is the most characteristic manifestation. The onset of the chronic neurologic form is insidious. Over the course of days or weeks, the patient comes to be easily fatigued and experiences heavy feelings in the legs, together with stiffness and aching in the muscles. In time the muscles become weaker, acutely painful, and then atrophic. The extensors of the foot are usually first affected, then the muscles of the calf and thigh. Pain followed by atrophy soon occurs in the muscles of the arms; the muscles of the trunk may be affected later. Associated with these signs and symptoms are toe drop, foot drop, and wrist drop, together with loss of reflexes, such as ankle kick and knee jerk. Paresthesias and anesthesias may be demonstrated, particularly over the lower extremities. Circumoral anesthesia may be present. Aphonia is sometimes a symptom. Walking naturally becomes difficult, and the patient can only shuffle about with a cane or is forced to hold on to objects about him to keep from falling. Evidences of neurologic involvement may fluctuate. In time, however, the patient becomes completely bedridden. Involvement of the cerebrum is absent.

All the while, weight loss will have been progressing and anorexia is usually persistent. Diarrhea may be more or less continuous. Evidences of cardiac involvement may accompany these neurologic disturbances or may occur suddenly in the absence of any evidence of involvement of the nervous system. The cardiac manifestations consist of palpitation, precordial pain, and dyspnea which may come on in paroxysms without any warning. On examination, the heart is found to be enlarged. Tachycardia is present. Prominent venous pulsations are noted in the neck. Edema is usually present. Blood pressure is not elevated, but the pulse pressure is increased. Venous pressure is elevated. Death may result suddenly, with or without exertion.

Beriberi in infants has been and continues to be a problem in the Far East. The disease occurs almost solely in breast-fed children whose mothers may or may not exhibit overt beriberi. Cases are most frequent in the first four months of life. Clinically, the course is one of rapidly progressing heart failure, which responds dramatically to thiamine administration.

In the mid-1930s, observers in large urban clinics in the Occident began to observe instances of cardiac and neurologic disease occurring predominantly in alcoholics. In some areas the prevalence of these forms of occidental beriberi, as these entities came to be called, was high. The clinical aspects of this form of heart disease are described in Chap. 143.

The symptoms and signs relative to neurologic involvement in alcoholics have the characteristics of a progressive polyneuritis with sensory and motor defects. Almost invariably the history of excessive consumption of alcohol and poor dietary intake is presented. In addition, such patients frequently exhibit manifestations of delirium tremens, Korsakoff's syndrome, or Wernicke's disease. To such examples of neurologic involvement in poorly nourished chronic alcoholics have been added other syndromes in recent years, such as amblyopia, central pontine myelinolysis, and cortical cerebellar degeneration. None of these, including Wernicke's disease, have ever been described in beriberi occurring in oriental peoples.

LABORATORY FINDINGS. Biochemical studies have been very significant in elucidating the role of thiamine in intermediary metabolism. Such techniques have not been particularly helpful in clinical medicine, however. Serum concentrations of pyruvate and lactate are elevated, particularly after the administration of carbohydrate. These values return to normal following therapy. Blood levels of thiamine pyrophosphate are reduced. Perhaps the most convenient assessment of thiamine nutriture is the amount excreted in the urine per 24 hr or the concentration of thiamine per Gm creatinine in casual urine samples. The latter method has been used extensively in nutrition surveys of population groups. Urine concentrations after administration of thiamine loads have been utilized to obtain information on tissue saturation. Assay for the transketolase activity of erythrocytes is of value. Studies of the concentration of thiamine in normal and diseased tissues have delineated the ranges to be expected in health and in a few thiamine-deficient subjects.

PATHOLOGY. From the above account of the clinical manifestations of beriberi, anatomic alterations might be expected in the nervous tissues and heart, and they are found. Post-mortem examinations performed on patients dying with neurologic manifestations of beriberi at the turn of the century in the Orient revealed myelin degeneration of the peripheral nerves, with loss of axoplasm. Lesions in the brain and spinal cord have not been reported from the Orient. Among the sporadic cases designated as neurologic beriberi encountered in the Occident, usually among alcoholics, lesions of peripheral nerves have also been described. More prominent, however, are changes in the brain. Alterations characteristic of Wernicke's

disease—bilateral hemorrhagic necrotic foci in the mammillary bodies, the hypothalamic nuclei, and midline structures—are found. Damage to the optic nerve and lesions in the spinal cord have been reported.

The heart is usually described as enlarged, but this increase in size is usually due to dilatation, although hypertrophy of the right ventricle has sometimes been noted. The myocardial fibers do not exhibit necrosis, although swelling and vacuolization may be prominent. No cellular infiltration is present.

PATHOGENESIS. Classic endemic beriberi, which has been observed for centuries in the Orient, clearly represents the reaction of the host, man, to a diet composed in large part of polished rice. Rice is the principal foodstuff of one-half or more of the inhabitants of the world. The introduction of power milling machinery at the end of the nineteenth century led to a great increase in beriberi in the Far East. When rice is highly milled, most of its vitamin content, such as thiamine, riboflavin, nicotinic acid, pantothenic acid, and pyridoxine, is removed. Lipids and minerals, such as calcium, iron, and iodine, which are present in the outer portions of the grain, are lost as well. The protein content of rice is somewhat low, though its quality is good.

Although the rice eater's diet is deficient in a number of nutrients, the principal manifestations of beriberi—the derangements in cardiac and neurologic function—appear to be related to thiamine deficiency. The therapeutic response of the patient, whether infant or adult, with cardiac beriberi to thiamine is good evidence for this relationship. The development of anatomic lesions in the heart of experimental animals deprived of thiamine is further proof for the relation of this vitamin to the integrity of the myocardium. The precise relationship of thiamine to maintenance of the integrity of the peripheral nervous system is less clear. Clinical response to thiamine is usually not dramatic, though this can be explained on the basis that damage is severe enough to have caused structural loss. Hence, regeneration is necessary if function is to be restored. Lesions of the peripheral nerves have been difficult to produce in experimental animals. The manifestations of Wernicke's disease may clear up dramatically after thiamine administration. Lesions similar to those observed in Wernicke's disease have been demonstrated in the brains of thiamine-deficient animals. The enigma of the absence of Wernicke's disease in the Orient (except among Western prisoners of war) and its presence in the Occident remains. The explanation for the edema is probably twofold: heart failure and protein malnutrition.

Thiamine has been implicated in three biochemical reactions. Thiamine pyrophosphate (cocarboxylase) is necessary for the decarboxylation of pyruvic acid, the opening step of the reactions that feed into the citric acid cycle. A second reaction in which thiamine plays a role is the oxidative decarboxylation of d-ketoglutaric acid, a later step in the citric acid cycle. A third reaction in which thiamine participates is the transketolase reaction, which is involved in the direct oxidation of glucose. These reactions are merely mentioned here to recall the importance of thiamine in intermediary metabolism in at least three places. Though biochemical lesions do occur in the thiamine-deficient organism, the precise relation of such defects to anatomic lesions is obscure.

DIAGNOSIS. In the Orient, the symptoms are characteristic enough. Certain simple tests are helpful: pain when the calf muscles are squeezed, anesthesia to pinprick over the anterior surface of the tibia, loss of patellar reflex, and inability to rise from the squatting position. The presence of pitting edema and manifestations of cardiac involvement help with the diagnosis when they are present.

The diagnosis of the single case in the Occident is more difficult. Here the dietary history, particularly if alcoholism has been present, is important. Evidence of neurologic involvement is usually the most prominent symptom.

To evaluate thiamine nutriture in groups of persons in both the Orient and the Occident, thiamine concentration in relation to creatinine content in casual urine specimens has proved of value.

TREATMENT. When there is cardiac involvement in infants or adults, beriberi becomes a medical emergency. The immediate administration of thiamine is obligatory. Intravenous administration of 10 to 20 mg thiamine, two or three times a day, is recommended. Oral doses of thiamine, 3 to 5 mg two or three times a day, should be adequate for the ordinary patient. In more chronic cases, particularly those with neurologic involvement, 2 or 3 mg per day should be sufficient. Naturally a balanced diet is also important.

PROGNOSIS. The response of infants and adults with cardiac beriberi in the Orient is one of the most dramatic in medicine. Cardiac symptoms improve rapidly. Diuresis begins within the first 12 hr. In the Occident such dramatic responses are not seen as often. When neurologic involvement is present, response to therapy is much more gradual since anatomic alterations in the peripheral nerves are usually present. The ophthalmoplegia, ataxia, and nystagmus of Wernicke's disease respond to thiamine, as do mental symptoms such as apathy and drowsiness. Amentia responds less rapidly.

REFERENCES

Food and Agriculture Organization, "Rice and Rice Diets," Rome, 1954.

Kinney, T. D., and R. H. Follis, Jr. (Eds.): Nutritional Disease: Beriberi, Fed. Proc., 17: Supp. 2, 3, 1958.

Vedder, E. B., "Beriberi," New York, William Wood & Company, 1913.

Victor M., and R. D. Adams: On the Etiology of the Alcoholic Neurological Diseases, Am. J. Clin. Nutrition, 9:379, 1961.

Williams, R. R.: "Toward the Conquest of Beriberi," Cambridge, Mass., Harvard University Press, 1961.

74 SCURVY
Richard H. Follis, Jr.

HISTORY. Although accounts of a disease which might be construed as scurvy are found in ancient writings, the first clear-cut descriptions appear in records of the Crusades. When the long sea voyages of discovery began toward the end of the fifteenth century, scurvy became commonplace and soon rated first among causes of disability and mortality in sailors. Scurvy on land appeared among military and civilian population groups as a result of the many European wars, which led to troop movements and civilian displacement. Causes of crop failure uncontrolled by man such as flood, drought, and blight have played a part.

In 1747 James Lind, a Naval Surgeon, deliberately studied the effects of "two oranges and one lemon given every day" on sailors with typical signs of scurvy: "putrid gums, the spots and lassitude, with weakness of their knees." The curative efficacy of these citrus fruits was clear.

Infantile scurvy began to receive attention after 1883, when Barlow described the syndrome as it is recognized today: the swollen, tense, exquisitely painful, flexed lower extremities; crepitus at the ends of the shafts of the bones; swollen, bleeding gums, particularly when teeth are present; and cutaneous hemorrhages. With increasing use of breast milk substitutes, scurvy became common in the urban areas of Europe and the United States at the turn of the century.

A disease of the growing bones of guinea pigs, precisely like that seen in children, was produced by dietary means in 1907. Investigators now had a way to assay antiscorbutic materials. Twenty-five years later, C. G. King and his associates, who were deliberately investigating the problem, isolated from lemon juice a biologically active crystalline material. This compound was later synthesized and is known today as ascorbic acid.

PREVALENCE. In previous times scurvy in adults was prone to occur in epidemiclike outbreaks. Today the situation is different. Scurvy is seen in isolated individuals, usually men living alone whose diet is grossly unbalanced and devoid of sources of ascorbic acid ("bachelor scurvy"). Hence, each year in urban clinics in the United States and Europe occasional examples of adult scurvy are encountered. Occasional cases of scurvy continue to appear in pediatric clinics. In developing countries, where malnutrition may be a serious problem, scurvy is uncommon.

CLINICAL FINDINGS. There are three principal manifestations of scurvy in the adult: swollen gums with loss of teeth, skin lesions, and pain and weakness in the lower extremities. The clinical course of the disease is best understood as a result of studies on volunteers in whom ascorbic acid deficiency has been deliberately produced. The first change, which may be observed after approximately 140 days, is prominence of the hair follicles, usually those over the back and thighs. This prominence is due to plugging of the lumens with an excessive amount of keratin. This leads to an impediment of hair growth so that the hair becomes coiled upon itself within the follicle. The epithelium surrounding each follicle soon becomes hyperemic. Red blood cells pass through the dilated capillary walls to lie free in the tissues. These soon disappear leaving deposits of pigment, so that the perifollicular area becomes discolored. Lesions in the mouth appear after approximately 200 days of deprivation. Reddening and swelling of the interdental papillae occur first, soon followed by hemorrhage. The time of appearance and degree of severity of the gum changes are related to the state of oral hygiene. The other manifestation of scurvy, pain and weakness in the extremities, is a subjective one which has been prominent in the experimental studies.

The clinical picture in children is much different from that observed in adults. The peak incidence is 8 months; few cases are seen after the first year. The most prominent sign on physical examination is tenderness of the lower extremities, which in addition are usually somewhat swollen. The leg is characteristically partially flexed. Involvement of the upper extremities is less common. The extremities are obviously painful; the child screams when approached. The costochondral junctions may be enlarged. Crepitus of the ankles or wrists may be felt. The gums are swollen and hemorrhagic when teeth are present but show little change before teeth erupt. Subcutaneous hemorrhages may be observed; these tend to be in the form of ecchymoses, not the pinpoint hemorrhages seen about the follicles in the adult. Follicular lesions are uncommon in children. Hemorrhages occur elsewhere: suborbital with proptosis, epistaxis, hematuria, or signs of subdural bleeding.

LABORATORY FINDINGS.

The concentration of ascorbic acid may be determined in samples of plasma or in the buffy coat layer. Zero levels may be present in the plasma of adults for months before tissue stores are depleted. The plasma level mirrors the recent intake of ascorbic acid. Even if minimal or zero concentrations of ascorbic acid are present in plasma, the clinical syndrome will likely not be present. When adults subsist on an intake of 10 mg ascorbic acid per day, the concentrations of the vitamin in the buffy coat average about 2 mg per 100 ml. In such instances no clinical evidence of scurvy is present. On a vitamin C–deficient diet, the ascorbic acid concentration in the buffy coat falls to 1 mg or less after 4 to 6 months. At these values clinical scurvy may become manifest.

Saturation or load tests may be of some help in evaluating ascorbic acid nutriture. When adequate amounts of the vitamin are being ingested, the urinary output will be relatively high, i.e., about 25 to 75 mg per 100 ml. Urinary output will be virtually zero when the body stores are depleted. If 200 mg ascorbic acid is administered each day and urinary excretion of the vitamin is small during the first 3 or 4 days, this indicates that the stores are reduced.

PATHOLOGY.

In adults studied at autopsy, the most conspicuous finding is the presence of generalized hemorrhage. The perifollicular lesions and ecchymoses noted clinically are conspicuous. In addition, extravasations of blood are found in the pericardial or pleural cavities, walls of the intestinal tract, bladder, renal pelves, and so forth. In young adults separation of the epiphyses or costochondral junctions may be present, as well as subperiosteal hemorrhage.

In children the most characteristic changes at autopsy are found in the skeleton. The periosteum has separated or may be easily stripped from the shaft of a bone; the costal or epiphyseal cartilages have separated from the shaft of the rib or a long bone. Microscopic examination at the cartilage shaft junction shows a dense "lattice" of spicules of calcified cartilaginous matrix, many of which have fractured. Little bone has formed on this "lattice," which, furthermore, has not been destroyed. In less advanced cases, fractures occur only at the edges or corners of the bone. Hemorrhage may be usually observed in the marrow or beneath the periosteum. As a result of decreased osteoid formation, the cortex and trabeculae of the shaft are reduced in thickness; i.e., osteoporosis is present. Aside from hemorrhages elsewhere—subdural, subpleural, subcutaneous, and so on—little else is found that is specific for scurvy. Rickets is frequently also present.

PATHOGENESIS.

Scurvy represents the reaction of particular hosts, whether man, other primates, or the guinea pig, to a lack of ascorbic acid in the dietary environment. Other species can synthesize the vitamin. Ascorbic acid is found in high concentrations in citrus and other fruits, leafy vegetables, tubers, most grasses, and sprouting plants. The vitamin content of human milk varies, since the mother is dependent on dietary sources. Milk from a well-nourished woman should contain 5 to 7 mg per 100 ml. Fresh cow's milk contains 1.0 to 2.6 mg per 100 ml; however, storage and sterilizing reduces this to virtually zero. Scurvy is virtually unheard of in breast-fed infants. On the other hand, the use of sterilized infant formulas prepared from cow's milk or proprietary foods may be expected to produce scurvy in infants if the diet is not otherwise supplemented with a source of ascorbic acid. Classic scurvy in adults results from lack of fresh plant foods in the diet.

Scurvy in human beings as in other primates and the guinea pig is, broadly speaking, a genetic disease, in that the tissues of these species appear to have lost their ability to synthesize ascorbic acid. The chemical steps in the formation of the vitamin are now well known:

a. D-glucuronate + TPNH + H⁺ →

$$\text{L-gulonate} + \text{TPN}^+$$

b. L-gulonate + DPN⁺ →

$$\text{L-gulonolactone} + \text{DPN}^+ + \text{H}^+$$

c. L-gulonolactone → L-ascorbate + H_2O

Liver and kidney tissues of all mammalian species so far studied can carry out reactions *a* and *b*. Only liver cells can form L-ascorbate via reaction *c*, but the hepatic tissues of man, other primates, and guinea pigs cannot carry this out.

The basic structural disturbance in scurvy is the failure of various types of connective tissue cells to form their respective collagenous matrices. Fibroblasts are unable to elaborate collagen; osteoblasts and odontoblasts do not synthesize osteoid and dentine, respectively. The lack of formation of these matrices explains the failure of wounds to heal, the changes in the growing bone of infants and children, and the alterations in the teeth of experimental animals. What is the underlying biochemical lesion? Collagen is a fibrous protein of fairly uniform amino acid composition and characteristic structural pattern when viewed with the electron microscope or studied by small- and wide-angle x-ray diffraction techniques. Collagen is characterized chemically by large amounts of glycine, proline, and hydroxyproline. The presence of the latter hydroxy amino acid and of hydroxylysine make collagen unique, since these amino acids are not found in other proteins. The precise biochemical events in collagen synthesis are not known. However, since collagen is a protein, it is likely that mechanisms similar to those utilized to form other proteins may be employed in its synthesis. First of all, an adequate supply of amino acids must be available to the specific collagen-forming cells, whether fibroblasts, osteoblasts, or odontoblasts. That amino acids, such as glycine or proline, labeled with C^{14} or H^3, enter the cytoplasm of such cells has been adequately demonstrated. Next, it would be expected that each of the necessary amino acids would be activated. Finally, the usual series of events in which transfer RNA and messenger RNA participate to ensure proper sequence formation on ribosomal RNA would result in a molecule of trophocollagen, the smallest unit of collagen, which has the dimensions of 3,000 × 14 Å. Hydroxyproline is not synthesized in the absence of ascorbic acid. This is most important when it is recalled that exogenous hydroxyproline is normally not incorporated into collagen. All the hydroxyproline in the basic collagen molecule is derived from the hydroxylation of proline in vivo. Precisely at what point in collagen synthesis hydroxylation of proline takes place is not clear at this time. It has been assumed that the trophocollagen molecule is released from the cytoplasm into the intercellular space and there polymerized into typical collagen fibrils, which have the electron-microscopic and other patterns of the adult molecule. The mechanism whereby the trophocollagen molecule is polymerized to mature collagen is not known. In ascorbic acid–deficient organisms, the connective tissue cells can proliferate. However, their microscopic appearance implies their functional impotency. Their cytoplasm is scanty, and virtually no stainable RNA is present. What this means in terms of altered synthetic mechanisms is obscure at this time.

The role of ascorbic acid in the structural integrity of blood vessels is not clear. Obviously, the characteristic perifollicular hemorrhages indicate a defect in the vascular wall. Under the biomicroscope, capillary dilatation may be observed. Since the integrity of collagen is affected as a result of ascorbic acid deficiency, it is possible that the blood vessels may lose the support provided by these fibers and hence become more liable to the effects of minor trauma.

Certain other metabolic defects may be observed as a result of ascorbic acid deficiency, though these are not usually considered part of the scurvy syndrome. One of the most interesting aspects of ascorbic acid function is its nonspecific relation to metabolism of the aromatic amino acids, phenylalanine and tyrosine. Premature infants deficient in ascorbic acid excrete relatively large amounts of parahydroxyphenyllactic acid and pyrohydroxyphenylpyruvic acid in the urine when excess phenylalanine and tyrosine are administered. The defect appears to be an inability to oxidize the side chain of tyrosine. Ascorbic acid is implicated in the secretion of the aqueous humor. The vitamin also plays a role in the metabolism of folic acid, i.e., in the transformation of this material to folacin (citrovorum factor).

A great deal has been written about the anemia of scurvy. Inasmuch as deficiency of iron, folic acid, and other nutrients may be present, it is difficult to ascribe a direct role to ascorbic acid.

DIAGNOSIS. The clinical features of full-blown scurvy in adults or infants are characteristic enough. A most important point to emphasize is the feeding history in infants. If an infant four to six months or older has been bottle-fed with boiled milk or milk substitutes from birth, or from shortly after, and has received no supplemental ascorbic acid in the form of orange juice or other materials, the possibility of scurvy should be seriously entertained. The feeding history of adults is likewise important because the disease is so often observed in individuals subsisting on diets obviously low in ascorbic acid content.

X-ray examination in the adult is not of particular help in diagnosing scurvy, save that one may see alterations in the lamina dura of the teeth. In infants, x-ray examination of the skeleton may be helpful. At the junction between the epiphyseal cartilage and shaft of the long bones, there may be a zone of increased density, which represents the area of excess spicules of calcified cartilaginous matrix, some of which may have fractured. There may also be defects, i.e., areas of rarefaction, at the corners of the bones, which result from fractures at the periphery of the junction between cartilage and shaft. The formation of spurs or projections of the periosteum about the margins of the cartilage are also characteristic. In addition, the bone may have a so-called "ground glass" appearance, which reflects the decrease in density due to diminished width of the cortices and size of the medullary trabeculae.

TREATMENT. In infants the administration of 3 oz fresh orange juice in single or multiple doses per day is advised. This may be sweetened with sugar. If orange juice is refused, twice the amount of tomato juice is the next choice. Synthetic ascorbic acid may be employed orally, 100 to 300 mg per day. There is little need for intravenous therapy. In view of the changes that have taken place in the skeleton, children in whom the disease is in the stage of healing should be handled as little and as gently as possible. It is not necessary to manipulate any bony deformities, nor should splints or casts be applied. Since infection is such a conspicuous accompaniment of scurvy, antibiotics are usually indicated.

Treatment in adults involves administration of orange juice or synthetic ascorbic acid in divided doses up to 500 mg per day. A diet rich in vitamin C should be initiated and continued in both children and adults.

PROGNOSIS. Under therapy gum lesions, if present in infants and in adults, begin to regress in 2 to 3 days. Periosteal shadows, resulting from new bone formation, begin to appear in the long bones of infants after approximately a week. Hemorrhages in the skin usually disappear in 2 to 3 weeks.

REFERENCES

Barlow, T.: On cases described as "acute rickets" which are probably a combination of scurvy and rickets, the scurvy being an essential and the rickets a variable element, Med. Chir. Trans., 66:159, 1883.

Gould, B. S.: Collagen Formation and Fibrogenesis with Special Reference to the Role of Ascorbic Acid, Int. Rev. Cytol., 15:301, 1963.

Hess, A. F.: "Scurvy, Past and Present," Philadelphia, J. B. Lippincott Company, 1920.

Medical Research Council: Vitamin C Requirements of Human Adults, Spec. Rep. Ser., no. 280, London, 1953.

Park, E. A., H. G. Guild, D. Jackson, and M. Bond: The Recognition of Scurvy with Special Reference to the Early X-ray Changes, Arch. Dis. Child., 10:265, 1935.

75 RICKETS AND OSTEOMALACIA
Richard H. Follis, Jr.

HISTORY. Rickets was brought to the attention of the medical world by the publication of Glisson's *De Rachitide* in 1650. Glisson described the now well-known physical signs of rickets: "swellings and knotty excresences about some of the joynts," "tumors in the tops of the ribs where they are conjoyned with gristles in the breast," "breast of a hen or capon," "crooked bones," and so on. The chemical basis for the skeletal deformities was established two centuries later when analyses revealed decreased mineral content of the bones of children with rickets and of adults with osteomalacia, for by this time softness of the bones in older persons had been recognized as the counterpart of rickets in children. By the

nineteenth century in Europe, and a little later in North America, rickets was very prevalent in urban areas. The disease was not truly understood until 1918, when Mellanby produced by dietary means a rachiticlike condition in dogs; this could be prevented by an antirachitic vitamin found in certain fats. During an extraordinarily productive decade, 1918–1927, the pathogenesis of rickets was virtually completely elucidated: the disease was readily produced and studied histologically in experimental animals; the importance of the concentrations of calcium and phosphorus relative to one another in the diet was demonstrated; the antirachitic vitamin was proved to be a specific compound, vitamin D, which by 1927 had been chemically identified; the role of ultraviolet radiation in activating a provitamin in foods and in the skin was demonstrated; deranged concentrations of calcium and phosphorus in the blood serum of rachitic children were described and found to return to normal after therapy with vitamin D; healing processes in the bones were followed roentgenographically and histologically; and in vitro calcification of rachitic bone was produced by suitable concentrations of calcium and phosphorus in the incubation medium.

PREVALENCE. The prevalence of rickets, judged clinically, is low today in the United States and in Europe. The most common type continues to be that due to vitamin D deficiency. However, abnormalities of calcium and phosphorus metabolism, that is, endogenous or conditioned rickets, are also seen. In developing countries today, the history of rickets in Europe and North America is repeating itself. In the large urban centers that are expanding so rapidly in Latin America, Africa, and Asia, rickets is being encountered more frequently.

Osteomalacia is uncommon in both developed and developing countries today. In the past, famine accompanying war, such as that which occurred in Central Europe after World War I, gave rise to many cases of osteomalacia, particularly in women. In north China, osteomalacia has been common as a result of low calcium intake, insufficient sunlight, and many pregnancies. A similar situation has been described in Muslim women in *purdah*. Virtually all cases of osteomalacia encountered today are due to some conditioning factor relative to abnormal calcium and phosphorus metabolism, such as poor absorption, excessive intestinal loss, or increased renal excretion.

CLINICAL FINDINGS. In the infant and child, the patterns the skeletal deformities take are influenced in large part by the age at which the disease becomes manifest, that is, whether the patient is in the recumbent stage, has begun to sit up, or can stand. When the infant is recumbent, the effects of pressure due to gravity tend to produce flattening of the skull, thorax, and pelvic girdle. If the patient sits up, one observes kyphosis, deformity of the forearms, and anterior bowing of the lower legs, if the extremities have been crossed or if the feet hang over the edge of a chair. When the child can walk, further vertebral and pelvic deformity may ensue, as well as curvatures of the lower extremities such as bow legs, knock knees, and even fractures.

The earliest sign of rickets is the appearance of softened areas in the skull, *craniotabes*. The bone may be readily depressed due to lack of rigidity, resulting from decreased deposition of inorganic materials. Craniotabes is not a specific sign of rickets, since it may be observed in other diseases such as osteogenesis imperfecta and hydrocephalus. There may also be thickening and/or bossing of the cranial bones, particularly the parietal or frontal structures. Costochondral swellings, or beadings (rachitic rosary), are one of the cardinal signs of rickets, though changes difficult to differentiate may be observed in scurvy as well. With the development of the rachitic rosary, the lateral configuration of the thorax becomes flattened; as a result, the sternum is pushed forward to form the so-called "pigeon breast." The ribs are deformed by inward stress at the points of attachment of the diaphragm and pulled inward to form Harrison's grooves. The volume of the thorax is reduced. Pulmonary ventilation may be seriously impaired by the resulting collapse of the lungs. Kyphosis of the lower thoracic and upper lumbar spine is found if the child has begun to sit up. This is functional, however, and disappears if the infant is suspended. Bilateral swellings of the wrists and ankles, particularly the former, are characteristic. The shafts of the long

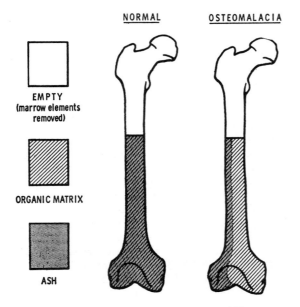

	NORMAL	OSTEOMALACIA
WEIGHT (gms)	300	180
VOLUME (cc)	500	500
DENSITY	.60	.36
WEIGHT ASH (gms)	180	60
PERCENT ASH	60%	33%
WEIGHT MATRIX (gms)	120	120

EMPTY (marrow elements removed)

ORGANIC MATRIX

ASH

Fig. 75-1. Chemical structure of normal bone compared with osteomalacic bone.

bones may be thickened. Fractures of the greenstick variety may occur. Curvatures, either outward (bow legs, genu varum) or inward (knock knees, genu valgum) are prominent. As noted above, bending of the lower leg may lead to anterior curvature. Twisting of the metaphysis may result in coxa vara.

Tetany may be present, usually when the rachitic changes are relatively slight. Tetany is uncommon when rickets is severe. Lowering of serum calcium concentrations may be sufficient to cause death.

Primary dentition is delayed; the order of tooth eruption may be abnormal. The enamel of the permanent teeth may exhibit pits or grooves if it has been developing while the disease was in progress. In severe cases the enamel may be virtually absent.

The clinical aspects of osteomalacia in adults are naturally not so striking as those seen in the growing child with rachitic deformities. The symptoms of osteomalacia usually begin as vague aches and pains in various parts of the skeleton: back, pelvis, chest (ribs), and extremities. Spontaneous fractures or collapse of vertebras may be prominent. Since these are usually painful, they call attention to the disease. Tetany may be encountered. If the disease has been going on for a long time, curvatures of the extremities may occur in association with fractures. Bone pain on pressure may be found on examination. Specific manifestations relating to an organ system are seen in patients with osteomalacia produced by conditioning factors such as chronic steatorrhea or chronic renal disease.

LABORATORY FINDINGS. In rickets, the serum calcium concentration is generally normal or at the lower limit of normal. Serum phosphorus values are reduced from the normal childhood level of 5 to 6 mg to 2 to 4 mg per 100 ml. In some individuals serum calcium and not phosphorus may be reduced. In premature babies both calcium and phosphorus concentrations may be lower than normal. In adults with osteomalacia it is usual for the serum calcium values to be normal or at the lower limit of normal, and the serum phosphorus concentrations are somewhat reduced from the normal adult levels of 3 to 4 mg per 100 ml. No biochemical methods for the determination of vitamin D are available. Bioassays have been carried out on occasion. In both children and adults alkaline phosphatase activity of the serum is generally elevated and remains so until some weeks after therapy has been instituted. In rickets of the vitamin D–deficiency type, aminoaciduria may be demonstrated. The increase in amino acid concentration of the urine results from an elevation of all amino acids. Similar abnormalities have been demonstrated in patients with osteomalacia.

PATHOLOGY. Before detailing the anatomic changes in rickets and osteomalacia, certain fundamental concepts concerning the chemical structure of normal bone in comparison with osteomalacic bone may help to clarify the basic defect (see Fig. 75-1). Let us take as an example a single bone, an entire femur from an adult white man, which has been cleaned of all adherent tissue, including periosteum. The total volume of this bone, as determined by displacement of water or millet seeds from a suitable receptacle, is 500 cc. The dry weight after fat, marrow cells, and blood vessels have been removed is 300 Gm. Hence, the whole bone density, according to the formula density equals mass divided by volume is 0.60. If the specimen is heated at 560°C, the residual material (ash) will weigh 180 Gm, or 60 per cent of the weight of the original dry specimen. The dry weight of the matrix of the original bone was therefore 120 Gm. To determine the absolute density of normal bone, a portion of moist material freed of other non-osseous elements is weighed in air and in water; the value of normal bone is usually about 1.8. If now we determine the whole bone and absolute densities of an osteomalacic femur of 500-cc volume, prominent differences are found. In the first place, the weight is reduced. For example, the whole dry bone weighs only 180 Gm, 120 Gm less than the normal. The whole bone density is therefore 0.36. When this dried whole bone is ashed, the weight of the resulting mineral is found to be 60 Gm, or only 33 per cent of the total dry weight. The matrix therefore has a weight of 120 Gm, the same as that found in the normal specimen of equal volume. Hence, in this hypothetical example, the matrix content is unchanged, although the amount of mineral is reduced to one-third normal, from 180 to 60 Gm. Obviously, the matrix may be increased or decreased, depending on the degree of osteoblastic activity. The matrix content of normal and osteomalacic bone in this example was kept constant to emphasize that the primary defect is one of change in mineral content. If now a piece of osteomalacic bone is weighed in air and water, its absolute density will be found to be reduced; that is naturally to be expected, since much of the density of bone results from the presence of hydroxyapatite.

Defective deposition of lime salts in the cartilage matrix of the growing ends of the bones is the microscopic hallmark of rickets. The bony trabeculae have prominent borders of osteoid, i.e., matrix that does not contain inorganic material. Osteoblastic activity may be normal but is usually accelerated, as evidenced by increased cells and osteoid. In some cases, particularly those of a severe chronic nature, evidence of excessive destruction of bone formed before the disease began or of newly produced osteoid may be observed; i.e., there is *osteitis fibrosa*, which may be defined as the presence of osteoblasts in resorption spaces and an associated proliferation of excessive amounts of connective tissue fibers. When malnutrition is extreme, there may be little growth, with the result that the bony trabeculae are reduced in size; osteoporosis may overshadow the rickets. The degree of involvement of the different parts of the skeleton is related to the rate of growth of the particular bone being studied. Since the anterior ends of middle ribs grow fastest, the disease will be most marked here. For the same reason, the epiphyses about the knee,

shoulder, and wrist will show more change than the opposite ends of these particular bones. Since osteomalacia is rickets in adults, in whom epiphyseal growth has ceased, the only change in osteomalacia is found in bone cortex and trabeculae, where the most conspicuous microscopic alteration is the presence of osteoid.

As healing of rickets occurs, inorganic material appears in the matrix about the most recently matured hypertrophic cartilage cells (Muller's line). Healing of osteomalacia is evinced by the disappearance of osteoid borders.

A fairly constant finding in cases of long-standing rickets and osteomalacia is enlargement of the parathyroid glands, as a result of increase in size and number of the cells.

In cases of classic vitamin D–deficiency rickets, little besides bone lesions is found at autopsy, save, of course, the cause of death: acute or chronic infectious disease, congenital disturbances, trauma, and so on. In instances of conditioned rickets or osteomalacia, disease of the gastrointestinal tract may be found, or obstruction of the bile or pancreatic ducts. Studies of the kidney may reveal abnormalities in the structure of the nephron, that is, the shortening of the tubules that has been observed in cases of phosphate diabetes with aminoaciduria. Chronic renal disease in the form of glomerular, vascular, or pyelonephritis may be present.

PATHOGENESIS. Rickets may be defined as a disease of the developing skeleton characterized by decreased concentration of the mineral component, hydroxyapatite, in the organic matrices of cartilage and bone (osteoid). Osteomalacia is rickets in the adult, and since cartilage growth has ceased, it may be defined as a skeletal disease in adults characterized by a decreased concentration of hydroxyapatite in bone matrix.

What is the cause of this disturbance in deposition of hydroxyapatite in the organic matrices of cartilage and bone? The defect immediately responsible is altered concentrations of calcium and phosphorus in blood plasma. First, however, it will be necessary to review briefly certain pertinent aspects of the normal calcification processes in cartilage and bone matrices. The first well-established principle is that certain humoral concentrations of calcium and phosphorus are necessary if these materials are to deposit as hydroxyapatite crystals in the matrices of cartilage and bone. This principle was introduced in the 1920s and with some modification, consisting in the realization that only a portion of the circulating calcium is ionized, has stood the test of time. On purely empirical grounds, the product of the serum calcium and phosphorus concentrations has been used to indicate whether rickets might or might not be present. If the product in children is above 40, the disease is likely not to be present. With products under 30, rickets is almost invariably present. The range 30 to 40 is the doubtful area. This product is of little value in adult disease. The second principle concerning calcification mechanism is that if hydroxyapatite deposition is to occur in cartilage and bone matrices, the cells responsible for forming these materials must elaborate new matrices, of which the most important organic component is collagen. Rickets does not occur if cartilage or bone is not growing. It is not necessary to discuss the hypotheses concerning the intimate details of the calcification mechanism (see Chap. 226), save to recall that calcification takes place in a very particular area in the matrices of costal and epiphyseal cartilages and nowhere else. Also, calcification occurs only in a specific type of collagenous matrix, such as osteoid or dentine, and under normal circumstances is not found in other collagenous tissues. Finally, the activities of the osteoblasts and odontoblasts undoubtedly determine whether or not calcification will occur in their matrices, providing, of course, concentrations of calcium and phosphorus in the circulating fluids are propitious.

Classic rickets is a deficiency disease due primarily to a lack of endogenous or exogenous vitamin D. Vitamin D plays an important role in maintaining the concentrations of calcium and phosphorus in the blood plasma at levels suitable for their deposition in cartilage and bone matrices. Endogenous vitamin D is derived from a provitamin, 7-dehydrocholesterol, which is present in human epidermis. Radiations in the ultraviolet region between 250 and 312 mμ, with a peak region from 296 to 310 mμ, effectively promote conversion of 7-dehydrocholesterol into the active form, which is called vitamin D_3. Similar irradiation of ergosterol, derived from yeast and plants, yields activated ergosterol or vitamin D_2 (calciferol). Human skin may be irradiated in vivo or in vitro; as far as vitamin D_2 formation is concerned, the effect is the same. It has been estimated that irradiated human skin contains approximately 10 IU vitamin D_3 per square centimeter.

The demonstration that rickets could be healed by ultraviolet radiation helped to explain the geographic distribution of rickets, which had been recognized but poorly understood for a number of years. It is now clear that the absence of rickets in persons living out of doors in the tropics is due to the abundance of ultraviolet light from the sun, which activates the endogenous provitamin in the skin. The amount of ultraviolet radiation furnished by the sun decreases as one proceeds north or south from the Equator, particularly as one passes the Tropics of Cancer or Capricorn. The intensity of ultraviolet radiation is greatest when the sun is directly overhead. As the angle of the sun to the earth decreases, the intensity of the ultraviolet radiation decreases. This accounts for seasonal variations. Other factors affecting intensity are water vapor, smoke, or dust in the atmosphere, since these absorb ultraviolet rays. In addition to direct sunshine, appreciable reflection of ultraviolet light from clouds and the atmosphere (skyshine) occurs. Being reflected, skyshine is directed at various angles and is present when direct sunlight is not; moreover, it appears earlier in the morning and remains longer in the evening than direct sunlight. Ultraviolet rays will not pass through ordinary window glass.

Vitamin D occurs only in very small amounts in common foods such as cereal grains, vegetables, and fruits. Liver, butter fat, and egg yolk contain some (8 to 20 IU per 100 Gm). Human and cow's milk are poor sources. Most marine fish contain appreciable amounts, liver oils being particularly high in vitamin D content. Cod liver oil contains 8,500 IU per 100 ml and halibut liver oil averages 60,000 IU per 100 ml. Irradiated ergosterol (viosterol) contains 1,000,000 IU per 100 ml. Milk fortified with vitamin D is available in the United States and other countries. In the United States the level of fortification is 400 IU per quart.

In the absence of endogenously produced or exogenously available vitamin D, certain important disturbances in serum concentrations of calcium and phosphorus occur. The role of vitamin D in calcium absorption is well-established. When vitamin D is lacking from the diet, excessive amounts of calcium are lost in the stools; this defect is corrected by administration of vitamin D. The vitamin has been shown to enhance the passage of radioactive calcium through isolated intestinal loops of rats in vivo or segments of small intestine in vitro. It has been postulated that vitamin D enhances an active transport system for the passage of calcium into the mucosal cell and its subsequent removal into blood vessels. If calcium absorption is decreased, one might expect to find reduced serum calcium levels. This is observed, but it is the exception rather than the rule. Increased activity of the parathyroids has been invoked to explain the normal and seemingly misleading serum calcium values in rickets. When calcium absorption is impaired by vitamin D deficiency, the lowered serum calcium promotes the release of parathormone, which raises the level of serum calcium. Enlargement of the parathyroids is commonly found at autopsy in cases of severe rickets and osteomalacia. Osteitis fibrosa, i.e., evidence of excessive bone destruction, is common in such cases.

The effect of vitamin D deficiency on calcium absorption has a secondary effect on phosphorus metabolism. With the enhanced loss of calcium from the intestines, phosphorus is excreted in combination. The increased parathyroid activity just referred to will also have an effect on phosphorus balance, which is reflected in increased phosphorus concentration in the urine as a result of diminished tubular resorption. The characteristic derangement found in vitamin D–deficiency rickets is reduced serum phosphorus concentration. The normal value of 5 to 6 mg per 100 ml in the child falls to level of 1 to 3 mg per 100 ml. Phosphorus is lost in the stool, but larger quantities are excreted in the urine. The typical chemical findings of normal or somewhat lowered calcium concentrations and decreased phosphorus values are explained as follows: vitamin D lack → diminished calcium (and phosphorus) absorption → hypocalcemia → parathyroid stimulation → normocalcemia → hyperphosphaturia → hypophosphatemia.

The situation is not really as simple as this; numerous aspects are not clear. The role of secondary hyperparathyroidism needs further investigation, for in addition to its effect on phosphorus excretion and bone destruction, this hormone also appears to affect calcium absorption in the intestine. In addition, it is thought by some that vitamin D has a direct effect on the intestinal absorption of phosphorus, on the renal excretion of phosphorus, on the metabolic activities of bone cells, and on the hypercalcemic response to exogenous parathormone.

A rise in serum alkaline phosphatase activity is a fairly consistent finding in cases of rickets and osteomalacia. Serum citrate concentrations and the excretion of this metabolite in urine are decreased in rickets. Following the administration of vitamin D, citrate levels in serum and urine increase. Citrate concentrations are reduced in rachitic bone, although the significance of these changes is not clear. Finally, vitamin D appears to have a direct effect on increasing the tubular resorption of amino acids since aminoaciduria is encountered in rachitic subjects.

After the relationship of endogenous or exogenous vitamin D deficiency to rickets had been established, it soon became apparent that derangements in calcium and phosphorus metabolism might be associated with disturbances in intake, absorption, or excretion of these two elements. Hence, a number of forms of endogenous or conditioned rickets and osteomalacia are recognized and must be differentiated from classic vitamin D deficiency rickets. These can be broadly classified by whether the abnormality is due to a defect in intake, absorption, or excretion of vitamin D, calcium, or phosphorus (Table 75-1).

Vitamin D Deficiency. Vitamin D deficiency can occur from lack of endogenous production in the skin or from failure to ingest sufficient quantities. In the presence of adequate intake, any situation that may impair absorption of fat will decrease absorption of this fat-soluble vitamin. Celiac disease in children, sprue in adults, loss of pancreatic secretions, obstruction of the biliary system, or the various entities that lead to the malabsorption syndrome in adults may impair vitamin D absorption.

Calcium Deficiency. In certain areas of the world calcium intake may be low, and as a result of inadequate sunlight, coupled with loss of calcium associated with numerous pregnancies, calcium deficiency with attendant osteomalacia may be encountered.

The absorption of calcium is affected by certain factors operating within the lumen of the intestinal tract. Protein appears to promote calcium absorption. The pH of the intestinal contents is important; acidity enhances the passage of calcium through the mucosa. Certain materials that form insoluble compounds or complexes with calcium, such as large amounts of oxalate or phosphate and, in particular, phytate (inositol hexaphosphoric acid), which is a constituent of

Table 75-1. THE PATHOGENESIS OF RICKETS AND OSTEOMALACIA

I. Vitamin D deficiency
   A. Defective endogenous formation in skin
   B. Exogenous dietary deficiency
   C. Decreased absorption:
      1. Malabsorption syndromes
      2. Absence of bile or pancreatic juice
II. Calcium deficiency
   A. Dietary deficiency
   B. Poor absorption (vitamin D deficiency)
   C. Insoluble complex formation
   D. Increased pH of intestinal contents
   E. Steatorrhea and malabsorption syndromes
   F. Idiopathic hypercalciuria
   G. Chronic renal disease
   H. Renal tubular acidosis
   I. Pregnancy and lactation
   J. Excessive sweating
III. Phosphorus deficiency
   A. Dietary deficiency
   B. Formation of insoluble complexes
   C. Malabsorption syndromes
   D. Phosphate diabetes (vitamin D–resistant rickets)
   E. Fanconi syndrome
      1. With glycosuria
      2. With glycosuria and aminoaciduria
      3. With cystinosis
      4. With glycinuria
      5. Associated with heavy-metal toxicity
      6. Associated with Wilson's disease
      7. Associated with multiple myeloma
      8. Associated with neurofibromatosis
      9. Lowe's syndrome
IV. Miscellaneous
   A. Hypophosphatasia

many cereal grains, may lead to excessive loss in the stool. The presence of large amounts of fatty acids will lead to the formation of calcium soaps, which will be excreted as such.

The syndrome of *idiopathic hypercalciuria* is characterized by excretion of large amounts of calcium in the urine and, as a result, the presence of urinary calculi. Calcium loss may be severe enough to lead to rickets or osteomalacia.

Chronic glomerulotubular disease may be accompanied by clinical rickets in children (renal rickets) and by microscopic evidences of osteomalacia in adults. Among the many metabolic alterations associated with chronic renal disease, hypocalcemia and hyperphosphatemia are commonly present. The cause of these derangements is not clear. Some have considered that tubular disease leads to acidosis, which is then followed by hypercalciuria and hypocalcemia. The latter leads to hyperplasia and increased secretory activity of the parathyroids. Hence, in addition to evidences of defective calcification of bone matrix, osteitis fibrosa is frequently present on microscopic examination of the bones.

Another metabolic defect associated with excessive calcium excretion is the *renal tubular acidosis syn-*

drome (*Lightwood's syndrome*). This generally begins in infancy. The primary difficulty is inability to produce urine of normal acidity. The urine, which is increased in volume, is alkaline or only slightly acid with a fixed specific gravity. Acidic metabolites are excreted with fixed base, so that losses of sodium, potassium, and calcium occur. The acidosis is characterized by low plasma bicarbonate, increased plasma chloride, and sometimes decreased plasma inorganic phosphorus. Nephrocalcinosis is the rule; the calcification affects the medullary portion of the kidneys. Hypocalcemia is generally present. Defects in calcification of the skeleton may be a clinical feature of this syndrome. It has been suggested that the basic defect is related to the mechanism whereby hydrogen ions from the renal tubular cells are exchanged for sodium, potassium, calcium, and other cations in the glomerular filtrate.

Phosphorus Deficiency. Although lack of dietary phosphorus may lead to rickets in experimental subjects, it is unlikely that this is of any clinical significance in man. However, absorption of phosphorus may be impaired by the formation of insoluble complexes with cations such as calcium, magnesium, or iron. Phosphorus loss is a prominent feature of the malabsorption syndrome.

The most important metabolic derangement that will be discussed here as a primary phosphorus deficit was referred to when first described as "vitamin D–resistant rickets." The clinical picture is identical with that seen in vitamin D–dietary–deficient rickets. The biochemical alterations and anatomic changes in the skeleton are identical. The early interpretation of this syndrome was, as the term indicates, rickets refractory to ordinary doses of vitamin D. In recent years the term *phosphate diabetes* has been applied to this syndrome, since the principal defect appears to be an inability of the tubular epithelial cells to resorb phosphate unless large, even toxic, amounts of vitamin D are administered. Not all workers agree with this concept, however. This disease has a definite hereditary background and is usually transmitted as a sex-linked dominant character. Females are more often affected than males. The disturbance becomes apparent during the first year of life, with development of increasing bony deformities and growth retardation. Laboratory studies reveal hypophosphatemia and increase in serum alkaline phosphatase activity. Diagnosis is made when therapy with conventional amounts of vitamin D fail to cure the skeletal deformities or raise the level of serum phosphorus concentration.

Sometimes phosphate diabetes is accompanied by defects in tubular reabsorption of other metabolites, such as glucose and amino acids. This syndrome, which generally goes under Fanconi's name, is regarded as one in which anatomic or functional defects in the proximal renal tubule lead to failure to resorb phosphate, glucose, and amino acids. In addition, other functions involving absorption of water, acidification, and potassium reabsorption may be deranged. *Fanconi syndrome* has come to include a number of distinct clinical entities, which can be classified into nine different categories (Table 75-1). The one of most serious import in children is that associated with cystine deposition in the tissues. This has a progressive unfavorable course. Abnormalities in phosphorus metabolism accompanied by aminoaciduria have been described in children and adults with heavy-metal poisoning (lead, cadmium, and uranium), Wilson's disease, multiple myelomatosis, and neurofibromatosis. In addition, a syndrome described initially by Lowe et al. is accompanied by rickets, mental retardation, glaucoma, chronic acidosis, glycosuria, aminoaciduria, and hypophosphatemia.

Miscellaneous. Included in the miscellaneous group for purposes of differential diagnosis is *hypophosphatasia*, since one of its characteristics is defective mineralization of bone. Abnormalities that set it apart are biochemical in nature: diminished alkaline phosphatase activity in serum and tissues, and increased urinary excretion of phosphorylethanolamine. This disease is genetically determined. Its pathogenesis is uncertain. One suspects some intrinsic defect in the calcification mechanism.

DIAGNOSIS. For the diagnosis of rickets, one relies on the clinical picture as already outlined, biochemical abnormalities, and x-ray changes. The clinical and biochemical alterations need no further discussion. On x-ray examination, certain fairly characteristic changes are found at the cartilage-shaft junctions of the long bones as well as in the shafts. In the former area the changes consist of *cupping* and *spreading* of the ends of the shaft, particularly the lower ends of the radius and ulna. Cupping means that the end of the shaft has become concave due to weakness and fanning out of the epiphyseal cartilage laterally. This same alteration may lead to spreading as the shaft becomes broadened due to the pushing out of the weakened cartilage. Another alteration is *fringing*, which consists of threadlike shadows extending from the metaphysis into the cartilage, as a result of alterations in the calcification pattern of the metaphysis. A further change is *stippling*, which means that the outer end of the shaft has an irregular or spotted appearance, which is due to the irregular deposition of inorganic materials in this area. In the shaft one may observe coarsening of the trabecular pattern and more feeble shadows cast by the cortex and trabeculae due to deficient deposition of inorganic materials, as well as increased destruction. The cortex may appear extremely thin or even absent. As many as five or six cortical shadows may appear after treatment has been instituted.

For x-ray diagnosis of osteomalacia, radiolucent zones or bands have been recognized in patients with this disease for many years. First described by Looser, these lesions were given prominence by Milkman. The term *Milkman's syndrome* is sometimes used to refer to ribbonlike zones of symmetric decalcification in the bones. These are characteristic of osteomalacia and calcify after therapy with vitamin D. Hence, it seems unnecessary to set apart this group of cases.

TREATMENT. In discussing the treatment of rickets and osteomalacia, it will be best to discuss prevention first. For infants, particularly premature babies, the administration of 400 to 800 IU vitamin D is recommended during the first few years of life; 400 units should be available during the winter months throughout childhood. It will be recalled that 1 qt enriched milk contains 400 IU vitamin D. There appears to be much individual variation in need for vitamin D. Some individuals appear to need very little, if any, yet still have normal skeletons; in others, "normal" amounts of vitamin D may be toxic. The curative dose for the ordinary case of rickets is approximately 1,200 IU; one may expect to see healing effects in the x-ray by approximately the third week. If the disease is especially severe, the dose may be increased to 5,000 to 20,000 IU. In developing countries, because of difficulties in administration, some pediatricians prefer to administer a massive oral dose, 300,000 to 600,000 IU, or a parenteral dose of 600,000 IU.

Treatment of the conditioned forms of rickets and osteomalacia requires much larger amounts of vitamin D, ranging from 50,000 to 250,000 IU per day. The lower dose is usually employed initially with increases until x-ray evidences of healing are seen. It is well to follow the patient's serum and urinary calcium concentrations when large amounts of vitamin D are used.

PROGNOSIS. The prognosis of rickets with regard to life is excellent, save in those cases in which the thorax has been so weakened as to jeopardize pulmonary ventilation. As a rule, deformities will always diminish. Severe skeletal defects usually persist in adult life, though marked deformities in infants may completely disappear. When rickets persist into the third and fourth years, deformities are usually permanent.

In cases of ordinary vitamin D–deficiency rickets the biochemical defects disappear with therapy. Cases of conditioned rickets or osteomalacia due to alimentary defects have good prognosis. In patients with renal defects it may be more difficult to revert to normal, since the underlying disease may not be particularly amenable to therapy. Chronic renal disease of one type or another, particularly when associated with intra- or extrarenal calcification naturally has a poor prognosis. The entire group is so varied that it is difficult to make an inclusive statement.

Hypervitaminosis D

Soon after crystalline vitamin D became available, evidences of untoward effects began to be reported in animals and human beings receiving amounts ranging from 50,000 to 100,000 IU or more daily. During the ensuing years, such reports have continued to accumulate. Poisoning has resulted either from empirical treatment by physicians of a wide variety of diseases, particularly arthritis and skin disturbances, with excessive amounts of the vitamin or from ignorance of the public. Of particular interest to the pediatrician has been the syndrome of hypercalcemia in infancy, reported during the past decade. Here, much smaller amounts of vitamin D appear to be responsible (2,000 to 4,000 IU).

Clinically, the individual poisoned with vitamin D may complain of weakness, fatigue, lassitude, anorexia, nausea, and vomiting. Severe polyuria, polydipsia, and nocturia may all be present. In children, growth failure may occur. On examination, small yellowish deposits may be found beneath the fingernails, along the outer borders of the lips, and scattered over the skin. Such deposits are also seen in the cornea and conjunctiva. Biopsy confirms their inorganic nature. Laboratory examination reveals an elevation in serum calcium concentration. Serum phosphorus concentration is also elevated. Alkaline phosphatase activity of the serum is generally decreased. Serum nonprotein nitrogen values may be elevated. Serum potassium values may decrease. Alkalosis may be present. Protein and casts may be found in the urine, which has a low specific gravity. The passage of gravel is sometimes reported. Changes associated with hypercalcemia may be observed in the EKG. Autopsies show widespread deposits of calcium phosphate crystals throughout the tissues, particularly the kidneys, but also in the heart, lungs, and stomach. It is imperative to stop ingestion of the vitamin. Even so, hypercalcemia may persist for some time, and evidences of renal damage may be prolonged. The deposits of inorganic materials in the skin and eye slowly disappear.

REFERENCES

Albright, F., and E. C. Reifenstein, Jr.: "The Parathyroid Glands and Metabolic Bone Disease," Baltimore, The Williams & Wilkins Company, 1948.

Dent, C. E., and H. Harris: Hereditary Forms of Rickets and Osteomalacia, J. Bone & Joint Surg., 38B:204, 1956.

Follis, R. H., Jr., E. A. Park, and D. Jackson: The Prevalence of Rickets at Autopsy during the First Two Years of Age, Bull. Johns Hopkins Hosp., 91:480, 1952.

Harrison, H. E.: Vitamin D and Calcium and Phosphate Transport, Pediatrics, 28:531, 1961.

Hess, A. F.: "Rickets, Including Osteomalacia and Tetany," Philadelphia, Lea & Febiger, 1929.

Howard, J. E., and W. C. Thomas: Clinical Disorders of Calcium Homeostasis, Medicine, 42:25, 1963.

Park, E. A.: Observations on the Pathology of Rickets with Particular Reference to the Changes at the Cartilage-shaft Junctions of the Growing Bones, Harvey Lect., 34:157, 1928–29.

Winters, R. W., J. B. Graham, F. F. Williams, V. W. McFalls, and C. H. Burnett: A Genetic Study of Familial Hypophosphatemia and Vitamin D Resistant Rickets with a Review of the Literature, Medicine, 37:97, 1958.

76 XEROPHTHALMIA AND OTHER MANIFESTATIONS OF VITAMIN A DEFICIENCY

Richard H. Follis, Jr.

HISTORY. Inability to see in subdued light, called *night blindness*, and dryness, haziness, and spontaneous necrosis of the cornea are abnormalities which have been recognized for many years. Over a century ago, Bitot called attention to the simultaneous occurrence of night blindness and lesions of the conjunctiva. By the turn of the century, Mori had suggested that ocular lesions in Japanese children might be related to a lack of fat in the diet. Soon a fat-soluble material (later to be called vitamin A) was shown to enhance the growth of rats and prevent the development of ocular lesions that histologically resembled those which had been observed in man. During the second decade of this century, investigators in Denmark clearly established the relationship of vitamin A to xerophthalmia in children. In 1930 carotene was demonstrated to be provitamin A. Vitamin A was chemically identified in 1931 and synthesized in 1936.

PREVALENCE. Today the areas of greatest prevalence of endemic vitamin A deficiency are found in Indonesia, particularly Java and parts of Sumatra, India, the Near East, and North Africa. Isolated instances of conditioned vitamin A deficiency have been described in Europe and the United States.

CLINICAL FINDINGS. The term *xerophthalmia* is used here in an inclusive sense to refer to certain anatomic abnormalities of the eye resulting from vitamin A deficiency. The lesions usually exhibit a definite sequence of stages in development. The initial change, which is called *xerosis* (*xerosis epithelialis conjunctivae*), consists of dryness and opacity of the bulbar conjunctiva. Secretion of tears is decreased. At the lateral margin of the cornea, a triangular-shaped accumulation of sticky secretion may appear. This is the *Bitot spot,* which resembles a plaque or pseudomembrane filled with bubbles; that is, it has a foamy appearance. This material is difficult to scrape off. Fine pigmentation may also be present throughout the conjunctiva. These alterations are either accompanied or soon followed by haziness and dryness of the cornea (*xerosis corneae*). Secretion of tears is impaired. The tarsal glands along the eyelid are frequently enlarged. Photophobia may be marked. The most serious consequence is the appearance of small epithelial erosions. These soon become infected and enlarged. If this ulceration continues, destruction of the cornea (*keratomalacia*) occurs, a process that may be extremely rapid. Naturally, destruction of the cornea is followed by prolapse of the lens and other contents of the anterior chamber. Panophthalmitis is inevitable. Eyesight is irrevocably lost. In children in developing countries, overt signs of malnutrition may be present, particularly those of kwashiorkor.

As already noted, visual acuity in subdued light is reduced as a result of vitamin A deficiency. This disturbance is called night blindness. Two other terms, *nyctalopia* and *hemeralopia,* have been used to refer to this condition. Nyctalopia means an inability to see in subdued light. Hemeralopia refers to a decrease in vision that follows exposure to bright light. Defective ability to see in subdued light may be established by certain tests; however, these are difficult to perform under routine conditions and are particularly unsuited for children. An instrument, the electroretinogram, has been developed for objective testing.

The nonocular manifestations of vitamin A deficiency are not conspicuous and are usually obscured by signs of general malnutrition or the presence of some conditioning disturbance, such as obstruction of the pancreatic or biliary ducts, which may lead to poor absorption of the vitamin. Tracheitis, bronchitis, and pneumonia are the commonest clinical manifestations.

LABORATORY FINDINGS. Vitamin A nutriture may be assessed by determining the carotene and/or vitamin A content of blood serum. Values are expressed in International Units (IU) or micrograms per 100 ml. One IU is equivalent to 0.3 μg vitamin A or 0.6 μg carotene. Vitamin A concentration is decisive; carotene values may be misleading, since other pigments may be present. Serum values for carotene and vitamin A are usually considered to be normal if over 40 and 20 μg per 100 ml, respectively. When values for carotene and vitamin A fall below 20 and 10 μg per 100 ml, respectively, the deficient state is probably present. Valuable information on vitamin A nutriture among population groups has been obtained from analyses of liver tissue. For instance, among well-nourished groups in Great Britain, values averaging 450 IU per Gm have been obtained. In contrast, data derived from Chinese subjects indicate much lower levels, averaging 79 IU per Gm.

PATHOLOGY. The tissues chiefly affected are epithelial in nature, principally those which ordinarily are not keratinized. These include the lining epithelium of the upper and lower respiratory passages, genitourinary tract, eye and paraocular glands, salivary glands, accessory glands of the tongue and buccal cavity, and pancreas. The fundamental change is metaplasia of the normal nonkeratinized lining cells into a keratinizing type of epithelium. The cornea becomes dry, wrinkled, and hazy due to intrinsic changes as well as to lack of tears as a result of obstruction of the ducts. The ciliated epithelium of the respiratory tract is replaced by a keratinizing lining so that the important mechanical effects of the cilia are lost. The basal cells in all areas retain, however, their potentiality for reverting to normal if their supply of vitamin A is restored.

At autopsy other changes may be found that are responsible for conditioned vitamin A deficiency. For instance, obstruction to the biliary tract or pancreatic duct may interfere with fat absorption. Liver disease may have interfered with storage.

PATHOGENESIS. At least two forms of vitamin A alcohol are known (A_1 and A_2), together with acid and aldehyde derivatives. The vitamin As are intimately related to provitamins, the carotenes, and certain other pigmented compounds. A part of ingested carotene is absorbed by the cells of the intestinal mucosa and transformed into vitamin A. Bile is important in this process. Vitamin A is usually present in ester form in foods; it is hydrolyzed in the intestinal tract and absorbed as the alcohol (*retinol*). Within the cells of the intestinal mucosa, vitamin A is esterified, usually with palmitic acid, and transported via the thoracic duct as the ester to the liver, where it is stored. As needed, vitamin A ester is hydrolyzed to the alcohol and transported, attached to plasma protein, to the tissues. Vitamin A aldehyde (*retinal* or *retinene*) is found in the retina and is important in the visual process. The interrelations between alcohol, acid, and ester forms of vitamin A have been greatly clarified. It is possible that vitamin A acid (*retinoic acid*) may be the "active form." The alcohol (retinol) is converted to aldehyde (retinal or retinene). The latter may be converted to the acid by an enzyme in the liver. The reverse reaction, i.e., acid to alcohol or aldehyde, does not appear possible. The acid is more effective for growth in experimental animals than is the aldehyde. The acid is not active in the visual process.

The greatest concentration of vitamin A in man is found in the liver. Concentrations are also appreciable in kidneys, adrenals, lungs, and, naturally, the retina. Fat depots contain a small amount of the vitamin.

Vitamin A deficiency may result from an insufficiency of this vitamin or its precursors in the diet or because of some process which interferes with absorption from the intestinal tract, transport, or storage in the liver. Obstruction of the biliary tract or pancreatic ducts in children or adults may lead to diminished absorption of vitamin A. Diarrhea and the various types of malabsorption syndromes are accompanied by vitamin A malnutrition. Of particular importance is the interrelation of vitamin A and protein nutrition, since vitamin A alcohol appears to be transported by plasma albumin. Transport to and mobilization from the liver may be impaired as a result of protein malnutrition. Since vitamin E has a sparing effect on vitamin A, the former may be an important consideration in infants in whom vitamin E serum levels tend to be low.

The intricate reactions whereby vitamin A enters into the visual process may be briefly summarized. Vitamin A aldehyde (retinal or retinene) is found in the retina bound to a protein called *opsin*. Together these form the compound *rhodopsin*, the red pigment of the retinal rods. Under the influence of light, *rhodopsin* breaks down into its two components, thereby initiating a nerve impulse. The presence of isomeric forms makes the reaction even more complicated than that just summarized, particularly with respect to the resynthesis of rhodopsin. Vitamin A is also concerned with cone vision.

How vitamin A maintains the integrity of epithelial structures remains a mystery. Vitamin A appears to be implicated in the metabolism of intracellular structures, the lysosomes, in mucopolysaccharide metabolism, and in steroid hormone formation.

DIAGNOSIS. The presence of dryness, haziness, or increased pigmentation of the cornea should arouse suspicion, particularly if both eyes are affected. A history of night blindness may be helpful. Bitot's spots, though not specifically pathognomonic, should make one consider the diagnosis. Laboratory studies in individual cases are not particularly helpful. It is highly important to make the diagnosis as quickly as possible. Xerophthalmia should be considered a medical emergency and therapy instituted immediately.

THERAPY. Oral administration of 500,000 IU vitamin A daily as the palmitate or acetate for 3 or more days is recommended. In addition, it may be well to administer similar-sized doses intramuscularly. The diets of children with vitamin A deficiency are usually also lacking in other nutrients and hence should be improved, particularly with respect to protein.

PROGNOSIS. The outcome as far as sight is concerned will depend on the degree of involvement of the ocular structures before therapy is instituted. If only clouding of the cornea has occurred, prognosis is excellent. However, if perforation and infection of the anterior chamber have taken place, restoration of sight is virtually unknown.

Hypervitaminosis A

The ingestion of large amounts of vitamin A, in doses ranging from 75,000 to 500,000 IU daily to infants or adults, results in a variety of signs and symptoms that sometimes may be extremely confusing, particularly if a history of ingestion has not been elicited. Ignorance is usually the reason for taking excessive amounts of vitamin A.

In infants, the effects of acute toxicity are drowsiness, vomiting, and bulging of the fontanels as a result of increased intracranial pressure. More chronic evidences of toxicity include failure to gain weight, alopecia, coarseness of hair texture, hepatomegaly, and evidences of bone pain. X-ray examination of the skeleton reveals characteristic areas of periosteal new bone formation, particularly prominent in the shafts of the long bones.

In adults, headache, blurred vision or diplopia, nausea, and vomiting all may be present. Bone pain and osseous changes similar to those occurring in children may be observed. In addition, calcification of ligaments and tendons may be seen on x-ray examination. Peeling of the skin, neuritis, fissures and sores at the corners of the mouth, coarsening of the skin, alopecia, and localized areas of hyperpigmentation of the epidermis are common. As might be expected, the level of vitamin A in the serum is elevated, values as high as 2,000 μg per 100 ml have been reported. Fortunately, the prognosis is good when vitamin A ingestion halts.

Mention should be made of *carotenemia*, because it may be confused with jaundice. When large amounts of carotene-containing foods are ingested, the blood plasma may contain a high enough concentration of pigment to impart a yellowish color to the skin (especially the palms of the hands and the nasolabial folds) but not the conjunctivas.

REFERENCES

McLaren, D. S.: "Malnutrition and the Eye," New York, Academic Press, Inc., 1963.

Medical Research Council: Vitamin A Requirements of Human Adults, Special Report Series no. 264, 1949.

Moore, T.: "Vitamin A," New York, Elsevier Publishing Company, 1957.

Oomen, H. A. P. C.: An Outline of Xerophthalmia, Int. Rev. Trop. Med., 1:131, 1961.

77 MISCELLANEOUS DEFICIENCY STATES

Richard H. Follis, Jr.

HYPONATREMIC STATES. As a result of feeding experiences in animals, the nutritionist has been aware of the need for sodium in the diet for many years. Historically, states of sodium deprivation were first recognized to accompany the diarrheal diseases of infancy and to result from excessive sweating. Later came the important relationship of sodium loss to the pathogenesis of Addison's disease. Terms such as *low sodium syndrome* and *low salt syndrome* have been applied to patients with states of hyponatremia of varied etiology. It is clear, however, that hyponatremia does not necessarily imply tissue sodium depletion. Some would prefer not to think of a specific hyponatremic syndrome. Certain clinical effects that may be associated with hyponatremia are weakness, apathy, semicoma, confusional states, nausea, anorexia, vomiting, cramps in the muscles of the extremities, evidences of circulatory failure with hemoconcentration, and uremia. None of these symptoms is particularly specific. All are usually overshadowed by the more serious effects produced by the underlying disease process. In Table 77-1 are summarized mechanisms whereby hyponatremic states may come about.

HYPOKALEMIC STATES. Reduction in serum potassium concentration may occur under a variety of conditions. The most conspicuous symptoms related to potassium deprivation are anorexia, nausea, muscle

Table 77-1. THE PATHOGENESIS OF HYPONATREMIC STATES

I. Decreased intake
  A. Experimental dietary restriction
  B. Dilution of extracellular fluid
    1. Intravenous sodium-low solutions
    2. Following trauma or surgical procedures
    3. Starvation
    4. Congestive heart failure
II. Internal loss (with removal)
  A. Edema, ascites, hydrothorax
III. External loss
  A. Renal
    1. Diuresis, especially with diuretic agents
    2. Renal disease
    3. Hormonal effects
      a. Adrenal: Addison's disease
      b. Pitressin
  B. Gastrointestinal tract
    1. Vomiting, suctional gastric drainage
    2. Diarrhea
    3. Fistulas
  C. Skin
    1. Sweat
    2. Burns
  D. Hemorrhage

weakness, and mental depression. Confusional states, shallow respirations, and abdominal distension as a result of paralytic ileus may be observed. Signs of the hypokalemic state are principally referred to the cardiovascular system. Such include irregular pulse, fall in blood pressure, and nonspecific alterations in the electrocardiogram. At autopsy certain characteristic lesions have been described, such as necrosis of cardiac and skeletal muscle fibers and extreme vacuolization of the renal tubular epithelium.

The various mechanisms whereby conditioned potassium deficiency may occur are summarized in Table 77-2. It is important to realize that hypokalemia is

Table 77-2. THE PATHOGENESIS OF HYPOKALEMIC STATES

I. Decreased intake
  A. Experimental restriction
  B. Starvation, followed with inadequate repletion
  C. Dilution of extracellular fluids with potassium-low solutions
II. Excessive renal loss
  A. Diuresis, especially with diuretic agents
  B. Acidosis (diabetes mellitus)
  C. Renal disease
  D. Hormone effects
    1. Hypophysis (ACTH): trauma
    2. Adrenal: aldosterone; cortisone; cortisol
III. Loss from gastrointestinal tract
  A. Vomiting, suctional drainage
  B. Diarrhea of any type
IV. Loss in sweat
V. Excessive transfer to cells
  A. Glycogenesis (treatment of diabetic acidosis mellitus)
  B. Familial periodic paralysis

not necessarily synonymous with intracellular potassium depletion.

THE LOW MAGNESIUM SYNDROME. Like deficiencies of sodium and potassium, magnesium depletion may occur from deficient intake, poor absorption, and increased renal excretion. A syndrome characterized by vertigo, weakness, distension, positive Chvostek sign, and convulsive seizures with or without tetany has been ascribed to a decrease in serum concentration of magnesium (see Chap. 45).

ARIBOFLAVINOSIS. During the studies that elucidated the pathogenesis of pellagra, it became clear that riboflavin deficiency contributed to certain manifestations of the syndrome. This viewpoint was further strengthened by observations on human subjects deprived of riboflavin. The principal manifestations of the experimentally produced syndrome are angular lesions and cheilosis, scrotal dermatitis, and seborrheic dermatitis. No glossitis or neurologic abnormalities have been noted. Such signs are similar to the clinical manifestations of a naturally occurring syndrome in man, which has been called *ariboflavinosis*. This syndrome is characterized by macerated lesions at the angles of the mouth, which may progress to linear fissures. In addition, a greasy erythema develops in the nasolabial region and is sometimes seen about the eyes and ears. In severely affected persons changes of the eyelids may be prominent. Response to riboflavin may be dramatic. It should be recalled that angular lesions are not a specific manifestation of riboflavin deficiency (see Chap. 66). On the basis of nutritional surveys in various parts of the world, riboflavin deficiency determined by decreased excretion of this vitamin in the urine, appears to be widespread. The public health significance of this is not clear.

VITAMIN B$_6$ DEFICIENCY. Experimentally produced and naturally occurring vitamin B$_6$–deficiency disease has been observed in both infants and adults. When babies are maintained experimentally on a vitamin B$_6$– deficient diet, convulsions and anemia develop. Conversion of tryptophan to N-methyl nicotinamide is impaired. These abnormalities are corrected by the administration of vitamin B$_6$. Pyridoxine deficiency has been studied experimentally in adults to whom the antagonist deoxypyridoxine has been administered. The symptoms consist of anorexia, nausea, and drowsiness. The most striking signs are an erythematous scaling of the nasolabial area, angular lesions of the mouth, and, in some individuals, hyperesthesia, anesthesia, and loss of position and vibratory senses. A mild normochromic, hypoplastic anemia develops. Iatrogenic neuritis has been frequently observed in patients receiving isoniazid, a pyridoxine antagonist, for tuberculosis.

Several reports have called attention to a convulsive syndrome in infants who had received a liquid proprietary formula of low vitamin B$_6$ content. Increase in the excretion of xanthurenic acid and N-methyl nicotinamide after a tryptophan load test was demonstrated. Administration of vitamin B$_6$ cured the syndrome.

A number of cases of a microcytic hypochromic anemia that responds partially to vitamin B$_6$ therapy are now on record (Chap. 111).

PANTOTHENIC ACID DEFICIENCY. The only possible examples of naturally occurring pantothenic acid deficiency so far described have been those cases of the "burning foot" syndrome that respond to therapy with this vitamin. The "burning foot" syndrome was frequently observed in prisoners in the Far East during World War II. Subjectively numbness, pins and needles, or tingling of the toes and feet were noted. After a few weeks, the paresthesia changed to a dull boring pain in the toes and soles of the feet, usually becoming worse at night. Reflexes were preserved. In some patients the administration of calcium pantothenate was reported to be beneficial.

A pantothenic acid–deficient diet, to which the antagonist ω-methylpantothenic acid, was added, has been administered to human subjects. A syndrome characterized by feelings of malaise, fatigue, headache, insomnia, nausea, and vomiting was reported. Numbness and tingling of the hands and feet and weakness of the extensor muscles were present. The eosinopenic response to ACTH was lost, and increased sensitivity to insulin developed. These symptoms and signs responded to the administration of pantothenic acid.

VITAMIN E DEFICIENCY. Since vitamin E is a fat-soluble material, poor absorption occurs where lipid absorption is defective, as with decreased or absent biliary and pancreatic secretions and disease of the intestinal tract. Tocopherol deficiency has been observed in infants with congenital biliary atresia and cystic fibrosis of the pancreas. Foci of necrosis of striated muscle fibers such as those seen in the vitamin E–deficient experimental animal have been observed in a few infants dying from diseases associated with poor fat absorption.

VITAMIN K DEFICIENCY. Dietary lack of this vitamin is rare. Being a fat-soluble vitamin, the absorption of vitamin K is impaired in the absence of biliary and pancreatic secretions and in the presence of intestinal disease. In liver disease the metabolism of this vitamin is deranged.

ESSENTIAL FATTY ACID DEFICIENCY. Clinical effects of deficiency of essential fatty acids in man have only been observed under fairly stringent laboratory conditions. Skin lesions have been observed in infants maintained on low-fat diets. These consist of dryness and scaling and are relieved when linolenic acid itself or foodstuffs containing it are administered. Much interest centers on the relationship of essential fatty acids to cholesterol metabolism, for it has been shown that the administration of vegetable oils containing unsaturated fatty acids lowers serum cholesterol and phospholipid levels in human subjects. The possible importance of this in the pathogenesis of atherosclerosis has attracted much attention.

78 OBESITY
George W. Thorn
and Philip K. Bondy

Obesity occurs when the caloric intake exceeds the energy requirements of the body both for physical activity and for growth. As a result there is an accumulation of fat, which is stored in the adipose tissue. The excessive tissue may be distributed generally over the body, or it may be localized. The factors controlling the location of the fat are not all known, but pituitary, thyroid, adrenal, and sex hormones play an important role. Obesity is a serious and common disease in those countries in which a combination of generous food supplies and sedentary occupations readily permits the assimilation of more food than is necessary. The excessive deposition of fat is associated with an increased incidence of degenerative diseases such as atherosclerosis, diabetes, and arthritis; indeed, the only common cause of death that does not strike earlier in the obese than in the lean population is suicide! The ill effects of obesity can be prevented and, to some extent, repaired by weight reduction. The treatment of obesity is one of the most serious problems in preventive medicine in the United States today.

ETIOLOGY. Under normal circumstances there is a very exact adjustment of food intake to body requirements. Unfortunately, in certain individuals this adjustment is deranged, and intake becomes excessive. The cause of the derangement is not understood, but several factors are important.

Familial and cultural eating habits are firmly implanted at an early age. In groups in which great emphasis is placed on food, there is a tendency to overeat. Sometimes the cultural pattern equates success with obesity (witness the common caricature of the obese banker) and thus encourages the ambitious person to achieve a comfortable corpulence. Moreover, when activity patterns change, eating habits may remain constant, so that the man who has previously been physically active may fail to reduce his caloric intake when he suddenly changes to a sedentary occupation. This tendency may be reinforced by the gradual decline of metabolic rate and of muscle activity, which ordinarily accompanies aging.

Certain individuals may have increased appetite for psychologic reasons. Such persons use food as a substitute for the satisfaction they should obtain from other emotional sources. In this respect, they are similar to alcoholics, who use alcohol as a substitute for such normal sources of satisfaction as their friends, their families, or success in their work.

It has been known for years that lesions involving the hypothalamus may lead to obesity. Experimental damage to the ventromedian nuclei of the hypothalamus, or of adjacent tracts, produces an increase in body weight of as much as 400 per cent. This increase is a result chiefly of increased caloric intake, but reduced physical activity may also play a part. When calories are restricted, hypothalamic-obese animals lose weight in a normal fashion. If unlimited calories are made available, the rapid weight gain lasts for only a short time; the animals then reach a plateau of weight at which they remain indefinitely. Hypothalamic lesions resulting from trauma or infectious processes may be a cause of obesity in rare instances. In view of the experimental relationship of the hypothalamus to hyperphagic obesity, it is commonly believed that control of appetite resides in the hypothalamus.

It is therefore clear that the basic cause of obesity is a derangement of the appetite-controlling mechanisms, permitting the assimilation of more food than is needed. It has been claimed that certain individuals are more efficient than others in their ability to digest, absorb, and utilize food and therefore that they become obese at lower caloric intakes than might be expected. Extensive balance studies on such patients have never substantiated this explanation; at equivalent levels of physical activity and basal metabolism, there seems to be little variation in the required caloric intake. It has been shown that young obese patients, when tilted rapidly to the vertical position, exhibit an impaired rise in serum unesterified fatty acids, in contrast to control subjects of normal weight. Gordon and his colleagues believe that some obese patients have a specific block in the utilization of fatty acids by peripheral tissues that can be removed by administration of triiodothyronine.

A careful history of the time and manner of onset of obesity may provide a clue to prognosis and etiology. Patients who have been oversized from birth are more likely to resist treatment than those who gained weight later in life; and the prognosis of a patient 10 per cent over ideal weight is better than that of one who is double normal weight.

Adipose tissue imposes a double load on the organism—a physical increase in the work that must be done in order to move about, and a metabolic increase in the amount of nutriment, oxygen, and blood needed to maintain the metabolism of the adipose tissue cells. Consequently, the addition of a given caloric increment to the diet of a person previously in equilibrium does not produce a continuous and infinite increase in body weight. After an appropriate amount of adipose tissue has been deposited, the additional caloric requirement imposed by the new tissue balances the added calories and the weight once again stabilizes at a higher level. This fact may explain in part the fact that weight gain tends to be rapid at first and later reaches equilibrium.

PATHOLOGY. The only pathologic lesion directly attributable to obesity is the presence of excessive amounts of adipose tissue. This tissue occurs chiefly in the subcutaneous areas, omentum, mesentery, and in the fat pads normally present around the kidneys and in the epicardium. The composition of the adipose tissue in obesity is identical with that found normally in smaller quantities in the same areas. It consists of clumps of fat cells, a special type of connective tissue cell that contains a relatively huge droplet of neutral fat displacing all other cell structures, together with supporting tissue such as blood vessels, lymphatic vessels, and fibrous tissue. Thus, although adipose tissue has a very high content of neutral fat, it also contains water, protein, and even small amounts of glycogen. A number of secondary pathologic changes are often seen in obese patients. These include premature atherosclerosis, fatty infiltration of the liver, and traumatic skeletal changes such as hypertrophic arthritis.

CLINICAL PICTURE. Obesity itself produces no symptoms, but the mechanical load of the excessive adipose tissue causes a series of secondary difficulties, which may cause symptoms. These include postural adjustments that ultimately may cause backache and painful knees and feet, and also circulatory embarrassment with dyspnea, easy fatigability, and orthopnea. Severe obesity is also frequently associated with menstrual disorders and infertility.

DIAGNOSIS. No arbitrary aids to diagnosis are comparable to the information that can be obtained by simple inspection of the patient. From the standpoint of longevity, the ideal weight is one at which the patient is sparingly covered with a thin layer of adipose tissue. As soon as he accumulates enough subcutaneous adipose tissue to present a roll of redundant subcutaneous fat, he must be considered obese.

TREATMENT. The only effective method of treating obesity is restriction of caloric intake below the energy requirement; this can usually be accomplished without reducing the intake of essential minerals, vitamins, and amino acids below the danger point.

Motivation. In no disorder is the prescription so simple and the possibility of cure so high as in the treatment of obesity. Why, then, is there so much discussion concerning the "best diet," such concerted effort to seek the "magic pill," such quackery and chicanery surrounding attempts to restore weight to normal? The answer is readily apparent: caloric restriction maintained over any appreciable length of time requires courage and self-discipline of the highest order. To attain success a patient must possess sufficient motivation to enable him to carry through a prolonged uncomfortable program of relative starvation. If the ingestion of large quantities of food has provided essential emotional and psychologic satisfactions, caloric restriction may be accomplished only by substituting other sources of satisfaction or by increasing understanding of the nature of the emotional disturbances and subconscious conflicts which form a basis for the patient's present situation. In all these considerations the physician's patience and understanding are important determining factors in the success of the program. There are a few patients whose obesity has resulted from long-continued, modest excess of intake of calories, without deep underlying emotional conflict or overt disturbances in metabolism

as the cause. For such as these it is simple to provide nutritional education and guidance. The number of such cases is diminishing rapidly as the appreciation of the dangers and difficulties which confront the obese individual becomes more widespread.

In general, motivation sufficient to sustain a patient in following the diet prescription arises from one or more of the following factors:

1. Pride in personal appearance
2. Symptoms of disordered physical function (shortness of breath, painful knees)
3. Fear of future diseases (diabetes, arteriosclerosis)
4. An attempt to avoid the antagonistic reaction or "pressure" manifested by friends, relatives, or business associates

Obviously the last factor is the least satisfactory and, if at all potent, almost invariably leads to resentment. The danger in this instance is intensified by the probability that disturbed interpersonal relationships with mother, father, sister, or employer may have played an important role originally in the genesis of obesity. The submission to authority under these circumstances, while occasionally successful in accomplishing the immediate end (weight loss), may ultimately result in the development of much more serious emotional conflicts.

Although the presence of organic disease or the fear of its development may provide strong motivation for weight reduction, the fact that patients may have used the satisfaction derived from food as an important aid in meeting life's problems may create a serious conflict. On the one hand, there is fear of the physical consequences if weight is not reduced; on the other, the patient must face the loss of a necessary source of satisfaction. In some individuals who are incapable of making a reasonable, healthy adjustment to this predicament, the long-range effect of diet restriction may exert a detrimental effect on the underlying disease despite immediate benefits associated with weight loss.

Obese patients vary greatly in the ease with which dietary restriction enables them to lose weight. In instances in which only moderate restriction is necessary, success is almost certain with reasonable motivation, whereas patients requiring severe caloric restriction for prolonged periods need the strongest motivation. The skill with which the physician is able, on the one hand, to estimate the degree of dietary restriction which will be necessary and, on the other, to encourage the forces conspiring to motivate the patient will determine his success or failure in a therapeutic program.

It must be apparent that the "aura" which surrounds many diet fads and programs represents an attempt to fortify the patient's motivation. One of the important aspects of the "cults" and "spas" is the reinforcement of resolution associated with constant supervision in a setting of group enterprise. Interest, pride, and cooperation are stimulated by the discussions which occur in conjunction with "classes" of patients on a

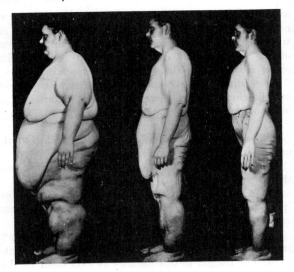

Fig. 78-1. Gradual weight reduction by diet alone in a 28-year-old woman with obesity due to overeating. Excess subcutaneous and connective tissue had to be removed surgically after a loss of 120 lb.

similar regimen. The discussion of personal problems which may have arisen in conjunction with the application of the dietary program is helpful. For ultimate and permanent success, however, the individual must not become too dependent on the group. A physician in private practice may strengthen motivation by having certain of his patients on weight-reducing programs meet in his office in a group. This also offers the possibility of providing dietary instruction more efficiently. It is not, however, a substitute for individual attention. Since the emotional support supplied by the physician is most important during the early days of the diet, patients should be seen very frequently at first—probably once a week. Only when secure patterns of dietary restriction have been well established can visits become less frequent. Even when a normal weight level has been established, patients require continuing observation and support. It is depressingly common to have a patient return some months after having achieved a reasonable weight, once again obese and repentant. Constant support from the physician may prevent some lapses of this sort.

Dietary Prescription. In order to lose weight, the patient must assimilate fewer calories than he burns. The physician, in prescribing the diet, must have some concept of the total caloric requirement of the patient; and, in addition, he must know both the minimum nutritional requirements which the restricted diet must meet and the patient's dietary habits and prejudices. The use of a "standard" reducing diet is, therefore, not wise. In calculating the diet, at least 1 Gm protein per kilogram ideal weight should be included. Fats and carbohydrate should then be used to achieve the desired caloric level. The dietary habits of the patient

should be consulted and the diet designed to resemble the patient's normal food preferences as closely as possible.

The caloric prescription depends on many factors—height, weight, level of physical exertion, basal metabolic rate, and rate of desired weight loss. Although in some instances weight reduction can occur at intakes as high as 2500 Cal per day, the usual prescription is for 1800 Cal or less.

In deciding the proper caloric intake the physician must be empiric. Every patient is anxious to attain his ideal weight at the earliest possible moment. It is essential for the physician to decide the rate of weight loss which is most desirable for an individual patient. He must not be influenced unduly by his patient's demands. He must explain the advantages of a relatively slow rate of weight loss; he must point out that great weight loss may be accomplished over a prolonged period by moderate methods and that undue dietary restriction may be fraught with real dangers to health.

In most instances it is best to lose weight gradually rather than suddenly. A slow rate of weight loss allows better adjustment of the body and is a protection against nutritional deficiencies. There is opportunity for tissue to regain some of its elasticity, and the psychic and physical disturbances which occur with redundant folds of skin may be prevented (Fig. 78-1). Weight reduction should certainly proceed at a slow rate in the elderly, in the very young, and in pregnant and lactating women. Weight loss on a given caloric-deficient diet proceeds more rapidly in the first weeks than later. This is in part because of the compensatory fall in basal metabolic level which develops as dietary restriction is prolonged, and in part because of the early loss of relatively large quantities of minerals and water.

Total caloric intake should therefore be adjusted to produce a weight loss of 1 to 2 lb per week after the first 2 weeks. It should be remembered that very obese individuals may lose safely at a greater rate than this, that growing children should lose more slowly than this, and that patients with cardiac insufficiency may lose large quantities of salt and water which should not be interpreted as tissue loss.

Most patients with moderate activity will lose satisfactorily on a 1200- to 1500-Cal intake. Some patients may have to be restricted to 1000 Cal or less. There is no real justification for diets under 800 Cal for ambulatory patients. Failure to lose weight on a diet prescription of 800 to 1000 Cal almost invariably means that the diet formula has been misunderstood or is not being followed. For short periods of time a diet of 500 to 600 Cal may be given, but the potential dangers of such rigid restriction should be appreciated.

Many excellent articles have been written with a view toward helping the physician and patient attain this end. In these discussions the advantages of bulk, the satiation value of foods high in protein, and the preparation of tasty foods of low caloric value are discussed at length. The means by which the diet is manipulated should not be confused with the end, which is only caloric restriction with the preservation of optimum essential food constituents.

Of great help to physician and patient during the early period of dietary regulation is the maintenance of a diary in which the patient writes down each article of food which he eats along with the approximate quantity. This should be checked over carefully by physician and patient together. Such a record is invaluable in suggesting necessary changes in diet, in rearranging meals and feedings, and in providing a simple means of detecting errors of omission as well as commission.

There is universal agreement that, in addition to caloric restriction, it is desirable to maintain a relatively high protein intake. Such a regimen reduces the negative nitrogen balance and prevents specific amino acid deficiencies which are more likely to occur in the presence of calorie-deficient diets. A high protein diet takes advantage of the specific dynamic action of protein, preventing to some extent the fall in metabolic rate which follows restriction of caloric intake. An adequate protein intake assists in maintaining a more constant blood sugar level, thus avoiding the relative hyperglycemia immediately after a predominantly carbohydrate meal and the relative "hypoglycemia" 2 to 3 hr later. Protein foods have increased "satiety" value. This, no doubt, is due, in part at least, to the increased specific dynamic action of proteins and the facilitation of gluconeogenesis.

Shifts in salt and water metabolism often induce relatively wide fluctuations in body weight from day to day. It is therefore preferable for patients to weigh themselves once weekly. This minimizes the effects of daily fluctuations and gives a true picture of the actual overall effect of the dietary regimen. The fact that rapid shifts in body weight usually reflect alterations in salt and water intake or loss is taken advantage of by unscrupulous individuals who advertise "how to lose 12 lb in 12 days!" Physicians may take advantage of the effect of salt restriction in encouraging patients temporarily, since this will, of course, greatly increase the rate of weight loss. However, the disappointment which follows the slower rate of loss after a week or so on this regimen usually offsets its psychologic advantages. Physiologically, there is little advantage, and indeed some danger, in restricting unnecessarily the intake of sodium chloride on a weight-reduction program, unless edema or excess fluid retention is present. *Under no circumstances should water intake be restricted,* since dehydration is undesirable in a prolonged dietary regimen, and since edema is not effectively controlled by water restriction.

In female patients with active ovarian function, it is helpful to point out that weight gain normally occurs during the 10 days prior to the onset of menstruation, since patients who maintain their diet carefully may be disappointed to observe no weight loss during the premenstrual period. This periodic reten-

tion of salt and water adjusts itself automatically by a subsequent diuresis and increased rate of weight loss at the end of the cycle.

Total starvation or near total starvation, i.e., 200 to 300 Cal per day, has some support as a rapid means of weight reduction. Its advantages lie in the stimulation this vigorous program exerts on all fat-mobilizing mechanisms in the body, and the encouragement rapid weight loss provides for a more persistent effort at moderate caloric restriction over the long term. Patients must appreciate the fact, however, that only a small proportion of the weight lost during the first few days of total starvation is adipose tissue and that a major proportion is salt and water, which will be retained again with resumption of food intake. In general, prolonged periods of total starvation are undesirable, but short periods may be a very useful adjunct to a dietary program. Certain patients will prefer 1 day a week of total or near-total starvation as a means of attaining a significant caloric reduction in conjunction with moderate restriction of calories during the remainder of the week. With rigid dietary restriction there occurs a decrease in renal clearance of water and a rise in serum uric acid. In patients with familial hyperuricemia or with a known gouty history it is desirable to prescribe a uricosuric agent such as probenecid (Benemid), 0.5 to 1.0 Gm daily, during periods of dietary restriction.

Exercise. Increased physical exercise is excellent for improving general health and body "tone" in individuals without serious organic disease. Patients should be informed, however, that it requires a great deal of exercise to assist appreciably in weight loss. Thus, if food intake is held constant (and this may present difficulties with increased exercise), playing 18 holes of golf may utilize 800 to 1000 extra calories. Exercise is helpful, and its value should not be underestimated, but the quantitative aspects should be carefully discussed with each patient. There are dangers in excessive exercise by patients on a diet with rigidly restricted caloric intake.

Vitamin and Mineral Supplements. Emphasis should be placed on a well-rounded, nutritious diet, since there may be essential factors of which we are not now cognizant. In addition, it is wise to provide an adequate supplement of the known vitamins. This is most easily accomplished by giving daily one or two of the readily available multivitamin tablets. Patients should know that it is vital for their good health that they abide by the restrictions imposed but that they also eat *all* the diet which they are permitted.

Only two mineral replacements need to be considered—calcium and iron. The indication for these is greatest during periods of growth and pregnancy. Because skimmed milk is permissible in large amounts on most weight-reduction diets, it is usually unnecessary to prescribe additional calcium unless the patient cannot drink milk. Under these circumstances, calcium lactate in dosage of 0.3 Gm three times a day will supply ample calcium. Iron supplementation is neces-

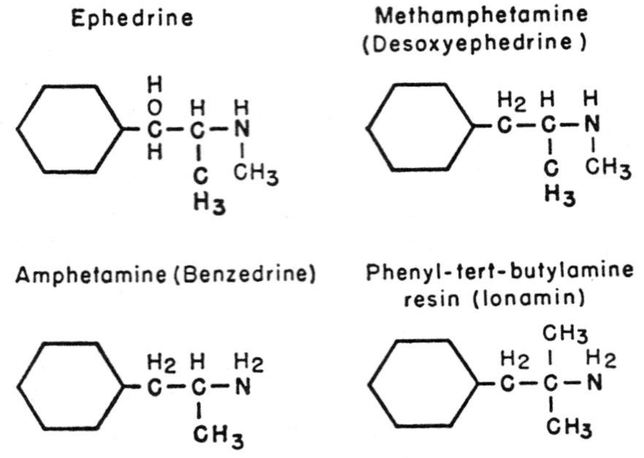

Fig. 78-2. Amphetamine and congeners.

sary only in pregnancy, in growing children, and in patients suffering from iron-deficiency anemia.

Appetite Depressants. Depression of appetite by a pharmacologic agent can facilitate weight loss, although it is apparent that as soon as the pharmacologic effect wears off, or the medication is discontinued, appetite will return and weight gain will recur unless the patient's inherent capacity to control his food intake has been altered fundamentally. That the pharmacologic agent used for these purposes be devoid of serious toxic side effects is axiomatic.

CENTRAL DEPRESSION OF APPETITE. Unfortunately there is no pharmacologic agent available at this time which acts primarily by depressing the "appetite center." This type of depression is seen regularly in disease states such as hepatitis and uremia and as a toxic manifestation of drugs such as digitalis. It will be of considerable clinical interest to observe whether or not it is possible to develop a pharmacologic agent which will effectively reduce appetite through its centrally mediated action without at the same time inducing some degree of nausea or general feeling of ill health.

SUBSTANCES WHICH DEPRESS APPETITE BY INDUCING A SENSE OF WELL-BEING. Amphetamine and its derivatives are the prototype of this group of substances. These agents are commonly referred to as "anorexigenic" or "anorectic." There is no evidence to show, however, that their action results from a depression of the "appetite center." As a result of stimulation, or a "lift," the patient's drive toward overeating may be significantly modified and as far as he is concerned, the over-all effect of the drug is "appetite-depressing." Obviously, drugs which create such a state of euphoria may lead to habituation in certain individuals.

Amphetamine and its derivatives have been shown to depress food intake in man as well as in experimental animals. Patients experience a sense of well-being after the ingestion of these drugs, and it is thought that the reduction in appetite is a consequence of distraction. At least in the hyperphagia which follows frontal lobotomy, no depression of appetite is induced by amphetamine or its congeners.

At present there is a large number of derivatives of amphetamine sulfate (Benzedrine) and closely related compounds available for clinical use, for example, dextroamphetamine sulfate (Dexedrine), levoamphetamine sulfate and phosphate, levoamphetamine alginate (Levonor), methamphetamine hydrochloride (Amphodroxyn, Desoxyephedrine, Desoxyn, Desyphed, Dexoval, Desoxyfed, Drinalfa, Efroxine, Methedrine, Norodin, Semoxydrine, Syndrox), phenylpropanolamine (Propadrine), phenmetrazine (Preludin), phenyl-tert-butylamine resin (Ionamin), and diethylpropion (Tenuate and Tepanil).

Although it is unfortunate that manufacturers avoid or disclaim the relationship of many of these substances with amphetamine, the fact is that the structural formulas differ very little (Fig. 78-2). The dextro form of amphetamine differs in its pharmacologic action from the levo form in that the cephalotropic effect is enhanced and the cardiovascular actions are less intense. However, this fact suggests that the dextro form might be expected to cause anxiety, restlessness or sleeplessness at the same dosage level. The action of methamphetamine differs little from dextroamphetamine except in its somewhat enhanced cardiovascular effects. Since phenylpropanolamine may be sold without prescription, it has become a common ingredient of many weight-reducing tablets (Didol, Rx 1121). Although if given in adequate dosage phenylpropanolamine may reduce appetite, in the usual dosage found in most weight-reducing tablets (25 mg or less) it is no more effective than a placebo. Phenmetrazine, although subjected to intensive study and claimed to be quite different, is a typical congener of amphetamine with the effectiveness of dextroamphetamine. Phenyl-tert-butylamine resin is advertised as not being an amphetamine drug, although it clearly belongs to the amphetamine series, as a study of its structural formula indicates (Fig. 78-2).

The usual dosage of amphetamine sulfate (Benzedrine) or dextroamphetamine sulfate (Dexedrine) is 5 mg given 30 to 60 min before meals. It may be necessary in some patients to omit the evening dose because of increased nervousness or sleeplessness. Long-acting preparations which can be given in a single dose of 10 to 15 mg each morning are also useful. These substances may prove helpful for some patients during the early weeks of restricted food intake.

Although serious reactions are rarely encountered with amphetamine and its congeners, the physician must be alert to the sympathomimetic effect of these agents in causing a rise in blood pressure, increased cardiac rate and work, and the possible development of cardiac arrhythmias. Since tolerance to these drugs develops relatively rapidly, their usefulness is short-lived unless the dosage is increased. As noted above, habituation has been reported for some of these substances.

BULK PRODUCERS. Repeated attempts have been made to satiate the appetite by means of bulk of low caloric content. Leafy vegetables such as cabbage, spinach, and lettuce are helpful in many patients and constitute an important element in most low-caloric diets. Addition of calorie-free bulk to the diet does not automatically displace calorie-containing food unless specific restrictions are prescribed. Because of the significant reduction in fat content of the diet, patients may experience constipation; for this reason bulk producers such as Colace, 50 to 200 mg daily, and agar may be required.

Metabolic Stimulants Including Hormones. Repeated efforts have been made to discover a nontoxic agent which would maintain a normal metabolic level in the face of weight loss. Dinitrophenol has had the widest use. The consensus today is that its undesirable toxic side reactions make its use unjustified.

In most instances, substances of this type are being employed by physicians or patients in an attempt to induce *weight loss without caloric restriction*. To do this, it is obviously necessary to raise basal metabolic level *above normal*. There is no known substance which can be used safely to increase metabolic level above normal for prolonged periods of time without danger of toxicity.

In the mind of the lay public, "hormones" are the most important cause of obesity and are hopefully considered to be its cure. The well-informed physician recognizes to what a small extent disturbances in hormone secretion are primarily responsible for obesity and how futile most types of hormone therapy are as cures of obesity.

No pituitary preparation now available is useful in weight reduction. Male and female gonadal hormones and adrenal cortical hormones have no place in therapy unless specific deficiency of these hormones exists. Thyroid therapy has received wide application and merits special discussion.

Thyroid therapy is effective substitution therapy in patients with hypothyroidism. Unfortunately, however, the number of patients with hypothyroidism among the obese is relatively small. Thyroid therapy has a definite and sustained effect on the metabolism of the hypothyroid case. Complete thyroid deficiency may require 0.2 Gm thyroid (USP) daily; 0.1 Gm thyroid (USP) daily should be adequate for milder cases. A given dose of thyroid will produce a predictable rise in basal metabolic rate in a patient with hypothyroidism, and a daily dose of thyroid will maintain the increase in basal metabolic rate indefinitely. It appears that certain patients with obesity can tolerate rather large doses of thyroid without undue symptoms but with sufficient increase in metabolic rate to assist appreciably in their weight-reduction program.

Maintenance of Ideal Weight. Patients should understand thoroughly when they undertake a reduction diet that, in all probability, some degree of dietary restriction or discretion will be necessary permanently after ideal weight has been attained. The degree of dietary restriction is best attained by establishing the custom of weighing in each morning and adjusting the day's intake of food to the changes in body weight. It may be necessary at this time for the physician to review the comparative caloric content of certain foods which may have been withheld during the diet regimen. It is usually desirable to discuss in detail the calories contained in alcoholic beverages.

Once ideal weight has been attained, a patient should be encouraged to visit his physician every 3 to 6 months for examination and advice. The continued interest of the physician is of paramount importance to the health and happiness of his patient.

REFERENCES

Gordon, E. S., E. M. Goldberg, J. J. Brandabur, J. B. Gee, and J. Rankin: Abnormal Energy Metabolism in Obesity, Trans. Assoc. Amer. Physicians, 75:118, 1962.

Kekwick, A.: On Adiposity, Brit. Med. J., Aug. 6, 1960, p. 407.

Modell, Walter: Status and Prospect of Drugs for Overeating, J.A.M.A., 173:1131, 1960.

Rosenberg, B. A.: A Double-blind Study of Diethylpropion in Obesity, Am. J. Med. Sci., 242:201, 1961.

Section 2

Hormonal Disorders

79 GENERAL CONSIDERATIONS AND MAJOR SYNDROMES

George W. Thorn

INTRODUCTION

Isolation, purification, identification, and synthesis of new hormones continue at a rapid rate, and it is reasonable to assume that within the near future those few remaining unidentified principles will also succumb to the technical advances of chemistry and biophysics. Noteworthy among recorded achievements are the determination of the structure and amino acid sequence of adrenocorticotropin, melanocyte-stimulating hormone, and insulin; the synthesis of posterior pituitary hormone and a host of adrenal and gonadal steroid hormones; and the identification and isolation of several new thyroid substances. Coupled with these chemical advances is a rapidly expanding body of knowledge concerning the regulation of hormonal secretion and the precise locus of hormonal action. Although this latter field has barely been opened, the effect of insulin on permeability to certain sugars, the mechanism whereby estrogens provide energy for the growth of their target organs, and the physical modification of mitochondrial particles by thyroxin illustrate the type of information rapidly becoming available.

It is now generally agreed that hormones do not initiate new events in the complicated biochemistry of metabolic processes, but rather produce their effects by regulating enzymatic and other chemical reactions already present. In view of the relatively large number of hormones, their diverse chemical structures, and their multiple sites of action, it can be assumed that scarcely a single important metabolic event can escape the effect of their primary or secondary action. From this one may conclude that a true understanding of any disease process or physiologic disorder must encompass an appreciation of the possible etiologic role of hormones and the factors regulating their synthesis, release, and degradation. In this regard, one can point to such widely diverse actions as the effect of catechol amines (adrenal medulla) on brain metabolism and psychologic behavior; the effect of adrenal steroids on the inflammatory reaction associated with infection, trauma, surgery, or burns; the effect of insulin on adipose tissue metabolism; and the importance of growth hormone on the fabrication of body proteins.

MECHANISMS OF ENDOCRINOPATHIES

Characteristically, endocrine abnormalities arise as a consequence of increased or decreased hormone secretion. In the majority of patients, the clinical manifestations derive from an excess of or deficiency of the *normally* secreted hormone. However, in certain syndromes, such as some cases of adrenal virilism, the endocrinopathy may result from secretion of an abnormal hormone. In addition, hormonal disorders may result from aberrations in the metabolism or degradation of hormones. For example, a deficiency of plasma proteins may decrease the quantity of hormone-carrying protein in the blood and hence modify significantly the balance between "free" and "bound" thyroid hormone; liver disease may alter the conjugation or degradation of steroid hormones, giving rise to abnormal blood and tissue hormone levels. In such types of abnormalities, however, serious endocrine disorders will result only if the "servo-regulating" mechanism, or feedback response, fails to stimulate the appropriate reaction in the trophic gland. Endocrine abnormalities may also develop when local tissues are unable to respond to a normal hormonal level. For example, localized myxedema over the tibia may occur in the presence of thyrotoxicosis or euthyroidism; in cases of pseudohypoparathyroidism, the abnormali-

ties observed in hypoparathyroidism occur despite the presence of normal parathyroid glands. In some endocrinopathies, heightened tissue susceptibility to hormone action is the determining factor in the genesis of the syndrome, for example, hirsutism in young women with a minimal abnormality in androgenic steroid secretion, or extreme degrees of hyperpigmentation observed in patients with early adrenal insufficiency and increased melanin pigmentation on a racial basis.

Hormonal secretions in general show wide fluctuations throughout the 24-hr period, periods of high activity often alternating with those of reduced secretion; for example, in the early morning the level of adrenal cortical secretory activity is high. Evidence is accumulating that endocrinopathy may result from a loss of cyclic diurnal pattern due to a more or less constant hormonal elaboration throughout the day and night, resulting in only a slight increase, if any, in total secretion. Two important considerations have been derived from these observations: (1) Interpretation of single determinations of hormone content—of blood, tissues, or urine—reflecting instantaneous or relatively short collection periods may be unreliable; for final evaluation, repeated determinations, longer collection periods, or isotopic "turnover" studies may be required. (2) Clinical application of the cyclic method of hormone administration has been quite successful in minimizing undesirable hormone side effects while maintaining control of the underlying disease process.

DIAGNOSTIC APPROACH TO ENDOCRINE ABNORMALITIES

The suspicion that an endocrine abnormality may play a role in a patient's illness will often derive initially from the gross physical appearance of the patient, as in myxedema, hyperthyroidism, pituitary dwarfism or gigantism, acromegaly, hypogonadism, carotenemia (diabetes mellitus or hypothyroidism), Addison's disease, Cushing's syndrome, and the adrenogenital syndrome. Although a careful history and physical examination will in most instances provide presumptive evidence of an underlying endocrine disorder, the definitive diagnosis will almost invariably depend upon the values obtained from laboratory examinations. Here, accuracy in diagnosis depends upon the specificity of the laboratory test, its precision and its reproducibility, the care and understanding with which specimens are collected, and the reliability of the laboratory that carries out the procedures. In the past, endocrine abnormalities were established for the most part on the basis of nonspecific laboratory examinations such as the basal metabolic rate; roentgenograms; glucose tolerance test; and blood sugar, calcium, sodium, and potassium determinations. Today, tests of endocrine dysfunction are employing more and more frequently measurement of the specific hormones under consideration, for example, protein-bound iodine level, blood and urinary steroid values, urinary gonadotropins, and blood ACTH or insulin levels. It is essential for the practicing physician to realize, however, that a single determination of a specific hormone (in blood, urine, or tissue) does not necessarily estab'ish or exclude an endocrine abnormality. The addition of hormonal "turnover" or "secretory" measurements by means of isotopic techniques represents a great step forward. The use of stressful situations or specific substances such as ACTH (adrenocorticotropin) for the adrenal, thyroid-stimulating hormone (TSH) for the thyroid, and glucose for the detection of early diabetes permits one to test the functional reserve of these endocrine systems and thereby facilitates the diagnosis of potential endocrine deficiency at a time when prophylactic measures may prove effective. In the succeeding chapters, particular attention will be devoted to indicating the usefulness and limitations of diagnostic methods and the degree of specificity attached to the procedure. Because of its great practical importance, the source of common errors related to these determinations will also be emphasized.

ENDOCRINE SYNDROMES

Although secretions of the endocrine glands govern widespread metabolic activities throughout the body, from the viewpoint of the internist, major endocrine disorders present over and over again as a limited number of syndromes. These will be reviewed briefly in relation to the cardinal manifestations of disease.

WEAKNESS AND INCREASED FATIGABILITY (see also Chap. 43). These are without doubt the most frequent presenting symptoms of adult patients seeking assistance from the internist or general practitioner. Although in the majority of instances these complaints derive primarily from emotional or psychologic disturbances, underlying organic disease must always be considered. When endocrine abnormalities are suspected, one should inquire first whether the symptoms have been accompanied by *weight loss*—if so, adrenal cortical insufficiency, hyperthyroidism, and diabetes mellitus should be considered. Adrenal cortical insufficiency, if present, should be accompanied by some increase in pigmentation, hypotension, gastrointestinal disturbances, and perhaps salt craving. Hyperthyroidism would be suggested by goiter, eye changes, tremor, intolerance for heat, etc., and diabetes mellitus by polyuria and polydipsia.

Without weight loss, but with symptoms of weakness and fatigability, one would consider hypothyroidism, hypopituitarism, hyperparathyroidism, and hyperaldosteronism. The first of these is characteristically associated with delayed reflexes, intolerance to cold, dry skin, and carotenemia. Hypopituitarism is suggested by oligomenorrhea or amenorrhea in the female, impotence in the male, decreased tolerance to cold, hypoglycemic episodes, and hypotension. Hyperparathyroidism is suggested by the association of bone pain, renal calculi, and polyuria. Hyperaldosteronism

might be accompanied by significant hypertension, demonstrable muscular weakness, polyuria, and electrocardiographic changes that suggest potassium depletion.

MENSTRUAL IRREGULARITIES (see also Chap. 21). In addition to pregnancy and local disease of the uterus, menstrual irregularities are associated with four major endocrine disturbances: (1) *primary ovarian failure,* prior to natural menopause and characterized by hot flashes, gain in weight, increased emotional instability, and elevated urinary values of follicle-stimulating hormone; (2) *secondary ovarian failure,* associated with reduced or absent urinary gonadotropins and evidence of other target gland deficiencies, i.e., thyroid and adrenal; (3) *hypothyroidism,* in which menorrhagia as well as oligomenorrhea frequently occur; (4) *adrenogenital syndrome,* in which oligomenorrhea or amenorrhea is seen in combination with increased muscular development, hirsutism, and other signs of masculinization.

HIRSUTISM (see also Chap. 34). Increased body hair in females and decreased scalp hair in both sexes is a frequent disorder for which patients seek medical attention. Unfortunately, to date, most female patients with increased hair do not have a demonstrable excess of adrenal or ovarian androgens. Increased androgenic secretion should be considered when *hirsutism* is associated with menstrual irregularities and amenorrhea, or with other evidence of virilism, i.e., increased muscular development and increased size of clitoris.

Although loss of scalp hair and baldness is almost never due to a specific endocrinopathy, a receding hair line in female patients associated with *increased* body hair should always suggest excessive androgenic hormone secretion of adrenal or gonadal origin. Thinning of the hair is frequent in patients with Cushing's syndrome, hypothyroidism, or hypopituitarism. It is rare, however, to observe disturbances in hair growth as a manifestation of serious endocrine abnormality in the absence of rather well-defined signs and symptoms of adrenal, pituitary, or gonadal dysfunction.

IMPOTENCE AND DECREASED LIBIDO (see also Chap. 22). Although these cardinal manifestations of functional disorder are a frequent basis for medical consultation, they are rarely due primarily to endocrinopathies. In addition to primary disease of the generative organs, however, *anterior pituitary deficiency,* especially associated with chromophobe adenomas, should be considered. Evidence of local tumor (changes in vision, headache, etc.) and associated target gland deficiencies (adrenal, thyroid, and gonadal) should be sought. Patients with diabetes mellitus will often exhibit both impotence and decreased libido, but in most instances this occurs after the disease has been present for some time.

OBESITY (see also Chap. 78). Obesity suggests the possibility of an underlying endocrine disturbance, which in practice rarely is causative. However, two serious disorders must be considered in patients with marked, generalized obesity. The first is diabetes mellitus, and this should be investigated with a post-prandial glucose determination and a glucose tolerance test, if fasting blood glucose levels are within the normal range and if sugar is not present in the urine. The second serious disorder is insulinoma. Hunger, increased appetite, and weight gain are characteristic of patients with insulinoma as well as those with "reactive" hypoglycemia. The former experience greatest hunger and symptomatology after prolonged fast, the latter shortly after eating, particularly a meal of high carbohydrate content. In both instances appetite and food intake are stimulated by absolute or relative hypoglycemia, and the vicious cycle is continued.

Hypothyroidism and mild hypopituitarism may be associated with moderate obesity. The final diagnosis of the former will require laboratory tests of thyroid function; the latter requires tests for the adequacy of target gland function.

Gross obesity in Cushing's syndrome is rare—what is more common is loss of adipose tissue in the extremities with an increase in abdominal fat pad, striae, and "buffalo hump."

There is no doubt that castration or ovarian failure predispose to obesity. This is not only well-established in man but of practical significance to poultry and cattle raisers. However, in young women there often occurs a reversal of this cycle; namely, rapid weight gain secondary to excess food intake, stress, and anxieties, which may be *followed* by oligomenorrhea or amenorrhea. Whether the weight gain itself is of primary importance in the genesis of the ovarian dysfunction, or whether weight gain and altered gonadal function are both secondary to changes in the hypothalamic centers is not known. However, it is well-established that with improvement in emotional status and with weight loss, normal ovulation and menstruation will often ensue. In contrast, primary ovarian failure from organic disease is usually attended by hot flushes and other evidence of vasomotor instability as well as by elevated urinary gonadotropin levels.

HYPERTENSION (see also Chap. 132). Hypertension is another frequent disorder encountered in medical practice that should suggest an underlying endocrine abnormality. The hypertensive patient with minimal abnormalities in urinary constituents but with polyuria and nocturia suggests hypokalemia (hyperaldosteronism) or hypercalcemia (hyperparathyroidism). Clinically the hypokalemic patient with *hyperaldosteronism* rarely presents with the malignant form of hypertension and characteristically exhibits neuromuscular weakness. The electrocardiogram will often reveal changes consistent with potassium depletion, whereas serum sodium concentration is usually *elevated*. The problem is to exclude hypokalemia induced by diuretic administration, especially the thiazides, and the ensuing secondary hyperaldosteronism.

The patient with hypertension, polyuria, and hypercalcemia associated with *hyperparathyroidism* will frequently give a history of urinary calculi or bone pain. He may also present the stigmas of psychoneurosis

as a consequence of sustained hypercalcemia. Band keratopathy is rare except with long-continued elevated serum calcium level. A palpable tumor in the neck, unfortunately, is usually a thyroid nodule.

Two characteristic findings in patients with hypertension secondary to *pheochromocytoma* are the cyclic nature of hypertension in the classic syndrome and the absence of obesity. Unfortunately, most tumors secrete predominantly norepinephrine; hence, the textbook picture of tachycardia, nervousness, sweating, and glucosuria is infrequent. Catechol amine excretion may be within normal values between episodes.

Hypertension and moderate obesity, particularly of the truncal type, suggest the possibility of underlying Cushing's syndrome. This possibility is greatly increased if diabetes mellitus, easy bruisability, and pink abdominal striae are present. Every hypertensive patient with diabetes mellitus should be screened for adrenal overactivity. The simplest test is a direct eosinophil count. With a count of more than 100 per cu mm, Cushing's syndrome can be reasonably excluded; with a value under 50, definitive tests should be carried out (Chap. 84).

Hypertension as an early manifestation of diabetes mellitus is uncommon. However, since hypertensive-vascular disease is such a frequent complication of diabetes mellitus, hypertensive patients—especially those who are obese—should have postprandial blood glucose determinations evaluated and glucose tolerance tested.

Hypertension as a manifestation of *adrenogenital syndrome* should be considered in young subjects with associated evidence of virilism.

ABNORMALITIES IN GROWTH (see also Chaps. 80 and 82). Abnormalities in growth, particularly in children, are associated with *hypothyroidism* and *cretinism*. The latter must be detected within the first few weeks after birth if serious damage to the central nervous system is to be prevented. All babies with *persistent* umbilical hernia should be screened for possible *hypothyroidism*. Untreated diabetes mellitus will result in retarded growth as will excess cortisol and androgen secretion. Long-standing renal disease will impair skeletal growth and mimic an endocrinopathy because of the frequent coexistence of secondary hyperparathyroidism.

Closely related to abnormalities in growth among adolescent boys is the problem of undescended testes. A conservative approach is urged, and the reader is referred to Chap. 89 for details as to the management of this important problem.

Other cardinal signs that should call attention to possible endocrine abnormalities include the following:

1. Changes in the skin (see also Chap. 108). Dryness in hypothyroidism and Addison's disease; thin, atrophic skin with "wrinkles" in pituitary and gonadal failure; easy bruisability in Cushing's syndrome; moist, fine, warm skin in hyperthyroidism; coarse, reduplicated skin in acromegaly; hyperpigmentation in Addison's disease.

2. Arthropathies (see Chap. 232) are not infrequent in acromegaly, gigantism, myxedema, and primary gonadal failure.

3. Tetany and convulsive seizures (see Chap. 52) may indicate hypoglycemia (insulinoma, reactive hypoglycemia, Addison's disease, hypopituitarism), hypocalcemia (hypoparathyroidism), or hypokalemia (hyperaldosteronism, Cushing's syndrome).

4. The presence of edema (see Chap. 16) should suggest hypothyroidism or myxedema as well as secondary hyperaldosteronism and Cushing's syndrome.

5. Psychologic abnormalities (see Chap. 42) are frequently observed in Addison's disease and Cushing's syndrome as well as in hypopituitarism, hypothyroidism, hyperthyroidism, hyperparathyroidism, and acromegaly.

IATROGENIC ENDOCRINOPATHIES

With the general use of the corticosteroids, thyroid, and the sex hormones as nonspecific therapeutic agents, new and difficult problems present themselves to the internist and endocrinologist. One may be faced on the one hand with iatrogenic Cushing's syndrome, hyperthyroidism, or virilism—or severe adrenal insufficiency or hypothyroidism if hormone therapy is discontinued rapidly or completely. Special problems relating to these phenomena will, because of their seriousness, be discussed at length in relation to each of the specific hormones so implicated. The use of hormones as nonspecific therapeutic agents, while offering great promise in many serious and often fatal diseases, is fraught with difficulties and requires, in addition to a thorough knowledge of the endocrine preparations a comprehension of their physiologic and pharmacologic effects, the exercise of sound judgment on the part of the physician, and complete cooperation on the part of the patient. Without these the end result accompanying endocrine pharmacotherapeutics may be more disabling than the untreated cause of the primary disease.

80 DISEASES OF THE ANTERIOR LOBE OF THE PITUITARY GLAND

Don H. Nelson and George W. Thorn

The pituitary gland lies at the base of the brain in a bony cavity, the sella turcica, within the sphenoid bone. The normal gland measures $10 \times 13 \times 6$ mm and weighs approximately 0.6 Gm. Anatomically it is divided into the anterior lobe, which constitutes three-quarters of the weight of the gland, a rudimentary intermediate lobe, and a posterior or neural lobe. The classic histology of the anterior lobe divides the cells into three types, depending on the presence and staining characteristics of the intracellular granules. These are the chromophobes, which are agranular, the eo-

sinophils and the basophils, in the proportions of approximately 52, 37, and 11 per cent, respectively. More detailed studies suggest that some of the agranular cells may contain fine acidophilic and basophilic granules; hence the term "amphophils."

The anterior lobe secretes a variety of peptide hormones, of which six are clearly defined. Growth hormone (HGH) has a generalized somatic effect on growth; adrenocorticotropin (ACTH) stimulates the secretory activity of the adrenal cortex; thyroid-stimulating hormone (thyrotropin, TSH) stimulates the formation and release of thyroid hormones; follicle-stimulating hormone (FSH) stimulates growth of the graafian follicle and estrogen secretion in the female and spermatogenesis in the male; luteinizing hormone (LH) initiates ovulation and luteinization of the mature follicle in the female; in the male, this hormone is the testicular interstitial cell-stimulating hormone (ICSH), responsible for male hormone secretion. Prolactin or lactogenic hormone (LtH) is responsible for secretion of milk by the properly developed mammary gland. Although production of the melanocyte-stimulating hormone (MSH) is classically ascribed to the intermediate lobe, this hormone may also be a secretion of the anterior lobe.

According to classic concepts, the chromophobe cells are considered to be nonsecretory, the eosinophilic cells responsible for secretion of GH, LH, and LtH, and the basophilic cells producing ACTH, TSH, and FSH. Such a simple classification, however, does not now seem probable; some pituitary tumors associated with Cushing's syndrome have been found to be composed of chromophobe as well as eosinophilic cells, although the largest number are small basophilic tumors. Similarly, eosinophilic tumors are most often associated with increased growth hormone production, but tumors of other cell types may occasionally be responsible.

PITUITARY TUMORS

Pituitary tumors account for approximately 10 per cent of all intracranial tumors. By far the commonest pituitary tumor is the chromophobe adenoma, which is usually nonsecretory in nature. Active pituitary tumors usually secrete only one pituitary hormone in excess. Tumors secreting GH, ACTH, MSH, TSH, and LtH have all been described, although the last three types of tumor are very rare. FSH- or LH-secreting tumors are notable by their absence.

In addition to producing the signs and symptoms of hormone excess, discussed in later sections on the specific hormones, these tumors may compress and destroy normal pituitary tissue within the sella turcica and produce hormonal deficiency states, or they may extend out of the sella turcica to compress the optic nerves, hypothalamus, and other nervous structures in the vicinity. Pressure on the optic chiasma most often involves the decussating nerve fibers supplying the nasal retinal fields and leads to loss of the temporal fields of vision and classical bitemporal hemianopsia. Further extension of the tumor may involve one or both optic nerves and result in loss of visual acuity and even in complete blindness. These tumors may also compress the hypothalamus and result in disturbances in sleep, temperature control, appetite, and autonomic nervous functions. Curiously, these tumors are not known to damage the supraopticohypophyseal tract to a degree to cause diabetes insipidus. Involvement of the third, fourth, and sixth cranial nerves is rare but may occur. Headache is a frequent complaint in patients with this condition and has no well-defined pattern.

Clinical evaluation of these patients should include roentgenograms of the skull and visual fields, ophthalmoscopic examination, spinal fluid examination (particularly for increased protein content), and pneumoencephalography, especially in patients with severe optic nerve compression, increased intracranial pressure, or signs of hypothalamic and brain involvement.

Therapy of pituitary tumors generally involves a choice between pituitary irradiation or surgery. Postponement of specific treatment is justifiable in occasional patients with small, localized chromophobe adenomas, in which case specific hormonal replacement therapy should be initiated and the patient carefully observed for signs of tumor growth and extension. Surgical resection of tumor tissue is indicated when there is rapid deterioration of vision, ventricular obstruction, or significant brain compression. Although surgery provides the greatest opportunity for arrest of tumor growth, there is a calculated morbidity and mortality, particularly with the large tumors extending outside the sella turcica.

Radiotherapy in tissue doses of 3,500 to 4,500 r is often associated with regression of the tumor and relief of local signs and symptoms. In these doses, normal pituitary tissue and surrounding nervous structures are unharmed. Some tumors recur and may require further x-ray therapy, or surgery. Further experience with such experimental techniques as cryohypophysectomy, high-voltage and proton-beam irradiation, and radioactive implantations offers hope for better methods of treating these tumors.

Hemorrhage into a tumor, so-called "pituitary apoplexy," often results in an acute catastrophe accompanied by severe headache, blindness, hypotension or shock, fever, and signs of meningeal irritation or brain involvement. Emergency treatment is required, which may include surgical aspiration of the sella turcica, use of adrenal steroids, and other supportive measures. Pituitary apoplexy may occur spontaneously and is occasionally observed following irradiation.

The craniopharyngioma, which is usually suprasellar in position, is the most common type of tumor involving the pituitary gland in childhood and thus the most common cause of prepuberal hypopituitarism. The tumor represents a secretory vestige of Rathke's pouch cut off from its origin in the roof of the pharynx and carried cephalad by the migrating pituitary anlage. The viscous, cholesterol-containing fluid of such suprasellar cysts is prone to calcification, which provides a useful diagnostic sign on x-ray examination. Although these tumors are more frequent in the younger age group, occasionally they are slow-growing and may not be clinically apparent until adult life. These patients often mature normally and come to the physician with an adult form of hypopituitarism. These tumors usually require surgical intervention. Other tumors which may involve the pituitary or the suprasellar area include meningiomas, epidermoid or dermoid tumors, primary or metastatic carcinomas, and granulomatous disorders such as sarcoidosis, gummas, tuberculomas, and Hand-Schüller-Christian disease.

GROWTH HORMONE

Growth hormone, unlike the other anterior pituitary hormones, does not have a specific "target organ" but has a generalized effect on all tissues and organs. This hormone has a molecular weight of 29,000, although there is some indication that an "active core" may be considerably smaller. Though once thought to be solely concerned with growth in the early years of life, growth hormone has been found to exert significant physiologic functions throughout life. It has been shown to facilitate amino acid transport and incorporation into protein, to mobilize free fatty acids from peripheral fat stores, and to reduce lipid synthesis. Growth hormone also causes renal retention and body storage of calcium, phosphorus, sodium, potassium, and nitrogen as part of its generalized anabolic action. It has an anti-insulin or diabetogenic action and, in large doses, can produce glucosuria, impaired glucose tolerance, and insulin resistance. Growth hormone is responsible for the elevated level of serum inorganic phosphorus and alkaline phosphatase observed in growing children.

Growth hormone is species-specific, and only primate growth hormone has been found to have significant physiologic effects in man and to be capable of stimulating growth in pituitary dwarfs.

Concentration of plasma growth hormone can now be determined with immunologic techniques, and elevated levels have been found in most patients with acromegaly. Significantly, growth hormone levels have been shown to increase following exercise, prolonged fast, and during hypoglycemia, which suggests a dynamic physiologic role for this hormone throughout life, in addition to its growth-promoting effects in childhood.

Growth Hormone Secreting Tumors

Marie, in 1886, first described the classical clinical manifestations of acromegaly. One year later, Minkowski reported a case with a pituitary tumor, and Benda subsequently showed that such tumors were eosinophilic in nature. In 1895, Brissaud and Meige suggested an association between gigantism and acromegaly, and Hutchinson subsequently reported the pathologic findings in three cases of gigantism associated with pituitary tumors. Acromegaly and gigantism are now recognized as identical disturbances of growth hormone secretion, differing only in the age of onset of the disorder.

Gigantism

Prior to puberty, excess growth hormone secretion results in a generalized overgrowth of the skeleton and soft tissues. Early in the course of the disorder, these patients are usually physically strong and alert. Later in the disease, however, pituitary insufficiency may develop, with its associated weakness and easy fatigability. Hypogonadism of the pituitary type develops during the course of the disease.

The underlying lesion is generally an eosinophilic or mixed cell adenoma of the anterior lobe which is usually visible radiologically. The condition, although rare, presents no difficulty in diagnosis and needs only to be differentiated clinically from the tall stature of primary gonadal failure. Persons with the latter condition exhibit the characteristic eunuchoid habitus and

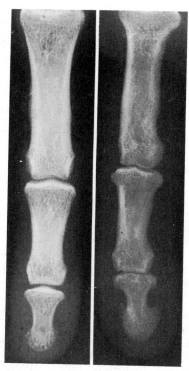

Fig. 80-2. Characteristic tufting or "arrowhead" appearance of the terminal phalanx in acromegaly (*right*). Normal phalanx for comparison (*left*). Note also the thickness of the acromegalic finger.

associated gonadal failure and, unlike the patient with gigantism, have increased titers of urinary follicle stimulating hormone characteristic of primary hypogonadism. Treatment of pituitary gigantism is similar to that for acromegaly.

Acromegaly

In adults, the same type of pituitary tumor producing excess growth hormone results in the clinical picture of acromegaly. The disease is usually first manifested by changes in facial features and overgrowth of the head, hands, and feet which may necessitate an increase in hat, glove, or shoe size (Fig. 80-1). In other instances, headache or visual disturbances from local effects of the expanding pituitary tumor may be the first indications of the disorder.

The fully developed syndrome is easily recognized, but in the earlier stages, comparison of serial photographs over a span of years may be extremely helpful in documenting a gradual and progressive change in features. The hands and feet are broad and greatly enlarged, the ends of the digits are square, and prognathism may be so marked as to interfere with mastication (Fig. 80-2). Arthritic manifestations are not unusual, and widespread osteoarthritic-like changes in the bones and joints are often demonstrable Patients with acromegaly are particularly subject to psycho-

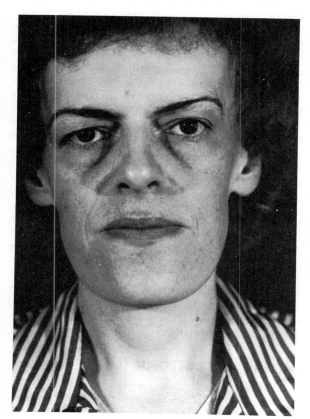

Fig. 80-1. A forty-four-year-old woman with arrested acromegaly. Onset of the disease occurred when patient was twenty-four years of age, when enlargement of the sella turcica was demonstrated. Following x-ray therapy of the pituitary no further progression of the disease has been observed.

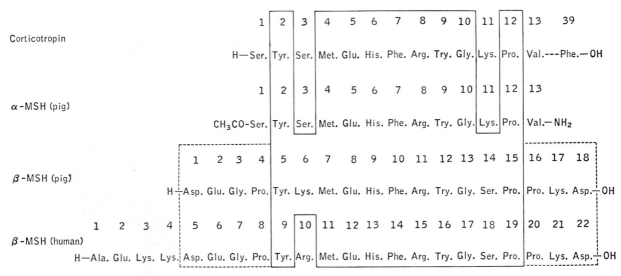

Fig. 80-3. Amino acid sequences of corticotropin and melanocyte-stimulating hormones (*Modified from I. Harris.*)

logic disturbances and almost always exhibit considerable emotional instability.

Among the associated endocrine disturbances, enlargement of the thyroid and an increased basal metabolic rate are frequently found. Hyperthyroidism, however, occurs in only a small percentage of cases. Although frank diabetes mellitus is present in only 10 to 15 per cent of these patients, glucose tolerance is impaired in the majority of patients during the active phase of the disease. Diabetes mellitus, when present, is typically mild but may be relatively resistant to insulin therapy. Libido may be increased at the onset but is lost subsequently, and gonadal atrophy may occur late in the disease. The course of the disease is usually one of benign chronicity, but fatal termination may occur as a result of cardiac failure, diabetic acidosis, local complications of the tumor, or unrecognized hypopituitarism.

DIAGNOSIS. Diagnosis is made by the typical changes in body configuration and the demonstration of pituitary tumor by x-ray or visual field defects. Because the skeletal changes are in large measure permanent, the real challenge in diagnosis is to determine whether there is continual hypersecretion of growth hormone, or whether a deficiency of growth hormone and perhaps of other hormones has resulted from pituitary destruction from pressure, hemorrhage, or earlier x-ray therapy. Activity of the process is implied by continued skeletal and soft-tissue growth, by the presence of diabetes mellitus or a significantly impaired glucose tolerance test, by an increased plasma level of growth hormone, by elevated levels of serum inorganic phosphorus and alkaline phosphatase, and by increased excretion of hydroxyproline in the urine. Patients with active acromegaly may show a hyperactive increase in urinary 17-ketosteroid excretion following intravenous ACTH while 17-hydroxysteroid excretion is normal.

There is one familial condition without evidence of increased growth hormone, the Touraine-Solenti-Golé syndrome, in which afflicted individuals present acromegalic features. Particularly suggestive of acromegaly in this condition are the skin changes; thus its common designation, pachydermoperiostitis (idiopathic hypertrophic osteoarthropathy). Although the fingers are often clubbed, the periosteal thickening of the bones is not what one would expect to see in acromegaly. The amount of growth hormone is of course not increased.

TREATMENT. Eosinophilic adenomas may respond to irradiation, but in general this form of therapy is not presently considered to be so effective as an ablative procedure of the pituitary gland. The presence of hypopituitarism must be suspected and the appropriate substitution therapy instituted (adrenal, thyroid, and gonadal hormones), particularly if surgery is contemplated. Because of the permanent disfigurement which acromegaly produces, the progress of the disease must be watched closely, particularly in women, and earlier surgical intervention should be considered in an attempt to minimize the cosmetic complications. Although successful therapy will not reverse the bony changes, the decrease in hypertrophy of the skin and subcutaneous tissues may produce an important improvement in appearance.

ADRENOCORTICOTROPIN (ACTH)

This hormone is a polypeptide composed of 39 amino acids with a molecular weight of approximately 4,500. The primary structure has been elucidated, and small quantities have been synthesized (Fig. 80-3).

The principal physiologic effect of this hormone is to stimulate the secretion of hydrocortisone from the adrenal cortex. Under the stimulus of ACTH, the adrenal gland also secretes corticosterone, aldosterone, estrogens, and certain so-called adrenal androgens. In the case of aldosterone, ACTH is not the chief controlling factor regulating its secretion. As part of its adrenal stimulating effect, ACTH promotes an increase in adrenal blood flow and hypertrophy of the gland. Certain extra-adrenal actions of ACTH of obscure physiologic significance include a lipid-mobilizing effect and a hypoglycemic action. ACTH has intrinsic melanocyte-stimulating activity because of similarities between its N-terminal amino acid sequence and the structure of MSH (Fig. 80-3).

Secretion of ACTH is regulated by the concentration of hydrocortisone in plasma and by various parts of the brain, particularly the ventromedial hypothalamus. Nerve cells in this area are thought to produce one or more peptide neurohormones, termed corticotropin-releasing factors (CRF), which are released into the pituitary portal circulation and stimulate the secretion of ACTH by the anterior pituitary cells. Higher centers of the brain may act to stimulate or inhibit ACTH secretion.

Central nervous system activity maintains a diurnal rhythm of ACTH secretion, which results in highest levels in early morning and lowest levels at night. There is a considerable increase in plasma ACTH concentration in adrenal insufficiency because of loss of the normal reciprocal relationship between plasma hydrocortisone concentration and ACTH secretion. Substantial increases in ACTH secretion occur during stress irrespective of the plasma steroid level. Prolonged administration of corticosteroids depresses the secretion of ACTH and results in adrenal atrophy indistinguishable from that observed in spontaneous hypopituitarism.

Cushing's Disease

In 1932, Cushing described the clinical disorder of pituitary basophilism associated with adrenocortical hyperplasia. This concept led to considerable controversy and a voluminous literature on the presence and significance of basophilic adenomas in patients with adrenocortical hyperfunction.

Relatively few patients with adrenocortical hyperfunction first come to the physician with definite enlargement of the pituitary gland; however, the incidence of pituitary tumor is significantly increased in those patients subjected to total adrenalectomy. Since bilateral total adrenalectomy has only been widely practiced for little more than a decade, it is possible that more patients will develop clinically evident pituitary tumors in due time. Curiously, most of the postadrenalectomy pituitary tumors have proved to be chromophobe adenomas. Eosinophilic and mixed-type tumors have also been found in Cushing's disease, but the largest number are associated with small basophilic tumors or hyalinization of the basophils.

Although not widely available, biologic tests for the measurement of ACTH in plasma, and more recently immunoassay techniques, may be of value in establishing the cause of adrenocortical hyperfunction. The finding of an elevated plasma ACTH level suggests a pituitary origin, but such an elevation may also be found in patients who have nonendocrine carcinomas that also secrete ACTH-like substances. In a series that we have undertaken, an elevated plasma ACTH level was found more often in those patients with a nonendocrine tumor, e.g., in the lung or pancreas, than in patients with Cushing's syndrome and adrenal hyperplasia. In an adrenalectomized patient with Cushing's disease, an abnormal elevation in ACTH, exceeding the level observed in Addison's disease or in patients adrenalectomized for other diseases, is highly suggestive of an ACTH-secreting pituitary tumor. These patients often show intense pigmentation of the skin which may be due to the MSH-like activity of ACTH referred to above or to actual secretion of MSH by the tumor.

Increased Plasma ACTH in Addison's Disease and Congenital Adrenal Hyperplasia

Elevated plasma ACTH levels are apparent within 24 hr of steroid withdrawal in patients with Addison's disease and fall to normal several hours after a physiologic dose of steroid. This excess production of ACTH is not pathologic and has not been associated with pituitary tumors. It may be, at least in part, responsible for the hyperpigmentation which occurs in this disease.

Patients with congenital adrenal hyperplasia also have elevated plasma ACTH level, because of a similar mechanism, deficient secretion of hydrocortisone. As far as is known, the pituitary gland is normal in this disease. The excess secretion of ACTH is also easily suppressed by physiologic doses of corticosteroids (see Chap. 84).

ACTH Secretion in Nonendocrine Tumors

A number of patients with Cushing's syndrome secondary to the release of ACTH-like substances from nonendocrine neoplasms has been reported. Carcinoma of the lung is the most frequent type of tumor associated with this syndrome. The exact nature of the polypeptide hormone released by such tumors is not known, although its adrenal cortical stimulating capacity has been demonstrated. It is possible that neoplastic tumors could also secrete an ACTH-releasing factor which would in turn stimulate the secretion or release of ACTH. The latter could be detected biologically by its effectiveness in the presence of an intact pituitary-adrenal system and its ineffectiveness in the absence of the anterior pituitary gland. To date, there is no evidence that these nonendocrine neoplasms secrete adrenal steroids; hence, removal of both adrenals should result in a cure of the Cushing's syndrome in circumstances which prevent the complete renewal of the primary neoplasm.

THYROTROPIN (TSH)

Thyrotropin is a glycoprotein of approximately 26,-000 molecular weight. It stimulates the uptake of iodide by the thyroid gland and the synthesis and release of thyroid hormones. Continued stimulation results in hypertrophy of the gland and an increase in the vasculature. Thyrotropin deficiency results in glandular atrophy and depressed thyroid function. The administration of thyroid hormone depresses the secretion of thyrotropin and produces similar changes in thyroid function. There is good evidence that the ventral medial nuclei and paraventricular nuclei of the hypothalamus are involved in the control of TSH secretion, and that destruction of these areas depresses thyroid hormone synthesis.

The role of the anterior pituitary in the causation of primary hyperthyroidism is not clear. Although elevated levels of TSH in the blood of patients with hyperthyroidism have been reported, the results have not been consistently reproducible. A long-acting thyroid stimulator (LATS) has been demonstrated in the plasma of patients with hyperthyroidism. There is some evidence that LATS may actually be TSH complexed to a γ globulin or a distinct immune globulin free of TSH.

The anterior pituitary gland may also secrete an exophthalmos-producing substance which may be responsible for the ocular manifestations of exophthalmic goiter.

The occurrence of hyperthyroidism following hypophysectomy or pituitary stalk section suggests that TSH may not be essential for the development of hyperthyroidism. It does appear, however, that certain pituitary tumors may secrete excess TSH and result in thyroid hyperplasia and hypersecretion. Since TSH secretion may be increased by stimuli arising in the hypothalamus, it is thought that a mechanism acting through higher central nervous system centers may be related to the not-infrequent development of thyrotoxicosis following major emotional or psychic trauma. It is also probable that increased TSH secretion is involved in the hyperthyroidism associated with acromegaly.

GONADOTROPINS

The gonadotropins, FSH and LH, are large protein hormones of approximately 30,000 molecular weight. These hormones regulate the development, reproductive functions, and hormonal secretions of the ovary and testicle. Prolactin (LtH) is also classed as a gonadotropin; however, its primary action is on the mammary gland and though it may be luteotrophic (i.e., sustaining the function of the corpus luteum) in lower animal species, this action has not been shown to be of physiologic significance in man.

The secretion of gonadotropins is influenced by the rate of sex hormone production and by certain areas of the hypothalamus. Castration increases and estrogens decrease the secretion of FSH, probably by modifying the hypothalamic centers which control FSH secretion by the anterior pituitary. The secretion of LH is also increased by castration but is less sensitive to inhibition by estrogens. Progesterone depresses LH secretion in some species. Testosterone is a poor inhibitor of FSH secretion but does block the secretion of LH.

Secretion of LH has been clearly shown to be regulated by the posterior hypothalamus. This area is also important in prolactin secretion, probably by producing a hormone that inhibits the production and release of LtH by the anterior pituitary. Lesions in this area block LH secretion and result in enhanced secretion of prolactin and pathologic lactation.

Gonadotropins are not found in the urine until puberty. Thereafter, they are present in significant quantities throughout life, with peaks of excretion appearing at the time of ovulation and greatly increased levels occurring after the menopause or following castration. Although relatively crude, the bioassay for urinary gonadotropins (FSH assay) is still the only direct assay of a pituitary hormone in general use and widely available in clinical medicine. The assay is not specific for FSH, since even small quantities of LH appear to be necessary for the biologic action of FSH. Low urinary FSH levels are occasionally found in normal individuals, and several determinations are necessary for accurate clinical evaluation.

Chorionic gonadotropin (HCG) is derived from the placenta and appears in the urine in large quantities during pregnancy. Preparations from human pregnancy urine are available for clinical use. This hormone has predominantly an LH action and is used clinically to stimulate Leydig cell function and ovulation (Chap. 90).

SEXUAL PRECOCITY. No definite pituitary disorders are associated with increased secretion of LH or FSH. There are cases of isosexual precocity, often familial, in which premature but normal sexual development occurs, probably on the basis of early maturation of central nervous system centers regulating gonadotropin formation and release. Lesions of the hypothalamus or pineal gland also may result in premature secretion of gonadotropic hormones and precocious puberty (Chap. 93).

GALACTORRHEA. Abnormal lactation is sometimes observed in patients with acromegaly or chromophobe adenomas and also may occur after pituitary stalk section. A condition associated with persistent postpartum lactation and amenorrhea is referred to as the Chiari-Frommel syndrome. The galactorrhea in these disorders is most likely the result of excess prolactin secretion. If a pituitary tumor is found, it should be treated. In the absence of evidence of a tumor, galactorrhea may be suppressed by estrogen administration.

PANHYPOPITUITARISM

PREPUBERAL. Prepuberal panhypopituitarism, which was first described in 1871 by Lorrain, is a rare condition usually associated with suprasellar cyst or craniopharyngioma. The disease is characterized by dwarfism and subnormal sexual development but normal mentality. The impairment of growth is symmetric and the body proportions are normal. As in other cases of hypopituitarism, the skin often has a pale yellowish appearance and increased wrinkling. Sexual maturation is delayed, and in rare cases there may be obesity from hypothalamic involvement. Diabetes insipidus is not an infrequent accompaniment.

If the tumor is of sufficient size to affect the optic chiasma, there may be bitemporal hemianopsia or complete blindness. X-ray studies reveal delayed fusion of the epiphyses, suprasellar calcification, and, often, destruction of the sella turcica. The condition must be distinguished from genetic dwarfism and from hypothyroidism. Genetic dwarfs have normal pituitary function and development of the epiphyses in keeping with chronologic age. Hypothyroid children have subnormal mentality, infantile body proportions, dwarfism, and the characteristic epiphyseal dysgenesis.

Treatment with cortisone, thyroid, and sex hormones, described in more detail in the next section, should be instituted, with dosage adjusted for body size and age. Although limited by the availability of material, human or monkey growth hormone in doses of 1 to 3 mg weekly has had considerable success in producing growth in these patients. Because of the psychologic and sociologic importance of reaching normal stature, every attempt should be made to obtain such therapy for these patients if the epiphyses have not closed. Growth hormone from nonprimate sources has had no effect on growth in human beings.

POSTPUBERAL PANHYPOPITUITARISM. The common causes for panhypopituitarism in the adult include chromophobe adenoma, post-partum pituitary necrosis, craniopharyngiomas, and the end stages of acromegaly. Less common lesions include gliomas, basilar meningitis, head injuries associated with hemorrhage into the pituitary or the suprasellar region, and granulomatous disorders such as sarcoidosis and Hand-Schüller-Christian disease.

Post-partum pituitary necrosis (Sheehan's syndrome) is due to extensive thrombosis of the pituitary circulation during delivery, usually associated with uterine hemorrhage but occasionally developing after a bout of hypotension without blood loss. Characteristically, these patients fail to lactate in the puerperium and do not have a recurrence of menstrual function. The association of these signs should always suggest this diagnosis. There follows the insidious onset of a host of vague symptoms, including asthenia, lethargy, loss of libido, loss of axillary and pubic hair, and cold intolerance (Fig. 80-4). Some patients appear quite healthy and often are classified as psychoneurotic until the true diagnosis is revealed. Others gradually lapse into a far-advanced state of anterior pituitary insufficiency involving gonadal, thyroid, and adrenal function in approximately that order of development. Physical signs consist of bradycardia, hypotension, loss

of axillary, pubic, and scalp hair, premature wrinkling and pallor of the skin, which is fine and atrophic, and a general loss of secondary sex characteristics, with atrophy of the breasts and genitalia.

Irrespective of the cause of panhypopituitarism, the secondary effects on the endocrine glands are similar. There is marked atrophy of the thyroid, adrenals, and gonads. Interference with growth occurs if the lesion appears prior to epiphyseal closure. The pituitary gland has a large reserve, and substantial amounts of pituitary tissue must be damaged before significant hormone deficiency develops. Not all patients develop hypofunction of all three target glands; isolated gonadal failure is relatively common, or gonadal failure may be associated with either thyroid or adrenal insufficiency. Isolated deficiency of TSH or ACTH secretion has been described in rare instances.

LABORATORY FINDINGS AND DIFFERENTIAL DIAGNOSIS. Laboratory findings reflect decreased function of the target endocrine glands. Thus, the serum protein-bound iodine and thyroidal radioiodine uptake are low, and there is a decrease in the basal metabolic rate. The level of serum cholesterol, unlike that in primary myxedema, is rarely elevated, despite lowered thyroid function. Levels of urinary 17-ketosteroids, 17-hydroxycorticosteroids, and 17-ketogenic steroids are depressed, and urinary gonadotropins are subnormal or absent. Blood levels of ACTH and growth hormone are depressed, but these tests are not generally available for the diagnosis of the condition. A normochromic anemia is often present, and there may be leukopenia and relative lymphocytosis in the presence of adrenal insufficiency. Fasting hypoglycemia is rarely found but may occasionally be severe enough to produce coma. The serum sodium concentration is usually normal, but hyponatremia may occur during periods of stress. The serum potassium level, however, is usually normal, in contrast to that in the patient with Addisonian crisis.

The diagnosis of hypopituitarism is generally not difficult to establish once it is suspected, but because

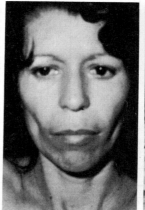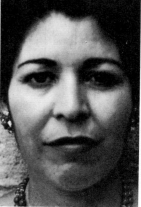

Fig. 80-4. Photographs of a forty-year-old woman when first seen for hypopituitarism (Sheehan's syndrome) and after 6 months' therapy.

of the insidious onset and the variable signs and symptoms, the disorder may escape detection for many years. These patients often come to the physician with acute medical emergencies associated with infection or trauma and fail to respond normally to the usual therapeutic measures. In such instances, clinical evidence of gonadal, thyroid, or adrenal insufficiency should be sought; if present, it will quickly suggest the diagnosis.

Patients with pituitary myxedema must be differentiated from those with primary thyroidal failure. Patients with the pituitary form often do not appear to be so myxedematous as those with primary hypothyroidism. An enlarged thyroid gland is indicative of primary hypothyroidism, since the thyroid is atrophic in hypopituitarism. In the absence of clear evidence of a primary thyroid disorder such as might result from radioiodine therapy, thyroidectomy, or thyroiditis, pituitary insufficiency should be ruled out in every patient with hypothyroidism. The response to TSH is helpful in differentiating primary from pituitary hypothyroidism. In contrast to the lack of response to TSH in the patient with primary hypothyroidism, a marked increase in the protein-bound iodine and the radioiodine uptake will be produced in the patient with the pituitary type of hypothyroidism by the administration of 10 units of TSH intramuscularly daily for 2 days. Some patients with pituitary myxedema may not respond to TSH, probably because of advanced thyroidal atrophy.

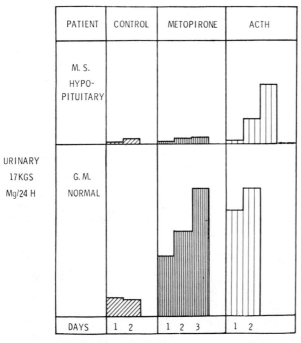

Fig. 80-5. Response of urinary 17-ketogenic steroids in a hypopituitary patient (M.S.) and a normal subject (G.M.) to Metopirone (750 mg every 6 hr for 48 hr) and ACTH (40 units intravenously over 8 hr on two or three successive days). Note the lack of response to Metopirone and delayed response to ACTH in the hypopituitary patient.

The patient with adrenal failure secondary to pituitary disease will show an increase in the 24-hr urinary excretion of 17-ketosteroids, 17-hydroxycorticosteroids, and 17-ketogenic steroids with administration of ACTH. These patients often do not respond to a single day's infusion of ACTH, but administration of 40 units intravenously over an 8-hr period on three or four successive days characteristically will reveal a stepwise increase in steroid excretion by the third or fourth day of administration. Hypopituitary patients secrete near-normal quantities of aldosterone and thus are usually in sodium balance. Hyponatremia, when it does occur, however, may be due to sodium depletion as well as to extracellular dilution.

Measurement of urinary steroids following the administration of 2-methyl-1,2 bis-(3-pyridyl)-1-propane [SU 4885 (Metopirone)] provides a particularly useful index of the ability of the pituitary gland to increase ACTH secretion. This compound inhibits the 11-hydroxylation of the steroid molecule in the adrenal gland and leads to decreased secretion of 17-hydroxycorticosterone (hydrocortisone) and increased secretion of 17-hydroxy-11-deoxycorticosterone (substance S). The hydrocortisone deficiency results in increased ACTH secretion from the anterior pituitary gland, a marked increase in the adrenal secretion of substance S, and a resultant increase in the urinary excretion of 17-hydroxycorticosteroids and 17-ketogenic steroids. Patients with normal pituitary-adrenal function will show an increase in these urinary steroids with this drug, but patients with either primary or secondary adrenal insufficiency will fail to demonstrate such an increase in urinary 17-hydroxycorticosteroids (Fig. 80-5). This test is of particular value in assessing pituitary ACTH reserve in patients who have normal or only slightly depressed basal urinary steroid levels. It is a hazardous test in patients with obvious deficiency in adrenal steroid secretion and can induce adrenal crisis in patients with primary adrenal insufficiency or those with adrenal atrophy secondary to deficient ACTH production.

Hypogonadism secondary to pituitary disease is characterized by decreased or absent urinary gonadotropins, in contrast to the increased titers found in primary gonadal failure. The prolonged amenorrhea observed in many patients with chronic illness and especially in those with anorexia nervosa is often confused with that due to panhypopituitarism. Urinary gonadotropin concentration may be low in these patients, but adrenal and thyroid function is usually normal. Thus, detailed study of each target gland will often be necessary to establish or rule out pituitary insufficiency in patients with obscure hypogonadism, hypothyroidism, or hypoadrenalism.

Other physiologic tests which have been employed in the past in establishing a diagnosis of hypopituitarism, such as the insulin tolerance test and the water test, are both nonspecific and life-threatening and should be carried out, if at all, only under close supervision.

Patients with pituitary-adrenal insufficiency excrete administered water at a depressed rate, similar to the rate of excretion in patients with primary adrenal failure; however, this test may be falsely positive in the presence of renal, hepatic, or cardiac disease. These patients are likely to develop water intoxication during the test and should be carefully observed for this complication and treated accordingly.

TREATMENT. The use of pituitary hormones would be true replacement therapy for panhypopituitarism. However TSH and ACTH must be given daily by intramuscular injection, and pituitary gonadotropins cannot be used successfully for any prolonged period because of the tendency to antibody formation. In practice, excellent results are obtained by oral replacement therapy with the target gland hormones. Thyroxin should be given at first in a dose of 0.05 mg a day, with the amount gradually increased over a period of several weeks to a total daily dose of 0.2 to 0.3 mg. Cortisone acetate should be initiated at a level of 5 to 10 mg per day and increased to 15 to 30 mg as needed. Since the administration of thyroid hormone alone in a patient with associated pituitary-adrenal insufficiency may precipitate a serious adrenal crisis, it is important to initiate cortisone therapy prior to or at least simultaneously with thyroxin therapy in these patients. Salt-retaining hormone therapy is generally not needed, but if required, can be achieved with the oral administration of 0.05 to 0.1 mg fluorohydrocortisone daily or at intervals of 2 to 3 days.

A long-acting testosterone preparation should be given intramuscularly in doses of 100 to 200 mg every 2 to 4 weeks to male patients; proportionately smaller doses are often beneficial in female patients. In the female patient, estrogens may be given daily by mouth or at intervals of 2 to 4 weeks by injection. If desired, cyclic therapy with estrogens and progesterone may be given to induce artificial menstrual function.

It should be emphasized that hormonal therapy is intended only to provide normal replacement of physiologic levels for proper body function. Although the harmful effects of large-dose corticosteroid administration may not be observed with this schedule, psychic disturbances of various kinds are occasionally noted in patients suddenly exposed to full replacement therapy after a long period of adrenal or thyroid hormone deficiency. Another problem often noted is that of excessive appetite in some patients receiving even small doses of cortisone. In this instance, it may be necessary to institute a restrictive diet or to decrease cortisone dosage to bare minimum levels.

OTHER SYNDROMES OF POSSIBLE PITUITARY ORIGIN

Froehlich's syndrome and the *Laurence-Moon-Biedl syndrome* are two disorders associated with failure of gonadal development in which disturbances in anterior pituitary gonadotropin secretion are postulated. However, no consistent lesions have been observed in the anterior pituitary, and it is thought that the primary disturbance is in the hypothalamus.

Froehlich's syndrome is associated with adiposity and sexual infantilism. In addition to truncal obesity, there are underdevelopment of the gonads and an absence of the secondary sex characteristics. The condition may be associated with mental retardation, visual disturbances, diabetes insipidus, and impaired skeletal growth. It is important to differentiate between cases of Froehlich's habitus (obesity and apparently delayed genital development) and true Froehlich's syndrome. The former condition is often observed in normal prepuberal boys who may have normal sex organs hidden in the adipose tissue. With the onset of puberty, these boys develop normally and often lose their adiposity and assume normal adolescent body proportions. Froehlich's syndrome may be associated with tumors or other disorders of the hypothalamic-pituitary area. The obesity may be caused by damage to hypothalamic centers regulating appetite.

The Laurence-Moon-Biedl syndrome is a hereditary disease characterized by adiposity, genital atrophy, mental retardation, skull deformities, retinitis pigmentosa, and associated congenital malformations such as polydactyly and syndactyly. Fewer than 100 cases have been reported, and there is no evidence of pituitary lesions in these patients. The adiposity and genital atrophy are assumed to be caused by hypothalamic-pituitary dysfunction.

INTERMEDIATE LOBE OF THE PITUITARY GLAND

The intermediate lobe of the pituitary gland is the probable site of production of melanocyte-stimulating hormone (MSH). Two types of MSH have been identified. Alpha-MSH is a polypeptide composed of the same 13 amino acids found in the N-terminal position of ACTH (Fig. 80-3). Human β-MSH contains 22 amino acids and is closely related structurally to α-MSH as well as to ACTH. Because of the common N-terminal sequence, ACTH preparations have intrinsic melanocyte-stimulating effects; however, pure MSH does not stimulate adrenal cortical secretion. It is of interest that cortisone administration may suppress MSH as well as ACTH secretion from the pituitary gland.

There have been descriptions of MSH-secreting tumors of the pituitary gland. These rare tumors are associated with a generalized increase in pigmentation similar to that observed in patients with pituitary tumors following adrenalectomy for Cushing's syndrome. The hyperpigmentation observed in patients with Addison's disease may be due to increased production of MSH as well as ACTH. Increased MSH secretion may also be responsible for the hyperpigmentation observed in some cases of hyperthyroidism, biliary cirrhosis, sprue, and other chronic diseases. Conversely, it is probable that the decreased pigmentation often apparent in patients with panhypopituitarism is due to decreased production of MSH.

REFERENCES

Antoniades, H. N.: "Hormones in Human Plasma," Boston, Little, Brown and Company, 1960.

Harris, I.: Chemistry of Pituitary Polypeptide Hormones, Brit. Med. Bull., 16:189, 1960.

Knobil, E., and J. Hotchkiss: Growth Hormone, Ann. Rev. Physiol., 26:47, 1964.

Lerner, A. B.: Hormonal Control of Pigmentation, Ann. Rev. Med., 11:187, 1960.

Liddle, G. W., D. Island, and C. K. Meader: Normal and Abnormal Regulation of Corticotropin Secretion in Man, Recent Progr. Hormone Res., 13:125, 1962.

Nelson, D. H., J. W. Meakin, and G. W. Thorn: ACTH-producing Pituitary Tumors Following Adrenalectomy for Cushing's Syndrome, Ann. Internal Med., 52:560, 1960.

Poppen, J. L.: Changing Concepts in the Treatment of Pituitary Adenomas, Bull. N.Y. Acad. Sci., 39:21, 1963.

Wolstenholme, G. E. W., and C. M. O'Connor: "Human Pituitary Hormones," Ciba Foundation Colloquia on Endocrinology, vol. 13, Boston, Little, Brown and Company, 1960.

81 DISEASES OF THE NEUROHYPOPHYSIS

*Joseph F. Dingman
and George W. Thorn*

Oliver and Schaefer in 1894 demonstrated a pressor effect of pituitary extracts, and in 1897 Howell showed that the pressor principle resided in the posterior lobe. The oxytocic action of posterior pituitary extracts was described by Dale in 1909 and the antidiuretic action by von den Velden in 1913. Fisher, Ingram, and Ranson in 1938 demonstrated a functional relationship between certain hypothalamic nuclei and the posterior pituitary. The studies of Scharrer and Scharrer since 1928 concerning the secretory activity of nerve cells (neurosecretion), the demonstration by Bargmann in 1949 of secretory granules in the neurones of the supraoptic and paraventricular nuclei of the hypothalamus, and the successful synthesis of oxytocin and vasopressin by du Vigneaud and coworkers represent important advances in current understanding of the endocrine functions of the neurohypophysis.

General Considerations

The principal effects of posterior pituitary extracts are to enhance the reabsorption of water by the renal tubules (antidiuretic effect); stimulate uterine contraction (oxytocic effect); promote the secretion of milk from the lactating breast (milk-ejecting effect); and, only in anesthetized mammals, produce a rise in blood pressure (vasopressor effect). The neurohypophyseal hormones are vasopressin (antidiuretic hormone, ADH) and oxytocin. The former is predominantly responsible for pressor and antidiuretic actions, whereas the latter is most potent in uterine stimulation and milk ejection. The neuroendocrine unit responsible for production and secretion of these hormones has been designated the neurohypophysis (Fig. 81-1), which includes the neurones of the supraoptic and paraventricular nuclei of the anterior hypothalamus, the axones that form the supraopticohypophyseal tract,

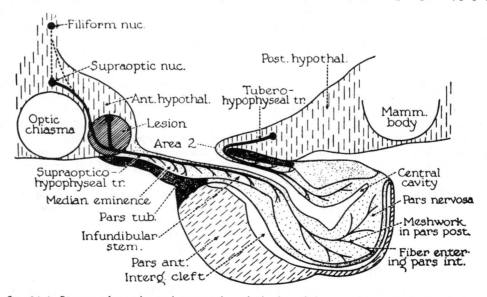

Fig. 81-1. Diagram of a midsagittal section through the hypothalamus and hypophysis. The broken lines indicate proposed filiform-supraoptic connections and the tractus paraventricularis. The obliquely striped circle indicates the position of a typical lesion designed to produce diabetes insipidus. (Fisher, Ingram, and Ranson: "Diabetes Insipidus and the Neuro-Hormonal Control of Water Balance," Fig. 2, Ann Arbor, Mich., Edwards Brothers, Inc., 1938.)

and the posterior lobe of the pituitary body, the pars nervosa, in which the axone endings terminate.

Classic concepts of the endocrine function of the neurohypophysis ascribed the role of hormone production to parenchymatous secretory cells in the posterior lobe; however, an impressive body of evidence has been accumulated to show that the hormones are actually secreted by the neurones of the supraoptic and paraventricular nuclei. Gomori's chromalum hematoxylin stain for the beta cells of the pancreatic islets demonstrated the presence of secretory granules within the cytoplasm of these neurones. These granules migrate along the axones and accumulate in the perivascular axone end-plates in the posterior pituitary. The bulk of neurohypophyseal hormone is contained in the posterior lobe and only a small fraction of total activity is found in the tuber cinereum, stalk, and hypothalamic nuclei. The posterior pituitary then serves mainly as a reservoir of hormone readily available for rapid release into the systemic circulation.

Removal of the posterior lobe will lead to hormonal deficiency only if most of the axones of the supraopticohypophyseal tract are severed and retrograde degeneration of the hypothalamic neurones occurs. With severance of the stalk close to the posterior pituitary body, short axones terminating at a higher level may escape injury and the remaining viable neurosecretory cells apparently can maintain secretion and release of hormones, probably into the vessels of the stalk and the hypothalamus.

The physiologic significance of the peculiar anatomic location of this neurosecretory organ, in which hypothalamic neurones extend their processes over relatively great distances into the posterior pituitary, is obscure. Such an arrangement may have been necessary, teleologically, in order to provide a ready route for hormone release into the systemic circulation through the highly vascularized posterior pituitary. In addition, posterior lobe extracts contain one or more hypothalamic neurohormones, which regulate the release of ACTH from the anterior pituitary (corticotropin-releasing factor, CRF), and oxytocin may play a role in regulating the secretion of prolactin (lactogenic hormone). Thus, the neurohypophysis may provide an important link between the central nervous system and the secretion of anterior pituitary tropic hormones which so profoundly influence the body economy.

In view of this evidence, consideration of the posterior pituitary as an endocrine gland warrants revision, and reference should be made to the neurohypophysis when discussing this endocrine system. However, the terms posterior pituitary gland and posterior lobe hormone are still in common usage at the present time.

Nature of Neurohypophyseal Hormones

Extracts of the neurohypophysis are assayed biologically with reference to oxytocic, vasopressor, and antidiuretic activities. One international USP or BP unit is defined as the activity of 0.5 mg of an international standard bovine posterior pituitary powder. In crude extracts of the posterior lobe the biologic activity appears to reside in a homogeneous protein or polypeptide fraction having a molecular weight of the order of 30,000 and an isoelectric point of pH 4.8. Such fractions show approximately equal vasopressor and oxytocic activities in terms of the reference powder, of the order of 16.6 IU per milligram. It has not been conclusively established whether this protein represents the natural secretion of the neurohypophysis or whether vasopressin and oxytocin loosely bound to the protein by electrostatic forces are released in a free form into the circulation.

Using modern technics of ion exchange chromatography and countercurrent distribution, highly purified preparations of vasopressin (600 IU per milligram) and oxytocin (500 IU per milligram) have been obtained from posterior lobe extracts. Both vasopressin and oxytocin contain eight amino acids and 3 moles of ammonia. The peptide structure of each hormone has been determined, and both hormones have been successfully synthesized by de Vigneaud and his coworkers, representing a milestone in peptide chemistry and hormone research. Both hormones are composed of five amino acids arranged in the form of a ring closed by the disulfide linkage of cystine, with a side chain of three amino acids. Oxytocin contains cystine, tyrosine, isoleucine, glutamine, and asparagine in the ring, with proline, leucine, and glycinamide in the side chain (Fig. 81-2). Vasopressin differs from oxytocin

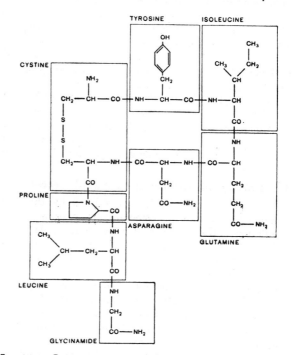

Fig. 81-2. Oxytocin. (B. Berde: "Recent Progress in Oxytocin Research," Fig. 1, Springfield, Ill., Charles C Thomas, Publisher, 1959.)

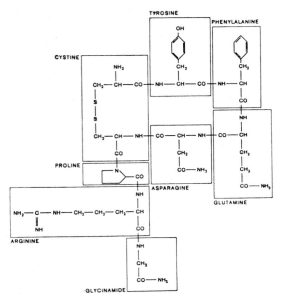

Fig. 81-3. Vasopressin. (B. Berde: "Recent Progess in Oxytocin Research," Fig. 2, Springfield, Ill., Charles C Thomas, Publisher, 1959.)

by only two amino acids. Phenylalanine replaces isoleucine in the ring, and leucine in the side chain is replaced by arginine (human, beef vasopressin, Fig. 81-3) or lysine (hog vasopressin). The molecular weight of oxytocin is 1,007 and of arginine vasopressin, 1,084. Both are ampholytes, oxytocin having an isoelectric point of pH 7.7, and arginine vasopressin being considerably more basic, with an IP of pH 10.9.

Oxytocin has been shown to possess slight but definite pressor and antidiuretic effects, whereas vasopressin contains not only equal pressor and antidiuretic activities but also significant intrinsic oxytocic and milk-ejecting properties. Partially purified posterior pituitary preparations available commercially include Pitocin (oxytocin) and Pitressin (vasopressin), each fraction being slightly contaminated by the other in pharmaceutical preparations. Synthetic oxytocin (Syntocinon) is now available, and synthetic lysine vasopressin should soon become available for clinical use.

Physiology of Neurohypophyseal Secretion

Secretion of vasopressin is regulated by the total solute concentration or osmolality of plasma (osmoregulation), the intravascular or extracellular fluid volume (volume regulation), and by central nervous system activity (neural regulation). The osmoregulatory mechanism is exquisitely sensitive to slight changes in plasma osmolality. Dilution of the plasma solutes by administration of water inhibits the secretion of vasopressin, and rapid excretion of water by the kidneys ensues; secretion is restored when plasma osmolality returns to normal. An increase in plasma osmolality resulting from a deficit of water or a relative increase in the ratio of extracellular to intracellular solutes stimulates the secretion of vasopressin and

maximum conservation of water by the kidneys. This mechanism is probably the first line of defense in day-to-day preservation of water balance and is mediated principally by changes in the concentration of sodium in the extracellular fluid.

A poorly understood auxiliary mechanism regulating vasopressin secretion, which may be more important than plasma osmolality, especially in pathologic conditions, is the influence of the volume of the body fluids on neurohypophyseal function. Thus, the antidiuresis of quiet standing, hemorrhage, venous congestion, etc., is probably mediated through an alteration in the volume of blood flowing to the neurohypophysis or by an overall contraction of effective blood volume leading to stimulation of the hypothalamic nuclei by ill-defined afferent nervous pathways. There is some evidence that stretch receptors in the wall of the right atrium sensitive to volume or pressure changes may initiate afferent vagal impulses to the hypothalamus regulating vasopressin release.

Of the two vascular modalities, osmolality and volume, the former apparently operates effectively in most normal situations by retaining or releasing body water to suit the needs of the body. However, in pathologic conditions characterized by a decrease in intravascular or extracellular fluid volume or in cardiac output, volume regulation supersedes osmoregulation. In this situation, vasopressin secretion may persist despite the simultaneous occurrence of hypotonicity. A primary decrease in osmolality, such as that seen in the hyponatremia of Addison's disease, salt-losing nephritis, or long-standing congestive heart failure, would severely deplete body water if osmolality were the only factor governing vasopressin secretion. A regulator of secretion sensitive to the volume of the body water or the fullness of the vascular compartment or both would protect against desiccation and vascular collapse in these situations, the body giving up an optimal osmotic state for the vital requirements of the tissues for water. This antidiuretic mechanism, although protective in nature, may lead to serious complications, particularly in disorders already characterized by fluid retention and edema, since persistent water retention in salt-restricted subjects may lead to severe hyponatremia, water intoxication, and further compromise of circulation and renal function (Chap. 60).

Since neurohypophyseal hormones represent secretions of the central nervous system, studies of the central neural control of the neurohypophysis have assumed great importance in neuroendocrine physiology. There is little doubt that the central nervous system has a dominant role in regulating vasopressin secretion. Secretion of vasopressin has been produced in man and monkeys by electrical stimulation of the hypothalamus and components of the "limbic system" including the hippocampus, the amygdala, the septal nuclei, and the mesencephalic reticular formation. Electrical stimulation of various areas of the cerebral cortex, however, has been shown not to evoke vasopressin release. These findings suggest that neural reflexes to the neurohypophysis may be transmitted primarily via the more primitive areas of the brain rather than through neocortical pathways.

The physiologic control of oxytocin secretion has not been well-defined. There is a widely held concept based on animal experiments that the neurohypophysis indiscriminately releases both vasopressin and oxytocin irrespective of the nature of the physiologic stimulus. Studies in lactating human subjects, however, suggest that independent regulatory mechanisms may exist for each hormone. Isolated secretion of vasopressin was observed with application of osmotic, vascular, and central neural (nicotine) stimuli; oxytocin secretion, not apparently accompanied by vasopressin release, occurred in response to suckling or mechanical distension of the mammary ducts.

Numerous centrally acting substances stimulate the neurohypophysis. These include emotional stresses such as fright, noise, and pain; fainting, which may also act through volume regulators; coitus, suckling, and changes in environmental temperature; and numerous drugs such as nicotine, acetylcholine, and many hypnotics and sedatives. Alcohol inhibits ADH secretion. Of the various hormones and endogenous substances, small doses of epinephrine inhibit and large doses stimulate the release of vasopressin, at least in animals. Ferritin, the iron-containing hepatic vasodepressor substance, and bradykinin have been shown to be antidiuretic by virtue of stimulating the neurohypophysis and the hydrocortisone-like adrenal steroids have been shown to inhibit vasopressin secretion (see below).

Thus, it is readily apparent that the neurohypophyseal hormones are secreted in diverse situations. Their importance in the body economy and in the pathogenesis or the complications of disease is poorly defined. Scientific study of neurohypophyseal function has been seriously limited by the fact that the concentrations of these hormones in human plasma is infinitesimally small, the estimated plasma concentration of vasopressin, for instance, being no more than 5 microunits or 10 $\mu\mu$g per milliliter.

Although the chemical structure of the neurohypophyseal polypeptides is known, their extremely low concentration in biologic fluids defies quantitative determination by any known analytic method. Because of this limitation, present physiologic knowledge is based upon demonstration of the known biologic effects of the hormones in the intact human being and biologic assay of plasma or urine in appropriate bioassay systems. These methods are far from ideal and are subject to the variability and lack of specificity of biologic methods in general.

Physiologic Actions of Neurohypophyseal Hormones

VASOPRESSIN (ADH). The pressor and antidiuretic activities of vasopressin are properties of a single mole-

cule. The antidiuretic action is of profound importance in regulating water balance. The current hypothesis as to the mechanism of action of vasopressin on water reabsorption by the kidney, based on experiments with various biologic membranes, such as frog skin and toad bladder, is that it renders the cells of the distal portions of the nephron permeable to water, permitting passive diffusion of tubular water along an osmotic gradient across the cell and into the peritubular vessels. The antidiuretic action of vasopressin is best demonstrated during water diuresis; *this effect represents the true physiologic role of the hormone on water metabolism, which is to prevent the bulk of the filtered water entering the distal tubular segment from escaping into the urine.* The effect of vasopressin during hypertonic urine flow is extremely variable and limited by the maximum rate of water reabsorption which the concentrating mechanism of the collecting tubules can achieve.

An interesting aspect of the studies of the action of vasopressin on biologic membranes has been the demonstration that this hormone has a pronounced effect on transport of sodium as well as water across cell boundaries. The effect of vasopressin on sodium excretion by the kidney is, however, extremely variable and depends upon experimental conditions. It is probable that vasopressin does not have a direct effect on sodium excretion and that any observed change in sodium balance is secondary to the modifying influence of this hormone on the total volume and distribution of body water.

Vasopressin has been shown to exert a pressor effect in persons with postural hypotension, and large intravenous doses may also produce transient increases in blood pressure even in normal man. The significance of this observation in relationship to blood pressure regulation in normal persons is unknown. Generally, posterior lobe preparations used therapeutically in man have no consistent effect on blood pressure, probably because of compensatory adjustments elsewhere in the circulation.

OXYTOCIN. Recent studies with purified and synthetic oxytocin have significantly advanced understanding of the role of this hormone in uterine function and milk secretion. Oxytocin has been shown to be the hormonal substance of posterior lobe extracts responsible for release of milk from the lactating breast, as little as 0.5 units, or 1 μg, synthetic hormone producing a copious flow of milk within 30 sec of intravenous injection. Synthetic oxytocin has also been used successfully to initiate labor, and as previously mentioned, there is some evidence that oxytocin stimulates or sustains the secretion of prolactin by the anterior pituitary. Oxytocin, therefore, appears to play a very important and fundamental role in reproduction. Vasopressin also possesses oxytocic and milk-ejecting properties but is much less potent than oxytocin in this regard.

Other effects of oxytocin that warrant consideration include its marked but evanescent vasodepressor action demonstrable both in human beings and experimental animals and its effect on water excretion and renal function. In appropriate experimental situations, oxytocin has been shown to antagonize the antidiuretic action of vasopressin and to increase renal plasma flow and sodium excretion. The latter effect is currently attributable to an action of the hormone on the brain, which is abolished by hypophysectomy or the induction of diabetes insipidus. The demonstration that some of the actions of oxytocin are directly opposed to those of vasopressin implies a physiologic system for regulation of the volume and composition of the body fluids as well as the arterial pressure under the control of the central nervous system and the hypothalamus, which, although obscure at this time, may prove to be of clinical significance in the future.

Adrenocortical-Neurohypophyseal Relationships

Ever since crude cortical extracts were found to protect against water intoxication and enhance the diuretic response to water administration, the interaction of adrenal steroids and ADH on water metabolism has been studied extensively. Hydrocortisone, the principal glucocorticoid secreted by the human adrenal cortex, has been shown to suppress the reactivity of the neurohypophysis to neural stimulation and to elevate the osmolal threshold for ADH release. A transient water diuresis is often observed within the first few hours of hydrocortisone administration, which may be related to an acute decrease in vasopressin secretion.

The resulting loss of body water would lead to relative hypertonicity of the body fluids and reactivation of vasopressin release via osmoregulatory pathways, even though blockade of neural pathways for ADH secretion may persist. The physiologic significance of this effect of hydrocortisone on the secretion of a hormone of prime importance in regulating water metabolism has not been delineated, but it may represent a hormonal mechanism for independently regulating the body content of sodium and water.

The adrenal steroids have not been shown to modify the antidiuretic effect of vasopressin in man. Thus, the diuretic effect of adrenal steroids is probably mediated not through a direct effect on the renal tubular reabsorption of water but by an indirect pathway involving inhibition of neurohypophyseal hormone secretion and a decrease in antidiuretic hormone action on the kidney.

In patients with partial neurohypophyseal insufficiency, a more complete state of diabetes insipidus can be induced with hydrocortisone administration, and a greater loss of solute-free water from the kidney occurs. Patients with a complete absence of vasopressin secretion do not have a true water diuresis with adrenal hormone administration. Since these hormones, at times, increase solute excretion by the kidney, there may be a concomitant increase in water excretion because of an inability of the kidney, in the absence of vasopressin, to increase solute concentration of the urine.

Adrenal steroids affect water metabolism in several other ways. Prolonged steroid therapy may occasionally result in extensive potassium depletion and the development of kaliopenic nephropathy associated with isosthenuria and a two- to threefold increase in urine flow. Very rarely, adrenal steroids may produce a striking polydipsic syndrome with urine volumes as high as 15 to 20 liters per 24 hr. Steroid effects on thirst-regulating centers in the anterior hypothalamus or other parts of the brain may be implicated in this disorder.

The adrenal steroids thus appear to influence water metabolism in man (1) by inhibiting the central neural control of vasopressin secretion and decreasing vasopressin action on the kidney; (2) by increasing solute excretion and the obligatory excretion of water in patients with vasopressin deficiency; (3) by producing the sensation of thirst, possibly by an effect on hypothalamic and other central nervous system thirst centers; (4) by producing potassium deficiency and kaliopenic nephropathy.

Vasopressin Deficiency—Diabetes Insipidus

Diabetes insipidus is a chronic symptom complex characterized by the passage of large quantities of pale, dilute urine, with secondary polydipsia. It results from a defect in the chain of events by which vasopressin is released from the neurohyophysis and acts on the cells of the renal tubules. The classic anatomic and physiologic studies of Fisher, Ingram, and Ranson, revealed that the disease may be caused by interference with the functional integrity of the neurohormonal unit comprising the supraoptic and paraventricular nuclei of the hypothalamus, the supraoptico hypophyseal tract, and the posterior lobe of the hypophysis. The full-blown disease occurs only when the tract is interrupted close enough to the hypothalamus to cause degeneration of at least 85 per cent of the supraoptic and paraventricular neurones. There is also a relatively rare disorder, nephrogenic diabetes insipidus, which is mostly familial. This disorder may be due to a hereditary refractoriness of the renal tubules to vasopressin, and it is presumed that there is no neurohypophyseal disease in this group.

The incidence of classic diabetes insipidus following hypophysectomy may be significantly diminished if damage to the supraoptic neurones is minimized by careful severance of the pituitary stalk as close to the pituitary gland as possible. The polyuria of hypophysectomized human beings has been shown to vary with the magnitude of vasopressin deficiency. Patients who lack this secretion demonstrate persistent polyuria despite withdrawal of adrenocortical replacement therapy. These observations illustrate the important role of vasopressin in determining the rate of water excretion and corroborate the concept that the diuretic effect of adrenal steroids is mediated indirectly through an effect on vasopressin secretion. The adrenal steroids may increase urine volume in such patients, however, by increasing solute excretion.

The thyrotropic and growth hormones of the anterior pituitary are necessary to maintain polyuria, probably by influencing the nutritional state and solute turnover as well as by sustaining renal function. A peripheral antagonism of vasopressin by thyroid hormone has been demonstrated, but this effect may not be a direct one.

INCIDENCE. Diabetes insipidus is a rare disease, with a slightly greater incidence in youth and in males. In 1924 Rowntree reported 10 and 16 cases, respectively, in two series of 100,000 admissions to the Mayo Clinic. With the advent of hypophysectomy in recent years for the treatment of far-advanced breast carcinoma and other serious disorders, the disease is becoming much more prevalent in the general hospital population.

ETIOLOGY. As shown by Fink's pathologic studies in 107 cases, the great majority of instances of this disease are due to anatomic lesions involving the hypothalamic-hypophyseal system and, hence, presumably interfering with vasopressin production. In clinical practice, it will often be impossible to elicit any other evidence of such a lesion; while the label *idiopathic* may be justifiable for such cases antemortem, the finding of an anatomic lesion at autopsy generally may be predicted.

PATHOLOGY. The primary pathologic processes associated most frequently with the syndrome have been tumors of the diencephalopituitary region, basilar meningitis, sarcoidosis, and the histiocytic disorders. Transitory and occasionally permanent polyuria may follow severe head injuries. Pathologic changes consist of those due to the primary disorder, such as tumor, brain injury, and inflammation, and secondary changes in the urogenital tract, such as dilatation and hypertrophy of the bladder with megaloureter.

CLINICAL PICTURE. The chief symptoms of diabetes insipidus are polyuria and polydipsia. The loss of large amounts of pale, dilute urine, occasionally as much as 15 to 29 liters per day, results in dehydration and, consequently, in such related symptoms and signs as dry skin, constipation, and an intense, almost insatiable thirst. Water deprivation to the limit of tolerance does not prevent polyuria, nor does it lead to a significant increase in urine concentration. Thus, in this disease, polydipsia is secondary to polyuria, in contrast to patients with psychogenic polydipsia, who pass large quantities of urine as an aftermath of a large fluid intake. In patients with diabetes insipidus, no consistent physical or chemical changes are noted other than those of dehydration. However, there may be symptoms referable to the localized disease process causing the syndrome.

The role of trauma in the production of diabetes insipidus deserves special comment, since the polyuria that sometimes follows head injury is not infrequently transient, as contrasted with the chronicity of most other forms of the disease. A similar syndrome may develop subsequent to cerebrovascular accidents or intracranial surgery, and in association with other forms of cerebral disease. When the full-blown syndrome develops under these conditions, serious dehydration may occur before the diagnosis is suspected, particularly in the incontinent patient or in the patient with clouded sensorium who is unable to request or partake of an adequate volume of fluids. The dehydration, which is due principally to water loss, may be accentuated by the administration of isotonic saline or solutions containing large amounts of protein. Such large solute loads will aggravate the renal loss of water in these patients because of an inability of the kidney to increase the solute concentration of the urine in the absence of vasopressin.

DIAGNOSIS. The symptoms plus the large urine volume, with specific gravity below 1.010 and urinary osmolality less than that of plasma, unassociated with a history or other findings of diabetes mellitus or of chronic renal disease, will quickly suggest diabetes insipidus. Since this diagnosis commits the patient to sustained replacement therapy for an indefinite period, it is not to be made lightly, and the clinical impression should be supported by careful studies made under hospital conditions. All cases of diabetes insipidus, moreover, should be studied carefully for active intracranial lesions, which should be presumed to be present until proved otherwise. Thus, examination should include, in addition to the differential tests of water excretion outlined below, a study of the spinal fluid, roentgenograms of the skull and chest (metastatic disease), electroencephalogram, serologic test (syphilis), the serum protein level, sternal marrow aspiration (multiple myeloma), and visual fields.

DIFFERENTIAL DIAGNOSIS. The syndrome must be differentiated from psychogenic polydipsia, chronic nephritis, and diabetes mellitus as well as from the polydipsia and polyuria so characteristically associated with the hypochloremic alkalotic syndrome and the hypercalcemia of hyperparathyroidism and vitamin D intoxication. Chronic nephritis may be excluded by the absence of protein or formed elements in the urine, a normal blood urea nitrogen level, and normal kidney function tests. Often the most difficult differential diagnosis is that between diabetes insipidus and psychogenic polydipsia. Other procedures helpful in making a differential diagnosis are the following:

1. Dehydration for 8 to 12 hr should be performed cautiously during the day, with close observation of the patient for signs of vasomotor collapse, which can occur with sudden severe dehydration. An inability to increase the specific gravity and osmolality of the urine to hypertonic levels is characteristic of diabetes insipidus and serves to differentiate this syndrome from psychogenic polydipsia but not from chronic nephritis. Great care must be taken in suspected psy-

chogenic cases to be certain that the patient does not have access to water or other fluids.

2. Alleviation of symptoms will follow repeated small doses of aqueous vasopressin, i.e., 5.0 units intramuscularly every 3 to 4 hr. This differentiates diabetes insipidus from chronic nephritis but not from psychogenic polydipsia. The possibility of vasopressin-resistant diabetes insipidus must always be kept in mind, since 5 to 15 per cent of cases of diabetes insipidus fall into this category.

3. Secretory function should be tested. Since the secretion of vasopressin can be initiated by either neurogenic or osmotic stimuli, both the hypothalamic neurones and the osmoregulators must be stimulated in turn for the integrity of this neurohormonal unit to be properly evaluated. In addition, the adequacy of renal tubular responsiveness to vasopressin must also be measured to understand fully the nature of the polyuria. The functional integrity of the neurohypophyseal-renal system may be evaluated within a few hours by serial intravenous injections of nicotine, hypertonic saline solution, and vasopressin under constant water-loading conditions. Acute changes in urinary osmolality and free water clearance (C_{H_2O}) during water diuresis reflect the action of vasopressin on the renal tubular reabsorption of water and may be regarded as a useful index of the secretory capacity of the neurohypophysis.[1]

TECHNIQUE. The patient is hydrated with 20 ml water per kg body weight over 30 to 60 min. Preliminary dehydration is unnecessary and may be dangerous. Urine is collected at 15- to 30-min intervals by spontaneous voiding if at all possible or else through an indwelling catheter. In the latter case, it is worthwhile to administer 0.5 Gm tetracycline by mouth several hours before catheterization to prevent urinary tract infection. A constant state of hydration is maintained by oral or intravenous administration of

---

[1] The urine volume, V, is equal to the algebraic sum of the osmolal clearance, C_{osm}, and the free water clearance, C_{H_2O}.

$$V = C_{osm} + C_{H_2O}$$

$$C_{osm} = V \frac{\text{total solute conc. urine}}{\text{total solute conc. plasma}}$$

C_{osm} represents the volume of water required to contain the urinary solutes in a solution isosmotic with plasma. C_{H_2O} represents the net excess or deficit of water beyond the osmolal clearance; it will be positive during a water diuresis and negative when urine is concentrated by the abstraction of solute-free water, as in antidiuresis. C_{H_2O} usually parallels urine flow during water diuresis studies, since osmolal clearance remains relatively constant. This index is particularly useful in determining the changes in water excretion occurring with the solute diuresis usually observed with hypertonic saline administration. Not infrequently, a large increase in C_{osm} may mask a concomitant decrease in C_{H_2O}. In this instance, urinary flow may fall only slightly or may actually increase, even though an increase in water reabsorption may be under way under the influence of released vasopressin.

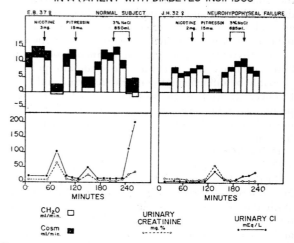

Fig. 81-4. See text and footnote. Patient, J. H., a nonsmoker, was given twice the usual dose of nicotine.

a volume of fluid equal to that excreted during the preceding collection period. When a sustained high rate of urine flow is reached (over 5 ml per min), 1.0 mg nicotine in solution is injected intravenously over a period of 0.5 to 2 min. The dose of nicotine is gradually increased by 0.5 to 1.0 mg at intervals of 30 min until a clear-cut antidiuretic response ensues or symptoms of nicotine intoxication (i.e., vertigo, nausea, vomiting) preclude further administration. As an alternative, the subject can smoke one to three cigarettes rapidly and with deep inhalation.

The normal antidiuretic response to nicotine, which occurs within 15 to 30 min after injection, is a decrease in urine flow and free water clearance, accompanied by an increase in urinary creatinine, chloride, and total solute concentrations (Fig. 81-4). Patients with diabetes insipidus usually do not show a fall in water excretion with normal doses of nicotine; however, some may have a minimal antidiuretic response with much larger amounts (5 to 6 mg nicotine base), which may be due to residual neurohypophyseal activity or transient hemodynamic effects on the kidney. When urine flow returns to control levels, 15 to 25 milliunits aqueous vasopressin is injected intravenously. The response to vasopressin differentiates renal disease from true diabetes insipidus.

The administration of water is discontinued with the vasopressin injection to decrease the volume of retained water in preparation for the intravenous administration of hypertonic saline solution, since excessive hydration may abolish the osmotic response by diluting the hypertonic saline as it enters the circulation. When the antidiuresis to vasopressin is completed, 3 per cent saline (10 ml per kilogram) is infused rapidly over 30 to 45 min. In normal persons a marked antidiuretic response will occur during the infusion or within the following 60 min. In patients with diabetes insipidus, this antidiuresis does not occur and a rise in free water clearance is frequently observed due to the associated solute diuresis (Fig. 81-4). Patients with psychogenic polydipsia demonstrate normal antidiuresis to the hypertonic saline infusion, but, curiously, many do not respond normally to nicotine, suggesting some derangement in hypothalamic function and neural regulation of vasopressin release in this disorder.

The response to nicotine, to hypertonic saline solution, and to vasopressin may be used to differentiate the locus of the functional disturbance responsible for the polyuria, i.e., hypothalamus, osmoregulators, and renal tubules. Patients with vasopressin-deficient diabetes insipidus classically do not respond to hypertonic saline. However, certain patients with diabetes insipidus apparently have secreting neurohypophyseal tissue that responds to normal doses of nicotine but not to hypertonic saline solution. Post-mortem studies on one such patient with metastatic breast carcinoma demonstrated an abundance of secretory granules within the neurones of the intact supraoptic nuclei, but the posterior pituitary and stalk were devoid of neurosecretion and completely destroyed by tumor. This phenomenon suggests that isolated posterior pituitary damage may lead to a selective failure of the osmoregulatory control of vasopressin secretion and a clinical syndrome of vasopressin-deficient diabetes insipidus despite the presence of functioning neurohypophyseal tissue.

TREATMENT. Treatment of diabetes insipidus may be divided into two phases: (1) correction of the underlying intracranial difficulty, if present; (2) replacement therapy with vasopressin, which usually must be continued throughout life.

Pitressin is a partially purified vasopressin fraction obtained from animal posterior lobes supplied as an aqueous solution in 0.5- and 1-ml ampuls with a strength of 20 IU pressor activity per milliliter. The quantity of Pitressin required to ameliorate polyuria is very small (0.1 to 0.2 ml), but the evanescent action of the aqueous preparation necessitates repeated injections at 3- to 4-hr intervals, making this form of treatment impractical for prolonged periods. Synthetic lysine vasopressin solution for parenteral use is comparable in action to aqueous Pitressin.

Nasal insufflations of dried posterior pituitary powder (supplied in 5- and 30-Gm bottles) every 3 to 6 hr accomplish the same purpose and are more easily administered, but some patients develop a chronic rhinopharyngitis and even gastritis from swallowed powder. Systemic allergic reactions are rare but have been observed.

A synthetic lysine vasopressin solution containing 50 pressor units per milliliter in 5-ml plastic spray vials is available for intranasal use as a spray or as drops. Its activity is as rapid and as prolonged as posterior lobe powder, but this preparation has the decided advantage of eliminating the local or systemic allergic reactions to the foreign protein in posterior pituitary preparations of animal origin. This material currently is the treatment of choice for ambulatory patients.

Pitressin tannate in oil is supplied in 1-ml ampuls with a strength of 5 IU per milliliter. This preparation provides relatively prolonged hormonal action; a single injection is usually effective for 24 to 72 hr. A test dose of 0.3 to 0.5 ml (1.5 to 2.5 IU) should be given initially to determine the effectiveness of treatment and to guard against the serious, but fortunately rare, occurrence of excess fluid retention and water intoxication in particularly sensitive individuals. For practical purposes chronic treatment with 1.0-ml doses of hormone should be tried and the frequency of injection gauged by the recurrence of polyuria. Most patients will retain 1 to 2 kg water following an injection, and the dissipation of effective hormone levels will be attended with a sudden polyuria and loss of body weight before onset of polydipsia. In general, injections should be timed to coincide with the onset of polyuria in order to prevent marked fluctuations in body water content and fluid compartmental shifts. Abnormal fluid retention may be mitigated by instructing the patient to guard against excessive fluid ingestion after treatment. The hormone is preferably given in the evening to ensure a restful night. *It is very important to instruct the patient to warm the vial and to shake it thoroughly, since the active material has a tendency to precipitate out in the vial.* This is the commonest cause of so-called "vasopressin resistance."

Occasionally, patients with vasopressin-sensitive diabetes insipidus may develop resistance to the action of the hormone, in some cases accompanied by allergy either to the hormone or to the oily menstruum. Allergy to the latter may be easily corrected by use of a different medium, and hormone allergy may be overcome by desensitization. Vasopressin resistance is also observed in patients with hypokalemia and hypercalcemia or hypercalciuria, either of which blocks the full action of ADH on the renal tubules. Serum and urinary calcium and potassium measurements should be made in all patients with vasopressin-resistant polyuria and appropriate investigations and treatment carried out.

Both chlorothiazide and hydrochlorothiazide have been shown to increase free water reabsorption in diabetes insipidus. These drugs, however, will decrease urine flow by no more than about 30 to 50 per cent, and most patients usually will continue to require vasopressin therapy as well to prevent abnormally large urine volumes. The thiazide derivatives may have their greatest usefulness in lessening polyuria in the rare form of vasopressin-resistant diabetes insipidus. The average daily dose of chlorothiazide is 0.5 to 1.0 Gm and of hydrochlorothiazide, 0.05 to 0.1 Gm given in divided doses. Since the thiazides may produce potassium depletion, which can impair the concentrating ability of the kidney, it is worthwhile to administer 1.0 to 2.0 Gm KCl by mouth with each dose of thiazide drug. The prognosis of this chronic deficiency syndrome is determined by the outcome of the initiating disease process. Patients with isolated neurohypophyseal atrophy can lead a normal life with regular treatment.

Excess of Antidiuretic Hormone

Abnormally elevated levels of antidiuretic substances in blood and urine have been reported in a variety of disease states associated with edema or defects in water diuresis, including cardiac failure, cirrhosis with ascites, nephrosis, and Addison's disease. While the hypothesis that excessive antidiuretic activity may be responsible for the water retention observed in edematous patients is quite attractive, proof has not been clearly established. It is generally agreed that patients with these disorders do not show excessive sensitivity to or delayed inactivation of administered vasopressin. Some studies with nicotine stimulation of endogenous vasopressin secretion in patients with edema have yielded normal results, but some patients whose disease is associated with severe hyponatremia have shown enhanced neurohypophyseal response to nicotine and other stimuli. Many of the studies that minimize a role of vasopressin in edema formation are based upon data observed in patients in equilibrium with their fluid retention who can excrete water loads, albeit at a somewhat depressed rate. It is obvious that vasopressin release mechanisms should be evaluated during the active phase of edema formation, but studies have been hampered by the fact that such patients frequently cannot excrete administered water, which automatically vitiates the only reliable biologic end point of vasopressin action, i.e., antidiuresis. Further advances in this field will depend upon the development and application of precise and reliable methods for measuring vasopressin levels in the plasma.

The level of vasopressin in the body fluids need not necessarily be increased to account for water retention, since even physiologic amounts effectively halt a water diuresis. The abnormality in water metabolism may be primarily related to a *persistence* of vasopressin secretion despite the presence of excess body water or hypotonicity, both of which normally should induce water diuresis. It appears that the distribution rather than the total quantity of body water may determine the secretory activity of the neurohypophysis, and more extensive studies of the precedence of volume versus osmolal regulation of vasopressin secretion should shed more light on the nature of fluid retention in these disorders.

The above discussion is particularly pertinent in understanding the nature of the antidiuretic factors responsible for the *inappropriate ADH syndrome*, described in patients with oat cell carcinoma of the lung, acute intermittent porphyria, various central nervous system disorders, etc. Antidiuretic assays of whole plasma and urine purport to show increased ADH levels in several patients. The situation is made more complex by the finding of antidiuretic activity in extracts of the primary lung tumor and hepatic metastases in one patient. These antidiuretic substances have not been confirmed as ADH, however; the bioassay methods employed are not specific for vasopressin and may be interfered with by vasoactive peptides other than ADH in the biologic extracts or by a nonspecific release of ADH by the assay animal following injection of noxious substances or heterologous tissue extracts.

The interrelationships between neurohypophyseal secretion and the adrenal secretion of aldosterone are not well-defined. Patients with aldosterone-secreting tumors do not usually develop edema, and normal subjects treated with aldosterone have been shown to escape readily from sodium and water retention. Furthermore, patients with diabetes insipidus will retain sodium with aldosterone therapy but will not retain isosmotic quantities of water unless they receive vasopressin simultaneously.

Aldosterone secretion may be inhibited by expansion of body fluids despite the presence of hyponatremia. In this respect, the regulation of aldosterone secretion resembles that for vasopressin secretion, the influence of fluid volume having precedence over osmolal concentration. It is probable that there is an intimate physiologic interrelation between aldosterone, which governs sodium metabolism, and vasopressin, which regulates water metabolism. Both vasopressin and aldosterone are probably necessary for the isosmotic retention of fluid, and persistent secretion of both hormones could be responsible for the development of edema in patients with fundamental derangements in circulation.

REFERENCES

Berde, B.: "Recent Progress in Oxytocin Research," Springfield, Ill., Charles C Thomas, Publisher, 1959.

Dingman, J. F., K. Benirschke, and G. W. Thorn: Studies of Neurohypophyseal Function in Man: I. Diabetes Insipidus and Psychogenic Polydipsia, Am. J. Med., 23:226, 1957.

——, and R. H. Despointes: Adrenal Steroid Inhibition of Vasopressin Release from the Neurohypophysis of Normal Subjects and Patients with Addison's Disease, J. Clin. Invest., 39:1851, 1960.

——, and J. Hauger-Klevene: Treatment of Diabetes Insipidus: Synthetic Lysine Vasopressin Nasal Solution, J. Clin. Endocrinol. & Metab., 24:550, 1964.

du Vigneaud, V.: Trail of Sulfur Research: From Insulin to Oxytocin, Science, 123:967, 1956.

Fink, E. B.: Diabetes Insipidus: A Clinical Review and Analysis of Autopsy Reports, Arch. Pathol., 6:102, 1928.

Scharrer, E., and B. Scharrer: Hormones Produced by Neurosecretory Cells, Recent Progr. Hormone Research, 10:183, 1954.

Schwartz, W. B., D. Tassel and F. C. Bartter: Further Observations on Hyponatremia and Renal Sodium Loss Probably Resulting from Inappropriate Secretion of Antidiuretic Hormone, New England J. Med., 262: 743, 1960.

Verney, E. B.: Absorption and Excretion of Water, Brit. Med. J. (Lancet), II:739, 1946.

82 DISEASES OF THE THYROID

Herbert A. Selenkow
and Sidney H. Ingbar

Diseases of the thyroid gland are manifested by either increases in gland size (goiter, neoplasm), alterations in hormonal secretion, or both. Changes in gland size and weight (normally 15 to 35 Gm) are associated with toxic or nontoxic goiter, adenomas, thyroiditis, or malignancies. Symptoms may arise from local compression in the neck and superior mediastinum, from disturbances in hormonogenesis resulting in hypothyroidism or hyperthyroidism, or from malignancy. Alterations in thyroid hormone secretion produce a wide variety of anatomic, physiologic, and metabolic effects, characteristic of which are increased oxygen consumption (hypermetabolism) from excessive secretion and decreased oxygen consumption (hypometabolism) from thyroid insufficiency.

In 1891, Murray, an English physician, administered thyroid substances to a myxedematous patient, who subsequently improved remarkably. The material employed was a glycerin extract obtained from sheep thyroids. Magnus-Levy, in 1895, observed that administration of thyroid extract to patients with hypothyroidism was followed by an increase in basal metabolic rate. In 1896, Baumann obtained an acid hydrolyzate of thyroid tissue in powder form that contained 10 per cent iodine, thus establishing the high iodine content of this hormone. Oswald, 8 years later, prepared iodothyroglobulin, thus indicating that thyroid hormone was a protein substance. Thyroxin was first isolated by Kendall in 1915 and subsequently synthesized by Harington and Barger in 1927. The potent homolog of thyroxin, 3,5,3'-triiodothyronine, was isolated chromatographically from plasma and thyroid tissue and identified simultaneously in 1952 by Gross and Pitt-Rivers and by Roche, Lissitsky, and Michel.

ANATOMY AND EMBRYOLOGY. The human thyroid originates embryologically from an invagination of the pharyngeal epithelium with some cellular contributions from the lateral pharyngeal pouches. Progressive descent of the midline thyroid anlage gives rise to the thyroglossal duct, which extends from the foramen cecum at the base of the tongue to the isthmus of the thyroid. Remnants of tissue may persist along the course of this tract as "lingual thyroid," as thyroglossal cysts and nodules, or as a structure contiguous with the thyroid isthmus called the *pyramidal lobe.* The cephalad portion of the pyramidal lobe in adults is usually a vestigial structure consisting of a thin fibrous cord. The remnant close to the thyroid isthmus may contain significant amounts of thyroid tissue that can be identified by careful palpation as the pyramidal lobe. This lobe usually extends from the thyroid cartilage to the thyroid isthmus and is more commonly located to the left than to the right of the midline. Hypertrophy of this lobe is found in disorders of diffuse thyroid enlargement such as hyperthyroidism, diffuse hyperplasia of adolescence or pregnancy, and in lymphoid thyroiditis. Ectopic thyroid tissue may occur rarely in the trachea or esophagus.

The human fetal thyroid becomes detectably functional around 14 to 16 weeks and during the latter part of gestation develops the capacity to synthesize and secrete thyroid hormones. The extent to which fetal requirements for thyroid hormones are met by secretion from the maternal or fetal thyroid is not clear. The thyroid gland enlarges progressively during fetal development and neonatal life and reaches the adult size of about 20 to 25 Gm. The precise weight of the "normal" adult thyroid gland varies considerably with geographic, genetic, and environmental factors (see Chap. 71).

BIOCHEMICAL PHYSIOLOGY. The hormonal activity of the thyroid gland is controlled mainly by the thyrotropic or thyroid-stimulating hormone (TSH) of the anterior pituitary gland (see Chap. 80). Release of TSH from the pituitary is regulated, at least in part, by hypothalamic centers and generally depends upon the quantity of thyroid hormones available to the tissues. A reduction in the availability of thyroid hormones stimulates TSH output, which, in turn, tends to increase the secretion and size of the thyroid gland. Conversely, in normal persons, an excess of available thyroid hormones tends to depress secretion of TSH and so, in turn, to reduce thyroid activity and size. Certain chemical compounds, as well as congenital or acquired enzymatic defects within the thyroid, reduce hormonal secretion and thus lead to goiter formation (goitrogenesis) by permitting increased TSH secretion. Conversely, thyroid hormones inhibit secretion of TSH and thus act as antigoitrogenic agents.

Pathways of iodine metabolism are schematically represented in Fig. 82-1. Approximately 100 to 200 μg dietary iodide are absorbed daily via the gastrointestinal tract. Circulating inorganic iodide is usually present in serum in minute amounts of the order of 1.0 μg per 100 ml. This ionic iodide is available to the thyroid, kidneys, and exocrine glands. That portion not concentrated by the thyroid is rapidly cleared by the kidneys. Iodide extracted by the exocrine glands is recirculated via intestinal resorption. The intrathyroidal processes leading to synthesis and secretion of thyroid hormones may be divided into four sequential stages (Fig. 82-2). Iodine in the plasma is available to the thyroid gland for hormonal synthesis only in the inorganic ionic form. This is derived from two major sources, the peripheral degradation and deiodina-

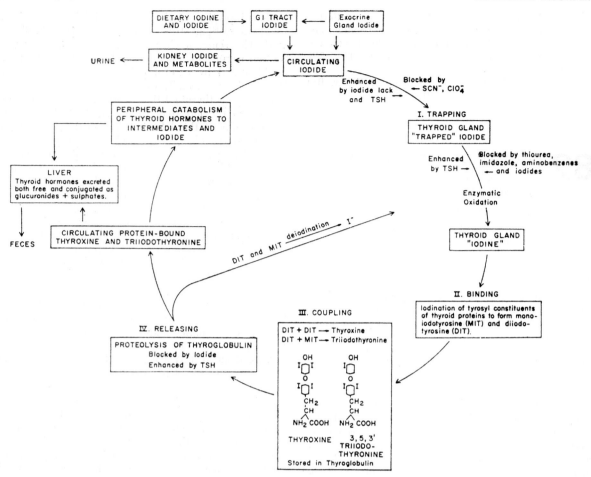

Fig. 82-1. Simplified schematic representation of pathways of iodine metabolism.

tion of hormonal as well as nonhormonal iodinated compounds and, more importantly, the diet. In most areas of the world, the dietary intake of iodine is sufficiently low so that the concentration of iodide in plasma is well below 1 μg per 100 ml. The first step in hormonal biosynthesis is maintenance by the thyroid of an iodide store in which the concentration of iodide is many times that in the plasma. Thyroid/serum gradients may vary from 10 to 500, or more, under varying physiologic conditions. This high level of "trapped" iodide is maintained by an active transport mechanism, is increased directly by TSH or indirectly via low thyroidal iodine stores, and provides a concentrated substrate for subsequent stages in thyroid hormone synthesis. Next, through a reaction apparently mediated by an intrathyroidal peroxidase, iodide is oxidized to a higher valence form, possibly iodine or hypoiodite. This highly reactive form of iodine exists only momentarily, as it combines rapidly with tyrosyl groups in thyroid proteins to form monoiodotyrosine (MIT) and diiodotyrosine (DIT). These iodotyrosines then undergo oxidative coupling, possibly again through the mediation of a thyroidal peroxidase, to yield a variety of iodothyronines, including thyroxin

and 3,5,3'-triiodothyronine. The latter compound (hereafter referred to as triiodothyronine) and thyroxin are the major hormonally active products secreted by the thyroid gland. These, as well as the other iodinated amino acids, are formed within the thyroglobulin molecule and stored as such in the thyroid follicle. Under physiologic conditions, thyroglobulin does not enter the circulation. Secretion of hormonally active materials requires hydrolysis of thyroglobulin by a group of thyroidal proteases and peptidases. The thyroid hormones released by proteolysis of thyroglobulin are free to enter the blood stream, whereas mono- and diiodotyrosine are prevented from entering the circulation by action of an iodotyrosine deiodinase, which removes their iodide. This iodide is in part reutilized for synthesis of hormone and in part lost from the thyroid gland by release into the circulation.

The foregoing reactions are subject to inhibition by a variety of chemical compounds. Such agents are generally termed *goitrogens*, since, by virtue of their ability to inhibit hormonal synthesis, they induce goiter formation. Certain inorganic anions, notably perchlorate and thiocyanate, inhibit the iodide transport

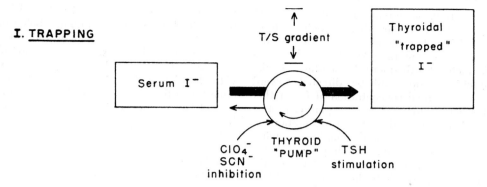

I. TRAPPING

II. BINDING

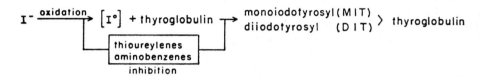

III. COUPLING

$$2 \text{ DIT} \longrightarrow \text{thyroxinyl} \qquad (T4)$$
$$1 \text{ MIT} + 1 \text{ DIT} \longrightarrow \text{triiodothyroninyl (T3)} \Big\rangle \text{ thyroglobulin}$$

IV. RELEASING

$$T4-T3-MIT-DIT-\text{thyroglobulin} \xrightarrow[\text{thyrotropin activated}]{\text{enzymatic hydrolysis}} \nearrow T4 + T3 \text{ (plasma)}$$
$$\searrow MIT + DIT \text{ (thyroid)}$$

$$MIT + DIT \text{ (thyroid)} \xrightarrow[\text{deiodinase}]{\text{tyrosine}} \text{tyrosine} + I^- \text{ (recycled)}$$

Fig. 82-2. Sequential stages of intrathyroidal synthesis and secretion of thyroid hormones.

mechanism and thus either prevent thyroid cells from concentrating iodide or release thyroidal iodide into the circulation. The goiter and hypothyroidism that follow chronic depletion of intrathyroidal iodide, such as these agents induce, can be prevented or relieved by doses of iodide sufficiently large to enable adequate quantities to enter the gland by simple diffusion. The commonly employed antithyroid agents, such as the derivatives of thiourea and mercaptoimidazole, exert more complex actions upon pathways of hormonal biosynthesis. These agents, as well as certain aniline derivatives, inhibit the initial oxidation (organic binding) of iodide, decrease the proportion of diiodotyrosine relative to monoiodotyrosine, and block coupling of iodotyrosines to form the hormonally active iodothyronines. The latter reaction is the most sensitive to inhibition by these agents. It is therefore possible for the synthesis of hormonally active iodothyronines to be decreased greatly although the total incorporation of iodine by the thyroid is inhibited but little. Excessive concentrations of intrathyroidal iodide, such as

follows acute administration of large quantities of iodide, also inhibit these oxidative reactions. Normally, this effect is transient; however, in a few peculiarly sensitive individuals, the antithyroid effect of iodide may persist and lead to development of goiter and myxedema. Pharmacologic quantities of iodide can also inhibit proteolysis of thyroglobulin. This effect is most readily demonstrable in hyperfunctioning thyroids and is responsible for the rapid ameliorative action of iodides in thyrotoxicosis.

In the blood stream, thyroxin and triiodothyronine are almost entirely bound to plasma proteins. Electrophoretic analyses indicate that thyroxin is bound primarily to an interalpha-globulin termed *thyroxin-binding globulin*, or TBG, and to a prealbumin, *thyroxin-binding prealbumin*, or TBPA. Thyroxin is bound secondarily to albumin and perhaps to a beta-globulin. The interaction between thyroxin and its binding proteins conforms to a reversible binding equilibrium in which the majority of the hormone is bound and a very small proportion (normally less than

0.1 per cent) is free. Since only the free or unbound hormone is available to tissues, the metabolic state of the patient will correlate more closely with the concentration of free hormone than with the total concentration of hormone. Furthermore, homeostatic regulation of thyroid function will be directed toward maintenance of a normal concentration of free rather than total hormone. Thyroid hormone–plasma protein interactions are sometimes disturbed by alterations in the concentration or avidity of the binding proteins. An increase in binding activity, for example, will lower the concentration of free hormone and decrease the quantity of hormone available to the tissues. Total hormonal concentration will then increase until the concentration of free hormone is restored to normal. Converse changes will occur when the binding of thyroxin by plasma proteins declines. Primary changes in hormonal binding, therefore, will result in qualitatively similar changes in the total concentration of hormone but, in general, will not influence the metabolic state of the patient ultimately. The binding activity of TBG is increased in normal pregnancy, during the administration of estrogens, and in patients with estrogen-secreting tumors. Binding activity of TBG in plasma is decreased in patients given androgenic or anabolic steroids, in nephrosis (where substantial quantities of TBG are lost in the urine), and in patients receiving hydantoins that are competitive inhibitors of thyroxin binding by TBG. Rarely, the binding activity of TBG may be either increased or virtually absent for unknown reasons. Such idiopathic disorders of hormonal binding appear to be familial. The thyroxin-binding activity of TBPA is not known to be increased in any disorder, but it is decreased in patients with a wide variety of systemic diseases and by competitive inhibitors such as salicylates, dinitrophenol, and their congeners.

Thyroid hormone–plasma protein interactions are also disturbed by primary alterations in the concentration of hormone in blood, such as occur in hyper- or hypothyroidism. Since the activity of thyroxin-binding proteins is generally unchanged, the concentration of free hormone will vary directly with the total concentration. Since such changes in circulating hormone usually result from intrinsic thyroidal disease, homeostatic mechanisms cannot restore the concentration of free hormone in the circulation to normal. Primary changes in thyroidal function are therefore associated with persistent changes in the concentration of both total and free hormone and, therefore, with alterations in the metabolic state of the patient.

Because the free thyroid hormone in the blood represents only a very small proportion of the total, even in abnormal states, the concentration of protein-bound hormone will closely reflect the total concentration of hormone in the blood. This is generally measured as the protein-bound iodine, PBI, in the serum. Direct measurement of either the proportion or the total concentration of unbound thyroid hormone in plasma can be performed by dialysis techniques, but such measurements are not at present generally available. An indication of the proportion of unbound hormone can be obtained, however, by adding labeled thyroid hormones to plasma and determining the extent to which they are removed by adsorption to an indifferent, particulate material capable of competing for hormone with the plasma thyroxin-binding proteins. This principle forms the basis for such tests as the in vitro uptake of labeled thyroid hormones by red blood cells or by anion exchange resins. These tests reflect, but do not measure directly, the proportion of unbound hormone in the plasma.

Triiodothyronine is not bound by TBPA and is bound by TBG only weakly. As a consequence, the unbound proportion of triiodothyronine is normally eight to ten times greater than thyroxin. Triiodothyronine is, therefore, removed from the blood much more rapidly than thyroxin, which accounts for its failure to contribute materially to the total hormonal iodine concentration in the blood and possibly for its more rapid onset and offset of action. Its binding characteristics, however, do not account fully for the fact that it has a three- to fourfold greater metabolic potency than thyroxin when administered orally.

In the normal individual, the metabolic state reflects a summation of the action of thyroxin, which contributes substantially to PBI, and of triiodothyronine, which does not. Therefore, when exogenous hormone is employed to treat hypothyroidism or to suppress endogenous thyroid function, a normal metabolic state will be associated with a slightly elevated PBI if thyroxin is used and with a subnormal PBI if triiodothyronine is employed.

DIAGNOSTIC LABORATORY TESTS. Availability of a variety of clinically useful laboratory tests makes possible accurate evaluation of the state of thyroid hormone economy under diverse clinical circumstances (Table 82-1). For simplicity, such tests may be divided into two major categories: *nonspecific* tests, which measure some metabolic effects of thyroid hormones within tissues, and *specific* tests, which measure some aspect of thyroid hormone economy such as synthesis, release, or transport.

The *basal metabolic rate*, BMR, measures oxygen consumption in the basal state and is expressed as a percentage of values found in normal individuals of the same age, sex, and body surface area. Nonthyroidal disorders that alter oxygen consumption must be excluded if this test is to be of diagnostic value. Febrile illnesses, leukemia, neoplasms, hypertension, congestive heart failure, aortic stenosis, diabetes, pheochromocytoma, chronic pulmonary insufficiency, polycythemia, or perforated ear drums may be associated with an increased BMR. The BMR is most helpful in following changes in oxygen consumption in the same individual during therapy. Similarly, the serum cholesterol, creatine tolerance test, photomotogram, and electrocardiogram are of ancillary but limited diagnostic value because of their nonspecificity. Fortunately, measures of thyroid activity that more directly reflect some aspect of thyroid hormone economy are now generally available.

Table 82-1. COMPARATIVE VALUES COMMONLY OBTAINED FOR TESTS OF THYROID FUNCTION IN VARIOUS CLINICAL SITUATIONS

Diagnostic and Clinical Status	24-hr I[131] uptake, %	Serum PBI,* μg/100 ml	Serum BEI,* μg/100 ml	BMR, % normal standard	RBC-T₃ uptake, %
Euthyroidism:					
Normal values..................	15–50	4–8	3–7	−15–+15	11.5–19 (male) 11–17 (female)
Pregnancy......................	Normal/high	High	High	+20–+25	Low
Iodide deficiency.................	High	Normal/low	Normal/low	Normal/low	Normal/low
Iodide therapy, 3.0 mg/day........	Low	High	Normal	Normal	Normal
Thyroid, USP, >120 mg/day.......	Low	Normal/high	Normal/high	Normal/high	Normal/high
L-thyroxin, >0.4 mg/day.........	Low	Normal/high	Normal/high	Normal/high	Normal/high
L-triiodothyronine, >0.1 mg/day....	Low	Low	Low	Normal/high	Normal/high
Congestive heart failure...........	Variable	Normal	Normal	Variable	Normal/high
Hyperthyroidism:					
Untreated......................	50–100	7–20	5–15	High	>19 (male) >17 (female)
Pregnancy......................	High	High	High	High	High
Iodide therapy, >2.0 mg/day.......	Low	>20	5–15	High/normal	High/normal
Thyroid, USP, >120 mg/day†......	>20	High	High	High	High
L-thyroxin, 0.4 mg/day†..........	>20	High	High	High	High
L-triiodothyronine, 0.1 mg/day†.....	>20	High	High	High	High
Antithyroid drug therapy (euthyroid)	Variable	Normal	Normal	Normal	Normal
Thyroiditis (acute):............	Low	Normal/high	Normal/high	Normal/high	Normal/high
Myxedema (primary):					
Untreated......................	0–15	0–4	0–3	−20–−50	Unreliable‡
Thyroid USP, 120 mg/day-euthyroid	Low	Normal§	Normal§	Normal	Normal
L-thyroxin, 0.4 mg/day-euthyroid...	Low	Normal/high	Normal/high	Normal	Normal
L-triiodothyronine, 0.1 mg/day-euthyroid.....................	Low	Low	Normal	Normal	Normal

* The presence of trace amounts of mercury in serum will render the values for the PBI and BEI factitiously low.
† Suppression test.
‡ The RBC-T₃ and Resin-T₃ tests are not generally valid in hypothyroidism because of overlap with normal values.
§ Some lots of thyroid, USP, and thyroglobulin preparations (Proloid) may give somewhat lower values for PBI and BEI than represented by metabolic status of the patient.

The *serum protein-bound iodine* (PBI) usually reflects the concentration of circulating thyroid hormone and represents an excellent diagnostic laboratory test for estimating thyroid function. Under abnormal circumstances, however, PBI may include iodinated materials of either endogenous or exogenous origin. These may be either proteins themselves or may be firmly bound to plasma proteins (usually serum albumin). Many of these abnormal products (but not most organic iodinated dyes) can be separated from true thyroid hormones by a butanol extraction procedure, with the result that butanol-extractable iodide, BEI, more closely reflects the concentration of circulating hormone than does PBI.

The *thyroidal I[131] uptake* indicates the *proportion* of ingested iodide accumulated by the thyroid gland. A normal value suggests a physiologic rate of hormone synthesis if it is assumed that the total quantity of iodide being metabolized is normal and that the iodide, once accumulated by the thyroid, is incorporated into active hormonal products. When body iodide stores are expanded, the I[131] uptake will almost invariably decrease although the patient remains metabolically normal. The converse will occur in iodide deficiency.

The *thyroid suppression test* has come into wide clinical usage. This test reflects the integrity of the pituitary-thyroid mechanisms that maintain homeostasis, as described in an earlier section. It is based on the fact that when normal homeostatic mechanisms are disrupted, exogenous thyroid hormone will not suppress the patient's thyroid function. Abnormal tests are therefore found in patients with thyrotoxicosis resulting from hormonal overproduction, whatever its cause. In addition, abnormal tests reflect the physiologic disturbance which, in Graves' disease, may exist in the absence of thyrotoxicosis. Examples occur in some patients whose hyperthyroidism has been treated and in some exhibiting solely the ophthalmic manifestations of Graves' disease (hyperophthalmic Graves' disease).

The *thyrotropin stimulation test* (TSH test) is useful to distinguish primary thyroidal failure, either complete or partial (decreased thyroid reserve) from thyroid hypofunction caused by inadequate TSH stimulation. The latter may result from either intrinsic pituitary disease or from pituitary suppression by exogenous hormone. An increase in radioactive iodine uptake of 10 to 15 per cent or more or a rise in serum PBI of more than 1.5 to 2.0 μg per 100 ml indicates that the thyroid gland can respond to exogenous TSH stimulation. The usual dosage of USP thyrotropin is 15 to 30 units given over a 24- to 48-hr period, 5 to 10 units each 12 to 24 hr. The second uptake test or PBI is obtained 24 hr after the last dose of TSH. Absence of a measurable response to TSH may be caused by several factors but is most commonly the result of primary thyroid failure.

Values for the 24-hr thyroidal radioactive iodine uptake, serum PBI, and BEI as well as the in vitro triiodothyronine uptake tests are listed in Table 82-1 for common clinical situations. Despite the specificity of these tests, numerous factors may alter their absolute value and yield a result inconsistent either with other results or with the clinical condition of the patient. Modification of test results by extraneous factors most commonly follows administration of iodine, in either organic or inorganic form. Here, high values for tests measuring serum iodine levels and low thyroidal uptakes of I^{131} are seen. Under such circumstances, the tests of hormonal binding (RBC-T_3 and Resin-T_3) are useful since they are not influenced by nonhormonal iodinated compounds. The presence of mercury in serum will produce factitiously low values for PBI and BEI but will not alter the binding tests. On the other hand, systemic disorders and drugs that alter protein binding also affect the values for the RBC-T_3 and Resin-T_3 tests. Liver disease, cachexia, pulmonary insufficiency, acidosis, estrogens, androgens, anticoagulants, and anticonvulsants produce deviations in the RBC-T_3 or Resin-T_3 tests that differ from the values expected from the patient's clinical status. When there is some apparent contradiction in the values for different tests, the explanation can usually be found by a careful history of drug ingestion and by a physiologic interpretation of the observed facts.

SIMPLE (NONTOXIC) GOITER

There is considerable confusion concerning the descriptive terms *endemic* and *sporadic goiter*. Endemic implies an etiologic factor or factors common to a particular geographic region. The term has been defined as the presence of generalized or localized thyroid enlargement in over 10 per cent of the population. The connotation of sporadic is that goiter arises in nonendemic areas as a result of a stimulus that does not affect the population generally. Since these terms fail to define or distinguish the causes of such goiters and since thyroid enlargement of diverse etiology may exist in both endemic and nonendemic regions, it seems prudent to employ a general term such as *simple* or *nontoxic goiter*. This all-inclusive

category can then be further subdivided into specific etiologic groups as defined by objective procedures. Simple or nontoxic goiter may be defined as any enlargement of the thyroid gland that does not result from an inflammatory or neoplastic process and does not lead to thyrotoxicosis or myxedema.

The historical and geographic aspects of simple goiter are discussed in Chap. 71.

ETIOLOGY. Although the causes of simple goiter are manifold, their clinical manifestations reflect the operation of a common pathophysiologic mechanism. Simple goiter results when one or more factors impair the capacity of the thyroid, in the basal state, to secrete sufficient quantities of physiologically active hormone to meet the needs of peripheral tissues. Under these conditions, secretion of thyrotropin (TSH) is enhanced, and this stimulates both glandular growth and the activity of all intrathyroidal reactions involved in synthesis and secretion of thyroid hormone. Such compensatory increases in functioning thyroidal mass and stimulation of cellular activity are sufficient to overcome mild or moderate impairments of hormonal synthesis and the patient remains metabolically normal although goitrous. When, however, impairment of hormonal synthesis is severe, compensatory responses are inadequate and the patient is both goitrous and more or less severely hypothyroid. Thus, the entity of simple goiter cannot be separated clearly, in the pathogenetic sense, from goitrous hypothyroidism. Specific causes of simple goiter are included in Table 82-2 and may exist with or without hypothyroidism.

PATHOLOGY. The histopathology of the thyroid in simple goiter will vary with the severity of the etiologic factor and the stage of the disorder at which the examination is made. In its initial stages, the gland will reveal a uniform hypertrophy, hyperplasia, and hypervascularity. As the disorder persists or undergoes repeated exacerbations and remissions, uniformity of thyroidal architecture is usually lost. Occasionally, the greater part of the gland may display a reasonably uniform degree of involution or hyperinvolution with colloid accumulation. More often such areas are interspersed with patchy areas of focal hyperplasia. Fibrosis may demarcate a variable number of nodules, which may be hyperplastic or involuted; these may resemble, but do not really represent, true neoplasms (adenomas). Areas of hemorrhage and calcification may be present.

CLINICAL PICTURE. In simple goiter, the clinical manifestations arise solely from enlargement of the thyroid, since the metabolic state of the patient is normal. In goitrous hypothyroidism, symptoms caused by thyromegaly are similarly present but are accompanied by signs and symptoms of hormonal insufficiency. Mechanical sequelae include compression and displacement of the trachea or esophagus, occasionally with obstructive symptoms if the goiter becomes sufficiently large. Superior mediastinal obstruction may occur with large intrathoracic goiters. Signs of compression can be induced in the case of large cervical goiters when the patient's arms are raised above the head (Pemberton's sign); suffusion of the face, giddiness, or syncope may result from this maneuver. Compression of the recurrent laryngeal nerve leading to hoarseness is rare in simple goiter and suggests neoplasm. Sudden hemorrhage into a nodule may lead to an acute, painful swelling in the neck and may produce or enhance compressive symptoms. Hyperthyroidism not uncommonly supervenes in long-standing multinodular goiter (toxic multinodular goiter). It is not known whether this represents the superimposition of Graves' disease upon a chronic nontoxic goiter or a separate disease entity.

The diagnosis of simple goiter can often be suspected on clinical grounds. However, other goitrous conditions such as forms of chronic thyroiditis, drug or iodide goiter, or primary thyroid neoplasms cannot always be excluded by the consistency, size, or symmetry of the enlargement. A careful history is important to determine the prevalence of thyroidal pain and tenderness, drug ingestion, rapid changes in size or hoarseness. High titers of circulating thyroglobulin antibodies suggest but do not necessarily indicate lymphoid thyroiditis (Hashimoto's struma). At times, needle biopsy of the thyroid is indicated to confirm or exclude the diagnosis of thyroiditis, but it should not be used if thyroid cancer is suspected.

TREATMENT. The object of treatment is to remove the stimulus to thyroidal hyperplasia, either by relieving external encumbrances to hormone formation or by providing sufficient quantities of exogenous hormone to inhibit TSH and thereby put the thyroid gland almost completely at rest. In disorders characterized by decreased thyroidal iodide stores, such as iodine deficiency or impairment of the thyroidal iodide-concentrating mechanism, small doses of iodide may prove effective. Occasionally, a known extrinsic goitrogen can be withdrawn. Most commonly, however, no specific etiologic factor can be detected, and suppressive thyroid therapy is required. For this purpose, desiccated thyroid in dosage usually ranging from 120 to 180 mg is the agent of choice. Purified hormones such as thyroxin or triiodothyronine are equally effective metabolically but may render it difficult to assess overdosage through measurement of the PBI. Suppression of endogenous thyroid function is most readily assesed by serial measurements of the 24-hr thyroidal uptake of I^{131}. Partial suppression is indicated when I^{131} uptake is reduced below control values and complete suppression when the 24-hr uptake falls below 10 per cent. Such measurements can be obtained at appropriate intervals and the dose of exogenous hormone gradually adjusted as needed to achieve maximum suppression. Occasionally, physiologic replacement doses of exogenous hormone will induce mild but usually transient symptoms of thyrotoxicity. In such patients, more prolonged intervals between dosage changes will usually permit achievement of full thyroid suppression without inducing symptoms of toxicity.

Reported results of therapy vary widely. There is general agreement that the early, diffuse, hyperplastic goiter responds well, with regression or disappearance in 3 to 6 months. In the authors' experience, the later, nodular stage responds less favorably, and significant reduction in gland size is achieved in approximately half the cases. Internodular tissue regresses more often than do nodules themselves. The latter may therefore become more prominent during treatment. After maximum regression of the goiter, suppressive medication may be reduced to minimal levels or at times withdrawn. In an unpredictable manner, goiter will in some cases remain relieved while in others it will recur. In the latter instances, suppressive therapy should be reinstituted and should be continued indefinitely. When treatment is initiated in patients in the childbearing ages, it should probably be continued through the menopause.

Surgical therapy of simple goiter is physiologically unsound, but it may occasionally be necessary to relieve obstructive symptoms, especially those which persist after a conscientious trial of medical therapy. Surgical exploration of nodular goiter may be indicated in some individuals when evidence suggests carcinoma. However, the suggestion that subtotal resection of multinodular, nontoxic goiter affords effective prophylaxis against the development of thyroidal carcinoma is unsound. If for some reason subtotal thyroidectomy has been performed, use of physiologic replacement doses of desiccated thyroid, 120 to 180 mg daily, is recommended to inhibit regenerative hyperplasia and further goitrogenesis.

HYPOTHYROIDISM

HISTORY. The concept that sporadic cretinism is caused by absence of the thyroid gland was first expressed by Dr. C. H. Fagge at Guy's Hospital in 1871. In 1874, Gull described adult myxedema, stating that it resembled cretinism but occurred in adult life. The term *myxedema*, or *mucous edema*, has been credited to Ord (1878). During the subsequent 4 or 5 years, the Reverdin brothers, of Geneva, and Kocher, of Berne, observed that following thyroidectomy for goiter there appeared what they termed *postoperative myxedema* or *cachexia strumipriva*.

INCIDENCE. Cretinism is rare. The incidence of myxedema (juvenile and adult) is estimated to be 1 in every 1,500 hospital admissions. Adult myxedema occurs about five times as frequently in women as in men and most frequently between the ages of thirty and sixty years.

ETIOLOGY. Hypothyroidism may be either primary (thyroid gland failure) or secondary (anterior pituitary failure) (Table 82-2). Primary hypothyroidism dating from birth results in a clinical picture characteristic of cretinism. Two varieties of cretinism can be distinguished, athyreotic and goitrous. In areas of endemic goiter, cretinism is common and is usually, but not invariably, goitrous. The sporadic cretinism of nonendemic areas is usually athyreotic but may be goitrous. In the latter patients, hereditary disorders

Table 82-2. CLASSIFICATION OF HYPOTHYROIDISM

I. Primary (sporadic and endemic)
    A. Nongoitrous
        1. Idiopathic
        2. Postablative (surgery, radiation)
        3. Postinflammatory
    B. Goitrous
        1. Congenital and hereditary defects
            a. Trapping
            b. Iodination
            c. Coupling
            d. Deshalogenation
            e. Releasing
            f. Maternal-induced (iodide, antithyroid compounds)
        2. Acquired
            a. Iodides (excess or lack)
            b. Drugs (thiocyanates, PASA, butazolidine, cobalt)
            c. Natural goitrogens (food, milk)
            d. Thyroiditis (Hashimoto's)
II. Secondary
    A. Pituitary failure
    B. Transport abnormalities
    C. Utilization defects (hypothetic)

of thyroid hormone biogenesis can often be distinguished. Deaf-mutism is a common accompaniment of cretinism and, when associated with goiter, has been termed *Penred's syndrome.*

The occurrence of primary thyroid deficiency later in life gives rise to the syndromes of juvenile and adult myxedema. Under these circumstances, inadequate production of thyroid hormones results from destruction of the thyroid gland by disease, atrophy, or ablative procedures (thyroidectomy, radioactive iodine therapy, or external radiation). Secondary hypothyroidism results from a deficiency of pituitary thyrotropin (TSH) and may occur at any age as a consequence of anterior pituitary failure (Chap. 80).

A classification of the more important pathophysiologic etiologies of hypothyroidism is presented in Table 82-2. The most frequent cause of spontaneous hypothyroidism is idiopathic atrophy of the thyroid gland. In children, this may result from developmental abnormalities. In adults, such atrophy may represent the final stage of an autoimmune response to thyroglobulin or other thyroid antigens and may therefore be related to one form of chronic thyroiditis, struma lymphomatosa (Hashimoto's struma). Circulating thyroid antibodies may be detected in a majority of patients with spontaneous hypothyroidism (see under Thyroiditis). Postthyroidectomy and postradiation hypothyroidism occur more frequently than the spontaneous varieties, and radioactive iodine therapy of hyperthyroidism is currently the most common cause of hypothyroidism. Occasionally, in patients who have undergone thyroid ablative procedures or have experienced chronic thyroid inflammation, thyroid function is not completely abolished but is insufficient to meet adequately the peripheral hormonal needs. Such patients, who may have mild symptoms of hypothyroid-

ism, can be distinguished by their failure to respond to TSH and have been described as having decreased thyroid reserve.

CLINICAL PICTURE. The general appearance of children with hypothyroidism varies considerably, depending on the age at which the deficiency begins and the promptness of replacement therapy. Signs and symptoms of cretinism may be clinically evident at birth or, more commonly, within the first several neonatal months, depending upon the completeness of thyroid failure. These children are dwarfed, stocky, and somewhat overweight, with a broad flat nose, eyes set apart because of failure of naso-orbital development, coarse features with thick lips, protruding tongue, pale mottled skin, poor muscular tone and intestinal activity, spadelike stubby hands with x-ray evidence of retarded bone age and epiphyseal dysgenesis, delayed eruption of teeth, and malocclusion resulting from macroglossia. In infancy, the characteristic facies, the hoarse cry, the large tongue, the "potbelly," and the presence of an umbilical hernia should call attention to the diagnosis of severe degrees of thyroid deficiency. Diagnosis and treatment at the earliest possible date in infancy are important since the extent of mental retardation may be related to the age at which treatment is instituted. Good results are obtained only when the diagnosis is established early and adequate therapy is instituted at once. If therapy is delayed, most of the clinical features of cretinism may still be reversed but some degree of mental retardation usually persists.

The adult and older child with myxedema have a typical facies, characterized by a dull, uninterested expression and puffy eyelids, often with alopecia of the outer third of the eyebrows. The skin of the face exhibits creamy pallor, and occasionally there is palmar yellowing. The changes in coloring result from anemia combined with carotenemia. The skin elsewhere on the body is dry and rough. The subcutaneous tissue is indurated and doughy because of interstitial fluid of high protein content. The hair is brittle and dry. There is swelling of the tongue and larynx and a halting, slurred, hoarse speech with slowing of physical and, seemingly, of mental activity. Anemia, constipation, and increased sensitivity to cold are present as well as increased capillary fragility, as evidenced by susceptibility to bruising. Women with myxedema during the active ovarian cycle usually note prolonged or excessive menstrual bleeding. Some patients with hypothyroidism complain of constant rhinorrhea, coryza, or deafness. There may also be arthralgia, symptoms indistinguishable from those of peripheral neuropathy, signs and symptoms of cerebellar disturbance, muscular weakness, or myotonia.

The cardiac silhouette is usually larger than normal, partially because of dilatation but mostly from pericardial effusion, which is commonly present. Rarely, the cardiac silhouette may be small; if so, pituitary myxedema should be considered. Thyroid tissue is rarely palpable except in the presence of chronic thyroiditis, endemic goiter, goitrogen ingestion, or goitrous cretinism. Skeletal growth is usually normal in the adult patient with myxedema, but in children or adolescents both growth and skeletal maturation are usually retarded significantly. The relaxation time of the deep tendon reflexes is characteristically slowed in patients with myxedema. Severe ileus with a picture of megacolon is also seen. Rarely, psychoses (myxedema madness) may dominate the clinical picture in patients with myxedema. Untreated patients with profound degrees of myxedema may exhibit hypothermic coma (myxedema coma), a serious and usually fatal complication. Some features of myxedema coma are related to respiratory depression and consequent CO_2 narcosis. Occasional hyponatremia, not responsive to glucocorticoids, is present and may represent a form of refractive dilutional hyponatremia. Hydrothorax, ascites, and pericardial effusions of high protein content are not uncommon.

DIAGNOSIS. Laboratory examinations in primary thyroid atrophy reveal a low basal metabolic rate, elevated serum cholesterol level, low plasma protein-bound iodine, depressed red blood cell uptake of labeled triiodothyronine, and decreased radioiodine uptake in the thyroid. Extraneous factors that may modify the plasma PBI level or the radioiodine uptake of the gland are enumerated in Table 82-1. In some varieties of goitrous hypothyroidism, the thyroid uptake of radioactive iodine may be increased. In those in whom I^{131} remains unbound, it may be discharged from the gland after administration of potassium thiocyanate or perchlorate.

It is noteworthy that the spinal fluid protein concentration may be elevated in patients with profound myxedema. There may be a significant normocytic or slightly macrocytic anemia as well as gastric achlorhydria. When losses of iron are excessive, such as may occur with menorrhagia, a picture of hypochromic anemia may predominate. The electrocardiograph may reveal a marked decrease in voltage with flattened or inverted T waves.

The signs and symptoms of mild or moderate hypothyroidism are less striking. The symptoms are similar to those in frank myxedema but are less severe. Such symptoms are, however, readily confused with those of many other organic or psychogenic disturbances. Even the BMR may be low for reasons other than the presence of thyroid disease. It is important, therefore, to establish the diagnosis of true, mild hypothyroidism on the basis of objective criteria. Such criteria may be met either by the finding of subnormal values for PBI or I^{131} uptake or, in the presence of marginal values for these tests, by their failure to increase after TSH.

Hypothyroidism secondary to anterior pituitary deficiency may present a picture indistinguishable from that of primary myxedema. However, the accumulation of subcutaneous fluid (myxedema fluid) is usually not so pronounced in patients with pituitary myxedema as in those with primary myxedema. Careful investigation will usually reveal associated gonadal and adrenocortical deficiency out of proportion to that seen in primary myxedema. In general, the serum cholesterol level is within, or close to, normal limits in patients with hypothyroidism secondary to anterior pituitary failure, whereas it is usually elevated in primary myxedema. Patients with primary myxedema respond readily and satisfactorily to thyroid replacement therapy. In contrast, administration of this hormone to patients with pituitary myxedema is usually less effective and may precipitate adrenal crisis. The administration of pituitary thyrotropic hormone (TSH), 10 to 30 USP units over a 24- to 72-hour period, to patients with pituitary hypothyroidism is usually followed in 24 to 48 hr by a rise in the thyroidal uptake of radioactive iodine and in serum protein-bound iodine.

DIFFERENTIAL DIAGNOSIS. Little difficulty will be experienced in diagnosing classic cretinism or juvenile and adult myxedema. Occasionally, a mongoloid infant may be confused with a cretin. However, the characteristic mongoloid eyes, hyperextensibility of the finger joints, and normal skin and hair texture distinguish the mongoloid imbecile from the hypothyroid cretin. Chronic nephritis and especially nephrosis may simulate myxedema. This is particularly true of the chronic uremic patient with retarded mental acuity and characteristic facial expression. In nephrosis, the basal metabolic rate is usually below normal as is the level of the serum protein-bound iodine. Since the nephrotic patient may also exhibit anemia, hypercholesterolemia, and anasarca (simulating myxedema fluid), the differential diagnosis may be confusing. However, the uptake of radioactive iodine is usually normal in nephrotic patients, and the low level of serum protein-bound iodine is caused by a decrease in thyroxin-binding proteins in the blood, resulting from proteinuria. The hyperactive deep tendon reflexes of the uremic patient, as contrasted with the slowed relaxation phase of the reflexes in patients with myxedema, may aid in distinguishing the two conditions. Not infrequently hypothyroid patients exhibit anemia and clinically resemble patients with pernicious anemia. Though usually separate, myxedema and pernicious anemia may coexist; recent evidence suggests that they may share related immunologic abnormalities.

Patients with secondary hypothyroidism, because of attendant adrenocortical failure, must be distinguished carefully from patients with primary myxedema. Urinary 17-ketosteroid and 17-hydroxycorticoid excretion may be reduced in both conditions, and the response to the 2-day ACTH test may occasionally be misleading in differentiating these conditions (see Chap. 80). The finding of elevated levels of urinary FSH, a normal water-loading test, and a good response to metyrapone (SU-4885) helps distinguish primary myxedema from anterior pituitary failure. Although the patient with Addison's disease is frequently hypometabolic, absence of excessive pigmentation, a normal water-loading response, and low values for PBI and radioactive iodine uptake help distinguish myxedema from Addison's disease.

Table 82-3. APPROXIMATE EQUIVALENT DOSES OF
VARIOUS THYROID PREPARATIONS

Preparation	Average daily oral maintenance dose, mg*	Serum PBI†
Thyroid, USP	120–180	Normal
L-thyroxin	0.3 –0.4	Slightly elevated
L-triiodothyronine	0.075–0.125	Depressed
Diotroxin (British), 90% thyroxin, 10% triiodothyronine	0.25 –0.35	Slightly elevated

* Infants and children require proportionately larger doses of thyroid preparations than adults.

† Serum levels of PBI vary according to preparation used and may not be a direct measure of thyroid hormone effect (see text).

TREATMENT. Desiccated thyroid (thyroid, USP) is the most commonly used preparation and is usually administered in 30-, 60-, 120-, or 180-mg tablets. Its major disadvantage is inadequate standardization of hormonal content. Sodium L-thyroxin is available as 0.05-, 0.1-, 0.2-, and 0.3-mg tablets (Synthroid), and sodium L-triiodothyronine is marketed in 0.005- and 0.025-mg tablets. The British have introduced a physiologic combination of 90 per cent thyroxin and 10 per cent triiodothyronine (Diotroxin) which is chemically pure and represents a combination of thyroid hormones in proportions said to be secreted in normal individuals. The average daily maintenance dosages of these preparations are listed in Table 82-3. Some commercially available lots of USP thyroid, as well as some lots of a thyroglobulin preparation (Proloid), give levels of PBI lower than anticipated by the patient's metabolic status. This is presumably a result of increased proportions of triiodothyronine to thyroxin in these preparations.

In all instances, except perhaps in myxedema coma, it is desirable to institute therapy with relatively small doses of a thyroid substance since sudden changes in metabolic level may induce undesirable psychologic or cardiovascular disturbances, especially in elderly patients. The occurrence of angina pectoris or congestive heart failure during therapy for myxedema is an indication to proceed with caution since rapid changes in metabolic rate may precipitate as well as increase the severity of these conditions. In adults, one may begin with a dose of 15 mg USP thyroid or less per day, gradually increasing the dosage at weekly or biweekly intervals. In patients over forty or fifty years of age, thyroid therapy should be given cautiously with longer intervals between increments in dosage. The usual daily dose of desiccated thyroid necessary to maintain an athyreotic patient in euthyroidism is 90 to 180 mg. In the presence of any evidence of cardiovascular disease, the total dosage should not exceed 30 to 60 mg daily until the patient has been followed for several weeks at this level. The maximum effect from a given dosage level will not be obtained for at least 7 to 10 days, and thyroid hormone action will persist for several weeks after the last dose. It is not necessary to give desiccated thyroid more than once daily. Because of its relatively more rapid onset and shorter duration of action, triiodothyronine may be given in divided doses.

In many patients, generalized muscular aching follows initiation of therapy regardless of the dosage of thyroid hormone, and occasionally coryza is noted. It is essential in patients with cretinism or juvenile myxedema to maintain therapy at close to toxic levels in order to ensure the desired growth response. The requirement for optimum bone growth appears to be higher than that usually needed for satisfactory maintenance of the overall clinical status. Children need somewhat more thyroid in proportion to their size than do adults. Dosage usually must be adjusted according to clinical evaluation of the effects obtained, at the same time avoiding symptoms of overdosage such as tachycardia, irritability, continuous weight loss, diarrhea, or sweating. In panhypopituitarism, thyroid hormone therapy should *not* be instituted until after adrenocortical replacement therapy has been initiated. The initial dose of desiccated thyroid should be small and increased gradually by 15-mg increments at 3-week intervals.

It should be noted that patients with untreated myxedema, like patients with Addison's disease, are extremely sensitive to the pharmacologic actions of many drugs such as narcotics, barbiturates, and tranquilizers as well as to most stressful situations such as operations. Patients with myxedema coma should be treated with parenteral triiodothyronine, adrenocortical steroids, artificial respiration (if CO_2 narcosis exists), and correction of any electrolyte disturbances.

HYPERTHYROIDISM

The terms *hyperthyroidism* and *thyrotoxicosis* usually denote the complex of physiologic and biochemical disturbances that result when the tissues are exposed to excessive quantities of thyroid hormones. This occurs most commonly in association with diffuse hyperplasia of the thyroid gland often accompanied by specific ophthalmic abnormalities and is usually designated *Graves' disease.* It is also termed *Parry's* or *Basedow's disease.* It should be recognized, however, that hyperthyroidism may result from overproduction of thyroid hormone by a hyperfunctioning adenoma, multinodular goiter (Plummer's disease), or ectopic thyroid tissue. The peripheral features of hyperthyroidism also result when thyroid medication is taken in excess (thyrotoxicosis factitia). The following discussion will deal mainly with Graves' disease. In addition, features of other disorders that may produce hyperthyroidism will be discussed.

HISTORY. In 1786, Dr. Caleb Parry described a disease characterized by thyroid enlargement, dilatation of the heart, palpitation, exophthalmos, and nervous as well as menstrual symptoms. Graves and

Basedow, between the years 1835 and 1843, published treatises independently on the syndrome that now bears their names. That hyperthyroidism was the fundamental disorder in Graves' disease was formulated by Möbius in Germany in 1887. The use of iodine in the treatment of thyrotoxicosis was popularized by Plummer. Recent advances in the medical therapy of hyperthyroidism include the introduction in 1942 of antithyroid substances such as derivatives of thiourea and imidazole. Radioactive iodine, introduced in 1942, now occupies a prominent position as a therapeutic agent in the treatment of thyrotoxicosis.

INCIDENCE. Graves' disease is a relatively common disorder, which may occur at any age, but especially in the third and fourth decades. The disease is much more frequent in women than in men. In nongoitrous areas the ratio of predominance in females may be as high as 8:1. In endemic goitrous areas the ratio is smaller. Hyperthyroidism is comparatively rare in children. When it occurs, there is usually a diffuse goiter free of nodules.

ETIOLOGY. Basic to Graves' disease is a derangement of those homeostatic mechanisms which normally adjust thyroidal secretion to meet the physiologic needs of peripheral tissues. In the past, it had been suggested that this was a result of overproduction of pituitary thyrotropin, but convincing evidence of this was lacking. More recently, interest has been focused on the possibility that other thyroid stimulators, possibly not of pituitary origin, may be responsible for the major manifestations of this disease. The role of emotional factors in initiating Graves' disease has long been recognized, but the manner by which this is mediated is unknown.

PATHOLOGY. In Graves' disease the thyroid gland is diffusely enlarged bilaterally, soft, and vascular. The essential pathology is that of parenchymatous hypertrophy and hyperplasia, characterized by increased height of the epithelium and redundancy of the follicular wall, giving the picture of papillary infoldings and cytologic evidence of increased activity. Such hyperplasia is usually accompanied by lymphocytic infiltration. In hyperthyroidism associated with nodular goiters (Plummer's disease), the major part of the thyroid tissue shows colloid involutional changes with hyperplastic paranodular areas that exhibit the functional changes responsible for the hyperthyroidism. This type of gland is thought to represent the end stage of an involuted nodular goiter and is erroneously termed *toxic adenoma*. True thyroid tumors (adenomas) that produce hyperfunction occur only rarely; in these, the paranodular tissue is inactive. Following iodine medication, there is colloid storage, which sometimes causes enlargement and increased firmness of the gland. Graves' disease is associated with generalized lymphoid hyperplasia and infiltration. Thyrotoxicosis may lead to degeneration of skeletal muscle fibers, enlargement of the heart, fatty infiltration or diffuse fibrosis of the liver, decalcification of the skeleton, and loss of body tissue (including fat depots, osteoid, and muscle).

CLINICAL PICTURE. Common manifestations of Graves' disease include exophthalmos, goiter, fine tremor (especially of the extended fingers and tongue), increased nervousness as well as emotional instability, excessive sweating and heat intolerance, palpitations, and hyperkinesis. Loss of weight and of strength usually exist, often despite increased appetite. Hyperdefecation and occasionally anorexia, nausea, and vomiting may occur. Dyspnea, paroxysmal arrhythmias, and, in individuals over the age of forty, cardiac failure not infrequently occur. Oligomenorrhea and amenorrhea are commoner than menorrhagia. In general, nervous symptoms dominate the clinical picture in younger individuals, whereas cardiovascular and neuromuscular symptoms predominate in older subjects.

The skin is warm and moist with a velvety texture, and palmar erythema is often found. The hair is fine and silky. Occasionally, increased loss of hair from the temporal aspects of the scalp may be noted. Excessive melanin pigmentation is not uncommon. Ocular signs include a characteristic stare with widened palpebral fissures, blinking, lid lag, failure of convergence, and failure to wrinkle the brow on upward gaze. These signs are thought to result from sympathetic overstimulation and usually subside when the thyrotoxicosis is corrected. The *infiltrative ophthalmopathy* characteristic of Graves' disease will be discussed in a later section.

The diffuse toxic goiter may be asymmetric and lobular. A bruit heard best directly over the gland is not found invariably. When heard, it usually signifies that the patient is thyrotoxic but may also rarely be present in association with other disorders in which the thyroid is markedly hyperplastic. Venous hums and carotid souffles should be distinguished from true thyroid bruits. A hyperplastic pyramidal lobe of the thyroid may often be palpable if carefully sought.

Cardiovascular findings include a wide pulse pressure, sinus tachycardia, atrial arrhythmias (especially atrial fibrillation), systolic murmurs, increased intensity of the apical first sound, cardiac enlargement, and, at times, overt heart failure. A to-and-fro, high-pitched sound may be audible in the pulmonic area and may simulate a pericardial friction rub (Means-Lerman scratch).

DIAGNOSIS. When severe, Graves' disease (as well as other thyrotoxic disorders) is so striking that the diagnosis presents little difficulty. Goiter, eye signs, loss of weight despite good appetite, tachycardia, sweating, psychic instability, tremor, increased basal metabolic rate, high serum PBI and BEI, increased red cell or resin uptake of radioactive triiodothyronine, and a rapid, increased thyroidal uptake of radioiodine all serve to establish the diagnosis (Table 82-1).

In a few patients the clinical picture may be one of apathy rather than of hyperactivity, and the basal metabolic rate elevation may be relatively slight. In such instances the clinical detection of underlying thyrotoxicosis is difficult, but the thyroidal uptake of radioactive iodine and the serum protein-bound iodine levels are usually diagnostic. A barium swallow may be helpful in demonstrating displacement of the esophagus or trachea by substernal enlargement of the thyroid. All patients with unexplained cardiac failure or irregularities in rhythm, especially supraventricular tachycardias, should be surveyed carefully for underlying thyrotoxicosis. In patients with pre-existing cardiac disease, even mild thyrotoxicosis may induce severe disability. The circulation time may be rapid or normal in the presence of an elevated venous pressure, and the response to digitalis is usually poor.

Although eye signs are important, it should be recognized that infiltrative ophthalmopathy may occur antecedent to or in the absence of thyrotoxicosis. Prominent eyes and wide palpebral fissures without infiltrative ophthalmopathy occur normally in some individuals. Proptosis and occasionally mild degrees of conjunctival hyperemia are seen in advanced uremia, Cushing's syndrome, cirrhosis of the liver, and malignant hypertension; in such instances, thyroid function is normal and the ophthalmopathy is not of thyroidal origin.

DIFFERENTIAL DIAGNOSIS. Signs and symptoms in a number of nonthyroidal disorders may simulate certain aspects of the thyrotoxic syndrome. Anxiety is a prominent feature of hyperthyroidism, and there is thus some overlap in the symptomatology of this disorder with pure anxiety states of emotional origin. Such symptoms as tachycardia, tremulousness, irritability, weakness, and fatigue are common to the anxiety of both disorders. In anxiety of emotional origin, however, the peripheral manifestations of excessive thyroid hormones are absent; thus, the skin of the extremities is usually cold and clammy rather than warm and moist. Weight loss, when present in emotional anxiety, is characteristically accompanied by anorexia, whereas in hyperthyroidism it is generally but not invariably accompanied by excessive appetite. Hyperthyroidism can occasionally be confused with such disorders as metastatic carcinoma, cirrhosis of the liver, hyperparathyroidism, sprue, and neuromyopathies such as myasthenia gravis and periodic paralysis. These conditions may be mimicked by hyperthyroidism or, rarely, may coexist with it. Sympathetic activity in thyrotoxicosis may result in an overlap of signs and symptoms with those of pheochromocytoma, including heat intolerance, excessive perspiration, tachycardia with palpitations, and a hypermetabolic state, which may often be severe. In all the above disorders, as well as other conditions considered in the differential diagnosis of hyperthyroidism, careful evaluation of one or more of the specific laboratory procedures previously described will usually distinguish hyperthyroidism from the others.

Hyperthyroidism is a disorder of so many diverse clinical manifestations that it may masquerade as one of many seemingly unrelated disorders. Signs and symptoms directing the physician's attention to gastrointestinal, cardiovascular, or neuromuscular diseases are not infrequent, particularly in older individuals. This differential diagnosis is extremely important in patients with heart disease in whom thyrotoxicosis must be considered in the etiology of atrial fibrillation and congestive heart failure. Subacute bacterial endocarditis, myocarditis, pericarditis, acute rheumatic fever, and coronary heart disease may be mimicked by uncomplicated hyperthyroidism.

COMPLICATIONS. A number of severe complications may result from the profound metabolic effects of hyperthyroidism or from other aspects of Graves' disease. As these require special consideration and treatment, they will be dealt with separately.

Thyrotoxic Crisis

The clinical picture of thyrotoxic crisis or storm is that of a fulminating increase in all the signs and symptoms of thyrotoxicosis. In the past, this disturbance was most often observed postoperatively in patients poorly prepared for surgery. However, with the preoperative use of antithyroid drugs and iodide and with appropriate measures directed to control of metabolic factors, weight, and nutritional status, postoperative thyrotoxic crisis should not occur. At present, so-called "medical storm" is more common and occurs in untreated or inadequately treated patients. It is precipitated by surgical emergency or complicating medical illness, usually sepsis. The syndrome is characterized by extreme irritability, delirium or coma, hyperpyrexia to 106°F or more, tachycardia, restlessness, hypotension, vomiting, and diarrhea. Rarely, the clinical picture may be more subtle, with apathy, severe prostration, and coma with only slight elevation of temperature. Such postoperative complications as sepsis, septicemia, hemorrhage, and transfusion or drug reactions may mimic thyrotoxic crisis. It is thought that in certain patients thyrotoxic crisis is associated with or precipitated by adrenocortical insufficiency. The possibility of this complication gains support from evidence indicating increased adrenocortical hormone requirements in thyrotoxicosis and from evidence indicating reduced adrenocortical reserves in this disorder.

Treatment of thyroid crisis should include the intravenous administration of large quantities of hypertonic glucose, hydrocortisone and iodide, the intramuscular administration of B-complex vitamins, particularly thiamine, and, where indicated, reserpine. Large doses of antithyroid drugs should be continued or instituted. The patient should be placed in a cooled, humidified oxygen tent and the hyperpyrexia treated as indicated. Full digitalization should be employed only in the presence of cardiac failure. If shock exists, intravenous pressor agents may be employed with extreme caution since patients with hyperthyroidism are particularly sensitive to pressor amines.

Ophthalmopathy

The clinical signs associated with the ophthalmopathy of Graves' disease may be divided into two components: the spastic and the mechanical. The former includes the stare, lid lag, and lid retraction that accompany thyrotoxicosis and account for the "frightened" facies and classic eye signs previously described. These findings need not be associated with actual proptosis and usually return to normal after appropriate correction of thyrotoxicosis. The mechanical component includes proptosis of varying degrees with ophthalmoplegia and congestive oculopathy characterized by chemosis, conjunctivitis, marked periorbital swelling, and the resultant complications of corneal ulceration, optic neuritis and optic atrophy. These changes are associated with and may result from an increase in retrobulbar volume and pressure produced by accumulation of fat, water and inflammatory cells in the retroorbital connective tissue and ocular musculature. When exophthalmos progresses rapidly and becomes the major concern in Graves' disease, it is usually referred to as *progressive* and, if severe, *malignant* exophthalmos. Such descriptive terms as infiltrative, pituitary, or endocrine ophthalmopathy have not added to our understanding of the disorder. The term *exophthalmic ophthalmoplegia* refers to the ocular muscle weakness that so commonly accompanies this disorder and results in strabismus with varying degrees of diplopia. Exophthalmos may be unilateral early in the course of the disorder but usually progresses to symmetric involvement. It must be differentiated from retrobulbar tumors of various types as well as from a rare granulomatous disorder, *pseudotumor oculi*. Exophthalmos can be familial, is more common in some ethnic groups, and is seen in other endocrine disorders such as Cushing's syndrome and acromegaly, as well as in uremia, malignant hypertension, severe aortic stenosis, and superior mediastinal obstruction. Where doubt as to the cause of exophthalmos exists, an abnormal thyroid suppression test affords strong presumptive evidence that the oculopathy takes its origin in Graves' disease.

It is probable that the ophthalmopathy of Graves' disease results from some factor or factors of the anterior pituitary gland or the hypothalamus, although the genesis of this disorder is not known definitely. The exophthalmos may stabilize or decrease after treatment of hyperthyroidism but usually follows a course independent of the therapeutic metabolic response. Rapid progression of exophthalmos with marked chemosis and edema is generally a grave prognostic sign and should serve as a warning that progressive eye changes may be anticipated. In treating this type of exophthalmos it is important to bring the thyrotoxicosis under control gradually and to prevent the development of hypothyroidism. Subtotal thyroidectomy or radioactive iodine therapy early in the course of this disease may enhance the progression of exophthalmos. Although there appears to be little difference in the incidence of progressive eye changes following the various forms of therapy of hyperthyroidism, antithyroid drug therapy seems to be the least provocative of severe or malignant exophthalmos. The long-continued administration of thyroid to forestall hypothyroidism may favor the regression of exophthalmic changes.

Application of ophthalmic hydrocortisone, 5 mg per milliliter, locally every 2 hr, may produce symptomatic improvement and slight regression of the chemosis. Use of tinted glasses and methylcellulose eye drops may afford some protection against irritation from dust or wind. Hydrocortisone, cortisone, or ACTH given systemically in high dosage may be helpful temporarily but should be used only in selected cases. Elevation of the head of the bed during sleep, a low sodium diet with added diuretic therapy, and cold compresses or pressure dressings applied to the eyes may be beneficial occasionally. X-ray irradiation to the orbit or pituitary has been successful in some instances. Tarsorrhaphy may be beneficial in protecting the cornea during sleep and in helping contain the exophthalmos. Corneal ulcerations must be treated vigorously. In cases that appear to progress despite all therapy, orbital decompression by surgery may be necessary ultimately to preserve the patient's vision.

Localized or Pretibial Myxedema

Localized myxedema, a circumscribed deposition of mucinous material in the deeper layers of the skin over the lower portions of the legs or dorsa of the feet, occurs in patients with past or present Graves' disease and is not a manifestation of hypothyroidism. The affected area of skin may be pruritic with increased pigmentation, hirsutism, and a *peau d'orange* appearance that is sharply delineated from the normal skin. The clinical course resembles that of exophthalmos, with which it is associated frequently. It may also be associated with clubbing of the fingers. About half the cases occur during the active stage of thyrotoxicosis, and in the remainder the lesions develop after treatment. The activity of the disorder is usually self-limited. No form of therapy is entirely satisfactory, although the local injection of hyaluronidase or hydrocortisone has been beneficial transiently in some cases.

Thyrotoxic Heart Disease

The cardiac manifestations of hyperthyroidism have been described. Many elderly patients may exhibit obvious cardiac disease but without the usual clinical appearance of hyperthyroidism. These thyrocardiac patients have been called *apathetic* or *masked*. Occasionally they represent difficult diagnostic problems but if one maintains a constant awareness of thyrotoxicosis in patients with heart disease, the correct diagnosis is almost always suspected. In these patients hyperthyroidism is usually associated with a toxic multinodular goiter. Although the basal metabolic rate may not be grossly abnormal, the plasma protein-bound iodine (in the absence of antecedent mercurial therapy) and the radioactive iodine uptake of the thyroid are usually diagnostic.

In patients with cardiac decompensation and thyrotoxicosis, the cardiac output is frequently above normal, with a rapid or normal circulation time in spite of an elevated venous pressure. This condition is one of several examples of so-called "high-output failure." Even though elevated, the cardiac output is unable to satisfy the high metabolic requirements of the body, and thus heart failure occurs. It is probably wise to obtain such thyroid studies as the protein-bound iodine and the radioactive iodine uptake in all patients with atrial fibrillation or congestive heart failure of undetermined etiology, since the finding of thyrotoxicosis affords a remediable form of cardiac disease.

Evidence suggests that the production of hypothyroidism and, consequently, hypometabolism is beneficial in appropriately selected *euthyroid* patients with congestive heart failure from any cause or in those with angina pectoris or intractable supraventricular tachycardia. This hypothyroidism may be produced readily by the administration of radioactive iodine.

Thyrotoxic Myopathy

Weakness, impairment of muscular function, and wasting of varying severity often accompany thyrotoxicosis and may suggest the presence of a primary muscular disorder. In certain patients, severe myopathy may be the dominant feature of thyrotoxicosis. Creatinuria is present under these circumstances, as it is in nonthyrotoxic myopathies. Myasthenia gravis and periodic paralysis occur more commonly with, or may be exacerbated by, thyrotoxicosis. A moderately beneficial response to prostigmine and related drugs may occur in thyrotoxicosis and does not of itself indicate the presence of myasthenia gravis (see Chap. 224).

Thyrotoxic Bone Disease

Skeletal demineralization is a not uncommon manifestation of thyrotoxicosis and is associated with hypercalciuria and hyperphosphaturia even when loss of bone salts is not demonstrable radiologically. Serum calcium, phosphorus, and alkaline phosphatase levels are usually normal. In some patients, however, serum calcium and alkaline phosphatase may be elevated. The latter findings may be purely a manifestation of uncomplicated thyrotoxicosis rather than associated hyperparathyroidism, but at times the two diseases coexist. Clinically, significant degrees of skeletal demineralization are rarely seen except in elderly patients in whom thyrotoxicosis may accentuate the effects of preexisting osteoporosis (see Chap. 227).

TREATMENT. Graves' disease is a disorder often characterized by cyclic phases of exacerbation and remission. Occasionally, patients with mild forms of the disease may recover spontaneously. This characteristic of Graves' disease has important implications in the choice of and response to therapy.

There are two major approaches to the treatment of hyperthyroidism; both are directed to limiting the quantity of thyroid hormones the gland can produce. The first major therapeutic category, the use of antithyroid agents, interposes a chemical blockade to

hormone synthesis, the effect of which is operative only as long as the drug is administered. Thus, the agents can control successfully a single phase of active thyrotoxicity but probably will not prevent exacerbation at some subsequent period. The second major approach is ablation of thyroid tissue, thereby limiting hormone production. This may be achieved either surgically or by means of radioactive iodine. Since these procedures induce permanent anatomic alterations of the thyroid, they can control the individual active phase and are more likely to prevent recurrence of thyrotoxicity during a later exacerbation.

Each major mode of therapy has advantages and disadvantages, indications and contraindications. The latter are more often relative than absolute. In general, a trial of long-term antithyroid therapy is desirable in children, adolescents, young adults, and pregnant women, but it may also be employed in older patients. Indications for ablative procedures include relapse or recurrence following drug therapy, a large goiter, drug toxicity, and failure of the patient to follow a medical regimen or to return for periodic examinations. Subtotal thyroidectomy is usually elected for patients under the age of forty in whom ablative therapy is required. With older patients, radioactive iodine is clearly the ablative procedure of choice, as it is for patients who have had previous thyroid surgery or those in whom serious systemic disease contraindicates elective surgery.

In those patients selected for long-term antithyroid therapy, satisfactory control can almost always be achieved if a sufficient dosage of the drug is administered. Most patients can be managed successfully by propylthiouracil, 100 mg every 8 hr. Methimazole is at least as effective as propylthiouracil when administered in one-tenth the dosage. Once euthyroidism is achieved, the initial daily dosage may be reduced to the smallest doses that control the thyrotoxicosis fully. In many clinics, however, the initial dose is continued and is supplemented with 120 to 180 mg USP thyroid or its equivalent in synthetic thyroid preparations. By this latter regimen, hypothyroidism resulting from overdosage of antithyroid drugs can be prevented. This is especially important in pregnant patients. Furthermore, the undesirable consequences of hypothyroidism, such as enhancement of oculopathy and enlargement of the goiter, may thereby be forestalled. The precise duration of therapy is difficult to predict in the individual patient and may be a function of the spontaneous course of the disease itself. If this is the case, the longer the course of therapy, the more likely it is that the patient will remain well when the drug is discontinued. In general, however, an 18- to 24-month course is usually employed. A normal suppressive response to exogenous thyroid hormone when the antithyroid compound is discontinued indicates that the patient is likely to remain well for some time. Following a regimen of this type, approximately 50 per cent of patients will remain well for a prolonged period or indefinitely.

During the treatment of hyperthyroidism occurring

with pregnancy, the basal metabolic rate should not be maintained at a lower value than is physiologic for that particular trimester in order to assure a normal thyroid status in the fetus. During the last trimester of pregnancy the basal metabolic rate should be maintained usually between +25 and +30 per cent, and the plasma protein-bound iodine level will remain usually around 7 to 10 μg per 100 ml. The use of thyroid replacement therapy is especially efficacious when antithyroid compounds are employed in the treatment of hyperthyroidism during pregnancy.

Leukopenia is the principal undesirable side effect of antithyroid drugs. Mild transient leukopenia may occur in approximately 10 per cent of patients treated and is not necessarily an indication for discontinuing therapy. When the absolute number of polymorphonuclear leukocytes reaches 1,500 or less, antithyroid medication should be discontinued. Allergic rashes and drug sensitivity develop in a small percentage of patients. These may disappear with antihistamine therapy at the same or reduced dosage of antithyroid agent, but it is probably preferable, when sensitivity reactions occur, to change to another drug. On rare occasions (in less than 0.2 per cent), agranulocytosis may occur. This may be sudden in onset.

Iodides inhibit the release of thyroid hormones from the thyrotoxic gland, and their ameliorative effects occur more rapidly than those of antithyroid compounds. However, response to iodides is often incomplete and transient. Furthermore, by expanding the thyroidal stores of hormone, iodides may prolong greatly the latency of response to subsequently instituted antithyroid therapy. Therefore, in the medical therapy of hyperthyroidism, iodides are mainly useful as an adjunct to other therapeutic measures in those cases in which rapid control of thyrotoxicosis is mandatory. Only rarely will contraindication to other forms of therapy dictate the use of iodides alone.

Radioactive iodine (I^{131}) affords a relatively simple, effective, and economic means of treating thyrotoxicosis. Its major advantage is that it can produce the ablative effects of surgery without the immediate operative and postoperative complications. Among the late complications, hypothyroidism may occur somewhat more commonly after radioiodine than after surgery, but this sequela is readily treated.

Other undesirable late effects of radioisotopic therapy remain to be evaluated, but current evidence suggests that for the most part serious complications will not be significant. Many physicians prefer to reserve radioiodine therapy for patients over forty years of age, thinking that it is currently not justifiable to administer an agent of undetermined radiation potentialities to younger persons, particularly those of childbearing potential. Patients with recurrent thyrotoxicosis following surgery, those who refuse surgery, or those who have complicating illnesses contraindicating surgery are excellent candidates for radioiodine therapy. The usual therapeutic dose for diffusely enlarged thyroid glands ranges between 120 to 140 μc per estimated Gm thyroid tissue (approximately 4 to 8 mc

total dose). Nodular goiters may require somewhat larger doses, usually 8 to 12 mc. Repeated doses are sometimes required, and these may be given at intervals of 3 to 6 months, and until euthyroidism is achieved.

Radiation thyroiditis from radioiodine may contraindicate its use in patients with large substernal goiters likely to induce respiratory embarrassment upon swelling. Patients exhibiting severe hyperthyroidism, heart failure, or progressive ophthalmopathy may first be rendered euthyroid by the use of methimazole or propylthiouracil; by discontinuing antithyroid treatment for 2 or 3 days, or longer, and then administering radioactive iodine, a good therapeutic response may be obtained and the potential complication of radiation thyroiditis avoided.

Before radioactive iodine was introduced, subtotal thyroidectomy was the classic form of ablative therapy and it is still widely employed in younger patients in whom antithyroid therapy is unsuccessful. Although precise preoperative programs differ, several general principles should be emphasized. Patients should first be rendered fully euthyroid by means of antithyroid agents. Only then should iodides (5 to 10 drops of Lugol's solution 3 times a day for approximately 2 weeks) be administered concomitantly to effect an involutional response in the gland. Antithyroid drugs should not be discontinued merely because treatment with iodides is instituted.

Hazards of subtotal thyroidectomy include immediate operative complications such as anesthetic accidents, hemorrhage sometimes leading to respiratory obstruction, and hypoparathyroidism. As time progresses, wound infection, cord paralysis, and hypothyroidism may occur. In experienced hands, surgery is an effective and relatively safe mode of therapy in which postoperative recurrences are relatively uncommon.

THYROID NEOPLASMS

ADENOMAS. True adenomas, as contrasted with localized adenomatous areas, are encapsulated and usually compress contiguous thyroid tissue. Such adenomas are generally present in the thyroid gland but may also occur ectopically. They vary greatly in size and histologic characteristics. Adenomas are often classified into three major types: papillary, follicular and Hürthle cell. The follicular adenomas can be subdivided according to the size of the follicle into colloid or macrofollicular, fetal or microfollicular, and embryonal varieties. There is considerable variation in physiologic differentiation as judged by their ability to concentrate radioiodine. Generally, the more highly differentiated adenomas (follicular) are most likely to mimic the function of normal thyroid tissue. Functioning adenomas are usually independent of TSH stimulation and may produce sufficient thyroid hormone to suppress completely the activity of the remainder of the thyroid gland. Ultimately, production of hormone by the adenoma may be sufficient to produce thyrotoxicosis (toxic adenoma). Such lesions can be dis-

Table 82-4. CLASSIFICATION OF THYROID TUMORS

I. Tumors of low malignancy
   A. Adenomas with blood vessel invasion
   B. "Histologic carcinoma" (small tumors found incidentally at operation; without symptoms, recurrence, or metastases)
   C. Papillary adenocarcinoma (occurs in young age group; lymphangioinvasive)
II. Tumors of moderate malignancy
   A. Nonpapillary, solid or alveolar, adenocarcinoma (occurs in older age group; hemangioinvasive; histologically the metastases may appear benign—"benign metastasizing struma")
   B. Hürthle cell adenocarcinoma (occurs in middle age group; usually locally invasive, occasional skeletal or pulmonary metastases)
III. Tumors of high malignancy (rare)
   A. Small-cell carcinoma (simplex)
   B. Giant-cell carcinoma
   C. Epidermoid carcinoma
   D. Fibrosarcoma
   E. Lymphoma

tinguished by isotopic scanning procedures, which reveal localization of radioiodide solely in the area of the adenoma ("hot nodule"). This uncommon disorder should not be confused with Graves' disease. When the toxic adenoma is ablated by surgery or radioiodine, the remainder of the thyroid tissue almost always resumes entirely normal function. The incidence of adenomas varies considerably and is usually increased in areas of endemic goiter. The etiology of true encapsulated adenomas is unknown and probably differs from that of adenomatous goiter. As in other organs, the role of benign adenomas as forerunners of carcinoma is uncertain.

Ectopic thyroid tissue, both encapsulated and nonencapsulated, can occur along the thyroglossal tract from the base of the tongue to the diaphragm. Lingual goiters, thyroglossal duct cysts, pyramidal lobe adenomas, and both esophageal and tracheal rests have been described. Ectopic thyroid tissue in the ovary (struma ovarii) may produce thyroid hormone and has been alleged to cause thyrotoxicosis. Use of isotopic scanning techniques can be helpful in diagnosing ectopic thyroid tissue if it is sufficiently differentiated to concentrate radioiodine.

CARCINOMA. Cancers of the thyroid gland are pathologically pleomorphic and seldom of a pure type. Definitive pathologic classification is difficult, and the degree of malignancy as determined histologically is not necessarily consistent with the clinical course of the disease. A modification of Warren's classification is given in Table 82-4.

From a clinical point of view, primary thyroid carcinomas are of three major types: (1) A small number are highly anaplastic and histologically undifferentiated. These are often quite malignant and for the most part not amenable to surgical or radiation therapy. (2) A similarly uncommon type is the follicular carcinoma, whose structure so closely mimics that of normal thyroid tissue that it has been termed *benign*

metastasizing thyroid carcinoma. This variety has a predilection for metastases to bone and is often first discovered radiologically or when a metastatic lesion is biopsied. (3) The largest number of thyroid cancers present with varying degrees of differentiation. The most common of these is papillary adenocarcinoma, which is generally of low virulence, metastasizes to regional lymph nodes, and is the most amenable to therapy.

DIAGNOSIS AND MANAGEMENT. The diagnosis and management of malignancies of the thyroid gland present several problems, each of which must be taken in proper perspective. In the past, statistical analyses of the incidence of thyroid cancer in surgical specimens led to a concept upon which was based the rationale for surgical removal of thyroid nodules in the prophylaxis or therapy of thyroid cancer. This concept proposes that goiters be removed surgically to prevent cancer and is predicated upon the finding of a high incidence of cancer in goiters containing either a single nodule or multiple nodules. Recent reappraisal of this concept has shown that, although the incidence of thyroid cancer in surgical specimens appears to be increasing, the actual incidence of thyroid cancer in the general population is quite low, somewhere in the range of 2.5 cases per 100,000 population per year. This is in contrast to the high incidence of nodular goiter in the population. The death rate from thyroid cancer is quite low, probably less than 0.6 per 100,000 population per year. The low death rate from this disease has suggested that the high incidence of carcinoma in surgical specimens results from effective selection of high-risk patients and that the pathologic criteria of thyroid malignancy may not truly reflect the natural history of this lesion.

Signs and symptoms most suggestive of thyroid cancer are rapid and progressive growth (not to be confused with overnight enlargement of a nodule, which is usually the result of hemorrhage or infarction), hoarseness caused by recurrent laryngeal nerve paralysis, presence of lymph node enlargement in the neck or supraclavicular area, or fixation of the thyroid gland to contiguous structures. Hyperthyroidism or hypothyroidism is rarely associated with thyroid cancer. Needle biopsy of the thyroid is contraindicated in the diagnosis of thyroid malignancy because of the tendency of these neoplasms to "seed" in the incised area.

The relative degree of functional differentiation can be determined by use of the scintigram obtained after administration of radioactive iodine. The degree of I^{131} uptake in the nodule can thus be determined and compared to that present in the normal tissue. In this manner, thyroid nodules may be divided arbitrarily into "hot" or "cold," depending upon whether or not they take up more or less I^{131} than the normal portions of the gland. Generally speaking, the "cold" nodules have a greater likelihood of being malignant because of their lesser function. However, it must be remembered that many benign nodules and cysts are likewise "cold" and that this test should not be used as the sole determinant of malignancy or operability. There appears to be some etiologic relationship between radiation therapy directed to the head and neck regions of children and young adults and the later development of thyroid cancer.

Conservative treatment of most thyroid malignancies is a growing trend in the approach to this problem. Such conservatism stems from several factors. First, thyroid cancer of high degrees of malignancy usually progresses so rapidly that it is frequently beyond any form of treatment at the time diagnosis is established. Second, nodular goiter is common while carcinoma of the thyroid is rare; hence, indiscriminate operation on all nodular goiters in the hope of uncovering the occasional malignancy may result in a greater morbidity and mortality than would be produced by the carcinoma if left untreated. However, as indicated above, a presumptive diagnosis of carcinoma in the thyroid can usually be made with a reasonable degree of accuracy on the basis of the criteria previously mentioned. Therefore, it should be possible to select a group of high-risk patients in whom surgery may be indicated. When such a high-risk patient is young, most authorities agree that surgery should be performed. There is less agreement as to the benefits of surgery when similar lesions are detected in older patients. When, at surgery, a carcinoma is found, block excision with a generous portion of surrounding normal tissue is recommended. Removal of lymph nodes in which cancer is obviously present is justified. In addition, selected nodes from areas of drainage should be removed to provide information concerning the extent and localization of distant metastases. Radical neck dissections do not appear to be justified at this time.

Although ablation of thyroid carcinoma with large therapeutic doses of radioactive iodine is theoretically possible and has been used occasionally, instances are rare in which the primary or metastatic lesions concentrate sufficient radioiodine to make this possible. External radiation may be helpful especially when metastases are localized to a single accessible area.

Currently, the use of suppressive doses of exogenous thyroid hormone to inhibit tumor growth is being explored. Because of the virtual absence of serious side effects from such medication (120 to 240 mg USP thyroid daily), all patients with thyroid cancer, regardless of whether or not surgery has been undertaken, should be treated with thyroid suppression.

THYROIDITIS

Thyroiditis is a comparatively rare disease. It may be specific (suppurative or nonsuppurative), nonspecific (acute or subacute), or chronic (Hashimoto's or Riedel's struma).

SPECIFIC THYROIDITIS. This condition may be caused by almost any known pathogenic organism, pyogenic or nonpyogenic, and is relatively rare compared to the nonspecific varieties. It may occur after infection of the mouth, pharynx, upper respiratory tract, or cervical lymph nodes. Very rarely tuberculosis, actinomycosis, syphilis, or infection with pyogenic organisms

may result in single or multiple abscesses. Classically, redness, swelling, and tenderness of the skin over the thyroid occur together with fever and other systemic signs of infection. Treatment consists, for the most part, of specific antibiotic or chemotherapeutic agents along with surgical drainage where indicated.

NONSPECIFIC THYROIDITIS. This variety of thyroiditis is of unknown etiology, is probably not an autoimmune disorder, and may be viral in origin. It is usually self-limited, with repetitive episodes of progressively less severity. It is seen predominantly in middle-aged women and rarely progresses to hypothyroidism. The most common form of acute or subacute thyroiditis is associated histologically with giant-cell formation (de Quervain's thyroiditis). The onset of symptoms may be dramatic and often seems to follow an upper respiratory tract infection. There is usually progressive swelling and tenderness in the thyroid gland, with radiation of pain to the ears or jaw associated with systemic manifestations of fever, nervousness, myalgia, and headache. Laboratory investigation often shows an elevated sedimentation rate, a normal or low leukocyte count, and a slightly increased PBI and BMR. The thyroidal I^{131} uptake is characteristically depressed but may at times be normal. Each lobe of the thyroid can be affected separately, but the entire gland is involved as the disease progresses. A needle biopsy is helpful if the diagnosis is not clear and may be necessary to differentiate thyroiditis from hemorrhage or from a suppurative process.

Therapy should be conservative, since complete spontaneous recovery is the general rule. Hypothyroidism only rarely results from this inflammatory process. Rest, fluids, and aspirin with mild analgesia, if necessary, usually suffice. When symptoms are severe, a short course of steroid therapy, 50 mg cortisone or its equivalent every 6 hr), usually will reduce them, but they often return upon withdrawal of the steroid. X-ray therapy in doses of 300 to 400 r has been reported to be efficacious rapidly in this disorder.

CHRONIC THYROIDITIS. Two varieties of chronic thyroiditis of undetermined etiology may be diagnosed histologically: *Hashimoto's* struma (struma lymphomatosa, lymphadenoid goiter) and *Riedel's struma.* Struma lymphomatosa, the more common of the two, occurs predominantly in middle-aged women. It is characterized by a firm, rubbery, lobular swelling of the thyroid, simulating multinodular goiter. The serum of patients with this disorder may contain increased amounts of gamma-globulin, and the thymol turbidity and cephalin flocculation tests may be abnormal.

In the early stages of this disorder, the patients are metabolically normal, and thyroid function studies are either normal or may reveal a slightly elevated I^{131} uptake. Occasionally there are abnormal, noncalorigenic, iodinated proteins in the blood. As a result, the PBI may be inordinately high compared to the metabolic state of the patient. Since these iodoproteins are not butanol-soluble, the BEI will provide a more accurate indication of the patient's metabolic state. Such dissociation of the PBI and BEI, although occasionally seen in other nontoxic goiters, most commonly occurs in Hashimoto's disease. Ultimately, hypothyroidism results from replacement of the functional thyroid structures by lymphoid or fibrous tissue. At this time, the serum protein-bound iodine and the 24-hr radioactive iodine uptake are usually low, and there is often no response in these indices to TSH administration.

Of particular interest in this disorder is the detection of circulating autoantibodies to thyroglobulin as well as to cellular antigens. A variety of antibodies has been described, certain of which may be measured by gel diffusion or fluorescent antibody techniques or by the tanned erythrocyte hemagglutination assay. It has been postulated that Hashimoto's struma is an example of an autoimmune disease in which the damaging effects of the antigen-antibody combination in the thyroid gland lead to destruction of functional thyroid tissue. Detection of circulating antibodies to thyroglobulin is not specifically diagnostic of Hashimoto's struma, however, since they may be found in other thyroidal disorders.

Diagnosis of Hashimoto's struma is suspected on clinical grounds when nodular goiter is present with hypothyroidism. Definitive diagnosis depends upon histologic confirmation, which may be obtained by needle biopsy and by the presence of high titers of thyroglobulin antibody. Treatment consists of replacement doses of 120 to 180 mg USP thyroid daily to correct or avoid hypothyroidism and, in some patients, to reduce the size of the goiter. When Hashimoto's disease is first diagnosed following subtotal thyroidectomy, it is particularly important to institute thyroid substitution therapy to avoid the unusually common postoperative consequences of hypothyroidism.

Riedel's struma produces a firm, ligneous swelling of the thyroid, which may involve surrounding neck structures. This disorder is exceptionally rare and must be differentiated from thyroid neoplasia.

REFERENCES

Forester, C. F.: Coma in Myxedema: Report of a Case and Review of the World Literature, A.M.A. Arch. Int. Med., 111:734, 1963.

Hazard, J. B.: Thyroiditis: A Review, Am. J. Clin. Path., 25:289; 399, 1955.

Ingbar, S. H., and N. Freinkel: Hypothyroidism, Disease-a-Month, Sept., 1958.

——: Physiological Considerations in Treatment of Diffuse Toxic Goiter, A.M.A. Arch. Int. Med., 107:932, 1961.

Lindsay, S.: "Carcinoma of the Thyroid Gland," Springfield Ill., Charles C Thomas, Publisher, 1960.

McGill, D. A., and S. P. Asper, Jr.: Endocrine Exophthalmos. A Review and a Report on Autoantibody Studies, New England J. Med., 267:133, 188, 1962.

Means, J. H., L. J. DeGroot, and J. B. Stanbury (Eds.): "The Thyroid and Its Diseases," 3d ed., New York, McGraw-Hill Book Co., Inc., 1963.

Pitt-Rivers, R. (Ed.): "Advances in Thyroid Research," London, Pergamon Press, 1961.

——, and W. R. Trotter (Eds.): "The Thyroid Gland," vols. 1 and 2, London, Butterworth & Co., Ltd., 1964.

Selenkow, H. A., and C. S. Hollander: Physiologic, Pharmacologic and Therapeutic Considerations in Surgery for Hyperthyroidism, Anesthesiology, 24:425, 1963.

Veith, F. J., J. R. Brooks, W. P. Grigsby, and H. A. Selenkow: The Nodular Thyroid Gland and Cancer: A Practical Approach to the Problem, New England J. Med., 270:431, 1964.

Werner, S. C. (Ed.): "The Thyroid," New York, Harper & Row, 1962.

83 DISEASES OF THE PARATHYROID GLANDS

Daniel S. Bernstein
and George W. Thorn

The parathyroid glands were first recognized as separate structures and described by Sandstrom in 1880. Shortly thereafter Gley (1881) and others performed extirpation experiments demonstrating that tetany ceased with the intravenous injection of calcium. Further proof of the endocrine nature of these glands followed from the preparation of parathyroid extracts by Collip in Canada, and by Hanson and Berman in the United States, and from the demonstration that these extracts could induce elevation of plasma calcium.

ANATOMY AND PHYSIOLOGY OF THE PARATHYROID GLANDS

ANATOMY. The parathyroid glands originate from the posterior halves of the third and fourth pairs of pharyngeal pouches. Therefore, like the thyroid, the parathyroids are entodermal in origin. In man the parathyroids are reddish- or yellowish-brown and are flattened, ovate, or pyriform bodies located on the posterior surfaces of the lateral lobes of the thyroid. There are normally 4 glands. The number may vary from 2 to 10, and their location is extremely variable. They have been found within the thyroid gland, in the mediastinum, and in scattered regions of the neck. The average size of a human parathyroid gland is $5 \times 3 \times 3$ mm, and the combined weight of 4 glands averages about 120 mg.

In the adult, the parathyroid gland contains chief cells and oxyphil cells. The chief cells are more numerous and are the source of the parathyroid hormone. These cells are 6 to 8 μ in diameter and contain glycogen. The oxyphil cells appear in the human gland at about the tenth year of life. They contain no glycogen, and their nuclei are somewhat pycnotic. They may represent a more mature or inactive chief cell. Another cell, the large water-clear cell (*wasserhelle* cell) derived from the chief cell, is the commonest cell type observed in hypertrophy and hyperplasia of the parathyroids.

EFFECTS OF PARATHYROID HORMONE. The function of parathyroid hormone is to maintain a normal level of plasma calcium. In the normal human being, the hormone performs this action so well that the plasma calcium varies only slightly from time to time even though the entry and egress of calcium to and from the body may vary widely. This regulation is mediated by an effect on the skeleton, the largest reservoir of calcium in the body. The significance of the phosphaturic effect of parathyroid hormone is unknown, although it may be a factor in stabilizing the plasma calcium.

Bone. The mechanism by which parathyroid hormone releases bone calcium to the extracellular fluid is unknown. It appears, however, that the hormone not only affects the relatively stable fraction of bone mineral, but also causes dissolution of bone matrix. The mobilization of bone mineral is a product of bone cellular metabolism, perhaps secondary to osteoclastic resorption and changes in bone mineral solubility produced by metabolic organic acid end products of bone cellular metabolism.

There is little doubt now that the action of parathyroid hormone on bone is a direct one. Bone tissue culture implants can be seen actively to resorb bone after minute amounts of parathyroid hormone are added. Parathyroid glands transplanted directly to bone cause local resorption around the area of transplantation. Histologically, the end product of parathyroid hormonal activity is a cystic space in the bone filled with fibrous tissue, i.e., osteitis fibrosa cystica. Any theory explaining the action of parathyroid hormone on bone must account for this pathologic picture.

Urinary Inorganic Phosphate. Since the advent of a more purified parathyroid preparation, arguments over the major site of the phosphaturic action of the hormone have been, for the most part, resolved. It is apparent that the hormone inhibits the well-documented process of renal tubular reabsorption of phosphate. There is, however, a small group who maintain that the hormone causes an increase in tubular secretion of phosphate, although the evidence for this process of tubular secretion of phosphate is scanty. The site in the kidney for tubular phosphate absorption is the proximal tubule, and the hormone exerts its effect on this function with little, if any, action on glomerular filtration rate.

Urinary Calcium. Renal handling of calcium is a complex process complicated by an interrelationship with sodium excretion. Calcium is probably actively resorbed from the distal tubule, although there may be some passive diffusion of calcium in the proximal tubule. In human beings with hypocalcemia, it appears that the TR Ca^{++} (TR = tubular reabsorption, Ca = calcium) is decreased. When parathyroid hormone is given, the TR Ca^{++} increases somewhat, although the evidence for this has not been sufficiently documented as yet. It would fit the scheme that parathyroid hormone tends to maintain the plasma Ca^{++} level within narrow limits. Excessive calcium loads presented to the kidney cause increased excretion of sodium, and vice versa, although mechanisms are not

well understood. One may conclude that the majority of investigators now feel that parathyroid hormone effects an increase in the renal tubular reabsorption of calcium, although additional evidence is needed to substantiate this hypothesis.

Gastrointestinal Absorption and Secretion. The effect of parathyroid hormone on the intestinal transport of calcium is probably to increase the amount of calcium absorbed against the mucosal-serosal gradient. The experimental evidence for this effect is disputed, and, even if substantiated, probably is of such small magnitude as to be relatively insignificant in affecting the overall calcium balance.

Lactation. It has been postulated that parathyroid hormone controls the amount of calcium in breast milk in animals, although there are no data regarding this point in human beings. Experimentally, parathyroidectomy in a lactating animal increases the calcium content of breast milk and parenterally administered parathyroid extract given to such animals will restore the calcium content by reducing the amount of calcium secreted by the tubular epithelium of the breast. Therefore, parathyroid hormone may act to conserve blood calcium not only by its action on bone, kidney, and gut, but also on another portal of egress of calcium, the breast.

Lens. It has long been recognized that the incidence of cataracts is high in untreated hypoparathyroidism. Some experimental evidence suggests that the lens calcium is increased in hypoparathyroidism at a time when extracellular fluid calcium is reduced. Incubation of the lens in vitro with parathyroid hormone can reduce the lens calcium.

In summary, parathyroid hormone has an effect on any organ system involved in the handling of calcium. This action, at any specific site, is designed to maintain a constant level of plasma calcium. The exact manner by which the parathyroid hormone exerts its effects on single organ systems remains an enigma, however, and a fertile field of future research.

Parathyroid Hormone. In recent years major progress has been made in purifying parathyroid hormone. The purest preparation has been made by phenol extraction of bovine parathyroid glands and subsequent purification by gel filtration. Various estimates of the molecular weight range from 8,400 to 9,400. All the common amino acids, with the exception of cystine, 17 in number, are represented. Methionine accounts for the sulfur content of the polypeptide. The absence of cystine and the isolation of a single N-terminal amino acid, alanine, support the conclusion that the hormone is a single-chain polypeptide. Parathyroid extracts can be reversibly inactivated by oxidation (as by hydrogen peroxide) and the biologic activity restored or increased above preinactivation values by reducing agents (mercaptoethanol; cysteine). Other agents, such as heparin, oil, and gelatin, appear to stabilize the activity of the hormone. The active, purified hormone contains both calcium-mobilizing and renal-tubular-phosphate–blocking properties. Parathyroid extract is available commercially. Parathyroid extract, USP, is standardized by biologic assay so that 1 ml contains 100 to 120 USP units. The USP unit is defined as $\frac{1}{100}$ of the amount required to raise the plasma calcium level of a normal male dog weighing 10 to 12 kg by 1.0 mg per 100 ml within 16 to 18 hr after a single subcutaneous injection.

REGULATION OF PARATHYROID ACTIVITY. The parathyroid glands do not appear to be under direct control of a tropic hormone elaborated by the anterior pituitary, nor is there evidence of nervous control of their secretory activity. However, a number of observations point to an indirect relationship to other endocrine organs. Parathyroid hyperplasia has been reported in cases of acromegaly, Cushing's syndrome, Addison's disease, and pancreatic islet cell adenomas. Experimentally, hypophysectomy in animals causes some involution of the parathyroids, whereas growth hormone, adrenocorticotropin, crude anterior pituitary extracts, and adrenal steroids cause hyperplasia. It is possible that these changes are secondary to the alteration in serum mineral levels mediated by the pituitary, thyroid, adrenal, gonadal, and islet cell hormones. A number of cases of multiple tumors involving the anterior pituitary, pancreatic islet tissue, and the parathyroids have been reported. Since tumors of these glands are quite rare, their association can scarcely be explained as a matter of chance. Also the familial occurrence of multiple tumors of this type has been noted. Although unexplained, the association of these tumors is of clinical importance.

The parathyroid glands alter their production of hormone in response to change in the plasma level of ionized calcium. It is generally agreed that hormone production is stimulated by hypocalcemia and decreased by hypercalcemia. Hyperplasia of the parathyroids is found in those conditions in which there is a tendency toward a low plasma calcium level, namely, rickets (or osteomalacia), calcium deprivation, and renal insufficiency with acidosis. There is conflicting evidence concerning an increase in parathyroid hormone production in patients with hyperphosphatemia in the absence of hypocalcemia.

A new polypeptide hormone, *calcitonin*, has been found in thyroid extracts. This hormone is a plasma calcium–lowering agent. The duration of action is quite brief (15 to 20 min), and it is probably secreted only in response to a hypercalcemic stimulus. As yet, its activity has been shown only in dogs and rats. The mechanism of action whereby calcitonin exerts its effect is entirely unknown, but it may be significant for an understanding of the homeostatic mechanisms responsible for plasma calcium stability.

Newer methods of radioimmunoassay and complement fixation techniques give promise that levels of parathyroid hormone in blood and urine may soon be estimated in various clinical states. Endogenous parathyroid hormone secretion is probably very small and has, as yet, not been estimated. Changes in the plasma calcium, phosphate, and alkaline phosphatase levels are still the most reliable and important indicators of parathyroid function.

HYPOPARATHYROIDISM

HISTORY. One of the causes of tetany is total or extensive parathyroidectomy. Tetany received its name from Corvisart in 1852. MacCallum and Voegtlin in 1908 showed that the mechanism of this type of tetany was dependent upon hypocalcemia. The Swiss surgeons Reverdin and Kocher in 1882 described postoperative tetany after a complete thyroidectomy for goiter without realizing that the condition was due to parathyroid deficiency.

ETIOLOGY AND PATHOLOGY. Primary parathyroid deficiency is extremely rare, usually occurring in patients under the age of sixteen, but often persisting throughout adult life. In most instances, clinical evidence of parathyroid deficiency is secondary to thyroidectomy. During the past decade increased knowledge and experience in surgical techniques have decreased the incidence of permanent parathyroid deficiency secondary to thyroidectomy. Transient deficiency is not unusual and is attributed to trauma, edema, hemorrhage, and temporary interference with the blood supply to the remaining parathyroid glands. There have been no documented cases of hypoparathyroidism secondary to the administration of radioactive iodine in the treatment of thyrotoxicosis.

PATHOLOGIC PHYSIOLOGY. There is a pronounced disturbance of calcium and phosphate metabolism as reflected by plasma calcium levels as low as 2.5 mEq per liter (5 mg per 100 ml) and plasma inorganic phosphate levels as high as 3 to 4 mM per liter (9.3 to 12.4 mg per 100 ml). The decrease in calcium facilitates the transmission of impulses across the myoneural junction, which is responsible for much of the clinical picture.

CLINICAL PICTURE. The most striking symptom is an increased neuromuscular excitability resulting from a decrease in the plasma ionized calcium. The presenting complaint in most (70 per cent) of these patients is tetany or tetanic equivalents. Tetany is manifested by carpopedal spasm in which the stiff, hollowed hand with rigid fingers is flexed at the metacarpal-phalangeal, wrist, and elbow joints and the legs and feet are extended. The tetanic equivalents include tonic and clonic convulsions, laryngeal stridor (spasm) which may be fatal, paresthesias, numbness, muscle cramps, dysphagia, dysarthria, muscular palsies, and cardiac irregularities. Spasm may involve the smooth muscle of the eye, gastrointestinal tract, bladder, and blood vessels. About 40 per cent of these patients are seen because of epileptic seizures. The electroencephalographic findings in these patients suggest that occasionally underlying factors unrelated to plasma calcium levels play an important part in lowering the threshold for convulsive seizures. Mental changes are frequent and include anxiety, depression, increased irritability, and psychoses. Acute symptoms may be precipitated by infection, undue fatigue, menstruation, and emotional upsets and by an increase in the phosphate content of the diet. In some cases, the symptoms may be quite mild, varied, and even vague. Patients have manifested fatigue, muscular weakness, palpitations, numbness and tingling of the extremities, and other signs of latent tetany for as long as 30 years before a diagnosis of chronic hypoparathyroidism was established.

On examination, increased neuromuscular excitability may be demonstrated by contraction of the facial muscles in response to a light tap over the facial nerve in front of the ear (Chvostek's sign). This test is almost always positive in untreated hypoparathyroidism; however, it does occur occasionally in normal individuals. Dorsal flexion and abduction of the foot may be elicited by tapping the lateral surface of the fibula just below its head (peroneal sign). If the circulation to the arm is occluded by inflation of a blood pressure cuff above the level of systolic pressure, the hand may assume the typical position seen in carpopedal spasm within 3 min (Trousseau's sign). This sign is sometimes negative in marked hypoparathyroidism. Extensive tropic changes of the ectoderm may be seen. The hair is likely to be sparse, prematurely gray, and is occasionally absent in the axillary and pubic regions. Generalized or patchy erythema may be found. The skin is rough, dry, and scaling, and there may be papules, vesicles, or bullae. A number of skin diseases have been described in association with hypoparathyroidism, including moniliasis of the skin, nails, tongue, and mouth. However, no etiologic relationship has been established. The nails are deformed and brittle, showing transverse ridging. In children one finds evidence of faulty dentition, including pitting and ridging of the enamel. Cataracts are frequently present, their extent being related to the duration and severity of the hypocalcemia. Early lens changes, not apparent on ophthalmoscopic examination, can usually be found with the aid of a slit lamp. Papilledema has been observed. The electrocardiogram usually shows a prolongation of the Q-T interval. The density of the bone may appear normal or increased. Abnormalities of dentition, such as deformed or absent roots, may be helpful in determining the age of onset of the disease. The pronounced disturbance of calcium and phosphate metabolism is reflected by lowered plasma calcium and elevated plasma inorganic phosphate levels. The alkaline phosphatase is normal or low. Hypocalcuria may be present, as shown by a negative Sulkowitch test (see p. 442). The spinal fluid may be under increased pressure without other abnormalities. When this occurs in the presence of papilledema, the diagnosis of a brain tumor may be made incorrectly. In primary hypoparathyroidism, bilateral symmetric calcification of the basal ganglions is commonly seen on the skull film. Other areas, such as the cerebellum and choroid plexus, are occasionally calcified.

DIFFERENTIAL DIAGNOSIS. The principal causes of tetany are hypocalcemia and alkalosis. Of the nonparathyroid causes of hypocalcemia, rickets, osteomalacia, steatorrhea, and renal insufficiency are the most common. Recently, there has been described a new syndrome of "decreased tissue calcium with tetany." This condition is manifested by severe tetany with normal plasma levels of calcium, magnesium, potassium, and carbon dioxide content. It has been demonstrated by radioactive calcium studies that the tissue calcium pool is lower than normal and that treatment with vitamin D will tend to bring the level of calcium in this pool toward normal. Extreme caution must be employed since the difference between the therapeutic and toxic dose of vitamin D is narrow.

In rickets, osteomalacia, and steatorrhea, a low value for plasma calcium is almost invariably associated with a normal or low value for plasma phosphate. In late-stage renal insufficiency with hypocalcemic tetany, the elevation in plasma phosphate level is disproportionately higher than that which occurs with a given level of hypocalcemia in parathyroid tetany. Nitrogen retention, as evidenced by an elevated blood urea nitrogen or nonprotein nitrogen, is nearly always present and differentiates the two conditions. A lowered plasma magnesium can also produce tetany. Magnesium salts have been used to eliminate hypocalcemic tetany. Furthermore, the level of plasma potassium plays an important part in the clinical manifestation of hypocalcemic tetany. The relationship of these three ions in the serum as regards tetany can be formulated as follows: calcium $\times$ magnesium/potassium. This is especially important in the treatment of renal failure where all three of these ions are drastically altered.

In addition to general renal insufficiency, there are two specific tubular lesions to be considered. The first is a failure of reabsorption of certain amino acids (Fanconi syndrome, Chap. 96) in which there is increased excretion of phosphate and low-phosphate rickets, and the second is a rare selective failure of calcium reabsorption accompanied by metabolic acidosis and often by renal calcinosis.

Alkalosis causes tetany with no demonstrable change in the concentration of calcium in the plasma. Alkalosis may be due to hyperventilation, to prolonged vomiting of acid gastric contents, or to excessive alkali ingestion. With hyperventilation, the carbon dioxide *content* of the plasma is reduced; whereas with vomiting, and alkali ingestion, the carbon dioxide–combining power of the plasma may be increased greatly (see Chap. 61). Alkalotic tetany occurs most frequently in association with acute infection, particularly in children.

TREATMENT. The object of treatment is to increase and maintain the plasma calcium at an approximately normal level.

MANAGEMENT OF ACUTE HYPOPARATHYROIDISM. Immediate correction of hypocalcemia may be accomplished by intravenous injections of calcium gluconate (10 ml of a 10 per cent solution) or calcium chloride (10 ml of a 5 per cent solution or an intravenous drip

Table 83-1. CALCIUM-REGULATING COMPOUNDS

Type	Route of administration	Dosage	Effect on plasma calcium
Calcium gluconate (USP).....	Intravenous Intramuscular	5 to 20 ml of 10% aqueous solution (IV) 10 ml of 5% solution (1 to 2 times daily IM)	Immediate but of only short duration
Calcium chloride (USP).......	Oral Intravenous Oral	10 to 25 Gm daily 55 ml of 0.2% over 1 hr (IV) or 10 ml of 5% aqueous solution slowly (IV) 10 ml of 30% aqueous (2 to 3 times daily)	Immediate but of only short duration
Calcium lactate..............	Oral	10 to 15 Gm daily (as a clear solution)	Immediate but of only short duration
Dihydrotachysterol (AT 10)...	Oral	3 to 4 ml (1.25 mg per ml) daily initially; 1 ml (3 to 5 times weekly) as maintenance	Delayed, with a maximum in 48–96 hr. Prolonged effect
Calciferol (vitamin D$_2$)........	Oral	50,000 to 200,000 units daily (1.25 to 5 mg)	Delayed. Prolonged effect
Parathyroid.................	Subcutaneous or intramuscular	100 to 200 units in severe tetany and then 25 to 50 units every 6 to 12 hr. Not recommended maintenance	Moderately rapid, with maximum in 8 to 18 hr

of 500 ml of 0.2 per cent solution over a 1-hr period) (see Table 83-1). The effect is transitory, lasting only a few hours, and additional calcium may have to be administered. Caution should be exercised with patients on digitalis, since rapid infusion of calcium may cause cardiac arrest. Parathyroid extract injection may be instituted along with the infusion of calcium and will give more prolonged action (12 to 24 hr). Parathyroid extract is available in injectable form containing 80 to 120 USP units per milliliter. From 100 to 200 units should be administered intravenously. Administration should proceed slowly initially since anaphylactoid reaction may occur and necessitate discontinuance. From 25 to 50 units of parathyroid extract may be given every 6 to 12 hr during the acute phase of hypoparathyroidism.

Dihydrotachysterol should be administered in doses of 1 to 3 ml (1.25 to 3.75 mg) one to three times daily by mouth until calcium appears in the urine, as indicated by the Sulkowitch test. The dose is then adjusted to maintain a normal serum calcium level. Treatment may be continued with this preparation or with a cheaper but just as adequate preparation of calciferol (vitamin D$_2$). Supplementary calcium preparations should be given orally as soon as possible. Calcium chloride is most effective, since it forms an acid solution which favors calcium absorption and also contains a higher percentage of available calcium. It may be administered in doses of 10 ml of a 30 per cent solution, well diluted, three times a day after meals (see Table 83-1). A licorice syrup medium will conceal the taste of calcium chloride solution.

MANAGEMENT OF CHRONIC HYPOPARATHYROIDISM. The objective of therapy in chronic hypoparathyroidism is to reduce the plasma phosphate and raise the plasma calcium levels. This is best accomplished by a combination of dietary and drug therapy. The diet

should include as much calcium as can be tolerated, but there is nothing to be gained by reducing the amounts of phosphate in the diet unless it is eaten in excess. From 4 to 8 Gm of the various calcium salts shown in Table 83-1 should be given.

Parathyroid hormone is rarely used except in critical situations since it must be given daily and may be associated with local reactions. There is no evidence that antibodies will develop to chronically administered parathyroid hormone. It is almost always advantageous to administer vitamin D$_2$ (calciferol) in ranges of 50,000 to 150,000 units daily, in order to enhance plasma calcium levels. Dihydrotachysterol, a synthetic derivative of ergosterol, may also be used, but while its action is similar to vitamin D$_2$ in all respects, it is much more expensive and rarely must be resorted to in favor of vitamin D$_2$. When vitamin D$_2$ or AT 10 (dihydrotachysterol) is used in therapy, the plasma calcium should be determined at frequent intervals, because persistent hypercalcemia and hypercalcuria may lead to deleterious effects. Since vitamin D$_2$ or AT 10 will cause an increase in the urine calcium before affecting a rise in blood calcium levels, it is important to check the urine level of calcium often as well as the plasma calcium, either by total 24-hr calcium excretion or by the Sulkowitch test. The Sulkowitch solution has the following composition:

Oxalic acid.................	2.5 Gm
Ammonium oxalate..........	2.5 Gm
Glacial acetic acid..........	5.0 ml
Distilled water q.s. ad.......	150.0 ml

The test is performed by adding 5 ml of the reagent to 5 ml urine in a test tube and noting the speed of appearance and the density of the precipitate. The result is graded 0, 1, 2, 3, or 4 plus. Routine use of the test for a short time enables one to become familiar with a normal response. The calcium intake (e.g., quantity of milk) as well as marked concentration or dilution of the urine should be taken into account. A negative test after a week on a diet free of milk and cheese suggests hypocalcemia—less than 3.5 mEq per liter (7.0 mg per 100 ml)—and a 3 to 4 plus test suggests hypercalcemia—more than 5.2 mEq per liter (10.4 mg per 100 ml). Although this test can be run by the patient, it is important to check plasma levels from time to time. A 2 plus Sulkowitch reaction is the most desirable.

An adjunctive mode of therapy is the use of probenecid (Benemid) by mouth in doses ranging from 0.5 to 1.5 Gm (daily). This agent is most useful in treating the tetany seen directly after inadvertent surgical removal of the parathyroids but is of little help in the chronic treatment of hypoparathyroidism. Rarely can Benemid be used alone. It acts on the kidney, blocking the reabsorption of phosphate by the renal tubule in a similar manner to the way it blocks the tubular reabsorption of uric acid. If epilepsy is evident, Dilantin or other antiepileptic drugs should be employed.

PSEUDOHYPOPARATHYROIDISM

The first description of this rare condition was given by Albright and his coworkers in 1942. This disease presents the same clinical and chemical features as hypoparathyroidism, except that these patients have round faces and short, thick figures. Subcutaneous centers of ossification are seen. There is a characteristic shortening of some of the metacarpal and metatarsal bones as a result of early epiphyseal closure, so that a dimple rather than a knuckle shows upon clenching of the fist. Most of the patients show some degree of mental deficiency. Not all these characteristics are necessarily present; any one or a combination of them may be found. The apparent parathyroid deficiency in these patients appears to be due to a lack of end organ response. This is supported by the failure to respond to parathyroid extract, the finding of normal or hyperplastic glands where biopsy specimens have been obtained, and the failure to demonstrate antibodies to parathyroid hormone in the serum of patients in whom studies were done. The failure of these patients to respond to parathyroid extract need not be complete, and there are cases which have almost normal response to injected hormone.

It was suggested that the abnormalities seen in pseudo-pseudohypoparathyroidism and which are also found in pseudohypoparathyroidism are probably due to separate genetic factors, which may penetrate independently. Subsequent reports support this concept. Albright and his group have reported a case of a young woman with a rounded face, thickset figure, characteristic smile, shortened fingers and toes, and subcutaneous calcium deposits. However, the plasma calcium and phosphate levels were normal, and the Chvostek and Trousseau signs were absent.

DIAGNOSIS. Because of the frequent history of convulsions, the condition may be incorrectly labeled epilepsy. The symptomatology, chemical findings, and physical signs are those of hypoparathyroidism. The relative resistance to parathyroid extract as measured by failure to produce a phosphate diuresis (Ellsworth-Howard test) serves to distinguish it from hypoparathyroidism.

The Ellsworth-Howard Test. The test is performed as follows: The patient, in the fasting state, is given 2 ml (200 units) of parathyroid extract intravenously, and the urinary phosphate content is determined hourly for 3 hr prior to, and for 3 to 5 hr following, the injection. Occasional anaphylactoid reactions to the extract make slow and careful administration necessary. Parathyroid extracts are assayed by their effect on the plasma calcium level, and recent preparations have not been so effective in producing an increased phosphate excretion as those previously available. It is best to compare the response of the patient to that of a normal control given the same amount of hormone. The degree of phosphate diuresis induced by parathyroid hormone is dependent upon both the level of endogenous parathyroid secretion and the responsiveness of the phosphorus reabsorbing mechanism of the renal tubules. Following the injection of a standard amount of parathyroid extract, there is a five- to sixfold increase in urine phosphate in normal persons, a tenfold or greater increase in patients with hypoparathyroidism, and at the most a twofold increase in patients with pseudohypoparathyroidism (parathyroid hormone resistance). Patients with hyperparathyroidism show a variable response to the extract.

TREATMENT. The therapy is the same as that outlined under chronic hypoparathyroidism.

PRIMARY HYPERPARATHYROIDISM

HISTORY. Generalized osteitis fibrosa cystica, a generalized disease of bones, was described in 1891 by von Recklinghausen. Askanazy associated this condition with a parathyroid tumor in 1904, and in 1925 Mandl removed a parathyroid adenoma from a patient suffering from this disease and noted a remarkable improvement. The occurrence of hyperparathyroidism without bone disease was pointed out by Albright in 1934. The clinical and metabolic studies subsequently carried out by Albright, Bauer, Aub, and Cope are classic.

INCIDENCE. The exact incidence of the disease is unknown, but thanks to the work of Albright and his colleagues there has been a deliberate search for the disease, with a consequent increase in the frequency of diagnosis. The disease occurs most often in middle life, and about 70 per cent of the patients reported are women. It has been shown that hyperparathyroidism can exist without evident disease of bone and that skeletal involvement represents a relatively late development. Involvement of the urinary tract is much more common than bone disease in the United States, presumably because of the high calcium intake, and in several series of cases more than 5 per cent of all kidney stones have been associated with hyperfunction of these glands. Many cases of hyperparathyroidism in the United States are "masked" by insignificant or atypical alterations in plasma calcium and phosphate levels resulting from a high phosphate intake.

ETIOLOGY. Hypersecretion of the parathyroid glands may be caused by adenoma, hyperplasia, or carcinoma. The most common cause of primary hyperparathyroidism is an adenoma (90 per cent of cases), hyperplasia is rather infrequent, and carcinoma is rare.

PATHOLOGY. Adenomas are usually limited to one gland. Norris collected from the literature 322 cases of parathyroid adenoma, with only 20 cases (6.2 per cent) having multiple tumors. The pathologic overactivity of these tumors is not closely associated with their size. The adenomas are encapsulated, soft, orange-brown masses embedded in fat. They are occasionally lobular. The appearance, grossly, differs from that of the hyperplastic gland, which is irregular in shape and a darker, mahogany brown in color. The adenoma usually involves the entire gland but may involve only part of it. Adenomas are found in all the locations of the normal parathyroid glands. In one large series, 75 per cent were found in the mediastinum. All cell types may be present, forming cords, glands, and solid masses. Cyst formation is common.

In primary diffuse hypertrophy and hyperplasia all the glands are involved but not necessarily to the same extent. The glands show a uniformity of structure, with a predominance of very large *wasserhelle* cells and a tendency to gland formation. There is a good correlation of size to the degree of overactivity.

Carcinoma of the parathyroid gland is extremely rare, accounting for 1 per cent of functioning parathyroid tumors. They are generally larger than adenomas and in most cases have been clinically palpable. All these tumors have been associated with severe hyperparathyroidism with bone disease. They are generally slow-growing, tending to recur locally when excised, and are very resistant to x-ray therapy. Metastases to the regional lymph nodes, lungs, and liver may occur. There is evidence indicating that carcinoma may develop from an adenoma.

The skeletal lesions observed in conjunction with long-standing hyperparathyroidism are discuesd in Chap. 75, Osteomalacia and Rickets. Degenerative changes occur in the renal tubular epithelium, heart muscle, and gastric mucosa and are often followed by calcification. About 80 per cent of the cases show some evidence of renal damage such as nephrolithiasis, pyelonephritis, and calcium deposits in and around the tubules.

MINERAL LEVELS. Characteristically, the plasma calcium is elevated and may attain values as high as 10 mEq per liter (20 mg per 100 ml). The plasma inorganic phosphate level is reduced below 1 mM per liter (3.1 mg per 100 ml) unless renal damage has resulted in secondary phosphate retention. In the presence of a high phosphate intake, many patients with hyperparathyroidism have plasma phosphate levels which fall within normal limits, with minimal elevation in plasma calcium levels. The excretion of calcium and phosphate in the urine is increased. With extensive bone involvement, the alkaline phosphatase may reach levels as high as 20 to 30 Bodansky units.

CLINICAL PICTURE. The earliest symptoms rarely lead to a diagnosis. They may be recognized in retrospect as an accompaniment of hypercalcemia. The symptoms include muscular weakness, anorexia, nausea, and constipation. Polyuria and polydipsia accompany the excessive calcium, phosphate, sodium, and potassium excretion as well as the renal lesions, which cause a loss of the ability of the kidney to concentrate urine even before structural changes have occurred. Often the first indication of hyperparathyroidism is renal colic or a spontaneous fracture. Deafness, paresthesias, and bone pain have been observed, and weight loss may be marked. On examination one may find hypotonia, muscular weakness, calcific keratitis (band keratitis), skeletal deformities, fractures, and tumor masses, especially in the jaw (epulis). When bone disease is present, x-ray studies may show a generalized decrease in bone density, cysts, tumors, fractures, and deformities, which are most marked in the hands, long bones, vertebras, pelvis, skull, and jaw. Bone marrow depression is common, with anemia, leukopenia, and occasionally thrombocytopenia. Peptic ulcer occurs in many patients with this disorder.

DIAGNOSIS. Classic cases of chemical hyperparathyroidism with von Recklinghausen's disease (osteitis fibrosa generalisata or osteitis fibrosa cystica) are diagnosed easily from the clinical picture and the chemical findings of hypercalcemia, hypophosphatemia, hypercalcuria, and an increased plasma alkaline phosphatase (Table 83-2). It is important to carry out simultaneous calcium and total protein determinations, as marked hypoproteinemia (with accompanying decrease in calcium proteinate) may mask an increase in diffusible ionized calcium, the fraction of importance in this disease. It is also important to obtain plasma calcium levels on several occasions, particularly if the first determination is not elevated. While neither the protein nor the ionic fraction can be measured with ease directly, both can be estimated from the concentration of total calcium and total protein by use of the readily available nomogram of McLean and Hastings. Bone lesions may be absent or minimal when calcium and protein intake have been high or when the disease is relatively mild or of short duration. In such cases the plasma alkaline phosphatase level may not be elevated. The diagnosis of hyperparathyroidism should be carefully ruled out in all patients with renal stones. Lithiasis often occurs in mild cases in which no other symptoms are present and plasma mineral levels show minimal changes.

Although hypercalcuria occurs in the absence of hyperparathyroidism, particularly in patients with nephrolithiasis, it is helpful in establishing the **diagnosis**

Table 83-2. SUMMARY OF CHEMICAL FEATURES OF DISEASES WITH DISTURBED PLASMA CALCIUM AND PHOSPHATE

Disease	Serum			Urine		Feces*	
	Calcium	Phosphate	Alkaline phosphatase	Calcium	Phosphate	Calcium	Phosphate
Hyperparathyroidism..	Increased	Decreased	Normal or increased	Increased	Increased	Normal	Normal
Paget's disease........	Normal	Normal	Increased	Normal	Normal	Normal	Normal
Hypoparathyroidism...	Decreased	Increased	Normal	Decreased	Decreased	Normal	Normal
Renal insufficiency.....	Decreased	Increased	Normal or increased	Decreased	Decreased	Normal	Increased
Osteomalacia.........	Decreased or normal	Decreased	Increased	Decreased	Decreased	Normal or increased	Decreased
Senile osteoporosis	Normal	Normal	Normal	Normal	Normal	Normal	Normal
Multiple myeloma.....	Normal to increased	Normal	Normal	Normal to increased	Normal to decreased	Normal	Normal
Milk-alkali syndrome..	Increased	Normal to increased	Normal	Normal to decreased	Normal to decreased		
Vitamin D intoxication	Increased	Increased	Normal	Increased	Decreased	Decreased	Decreased
Metastatic carcinoma..	Normal to increased	Normal	Normal to increased	Increased	Normal		
Sarcoidosis..........	Increased	Normal to increased	Normal to increased	Increased	Decreased	Decreased	Decreased
Hyperventilation (alkalosis).........	Normal	Normal	Normal	Normal	Normal		

* On low-calcium diet.

from other causes. If after 7 to 14 days on a diet of 200 mg calcium the patient excretes more than 200 mg calcium in the urine in 24 hr, hypercalcuria is present. In the presence of avitaminosis D or renal insufficiency, hypercalcuria may not be found in hyperparathyroidism. An approximation of the urinary calcium concentration may be made with the Sulkowitch test.

The early diagnosis of hyperparathyroidism in the absence of renal and skeletal lesions may be extremely difficult, and several procedures have been devised to facilitate diagnosis.

Intravenous Calcium Test. When a calcium load is administered intravenously, the normal individual responds with a rise in the plasma phosphate level and a fall in the urinary phosphate excretion. This is due to the fact that calcium will "shut off" the parathyroids if the plasma level is high enough. Theoretically, patients with hyperparathyroidism should not show the decrease in urinary excretion of phosphate, but the results are often inconclusive. Patients with hypoparathyroidism show a marked phosphate diuresis, and this test is probably most useful in diagnosing true hypoparathyroidism.

Tubular Reabsorption of Phosphate. Parathyroid hormone decreases the tubular reabsorption of phosphate in the renal tubules, and it has been found that patients with hyperparathyroidism have a tubular reabsorption of phosphate which is distinctly lower than normal. This can be best demonstrated by giving these patients an oral phosphate load (1 mM phosphate per kg body weight, made up of buffered mono- and dibasic sodium phosphate at pH 7.4), following which the tubular maximal transport of phosphate can be calculated (expressed as tubular reabsorption of phosphate in micromoles per 100 cc glomerular filtration rate per minute). Normal values range from 110 to 150. It can be shown that when there is a normal inulin clearance, this type of determination is valid and is further evidence for the tubular blocking action for phosphate by parathyroid hormone.

Cortisone Test. The action of cortisone on the normal subject is to decrease the absorption of calcium from the gastrointestinal tract and to increase the urinary output of calcium. In those patients with sarcoidosis and hypercalcemia, multiple myeloma, vitamin D intoxication, infantile hypercalcemia with failure to thrive, and metastatic carcinoma with hypercalcemia, cortisone acetate (150 mg per day in divided doses for 10 days, or its equivalent) has been shown to lower the plasma calcium within a matter of a few days to 2 weeks. When the diagnosis of hyperparathyroidism is uncertain, this test can often help make the correct diagnosis since cortisone in most instances does not affect the hypercalcemia due to a parathyroid adenoma.

DIFFERENTIAL DIAGNOSIS. Careful observation may be required to differentiate less typical cases from the following skeletal disorders.

Osteoporosis. This disease is characterized by a relative increase in bone resorption over bone formation, leading to an eventual decrease in bone mass and a negative calcium balance. It can arise from various hormonal disturbances such as hyperparathyroidism, hyperthyroidism, hyperadrenocorticism, and acromegaly, but it is considered most often to be of an idiopathic variety. Osteoporosis is frequently seen in women after the menopause and involves the spine and pelvis, very rarely the skull. Plasma calcium, phosphate and alkaline phosphatase levels, and the percentage of phosphate reabsorption by the renal tubules are generally within normal limits. The negative calcium balance can be reversed by the administration of estrogens or androgens, and it has also been shown that the balance can be made positive by the administration of large doses of calcium in the diet alone (see Chap. 227).

Osteomalacia. This implies failure to mineralize an otherwise normal matrix, seen especially in steatorrhea, vitamin D deficiency, and primary renal acidosis. Both plasma calcium and phosphate are decreased, while plasma alkaline phosphatase is increased. The urinary calcium excretion is decreased in the first two disorders and increased in the last.

Multiple Myeloma. This condition may show sharp demarcation of bone lesions by x-ray, with increased plasma and urine calcium, possible stones, a variable phosphate level, increased globulin, Bence-Jones protein (50 per cent), and plasma cells in the bone marrow. Even though massive bone disease may be seen by x-ray, the alkaline phosphatase usually remains within normal limits.

Metastatic Malignancies. These may present a variable x-ray picture, depending on whether the origin of the primary tumor is the breast, prostate, kidney, bronchus, or thyroid. Plasma calcium and alkaline phosphatase may be increased. An increase in the prostatic fraction of the total acid phosphatase is presumptive evidence for carcinoma of the prostate. The acid phosphatase may be elevated in other types of metastatic cancer to bone.

Renal Osteitis Fibrosa. In this condition there exists a history of onset of renal difficulties prior to skeletal changes. However, this differentiation is often extraordinarily difficult to ascertain. It should be stated that if an elevated plasma calcium level is found with severe long-standing renal disease, this is most likely due to primary hyperparathyroidism.

Sarcoidosis. It once was believed that the bone lesions seen as punched-out lesions in the hands and feet were responsible for the cases of hypercalcemia in association with sarcoid, but this has been shown not to be the case. Indeed, the association of hypercalcemia in sarcoidosis is rarely seen in those cases where the bones are involved. There is little doubt at present that the hypercalcemia is secondary to an increased sensitivity to vitamin D and that moderate exposure to bright sunlight is enough to induce hypercalcemia in the 20 to 30 per cent of those afflicted with sarcoid who have this sensitivity. The hypercalcemia responds rapidly to cortisone administration and serves to distinguish this disease from hyperparathyroidism in most instances. An increased globulin, pulmonary fibrosis, splenomegaly, hepatomegaly, and a positive Kveim test help to establish the diagnosis.

Other Skeletal Diseases. Gaucher's disease, Niemann-Pick disease, Hand-Schüller-Christian syndrome, Hodg-kin's disease, osteogenesis imperfecta, osteomyelitis, xanthomatosis, chronic radium poisoning, polycythemia vera, erythroblastosis, etc., may have to be considered in the differential diagnosis. A more complete discussion of these individual skeletal disorders is given in Part V, Sec. 12, Disorders of Bone.

Hypercalcemia Associated with Renal Insufficiency and Prolonged Milk or Alkali Ingestion. Burnett and his coworkers (1949) described a syndrome with many features common to primary hyperparathyroidism and secondary renal damage. The characteristic features in patients with this syndrome were a history of prolonged and excessive intake of milk and absorbable alkali, hypercalcemia without hypercalcuria or hypophosphatemia, marked renal insufficiency, calcinosis, and mild alkalosis. The differentiation of this syndrome from primary hyperparathyroidism may be very difficult because of the high incidence of ulcer symptoms in hyperparathyroidism. Treatment consists of a low-milk, low-alkali diet and a high fluid intake. The azotemia and hypercalcemia may diminish and the chemical imbalance may be restored to normal, but residual renal damage may persist.

Vitamin D Intoxication. Excessive vitamin D administration induces a clinical and pathologic picture similar to hyperparathyroidism. The symptoms of intoxication are those secondary to hypercalcemia and hypercalcuria already described. Recovery depends upon prompt diagnosis and upon the severity of the toxicity. Cortisone is the treatment of choice, as well as complete elimination of all sources of vitamin D, in moderate to severe cases of poisoning. The dosage of cortisone should range from 75 to 150 mg per day and should be maintained at this level until a normal plasma calcium is attained. The severe manifestations of the hypercalcemia will recede in a week to 10 days under such treatment, but other minor side effects, such as lassitude, weakness, and loss of appetite, may linger weeks or months before disappearing.

Hypercalcemia in Carcinoma without Metastases. Recently there have been numerous instances in which a picture resembling hyperparathyroidism was abolished by removing a cancer locally. These cases were not associated with any demonstrable bony metastases. The cause of the hypercalcemia is not evident, although it has been presumed that these tumors have secreted a substance with plasma calcium–raising properties. The cortisone test is often a useful tool in differentiating this cause of hypercalcemia from hyperparathyroidism.

Immobilization. Any patient with diffuse skeletal disease or chronic disease, if immobilized, can develop hypercalcemia and hypercalcuria, unless appropriate measures to prevent its occurrence are taken. No patient with Paget's disease should be put to bed for any long interval, since such a patient is especially prone to develop hypercalcuria.

Idiopathic Hypercalcemia of Infancy with Failure to Thrive. This is a new syndrome first described in Great Britain by Lightwood and his associates. These infants often have mental retardation, elfin facies, elevated cholesterol levels in the plasma, and hypercalcemia with all its secondary effects on the kidney and elsewhere. They will respond to cortisone or a diet devoid of vitamin D and calcium. It has been postulated that these children have an abnormal sensitivity to vitamin D similar to that found in sarcoidosis.

Idiopathic Hypercalcuria. There is a large group of stone formers who characteristically have hypercalcuria, low plasma phosphate, and normal plasma calcium. They may or may not have a lowered tubular reabsorptive rate for phosphate. Bone lesions and elevation of the alkaline phosphatase are absent. While the etiology of this syndrome is not clear at the present time, it is possible that these patients have a variant of hyperparathyroidism and they should be followed carefully. Should they develop hypercalcemia at any time in their clinical course, neck exploration for an adenoma should be considered seriously.

Other Causes of Hypercalcemia. Thyrotoxicosis has been described in association with hypercalcemia, although this is a rare phenomenon.

TREATMENT. Once the diagnosis of primary hyperparathyroidism is established, fluids should be forced, intake of calcium restricted, and surgical consultation obtained with a view toward neck exploration. Difficulty in locating the offending gland or glands because of inconstant anatomic positions, and because the non-involved glands show compensatory atrophy, may necessitate not only extensive but also repeated surgical exploration. Careful x-ray studies of the neck, including the esophagus and the mediastinum, may be helpful in attempting to locate the tumor before exploration, but they are often misleading. Removal of an adenoma or removal of all except a portion of one gland in case of hypertrophy and hyperplasia may be expected to cure the condition. When plasma alkaline phosphatase is markedly elevated, large quantities of calcium may be required postoperatively to prevent recurrent tetany since the bone will avidly remove calcium from the plasma in order to recalcify the bone lesions. The treatment of postoperative tetany is similar to that described in the treatment of hypoparathyroidism except that more vigorous treatment may have to be continued for some time to control the acute manifestations. A diet high in calcium and phosphate should be given postoperatively, but there is no need for increased doses of vitamin D over the normal intake unless there is a problem of chronic tetany. Under normal circumstances great improvement may be noted in the skeletal lesions as well as the renal function.

ACUTE HYPERCALCEMIC SYNDROME. Treatment of hypercalcemia caused by acute parathyroid intoxication or non-endocrine tumor constitutes an acute medical emergency. Acute parathyroid intoxication, with marked elevation of the plasma calcium level, occurs occasionally as a complication of hyperparathyroidism. It is characterized by weakness, lethargy, intractable nausea and vomiting, coma and sudden death. The same signs and symptoms can occur with hypercalcemia due to any cause such as vitamin D intoxication and malignant neoplasm. The successful treatment of severe hypercalcemia may be lifesaving. Oral or intravenous administration of phosphate has been recommended as the most effective medical therapy for the treatment of hypercalcemia. Orally, a solution composed of 1.0 M phosphate (0.8 mole Na_2HPO_4 plus 0.2 mole KH_2PO_4 per liter of distilled water) of which 10 to 20 ml diluted in water or juice is given t.i.d. Intravenously, one may administer 500 ml of 0.1 M phosphate (0.08 mole Na_2HPO_4 plus 0.02 mole KH_2PO_4 per liter) over a four-hour period, followed, if necessary, by an additional 500 ml. Inphos (Davies, Rose-Hoyt), a commercial preparation, is available for intravenous use. Chelating agents such as sodium ethylenediaminetetraacetic acid may help when given intravenously, but great care should be taken during their administration. Dialysis on an artificial kidney is of little benefit, since the plasma calcium will rise rapidly to predialysis levels following such a procedure.

SECONDARY HYPERPARATHYROIDISM

HISTORY. The existence of enlargement of the parathyroid glands secondary to another disease process in the body was first noted in 1905 by MacCallum in a case of nephritis. One year later, Erdheim noted similar findings in rickets, and since that time the syndrome of secondary hyperfunction of the parathyroids has been recognized.

INCIDENCE. As a complication of advanced renal disease, hyperfunction of the parathyroids is relatively common. In 1933 Pappenheimer and Wilens reported that in a series of 21 cases of nephritis the mean parathyroid weight was 50 per cent greater than in a control group.

ETIOLOGY. The most common cause of this condition is chronic, long-standing renal disease, as in glomerulonephritis and pyelonephritis. The term *renal rickets* does not apply to cases of secondary hyperparathyroidism and should be reserved for those cases seen most often in children where true rickets is secondary to prolonged and chronic renal disease and the supervening acidosis. Both secondary hyperparathyroidism and rickets have been described in the same patient as a complication of chronic renal disease. Reports of secondary hyperparathyroidism have been noted in a variety of diseases, such as osteogenesis imperfecta, Paget's disease, multiple myeloma, carcinoma with bone metastases, and pituitary basophilism.

PATHOLOGY. The parathyroid glands are enlarged diffusely and are hyperplastic. No single adenomas are visible. The cells are normal in size and easily differentiated from those seen in primary hyperparathyroidism. The former are principally chief cells with some increase in oxyphil cells, as opposed to the huge, water-clear cells of primary hyperparathyroidism due to hypertrophy and hyperplasia. The bone lesions are entirely similar to those seen in primary hyperparathyroidism, namely, generalized decalcification and bone cysts, with or without outright fracture.

PATHOLOGIC PHYSIOLOGY. It is unclear at the present time what the precise mechanisms for the development of parathyroid hyperplasia are in renal disease. It was believed that the presence of long-standing phosphate retention was the *sine qua non* for the development of the syndrome. It has been suggested by many that the metabolic acidosis secondary to renal disease may be the important factor in the development of a low plasma calcium level. The parathyroid glands respond to this lowering of the plasma calcium in a uniform manner by increasing their output of hormone in order to maintain normal plasma calcium values. If the acidosis persists, then parathyroid hyperplasia is induced. While this may not be the true explanation for the development of parathyroid hyperplasia secondary to renal disease, it is a more plausible one since it correlates very closely with the types of bone disease seen in response to primary renal disease.

CLINICAL PICTURE. The symptoms are usually those of the primary disease process before any evidence of hyperparathyroidism is noted. Classic glomerulonephritis or pyelonephritis, uremia, and evidence of renal insufficiency dominate the clinical picture. In children, dwarfism and pathologic fractures may be the presenting complaints.

DIAGNOSIS. The chemical findings of normal or low normal plasma calcium with hyperphosphatemia and high alkaline phosphatase, with the classic skeletal x-rays of bone cysts and generalized demineralization, lead to the diagnosis of parathyroid hyperfunction with renal disease. The history of early renal disease is often the only differential diagnostic point, since the primary cases are often complicated late in the disease by renal failure secondary to long-standing hyperparathyroidism. It is important to remember that an elevated plasma calcium level in the face of uremia indicates primary hyperparathyroidism.

TREATMENT. Of greatest importance is the correct diagnosis. Once this is accomplished, all therapy is directed at the primary disease and an attempt is made to correct the acidosis and to diminish the intake of phosphate by oral administration of aluminum hydroxide gel. The acidosis can be aided by administration of alkaline salts, such as sodium citrate. Attempts to elevate the plasma calcium by large amounts of vitamin D (calciferol, in doses of 50,000 to 150,000 units per day, or the equivalent in vitamin D_3 or dihydrotachysterol) are often indicated when the plasma calcium is reduced in order to suppress excessive parathyroid hormone secretion. However, this type of therapy is extremely dangerous and must be carefully regulated, since the difference between therapeutic and toxic doses of vitamin D is quite narrow. Certain patients with chronic renal disease and severe secondary hyperparathyroidism have had subtotal parathyroidectomy followed by vitamin D therapy. While the bone disease is strikingly cured by such means, the basic renal pathology is unaltered and the patients have ultimately died of uremia.

NONFUNCTIONING TUMORS OF THE PARATHYROID GLANDS

Nonfunctioning carcinoma of the parathyroids has been reported, but these cases have not been generally accepted because of the difficulty in establishing the origin of the tumor. Other nonfunctioning tumors include oxyphil adenomas (which may be burned-out primary adenomas), metastatic carcinoma, and cysts. Microscopic cysts are common in hyperplastic and adenomatous glands, whereas gross cysts are quite rare. Symptoms, when present, are due to pressure on local structures, including the recurrent laryngeal nerve. Most tumors have been found in the lower glands.

REFERENCES

Baker, W. H.: Abnormalities in Calcium Metabolism in Malignancy: Effects of Hormones, Am. J. Med., 21: 714, 1956.

Bernstein, D. S., and C. D. Guri: Hyperparathyroidism and Hypoparathyroidism: Preoperative and Postoperative Care, Anesthesiology, 24:448, 1963.

Bogdonoff, M. D., A. H. Woods, J. E. White, and F. L. Engel: Hyperparathyroidism, Am. J. Med., 21:583, 1956.

Bourne, G. H.: "The Biochemistry and Physiology of Bone," New York, Academic Press, Inc., 1956.

Bronsky, D., D. S. Kushner, A. Dubin, and I. Snapper: Idiopathic Hypoparathyroidism and Pseudohypoparathyroidism, Medicine, 37:317, 1958.

Castleman, B.: Tumors of the Parathyroid Gland, in "Atlas of Tumor Pathology," sec. 4, fasc. 15, Washington, D.C., Armed Forces Institute of Pathology, 1952.

Chambers, E. L., G. S. Gordan, L. Goldman, and E. C. Reifenstein, Jr.: Tests for Hyperparathyroidism: Tubular Reabsorption of Phosphate, Phosphate Deprivation, and Calcium Infusion, J. Clin. Endocrinol. & Metab., 16:1507, 1956.

Goldsmith, R. S., and S. H. Ingbar: Inorganic Phosphate Treatment of Hypercalcemia of Diverse Etiologies, New England J. Med., 274:1, 1966.

Heaney, R. P., and G. O. Whedon: Radiocalcium Studies of Bone Formation Rate in Human Metabolic Bone Disease, J. Clin. Endocrinol. & Metab., 18:1246, 1958.

Munson, P. L., P. F. Hirsch, and A. H. Rashjian: Parathyroid Gland, Ann. Rev. Physiol., 25:325, 1963.

Rasmussen, H.: Purification of Parathyroid Polypeptides, J. Biol. Chem., 235:3442, 1960.

Rodahl, K., J. T. Nicholson, and E. M. Brown, Jr.: "Bone as a Tissue," New York, McGraw-Hill Book Company, Inc., 1960.

Underdahl, L., L. B. Woolner, and B. M. Black: Multiple Endocrine Adenomas: Eight Cases Involving Parathyroids, Pituitary, and Pancreatic Islets, J. Clin. Endocrinol. & Metab., 13:20, 1953.

84 DISEASES OF THE ADRENAL CORTEX

David P. Lauler and George W. Thorn

INTRODUCTION

Thomas Addison's description in 1849 of a clinical syndrome resulting from destruction of the adrenal glands first attracted attention to these organs. Seven years later Brown-Séquard demonstrated that removal of both adrenals from experimental animals caused death soon after operation, whereas control animals subjected to a sham operation survived. Subsequent investigations established that the life-maintaining hormone was elaborated by cells in the cortex, since destruction of all medullary tissue was not accompanied by the classic signs and symptoms of adrenal insufficiency noted after complete removal of the glands.

Between 1927 and 1930, Hartman and his associates, Rogoff and Stewart, and Pfiffner and Swingle all independently described methods for preparing potent adrenal cortical extracts. During the following decade, crystalline steroid substances were isolated from these extracts by Kendall, by Grollman, and by Reichstein. In 1937, Steiger and Reichstein synthesized the first natural corticosteroid, 11-deoxycorticosterone, a year before it was identified in adrenal extracts. From 1940 to 1950, the synthesis of several 11-oxygenated compounds was achieved, including cortisone and hydrocortisone. The contributions of Sarett and his collaborator, Reichstein et al., and Kendall and his coworkers were outstanding in this regard. In 1954 aldosterone, the principal salt-retaining hormone of the adrenal was identified by Simpson and Tait in collaboration with the Swiss group under Reichstein. The chemical synthesis of pure *d*-aldosterone was achieved some years later. The decade 1954 to 1964 witnessed the isolation, identification, and synthesis of ACTH and the synthesis of substances such as amphenone and 2-methyl-1,2-bis-(3-pyridyl)-1-propanone (metyrapone), which are capable of interfering with the synthesis of hydrocortisone, and spironolactone, which can block the physiologic effects of aldosterone. Refinements in the ease and accuracy with which adrenal steroids and their metabolic products may be measured in biologic fluids have provided a tremendous stimulus to the study of physiologic as well as pathologic states of adrenal cortical function in man.

BIOCHEMISTRY AND PHYSIOLOGY

Steroid Nomenclature

The adrenal steroids contain as their basic structure a cyclopentanoperhydrophenanthrane nucleus consisting of three 6-carbon hexane rings and a single 5-carbon pentane ring (D). The carbon atoms are numbered in a predetermined sequence beginning with ring A (Fig. 84-1). The Greek letter Δ indicates a double bond, as does the suffix -ene. The position of a substituent below or above the plane of the steroid

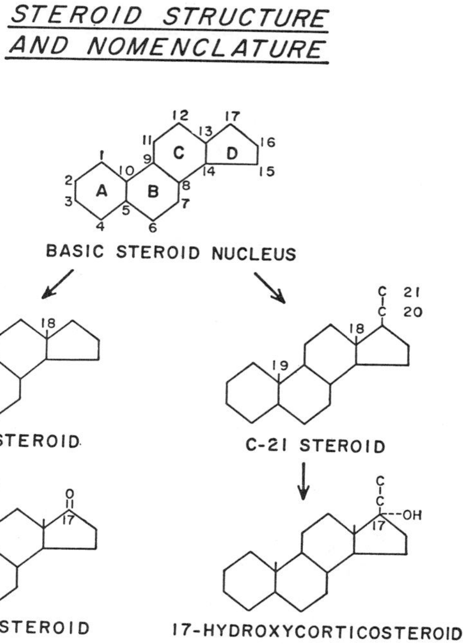

STEROID STRUCTURE AND NOMENCLATURE

Fig. 84-1. Basic steroid structure and nomenclature.

molecule is indicated by the letters α and β respectively. The α-substituent is drawn with a broken line (--OH), and the β-substituent is drawn with a solid line (—OH). The C_{19} steroids are those which have substituent methyl groups at positions C-18 and C-19. C_{19} steroids that also have a ketone group at C-17 are termed *17-ketosteroids*. These C_{19} steroids have predominant androgenic activity. The C_{21} steroids are those which have a 2-carbon side chain (C-20 and C-21) attached at position 17 of the D ring and, in addition, have substituent methyl groups at C-18 and C-19. C_{21} steroids that also possess a hydroxyl group at position 17 are termed *17-hydroxycorticosteroids* or *17-hydroxycorticoids*. The C_{21} steroids may have either predominant glucocorticoid or mineralocorticoid properties. *Glucocorticoid* signifies a C_{21} steroid with predominant action on intermediary metabolism, and *mineralocorticoid* indicates a C_{21} steroid with predominant action on the metabolism of the body minerals, sodium and potassium.

The major positions of substitution in the steroid molecule are at carbon atoms C-3, C-11, C-17, and C-21.

Biosynthesis of Adrenal Steroids

Cholesterol, derived from the diet and from endogenous synthesis via acetate, is the principal starting compound in steroidogenesis. The three major adrenal biosynthetic pathways lead to the production of glucocorticoids (cortisol), mineralocorticoids (aldosterone), and adrenal androgens (dehydroepiandrosterone) (Fig. 84-2).

GLUCOCORTICOID PATHWAY. Δ-5 pregnenolone is formed after cleavage of the side chain of cholesterol.

BIOSYNTHESIS OF ADRENAL STEROIDS

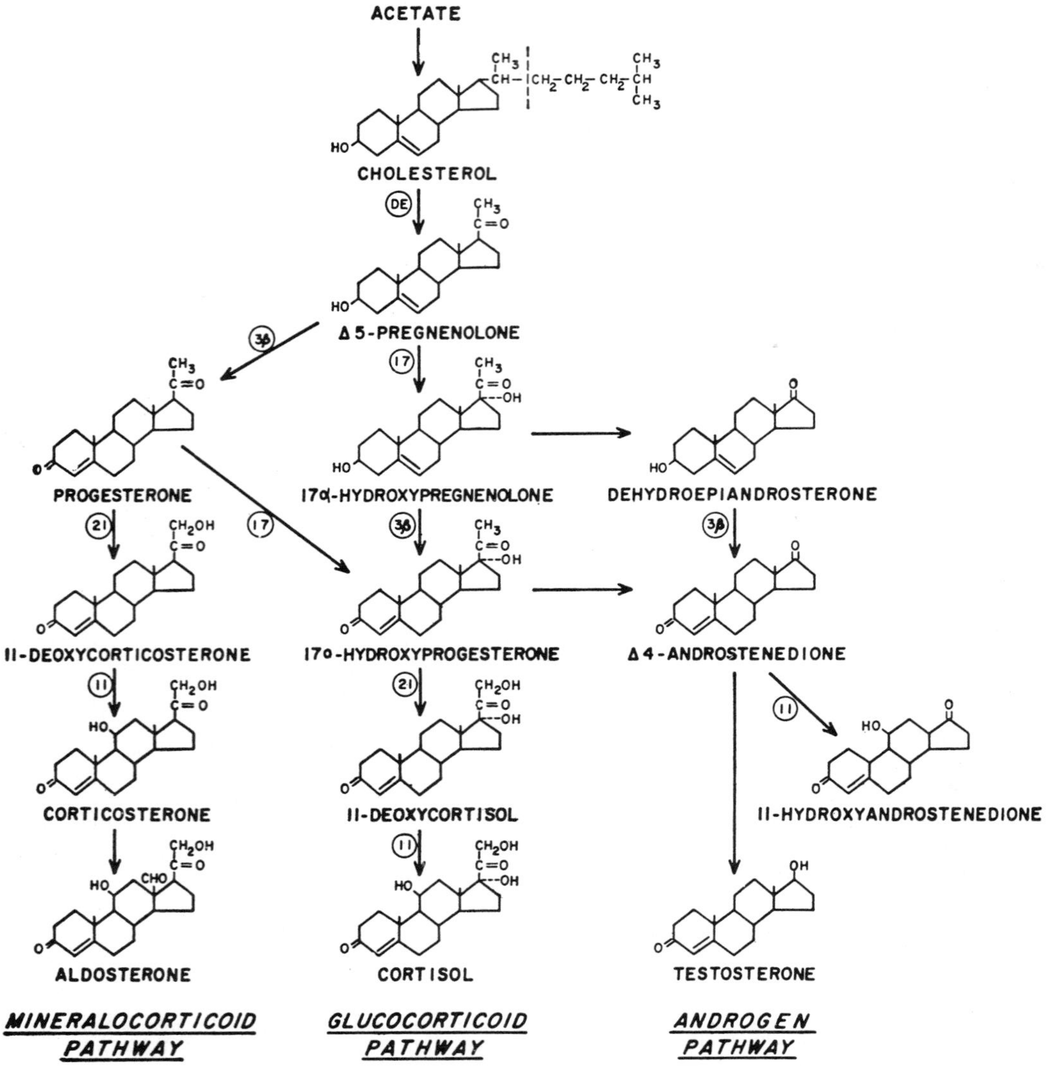

Fig. 84-2. Biosynthetic pathways for adrenal steroid production. Major pathways to mineralocorticoids, glucocorticoids, and androgens. Circled letters and numbers denote specific enzymes: (DE) = debranching enzyme; (3β) = 3β-ol-dehydrogenase with Δ4–Δ5 isomerase; (11) = C-11 hydroxylase; (17) = C-17 hydroxylase; (21) = C-21 hydroxylase.

Δ-5 pregnenolone is converted to progesterone by the action of the enzymes 3-β-hydroxy-dehydrogenase and Δ5,Δ4-isomerase. These enzymes transform the 3-β-hydroxy group of Δ-5 pregnenolone to a C-3-ketonic group and transform the double bond between C-5:C-6 of Δ5-pregnenolone to position C-4:C-5 of progesterone. A series of hydroxylations mediated by specific hydroxylating enzymes then occurs in sequential fashion at C-17, then C-21, and finally at C-11. With the introduction of a hydroxyl group at position C-17 of progesterone by the enzyme C-17 hydroxylase, 17α-hydroxy-progesterone is formed, which in turn has a hydroxyl group introduced at C-21 by the enzyme C-21 hydroxylase, producing 11-deoxycortisol

(Compound S), the major precursor of cortisol. Finally, a third hydroxyl group is introduced at the C-11 position of 11-deoxycortisol by the enzyme C-11 hydroxylase, to produce cortisol (Compound F, hydrocortisone), the major glucocorticoid. The chemical name for cortisol is 11-β,17-α,21-trihydroxy-4-pregnene-3,20-dione.

MINERALOCORTICOID PATHWAY. Progesterone after transformation from Δ5-pregnenolone is hydroxylated at C-21 to form 11-deoxycorticosterone. This steroid is then hydroxylated at position C-11 to form corticosterone (Compound B), the immediate precursor of aldosterone. With the introduction of an aldehyde group at position C-18 of corticosterone, the major mineralocorticoid *aldosterone* is formed. The chemical designation for aldosterone is $11\beta,21$-dihydroxy-18-aldo-4-pregnene-3,20-dione.

Note that 11-deoxycorticosterone differs from 11-deoxycortisol by the absence of a hydroxyl group at position C-17.

ANDROGEN PATHWAY. By the enzymatic action of 17α-hydroxylase, $\Delta5$-pregnenolone is converted to 17α-hydroxypregnenolone, which on cleavage of its C-20:C-21 side chain forms the 17-ketosteroid dehydroepiandrosterone. The $\Delta5,$-3 hydroxyl grouping of this compound is transformed to a $\Delta4,$-3 oxo- grouping by the enzymes 3β-hydroxydehydrogenase and $\Delta5,\Delta4$ isomerase to produce the 17-ketosteroid androstenedione. Androstenedione can undergo direct transformation to testosterone as a result of hydrogenation at position C-17 and androstenedione also is converted to 11β-hydroxy androstenedione by hydroxylation at position C-11. Note that the adrenal androgens require a preliminary hydroxylation at C-17 prior to their formation and, also, that 17-ketosteroids with an oxygen group at position C-11 are of adrenal origin.

Steroid Transport

Of the major adrenal steroids, only the transport of cortisol has been elucidated in detail. Cortisol after release into the systemic circulation occurs in the plasma in three forms: free cortisol, protein-bound cortisol, and cortisol metabolites. *Free* cortisol refers to that moiety which is neither protein-bound nor inactivated, and it is the physiologically active form of cortisol acting directly at tissue sites. It represents active steroid in transit, and at normal plasma cortisol concentrations of 10 to 15 μg per 100 ml, approximately 1 μg per 100 ml is "free" cortisol and the remainder is protein-bound. *Protein-bound cortisol* is that portion of cortisol which is loosely and reversibly bound to circulating plasma proteins. This cortisol-binding protein serves as a reserve buffer mechanism capable of binding excess cortisol when the plasma free cortisol level is high and, conversely, capable of releasing bound cortisol when the plasma free cortisol level is low. The two protein fractions capable of binding cortisol are albumin and a specific globulin fraction produced by the liver termed *corticosteroid-binding globulin* (CBG). CBG has a greater affinity for but a lesser total capacity to bind cortisol than does albumin. At normal blood levels approximately one-half the binding sites on CBG are saturated; as increased amounts of cortisol are released by the adrenal gland, the remaining binding sites on CBG become fully saturated and the excess cortisol then becomes in part bound to albumin while some also remains as additional free cortisol in the plasma. The CBG level may be increased by the administration of natural or synthetic estrogens. This induced rise in CBG is accompanied by a parallel rise in protein-bound cortisol with the result that plasma 17-hydroxycorticosteroids are elevated; however, the free cortisol plasma levels remain normal, and thus signs of cortisol excess do not appear. This effect of estrogens on steroid protein binding is most evident in pregnancy. A major difference from the administration of estrogens must exist, however, since in pregnancy cortisol secretion increases while the excretion of urine cortisol metabolites remains in the normal range.

Cortisol metabolites such as tetrahydrocortisol also circulate in the plasma. These metabolites are biologically inactive and bind only weakly with circulating plasma proteins.

Protein-binding of steroids also minimizes their loss by renal excretion since only unbound cortisol and its metabolites are freely filterable at the glomerulus.

Steroid Metabolism and Excretion

GLUCOCORTICOIDS. The principal glucocorticoids secreted by the normal adrenal gland are cortisol and corticosterone. The daily adrenal secretion of cortisol ranges between 15 and 30 mg with a pronounced diurnal cycle and that of corticosterone between 2 and 4 mg. Cortisol is distributed in a volume of body fluids approximating the total extracellular fluid space. The total plasma concentration of cortisol in the morning hours is approximately 10 μg per 100 ml, with more than 90 per cent of this cortisol appearing in the protein-bound fraction. The biologic half-life of cortisol is between 60 and 120 min. The plasma cortisol level is determined by the rate of adrenal gland secretion, the rate of inactivation, and the rate of excretion.

The major area of metabolism is the liver, where three transformations take place: saturation of ring A, hydroxylation at the C-20 position, and cleavage of the C-20:C-21 side chain. As a result of these metabolic transformations the steroids are inactivated. The initial saturation of the C-4:C-5 double bond in ring A by the introduction of two hydrogen atoms produces *dihydrocortisol,* an inactive compound (Fig. 84-3). Next, the C-3 ketonic group of dihydrocortisol is reduced by the further addition of two hydrogen atoms to form *tetrahydrocortisol* (THF). A rapid transformation of cortisol to cortisone occurs in the liver, where these two steroids are interchangeable. The cortisone so produced is likewise metabolized to *dihydrocortisone* and then to *tetrahydrocortisone* (THE). THE and THF are made water-soluble by conjugation in the liver with glucuronic acid at position C-3. This conjugation then permits greater urinary excretion of these compounds to occur. The second mechanism of inactivation, C-20 hydroxylation, is brought into play by the addition of two hydrogen atoms at C-20 to smaller amounts of THE and THF before their glucuronic conjugation. This reduction at C-20 forms *cortol* and *cortolone,* respectively, which after their conjugation are excreted in the urine. Lastly, approximately 5 to 10 per cent of the secreted cortisol is metabolized in the liver by the third mechanism of inactivation, cleavage of the C-20:C-21 side chain to

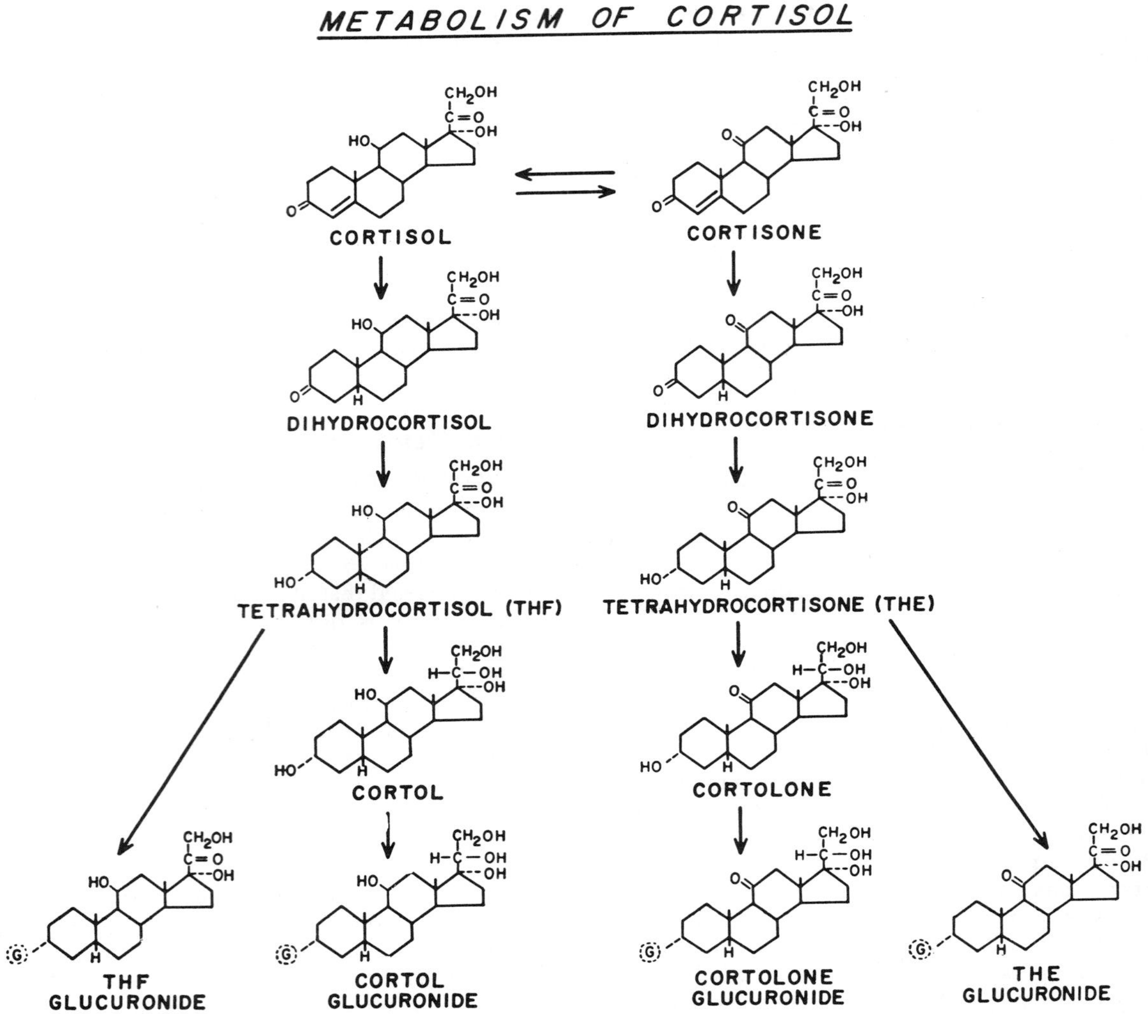

METABOLISM OF CORTISOL

Fig. 84-3. Metabolism of cortisol to tetrahydrocortisol, tetrahydrocortisone, cortol, and cortolone. Conjugation occurs with glucuronic acid at C-3 position. Note interconversion of cortisol and cortisone.

form the corresponding *11-oxy-ketosteroid*. The average amounts of cortisol and its metabolites excreted in the urine per 24 hr is as follows: free cortisol, 0.05 mg; glucuronides of THE and THF, 8 mg; glucuronides of cortols and cortolones, 3 mg; 17-ketosteroids derived from cortisol and cortisone, 1.5 mg.

The metabolism of corticosterone follows a similar plan as for cortisol.

MINERALOCORTICOIDS. The average daily secretion of aldosterone by normal subjects ranges between 50 and 250 μg. The plasma concentration of aldosterone ranges between 5 and 15 mμg per 100 ml. Aldosterone binds weakly with proteins, chiefly albumin, and as a result its volume of distribution is larger than that of cortisol and approximates 40 liters. The biologic half-life of aldosterone is approximately 30 min. Greater than 90 per cent of circulating aldosterone is inactivated during a single passage through the liver. Thirty to forty per cent of secreted aldosterone is in-

activated by ring A reduction in the liver, forming *tetrahydroaldosterone*, which after glucuronic acid conjugation is excreted in the urine. Ten to twenty per cent of secreted aldosterone is metabolized in the liver and in the kidney to a metabolite, not chemically identified, but referred to as the *acid-labile conjugate* of aldosterone, since on pH 1 acid hydrolysis the conjugate is hydrolyzed to yield aldosterone. This acid-labile conjugate of aldosterone is also referred to as the *3-oxo-conjugate*, since it is known that the 3-oxo- grouping is not irreversibly reduced, as it is in the tetrahydroaldosterone metabolite. The acid-labile conjugate is very rapidly excreted in the urine, with 90 per cent being excreted within 6 hr whereas comparable tetrahydroaldosterone excretion requires 24 to 36 hr. Aldosterone excretion is generally measured clinically using the pH 1 acid hydrolysis, and the excretion of the acid-labile conjugate in normal subjects with average salt intake ranges from 1 to 10 μg per

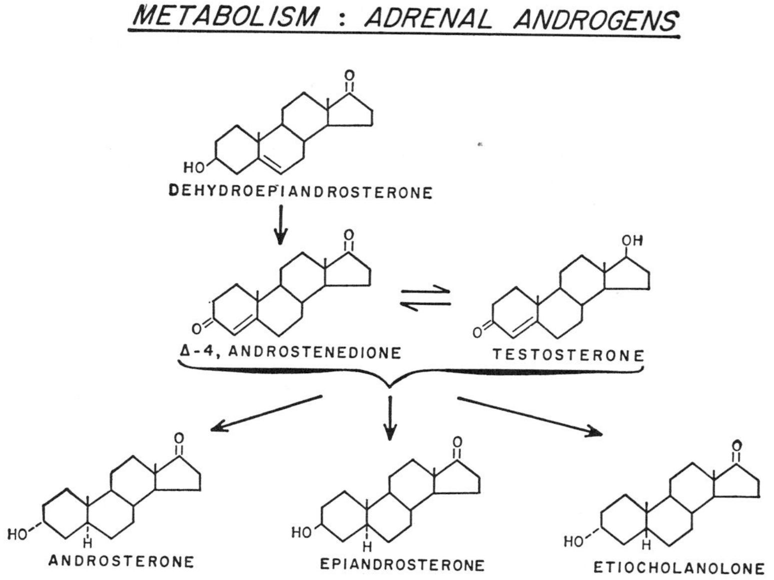

METABOLISM : ADRENAL ANDROGENS

Fig. 84-4. Adrenal androgens. Δ-4 androstenedione and testosterone contribute to the same metabolites.

day. The urine excretion of free aldosterone, that is, nonconjugated, nonreduced aldosterone, is between 0.2 and 0.6 μg per day. Aldosterone excretion exhibits diurnal variation with daytime excretion predominating.

ADRENAL ANDROGENS. The adrenal glands secrete approximately 15 to 30 mg daily of dehydroepiandrosterone (DHEA) and much smaller amounts of Δ-4 androstenedione and 11-β-hydroxyandrostenedione (Fig. 84-4). DHEA is conjugated in large part as a sulfate, both within the adrenal and in the liver, and is excreted in the urine as such. Δ-4 androstenedione is interconvertible with testosterone and shares with testosterone a common group of metabolites consisting of androsterone, epiandrosterone, and etiocholanolone. Two-thirds of the urine 17-ketosteroids in the male are derived from adrenal metabolites, and the remaining one-third comes from testicular secretion of testosterone. In the female, almost all urine 17-ketosteroids are derived exclusively from adrenal gland secretions.

ADRENAL ESTROGENS. The observations that bilaterally ovariectomized patients excrete estrone, estradiol, and estriol in the urine, which excretion is augmented by ACTH administration, suggest that the adrenal glands are capable of synthesizing estrogens. In addition, estrogenic "feminizing" adrenal tumors have been reported. Estradiol and estrone may be directly formed by transformation from the androgens, testosterone, and androstenedione, respectively.

ACTH Physiology (See Chap. 81)

The adrenal corticotropin hormone (ACTH) is a long-chain polypeptide containing 39 amino acids, and it is stored in and released from the anterior pituitary gland, where histologically it has been local-

ized to basophil cells. Approximately 50 mg of ACTH is stored in the anterior pituitary. ACTH stimulates the biogenesis and release of steroid hormones by the adrenal glands. It causes an increase in adrenal weight and a decrease in adrenal gland content of lipids, cholesterol, and ascorbic acid. The biologic half-life of ACTH is less than 10 min. The release of ACTH from the anterior pituitary gland is governed by a "corticotropin-releasing center" in the median eminence of the hypothalamus, which upon stimulation releases a chemical mediator (corticotropin-releasing factor, CRF) that travels via the pituitary-stalk portal blood stream to the anterior pituitary gland where it effects the release of stored ACTH (Fig. 84-5). CRF is thought to be a short-chain polypeptide whose release is facilitated by a large number of nervous stimuli including those arising from higher centers. The principal regulator of CRF release is the plasma free cortisol level, which by a negative feedback mechanism causes increased release of CRF when plasma cortisol level is low and a decreased release of CRF when plasma cortisol concentration is elevated. This servomechanism establishes the primacy of blood cortisol concentration and serves to buffer deviations in blood cortisol levels from a supposed optimal level.

Within minutes after the release of ACTH, increased concentrations of steroids are found in adrenal venous blood. The molecular basis of ACTH action has not been elucidated. Some suggest that ACTH accelerates the production of Δ-5, pregnenolone from cholesterol in a rate-limiting manner, whereas others have suggested that ACTH acts by increasing the formation and availability of adenosine-3',5'-monophosphate in the adrenal gland, which would lead to increases in the synthesis of reduced coenzymes needed for steroid biosynthesis. A major effect of ACTH is to

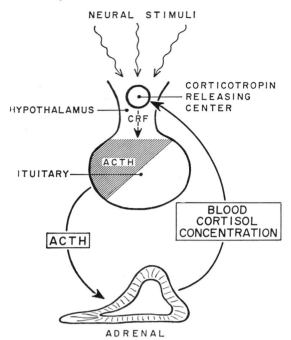

Fig. 84-5. Hypothalamic-pituitary-adrenal axis. CRF = corticotropin releasing factor.

increase the biosynthesis of adrenal proteins. ACTH administration to the rat results in a significant increase in adrenal weight, protein, and ribonucleic acid content within 24 hr. An effect on adrenal deoxyribonucleic acid is observed only after several days of hormone administration. Evidence has been obtained that suggests protein biosynthesis is an important, if not essential, part of the action of ACTH and possibly of other tropic hormones. ACTH apparently stimulates protein biosynthesis either by stimulation of messenger ribonucleic acid or by enzyme activation.

Glucocorticoid Physiology

The division of adrenal steroids into glucocorticoids and mineralocorticoids is somewhat arbitrary in that most glucocorticoids have some mineralocorticoidlike properties, and vice versa. The descriptive term *glucocorticoid* is applied to those adrenal steroids having a predominant action on intermediary metabolism. The principal glucocorticoid is cortisol (hydrocortisone). The actions of glucocorticoids on intermediary metabolism include their ability to increase hepatic glycogen content by increasing hepatic glucose synthesis. This is brought about by increasing the quantity of intermediary metabolites, especially those derived from glycogenic amino acids. Hepatic trapping and deamination of amino acids derived from peripheral supporting structures, such as bone, skin, muscle, and connective tissue, appears to be essential to the process. The increased mobilization of protein results in increased plasma amino acid levels and increased urinary nitrogen excretion. Glucocorticoids are capable

of directly increasing the level of specific hepatic enzymes, such as tryptophan pyrrolase and tyrosine-α-ketoglutarate transaminase. The elevated levels of these hepatic enzymes can influence the balance of serum amino acids, which in turn can be responsible for diminished protein metabolism and subsequent cytolysis of lymphoid tissues and muscle. Cortisol enhances the release of free fatty acids from adipose tissue during fasting or adrenergic stimulation. The action of cortisol on structural protein and adipose tissue varies considerably in different parts of the body. For example, depletion of protein matrix of the vertebral column may be striking, whereas long-bone structure may be affected only minimally; peripheral adipose tissue may diminish, whereas abdominal and interscapular fat may accumulate. Cortisol has a major effect on body water in both its distribution and its excretion. It subserves the extracellular fluid volume by a retarding action on the inward migration of water into cells. It affects renal water excretion in a dual manner by increasing the rate of glomerular filtration and by a direct action on the renal tubule, both of which summate to increase solute-free water clearance. Glucocorticoids, in general, will increase renal tubular sodium reabsorption and cause an increased urine potassium excretion. Cortisol is also necessary for normal vascular reactivity ensuring the response of vascular smooth muscle to circulating vasoconstrictor factors. Cortisol effects a diminution in circulating eosinophils, presumably by increased splenic and pulmonary sequestration. In addition, cortisol can effect lysis of lymphoid tissue. The integrity of personality is enhanced by cortisol, and emotional disorders are common with either excesses or deficits of cortisol. Lastly, cortisol is the major determinant of pituitary ACTH release by its direct effect on the hypothalamic corticotropin-releasing center.

Mineralocorticoid Physiology

Aldosterone is necessary for the homeostaic regulation of the total body stores of the principal cations, sodium and potassium. The *d*-isomer of aldosterone is the biologically active form. It acts predominantly on the distal renal tubule, causing increased sodium reabsorption in exchange for secreted potassium, as is evident by the renal retention of sodium and increased urine potassium excretion. This sodium-retaining action is also evident in salivary and sweat glands and in the gastrointestinal tract. As a result of sodium retention, there is maintenance of extracellular fluid volume since sodium is the principal osmotic determinant of this compartment. Aldosterone is important for the maintenance of extracellular fluid sodium content, and in its absence sodium migrates from the extracellular fluid into tendons and into cells and is lost via renal excretion.

The controlling mechanism for aldosterone release is not known. Evidence suggests that under conditions of extracellular volume depletion sensed by pressure-volume receptors located within the arterial system, a specific aldosterone-stimulating hormone is released, which in turn increases the adrenal secretion of aldosterone, with the result that additional sodium is conserved with consequent replenishment of the volume deficit. This would represent a feedback mechanism responsible for maintaining a normal extracellular volume, deficits and excesses of which would be appropriately nullified by this servosystem. It has been proposed that the renin-angiotensin system may function as such a mediator. Angiotensin is known to be a potent stimulating factor acting directly on the adrenal gland to effect increased release of aldosterone. As a corollary, it is postulated that the afferent arterioles of the cortical renal glomeruli may function as myogenic "stretch" receptors so that with decreased flow, additional amounts of renin are released from the juxtaglomerular cells. Renin is an enzyme that specifically transforms the basic α-2 globulin substrate angiotensinogen into angiotensin-I, an inactive decapeptide that is immediately acted upon by converting enzyme to form the biologically active octapeptide, angiotensin-II. Angiotensin-II is capable of stimulating the adrenal glands to release aldosterone, and the resultant sodium retention effects an increased circulating blood volume and blood flow through the afferent renal arterioles, thus dampening the initiating signal.

The renin-angiotensin system is not the only system capable of activating aldosterone release, since hemorrhage in the absence of kidneys will cause increased aldosterone secretion. This suggests that ACTH may play a physiologic role in aldosterone release under conditions of rapid acute volume depletion. In addition, the possibility of a completely independent neurophysiologic factor controlling aldosterone production after its release from the central nervous system has been suggested and has not been definitely excluded.

Androgen Physiology

The principal adrenal androgens in terms of quantitative secretion are dehydroepiandrosterone (DHEA), androstenedione, and 11-hydroxyandrostenedione. Of these, androstenedione is the major androgen, five times more active than DHEA. Testosterone, which is interconvertible with androstenedione peripherally and which has been isolated from the adrenal gland, exhibits an additional fivefold increase in androgenic potency when compared to androstenedione, pointing up that DHEA, androstenedione, and 11-hydroxyandrostenedione are biologically weak androgens. The release of adrenal androgens is stimulated by ACTH and not by gonadotropins. With ACTH stimulation urine 17-ketosteroids increase but to a much lesser extent than do urine 17-hydroxycorticoids. Part of this increment in 17-ketosteroid excretion is due to the metabolism of the increasing 17-hydroxycorticoids by the mechanism of C-20:C-21 side chain cleavage,

producing 11-oxy-17-ketosteroids. Adrenal androgens are suppressed by exogenous glucocorticoid administration as judged by decrements in urine 17-ketosteroid excretion. Additional specific control mechanisms for adrenal androgen release may exist independently of the ACTH system.

The major effects of these androgenic hormones are on protein metabolism and on secondary sexual characteristics. Androgens increase the synthesis of protein from amino acids, and this anabolic action leads to increased muscle mass and strength. Linear growth is accelerated by androgens prior to epiphyseal closure, which is hastened by androgen excess. The secondary sexual characteristics are affected through inhibition of the female characteristics (defeminization) and accentuation of the male characteristics (masculinization). These are seen clinically as hirsutism and virilization in the female with amenorrhea, atrophy of breasts and uterus, enlargement of the clitoris, deepening of the voice, acne, increased muscle mass, increased heterosexual drive, and receding hairline. In the male there is increased body and sexual hair and enlargement of the sexual organs.

The bioassay of androgens is based on the response of secondary and accessory sexual tissue to treatment with the hormones. Such methods include the increase in weight of the ventral prostate and seminal vesicle of the castrated rat and the increased weight and size of the comb of the castrated cock. The protein anabolic action of androgens may be bioassayed by the increase in weight of the levator ani muscle of castrated male rats. A clinical bioassay for androgens may be carried out utilizing a quantitative gravimetric determination of sebum production, which production is augmented by androgens.

LABORATORY EVALUATION OF ADRENAL CORTICAL FUNCTION

Blood Levels

Blood ACTH levels have been determined by bioassay preparations. One method commonly used consists of injecting intravenously an extract of the patient's plasma into an hypophysectomized animal and noting the increased production of steroids in the adrenal venous effluent. Such methods have established that the normal ACTH blood level is less than 1 milliunit per 100 ml plasma and that a diurnal cycle exists, with lower blood levels detectable in late afternoon and early evening. The method has proved reproducible for elevated values of plasma ACTH but is insensitive to low values.

The blood level of *17-hydroxycorticoids* is measured chemically, usually as Porter-Silber chromogens. The steroids thus measured are predominantly cortisol, both free and protein-bound, with much smaller amounts of unconjugated tetrahydrocortisol and tetrahydrocortisone included in the determination. By chromatography, cortisol may be isolated and determined separately. The normal morning plasma levels of 17-hydroxycorticoids range between 10 and 20 μg per 100 ml. These blood levels exhibit a marked diurnal pattern with highest values between 5 to 7 A.M. and lowest values at 6 P.M. in the evening, the evening values usually being less than half the early morning values.

Plasma *aldosterone* levels in patients on normal salt intake have been determined utilizing radioisotope dilution methods, and they range from 5 to 15 mμg per 100 ml. Diurnal variation has not been studied.

Testosterone in plasma has also been measured by isotopic means; the range for nonhirsute females is 30 to 100 and for males 400 to 1,000 mμg per 100 ml.

Urine Levels

The principal determinations are of urine 17-hydroxycorticoids, 17-ketosteroids, 17-ketogenic steroids, and free cortisol. The urine 17-hydroxycorticoids are determined as Porter-Silber chromogens, whereby these steroids react with the reagent phenylhydrazine to produce a characteristic color. This reaction is specific for steroids with a "dihydroxy acetone" C-17 side chain, that is, with hydroxyl groups on C-17 and C-21 and a ketone group on C-20 (Fig. 84-6). Therefore, this determination will include cortisol, cortisone, tetrahydrocortisol, tetrahydrocortisone, and 11-deoxycortisol but not cortols, cortolones, and pregnanetriol.

Normal values for 24 hr range from 1 to 10 mg per day, with daytime (7 A.M. to 7 P.M.). excretion exceeding night values (7 P.M. to 7 A.M.). It is of extreme importance that the completeness of any and all urine steroid collections be checked by urine creatinine determinations.

The urine 17-ketosteroids are those containing a ketone group at C-17, and two-thirds of these originate from the adrenal gland and the remainder from the testes. Their measurement depends on the Zimmerman reaction, whereby color is produced when 17-ketosteroids are condensed with *m*-dinitrobenzene. This reaction is specific for steroids with a ketone substituent with an adjacent unsubstituted carbon atom. The major urine 17-ketosteroids are dehydroepiandrosterone, epiandrosterone, androsterone, etiocholanolone, 11-oxoetiocholanolone, 11-hydroxyetiocholanolone and 11-hydroxyandrosterone (Fig. 84-7). Normal values for males range between 7 and 25 mg per day and for females between 5 and 15 mg per day. The diurnal pattern for 17-ketosteroid excretion is definite but less accentuated than that for 17-hydroxysteroids. Urine 17-ketosteroid values are highest in young adults and decline with age.

The total urine 17-ketosteroids may be subdivided into those having either an oxygen or hydroxyl substituent at position C-11 (11-oxy-17-ketosteroids) and those having no such groups (11-deoxy-17-ketosteroids). The *11-oxy-17-ketosteroids* include 11-oxoeti-

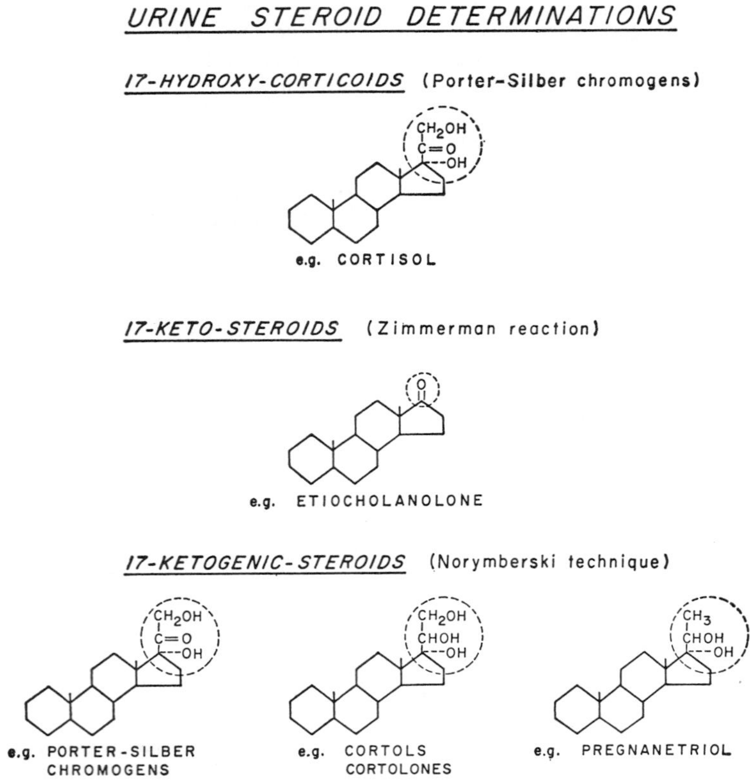

URINE STEROID DETERMINATIONS

17-HYDROXY-CORTICOIDS (Porter-Silber chromogens)

e.g. CORTISOL

17-KETO-STEROIDS (Zimmerman reaction)

e.g. ETIOCHOLANOLONE

17-KETOGENIC-STEROIDS (Norymberski technique)

e.g. PORTER-SILBER   e.g. CORTOLS   e.g. PREGNANETRIOL
      CHROMOGENS   CORTOLONES

Fig. 84-6. Key reactive groups (enclosed by dashed circle) in urine steroid determinations.

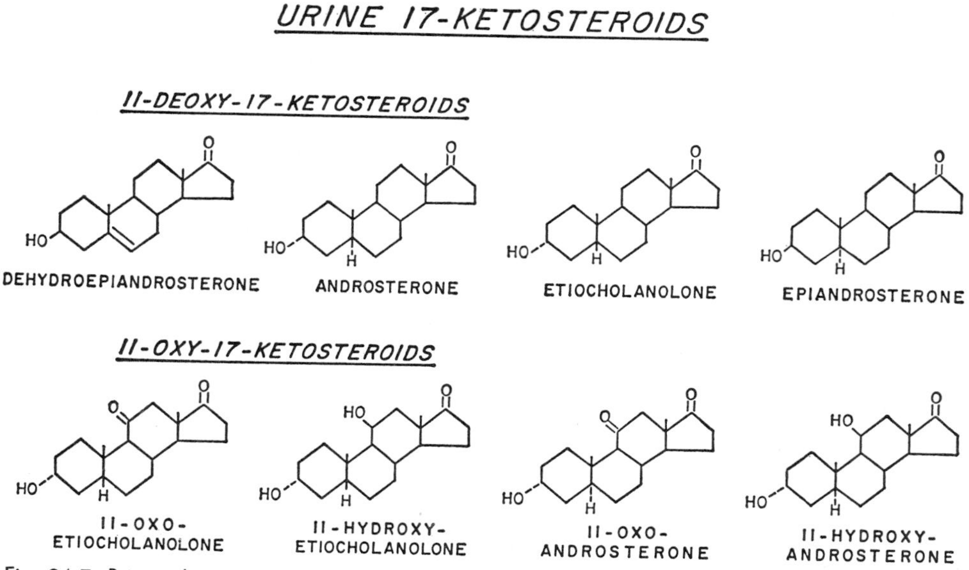

URINE 17-KETOSTEROIDS

11-DEOXY-17-KETOSTEROIDS

DEHYDROEPIANDROSTERONE   ANDROSTERONE   ETIOCHOLANOLONE   EPIANDROSTERONE

11-OXY-17-KETOSTEROIDS

11-OXO-   11-HYDROXY-   11-OXO-   11-HYDROXY-
ETIOCHOLANOLONE   ETIOCHOLANOLONE   ANDROSTERONE   ANDROSTERONE

Fig. 84-7. Principal urine 17-ketosteroids. 11-oxy-17-ketosteroids derived from the adrenal glands.

ocholanone, 11-hydroxyetiocholanolone, and 11-hydroxyandrosterone. These 11-oxo-17-ketosteroids are uniquely derived from the adrenal gland, since other tissues do not possess the enzymes for active C-11 hydroxylation, whereas the 11-deoxy-17-ketosteroids may arise from adrenal, testicular, and ovarian tissue.

Ketogenic steroids is a descriptive term for those C-21 hydroxycorticoids potentially capable of transformation into 17-ketosteroids in vitro. After the excreted 17-ketosteroids are reduced to noninterfering compounds, the side chains of C-21 hydroxycorticosteroids are oxidized to 17-ketonic groups, which then can be measured by the Zimmermann reaction as 17-ketosteroids. The Norymberski technique for ketogenic steroid analysis is specific for compounds containing the following groups: 17,21-dihydroxy-20-keto; 17,20,21-trihydroxy-; and 17,20-dihydroxy-21-deoxy-. It can be seen that the first of these groupings represents those compounds capable of reacting as Porter-Silber chromogens; the second, or trihydroxy, grouping would include the cortols and the cortolones; whereas the third, or 21-deoxy, grouping would include pregnanetriol. Thus urine 17-ketogenic steroid determination includes all steroids determined as 17-hydroxysteroids by the Porter-Silber method and in addition includes the cortols, cortolones, and pregnanetriol. The normal range for urine 17-ketogenic steroids is 5 to 20 mg per day.

The urine free cortisol may be determined by partition chromatography and represents biologically active unconjugated free cortisol. Normal subjects excrete less than 100 μg per day.

Steroid Secretion Rates

The basic assumption in the interpretation of urine steroid values is that excreted adrenal steroid metabolites (17-hydroxycorticoids, 17-ketogenic steroids) accurately reflect adrenal secretory rates of that steroid (cortisol). Measurement of the actual adrenal secretory rate of a given steroid would, of course, be preferable, and such methods are finding increasing clinical application. The adrenal secretory rate is calculated by the dilution an administered radioactive steroid undergoes as a consequence of the admixture of endogenously secreted nonradioactive steroid hormone with the exogenous radioactive steroid. In practice, a major metabolite of the steroid is isolated and purified by chromatography; from a determination of its specific activity (counts per minute per microgram of steroid) and knowledge of the specific activity of the administered steroid one may calculate by the dilution principle the actual amount of the steroid secreted by the adrenal gland during the period of urine collection (usually 24 hr). Such secretory rate determinations have been standardized for cortisol and aldosterone. The average daily cortisol secretory rate determined by such methods is 8 to 30 mg per day, and the average aldosterone secretory rate 50 to 250 μg per day. Estimates for the production of dehydroepiandrosterone by such methods have ranged from 15 to 25 mg per day.

Stimulation Tests

Within minutes after initiating an infusion of ACTH, increased cortisol levels are noted in adrenal venous blood. This responsiveness of the adrenal gland to ACTH is utilized as an index of the "functional reserve" of the gland to produce cortisol. Under maximal ACTH stimulation the cortisol secretion increases tenfold to 300 mg per day. Such maximal stimulation is obtainable only with prolonged ACTH infusions. For clinical purposes, the functional adrenal reserve for cortisol production is standardized with a shorter infusion time (8 hr). The standard intravenous ACTH test is performed by administering 50 units of aqueous ACTH in 500 ml normal saline intravenously over an exact 8-hr interval (from 8 A.M. to 4 P.M.) on two successive days and collecting the complete 24-hr urine output for analysis of creatinine, 17-hydroxycorticoids, (or 17-ketogenic steroids), and 17-ketosteroids. The patient may be ambulatory during this period. With such a method of testing an average increment of 15 mg (range, 5 to 25) has been noted in urine 17-hydroxysteroids on the first day of testing and an average increment of 25 mg (range, 15 to 35) on the second infusion day, by one commonly used method. Much smaller rises in urine 17-ketosteroid excretion are noted, with average increments of 4 to 8 mg per day on first and second day of testing, respectively. In the performance of the test the duration of the infusion must be strictly adhered to. Screening tests utilizing the intramuscular injection of ACTH (40 to 80 units twice daily) have been employed and offer the occasional advantage of ease of performance, but they have a more serious disadvantage in that the responses often vary because of irregular absorption of the ACTH from the injection site.

Suppression Test

The hypothalamic-pituitary ACTH release mechanism is sensitive to the circulating blood level of glucocorticoids. When such blood levels are increased in the normal individual the corticotropin-releasing center decreases its production of the corticotropin-releasing factor and consequently less ACTH is released from the anterior pituitary; secondarily, less steroid will be produced by the adrenal gland. The integrity of this feedback mechanism can be tested clinically by giving a potent glucocorticoid and judging suppression of the corticotropin-releasing center by analysis of urine steroid excretory values. A potent glucocorticoid such as dexamethasone is utilized in order that the administered compound may be given in such small amounts that it will not contribute significantly to the urine steroids to be analyzed. A standard method of testing is to administer 0.5 mg dexamethasone every 6 hr for two successive days while collecting 24-hr urine output for determination of creatinine, 17-hydroxysteroids, and 17-ketosteroids. In patients with a normal hypothalamic-pituitary ACTH release mechanism a fall in the urine 17-hydroxysteroid level to less than 2 mg per day on the second day of dexamethasone administration is seen. A normal response to such a suppression test implies that the adrenal glands are under the control of ACTH.

Test for Pituitary ACTH Reserve Capacity

Metyrapone [SU4885 (Metopirone)] is a drug that selectively inhibits the enzyme action of 11-beta-hydroxylase in the adrenal gland. As a result, the conversion of 11-desoxycortisol (Compound S) to cortisol is interfered with and increased amounts of 11-desoxycortisol accumulate while blood levels of cortisol decrease (Fig. 84-2). Since 11-desoxycortisol is a weak suppressor of the hypothalamic-pituitary axis, the anterior pituitary reponds to the declining cortisol blood levels by releasing larger quantities of ACTH in an attempt to stimulate the adrenal gland to release additional cortisol, which attempt, however, is thwarted by the metyrapone-induced enzymatic blockade. The metabolites of 11-deoxycortisol are excreted in increasing amounts in the urine, where they are measured as 17-hydroxycorticoids. Note that the adrenal glands must be capable of being stimulated by ACTH, since assessment of the response depends on adrenal steroid production.

The metyrapone (SU4885) response has been standardized for clinical evaluation of the reserve capacity of the anterior pituitary gland to release ACTH. Every 4 hr over a 48-hr period 750 mg metyrapone is administered orally, and daily urine collections for 17-hydroxycorticosteroids are obtained the day before testing, the two days of testing, and the day after the last dose of metyrapone. The peak response of increased urine 17-hydroxysteroid excretion may be seen on the day after completion of metyrapone administration, and normal individuals will respond with at least a doubling of their basal 17-hydroxysteroid excretion.

HYPERFUNCTION OF THE ADRENAL CORTEX

Distinct clinical syndromes are produced when excess amounts of the principal adrenal cortical hormones are secreted. Thus, excess production of the principal glucocorticoid cortisol is associated with Cushing's syndrome; excess production of the principal mineralocorticoid aldosterone with clinical and chemical signs of aldosteronism; excess production of adrenal androgens with adrenal virilism. As would be expected, these syndromes do not always occur in the "pure" form but may have overlapping features.

Cushing's Syndrome

From an analysis of the clinical and pathologic findings in a series of 12 patients, Harvey Cushing, in 1932, established a syndrome characterized by truncal obesity, hypertension, fatigability and weakness, amenorrhea, hirsutism, purplish abdominal striae, edema, glucosuria, and osteoporosis. As knowledge of this syndrome increased and as clinical tests of adrenal cortical function became standardized and readily available, the diagnosis of Cushing's syndrome has been broadened into the following classification:

CAUSES OF CUSHING'S SYNDROME

I. *Adrenal hyperplasia*, 70 per cent of cases
    A. Secondary to hypothalamic dysfunction

    B. Secondary to ACTH producing tumors
      1. Pituitary tumors
      2. Nonendocrine tumors (bronchogenic carcinoma)
  II. *Adrenal adenoma,* 15 per cent of cases
  III. *Adrenal carcinoma,* 10 per cent of cases
  IV. *Exogenous,* iatrogenic
    A. Prolonged use of glucocorticoids
    B. Prolonged use of ACTH

It is apparent that, regardless of etiology, all cases of Cushing's syndrome are due to increased production of cortisol by the adrenal gland. The majority of cases are due to *bilateral adrenal hyperplasia,* in which the adrenal gland weight usually exceeds the normal combined total weight of 10 Gm. Harvey Cushing originally postulated that the adrenal hyperplasia in these patients was attributable to the presence of pituitary basophilic adenomas. However, many cases are found without basophilic adenomas. Some are due to ACTH-producing chromophobe adenomas, but these cases represent a small fraction of the total. In the remaining cases attention has focused also on the elaboration of increased amounts of ACTH in the absence of pituitary tumors, possibly as a result of hypothalamic dysfunction, whereby the corticotropin releasing center is reset to respond to a higher level of circulating cortisol. Proof of such a theory awaits more sensitive methods for measuring ACTH blood levels and production rates than are currently available. Such cases of Cushing's syndrome due to adrenal hyperplasia, presumably due to excessive ACTH stimulation, always affect both adrenal glands.

In some 15 per cent of cases of Cushing's syndrome, unilateral *adrenal adenomas* are found. On occasion they may occur bilaterally. These adenomas may or may not function in autonomous manner; that is, they may or may not be independent of ACTH stimulation and control. In addition, approximately 10 per cent of cases of Cushing's syndrome are associated with *adrenal carcinomas,* most often unilateral and most often functioning autonomously. In those cases of Cushing's syndrome due to unilateral adrenal adenomas or carcinomas functioning independently of ACTH, atrophy of the contralateral gland is often found, attributable to suppression of ACTH release by the high levels of cortisol secreted by the tumors. A small number of patients with Cushing's syndrome are found to have *adrenal rest tumors,* that is, aberrant adrenal cortical tissue occurring outside the adrenal gland. These embryologic remnants may be in the perirenal area, ovaries, or testes and exhibit histologic features of hyperplastic or adenomatous changes.

Nonendocrine tumors secreting polypeptide fractions that have an ACTH-like action are also occasionally responsible for Cushing's syndrome secondary to bilateral adrenal hyperplasia. The major association of a nonendocrine tumor has been with primitive "oat-cell" carcinomas of the lung. Hypokalemic alkalosis is often prominent in such cases, whereas many of the distinctive physical findings usually associated with Cushing's syndrome may be absent.

Table 84-1. INCIDENCE OF SIGNS AND SYMPTOMS IN 35 CASES OF CUSHING'S SYNDROME, PER CENT

Typical habitus	97	Amenorrhea	77
Increased body weight	94	Cutaneous striae	67
Fatigability and weakness	87	Personality changes	66
Hypertension (above 150/90)	82	Ecchymoses	65
Hirsutism	80	Edema	62
		Polyuria, polydipsia	23
		Hypertrophy of clitoris	19

INCIDENCE. As steroid analyses have become more available, increasing numbers of patients with Cushing's syndrome are being detected among persons undergoing evaluation for such diverse entities as diabetes mellitus, hypertension, obesity, and osteoporosis. Many of these patients exhibit mild degrees of adrenal hyperfunction. The incidence of Cushing's syndrome in the female is three times that in the male. The most frequent age of onset is the third or fourth decade.

CLINICAL SIGNS AND SYMPTOMS. The frequency of clinical findings is listed in Table 84-1. From knowledge of the physiologic effects of glucocorticoids, many of the signs and symptoms logically follow. As a result of mobilization of peripheral supportive tissue, there is muscle weakness and fatigability, osteoporosis, and cutaneous striae. The latter involves a weakening and rupture of collagenous fibers in the dermis, thereby exposing the heavily vascularized subcutaneous tissues. Likewise, because of the loss of perivascular supporting tissue, there is easy bruisability and ecchymoses often appear at sites of mild trauma. The osteoporosis may be so severe that collapse of vertebral bodies and pathologic fractures of other bones are frequently encountered. As a result of increased hepatic gluconeogenesis from these mobilized precursors, there may be frank diabetes with polydipsia and polyuria. More frequently, with the presence of an adequate reserve of insulin, there is deposition of this excess glucose into fat depots. This is observed most notably in the upper face, the classic "moon" facies; in the interscapular area, the "buffalo" hump; and in the mesenteric bed, producing the classic "truncal" obesity (Fig. 84-8). The reason for this peculiar distribution of lipid is not known. The face also appears plethoric, even in the absence of any increase in red cell concentration. Hypertension is most always present, and frequently there are profound emotional changes ranging from irritability or emotional lability to severe depression, confusion, or even frank psychosis. Acne and hirsutism are frequent in female patients, the latter often appearing as a fine "downy" coat over the face, forehead, and upper trunk. Likewise in women patients, oligomenorrhea or amenorrhea is a frequent disturbance.

LABORATORY FINDINGS. With rare exceptions, plasma and urinary 17-hydroxycorticoid levels are elevated. Circulating eosinophils are below 100 cells per cu mm in 90 per cent of cases, and patients characteristically show a mild neutrophilic leuko-

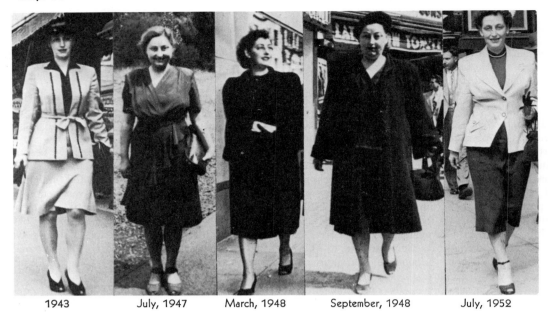

| 1943 | July, 1947 | March, 1948 | September, 1948 | July, 1952 |

Fig. 84-8. A 38-year-old woman with Cushing's disease: (1) patient before the onset of the disease, age 33; (2) patient 5 to 6 months after onset of symptoms, age 37; (3) improvement after x-ray treatment to the pituitary (2,800 roentgen units) and to the adrenal region (600 roentgen units); (4) return of the full-blown disease, just prior to admission to the Peter Bent Brigham Hospital; (5) remission after bilateral adrenalectomy.

cytosis. In spite of markedly plethoric facies, the hematocrit is usually within the normal range, but occasionally erythemia with higher hematocrits is encountered, particularly when the syndrome is associated with excessive production of 17-ketosteroids. Serum sodium concentration is usually normal; however, with marked excess secretion of cortisol, there may be hypokalemia, hypochloremia, and metabolic alkalosis. More than three-fourths of patients exhibit intermittent glucosuria, and nearly all have a decreased rate of disappearance of infused glucose from the circulation. Some patients may have frank diabetes necessitating insulin therapy. X-ray studies usually reveal generalized osteoporosis, most marked in the spine and pelvis, but also frequently including the skull, with disappearance of the lamina dura, and fractures are often seen in the ribs and vertebras. Intravenous pyelography and laminograms with or without retroperitoneal insufflation may demonstrate adrenal enlargement, particularly when an adenoma or carcinoma is the pathologic cause of the disease. Frequently, however, the truncal obesity makes radiologic interpretation difficult.

DIAGNOSIS. The diagnosis of Cushing's syndrome depends on the direct or indirect demonstration of increased cortisol production in the absence of stress. Once this is established, further testing is carried out to determine whether or not the excess cortisol production is being produced in an autonomous manner, since such knowledge will permit a more specific etiologic diagnosis.

For initial screening purposes, 24-hr urine 17-hydroxy- and 17-ketosteroid determinations are carried out, since values in excess of 10 mg per day for urine 17-hydroxysteroids (Porter-Silber) justifies further evaluation (Table 84-2). An ancillary screening procedure is to determine the diurnal excretion pattern for urine 17-hydroxysteroids by collecting urine between 7 A.M. and 7 P.M. and 7 P.M. to 7 A.M. The patient with Cushing's syndrome will generally excrete an equivalent or greater amount of the 17-hydroxysteroids in the night collection, in contrast to most normal subjects. Creatinine determinations are of critical importance to demonstrate the accuracy and adequacy of the collection procedure. An adult female excretes approximately 1,000 mg creatinine daily, with about 50 to 60 per cent found in the daytime collection; an adult male excretes approximately 1,800 mg daily. Day to day variation in creatinine excretion by the same patient should not exceed 20 per cent. If it is demonstrated that the diurnal cycle for steroid excretion is "reversed," that is, night urine 17-hydroxysteroids are almost equal to or greater than daytime excretion, one then knows that excessive cortisol is being released continuously "around-the-clock." These urine steroid determinations, which reflect the metabolites of cortisol, are indirect but adequate proof of excessive cortisol production. A direct method is available utilizing radioisotopic cortisol to determine the actual cortisol secretory rate, which in cases of Cushing's syndrome is in excess of 30 mg per day. Another method of direct confirmation of excess cortisol is the determination of the free cortisol in the urine, which reflects

Table 84-2. LABORATORY EVALUATION AND TESTING OF ADRENOCORTICAL FUNCTION IN NORMAL SUBJECTS AND IN PATIENTS WITH CUSHING'S SYNDROME*

	Plasma ACTH	Plasma cortisol	Cortisol secretory rate	Urine values	Control base line	Days of ACTH stimulation		Days of dexamethasone suppression, mg q 6h			
								0.5		2.0	
						1	2	1	2	3	4
Normal values	N	N	N	17-OH :	1–10	18–40	25–50	1–6	0–2	0–2	0–2
	N	N	N	17-KS :	5–25	15–30	20–40	6–18	5–15	4–12	4–8
Cushing's syndrome											
Hyperplasia..........	N–I	I	I	17-OH :	15	50	90	12	10	8	5
				17-KS :	20	50	90	18	15	12	10
Adenoma											
Complete autonomy	D	I	I	17-OH :	30	30	30	30	30	30	30
Incomplete				17-KS :	12	14	18	12	10	8	6
autonomy.......	N–D	I	I	17-OH :	15	50	90	15	15	12	10
				17-KS :	12	14	16	12	10	10	10
Carcinoma											
Adrenal..........	D	I	I	17-OH :	50	50	50	50	50	50	50
				17-KS :	60	60	60	60	60	60	60
Extra-adrenal (ACTH-producing tumor)	I	I	I	17-OH :	30	65	80	30	30	30	30
				17-KS :	25	55	70	25	25	25	25
Exogenous steroids (iatrogenic)	D	D	D	17-OH :	1	1	2	1	1	1	1
				17-KS :	4	5	6	5	4	4	4

* Clinical status charted vertically and *representative* values for steroid tests charted horizontally. 17-OH, 17-KS refer to 24-hr urine 17-hydroxycorticosteroid and 17-ketosteroid excretion. 17-KS base-line excretion higher in males than in females. All lab values given in milligrams per day. Urine ketogenic steroid values will be approximately twofold greater than those listed for urine 17-OH (except in adrenogenital syndrome). See text for normal blood steroid values. Note that only in the iatrogenic form of Cushing's syndrome are both the plasma ACTH and plasma cortisol levels decreased. ACTH stimulation causes brisk rise in *both* 17-OH and 17-KS in hyperplasia; disproportionate rise in 17-OH in adenoma; and no change in steroid excretion in adrenal carcinoma. Dexamethasone suppression is usually incomplete at the 2-mg daily dosage level in hyperplasia but complete with 8-mg dosage; incomplete at both 2- and 8-mg daily dosage in both adenomas and carcinomas with complete autonomy; incomplete in Cushing's syndrome secondary to extraadrenal ACTH-producing tumors. Abbreviations: N = normal; I = increased; D = decreased.

the active free cortisol in the blood. Normal persons excrete less than 100 μg daily of free cortisol, whereas patients with Cushing's syndrome may excrete up to ten times this amount. The sensitivity of this urine free cortisol test resides in the fact that only free cortisol of the plasma is freely filterable at the glomerulus, and thus increments in the plasma level of this biologically active form are magnified in terms of urine excretory values.

Owing to a marked diurnal variability plasma 17-hydroxycorticoid determinations are not meaningful when performed in isolated fashion, but demonstration that the expected normal fall in late afternoon blood levels does not occur is increasingly used as a diagnostic measure. Normally, the plasma level declines by half or more; if such a decrease is not noted, one assumes that continuous hypersecretion of cortisol is occurring.

An additional screening procedure involves the measurement of the plasma corticoid level at 8 A.M. and the total urinary excretion between 7 A.M. and 12 noon following the oral administration of 1 mg dexamethasone at midnight. Nugent et al. have shown that the 8 A.M. values for plasma corticoids in normal subjects who have received 1 mg dexamethasone at midnight rarely exceed 11 μg. We have included an analysis of the urinary steroid excretion from 7 A.M. to 12 noon on the same morning. The normal values for the 5-hr collection period should not exceed 2 mg hydroxysteroid (Porter-Silber method). Irregularities in urine collection can be obviated by calculating the ratio of milligrams of urinary steroid per milligrams of creatinine. The ratio for normal should not exceed .005 (5×10^{-3}).

Specific diagnosis of the type of lesion causing Cushing's syndrome can usually be made by the combined use of ACTH-stimulation and dexamethasone-suppression tests. Adrenal hyperplasia, whether caused by hypothalamic dysfunction or by an ACTH-producing tumor, is characterized by hyperreactivity to exogenous ACTH. The continuous stimulation of the hyperplastic glands by endogenous ACTH appears to "prime" the adrenals to this hyperactive response to exogenous ACTH testing. This hyperactive response is evidenced in the parallel rise of both urine 17-hydroxy- and urine 17-ketosteroids. Whereas adrenal cortisol production is suppressed in normal subjects given dexamethasone 0.5 mg every 6 hr for 48 hr, no suppression occurs in patients with bilateral adrenal hyperplasia given this dosage. Suppression of cortisol production in normal subjects is judged by a decrease in urine 17-hydroxysteroids to less than 3 mg per day, demonstrating that the hypothalamic-pituitary axis is appropriately responsive to increases in blood glucocorticoid levels, with a resultant decline in ACTH release. Lack of suppression in patients with adrenal hyperplasia given 2 mg daily of dexamethasone suggests that their hypothalamic-pituitary axis is "reset" to a higher blood level of glucocorticoids. On higher doses of dexamethasone (2 mg every 6 hr) suppression of urine 17-hydroxy-steroid levels to values less than half the base-line levels can be demonstrated, consistent with the view that the hypothalamic-pituitary axis in these patients is reset upward and responsive only to higher blood levels of glucocorticoids, at which point an appropriate decline in ACTH release does occur. The finding of a normal plasma ACTH level in these patients is an abnormal sign, since with the elevated blood cortisol levels one would expect a decreased blood ACTH level. On metyrapone testing patients with adrenal hyperplasia due to hypothalamic dysfunction will again demonstrate a hyperactive response. In patients with adrenal hyperplasia secondary to an *ACTH-producing tumor*, such as an oat-cell bronchogenic carcinoma, no suppression will occur after dexamethasone administration and an abnormally depressed metyrapone test results, since the ACTH production by the tumor functions in an autonomous manner.

In patients with Cushing's syndrome secondary to an *adrenal adenoma*, hyperreactivity to exogenous ACTH testing may or may not occur depending on whether the adenoma is functioning in an autonomous manner; if it is, it will be found ACTH-insensitive and thus fail to demonstrate a brisk rise in urine 17-hydroxycorticoids on ACTH stimulation. The diagnosis of adrenal adenoma is suggested by the disproportionate elevation in base-line urine 17-hydroxy-corticoids with only a modest rise in 17-ketosteroids. Those adenomas which function autonomously fail to suppress after administration of dexamethasone at either the 2- or 8-mg daily dosage schedule, whereas the ACTH-sensitive adenoma most often fail to suppress with the lower, 2-mg daily dosage but may demonstrate suppression at the higher, 8-mg daily

dosage. The variability of dexamethasone suppression testing is greater at the higher dose levels, and the distinction between adenomas and carcinomas is as a result less decisive. Another entity in the differential diagnosis is multinodular ("adenomatous") adrenal hyperplasia, which is an uncommon condition characteristically having features of both hyperplasia and of adenomas. Response to ACTH stimulation is abnormally brisk, but patients with multinodular adrenal hyperplasia most often do not show suppression after dexamethasone. Bilateral enlargement of the adrenals may be noted in such patients on x-ray, and some excrete high levels of 3β-hydroxy-$\Delta 5$-steroids.

Metyrapone testing is useful in differentiating adrenal tumors (adenoma or carcinoma) from adrenal hyperplasia, since the adrenal tumors by their autonomy suppress the ACTH-releasing capacity of the pituitary, with the result that on metyrapone challenge testing the pituitary fails to release ACTH in an appropriate manner and the usual rise in urine 17-hydroxycorticoids fails to occur. This finding of impaired response to metyrapone challenge separates adrenal tumors from adrenal hyperplasia, in which normal or hyperactive responses occur.

The diagnosis of *adrenal carcinoma* as a cause of Cushing's syndrome is suggested by markedly elevated base-line values of *both* urine 17-hydroxycorticoids and urine 17-ketosteroids. Adrenal carcinoma is usually resistant to both ACTH stimulation and dexamethasone suppression because of the autonomy of the tumor tissue itself and because of extreme atrophy of the normal remaining adrenal tissue. Virilization is often present. Functioning adrenal carcinomas that produce Cushing's syndrome are most often associated with elevated urine excretory values for the metabolites of the intermediates of steroid biosynthesis (such as tetrahydro-11-deoxycortisol) in addition to the cortisol metabolites, suggesting inefficient conversion of the intermediates to the final product. This is in contrast to Cushing's syndrome associated with adrenocortical hyperplasia, where the elevation of urine steroids is largely accounted for by cortisol metabolites.

Cushing's syndrome is being reported with increasing frequency in association with *nonendocrine tumors* producing an ACTH-like material in an autonomous manner, with the resultant development of adrenal hyperplasia. Approximately half these cases have been associated with the primitive small-cell type of bronchogenic carcinoma, and the remainder have been reported chiefly with tumors of thymus, pancreas, ovary, or thyroid. The onset of Cushing's syndrome is distinctively sudden in these patients, and this partly accounts for their failure to exhibit all the classic physical findings of the syndrome. Attempts to extract ACTH from these tumors have been most suggestive yet inconclusive. Since the tumors produce large amounts of ACTH-like material, base-line urine steroid values may be markedly elevated and skin pigmentation often is striking. Hypokalemic alkalosis due to excessive cortisol production is much commoner in these patients in comparison with cases of Cushing's syndrome due to other causes, and such a biochemical finding should accelerate diagnostic attempts to demonstrate nonendocrine tumors as the cause of Cushing's syndrome. Edema and hypertension are also seen with greater frequency in these patients. On testing, these patients will demonstrate a hyperactive response to ACTH stimulation but no suppression with dexamethasone and no increment in urine 17-hydroxycorticoid excretion after metyrapone administration. Plasma ACTH levels are most often markedly elevated in these patients, a helpful diagnostic finding, since plasma ACTH levels in other categories of Cushing's syndrome are at most modestly elevated.

Hyperpigmentation in patients with Cushing's syndrome always points to an extraadrenal tumor either in an extracranial location, as discussed in the previous paragraph, or occurring within the cranium. In the first 100 cases reported of Cushing's syndrome associated with pituitary tumors the majority had associated basophilic adenomas; chromophobe adenomas were in a distinct minority. Since this original series, chromophobe adenomas and carcinomas are being reported in much greater frequency than are basophilic adenomas. Basophilic adenomas do not cause enlargement of the sella turcica, whereas chromophobe tumors are the commonest cause of ballooning of the sella. Chromophobe tumors often are invasive and classically have been considered malignant. In cases of chromophobe tumors diagnosed at the onset of Cushing's syndrome the majority have been carcinomas, whereas almost all cases of chromophobe tumors occurring after bilateral adrenalectomy for Cushing's syndrome have been adenomas. The chief complaint of patients with chromophobe tumors is decreasing visual acuity, often with blurred vision and always with headaches. The chromophobe adenomas are asymmetric in growth, and as they progress upward, pressure on the optic nerve tracts results in visual field defects in most patients, with earliest losses occurring in the superior temporal quadrants; later a full bitemporal hemianopsia results. Headaches would appear to be caused by traction on surrounding dural structures or on the diaphragma sella. This association of pituitary tumors with Cushing's syndrome has generated interest as to whether all cases of adrenal hyperplasia may be caused by extraadrenal tumors and has led further to the speculation that chronic hypothalamic dysfunction may lead to the development of anterior pituitary tumors. A limitation to such interpretation has been the finding that approximately one-sixth of patients undergoing bilateral adrenalectomy for Cushing's syndrome have developed enlarged sella turcica and pituitary tumors, clinically evident only *after* the surgery, strongly suggesting that the loss of adrenal tissue, and consequent loss of the usual negative cortisol feedback on ACTH release, may be instrumental in the genesis of such tumors. Since intrasellar tumors may be present at an early stage in many patients *without* sellar enlargement, a decisive opinion as to their role in the genesis of, or in the sequelae of the surgical therapy of, Cushing's syndrome, must be withheld for further investigation. Clinically, all patients suspected of Cushing's syndrome must be carefully examined for visual field defects and enlargement of the sella turcica; if defects are found, further diagnostic procedures may be warranted, such as sellar tomography, pneumoencephalography, and angiography.

DIFFERENTIAL DIAGNOSIS. Patients with exogenous obesity, hypertension, and diabetes mellitus, occurring singly or in combination, present major problems in diagnosis. Extreme *obesity* is uncommon in Cushing's syndrome; furthermore, with exogenous obesity, the adiposity is generalized and not truncal. On adrenocortical testing, abnormalities, if noted in patients with exogenous obesity, are never extensive but only modest. Basal urine steroid excretion levels in obese patients are either normal or slightly elevated, a finding similar to their cortisol secretory values. Some patients demonstrate an increased percentage of conversion of secreted cortisol into excreted metabolites. Blood cortisol levels are normal and, of greater importance, a normal diurnal pattern in blood and urine levels is seen. On ACTH stimulation some of the patients will demonstrate a brisk response; however, most suppress easily with dexamethasone. It would appear that exogenous obesity may *cause* alterations in the secretion and metabolism of steroids, pointing up the secondary nature of altered steroid testing patterns sometimes encountered. These patients are best treated by a concerted weight reduction program with periodic retesting of adrenal function.

Patients with *hepatic disease,* notably cirrhosis, often with obesity, may exhibit some of the manifestations of Cushing's syndrome. The reason for this resides in their impaired ability to inactivate circulating steroids, owing to decreased hepatic blood flow, with the result that blood levels may increase but secretory rates generally are found in the normal range. The defect is in inactivation of steroids and not in excessive secretion, so therapy is initiated only for the underlying hepatic disease.

Iatrogenic Cushing's syndrome, induced by the administration of either glucocorticoids or ACTH, is indistinguishable by physical findings from the endogenous forms of adrenocortical hyperfunction. On occasion one may wish to rule out an underlying endogenous form of Cushing's syndrome that may be clinically magnified by exogenous therapy. This is accomplished by changing the patient's therapy to 1.0 mg dexamethasone daily while collecting baseline and diurnal split urine output for corticosteroid analysis. Patients with a pure exogenous form of Cushing's syndrome due to prolonged suppression of their hypothalamic-pituitary axis from administered steroid will demonstrate low base-line steroid excretion with predominant daytime excretion, a finding in distinct contrast to that in patients with endogenous Cushing's syndrome. Patients on long-term ACTH therapy, in addition to the features of Cushing's syndrome, may also present with melanodermia. The production of iatrogenic Cushing's syndrome is related both to the total steroid dose and to the duration of therapy. Also, patients on afternoon and evening doses of steroid develop Cushing's syndrome more readily and on smaller daily steroid doses than do patients on a steroid program limited to morning doses only. In addition, there appears to be a marked interpatient difference in the enzymatic disposition of administered steroid.

THERAPY. When an adenoma or carcinoma is suspected, adrenal exploration is performed, with excision of the tumor. Since cortisol production by the tumor generally causes atrophy of the contralateral gland, if an atrophied gland is noted on the initial side of exploration, the tumor must be on the opposite side. Because of this probable atrophy of the contralateral adrenal, the patient is prepared and treated pre- and postoperatively for total adrenalectomy even when a unilateral lesion is suspected, the routine being similar to that for an Addisonian patient undergoing elective surgery (Table 84-3). The possibility of chemically inhibiting adrenocortical hyperfunction due to carcinoma is under active investigation. The principal antitumor drug under evaluation is o,p′-DDD (2,2-bis[2-chlorophenyl,4-chlorophenyl]1,1-dichloroethane), an isomer of the insecticide DDT. o,p′-DDD originally was demonstrated to induce adrenal atrophy of the "cytotoxic type" in experimental animals. This drug suppresses cortisol production and decreases plasma and urine steroid levels. It also suppresses peripheral enzyme systems responsible for steroid

transformations. Daily dosage of o,p′-DDD has ranged from 2 to 8 Gm. Its cytotoxic action appears specific for adrenal glandular tissue, but histologic hepatic abnormalities have been reported. Almost all patients experience side effects of anorexia, diarrhea, or vomiting, and patients on long-term therapy must be observed closely for signs of adrenal insufficiency. In some patients dramatic regression of both tumor and metastases may occur, but long-term survival remains discouragingly limited. Predictability of expected response is poor. Investigation of this drug, however, has expanded the search for a more perfect chemical inhibitor of hyperactive adrenal tissue.

In patients with a severe form of Cushing's syndrome due to adrenal hyperplasia, with features of hypertension, overt diabetes, psychosis, and osteoporosis with pathologic fractures, and in the absence of an enlarged sella turcica, a complete total bilateral adrenalectomy is preferred. Since, as mentioned earlier, one-sixth of these patients develop pituitary tumors after surgery, pituitary irradiation is also indicated in any patient who develops increased pigmentation or in whom the sella turcica size increases postoperatively. In patients past the reproductive years pituitary irradiation may be carried out prophylactically in conjunction with complete adrenalectomy. It cannot be stressed too strongly that all patients with bilateral adrenalectomy must be followed diligently with periodic reexaminations for evidence of increasing sellar size or pigmentary changes.

If patients with adrenal hyperplasia are noted to have signs of pituitary tumor (melanodermia, increased sellar size, visual field defects), hypophysectomy is the operation of choice, particularly in individuals over the age of forty. A reversal of the

Table 84-3. STEROID THERAPY SCHEDULE FOR PATIENTS WITH CUSHING'S SYNDROME UNDERGOING ADRENALECTOMY*

	Steroid							
	Cortisone acetate (intramuscularly)		Cortisone acetate (orally)				Fluorohydrocortisone (orally)	Hydrocortisone infusion
	7 A.M.	7 P.M.	8 A.M.	12 M.	4 P.M.	8 P.M.	8 A.M.	Continuous
Day before operation........		100						
Day of operation............	100	50						300
Postoperative day 1.........	50	50						200
" 2.........	50	50						150
" 3.........	50	50						100
" 4.........	50	25	25	25	25	25		
" 5.........	50		25	25	25	25	0.1	
" 6.........			50	25	25	25	0.2	
" 7.........			25	25	25	25	0.2	
" 8.........			25	12.5	25	12.5	0.2	
" 9–14......			25	12.5	25		0.1	
" 15–21.....			25	12.5	12.5		0.1	
" 22–.......			25		12.5		0.1	

* Both intravenous and intramuscular routes are utilized to minimize hazards of infusion infiltration. All steroid doses are in milligrams.

biochemical steroid abnormalities occurs within 24 hr. The paranasal transsphenoidal surgical approach is becoming the method of choice. Cerebrospinal fluid rhinorrhea is a complication of this approach. Surgical hypophysectomy has the advantages of both completeness and rapidity of results, but the disadvantage of removing the tropic hormones for growth, gonads, and thyroid.

In patients with milder forms of adrenal hyperplasia without serious steroid-induced complications, several methods of approach are available such as unilateral adrenalectomy with or without pituitary irradiation, external or internal pituitary irradiation. Unilateral adrenalectomy without pituitary irradiation must be reserved for those patients with the mildest forms of adrenal hyperplasia, since the remaining adrenal undergoes immediate biochemical and later anatomic hypertrophy. Unilateral adrenalectomy in conjunction with pituitary irradiation can offset the disadvantage of the surgical procedure alone, and if the syndrome recurs, the remaining adrenal can then be removed. Subtotal adrenalectomy by itself is no longer indicated since, in addition to the problem of hypertrophy in the remaining remnant, these patients may be adrenal-insufficient without steroid replacement therapy and they rapidly become Cushingoid when receiving steroid replacement therapy, a most difficult management problem.

External pituitary irradiation with doses of 3,000 to 4,000 r, when carried out without concomitant surgical procedures, results in remission of Cushing's syndrome in less than one-third of cases. The total dosage that may be delivered is limited by possible damage to surrounding neural structures and by the loss of additional pituitary tropic functions. External pituitary irradiation is best utilized as an ancillary therapeutic approach preceding or following adrenal surgery.

Internal pituitary irradiation by the stereotaxic implantation of Yttrium[90] pellets via the transnasosphenoid route is increasingly used as an alternate form of pituitary ablation. Possible limitations of such therapy may arise once long-term evaluation of the effects of intrasellar radiation on perisellar structures (such as the internal carotid arteries) has been made.

If Cushing's syndrome redevelops after bilateral adrenalectomy, excessive stimulation of a remnant of adrenal cortical tissue must be occurring. In very rare instances an embryologic extra-adrenal remnant may be stimulated to produce excess cortisol. Surgical exploration has not been rewarding because of the difficulty in the identification of small adrenal cortical remnants. What is needed is an isotopic detection method whereby radioactive incorporation into the aberrant tissue could be monitored, and thus identification secured, at the operative field.

Aldosteronism

Aldosteronism is a syndrome associated with hypersecretion of the major adrenal mineralocorticoid aldosterone. *Primary* aldosteronism signifies that the stimulus for the excessive aldosterone production resides within the adrenal gland, whereas in *secondary* aldosteronism the stimulus is of extra-adrenal origin.

PRIMARY ALDOSTERONISM

The constellation of signs and symptoms of excessive inappropriate aldosterone production was first summarized by Conn in 1956. The disease results from an aldosterone-producing adrenal adenoma (Conn's syndrome) or, in some cases, an adrenal carcinoma; cases have occurred with adrenal hyperplasia, and in rare instances the disease has occurred in the absence of pathologic changes in the adrenal gland as judged by light microscopy.

The majority of cases (75 per cent) involve a unilateral adrenal adenoma, usually of small size and occurring with equal frequency on either side. It is twice as common in women as in men, presenting between the ages of thirty and fifty.

INCIDENCE. Primary aldosteronism is an uncommon disease. An estimated 400 cases have been reported worldwide in the first 10 years after its description. The incidence in unselected hypertensive patients is less than 0.5 per cent. Because of special diagnostic procedures involved, diagnosis has been largely restricted to symptomatic patients. With greater availability of these procedures an increased incidence may be seen.

SIGNS AND SYMPTOMS. The continual hypersecretion of aldosterone increases the renal distal tubular exchange of intratubular sodium for secreted potassium and hydrogen ions, with progressive depletion of body potassium and development of hypokalemia. Almost all patients have diastolic hypertension, usually not of marked severity, and complain of headaches. The hypertension is related in some unknown manner to the increased sodium reabsorption. *Potassium depletion* is responsible for the major complaints of muscle weakness and fatigue and is related to the effect of intra- and extracellular potassium ion depletion on muscle membrane. The muscle weakness is most striking in the legs and may progress to transient paralysis. Muscles innervated by cranial nerves are usually spared. Most patients have nocturnal polyuria due to a vasopressin-insensitive, potassium-depletion-induced nephropathy. The polyuria results from impairment of concentrating ability and is often associated with polydipsia. These patients may have electrocardiographic and x-ray signs of left ventricular enlargement secondary to their hypertension, and hypertensive retinopathy is often seen but papilledema is absent. Electrocardiographic signs of potassium depletion such as prominent U waves are often present. In the absence of associated congestive heart failure, renal disease, or preexisting abnormalities (such as thrombophlebitis), edema is characteristically absent in these patients.

In cases of long duration, potassium-depletion nephropathy becomes manifest with azotemia, often with superimposed bacilluria, and in some instances with congestive heart failure and edema.

LABORATORY FINDINGS. Laboratory findings are dependent on both the duration and the severity of the potassium depletion. On examination of the urine, negative to trace amounts of protein are found, sometimes with superimposed pyuria and bacilluria, presumably due to the predilection of potassium-depleted kidneys for infection. Urine specific gravity is low (less than 1.015), and an overnight concentration test with simultaneous vasopressin administration reveals impaired ability to concentrate the urine. Urine pH is often neutral to alkaline due to excessive secretion of ammonium and bicarbonate ions; potassium depletion may lower the maximal tubular transfer rate for bicarbonate. Urine 17-hydroxycorticosteroid and 17-ketosteroid excretion levels are always within the normal range in patients with aldosteronomas but may occasionally be elevated in those rare instances of primary aldosteronism due to adrenal carcinoma. Mild azotemia is an inconstant finding.

Serial blood sampling always reveals *hypokalemia* and usually a hypernatremia. Serial blood sampling is stressed. The hypokalemia may be severe (less than 3.0 mEq per liter) and reflects significant body potassium depletion, usually in excess of 300 mEq. *Hypernatremia* is due to both sodium retention and a concomitant water loss from polyuria. Serum bicarbonate may be elevated as a result of hydrogen ion loss into the urine and migration into potassium-depleted cells, with alkalosis then developing. The alkalosis is perpetuated with potassium deficiency since such deficiency increases the capacity of the proximal convoluted tubule to reabsorb filtered bicarbonate. This alkalosis predisposes to signs and symptoms of tetany. If hypokalemia is severe, serum magnesium levels will be reduced. In the absence of azotemia, serum uric acid concentration is normal.

Salivary sodium potassium ratios are reduced in the majority of cases, as is thermal sweat sodium concentration.

Total body sodium content is increased but not to the degree seen in edematous states. Total exchangeable sodium is moderately elevated, and total exchangeable body potassium is usually, but not invariably, reduced. The volume of extracellular fluid is expanded in most cases, with expansion of plasma volume in many. The expanded extracellular fluid volume is thought to be responsible for the reversed diurnal excretory pattern for salt and water many of these patients exhibit, with predominant salt and water excretion occurring during the night. Polyuria contributes to the nocturia.

DIAGNOSIS. The diagnosis of primary aldosteronism should be considered in all hypertensive patients exhibiting hypokalemia, particularly when associated with hypernatremia and alkalosis, in the *absence of diuretic therapy.*

The specific diagnosis of primary aldosteronism depends on demonstrating *autonomy* of aldosterone production, as judged by the evaluation of sodium and potassium excretion during base-line "balance" studies and during stimulation and suppression tests, preferably utilizing a direct measurement of aldosterone production such as determination of the aldosterone secretion or excretion rate. Since most cases of primary aldosteronism are due to tumors, most cases demonstrate partial or complete autonomy of function.

Base-line evaluation is carried out by placing the patient on a "normal" constant intake of sodium and potassium and obtaining periodic blood samples and daily urine collections for sodium and potassium. A normal daily intake of sodium and potassium may be taken as 80 to 100 mEq and 60 to 90 mEq, respectively. The patient with primary aldosteronism during this base-line evaluation will show an elevated rate of aldosterone secretion or excretion. Sodium "balance," with urine sodium output approximating intake, is rapidly achieved. Potassium "balance," which is a function of both aldosterone production and sodium intake, may or may not be "negative," with potassium excretion exceeding intake. Potassium excretion must always be judged in relation to the existing serum potassium concentration, since patients with potassium deficits incurred as a result of diarrhea, diuretic therapy, or decreased intake will show evidence of renal potassium conservation with urine potassium concentrations of less than 20 mEq per liter. Thus, patients with primary aldosteronism who always show urine potassium concentration greater than 20 mEq per liter are losing excessive amounts of urine potassium despite their hypokalemia. Such base-line evaluation lacks the specificity of suppression and stimulation testing designed to demonstrate autonomy of function.

Since volume expansion in normal subjects suppresses aldosterone production, *suppression testing* may be carried out in patients suspected of primary aldosteronism by volume expansion. This volume expansion is accomplished by dietary salt-loading. The patients are placed on a high-salt constant diet containing 200 mEq sodium and 60 to 100 mEq potassium per day while balance studies are carried out through daily urine collections. Serum potassium concentrations are measured daily. Such a program in patients *without* primary aldosteronism suppresses aldosterone secretory and excretory values to lower than normal by the fifth day; also, urine potassium excretion will not be excessive and serum potassium levels will not change. However, in patients *with* primary aldosteronism, aldosterone secretion or excretion rates are still elevated; that is, there is no suppression on salt-loading. Furthermore, the increased delivery of filtered sodium to the distal renal tubule results in increased renal potassium secretion with rapid development of negative potassium balance, in which urine potassium excretion exceeds intake. As a result of increasing potassium losses through the urine, hypokalemia develops or, if previously present, becomes more marked. Since hypokalemia may become severe, daily monitoring of serum potassium levels is mandatory and the testing phase should not be unduly prolonged. Since primary aldosteronism reflects excessive inappropriate adrenal secretion of the mineralocorticoid, in most patients with the disorder aldosterone production cannot be completely suppressed, and the condition is readily diagnosed by this testing program.

Aldosterone production is readily stimulated by salt restriction, a procedure that causes marked rises in aldosterone excretion in normal subjects. This is accomplished by giving a constant daily intake of 10 mEq sodium or less and 60 to 100 mEq potassium. Patients with complete autonomy of aldosterone production as a result of primary aldosteronism will show by the fifth day of salt restriction either no rise or a subnormal rise in aldosterone production. Some patients with primary aldosteronism and "incomplete" autonomy may exhibit a normal rise in aldosterone secretion but from *elevated* base-line values. As a result of less filtered sodium being delivered to the distal renal tubule, renal potassium wasting decreases and serum potassium reverts toward normal values in patients with primary aldosteronism.

The diagnosis of primary aldosteronism can be made with certainty in patients that show such inappropriate responses to base-line, suppression, and stimulation testing.

Salivary and sweat sodium concentrations, when reduced, are helpful in screening patients for primary aldosteronism, but these measures lack the specificity to be diagnostic. The findings of alkaline urine, reversed diurnal sodium excretion, expanded extracellular fluid, and impaired renal concentrating ability also are too nonspecific for diagnostic purposes but are helpful as ancillary measures.

Since aldosterone-producing tumors are quite small, intravenous pyelography and tomography studies characteristically fail to localize them. Urine 17-hydroxycorticoid and 17-ketosteroid excretion patterns are always normal unless the primary aldosteronism is due to adrenal carcinoma in which case both the metabolites of cortisol and of aldosterone may be elevated.

DIFFERENTIAL DIAGNOSIS. All patients with primary aldosteronism have hypertension, a finding that differentiates this condition from others with comparable renal potassium wasting but with normal blood pressures, such as renal tubular acidosis, hyperplasia of the juxtaglomerular complex, familial renal potassium wasting, and other renal tubular disorders such as the Fanconi syndrome.

Renal potassium wasting and hypertension may be seen with Cushing's syndrome, especially in those cases due to ACTH-producing nonendocrine tumors, but such cases are readily diagnosed by the finding of elevated urine 17-hydroxycorticoid levels, which elevation is not readily suppressible. The serum uric acid may be low in such cases as a result of steroid-induced uricosuria, whereas it is normal in patients with primary aldosteronism.

The major condition in which differentiation from primary aldosteronism is difficult is accelerated hypertension with or without a predisposing renal lesion such as renal arterial stenosis. Malignant hypertension with azotemia and papilledema is rare in primary aldosteronism; yet such accelerated hypertension may be associated with secondary aldosteronism as a result of increased renin release. The finding of *elevated blood renin* or angiotensin levels is diagnostic of secondary aldosteronism in such cases, since *renin and angiotensin blood concentrations are normal to below normal in patients with primary aldosteronism.* Hypertensive subjects often have a thiazide diuretic–induced hypokalemia, which may be separated out by the finding of elevated serum uric acid levels. All patients with accelerated hypertension and hypokalemia must be evaluated for unilateral renal disease; if such a diagnosis is confirmed, the diagnosis of primary aldosteronism is then excluded since the two entities are not known to coexist. Successful surgical correction or medical antihypertensive therapy in patients with unilateral renal disease may result in disappearance of aldosteronism.

In rare instances the biochemical signs of primary aldosteronism are duplicated by hypertensive patients ingesting large amounts of licorice, which has sodium-retaining properties, presumably due to its content of glycyrrhizinic acid.

ETIOLOGY AND PATHOGENESIS. Of all cases of primary aldosteronism 80 per cent are due to adrenal cortical adenoma, 15 per cent to adrenal cortical hyperplasia, and less than 5 per cent to adrenal carcinoma. Preoperative management centers around correcting potassium deficits by a low-sodium diet, potassium supplements, and aldosterone antagonists. If at the time of adrenal exploration an adenoma is found on the initial side, it is resected. However, if on complete mobilization of the gland a mass is not identified, exploration of the opposite adrenal is mandatory. In patients with adrenal cortical hyperplasia, complete total adrenalectomy is carried out. In the rare instances in which normal adrenal glands are identified, subtotal adrenalectomy is done. If potassium-depletion nephropathy is present, a renal biopsy is also performed to quantitate histologic changes. Renal biopsy by demonstrating the *absence* of juxtaglomerular hyperplasia can also serve as additional confirmation of the primacy of the aldosteronism.

Postoperatively, 80 per cent of patients are either cured or improved in regard to their hypertensive status. There is dramatic amelioration of the associated symptoms of aldosteronism. In a few patients azotemia, hyponatremia, and hyperkalemia develop during the immediate postoperative period, suggesting transient mineralocorticoid deficiency. Mineralocorticoid replacement therapy may be utilized in such cases, but such therapy is not mandatory since it has been found that the electrolyte imbalance is only transitory; however, azotemia may persist indefinitely.

SECONDARY ALDOSTERONISM

Secondary aldosteronism refers to the appropriate increased production of aldosterone by the adrenal gland in response to stimuli originating *outside* the gland. The actual adrenal aldosterone secretion rates are often higher in secondary aldosteronism than in primary. The *tropic hormone* or hormones for aldosterone release by the adrenal glands are not known with certainty. Pineal gland extracts in animals have been shown to be capable of causing increased aldosterone release; however, since salt and water metabolism is carried out effectively in pinealectomized animals, the pineal gland is thought to play, at most, a minor role. Exogenous ACTH has been shown to cause increased aldosterone excretion in man, but of a transient nature, suggesting that it may function as a tropic hormone only in acute situations. The tropic hormone responsible for chronic aldosterone release has not been elucidated. The ionic composition of adrenal arterial blood, when characterized by a low sodium and a high potassium concentration, also can elicit increased aldosterone release, but, again, such a mechanism appears to operate only in acute situations. The major stimulus for increased aldosterone release appears to be *volume depletion.* Any mode of volume depletion is an effective stimulus, such as hemorrhage, salt restriction, or diuretic therapy. Since volume deficits must be registered as pressure changes, evidence has been sought for the anatomic locus of a *volume-pressure receptor.* It would appear that such volume receptors are located within the arterial side of the circulation, since arterial hypovolemia is characteristic of the edematous states due to secondary aldosteronism. Edema is the cardinal physical finding of secondary aldosteronism and is absent in patients with primary aldosteronism. The reason why patients with primary aldosteronism do not sustain edema is that they are continually exhibiting the escape phenomenon. *Escape phenomenon* is the description given to the failure of normal patients to develop edema when given excessive amounts of parenteral aldosterone, since after an initial phase of sodium retention and extracellular fluid expansion, natriuresis ensues whereby they *escape* from the sodium-retaining properties of aldosterone and as a result remain free of edema. Patients with secondary aldosteronism, when given supplementary parenteral aldosterone, fail to exhibit the escape phenomenon and, on the contrary, become more and more edematous.

The *renin-angiotensin system* has been proposed as a system capable of governing aldosterone release. It is postulated that the afferent arterioles of cortical nephrons may act as pressure transducers by sensing the amount of "stretch" on their walls. If a volume deficit has been incurred and renal perfusion is decreased, there will be less myogenic stretch on the afferent arterioles and this will cause the contiguous juxtaglomerular cells to release additional quantities of *renin,* the enzyme that converts angiotensinogen to angiotensin-I, which in turn is very quickly acted upon by converting enzyme to form angiotensin-II. Angiotensin-II is then released into the systemic circulation via the renal veins and lymphatics. Angiotensin-II could then cause arteriolar constriction and could also directly stimulate the adrenal gland to release additional aldosterone. The released aldosterone would cause salt retention with concomitant volume expansion, which in association with the arterial pressure rise would increase the renal perfusion pressure, increase the stretch on the afferent arterioles, and thus "shut off" the stimulus to increased juxtaglomerular cell renin release. The finding of *increased* blood levels of renin in clinical states of secondary aldosteronism is consistent with this theory. Since most patients with edema and secondary aldosteronism do not have hypertension it is apparent that angiotensin cannot subserve a pressor role in these patients; this has been documented by the demonstration of increased pressor refractoriness to exogenous angiotensin in these patients. Since angiotensin-II is the most potent known chemical mediator for aldosterone release, the renin-angiotensin hypothesis has clinical merit. What is needed to delineate this hypothesis further is a method of determining the rate of angiotensin secretion.

Increased aldosterone secretion rates have been amply documented in patients who form edema as a result of either cirrhosis or the nephrotic syndrome. In congestive heart failure, however, elevated aldosterone secretion is a variable finding. The stimulus for aldosterone release in these clinical conditions appears to be *arterial hypovolemia.* Arterial blood volume may be depleted in cirrhosis as a result of decreased hepatic protein synthesis and protein loss into ascitic fluid; likewise, urine protein loses in the nephrotic syndrome may lead to arterial hypovolemia. Despite venous congestion, arterial hypovolemia may occur in congestive heart failure as a result of a failing cardiac output. The finding of normal aldosterone secretory rates in some patients with congestive heart failure requires explanation. It has been shown that approximately 95 per cent of the circulating blood aldosterone is removed from the plasma and metabolized or extracted by the liver during a single passage. The rate of removal of aldosterone from plasma is termed its *metabolic clearance rate,* and since aldosterone is almost exclusively "cleared" by the liver, hepatic blood flow will approximate the aldosterone clearance rate. Since the blood level of circulating aldosterone is presumed to be the critical factor in its biologic activity, it is to be appreciated that the blood level will be determined by both the aldosterone secretion rate and the rate of hepatic inactivation. Thus, in clinical states characterized by reduced hepatic blood flow, such as congestive heart failure, an increased blood circulating aldosterone level can occur and result in sodium retention, even though the secretion rate of the hormone is within the normal range.

The *steroid 17-spirolactones* [such as spironolactone (Aldactone)] are specific synthetic competitive inhibitors of aldosterone. They do not cause a natriuresis in the absence of aldosterone. They specifically block the distal renal tubular action of aldosterone, thereby causing natriuresis and potassium retention. In large doses, hyponatremia and hyperkalemia can occur. Since their action is limited to the distal tubule, they may be ineffective in severe sodium-retaining states because excessive sodium reabsorption in such patients occurs predominantly in the proximal tubule. The steroid 17-spirolactone aldosterone antagonists have been of limited value in the differential diagnosis of primary versus secondary aldosteronism.

Adrenal Virilism

The adrenal virilizing syndromes result from excessive productions of adrenal androgens, such as dehydroepiandrosterone and Δ-4-androstenedione. Similar to other states of adrenal cortical hyperfunction, the syndrome may result from hyperplasia, adenoma, or carcinoma. It also may arise in a congenital form, termed *adrenogenital hyperplasia,* due to enzymatic deficits. The adrenal virilizing syndromes may be associated with secretions of greater or smaller amounts of other adrenal hormones and may, therefore, present as a "pure" syndrome of virilization or a "mixed" syndrome associated with excessive production of glucocorticoid and some of the characteristics of Cushing's syndrome. In *congenital* adrenal hyperplasia the virilizing syndrome may be associated with either excessive or decreased secretion of mineralocorticoid or decreased production of glucocorticoid.

The enzymatic composition of the adrenal as determined by heredity (and perhaps other factors as well) determines the relative rate of synthesis of hormones with glucocorticoid activity and of hormones with androgenic activity.

Since in man hydrocortisone is the principal adrenal steroid regulating ACTH elaboration, and since ACTH stimulates both hydrocortisone and adrenal androgen production, it stands to reason that an enzymatic interference with hydrocortisone synthesis may result in the enhanced secretion of adrenal androgens. In severe congenital virilizing hyperplasia, the adrenal output of hydrocortisone may be so compromised as to cause clinical evidence of glucocorticoid deficiency despite anatomic adrenal hyperplasia. Conversely, a high hydrocortisone output as the result of primary adrenal pathology (adenoma) may inhibit ACTH secretion and thus result in a low adrenal androgen output.

INCIDENCE. Congenital bilateral adrenocortical hyperplasia is by far the most common adrenal disorder of infancy and childhood. It has also been described later in life, predominantly in women. Its appearance in postpuberal men would obviously not be as clinically apparent; nevertheless, it has been reported. The most common form of significant "noncongenital" adrenal virilization is that seen with bilateral adrenocortical hyperplasia and is most frequently associated with various degrees of excessive production of glucocorticoid hormone and the clinical signs and symptoms of Cushing's syndrome.

CLINICAL SIGNS AND SYMPTOMS. In the adult female, regardless of etiology, the clinical signs and symptoms are those anticipated from excessive androgen production. These include hirsutism, acne, increased sebum production, temporal baldness, deepening of voice, increased muscle mass and strength, decreased breast size, atrophy of the uterus, amenorrhea, enlargement of the clitoris, increased heterosexual drive, and development of a male habitus. The clinical distinction between excessive hair growth (hirsutism) and virilization is useful. Virilization signifies that multiple signs of androgen excess are present in addition to hirsutism, and one of the more easily recognized of these signs is hypertrophy of the clitoris. Hirsutism in the absence of other signs of virilization is uncommon in these patients. The virilizing syndromes are difficult to document in the adult male for obvious reasons.

Adrenal virilization secondary to *adrenal hyperplasia* is thought to be congenital in origin, with specific deficits in steroid hydroxylating enzymes. The most common enzymatic deficits are in either C-21 or C-11 hydroxylases or 3-β-ol-dehydrogenase. These enzymatic deficits may occur singularly or in combination. Adrenal virilization at birth is almost always due to congenital adrenal hyperplasia; however, the disease may not become apparent until many years later, and sometimes only in adult life. In the most common form of congenital adrenal hyperplasia, that due to impairment of *C-21 hydroxylation*, there will be reduced conversion of 17-hydroxyprogesterone to 11-deoxycortisol and thus reduced formation of cortisol from 11-deoxycortisol (Fig. 84-2). In addition to cortisol deficiency, there may or may not be an associated reduction in aldosterone secretion as a result of impaired C-21 hydroxylation of progesterone to 11-deoxycorticosterone, a precursor of aldosterone. Thus, with congenital adrenal hyperplasia secondary to C-21 hydroxylase deficiency, adrenal insufficiency will be present with or without an associated salt-losing tendency due to aldosterone deficiency. As a result of the C-21 hydroxylase deficit precursor products accumulate and are shunted into alternate pathways of metabolism, chiefly the androgen pathway, accounting for the production of excessive androgens. The accumulation of progesterone may also exaggerate any salt-losing tendency, since progesterone has an antialdosterone effect on renal tubular salt conservation. Since a cortisol deficiency exists, the adrenal glands become hyperplastic because of excessive ACTH stimulation.

With a *C-11 hydroxylase* deficiency a "hypertensive" variant of congenital adrenal hyperplasia develops with cortisol deficiency, since there is impaired conversion of 11-deoxycortisol to cortisol. Hypertension occurs because of the impaired conversion of 11-deoxycorticosterone to corticosterone, resulting in the accumulation of 11-deoxycorticosterone, a potent mineralocorticoid. Increased shunting again occurs into the androgen pathway.

With *3-β-ol-dehydrogenase* deficiency, there is impaired conversion of pregnenolone to progesterone with the result that pathways to both cortisol and aldosterone are "blocked" with shunting then occurring into the adrenal androgen pathway via 17α-hydroxy-pregnenolone to dehydroepiandrosterone.

Clinically adrenal virilism due to congenital adrenal hyperplasia manifests itself as *pseudohermaphroditism* of females and *premature virilization* of males. The age of onset of virilization is most probably prenatal after the fifth month of embryonic development. At birth there may be macrogenitosomia in the male infant and enlargement of the clitoris, partial or complete fusion of the labia, and sometimes a urogenital sinus in the female. If the labial fusion is nearly complete, the female infant will have external genitalia resembling a penis with hypospadias, changes consistent with female pseudohermaphroditism. Chromosomal sex can be determined by skin biopsy or examination of oral mucosal smears. Those infants with a salt-losing tendency often crave salt, and episodes of acute adrenal insufficiency are common. This salt-losing variant of congenital adrenal hyperplasia is often associated with vomiting, diarrhea, and hypotension. Hypertension is, of course, a key feature of the hypertensive variant of congenital adrenal hyperplasia and its severity may dominate the clinical picture. In the *postnatal period* from infancy through adolescence, congenital adrenal hyperplasia will be associated with virilization in the female and isosexual precocity in the male. The excessive androgens produced will result in accelerated growth before fusion of epiphyses occurs, with skeletal growth exceeding the chronologic age. With epiphyseal closure, which is hastened by excessive androgens, growth stops but truncal development continues, giving the characteristic appearance of a child of short stature with a well-developed trunk. Incomplete variants of congenital adrenal hyperplasia sometimes occur in adult life, with virilization occurring in the female. It is not apparent why the adrenogenital syndrome should be dormant until adult life. One possibility may be that only a partial deficiency of an enzyme system such as C-11 hydroxylase was inherited and that the production of androgens in adult life may further inhibit the action of this enzyme, with consequent overproduction of adrenal androgens.

DIAGNOSIS. The diagnosis of adrenal virilism due to *congenital adrenal hyperplasia* should be considered in all infants exhibiting "failure to thrive," particularly those having episodes of acute adrenal insufficiency or having sustained hypertension. The diagnosis is further suggested by the finding of hypertrophy of the clitoris, fused labia, or urogenital sinus in the female and isosexual precocity in the male infant. In infants and children with a *C-21 hydroxylation block*, increased urine 17-ketosteroid excretion is typically associated with an increase in the excretion of pregnanetriol, which is a metabolite of 17α-hydroxy-progesterone. These children will show low urine 17-hydroxycorticoid excretion levels and elevated levels of plasma ACTH. Ketogenic steroid excretion will be elevated since the depressed 17-hydroxycorticoid excretion is more than offset by increments in preg-

Table 84-4. LABORATORY EVALUATIONS AND TESTING OF ADRENOCORTICAL FUNCTION IN THEORETICAL CASES OF ADRENAL VIRILIZING SYNDROMES*

Syndromes	Plasma ACTH	Plasma cortisol	Cortisol secretory rate	Urine values		Control base line	Days of ACTH stimulation		Days of dexamethasone suppression, mg q 6h			
									0.5		2.0	
							1	2	1	2	3	4
Benign androgenic hyperplasia	N†	N	N	17-OH	:	7	20	35	4	2	1	1
				17-KS	:	17	35	50	10	5	4	3
Virilizing carcinoma	N–D‡	N–I	N–I§	17-OH	:	12	24	35	10	5	4	4
				17-KS	:	150	150	150	150	150	150	150
Virilizing adenoma	N	N	N	17-OH	:	8	17	30	6	4	3	3
				17-KS	:	150	160	170	150	140	130	120
Congenital adrenal hyperplasia	I	D	D	17-OH	:	3	12	20	3	4	5	5
				17-KS	:	40	60	90	25	20	15	10

* Clinical status charted vertically and representative values for steroid tests charted horizontally. 17-OH, 17-KS refer to 24-hr urine 17-hydroxycorticosteroid and 17-ketosteroid excretion. All lab values given in milligrams per day. Base-line urine 17-KS are either at upper limits of normal or slightly elevated in benign androgenic hyperplasia, whereas they are markedly elevated with virilizing carcinoma or adenoma. With ACTH stimulation, in benign androgenic hyperplasia, there is disproportionate rise in 17-KS; in virilizing tumors, there is no increment in 17-KS; in congenital adrenal hyperplasia, there is a rise in 17-KS (unless base-line 17-KS are very high). With dexamethasone suppression, in benign androgenic hyperplasia, there is complete suppression; in virilizing tumors, no suppression; in congenital adrenal hyperplasia, complete suppression.

† N, normal.

‡ D, decreased.

§ I, increcsed.

nanetriol excretion, which metabolite is included in the analysis. On testing with ACTH, the altered metabolic pathways are exaggerated with sharp rises occurring in 17-ketosteroid excretion and little or no rise in 17-hydroxycorticoid excretion (Table 84-4).

The diagnosis of a *salt-losing form* of congenital adrenal hyperplasia due to impaired C-21 hydroxylation is suggested by episodes of acute adrenal insufficiency with hyponatremia, hyperkalemia, dehydration, and vomiting. These infants and children often "crave" salt and exhibit laboratory signs of concomitant deficits in both cortisol and aldosterone secretion.

With the *hypertensive form* of congenital adrenal hyperplasia due to impaired C-11 hydroxylation, the precursor 11-deoxycortisol will accumulate. As a result, both urine 17-keto- and 17-hydroxycorticoid excretion may be elevated since 11-deoxycortisol would be included in the analysis of Porter-Silber chromogens. The diagnosis is secured by demonstrating increased amounts of tetrahydro-11-deoxycortisol in the urine with decreased amounts of tetrahydro metabolites of cortisol.

The finding of very high levels of urine dehydroepiandrosterone with low levels of pregnanetriol and of cortisol metabolites is characteristic of patients with congenital adrenal hyperplasia due to 3-β-ol-dehydrogenase deficiency. These patients also exhibit marked salt-wasting.

The adrenal virilizing syndrome in adults is most often due to noncongenital causes, namely, adrenal hyperpalsia or tumor. *Benign androgenic adrenal hyperplasia* refers to those patients with hirsutism with normal or slightly elevated urine 17-ketosteroids and normal 17-hydroxycorticosteroids. With ACTH stimulation there is a brisk rise in the urine 17-ketosteroids when compared to the 17-hydroxysteroids. Base-line 17-ketosteroids are easily suppressed on 2 mg daily of dexamethasone. An estimated one-third of patients with the polycystic ovarian syndrome and one-third of females with idiopathic hirsutism have findings consistent with benign androgenic adrenal hyperplasia. In adrenal cortical hyperfunction of Cushing's syndrome, both urine 17-ketosteroid and 17-hydroxysteroid base-line values will be elevated, the latter separating Cushing's syndrome from benign androgenic hyperplasia.

Adrenal adenomas and *carcinomas* may also cause a pure or mixed virilizing syndrome. Since adrenal androgens are weak androgens compared with gonadal androgens, adrenal virilization is characterized by large increments in urine 17-ketosteroids, often with less impressive clinical signs of virilism. Virilizing adrenal cortical adenomas are rare. They produce very high levels of urine 17-ketosteroids, often greater than 200 mg per day, and are associated with no rise or only a slight rise in urine 17-hydroxysteroids. They may or may not be sensitive to ACTH stimulation and likewise may or may not be sensitive to dexamethasone suppression. *Virilizing adrenal carcinomas* are the most common adrenal tumor causing virili-

Table 84-5. CAUSES OF HIRSUTISM IN FEMALES

1. Idiopathic
2. Familial
3. Ovarian
   a. Polycystic ovaries
   b. Tumor: arrhenoblastoma, hilus cell, adrenal rest
4. Adrenal
   a. Benign androgenic hyperplasia
   b. Congenital adrenal hyperplasia
   c. Virilizing carcinoma
   d. Virilizing adenoma
   e. Noncongenital adrenal hyperplasia (Cushing's)

zation. They are also associated with very high urine 17-ketosteroid excretion and may have normal 17-hydroxycorticoid excretion or a moderate rise in 17-hydroxysteroid excretion. They characteristically show no increase in steroid excretion upon stimulation with ACTH and also characteristically fail to suppress with dexamethasone administration. These tumors are often associated with marked virilization of sudden onset. The very high ketosteroid excretion of both virilizing adenomas and carcinomas is made up in large part of the weak androgen dehydroepiandrosterone, which has approximately 5 per cent of the androgenicity of testosterone. The clinical differentiation between virilizing adrenal adenoma and carcinoma is tenuous and cannot be made with certainty preoperatively.

DIFFERENTIAL DIAGNOSIS. The chief consideration in the differential diagnosis of adrenal virilization is virilization due to ovarian causes (Table 84-5). The low to slightly elevated urine 17-ketosteroid values associated with "idiopathic" hirsutism are in sharp contrast to the very high values with adrenal virilization. The hirsutism associated with polycystic ovaries is associated with other signs of virilization in 10 to 15 per cent of patients. The association of amenorrhea with bilaterally large ovaries suggests polycystic ovaries, although some polycystic ovaries are of normal size. Urine 17-ketosteroid excretion in polycystic ovarian syndrome is either normal or slightly increased and characteristically fails to exhibit normal suppression with dexamethasone administration. In some of these patients a modest rise in urine 17-ketosteroids is shown on ACTH administration and purified FSH preparations cause a rise in the 11-deoxy-17-ketosteroid fraction with no or little change in the urine 11-oxy-17-ketosteroids. Hirsutism in these patients is thought to be due to defective ovarian aromatization whereby the androgen precursors, Δ-4-androstenedione and testosterone, are not completely aromatized to the estrogens, estrone and estradiol, with the result that the blood level of the androgens will increase.

The most common *ovarian tumor* causing virilization is the arrhenoblastoma, but other ovarian tumors such as adrenal rest tumor, granulosa cell tumor, hilar cell tumors, and Brenner tumors have been associated with virilization. These masculinizing ovarian tumors may secrete testosterone as the major androgen, and the secretion of a few milligrams of testosterone, in view of its high androgenicity, can cause overt hirsutism. As a result, urine 17-ketosteroids are within the normal range in half these patients, and moderate elevations occur in the remainder. Urine base-line 17-ketosteroid excretion in excess of 40 mg per day is rare, with the exception of adrenal rest tumors. Urine 17-hydroxycorticoid excretion is normal. These ovarian tumors characteristically fail to suppress with dexamethasone; with the exception of adrenal rest tumors, they are largely independent of ACTH stimulation. Adrenal virilization due to *adrenal tumor* is characterized by high urine 17-ketosteroid excretion representing metabolites of weak adrenal androgens (such as dehydroepiandrosterone), whereas virilization due to ovarian tumors is characterized by normal or moderate elevation of urine 17-ketosteroids since the ovaries are secreting the extremely potent androgen, testosterone. The principal difference between biosynthesis of androgens by the ovaries and by the adrenals is that tropic control is exerted principally by gonadotropins in the former and by ACTH in the latter case.

Direct inspection of the ovaries by culdoscopy is a valuable means of differentiating between ovarian and adrenal causes of hirsutism. Polycystic ovaries have a characteristic "oyster" appearance, and varying degrees of bilateral enlargement may be seen. Unilateral ovarian enlargement suggests ovarian tumor. If on culdoscopic examination "normal" ovaries are found, this, of course, strengthens the probability of an adrenal etiology for virilization. Suprarenal and ovarian tomography, with or without contrast studies, is helpful in delineating this problem.

With the finding of isosexual precocity in young boys, in addition to congenital adrenal hyperplasia, one must consider the possibility of hyperplasia of adrenal rest tissue occurring in the epididymis or testes. These *testicular adrenal rests* secrete high quantities of ketosteroids and operate under ACTH control. The aberrant adrenal rest tissue usually causes bilateral testicular enlargement in contrast to the unilateral testicular enlargement with contralateral atrophy usually seen with true interstitial cell tumors. Further differentiation from interstitial testicular cell tumors is afforded by the insensitivity of the latter to ACTH stimulation.

TREATMENT. Treatment of adrenal virilism is dictated by the type of lesion suspected. The patients with *congenital adrenal hyperplasia* have the fundamental defect of cortisol deficiency with resultant excessive ACTH stimulation producing hyperplasia of the adrenal glands and causing additional "shunting" into the adrenal androgen pathway. Therapy in these patients consists of daily glucocorticoid (dexamethasone, prednisone, cortisone, etc.) administration to suppress pituitary ACTH secretion. In children, this not only suppresses urinary ketosteroid excretion but also ends virilization and the associated problems of hyperandrogenicity. The dosage schedule is governed by repetitive analysis of the urine 17-ketosteroids and by skeletal growth and maturation. Those children

born with abnormalities of external genitalia may require surgical correction of labial fusion, urogenital sinus, etc. Response of these children to steroid therapy is gratifying in that normal growth and development occur and the menarche and onset of spermatogenesis occur at the appropriate age. Many females with this disorder have married and borne children. Steroid therapy is indicated throughout the lifespan of these patients.

Some infants and children with the associated defect of salt-wasting require vigorous correction of salt deficits in conjunction with small doses of a potent mineralocorticoid such as 9α-fluorohydrocortisone.

In patients with adrenal virilization due to adrenal tumors, prompt surgical intervention with complete excision of the tumor is, of course, indicated. One cannot postpone surgical intervention in patients suspected of having virilizing adrenal adenomas since such adenomas are practically indistinguishable from adrenal carcinomas both clinically and biochemically. Preoperative localization of adrenal tumors is attempted with renal tomography and in some cases perirenal insufflation studies. Since "pure" virilizing adrenal tumors do *not* cause contralateral adrenal atrophy, thorough inspection and exploration of both suprarenal areas is mandatory. If metastases have occurred, one may consider the use of antitumor drugs such as *o,p′*-DDD with or without local irradiation. *o,p′*-DDD in some patients has been associated with striking regression in peripheral metastases paralleled by a decrease in urine 17-ketosteroid and 17-hydroxycorticoid excretion; however, long-term survival is rare. In some patients given a trial of *o,p′*-DDD, regression of metastases is not seen but a fall in urine 17-hydroxycorticoids occurs. The explanation resides in the fact that *o,p′*-DDD can alter the extra-adrenal metabolism of cortisol so as to decrease the metabolism and excretion of the usual metabolite, tetrahydrocortisol, causing the decrease in Porter-Silber chromogens; yet at the same time, there is increased conversion to and excretion of 6β-hydroxycortisol, a steroid not included routinely as a Porter-Silber chromogen because of its poor solubility in the preliminary extracting solvent (dichloromethane).

Adrenal Feminization

Adrenal feminization is an exceedingly rare entity and, when present, is almost always due to adrenal tumor. These adrenal tumors will cause feminization in the male with development of gynecomastia (often with breast tenderness), change in body habitus, testicular atrophy, feminizing hair changes, and loss of libido. They may occur in "pure" form, that is, with normal levels of urine 17-ketosteroids, or in "mixed" form, with feminization despite high 17-ketosteroid excretion. They are always associated in the male with increased excretion of estrogen metabolites, such as estrone and estradiol. These adrenal tumors secrete increased amounts of androstenedione, which undergoes conversion, either in the adrenal or peripherally in the liver, into the estrogens, estrone and estradiol. Some patients have had elevated urine values for pregnanetriol, suggesting that 11-β-hydroxylation may be impaired.

The majority of adrenal tumors causing feminization are carcinomas. They are most common in the age group twenty-five to forty-five. These tumors are almost always unilateral and occur with equal frequency on either side. In rare instances they have occurred in an extraadrenal locus such as the testis. The feminizing adrenal carcinomas are large tumors (several hundred grams) and often are easily palpable on physical examination, whereas feminizing adrenal adenomas are characteristically small tumors. Metastases occur most often to the liver and lungs. Feminizing adrenal tumors do not cause contralateral adrenal atrophy, which makes bilateral exploration mandatory if the initial adrenal explored is normal. Almost all cases of feminizing adrenal carcinoma are evident on suprarenal tomography studies. Patients with feminizing adrenal tumors usually have normal to moderately elevated 17-ketosteroid excretion levels. If the urine 17-ketosteroid excretion is greater than 100 mg per day, the diagnosis of a feminizing adrenal carcinoma is almost certain. Urine 17-hydroxycorticoid excretion is usually within the normal range or slightly elevated. Associated Cushing's syndrome is rare. ACTH stimulation causes little change in 17-ketosteroid excretion. The chemical determination of urine estrogen titers always demonstrates an elevated value. The elevated urine estrogen excretion level is principally due to increased estratriol and also to increments in estradiol and estrone. Since the estrogens produced by adrenal feminizing tumors are conversion products from androgen precursors, the amount of estrogens elaborated will depend both on the amount of androgen precursors formed and on the efficiency of the androgen-to-estrogen conversion process.

Radiotherapy has not been helpful in treatment. Despite operative intervention, most patients with adrenal feminizing carcinoma die within 3 years of diagnosis. With successful operative removal of feminizing tumors the urine estrogen titer falls; a failure of the titer to fall or a recurrence of elevated urine titers indicates functioning tumor tissue.

The diagnosis of adrenal feminization in the male is strongly suggested by the onset of gynecomastia associated with a flank mass. The additional finding of increased urine estrogen titers confirms the diagnosis. Gynecomastia may also be seen with *testicular tumors* (chorioepithelioma, Sertoli cell, seminoma, interstitial cell tumor) because of increased production by the tumors of chorionic gonadotropin with an associated elaboration of estrogens by the testes. Adrenal feminization in the female is more difficult to detect, but it has been reported.

HYPOFUNCTION OF ADRENAL CORTEX

Adrenal cortical hypofunction includes all conditions in which the secretion of adrenal steroid hormones

Table 84-6. CLASSIFICATION OF CAUSES OF ADRENAL INSUFFICIENCY

I. Primary adrenal insufficiency
   A. Anatomic destruction of gland (chronic and acute)
      1. Infection
      2. Invasion: metastatic, fungal, etc.
      3. Hemorrhage
      4. "Idiopathic" atrophy
      5. Surgical removal
   B. Metabolic failure in hormone production
      1. Virilizing hyperplasia, congenital (certain types)
      2. Enzyme inhibitors
         a. Specific: metyrapone
         b. Nonspecific: amphenone
      3. Cytotoxic agents: *o,p*'DDD
II. Secondary adrenal insufficiency
   A. Hypopituitarism due to pituitary disease
   B. Suppression of hypothalamic-pituitary axis
      1. Exogenous steroid
      2. Endogenous steroid from tumors after tumor removal
      3. Pharmacologic agents

falls below the requirements of the body. Various types of adrenal insufficiency are encountered and may be divided into two general categories: (1) those associated with primary inability of the adrenal to elaborate sufficient quantities of hormone and (2) those associated with a secondary failure due to a primary failure in the elaboration of ACTH (Table 84-6).

Chronic Adrenal Cortical Deficiency (Addison's Disease, Chronic Glucocorticoid Deficiency)

Addison's classic description of primary adrenal insufficiency in 1855, namely, "general languor and debility, remarkable feebleness of the heart's action, irritability of the stomach, and a peculiar change of the color of the skin," summarizes the dominant clinical features of the disease. Advanced cases usually cause little difficulty in diagnosis, but recognition of the disease in its earlier phases may present a real challenge. The disease, when unrecognized and untreated, carries an almost uniformly poor and frequently fatal prognosis. Early diagnosis is important since present-day therapy may provide complete correction of the metabolic derangement.

INCIDENCE. Primary adrenocortical insufficiency is relatively rare. It may occur at any age in life and affects both sexes with equal frequency. Because of increasing therapeutic use of exogenous steroids, secondary adrenal insufficiency is seen with increasing frequency.

CLINICAL SIGNS AND SYMPTOMS. Adrenocortical insufficiency is most frequently characterized by an insidious onset with slowly progressive fatigability, weakness, anorexia, nausea and vomiting, weight loss, cutaneous and mucosal pigmentation, hypotension, and occasionally hypoglycemia. These signs and symptoms compose the classic syndrome of Addison's disease; however, the spectrum may vary, depending on the

Table 84-7. LABORATORY EVALUATION AND TESTING OF ADRENOCORTICAL FUNCTION IN ADRENAL INSUFFICIENCY*

	Plasma ACTH	Plasma cortisol	Cortisol secretory rate	Urine values	Control base line	Days of ACTH stimulation			
						1	2	3	4
Primary:									
Complete	I†	D‡	D	17-OH :	0–2	0–2	0–2	0–2	0–2
				17-KS :	3–6	3–6	3–6	3–6	3–6
Incomplete	I	D	D	17-OH :	1–4	5–10	6–12	5–10	5–10
				17-KS :	5–7	7–10	8–12	7–10	7–10
Secondary:									
Complete	D	D	D	17-OH :	0–2	2–6	5–10	7–14	10–20
				17-KS :	0–6	4–8	5–8	6–10	8–15
Incomplete	D	D	D	17-OH :	1–4	5–10	7–14	10–20	20–30
				17-KS :	5–7	5–8	6–10	8–15	15–20

* Clinical status charted vertically and representative values for steroid tests charted horizontally. 17-OH, 17-KS refer to 24-hr urine 17-hydroxycorticosteroid and 17-ketosteroid excretion. All lab values given in milligrams per day. Note that plasma ACTH values are increased in primary forms and decreased in secondary forms. Note also that differentiation between primary and secondary forms on ACTH stimulation testing becomes greatest on day 3 and day 4 of stimulation.

† I, increased.

‡ D, decreased.

duration and degree of adrenal hypofunction, from a complaint of mild chronic fatigue to the fulminating shock associated with acute massive destruction of the glands in the type of syndrome described by Waterhouse and Friderichsen. Table 84-8 lists the incidence of symptoms and signs noted in cases of Addison's disease.

Asthenia is the cardinal symptom of Addison's disease. Early it may be sporadic, usually most evident at times of stress; as adrenal function becomes more impaired, the weakness progresses until the patient is continuously fatigued, necessitating bedrest. Even the voice may fail, so that speech finally becomes listless and indistinct.

Pigmentation is the most striking sign of the disease. It commonly appears as a diffuse brown, tan, or bronze darkening of both exposed and unexposed points such as elbows or creases of the hand and in areas normally pigmented such as the areolas about the nipples. In many patients, bluish-black patches appear on the mucous membranes. Some patients develop dark freckles, and occasionally irregular areas of vitiligo may appear paradoxically. As an early sign, patients may notice an unusually persistent tanning following exposure to the sun.

Arterial hypotension is also extremely frequent, and in severe cases blood pressures may be in the range of 80/50 or less. Postural accentuation is common, and syncope may occur.

Abnormalities of gastrointestinal function are not only extremely frequent but often are the presenting complaint. Symptoms may vary from mild anorexia with weight loss to fulminating nausea, vomiting, diarrhea, and various types of ill-defined abdominal pain, which at times may be so severe as to be confused with an acute surgical abdomen. Rarely a Landry's type of ascending paralysis with flaccid

quadriplegia and mixed sensory defects accompanied by ascending muscular weakness has been noted in conjunction with a high serum potassium level. In these instances, the electrocardiogram may reflect the hyperkalemia. In addition, patients with adrenal insufficiency frequently have marked personality changes, usually in the form of excessive irritability and restlessness.

LABORATORY FINDINGS. In the milder forms, sometimes called *partial* or *incomplete* Addison's disease, there may be no demonstrable abnormalities in any of the parameters measured in the routine laboratory, and even plasma and urinary steroid determinations may indicate values relatively low yet within normal range. However, definitive studies of adrenal stimulation with ACTH show abnormalities even in this stage of the disease. In the more advanced stages, levels of serum sodium, chloride, and bicarbonate are reduced while serum potassium is elevated. The hyponatremia is due to extravascular loss of sodium both into the urine (due to aldosterone deficiency) and from the vascular compartment into tendon, cartilage, and bone. This extravascular sodium loss depletes extracellular fluid volume and accentuates hypotension. The hyperkalemia is due to a combination of factors including aldosterone deficiency, impaired glomerular filtration rate, and acidosis. These patients may show marked reduction in heart size, and in about one-quarter of the patients suprarenal calcification is seen but is unfortunately not pathognomonic. The electrocardiogram may show nonspecific changes and the electroencephalogram a striking reduction and slowing of the predominant activity. The basal metabolic rate may be low, but other thyroid indices are usually normal. There may be a normocytic anemia, a relative lymphocytosis, and usually a moderate eosinophilia.

DIAGNOSIS. The diagnosis of adrenal insufficiency

requires demonstration either directly or indirectly of decreased cortisol production by the adrenal in the basal state (*complete* adrenal insufficiency) or the unmasking of decreased cortisol production only in the stimulated state (*incomplete* adrenal insufficiency) (Table 84-7).

In all cases of *complete* adrenal insufficiency the cortisol secretory rate is markedly decreased, and this may be ascertained indirectly by the finding of low to absent 24-hr urine 17-hydroxycorticoids and urine 17-ketosteroids. Because of the contribution of the male gonads to urine 17-ketosteroids, basal excretory values in complete adrenal insufficiency will be higher for males than females. With incomplete adrenal insufficiency, urine steroid excretion values overlap into the normal range; because of this, a diagnosis of adrenal insufficiency cannot be made solely on the values of basal urine steroid determinations. Plasma 17-hydroxycorticoid and free cortisol determination values are from zero to the lower range of normal. Aldosterone secretion is very low judged by isotopic secretory rate determinations, as are aldosterone excretory values. In patients with primary adrenal insufficiency plasma ACTH levels are elevated due to loss of the usual cortisol-hypothalamic feedback relationship, whereas in secondary adrenal insufficiency plasma ACTH values are low, a finding consistent with the absence of increased pigmentation in this latter group of patients.

The specific and definitive diagnosis of adrenal insufficiency can only be made with the ACTH stimulation test to assay the adrenal reserve capacity for steroid production. In addition, ACTH testing is helpful in establishing whether adrenal insufficiency is primary or secondary. In patients undergoing ACTH testing as a diagnostic method for adrenal insufficiency, saline should be utilized as the diluent for the ACTH to be infused, since on occasion patients may experience an acute febrile episode when glucose is used. An additional advantage of using saline diluent is that a clinical estimate of adrenal responsiveness may be made by the presence or absence of weight gain during the infusion period, weight gain commonly occurring when adrenal cortical function is intact. The potential dangers of ACTH testing in patients with limited adrenal reserves may be minimized by the prior administration of 1 mg of a potent steroid such as dexamethasone. The excretory products of 1 mg of this compound will not add appreciably to the amount of 17-hydroxycorticoids measured in the urine and therefore will not interfere with the test. For testing purposes, 50 units of ACTH is infused in the standard manner for 4 to 5 successive days with daily urine collections tested for creatinine, 17-hydroxycorticoid, and 17-ketosteroid levels. In patients with complete primary adrenal insufficiency ACTH stimulation will cause either no rise in steroid excretion or at most a rise in urine 17-hydroxycorticoids of less than 2 mg per day. A practical clinical aid is to determine the eosinophil count in these patients immediately before and after the ACTH infusion. Normal subjects with a base-line eosinophil count greater than 100 cells per cu mm will show a decrease of nearly 80 per cent in circulating eosinophils at the completion of the ACTH infusion, whereas patients with adrenal insufficiency will show a decrease of less than 25 per cent of their base-line values. The eosinophil count cannot be so utilized in patients receiving steroid therapy, such as dexamethasone, during ACTH testing or in patients with known parasitic eosinophilia.

In *incomplete* adrenal insufficiency, ACTH testing carried out on 4 to 5 successive days will result in subnormal increments in urine 17-hydroxysteroids, a response that demonstrates limited adrenal sensitivity to ACTH but characterized by a quantitative deficit in steroid excretion. A variant of this response is sometimes seen in which small increments in steroid excretion occur on the first 1 to 3 days of ACTH testing; then on the fourth and fifth days of testing the urine steroid levels actually decline, suggesting that the limited adrenal tissue had been maximally stimulated and had insufficient steroid reserve capacity. In patients with adrenal insufficiency secondary to *anterior pituitary hypofunction*, a "staircase" response in steroid excretion is seen on successive days of ACTH stimulation, signifying that the adrenals can respond to exogenous ACTH and that the deficit must reside in the failure to produce and/or release endogenous ACTH.

Patients on long-term steroid therapy, despite physical findings of Cushing's syndrome, develop adrenal insufficiency due both to prolonged suppression of the hypothalamic corticotropin-releasing center and to actual adrenal atrophy. Adrenal atrophy results from the loss of endogenous ACTH stimulation, which stimulus is prerequisite for maintaining normal adrenal size. Thus, it can be seen that these patients acquire two deficits, a loss of adrenal responsiveness to ACTH and a failure of pituitary ACTH release. These patients are characterized by low blood cortisol and ACTH levels, low base-line steroid excretion, and abnormal ACTH and metyrapone test results. On testing these patients with ACTH, one looks for the "staircase" response, with successive daily increments in steroid excretion; however, *prolonged ACTH testing* may be needed to elicit such a response. The urine steroid pattern, when adrenal reactivation does occur, often reveals increments in 17-hydroxycorticoids without parallel increments in 17-ketosteroids. Practically all patients with steroid-induced adrenal insufficiency will eventually respond to ACTH testing, but individual response time is most variable, ranging from days to months. Once such patients are shown to have reacquired adrenal sensitivity to exogenous ACTH, their ability to release endogenous pituitary ACTH must be determined. The standard metyrapone test is utilized for this purpose. For a valid metyrapone test, it must be previously documented that the patient's adrenal glands are sensitive to ACTH, since the metyrapone test response depends on adrenal responsiveness to

Table 84-8. INCIDENCE OF SYMPTOMS AND SIGNS IN 125 CASES OF ADDISON'S DISEASE, PER CENT

Weakness	99	Hypotension (below	
Pigmentation of skin	98	110/70)	87
Pigmentation of mucous		Abdominal pain	34
membranes	82	Salt craving	22
Weight loss	97	Diarrhea	20
Anorexia, nausea, and		Constipation	19
vomiting	90	Syncope	16
		Vitiligo	9

released ACTH. For this reason the test is *contraindicated* in patients with suspected or proved adrenal insufficiency. In patients with steroid-induced adrenal insufficiency, abnormal (low) metyrapone tests usually continue for several months after the adrenal glands have regained responsiveness to ACTH. In interpreting the metyrapone test it is useful to consider it as an endogenous ACTH stimulation test and compare the peak urine 17-hydroxycorticoid excretion with the maximal values previously obtained with exogenous ACTH stimulation.

Plasma ACTH levels help distinguish between primary and secondary adrenal insufficiency, since they are elevated in the former and decreased to absent in the latter.

Indirect tests of adrenal cortical function include (1) a delay in water excretion following an acute water load; (2) defective renal conservation of sodium when a low-sodium, high-potassium diet is imposed; (3) a tendency toward hypoglycemia during fasting and hypoglycemic unresponsiveness following the intravenous administration of insulin. Since ACTH is available for direct evaluation of adrenal cortical function, these procedures are *rarely* indicated; furthermore, in a patient with adrenal cortical insufficiency, water intoxication, sodium deprivation, or hypoglycemia may all be life-threatening situations.

DIFFERENTIAL DIAGNOSIS. Since weakness and fatigue are such common complaints, clinical diagnosis of early adrenal cortical insufficiency is frequently difficult (Table 84-8). However, mild gastrointestinal distress with weight loss, anorexia, and a suggestion of increased pigmentation make mandatory ACTH stimulation testing to rule out adrenal insufficiency, particularly before steroid treatment is begun. Weight loss is useful in evaluating the significance of weakness and malaise. Racial pigmentation in Negroes, Orientals, Indians, Spanish Americans, and Latins and in other diseases involving hyperpigmentation represent a major problem. These diseases include hemochromatosis, acanthosis nigricans, porphyria, thyrotoxicosis, polyostotic fibrous dysplasia, chronic metal poisoning (bismuth, lead, arsenic, silver), chronic malnutrition (starvation, anorexia nervosa, sprue syndrome, pellagra), progressive malignancy, chronic anemia, salt-losing nephritis with hypotension, renal tubular acidosis, scleroderma, excess nicotinic acid, and hepatic cirrhosis. In most cases, differentiation from Addison's

disease is not difficult, but when doubt exists, ACTH administration ordinarily provides clear-cut differentiation.

ETIOLOGY AND PATHOGENESIS. Addison's disease results from progressive adrenal cortical destruction, which must involve more than 75 per cent of the glands before clinical signs of adrenal insufficiency appear. The adrenal is a frequent site for chronic infectious diseases of the granulomatous variety, predominately tuberculosis but also including fungal infections such as histoplasmosis, coccidioidomycosis, and cryptococcosis. In previous years, tuberculosis was found at post mortem in 70 to 90 per cent of cases; however, the most frequent finding at present is *idiopathic* atrophy, and it has been suggested that an autoimmune mechanism may be responsible for this process. Rarely other lesions are encountered, such as bilateral tumor metastases, amyloidosis, or sarcoidosis.

The possibility that some patients may have primary adrenal insufficiency on an *autoimmune basis* has been strengthened by the finding that one-half of patients with Addison's disease have circulating adrenal antibodies, tested by the indirect Coons method. These antibodies appear species-specific but lack organ specificity. Certain of these patients also have additional circulating antibodies to thyroid or parathyroid tissue, a finding of interest because of the increased incidence of hypothyroidism and hypoparathyroidism in Addison's disease.

SCHMIDT'S SYNDROME. In 1926 Schmidt described two patients with nontuberculous Addison's disease and chronic lymphocytic thyroiditis. Subsequent reports have documented the association of thyroid insufficiency and Addison's disease and have in addition included studies of a number of patients with associated diabetes mellitus.

It is possible that further studies of patients with Schmidt's syndrome may prove valuable in unravelling the cause of spontaneous adrenal destruction.

TREATMENT. All patients with Addison's disease should receive specific hormone replacement therapy. Similar to the treatment of patients with diabetes, proper care also requires careful and persistent education in regard to the disease. Since the adrenal elaborates three general classes of hormone, of which two, glucocorticoids and mineralocorticoids, are of primary clinical importance, replacement therapy should correct both deficiencies. Cortisone (or hydrocortisone) is the mainstay of treatment; however, its mineralocorticoid effect, when it is given in sufficient dosage to replace the endogenous hydrocortisone deficiency, is inadequate for complete electrolyte balance; therefore, the patient usually requires other supplementary hormone. Cortisone dosage varies from 12.5 to 50 mg daily, with the majority of patients taking 25 to 37.5 mg in divided doses. Because of its direct local effect on gastric mucosa, patients are advised to take their cortisone with meals or, if this is impractical, with milk or an antacid preparation. In addition, the larger proportion of the dose (25 mg) is taken in the morning and the remainder (12.5 mg) in the late afternoon, to simulate somewhat the normal diurnal adrenal rhythm. Some patients may exhibit insomnia, irritability, mental excitement, and even frank psychosis soon after initiation of therapy; in these the dosage should obviously be reduced. Other indications for maintaining the patient on smaller amounts are the presence of hypertension, diabetes, or active tuberculosis.

Since, as mentioned earlier, this amount of cortisone or hydrocortisone fails to replace the mineralocorticoid component of the adrenal gland, supplementary hormone is usually needed. The simplest means is daily oral administration of 0.1 to 0.2 mg of 9α-fluorohydrocortisone. If parenteral administration is indicated, 2.0 to 5.0 mg of deoxycorticosterone acetate in oil can be given every day intramuscularly. An alternative method of therapy is an injection of 25 to 50 mg of deoxycorticosterone trimethylacetate in oil intramuscularly every 3 to 4 weeks, but as with the previous use of subcutaneous implantation of pellets of deoxycorticosterone which lasted for 8 to 10 months, most patients prefer the simplicity of daily oral administration of the 9α-fluorohydrocortisone.

Complications of cortisone therapy, with the exception of peptic disease, particularly ulcer or gastritis, are *extremely rare* in the dosage used in the treatment of Addison's disease. However, overtreatment with deoxycorticosterone preparations or 9α-fluorohydrocortisone is more frequent and may present as edema, hypertension, cardiac enlargement, or even congestive failure due to sodium retention. Overtreatment may also present as weakness, progressing to total paralysis, due to hypokalemia. In the management of patients with Addison's disease, regular measurements of body weight, serum potassium, heart size, blood pressure, and serial electrocardiograms are useful.

All patients with adrenal insufficiency, including bilaterally adrenalectomized patients should carry medical identification, should be educated and instructed in the parenteral self-administration of steroids, and should be registered with a national medical alerting system.

SPECIAL THERAPEUTIC PROBLEMS. During periods of intercurrent illness, the dose of cortisone or hydrocortisone should be increased to levels of 75 to 150 mg per day. When oral administration is not possible, parenteral routes should be employed. Likewise, before surgery or dental extractions, excess steroid should be administered. For a representative program of steroid therapy for an Addisonian patient or an adrenalectomized patient undergoing a major operation, see Table 84-9. The patients should all be advised of these facts and should carry an identification card bearing detailed instructions for the administration of steroid in case of acute illness or injury. Patients should also be advised to increase the dose of 9α-fluorohydrocortisone and add excess salt to their otherwise normal diet during periods of excessive exercise with sweating during extremely hot weather or during periods of gastrointestinal upsets. In spite of animal studies demonstrating an increased susceptibility to tubercular spread associated with excess steroid administration, patients with Addison's disease and tuberculosis may be maintained safely on 12.5 to 25 mg cortisone daily.

COURSE AND PROGNOSIS. Untreated Addison's disease characteristically runs a chronic and relentless course. In some patients, its advance is relatively slow, but in all patients the disease may rapidly deteriorate into adrenal crisis. With treatment, the prognosis of the disease is extremely favorable. In

Table 84-9. STEROID THERAPY SCHEDULE FOR ADDISONIAN PATIENT UNDERGOING A MAJOR OPERATION*

	Cortisone acetate (intramuscularly)		Cortisone acetate (orally)				Fluorohydro-cortisone (orally)	Hydro-cortisone infusion
	7 A.M.	7 P.M.	8 A.M.	12 M.	4 P.M.	8 P.M.	8 A.M.	Continuous
Routine daily medication....			25		12.5		0.1	
Day before operation........		50	25		12.5		0.1	
Day of operation...........	100	50						200
Postoperative day 1.........	50	50						100–150
" 2.........	50	50						50–100
" 3.........	50	50	25			25		
" 4.........	50		25	25	25		0.1	
" 5.........			25	25	25	25	0.1	
" 6.........			25	25	25		0.2	
" 7.........			25	12.5	25		0.2	
" 8.........			25	12.5	25		0.2	
" 9–13......			25	12.5	12.5		0.1	
" 14........			25	12.5			0.1	

* All steroid doses are given in milligrams.

fact, some of the degenerative vascular problems such as hypertension or congestive failure are more easily handled in an Addisonian patient compared to one with intact adrenals.

Acute Adrenocortical Insufficiency

Acute adrenocortical insufficiency may result from several processes. One of these, usually termed *adrenal crisis*, is a rapid and overwhelming intensification of chronic adrenal insufficiency. Another process involves an acute hemorrhagic destruction of both adrenal glands, usually associated with an overwhelming septicemia. A third, and probably the most frequent, cause of acute insufficiency results from the rapid withdrawal of steroids from patients with adrenal atrophy secondary to chronic steroid administration.

ADRENAL CRISIS

The long-term survival of patients with Addison's disease largely depends upon prevention and treatment of adrenal crisis. Consequently, the occurrence of infection, trauma (including surgery), gastrointestinal upsets, or other forms of stress requires an immediate increase in hormone. In previously untreated patients, preexisting symptoms are intensified. Nausea, vomiting, and abdominal pain may become intractable. Fever is frequently severe but may be absent. Lethargy deepens into somnolence, and the blood pressure and pulse fail as hypovolemic vascular shock ensues. In contrast, patients previously maintained on hormone therapy may not exhibit severe dehydration or hypotension until preterminally, at which time there is an extremely rapid decline.

Treatment is primarily directed toward the rapid elevation of circulating adrenal cortical hormone in addition to the replacement of the sodium and water deficit. Hence, an intravenous infusion of 1,000 ml 5 per cent glucose in normal saline containing 100 to 200 mg of any of several soluble hydrocortisone preparations is begun rapidly, with the first 250 ml infused in the first ½ to 1 hr and the remainder over the ensuing 4 to 8 hr. If the condition is extreme, immediate intravenous infusion of 100 mg hydrocortisone in the first few minutes is suggested, followed by a rapid infusion as described above. Epinephrine, 0.2 mg intravenously, may also be indicated. In any case, it is also advisable to administer 100 mg cortisone acetate intramuscularly in case the infusion becomes infiltrated or inadvertently stopped. If the crisis was preceded by prolonged nausea, vomiting, and dehydration, several liters of saline replacement is indicated. With large doses of steroid, as, for example, 200 mg cortisone or hydrocortisone, the patient receives a maximal mineralocorticoid effect, and supplementary deoxycorticosterone is superfluous. After the initial infusion, depending on the patient's condition, a second similar infusion may be given; if there has been marked improvement, the patient may be offered oral fluids and be given 50 mg cortisone acetate intramuscularly every 12 hr until gastrointestinal absorption is guaranteed, at which time the steroid can be given orally. Steroid dosage is then tapered over the next few days to maintenance levels, with reinstitution of supplementary mineralocorticoid if needed.

ADRENAL HEMORRHAGE

Adrenal hemorrhage (adrenal apoplexy) is usually associated with overwhelming septicemia (Waterhouse-Friderichsen syndrome); however, it may also occur in the absence of sepsis. Occasionally, massive bilateral adrenal hemorrhage results from birth trauma. The infant may either be stillborn or die soon after birth of shock and hyperpyrexia. Adrenal hemorrhage also occurs in patients with advanced hypertension and arteriosclerosis, during pregnancy, following idiopathic adrenal vein thrombosis, during convulsions in epilepsy or during electroconvulsive therapy, with excessive anticoagulant therapy, and after trauma or surgery. Pain in the flank and epigastrium is frequent, and if the hemorrhagic process ruptures into the abdomen, signs of peritoneal inflammation are present.

The adrenal hemorrhage associated with septicemia is most frequent with meningococcemia but is also seen with overwhelming infections due to pneumococcus, staphylococcus, or *Hemophilus influenzae*. The onset is often explosive, with a shaking chill, violent headache, vertigo, vomiting, and prostration. A petechial rash appears on the skin and mucous membranes and progresses rapidly to a confluent, extensive purpura. Large areas of skin may become grossly hemorrhagic. Body temperature may be subnormal but is usually markedly elevated. Circulatory collapse rapidly ensues, and death may occur within 6 to 48 hr. Specific diagnosis requires immediate identification of the organism. Frequently, the septicemia is so massive that organisms may be seen in peripheral blood smears or petechial scrapings. Time is not sufficient for determination of adrenal function; however, a plasma sample for later determination of 17-hydroxysteroid level may be of academic interest.

Treatment must be immediate and intensive. Control of the infection by vigorous administration of parenteral, preferably intravenous, antibiotics is indicated in addition to the steroid schedule delineated for adrenal crisis. Intravenous norepinephrine (4 to 8 mg per liter) may also be required to maintain vascular tone. Since shock may also be associated with massive septicemia without adrenal hemorrhage, one is never completely certain whether adrenal insufficiency is contributing to the patient's decompensation; however, the authors think that because of the increasing frequency of survival of patients treated with steroid, some degree of adrenal insufficiency, whether relative or absolute, is present and that steroid treatment is therefore indicated in all patients in whom there is fulminating septicemia associated with shock.

ADRENAL INSUFFICIENCY DUE TO METABOLIC FAILURE IN HORMONE PRODUCTION

This group of patients includes those with congenital adrenal hyperplasia and those receiving one of several pharmacologic agents which are capable of inhibiting hormone synthesis in the gland. These include Amphenone, which appears to inhibit synthesis of all hormones early in the sequence of reactions from cholesterol and concomitantly results in hypertrophy of the gland; various derivatives of diphenyl dichloroethane, of which the *o,p*-dichloro-derivative is the most active [*o,p'*-DDD (Perthane)] and causes atrophy and even necrosis of adrenal cortical tissue; and lastly, 2-methyl-1,2-bis-(3-pyridyl)-1-propanone (metyrapone, SU4885), a compound similar to the other two but more specific in that it selectively inhibits hydroxylation of the steroid nucleus at the 11-position. Amphenone and *o,p'*-DDD have been used to treat adrenocortical carcinoma.

Hypoaldosteronism

Patients with *isolated* aldosterone deficiency are rare. Such a deficiency accompanied by normal cortisol production has been reported as a congenital bio-synthetic defect; postoperatively following removal of aldosteronoma; during protracted heparin or heparinoid administration; in pretectal disease of the nervous system; in severe postural hypotension; and in association with complete heart block.

In severe cases urine sodium wastage is present on a normal salt intake, whereas in milder forms excessive urine sodium losses occur only during salt restriction. The patients always develop hyponatremia and hyperkalemia, the latter often to a severe degree.

A biosynthetic defect has been noted in some patients who are unable to transform the angular C-18 methyl group of corticosterone to the C-18 aldehyde grouping of aldosterone. This C-18 transformation requires first the formation of 18-hydroxycorticosterone from corticosterone, and then, secondly, dehydrogenation of the C-18 hydroxyl group to form the characteristic C-18 aldehyde group of aldosterone. These patients will manifest low to absent aldosterone secretion and excretion in association with elevated secretion and excretion values for corticosterone and 18-hydroxycorticosterone.

The feature common to all patients with hypoaldosteronism has been their inability to *increase* aldosterone secretion appropriately during severe salt restriction. An additional feature has been the reversal of the signs of salt wasting, hyponatremia and hyperkalemia, with the administration of potent mineralocorticoids. For practical purposes the oral adminis-

Table 84-10. ADRENAL PREPARATIONS

Commonly used name	Other names	Estimated potencies*	
		Glucocorticoid	Mineralocorticoid
Hydrocortisone	Cortisol, hydrocortone Compound F, 17-hydroxycorticosterone PREGN-4-ene-11β,17α,21-triol-3,20-dione	1	1
Cortisone	Cortone, compound E 11-dehydro-17-hydroxycorticosterone PREGN-4-ene-17α,21-diol-3,11,20-trione	0.8	0.8
DOC	Percorten, cortexone, 11-deoxycorticosterone PREGN-4-ene-21-ol-3,20-dione	0	15
Aldosterone	Electrocortin PREGN-4-ene-11β,21-diol-18-al-3,20-dione	0.3	400
Prednisolone	Meticortelone, Δ1-hydrocortisone PREGN-1,4-diene-11β,17α,21-triol-3,20-dione	4	0.25
Prednisone	Meticorten, Δ1-cortisone PREGN-1,4-diene-17α,21-diol-3,11,20-trione	4	0.25
Methyl prednisolone	Medrol, 6-methyl-Δ1-hydrocortisone	8–10	±
Triamcinolone	Aristocort, Kenacort 16α-hydroxy-9α-fluoro-Δ¹-hydrocortisone	5	±
Dexamethasone	Decadron, Hexadrol 16α-methyl-9α-fluoro-Δ¹-hydrocortisone	40	±
Fluorohydrocortisone	Florinef, Fluoro-F 9α-fluorohydrocortisone	10	300

* Relative milligram comparisons to cortisol, setting the glucocorticoid and mineralocorticoid properties of cortisol as 1. Sodium retention insignificant in usual doses employed of methyl prednisolone, triamcinolone, and dexamethasone.

tration of 9α-fluorohydrocortisone in a dose of 0.1 to 0.3 mg daily restores electrolyte balance.

NONSPECIFIC USE OF ACTH AND ADRENAL STEROIDS IN CLINICAL PRACTICE

The widespread application of ACTH and adrenal steroid therapy in many branches of medicine and surgery emphasizes the need for a thorough understanding of the metabolic effects of these agents if clinical use is to be most effective and if undesirable side reactions are to be minimized. Before instituting adrenal hormone therapy, a physician should weigh carefully the gains that can reasonably be expected versus the potentially undesirable metabolic actions of the particular hormone. Accurate appraisal will require familiarity with the reports of others in similar instances, a critical evaluation of the statistical significance of such reports, as well as a clear understanding of the chemical, physiologic, and psychologic changes that hormone preparations of this type are known to induce (Table 84-10).

Perhaps an approach to the problem presented by a particular patient may be facilitated by reviewing the specific considerations outlined in Table 84-11.

HOW SERIOUS IS THE UNDERLYING DISORDER? The use of any nonspecific or "symptomatic" pharmacologic agent must be weighed against the seriousness of the underlying disorder. Each pharmacologic agent has a "price tag," which must be evaluated carefully before a therapeutic program is begun. With the antibiotic agents this price tag may consist of the possibility of inducing drug-sensitivity reactions or the development of antibiotic-resistant strains of pathogenic organims; with the agents employed for hyper-

Table 84-11. CONSIDERATIONS PRIOR TO THE USE OF CORTICOSTEROIDS AS PHARMACOLOGIC AGENTS

1. How serious is the underlying disorder?
2. How long will therapy be required?
3. What is the anticipated effective dose range?
   a. To ameliorate symptoms?
   b. To suppress effectively the signs and symptoms of the disorder?
4. Is the patient predisposed to any of the known hazards of steroid therapy by virtue of having:
   a. Hypertension or cardiovascular disease?
   b. Peptic ulcer, gastritis, or esophagitis?
   c. Osteoporosis?
   d. Diabetes mellitus?
   e. Tuberculosis or other infections?
   f. Psychologic difficulties?
5. Which adrenal preparation is preferable?
   a. Choice of steroid preparation?
   b. ACTH versus steroids?
   c. Steroids by mouth versus steroids by injection?
6. Alternate day therapy.
7. Supplementary adjuvants employed to minimize metabolic disabilities.
8. A schedule for withdrawing corticosteroids.

tensive cardiovascular disease the price tag may consist of disturbing side effects referable to the autonomic nervous system. With the corticosteroids, effective therapy may be purchased at the risk of inducing undesirable side reactions such as peptic ulceration, osteoporosis, or psychologic abnormalities. Clearly, in a patient whose life is threatened by unexplained shock or in whom other measures have failed to modify the course of disseminated lupus erythematosus, the physician need not hesitate to employ massive steroid therapy. On the other hand, one should exercise restraint in administering suppressive steroid therapy to a patient with early rheumatoid arthritis who as yet has not received the possible benefits of physiotherapy and a well-organized program of general medical care.

HOW LONG WILL THERAPY BE REQUIRED? The problems which arise in connection with evaluating the seriousness of the underlying disorder naturally involve the expected or anticipated duration of therapy. Thus the use of intravenous hydrocortisone for 24 to 48 hr in the treatment of severe status asthmaticus or acute serum sickness or a drug reaction does not present the same problem as the treatment of chronic, lifelong asthma or psoriasis. In general, contraindications to steroids for severe, short-lived disorders will be few, whereas in suppressive therapy for chronic, persistent disorders one must envisage the serious problem presented by Cushing's syndrome, which results from prolonged ingestion of exogenous glucocorticoid.

WHAT IS THE ANTICIPATED EFFECTIVE DOSE RANGE? Hormone therapy may be employed in a relatively low dosage schedule calculated to achieve clinical improvement but not necessarily complete suppression of all signs and symptoms of the disorder. In the former case, 50 to 75 mg cortisone or hydrocortisone (or the equivalent amount of one of its derivatives) may be adequate to attain worthwhile clinical improvement, whereas 150 to 300 mg cortisone or hydrocortisone may be needed to suppress all evidences of activity of the disease. At the 50- to 75-mg dosage of cortisone or hydrocortisone, it might be feasible to embark on long-term therapy with minimal risk of serious complications resembling Cushing's syndrome, whereas at the 150-mg dosage level, relief of one disease may be attained only at the risk of inducing another (Cushing's syndrome). In general, doses of hydrocortisone or cortisone of 75 mg or less may be tolerated by most patients for prolonged periods of time with a minimum of underlying metabolic disabilities, whereas doses of cortisone or hydrocortisone of 100 mg or more will usually be associated with progressive metabolic aberrations. Dosage of cortisone or hydrocortisone in the range of 25 to 50 mg daily can, in all probability, be tolerated by most patients for life.

IS THE PATIENT PREDISPOSED TO ANY OF THE KNOWN HAZARDS OF STEROID THERAPY BY VIRTUE OF HAVING ANY OF THE FOLLOWING CONDITIONS? Hypertension or Cardiovascular Disease. In general, the sodium-retaining propensity of most adrenal steroid preparations requires that caution be used when they are given to patients with preexisting hypertension or cardiovascular or renal disease. The availability of preparations in which sodium-retaining activity is minimal (triamcinolone and dexamethasone), restriction of dietary sodium intake, and the use of resins, diuretic agents, and particularly supplementary potassium salts will permit the safe use of steroid therapy where important indications exist. Of course, in congestive failure or pericardial effusion associated with acute rheumatic activity or in patients with nephrotic edema, steroid hormone preparations may act as effective diuretic agents.

For all patients in whom prolonged steroid therapy is contemplated cardiovascular-renal status should be carefully evaluated, with a chest film for *heart size* and an electrocardiogram included.

Peptic Ulcer, Gastric, or Esophagitis. Patients with a history of gastric hypersecretion or peptic ulcer are likely to experience aggravation of their symptoms while receiving adrenal hormone therapy. It is not known for certain whether aggravation of peptic ulceration and complicating gastrointestinal hemorrhage reflect the increased gastric secretory activity so frequently associated with adrenal hormone therapy or whether the nitrogen-depleting effect of these hormones accelerates the process of ulceration and perforation. Antacid therapy and an ulcer diet are useful precautions in susceptible patients. *The development of anemia in a patient on ACTH or cortisone therapy should immediately suggest gastrointestinal bleeding,* and patients should be cautioned to note black or tarry stools. A clear-cut history of peptic ulcer is a contraindication to ACTH and cortisone therapy unless extreme precautions are taken.

Osteoporosis. All patients on prolonged cortisone-like steroid therapy are likely to develop some degree of osteoporosis. Obviously a considerable change in bone structure must occur before it is radiologically demonstrable. For this reason patients should have standard films of the spine and pelvis in order to establish the status of the bony framework before therapy and for comparative purposes later. Postmenopausal women and men and women of advanced age will be predisposed to the earlier development of serious changes of this type. The skin also participates in the depletion of body protein, becoming thin and atrophic and easily bruisable. It is possible that ACTH may cause less osteoporosis for a given level of steroid therapy because of a concomitant increase in adrenal androgen secretion. This possible advantage of ACTH over crystalline steroids is offset by the difficulty with which an exact pharmacologic dosage of endogenous steroid is maintained with the tropic hormone. Since corticosteroids, in general, exert an anti-vitamin-D-like action, all patients on adrenal steroids should receive a generous supplement of vitamin D, i.e., 1,500 IU daily. Supplementary calcium therapy in the form of calcium lactate, 1 Gm three times daily,

and estrogen and androgen therapy should be considered in those patients known to be susceptible to the catabolic action of adrenal steroids. Of course, the presence of any degree of osteoporosis a priori would constitute strong evidence against the desirability of prolonged high-dosage adrenal hormone therapy.

Diabetes Mellitus. Prolonged ACTH or cortisone-like steroid therapy may unmask latent diabetes mellitus and aggravate preexisting disease. For this reason a careful history is important to exclude familial incidence of diabetes, as well as an examination of the blood and urine for excess glucose levels. It is more valuable to carry out these examinations following a test load of carbohydrate. A convenient method consists in measuring blood and urinary glucose 2 to 3 hr after the ingestion of a breakfast containing approximately 100 Gm carbohydrate (see Chap. 86). Obviously the presence of frank diabetes mellitus or the demonstration of impaired glucose tolerance will affect the physician's decision to institute adrenal hormone therapy. However, if such therapy appears necessary or desirable in the presence of latent diabetes, the judicious use of supplementary insulin should be seriously considered. The insulin requirement of known diabetics will usually need to be increased with ACTH or cortisone-like therapy except in those rare instances in which the diabetic patient is suffering from some degree of insulin-protein reaction in which the antiinflammatory or antiallergic effect of cortisone enhances the metabolic effectiveness of the insulin sufficiently to balance off the diabetogenic action of the former.

Tuberculosis or Other Infections. Before prolonged steroid therapy is seriously entertained, it is imperative to exclude the presence of tuberculosis and other infections. Continued steroid therapy, without a specific antibiotic agent, can lead to serious spread of infection. A chest film is essential before prolonged steroid therapy is begun, and the desirability of cultures from the nose and throat and of the urine and feces, if symptoms point to any disturbances, is evident.

Psychologic Difficulties. From time to time steroid therapy may be complicated by severe psychologic disturbances, and, of course, less severe abnormalities are relatively frequent. In general, serious psychologic disturbances are more closely related to the patient's personality structure than to the actual dose of hormone, although, as might be anticipated, larger doses of hormone will be associated with more frequent serious reactions. At present there is no reliable method of determining beforehand a patient's psychologic reaction to steroid therapy. Patients with known psychologic difficulties undoubtedly experience more frequent and more severe disturbances. Further difficulty arises because previous tolerance of steroids does not necessarily ensure immunity from subsequent courses of therapy, and untoward psychologic reactions on one occasion does not invariably mean that the patient will respond unfavorably to a second course of treatment.

This is one area in which the physician must follow his patient carefully during the early period of steroid therapy and one in which he must take a responsible member of the patients' family into his confidence.

The foregoing considerations constitute important data on which the physician's ultimate decision for or against hormone therapy will rest.

WHICH ADRENAL PREPARATION IS PREFERABLE? Choice of Steroid Preparation. For practical purposes there is no clearly demonstrable qualitative difference among cortisone, hydrocortisone, prednisone, triamcinolone, and dexamethasone; the latter three groups of substances, however, have much less sodium-retaining effect in relation to their anti-inflammatory activity (Table 84-10).

Although the cost of medication may be reduced by prescribing generic names rather than brand or trade names, physicians should be aware that the steroid market has attracted unscrupulous pharmaceutical companies and that flagrant instances of inferior products have been detected among low-cost or "bargain" types of steroid preparations.

ACTH versus Steroids? In most cases, the only decision of major consequence is the possible use of ACTH rather than one of the adrenal steroid preparations. In general, it can be stated that adrenal steroid therapy is effective by mouth and can be regulated more accurately than ACTH therapy. The latter will fluctuate considerably in the amount of steroid produced from day to day, depending on the rate and extent of absorption of ACTH and on the state of the adrenal cortex. ACTH therapy does stimulate the secretion of adrenal androgens as well as hydroxysteroids. The former may have advantages in certain diseases, such as dermatomyositis, in which the adrenal androgens may prove helpful in maintaining the muscle mass while the inflammatory reaction is being suppressed by the 17-hydroxycorticosteroids. Combined androgen and corticoid therapy may, of course, attain the same objective. Sodium retention with ACTH has often been more marked than with cortisone or, particularly, with prednisone therapy.

There is little support for the belief that ACTH stimulates the production of naturally useful steroids qualitatively different from those available commercially. The use of ACTH, of course, presupposes a normally responsive adrenal cortex, an assumption that cannot always be verified in serious or prolonged disorders. Both ACTH and steroid administration induce pituitary inhibition. In addition, steroid therapy also induces adrenal suppression. For practical purposes ACTH is used to initiate a therapeutic response and to activate the adrenal cortex before steroid therapy is discontinued. It has, of course, a very important use in the diagnostic approach to disorders of adrenal function.

Steroids by Mouth versus Steroids by Injection. In acute emergencies such as brain tumor, allergic reactions, and shock, steroids will be administered intra-venously in large doses, i.e., 300 to 500 mg hydrocortisone or 10 to 20 mg dexamethasone in 24 hr. For patients on long-term steroid therapy who develop gastrointestinal bleeding or symptoms of peptic ulcer, in addition to the usual medical measures, it may prove helpful to administer the daily steroid requirement *intramuscularly*. This reduces the concentration of steroid reaching the gastrointestinal tract, without impairing the systemic effect.

"ALTERNATE DAY" THERAPY. It has been shown that twice the daily maintenance dose, given every other day, may minimize pituitary and adrenal atrophy as well as reduce the degree of Cushingoid changes. Such a schedule is well worth considering for any patient destined to receive corticosteroids for prolonged periods.

SUPPLEMENTARY ADJUVANTS EMPLOYED TO MINIMIZE METABOLIC DISABILITIES. Since the continued use of ACTH or adrenal steroids induces a hypokalemic, hypochloremic metabolic alkalosis, supplementary potassium therapy should be given daily to patients receiving these hormone preparations. Potassium may be given as an elixir of potassium chloride, 2 to 3 tsp three times daily with meals (4 mEq potassium per tsp). Potassium chloride has a great theoretical and practical advantage over "mixed" potassium salts, particularly those containing potassium bicarbonate or citrate. Renal insufficiency is the primary complication in which supplementary potassium medication must be monitored carefully.

Antacid therapy and an ulcer-type diet *should be instituted* for all patients on steroid or ACTH therapy who give evidence of past or present increased gastric acidity, peptic ulceration, or upper gastrointestinal bleeding.

In patients who will require long-term ACTH or steroid therapy, the attending physician should make repeated efforts to ascertain whether the major manifestations of the underlying disorder cannot be held in satisfactory abeyance with a reduced hormone dosage. The ultimate development of Cushing's syndrome and its serious complications may prove more disastrous 3 to 5 years hence than the disease for which steroids were initially prescribed. Therefore *any* reduction in hormone dosage, however small, may be important in postponing the day of reckoning.

It is often possible to effect a considerable reduction in steroid maintenance dosage, if very small decrements are made, such as 5 per cent per month. *Percentage* reduction should always be employed, as a reduction of 5 mg prednisone per day from a level of 100 mg to 95 mg is quite different from a reduction from 30 to 25 mg. It is also important for both patient and physician to appreciate the fact that steroid therapy in general creates some degree of "euphoria" and hence a tendency to addiction. Thus a reduction in steroid dosage will initially be accompanied by a decrease in "energy" or sense of well-being. This may reduce the patient's threshold for tolerating the symptoms of his underlying disease without necessarily representing a true exacerbation. With a very small percentage decrease in dosage and with reassurance by the physician and understanding on the part of the patient, it is remarkable what can be accomplished in reducing the steroid level over a prolonged period. Patients are extremely grateful for any help that they can be given in this direction, when the long-range threat of steroid-induced complications is carefully explained.

When carrying out a slow, gradual reduction in steroid dosage, it must be realized that a sudden exacerbation of the underlying process may occur in conjunction with an acute infection or unusual stress. Under these circumstances the steroid dosage must be increased immediately, but it can usually be reduced promptly to the former dosage level once the precipitating factor is alleviated.

A PROPOSED SCHEDULE FOR ATTEMPTING WITHDRAWAL OF ACTH OR CORTICOSTEROIDS FOLLOWING THEIR LONG–TERM USE AS PHARMACOLOGIC AGENTS. Corticosteroid therapy induces both pituitary and adrenal suppression, whereas ACTH therapy affects only the former. For practical purposes it should be assumed that the majority of patients on prolonged steroid therapy will ultimately regain sufficient pituitary-adrenal activity to meet everyday needs. Regardless of how far in the past prolonged steroid therapy was given, in case of emergencies such as surgery, injuries, and severe infections, *supplementary cortisol or cortisone should always be employed.* It will also be apparent that regardless of the stepwise manner in which complete withdrawal of steroids is accomplished, there must always be a period of relative hypoadrenalism before endogenous ACTH-adrenal activity is restored. This is a point that must be seriously considered in patients with systemic lupus or widespread skin diseases, in which temporary hypoadrenalism may precipitate a serious or life-threatening exacerbation and hence is contraindicated. In such patients, Addisonian maintenance therapy for the long term may be indicated. For those patients, however, in whom it would appear advantageous to withdraw steroid therapy, the following schedule is suggested. *Steriod medication should not be withdrawn* until a patient's daily requirement is less than 50 mg hydrocortisone, 10 mg prednisone, or 1 to 1.5 mg dexamethasone.

The patient's steroid is changed to dexamethasone in a dosage equivalent to that of the steroid being employed, i.e., 1 mg dexamethasone for each 30 to 40 mg hydrocortisone; 1 mg dexamethasone for each 5 to 8 mg prednisone.

After 3 to 5 days on dexamethasone alone, baseline 24-hr urinary hydroxysteroid levels are determined (dexamethasone at this dosage level does not add appreciably to urinary steroid values).

While dexamethasone therapy is continued, ACTH is added in relatively large doses, i.e., 50 units intravenously over 8 hr daily for 3 to 5 successive days, or 80 units intramuscularly twice daily until urinary hydroxysteroids have attained a value at least three times the normal base line.

With evidence of adequate adrenal cortical response, the maintenance dose of dexamethasone should be appropriately reduced and discontinued.

During this entire period the patient remains vulnerable to undue stress and must be protected on such occasions by administration of ACTH or an appropriate dose of glucocorticoid.

When a patient, being maintained on dexamethasone and being given ACTH in the larger dose as outlined above, fails to display a brisk adrenal response, he must be returned to a maintenance dose of steroid. ACTH can then be given intramuscularly two to three times weekly in a dose of 80 units in addition to the maintenance dose of steroid, and at a later date (4 to 6 weeks) the original schedule may be tried again. Failure to observe a satisfactory adrenal response on the second occasion implies, for practical purposes, permanent primary adrenalcortical insufficiency, and the patient should be treated as an Addisonian.

SUMMARY. Several general facts should be considered in the management of patients receiving prolonged steroid therapy.

1. There is real danger of inducing acute adrenal failure if steroid therapy is suddenly withdrawn. Furthermore, inadequate adrenal reserve may be present for a *prolonged* period after steroid therapy ends. Under these circumstances, patients must be warned about the additional risk of acute stress reactions such as injuries, operations, and infections. Both the patient and his doctor should be aware of this problem, and supplementary corticoid therapy should be readily available at all times.

2. Patients being maintained on a constant dose of steroid over a prolonged period should be protected by an increase in hormone therapy during a period of surgery or endocrine stress. It may be necessary to increase the basic dose of glucocorticoid by the equivalent of 100 mg of cortisone per day.

3. When steroids such as prednisone, which usually do not invoke appreciable sodium retention or edema are being used, one must be on the alert for more subtle evidences of overdosage during a prolonged therapeutic program. Special attention should be given to disturbance in the gastrointestinal tract, as indicated by the appearance of digestive symptoms or occult blood in the stool. Signs suggestive of bone pain due to the development of underlying osteoporosis should be carefully watched for.

4. All patients receiving prolonged steroid therapy should have periodic checks, which should include body weight, blood pressure, urine sugar, and appraisal of the cardiovascular, digestive, and skeletal systems. The possibility of the development of posterior subcapsular cataracts must be considered.

Adrenal hormone therapy constitutes a potent pharmacologic agent in the armamentarium of every practicing physician. As with all potent medicaments, a physician's responsibility must include an adequate knowledge of the pharmacologic actions of these agents as well as of the indications and contraindications for their use.

REFERENCES

Addison T.: On the Constitutional and Local Effects of Disease of the Suprarenal Capsules, London, D. Highley, 1855.

Beisel, W. R., V. C. DiRaimonde, and P. H. Forsham: Cortisol Transport and Disappearance, Ann. Internal Med., 60:641, 1964.

Cahill, G. F., Jr., and G. W. Thorn: The Diagnosis and Treatment of Addison's Disease Med. Clin. N. Am., 46:1191, 1962.

Carpenter, C. C. J., N. Solomon, S. G. Silverberg, T. Bledsoe, R. C. Northcutt, J. R. Klinenberg, I. L. Bennett, and A. M. Harvey, Jr.: Schmidt's Syndrome (Thyroid and Adrenal Insufficiency): A Review of the Literature and a Report of Fifteen New Cases Including Ten Instances of Coexistent Diabetes Mellitus, Medicine, 43:153, 1964.

Conn, J. W., and I. H. Louis: Primary Aldosteronism, a New Clinical Entity, Ann. Internal Med., 44:1, 1956.

Cushing, H.: The Basophil Adenomas of the Pituitary Body and Their Clinical Manifestations (Pituitary Basophilism), Bull. Johns Hopkins Hosp., 50:137, 1932.

Gabrilove, J. L., D. C. Sharma, H. H. Wotiz, and R. I. Dorfman: Feminizing Adrenocortical Tumors in the Male: A Review of 52 Cases, Medicine, 44:37, 1965.

Graber, A., R. L. Ney, W. E. Nicholson, D. P. Island, and G. W. Liddle: Natural History of Pituitary Adrenal Recovery Following Long-term Suppression with Corticosteroids, Trans. Assoc. Amer. Physicians, 77: 296, 1964.

Laidlaw, J. C., W. J. Reddy, D. Jenkins, N. A. Haydar, A. E. Renold, and G. W. Thorn: Advances in the Diagnosis of Altered States of Adrenocortical Function, New Engl. J. Med., 253:747, 1955.

Lipsett, M. B., W. D. Adell, L. E. Rosenberg, and Thomas A. Waldmann: Humoral Syndromes Associated with Nonendocrine Tumors, Ann. Internal Med., 61:733, 1964.

Luetscher, J.: Primary Aldosteronism: Observations in Six Cases and Review of Diagnostic Procedures, Medicine, 43:437, 1964.

Nugent, C. A., T. Nichols and F. H. Tyler: Diagnosis of Cushing's Syndrome, Arch. Int. Med., 116:172, 1965.

Paris, J.: On the Diagnosis of Addison's Disease and Cushing's Syndrome by Laboratory Methods, Proc. Mayo Clin., 39:26, 1964.

Ross, E. J.: Aldosterone and Its Antagonists, Clin. Pharm. & Therap., 6:65, 1965.

Soffer, L. J., A. Iannaccone, and J. L. Gabrilove: Cushing's Syndrome: A Study of 50 Patients, Am. J. Med., 30:129, 1961.

Strauss, J., and P. Pochi: The Human Sebaceous Gland: Its Regulation by Steroidal Hormones and Its Use as an End Organ for Assaying Androgenicity in Vivo, Recent Progr. Hormone Res., 19:385, 1963.

85 DISEASES OF THE ADRENAL MEDULLA

Roger B. Hickler
and George W. Thorn

Anatomy

Embryologically two cell types differentiate from a common stem cell, the sympathogonia of the primitive neuroectoderm, to form the adrenal medulla: the chromaffinoblast and the neuroblast, which mature into the chromaffin cell and sympathetic ganglion cell, respectively. These medullary cells are richly supplied with preganglionic fibers from the splanchnic nerves.

The chromaffin cell is so named because of its capacity to show brown intracytoplasmic granules on treatment with oxidants, a result of oxidation and polymerization of the catecholamine stored in the granules. Further histochemical studies suggest the presence of two different chromaffin cell types in the adrenal medulla, one for each of the two catecholamines. Chromaffin cells are widely dispersed in the body at birth, and the extraadrenal sites undergo progressive involution until puberty; the more persistent sites are the paraganglions, lying along the retropleural and retroperitoneal sympathetic chains, and the organs of Zuckerkandl, paired structures lying anterior to the lower abdominal aorta.

Diseases of the adrenal medulla involve benign and malignant neoplasms of its two cell types, the ganglion cell and the chromaffin cell. Identical tumors occur in extraadrenal sites of sympathetic ganglion cells and uninvoluted chromaffin cells and are predominantly retroperitoneal in location.

Physiology

The chromaffin cells of the adrenal medulla synthesize, store, and secrete epinephrine and norepinephrine. The biosynthesis of these hormones proceeds as follows: conversion of phenylalanine to tyrosine; oxidation of tyrosine to dopa (3,4-dihydroxyphenylalanine); decarboxylation of dopa to dopamine (3,4-dihydroxy-phenylethylamine); and oxidation of dopamine to norepinephrine; epinephrine is formed by methylation of norepinephrine. Epinephrine is the major hormone of the adrenal medulla, constituting 80 per cent of its stored content of catecholamine; the major source of norepinephrine is the postganglionic sympathetic neurone, where it acts as the neurotransmitter.

The catecholamines are stored in cytoplasmic granules in the medullary chromaffin cells, which also contain a high content of adenosine triphosphate. It has been suggested that hydrolysis of adenosine triphosphate in the granules by an adenosine triphosphatase disrupts the granules and permits release of the hormone, which is normally released by cholinergic preganglionic sympathetic nerve impulses. A number of agents can directly stimulate chromaffin cells or the adrenergic neurones to release catecholamines, including acetylcholine, nicotine, histamine, 5-hydroxytryptamine, tyramine, and reserpine. A number of physiologic stimuli cause an increase in the release of both epinephrine and norepinephrine, including severe muscular work, asphyxia and hypoxia, and hemorrhagic hypotension. Insulin hypoglycemia causes a selective release of epinephrine alone, favoring the concept of separate cells for the synthesis and separate control of the release of adrenomedullary epinephrine and norepinephrine.

The physiologic effects of the adrenomedullary hormones may be characterized as preparing the organism to meet an emergency situation. Both epinephrine and norepinephrine have a direct inotropic and chronotropic effect on the heart. However, the purely vasoconstrictor effect of norepinephrine results in diastolic and systolic hypertension, producing reflex slowing of the heart, so that cardiac output is generally unchanged or reduced. The net peripheral vasodilator effect of physiologic doses of epinephrine (due primarily to vasodilatation of resistance vessels of skeletal muscle) permits a rise in cardiac output, with widening of pulse pressure through a rise in systolic pressure; diastolic pressure may fall slightly. Cutaneous and renal vasoconstriction is common to both hormones. Both increase the rate and depth of respiration and stimulate the release into plasma of nonesterified fatty acids from neutral fat depots. Other metabolic effects characteristic of epinephrine and, to a lesser extent, of norepinephrine, include increased formation of active phosphorylase in liver and skeletal muscle, resulting in accelerated hepatic glycogenolysis and release of lactic acid from muscle. These effects lead to hyperglycema, increased oxygen consumption, and a high respiratory quotient.

More than half of intravenously administered catecholamine is metabolized within 2 min, and only 5 per cent is excreted as "free" catecholamine in the urine; a comparable percentage appears as conjugated catecholamine. Through the action of catechol-O-methyl transferase, widely dispersed in body tissues, the remaining 90 per cent of administered catecholamine is converted into the methoxy compounds (Fig. 85-1), of which about 40 per cent is metanephrine and normetanephrine (free and conjugated) and about 40 per cent is 3-methoxy-4-hydroxy mandelic acid (VMA). The latter is a product of the combined action of catechol-O-methyl transferase and monamine oxidase on epinephrine and norepinephrine.

Bilateral adrenalectomy results in very little depression of urinary catecholamines, since 80 per cent is normally norepinephrine, largely derived from

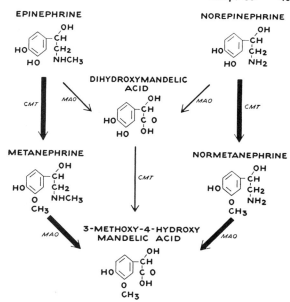

Fig. 85-1. The degradation of epinephrine and norepinephrine by catechol-O-methyl transferase (CMT) and monamine oxidase (MAO). All the above compounds appear in the urine in the free form or conjugated to glucuronide or sulfate. The heavier arrows indicate the major pathways. 3-Methoxy-4-hydroxymandelic acid is derived from epinephrine and norepinephrine.

sympathetic nerve endings. The ensuing loss of adrenomedullary hormones (primarily epinephrine) does not lead to any apparent deficiency, in contradistinction to the adrenocortical hormones, although serious hypotension has been observed in the immediate postoperative period despite adequate replacement of adrenocortical hormones.

PHEOCHROMOCYTOMA

The incidence of pheochromocytoma in a hypertensive population is approximately 0.5 per cent of patients screened for this tumor. The syndrome of paroxysmal hypertension due to this tumor was first described by Labe, Tinel, and Doumier in 1922, and C. H. Mayo was the first to report its successful operative removal with relief of hypertension in 1927.

PATHOLOGY AND SPECIAL CLINICAL ASPECTS. The comprehensive series of 76 cases reported from the Mayo Clinic permits some valid generalities about this rare tumor. The tumors ranged in weight from 1.2 to 700 Gm, although about half were 50 Gm or less. Tumor size did not correlate with severity of symptoms. The patients were divided into those with persistent and those with paroxysmal hypertension. The incidence of tumors with paroxysmal function and persistent function was equal. Two-thirds of the former occurred in women; no sex predilection was noted in the latter. The age range was twelve to seventy-seven years, averaging forty-five years in the paroxysmal group and thirty-nine years in the persistent group. On a basis of local invasion or distant metastasis, malignancy was four times as common in the group with persistent function, with a total incidence of 13 per cent for both groups. For the total of both groups the incidence of solitary unilateral adrenal tumor was 84 per cent, of multiple tumors 9 per cent, of bilateral adrenal tumors 6 per cent, and of solitary extraadrenal tumor 5 per cent.

Extraadrenal sites of pheochromocytoma are usually retroperitoneal (e.g., organs of Zuckerkandl) and may be as distant as the neck, thorax, and urinary bladder. Metastases, which may be functional, have occurred in liver, lungs, and central skeleton, as well as in paraaortic lymph glands. True polycythemia has been reported in association with the tumor, with return of the red cell mass to normal after successful surgery. Pheochromocytoma may coexist in members of the same family with other congenital disorders of the neuroectoderm, including multiple neurofibromatosis and central nervous system hemangioblastoma. Thyroid carcinoma has also been associated with familial pheochromocytoma. When a pheochromocytoma is present in a child, the hypertension is almost always sustained rather than paroxysmal and the tumor tends to be bilateral and to have a higher incidence of malignancy than in adults.

The tumors are round, frequently lobulated, and highly vascular. They may show hemorrhage and cystic degeneration, particularly large tumors. On section they appear brown or gray. Histologically they resemble the adrenal medulla; the nuclei are often multiple, cytoplasmic vacuolization is common, and dark staining with chromium salts is characteristic ("chromaffin reaction"). Malignant tumors are very difficult to distinguish from benign on purely histologic grounds.

CLINICAL MANIFESTATIONS. Three patterns are observed: (1) paroxysmal hypertension (intermittently secreting tumors); (2) persistent hypertension (sustained secretion by the tumor); and, less commonly, (3) the "metabolic syndrome" (predominant epinephrine secretion by the tumor), characterized by less severe hypertension in the presence of marked diabetes and hypermetabolism. However, considerable overlap between these groups occurs. Thus, about one-third of the patients with sustained hypertension will have superimposed paroxysmal attacks. Further, norepinephrine, the predominant secretion of most tumors, in excess can produce all the metabolic effects of smaller amounts of epinephrine.

In the presence of hypertension, the triad of headache, excessive perspiration, and palpitations is the clinical hallmark. Commonly associated manifestations are pallor, nervousness, tremor, nausea, vomiting, weakness, chest and abdominal pain, visual disturbances, marked weight loss, dyspnea, flushing, and dizziness. Bradycardia is found in approximately 20 per cent of the cases. Paroxysms are frequently spontaneous but may be precipitated by physical exertion, abdominal palpation, and emotional upset. They may

occur several times a day or at rare intervals and may last for a minute or for as long as a week. Blood pressure levels frequently exceed 250/150 mm during an attack. Cases of persistently secreting tumors may be difficult to distinguish from cases of essential hypertension, but hyperglycemia and hypermetabolism are found in approximately 50 per cent of the former as a distinguishing feature. A lean body habitus is characteristic of all patients with pheochromocytoma. The optic fundi tend to be benign in the paroxysmal group, but over half the patients in the persistent group will have grade 3 to 4 fundiscopic changes. Shock and renal failure may attend or follow an attack. During a paroxysm death may occur from pulmonary edema, ventricular fibrillation, or cerebral hemorrhage.

DIAGNOSIS. The diagnosis of pheochromocytoma may be strongly suspected on clinical grounds in a patient who proves to have essential hypertension, and it may be quite unsuspected in a patient regarded as having essential hypertension until it is discovered on routine laboratory screening. Thus, at some time, routine laboratory screening of *all* patients with significant hypertension is desirable for this potentially curable form of hypertension. Certainly, any of the clinical manifestations described above should raise suspicion. Other suggestive features may be cited: (1) a hypertensive patient under thirty years of age; (2) absence of a family history of hypertension; (3) presence of malignant hypertension; (4) tendency to postural hypotension; and (5) a hypertensive response to anesthesia or to therapy with ganglionic blocking agents and guanethidine. Incorrect diagnoses in the presence of a pheochromocytoma have included diabetes mellitus, thyrotoxicosis, anxiety neurosis, "vascular" headache, epilepsy, and hypertensive crises due to lead poisoning and porphyria.

Urinary Assay for Catecholamines and Their Methoxy Derivatives. In the study of patients for the possible presence of a pheochromocytoma, the determination of 24-hr urinary free catecholamines or their methoxy derivatives provides a safe and reliable basis for the diagnosis. Although bioassay techniques are useful for screening, chemical assay is becoming the standard approach. Current chemical methods for determining urinary free catecholamines involve modifications of the trihydroxyindole (THI) method of Lund. The urinary catecholamines are adsorbed on an alumina or resin column, eluted with acid, oxidized to form "chromes," which, in turn, are tautomerized in alkali to form strongly fluorescent trihydroxyindoles. Free epinephrine and norepinephrine are separately calculated from photofluorometric readings at different wave lengths. After acid hydrolysis to free the conjugated fractions, metanephrine (MN) and normetanephrine (NMN) are similarly measured by conversion to trihydroxyindoles or by oxidation to vanillin; in either instance the final product is read fluorometrically. VMA is measured by oxidation to vanillin, which may be read fluorometrically or combined with added indole and read colorimetrically. Simpler colorimetric and chromatographic assays for the methoxy derivatives are under evaluation.

With these techniques Crout, Pisano, and Sjoerdsma measured the levels for 24-hr urinary catecholamines and their methoxy derivatives in 23 patients with pheochromocytoma, controlled with a large group of patients with essential hypertension. The upper limits of normal in the control groups were (1) free catecholamines (epinephrine plus norepinephrine), 100 μg; (2) metanephrine plus normetanephrine, 1.3 mg; and (3) VMA, 6.0 mg. A diagnostic elevation above these values was found for all three determinations in 20 of the 23 tumor patients. Therapy with alphamethyl dopa will produce false elevations in the urinary free catecholamines because the fluorometric techniques detect the excreted drug as free hormone. The relative diagnostic merits of the three different indices is debated, and it is probable that any one of them, carefully done, will serve equally well.

Combined Pharmacologic and Chemical Approach. In a small percentage of patients, particularly during a normotensive period in those with intermittently secreting tumors, 24-hr urinary assay for catecholamines (or derivatives thereof) may not be clearly elevated into a diagnostic range. If suspicion is still strong on clinical grounds, the tumor may be provoked to secrete with 0.01 to 0.025 mg histamine base, given intravenously. This should be followed by the rapid injection of 5 mg phentolamine intravenously, should an alarming rise in blood pressure ensue. Blood may be drawn during the control period and at intervals of 2 min in the immediate posthistamine period for plasma assay for catecholamines, or a timed urine specimen (after prior emptying of the bladder) may be collected for a period of 6 hr for analysis for catecholamines or methoxy derivatives. The latter may be expressed as amount excreted per milligram of creatinine.

The upper limit of normal for plasma epinephrine and norepinephrine varies with the method employed (trihydroxyindole or ethylenediamine condensation) and must be established in a given laboratory to determine a diagnostic rise following histamine administration. The upper limit of normal for urinary catecholamines (epinephrine plus norepinephrine) is 0.05 μg per mg creatinine; for metanephrine plus normetanephrine, it is 2.1 μg per mg creatinine; for VMA, it is 9.5 μg per mg creatinine. Levels above these following histamine administration are diagnostic. If a spontaneous attack should occur while a patient is under observation, blood and urinary determinations should be made immediately (Fig. 85-2). The plasma ethylenediamine condensation method for plasma catecholamines is invalid in the presence of uremia. Specific dietary restrictions are necessary to avoid exogenous sources of interfering substances in the urine when measuring VMA (coffee, tea, nuts, cake, ice cream, bananas).

In the absence of facilities for bioassay or for these chemical determinations, the older pharmacologic tests

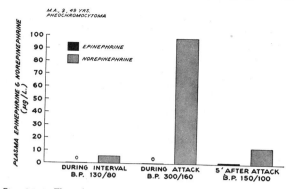

Fig. 85-2. The plasma epinephrine and norepinephrine levels before, during, and after a spontaneous paroxysm. The change in levels illustrates the intermittent secretory activity shown by some tumors and underlines the importance of obtaining samples for diagnostic purposes *at the height* of a spontaneous or induced attack.

must be employed, using the blood pressure response as a guide. Provocative tests with histamine are employed when the blood pressure is below 170/110 mm and should be compared with the cold pressor response for interpretation. False negative and positive results have been observed. If the blood pressure is 170/110 mm or above, intravenous phentolamine may be employed. A sustained fall of 35 mm or more systolic and 25 mm diastolic is considered diagnostic. False positive tests are frequently encountered, particularly in the presence of a number of agents commonly used in the treatment of hypertension. False negative results are rare. Fatalities have been reported following histamine and phentolamine administration in the presence of a pheochromocytoma.

An enhanced pressor response to intravenous doses of tyramine has been reported in six patients with pheochromocytoma in comparison with control subjects, and this may constitute a new and safer pharmacologic test. However, this test is strongly contraindicated in any patient receiving amine oxidase inhibitor therapy; the administration of tyramine may then precipitate a hypertensive crisis.

Localization of Tumor. While rarely palpable, a tumor mass may be detected on a plain film of the abdomen; tomography combined with an intravenous pyelogram may be more definitive. Presacral carbon dioxide insufflation and aortography have been useful; the latter is not without hazard. The analysis of catecholamines in plasma obtained by catheter at different levels in the venous system under fluoroscopic control has also been useful. Thoracic tumors, while rare, may be seen on a plain chest film.

Crout and Sjoerdsma report that the separate determination of urinary epinephrine and norepinephrine is of predictive value in tumor localization. If there is a significant elevation of epinephrine as well as norepinephrine (42 per cent of all cases), the tumor may be expected to lie in or adjacent to one of the adrenal glands in about 95 per cent of cases, or, rarely, in the organs of Zuckerkandl. If the urine contains elevated norepinephrine alone (58 per cent of all cases), the tumor will still be found in one of the adrenal areas in about two-thirds of the cases and in an extraadrenal location in the remainder. In only 6 per cent of patients of this type will the tumor be extraabdominal. In contrast to the normal adrenal medulla, the usually predominant secretion of norepinephrine over epinephrine by these tumors probably reflects a deficiency of N-methylating enzyme (due to anaplasia), necessary to convert norepinephrine into epinephrine.

TREATMENT. In patients in whom surgical resection cannot be performed, the regular oral administration of phentolamine or phenoxybenzamine has been reported to have controlled most of the disturbing symptoms for a period of many months. However, surgical removal is the treatment of choice for this potentially lethal disease. Since 96 to 97 per cent of all such tumors are located in the abdomen, a careful abdominal exploration through a generous transverse upper abdominal incision may be undertaken, even without the certain exclusion of a rare extraabdominal site. To avoid extremes of hypertension during induction of anesthesia and surgical manipulation, an intravenous drip of phentolamine is ready at all times. To avoid extremes of hypotension on clamping the blood supply of the tumor and following its removal, an intravenous drip of norepinephrine or other pressor amine is also prepared in advance. *Administration of whole blood or plasma on removal of the tumor may be of paramount importance in preventing postoperative shock, since a chronic reduction in blood volume is a consequence of the prolonged vasoconstriction attending the disease.*

Hyper- and Hypofunction of the Adrenal Medulla

There is one clear case report of hyperfunction in unilateral adrenal hyperplasia, resembling a pheochromocytoma in all clinical respects and cured by operative removal of the involved adrenal. Hypofunction of the adrenal medulla has been demonstrated in children with spontaneous idiopathic hypoglycemia. These individuals show no increase in urinary epinephrine during spontaneous or insulin-induced hypoglycemia.

NEUROBLASTOMA AND GANGLIONEUROMA

Tumors may develop from any of the mature cell types or their precursors which make up the sympathetic nervous system and the adrenal medulla.

The *neuroblastoma* consists of immature, undifferentiated neuroblasts and is highly malignant. Rare in adulthood, it is one of the commonest malignant tumors of infancy and early childhood and may be present at birth. It grows rapidly, forming a bulky mass in the flank and often displacing the kidney.

It metastasizes early to regional lymph nodes, liver, bones, and orbit. Metastasis to bone with new bone formation may be confused with Ewing's tumor, osteogenic sarcoma, and Hand-Schüller-Christian syndrome. The tendency to generalized lymphadenopathy may lead to confusion with lymphosarcoma. The prognosis is poor. Radical surgery followed by deep x-ray therapy may provide some cures. Farber reported 10 cures in 40 cases treated in this manner and followed over a 10-year period. It should be noted that in some of these children complete surgical removal of the tumor had not been possible.

The *ganglioneuroma* is formed from well-differentiated nerve cells and fibers and is benign. It occurs in older children and young adults as a small, well-encapsulated, slowly growing tumor and is usually an incidental finding at post-mortem examination. In children the association of ganglioneuroma and ganglioneuroblastoma with a clinical picture resembling the celiac syndrome has been observed. Chronic diarrhea, wasting, and abdominal distension are the most prominent symptoms, but hypertension associated with an increased urinary excretion of catecholamines may be found. Removal of the tumor is associated with remission of the hypertension and gastrointestinal symptoms.

CATECHOLAMINE METABOLISM IN NEUROBLASTOMA AND GANGLIONEUROMA. Studies in patients with ganglioneuroma and particularly neuroblastoma have shown not only elevated levels of norepinephrine in the urine but also increased excretion of its metabolites and biochemical precursors. In a study of 21 patients with neuroblastoma, Studnitz, Käser, and Sjoerdsma found increased amounts of each of the following compounds in over 85 per cent of cases: dopa; dopamine; norepinephrine; normetanephrine; and VMA. The diagnostic and prognostic usefulness of this phenomenon is apparent. Although some patients exhibit a modest blood pressure elevation, in contrast with pheochromocytoma, they usually do not exhibit signs of pressor amine overproduction, which also is in contrast with pheochromocytoma.

REFERENCES

Crandall, D. L., and R. T. Myers: Pheochromocytoma— Anesthetic and Surgical Considerations, J.A.M.A., 187: 12, 1964.

Crout, J. R., J. J. Pisano, and A. Sjoerdsma: Urinary Excretion of Catecholamines and Their Metabolites in Pheochromocytoma, Amer. Heart J., 61:375, 1961.

Engelman, J., and A. Sjoerdsma: A New Test for Pheochromocytoma, J.A.M.A., 189:81, 1964.

von Euler, U. S.: The Catecholamines. Adrenalin; Noradrenalin, in "Hormones in Blood," C. H. Gray and A. L. Bacharach (Eds.), New York, Academic Press, Inc., 1961.

Gifford, R. W., Jr., W. F. Kvale, F. T. Maher, G. M. Roth, and J. T. Priestlye: Clinical Features, Diagnosis and Treatment of Pheochromocytoma: A Review of 76 Cases, Proc. Mayo Clin., 39:281, 1964.

Horowitz, D., W. Louenberg, J. Engelman, and A. Sjoerdsma: Monamine Oxidase Inhibitors, Tyramine and Cheese, J.A.M.A., 188:1108, 1964.

Page, L. B., and G. A. Jacoby: Catechol Amine Metabolism and Storage Granules in Pheochromocytoma and Neuroblastoma, Medicine, 43:379, 1964.

Wolstenholme, G. E. W., and M. O'Connor (Eds.): "Adrenergic Mechanisms," Ciba Foundation Symposium, Boston, Little, Brown & Co., 1960.

86 DIABETES MELLITUS

Peter H. Forsham, Jurgen Steinke, and George W. Thorn

DEFINITION. Diabetes is a syndrome. Hereditary diabetes presents metabolic and vascular components, which are both probably interrelated. The metabolic syndrome is characterized by an inappropriate elevation of blood glucose, associated with alterations in lipid and protein metabolism, for which a relative or absolute lack of insulin is responsible. The vascular syndrome consists of nonspecific atherosclerosis and a more specific microangiopathy particularly affecting the eye and kidney.

The disease is important because of its high incidence throughout the world and because the treated diabetic individual has the potential for a nearly normal life-span.

HISTORY. Diabetes has been recognized from antiquity. Chinese medical writings mentioned a syndrome of polyphagia, polydipsia, and polyuria. Aretaeus (*ca* 70 A.D.) described the disease and gave it its name, meaning in Greek "to run through."

The study of the chemistry of diabetic urine was initiated by Paracelsus in the sixteenth century; however, he mistook the residue of the boiled urine for salt instead of sugar. Some 100 years later, Thomas Willis described the sweetness of the diabetic urine, "as if imbued with honey or sugar," which Dobson proved to be sugar. This led to a rational dietary approach, introduced by Rollo 20 years later. Morton (1686) noted the hereditary character of diabetes. In 1850, Claude Bernard demonstrated the increased glucose content of diabetic blood and recognized hyperglycemia as the cardinal sign of the disease. In 1869, Langerhans, still a medical student, described the islet cell formation in the pancreas, which now bears his name. Kussmaul characterized the air hunger and labored breathing of the patient in diabetic coma in 1874. The careful work by clinicians such as Bouchardat, Naunyn, von Noorden, Allen, and Joslin led to a significant therapeutic success with diet. Von Mering and Minkowski carried out their studies in 1889, demonstrating that dogs could be made diabetic by pancreatectomy. However, it took more than 30 years before Banting, Best, and Macleod were able to prepare an extract from dog pancreas capable of reducing an elevated blood glucose level. In 1936,

the first long-acting insulin was introduced by Hagedorn. The chemical structure of ox insulin was established by Sanger in 1953; Nicol and Smith described the chemical structure of human insulin in 1960. The basic unit contains two polypeptide chains united by disulfide bridges. In 1964, Katsoyannis and his associates completed the synthesis of both the A and the B chains of insulin and were able to combine both chains into biologically active material.

The accidental discovery of the hypoglycemic action of carbutamide by Franke and Fuchs in Germany, in 1955, and the earlier experimental work of Loubatieres in France initiated the use of oral hypoglycemic agents.

INCIDENCE. Diabetes mellitus is a disease of worldwide distribution. If it is more frequent in some countries than in others, it will have to be established when diagnostic criteria are agreed upon and uniformly controlled detection drives are executed. In the United States there are approximately 3 million persons with diabetes, close to 2 per cent of the population. Unless a cure or some preventive measure is found for diabetes, this number will continue to increase for the following reasons: (1) the life expectancy of the treated diabetic is close to normal, or is at least two-thirds that of the general population at a given age; (2) since more diabetics live long enough to have children, an increasing number of children will inherit the diabetic gene; and (3) obesity, which appears to precipitate diabetes among those predisposed to it, is also on the rise, thus allowing more potential diabetes to emerge.

The undiagnosed diabetic presents a major challenge to the practicing physician. Not infrequently diabetic symptoms are minimal, and the patient does not seek medical advice. In the United States, approximately 50 per cent of the 3 million diabetics are unidentified. Because early treatment prolongs life, these undiagnosed diabetics must be found. As it is impossible to test the entire population, it is advisable to concentrate on those individuals with a predisposition for the disease. They are (1) relatives of known diabetics, among whom diabetes is 2½ times more frequent than in the general population; (2) obese persons, since 85 per cent of diabetic patients are, or were at one time, overweight; (3) persons in the older age groups, as four out of five diabetics are over forty-five; and (4) mothers delivered of large babies, since the birth of a large infant may be an indication of maternal prediabetes.

Apart from these high-risk groups, routine testing for diabetes should be performed whenever a new patient visits a physician's office or is admitted to a hospital. Furthermore, it would be highly desirable to include testing for diabetes in preemployment examinations and to continue tests for employees at yearly intervals thereafter.

INHERITANCE. It is well-established that diabetes mellitus is inherited; the *mode* of inheritance is still under discussion.

The acceptance of heredity for diabetes is based on the greater frequency of diabetes among blood relatives of known diabetics. The pattern of inheritance is characterized by (1) a more frequent occurrence in the mates of identical than of non-identical twins; (2) the equilateral transmission of the trait by either affected parent; and (3) the susceptibility of both sexes. However, genetic study is complicated by the fact that susceptibility to diabetes is inherited, but the disease itself may not become apparent clinically for years. Genetic studies are based on occurrence of clinical diabetes (phenotype), not on presence of the genetic predisposition (genotype), for the latter cannot be detected at the present time. It is possible that the diabetic trait may be dominant and the manifest diabetic disease recessive. There is further confusion because diabetes is a syndrome; for example, chronic pancreatitis may be associated with hyperglycemia indistinguishable from that observed in genetic diabetes. This could lead to false designation of an individual as affected with genetic diabetes. Diabetes has a variable age of onset (youth onset and maturity onset), each with a characteristic clinical pattern. This has led, on the one hand, to the hypothesis of multifactorial inheritance and to the hypothesis that the mode of inheritance in juvenile diabetes is homozygous, whereas the hereditary factor in maturity onset diabetes is heterozygous. On the other hand, Steinberg has reviewed all available genetic data and expressed the belief that diabetic inheritance is consistent with homozygosity for a recessive gene at a single locus, with variable penetrance.

ETIOLOGY. Hereditary Diabetes (Idiopathic, Spontaneous, Essential, Primary).

1. Growth-onset (juvenile) type. A positive family history of diabetes is present in 20 per cent of these children at time of diagnosis; however, after 20 years of disease, a positive family history can be obtained in almost 60 per cent. Diabetes occurs equally in both sexes, childhood obesity does not seem to play a role, and infections precede diabetes in 10 per cent of cases. The most common finding is a spurt of linear growth just before clinical diabetes develops. This would point to excess growth hormone as an important factor in precipitating clinical diabetes. In experimental diabetes, injection of purified growth hormone will produce permanent diabetes in the dog (metahypophyseal diabetes). However, thus far, measurements of growth hormone in the plasma of juvenile diabetics have given discrepant results.

2. Maturity-onset (adult) type: As in growth-onset diabetes, heredity is important; however, in addition, the presence of obesity is of paramount significance, though it should not be inferred that all obese individuals are potential diabetics. Recently the relationship of obesity to diabetes has appeared in a new light. Vallance-Owen has presented evidence that the diabetic trait may manifest itself as an anti-insulin factor, present in serum of subjects susceptible to diabetes. As this factor migrates with albumin on electrophoresis, it has been designated *synalbumin*. This factor reduces the action of insulin selectively on muscle tissue but not on adipose tissue. Therefore, glucose, excluded from entering muscle, will produce hyperglycemia, which, in turn, triggers pancreatic insulin release, resulting in deposit of excess glucose in adipose tissue. Under these circumstances, an individual may become obese because he is predestined to become diabetic. Obesity in this interpretation is a prediabetes sign.

Pregnancy also seems to exert a definite diabetogenic action in women so predisposed. Initially, diabetes may become apparent only during pregnancy and disappear following delivery; rarely it remains; frequently, years later, permanent diabetes develops. There is evidence that hormonal anti-insulin factors of placental origin and marked destruction of endogenous insulin by the placenta may play a role in precipitating diabetes. It is speculated that the higher frequency of diabetes in adult females may be due to pregnancies and obesity.

Nonhereditary (Secondary) Diabetes. Secondary diabetes may arise from any one of several causes for which a definite etiology for carbohydrate intolerance can be established. It may follow surgical removal of the pancreas, destruction of the pancreas by carcinoma, severe pancreatitis, or damage of the islets by iron deposits in hemochromatosis.

Recently, the diabetogenic action of certain diuretics of the benzothiadiazine type has been noted. There is some evidence that these drugs mediate such mechanism by inhibiting pancreatic insulin release. This effect is reversible, contrary to the damage produced by the administration of alloxan. In addition, overactivity of the pituitary (acromegaly), adrenals (pheochromocytoma, Cushing's disease), or thyroid gland (Graves' disease) may result in diabetes, usually reversible once the primary disease is corrected. Growth hormone mediates its diabetogenic action by decreasing peripheral glucose utilization; excess epinephrine causes increased hepatic glycogenolysis, the steroids act by increasing hepatic gluconeogenesis, and thyroxin increases hunger and food intake and generally heightens the level of metabolic activity.

Liver disease is often associated with mild diabetes, though severe liver disease may lead to hypoglycemia. Infection of any sort will impair glucose tolerance and may unmask the tendency to diabetes. The diabetogenic mechanism of infection is probably nonspecific and consists of elevated levels of corticosteroids, fever that increases the general metabolic load, and possibly acidosis, which decreases the effectiveness of circulating insulin. In rare instances inflammation of the pancreatic islets takes place.

Regardless of what precipitates secondary diabetes, the common denominator in all these factors is hyperglycemia, with resulting stimulation of insulin secretion. This serves to put a constant strain on the beta cells, with eventual exhaustion of the insulin reserve.

PATHOLOGY. Pancreas. With the use of special stains with the light microscope and with the availability of the electron microscope, it now appears very likely that almost all diabetic patients exhibit a correlation between severity of their diabetes, on the one hand, with reduced total mass of beta cells and degree of beta cell degranulation, on the other. These two factors correlate with the amount of extractable pancreatic insulin. Generally speaking, after several years of established clinical diabetes, the patient with youth-onset diabetes shows essentially no extractable pancreatic insulin, whereas the pancreas of the adult-onset diabetic still contains some insulin, approximately half that found in control pancreases. Patients with maturity-onset diabetes studied at autopsy reveal a significant incidence of hyalinization of pancreatic islets. It has been suggested that this material is related to amyloid (Lacy).

Of special interest is the finding that some juvenile diabetics who come to autopsy shortly after clinical onset of diabetes show large islets of Langerhans. This would support the concept that the *initial* lesion is not decreased insulin production by the pancreas.

There is also the admittedly rare patient with recent onset of diabetes whose pancreatic islets indicate lymphocytic infiltration (insulitis), a lesion again found only in young diabetics. This raises the possibility of an autoimmune mechanism, at least in some patients.

Blood Vessels. Atherosclerosis in the diabetic patient is not different from that commonly observed, but it is equally present in both sexes and occurs more frequently earlier in life and is also more severe. In addition, these patients usually have small-vessel disease, or microangiopathy; its initial lesion is a thickened basement membrane.

Retina. Microaneurysms, hemorrhages, and exudates are frequently seen in patients with long-standing diabetes. Proliferative retinopathy is found almost exclusively in severe juvenile diabetes of long duration. There are strands of fibrous collagenous tissue and frequently around the optic disk formation of new blood vessels. If hemorrhage occurs in the vitreous, scar tissue will form, which, upon retracting, may produce retinal detachment. Frequently, there is also a striking dilatation of venules. In proliferative retinopathy, a secondary hemorrhagic glaucoma is often the final step leading to total blindness.

A better understanding of the mechanism of early vascular changes has been made possible by the introduction of the in vitro trypsin digestion of the flattened retina, thus making it possible to eliminate nonvascular components. Cogan and Kuwabara describe two types of vascular cells, the endothelial and the mural cell. In diabetics, there is a specific loss of mural cells, resulting in loss of tone with formation of microaneurysms and some diffuse distension with consequent ischemia of adjacent areas. This theory is supported by in vivo findings employing fluorescein, injected intravenously, in the general circulation, followed by serial photographs of the fundus. In diabetics, there is not only delayed emptying but also leakage of the dye from blood vessels in areas where exudates and hemorrhages are occurring.

Kidney. Specimens for histologic study can be obtained by open or percutaneous biopsy or, of course, at autopsy. The specific diabetic lesion is the nodular glomerulosclerosis described by Kimmelstiel and Wilson. The lesions consist of PAS-positive basement-membranelike material, believed to accumulate first in the mesangial region. With time, nodules form. As the disease advances, the basement membrane of the glomerular loops becomes diffusely or focally thickened and the effects of arterial and arteriolar sclerosis become manifest. The combination of these three lesions constitute diabetic nephropathy and manifests itself clinically with proteinuria, edema, and hypertension. Pyelonephritis, a frequent complication, is a local manifestation of the generalized increased susceptibility to infection.

Link Between Metabolic and Vascular Changes in Diabetic Patients. Some of the pathologic changes observed in diabetic patients are obviously secondary to hyperglycemia, lipemia, and varying degrees of ketosis. Hyperglycemia results in deposition of glycogen in the renal epithelium, especially in the proximal convoluted tubule and the loop of Henle, where it is directly correlated to the glucose concentration in the urine. Hyperglycemia also results in deposition of glycogen in non-insulin-dependent organs such as skin (pruritus), heart muscle, iris, and ciliary bodies of the eye. The liver of the diabetic patient, except in terminal stages, contains normal amounts of glycogen; however, the distribution may be abnormal within the nuclei of the hepatic parenchymal cells. Occasionally the liver is enlarged and infiltrated with fat, mainly in untreated or poorly treated diabetics.

The relationship between derangement of intermediary metabolism and microangiopathy has not been clarified and is the subject of controversy. Except for the patient with mild diabetes, perfect control is impossible to achieve in the immediate postprandial state and therefore most patients present varying shades of insufficient control.

Biochemically it is possible that excessive synthesis of mucopolysaccharides from glucose, via an insulin-independent pathway, leads to derangement of the basement membrane, with secondary infiltration by materials from the blood stream. It has been questioned whether such a derangement is necessarily the consequence of an abnormal glucose metabolism or if both the level of blood glucose and the state of the basement membrane could be influenced by a third factor. It is useful, therefore, to distinguish a vascular from a metabolic component.

PATHOLOGIC PHYSIOLOGY. In all likelihood the diabetic syndrome develops as a consequence of an imbalance between insulin production and release, on the one hand, and hormonal or tissue factors modifying the insulin requirement, on the other.

Insulin is absolutely lacking in those forms of secondary diabetes where destruction or removal of the pancreas has taken place. Similarly, growth-onset diabetes is characterized by an absolute insulin deficiency. There is essentially no extractable pancreatic insulin, no response to oral hypoglycemic agents of the sulfonylurea type, a marked tendency to ketoacidosis, and therefore absolute dependence on exogenous insulin for survival. It is assumed that diabetes in the child begins when the pancreatic production of insulin declines. This classic concept has been challenged by the following observations: (1) At least one-third of all juvenile diabetics will develop a phase of remission, usually within three months after the acute onset of the disease. If present, the remission may last from several days to several months; it rarely exceeds 1 year. Often during such a remission no insulin treatment is necessary, and a glucose tolerance test may be normal. This suggests strongly that at least initially the pancreas of the diabetic child has a potential recuperative power. Nevertheless, after this remission the juvenile diabetic progresses rapidly to total insulin deficiency. (2) Juvenile diabetics who have suffered accidental death shortly after onset of diabetes have been found to have an almost normal pancreatic insulin content, and on histologic examination larger than normal islets were found. (3) Measurement of serum insulin at an early stage of manifest diabetes has demonstrated that insulin is present in blood, although its activity may be masked. Methods for measurement of serum insulin which have found some degree of acceptance are the rat diaphragm assay, the rat adipose tissue assay, and an immunochemical technique. The first two are in vitro biologic methods in which the response of surviving isolated tissue to insulin present in serum is tested; the last technique is based upon reaction of the circulating insulin molecule with an insulin antibody. In juvenile diabetes of several years' duration none of these techniques detects any circulating endogenous insulin.

The patient with adult-onset diabetes develops his disease considerably more slowly. At the early stage no symptoms may be present, and diagnosis is made by glucose tolerance test or by discovery of elevated glucose levels 1 or 2 hr postprandially. Measurement of serum insulin by any of the above-cited methods may indicate close to normal levels; however, the insulin response to administered glucose is abnormal in that it occurs late. This is felt to be responsible for the elevated blood glucose 1 to 2 hr postprandially. As insulin release increases with the rising blood glucose, the blood glucose declines; with excess insulin, the blood glucose may fall precipitously, provoking the symptoms of reactive hypoglycemia between the *third and fifth hour* postprandially. As the disease progresses further, the insulin release becomes less pronounced, the episodes of reactive hypoglycemia tend to disappear, and finally the amount of circulating insulin is insufficient to return the blood glucose to normal levels between meals. In maturity-onset diabetes the pancreatic insulin reserve is decreased, but rarely totally absent. Thus the occurrence of diabetic ketoacidosis is uncommon.

Although in many patients the contrast between growth-onset and maturity-onset is initially at least quite sharp, there are crossovers between these two types and the above comments must be considered only as generalizations.

METABOLISM IN DIABETIC PATIENTS. Regardless of the type of diabetes, by definition, the cardinal sign is hyperglycemia frequently associated with glycosuria. The hyperglycemia has two components: hepatic overproduction and peripheral underutilization. The source of the glucose released from the liver is dietary carbohydrate, liver glycogen, and gluconeogenesis from protein. Underutilization of glucose in the peripheral tissue takes place mainly in adipose tissue and muscle, both of which are insulin-sensitive, and is attributed to a lack of circulating biologically effective insulin. Impaired glucose uptake by muscle leads to loss of muscle glycogen and release of amino acids for gluconeogenesis; the clinical symptom is fatigue. Impaired glucose uptake by adipose tissue causes impaired triglyceride synthesis with increased triglyceride breakdown, and the resulting free fatty acids and glycerol are released into the blood stream. The clinical sign is weight loss. In the liver, the fatty acids are metabolized to ketone bodies. Although they can be utilized by certain tissues, they are formed in excess in the diabetic person. They accumulate in the blood and lead to ketonuria. As they are strong acids, it is necessary for the kidney to excrete a fixed base with them, leading to both sodium and potassium loss. Therefore, the diabetic organism loses glucose, water, ketone bodies, and base. This will result in dehydration, ketoacidosis, and weight loss and in extreme cases may proceed to diabetic coma and death.

MECHANISM OF INSULIN ACTION. The exact mechanism by which insulin acts remains unknown. However, it is well established that tissues vary widely in sensitivity and responsiveness to insulin. Furthermore, it is likely that the mechanism of insulin action differs in different tissues. For example, in muscle and adipose tissue, insulin probably acts on cell membrane permeability and so facilitates the entry of glucose into the cell. On the other hand, liver cells exhibit no demonstrable permeability barrier to glucose. The insulin effect on liver appears to be on the phosphorylating mechanism. It has recently been suggested that the liver contains two enzymes for phosphorylation of glucose, hexokinase and glucokinase. Hexokinase is insulin-*independent* and glucokinase is insulin-*dependent*. In addition, it is probable that insulin alters the hepatic glucose output, particularly when glucose is being released as a result of glycogenolysis. It has been demonstrated that apart from its effect on glucose metabolism, insulin also exerts an accelerating effect on incorporation of amino acids in the protein of skeletal muscle. Tissues in which metabolism proceeds independently from insulin are the brain, red blood cells, and some epithelial tissues such as intestinal mucosa, renal tubules, and skin.

DIAGNOSIS. The diagnosis of diabetes mellitus is frequently suggested by a history of polydipsia, polyuria, and polyphagia, associated with weight loss. A clinical suspicion of diabetes is confirmed by finding glucose in the urine *and* by detecting an abnormally elevated blood glucose. If hyperglycemia is associated with glycosuria *and* with ketonuria, the diagnosis of diabetes mellitus is certain.

In the patient without any obvious symptoms suggestive of diabetes, the following procedures are recommended as screening tests for diabetes. By far, the simplest test is to obtain a urine specimen 1 to 2 hr after a heavy carbohydrate meal. However, in certain persons with an elevated renal threshold, the blood glucose may be elevated without being associated with glycosuria; furthermore, the finding of urinary sugar alone is not diagnostic of diabetes. Therefore, determination of blood glucose not only is preferable as a screening procedure but is mandatory to establish the diagnosis of diabetes. It can be measured in the fasting state or 1 or 2 hr after a meal.

Fasting Blood Glucose. The normal range for fasting blood glucose as measured by the Somogyi-Nelson technique or by the autoanalyzer is between 70 and 100 mg per 100 ml whole blood. An elevated fasting blood sugar is highly suggestive of diabetes; on the other hand diabetes can never be ruled out by presence of a normal fasting blood sugar. Therefore, it is advisable to obtain a blood sugar determination 1 or 2 hr after a meal which has contained approximately 100 Gm carbohydrates, as indicated in Table 86-1, or a regular breakfast to which 50 Gm glucose have been added. A 1-hr value of 160 mg per 100 ml or higher is highly suspicious of diabetes; so is a 2-hr value above 120 mg per 100 ml. If the level is borderline, or especially if one wishes definitely to rule out diabetes, then a formal 3-hr glucose tolerance test is indicated.

Oral Glucose Tolerance Test. Following a fasting blood glucose determination, 100 Gm glucose (available commercially in solution) is given and the blood glucose measured at ½ hr, 1 hr, 2 hr, and 3 hr; the urine is examined for the presence of sugar. The following are considered normal values obtained with venous blood as measured by the Somogyi-Nelson method: Fasting, 100 mg per 100 ml; ½ hr (or peak value), 160 mg; 1 hr, 160 mg; 2 hr, 120 mg; and 3 hr, 100 mg per 100 ml. There should be no glucose in the urine at any time. The result of the glucose tolerance test in an apparently healthy subject is influenced by at least three factors: diet, physical activity, and age. It is mandatory that the patient be on a preparatory diet containing 250 to 300 Gm carbohydrate for 3 days before testing; otherwise a decreased carbohydrate tolerance can be observed, known as *starvation diabetes.* Physical inactivity also decreases carbohydrate tolerance, and therefore prolonged bed rest may give false positive results. Finally, age exerts an effect on glucose tolerance. Although

Table 86-1. 100-GM CARBOHYDRATE BREAKFAST

Food	Quantity	Carbohydrate, Gm
Orange juice.........	8 oz	24
Cooked cereal........	4 oz ⎫	
or		16
Dry cereal...........	1 oz ⎬	
Bread...............	2 slices	32
Egg.................	1	
Butter..............	2 pats	
Milk................	6 oz	9
Cream..............	3 oz	4
Sugar..............	3 tsp	15
Coffee or tea........	ad lib.	
		100

standards are not available for individuals of different decades, especially over the age of fifty, Fajans suggests that between the ages of fifty and fifty-nine the 2-hr level can be considered normal up to 130; between the ages of sixty and sixty-nine, up to 140; between the ages of seventy and seventy-nine, up to 150; and above age eighty, above 160 mg per 100 ml. Additional factors known to affect glucose tolerance are fever, infection, endocrinopathies, liver disease, myocardial infarction, cerebral vascular accidents, and certain medication such as diuretics of the benzothiodiazine type.

Intravenous Glucose Tolerance Test. As intestinal absorption of glucose may interfere with a glucose tolerance test, it is occasionally desirable to perform an intravenous glucose tolerance test. This is especially indicated if there is a history of gastrointestinal surgery. Accelerated intestinal absorption of glucose, as in the "dumping syndrome," may result in a diabetic-type oral glucose tolerance curve; however, the intravenous glucose tolerance may be well within normal limits.

The dose of glucose is 0.5 Gm per kg body weight as a 25 per cent solution. It is administered intravenously within 2 to 4 min, and blood is collected every 10 min for 1 hr. Under these conditions, the rate of blood glucose decreases in an expotential manner, and the glucose disappearance can be calculated. Disappearance rate $= 70/t\frac{1}{2}$, where $t\frac{1}{2} =$ number of minutes it takes for the blood glucose to fall 50 per cent. In normal individuals it usually exceeds 1.5 per cent of the administered dose per minute, and values below 1 per cent are clearly diabetic.

If glucose tolerance tests are performed routinely in a large hospital population, many patients afflicted with chronic diseases like rheumatoid arthritis, cancer, or amyotrophic lateral sclerosis may exhibit impaired glucose tolerance curve without any clinical evidence of diabetes. Because many of these patients with "chemical diabetes" will not progress to a state of overt clinical diabetes, one has to be careful not to overdiagnose diabetes.

Cortisone Glucose Tolerance Tests. Fajans and Conn have proposed performing the oral glucose tolerance test after priming with cortisone in an attempt to establish the diagnosis of chemical diabetes at a time when the conventional oral glucose tolerance test is still within normal limits. The technique consists of administering 50 mg cortisone acetate 8 and 2 hr before the glucose tolerance test. The cortisone glucose tolerance test detects carbohydrate intolerance earlier than the standard oral glucose tolerance test; however, it remains to be established whether it can be employed as a reliable means of detecting the "diabetic trait."

Intravenous Tolbutamide Response Test. This test measures the response of the pancreatic beta cells to tolbutamide, by releasing endogenous insulin. It represents an alternative diagnostic procedure to the standard oral glucose tolerance test, especially for *early* diabetes mellitus.

TECHNIQUE. The same precautions as for the oral glucose tolerance need to be observed, including a preparatory diet. After an overnight fast, the patient is given sodium tolbutamide intravenously, 1 Gm dissolved in 20 ml sterile water. Blood specimens for glucose are obtained before the test and 20 and 30 min after the midpoint of the injection.

INTERPRETATION. This is based upon the decline of blood glucose after tolbutamide as a percentage of the preinjection fasting value. Almost all nondiabetic subjects will exhibit a fall in blood glucose concentration to less than 75 per cent of the preinjection level at 20 min. Definite diabetes is indicated by failure to decline to less than the 90 per cent level at the 20-min and 77 per cent at the 30-min specimen. In-between levels indicate varying degrees of probable diabetes.

DISCUSSION. The occurrence of hypoglycemia is not uncommon, and as this test may be hazardous in the older patient with coronary artery disease or cerebral vascular disease, it should be terminated after the 30-min specimen with a drink containing sugar. It is also possible that the tolbutamide test is less sensitive than the oral glucose tolerance test and, therefore, should not be used as the only test to exclude diabetes. Its main advantage is to verify by a different approach a borderline abnormal oral glucose tolerance test.

DIFFERENTIAL DIAGNOSIS OF GLYCOSURIA (See Chap. 87). The presence of glucose in the urine should be considered to indicate diabetes until an alternate diagnosis can be definitely established. Glycosuria may indicate a low renal threshold, which is present in pregnancy, in patients with chronic renal disease, and in patients with idiopathic renal glycosuria. In the latter, glucose is present in most urine specimens, including a second voided specimen after an overnight fast, but the glucose tolerance test is normal. The transient glycosuria that occurs occasionally in apparently healthy persons under conditions of stress or infection or following ingestion of a high-carbohydrate meal is usually associated with an abnormal glucose tolerance test and, therefore, indicates chemical diabetes.[1]

Melliuria Other Than Glycosuria. It is advisable for every patient with glycosuria to have his urine tested by a nonspecific reduction method (Clinitest) and by one of the enzymatic specific tests for glucose (Testape, Clinistix). By these simple techniques, nonglycosuric melliturias can be suspected.

Lactose is found in the urine of lactating women, but not as a rule in appreciable quantities before the third trimester of pregnancy. Occasionally, fructose may be found if large quantities of fruit have been ingested. Pentosuria and fructosuria are rare inborn errors of metabolism.

CLINICAL PICTURE. Three general types of diabetic patients can be distinguished: the juvenile, the adult-onset, and the patient with secondary diabetes.

Growth-onset Type. The growth-onset type of diabetes is characterized by a rapid onset with symptoms such as polydipsia, polyuria, polyphagia, loss of weight and strength, marked irritability, and not infrequently recurrence of bed-wetting. The diabetes is apt to be of the unstable or brittle type, being quite sensitive to the administration of exogenous insulin and easily influenced by physical activity. The patient is prone to ketoacidosis. For adequate treatment, diet and insulin therapy are mandatory. Since the introduction of insulin therapy, diabetic ketoacidosis has been markedly reduced as a major cause of death; the treated patient has a life expectancy of at least two-thirds of the normal population at the same age; the cause of death is now predominantly cardiovascular and renal. Diagnosis of diabetes in the growth-onset type patient is usually not difficult. However, occasional children and adolescents have asymptomatic diabetes demonstrable only by glucose tolerance test. In these patients the disease appears to progress very slowly.

Maturity-onset Type. The maturity-onset diabetic patient has a less stormy beginning. As a matter of fact, symptoms are minimum or absent. The chief complaint may be moderate weight loss; occasionally weight gain. There may be some nocturia. A female patient might consult her gynecologist because of vulvar pruritis. Frequently, however, the patient seeks medical attention because of complications. As a consequence of blurred or decreased vision, the patient may see an ophthalmologist first, who may diagnose diabetic retinopathy. Fatigue and anemia may be caused by fairly advanced diabetic nephropathy. Diabetic neuropathy may present as paresthesias, loss of sensation, impotence, nocturnal diarrhea, postural hypotension, or neurogenic bladder. Not infrequently, the patient presents with an ulcer or gangrene of his toes or heel and on examination has a pulseless or painless foot. Thus the patient with maturity-onset diabetes usually

---

[1] Chemical or asymptomatic diabetes: no diabetic symptoms but an abnormal glucose tolerance test with a normal fasting blood glucose.

does not present with the dramatic, acute metabolic syndrome observed in the juvenile patient but rather with a chronic vascular syndrome. It is therefore important to suspect diabetes as an underlying disease under a wide variety of circumstances.

Secondary Diabetic Syndrome. Chemical diabetes or clinical diabetes may be associated with cancer of the pancreas, pancreatitis, hemochromatosis, acromegaly, Cushing's syndrome, thyrotoxicosis, pheochromocytoma, or lipoatrophic diabetes. The latter extremely rare syndrome is characterized by absence of subcutaneous fat tissue, hepatomegaly, hyperlipemia, and hyperglycemia resistant to insulin but no tendency to develop ketosis.

TREATMENT. The aims of managing diabetes are (1) correction of the underlying metabolic abnormalities by diet, oral hypoglycemic agents, or insulin; (2) attainment and maintenance of ideal body weight; and (3) prevention, or at least delay, of complications commonly associated with the disease.

Successful therapy will depend upon the thoroughness with which the physician understands the particular problems in each individual case, upon how well the patient has been instructed, and upon how conscientious the patient is about following instructions.

On initiating treatment of a patient with diabetes, it is essential to be certain that there is no active focus of infection, as infection will aggravate the diabetic state. Infection of the urinary tract should be looked for particularly, and a chest x-ray is imperative. It is also advisable to obtain careful baseline evaluations of the state of the cardiovascular, nervous, and renal systems and of the eyegrounds to serve as subsequent points of reference.

Diet. Dietary treatment of diabetes still constitutes the basis for management. The principal considerations in designing diabetic diets are as follows: (1) the basic nutritional requirements of a patient with diabetes are the same as those of a nondiabetic patient; (2) protein intake must be sufficient for tissue anabolism; (3) an optimum intake of vitamins and minerals should be assured; (4) the diet should be varied and palatable.

The Basic Caloric Requirement. This is dictated by the desirable or ideal weight, the age, and the occupation of the patient. If he is obese, the diet will be restricted in calories; if the patient is undernourished, the diet initially will exceed the basic caloric requirement. The desired weight is calculated from the height, taking frame size into consideration. For an approximate calculation of the basic caloric requirement, the ideal weight is multiplied by 10. Example: A patient's ideal weight is 180 lb, his total caloric requirement will be 1800 Cal. Additional calories should be allowed according to the patient's occupation and activities. Calories may be reduced for patients over fifty years of age who are less active.

Partition of Calories. The average American diet consists of carbohydrate, 40 to 45 per cent; protein, 15 to 20 per cent; and fat, 35 to 40 per cent. The diabetic diet can approximate this distribution. The caloric value of carbohydrate and protein is approximately 4 Cal per Gm and of fat, 9 Cal per Gm.

CARBOHYDRATE. To prevent acetonuria, a minimum of 1 Gm per lb body weight is necessary, or in the example of the patient weighing 180 lb, 180 Gm. This minimum requirement should be increased if indicated by occupation or during the growth period in children. It is obvious that regulation of diabetes will be simpler with a greater number of feedings involving smaller quantities of carbohydrate than with three large meals. In particular, diabetic patients receiving insulin or oral hypoglycemic agents should receive a midafternoon and bedtime snack in order to minimize fluctuation of the blood glucose.

PROTEIN. A *minimum* of 0.5 Gm per lb body weight is indicated. This is increased during pregnancy and during childhood and decreased only in the presence of azotemia.

FAT. Although fat can be metabolized without the direct influence of insulin, dietary fat, together with other factors such as decreased physical activity, seems to play an important role in the pathogenesis of atherosclerosis; therefore, fat intake should be kept to a minimum. The amount prescribed is calculated by subtracting calories allowed for carbohydrate and protein from the total caloric requirement.

Table 86-2. FOOD EXCHANGES

LIST 1. MILK[1]
Calories 170, Carbohydrate 12 Gm, protein 8 Gm, fat 10 Gm per serving.

Food	Approximate measure 1 exchange	Weight, Gm
Milk, plain............	1 cup (8 oz)	240
Milk, evaporated......	½ cup	120
Milk, powder, skim[2]....	⅓ cup (5⅓ tbsp level)	48
Milk, powder, whole...	½ cup (8 tbsp level)	35
Buttermilk[2]..........	1 cup	240
Milk, skim[2]..........	1 cup	240

LIST 2. VEGETABLES
One or more fat exchanges from the diet allowance may be used to season the vegetables.
Carbohydrate 7 Gm, protein 2 Gm, fat negligible.
One exchange equals ½ cup.

Beets	Peas, green	Squash, winter
Carrots	Pumpkin	Turnip
Onions	Rutabagas	

[1] Modified from Meal Planning with Exchange Lists. Obtainable from the American Diabetes Association, Inc., New York, N.Y.

[2] Add 10 Gm fat (2 fat exchanges). Most commercial buttermilk is skimmed. Check local supplies.

All other vegetables, except those listed under Bread Exchanges, contain negligible carbohydrate, protein, and fat. They may be used as desired.

Table 86-2. FOOD EXCHANGES (*Continued*)

LIST 3. FRUITS

Fresh, cooked, canned, or frozen *unsweetened*. Carbohydrate 10 Gm per exchange; protein and fat negligible.

Fruit	Approximate measure 1 exchange	Weight, Gm
Apple, 1 small............	2″ diameter	80
Applesauce..............	½ cup	100
Apricots, dry...........	4 halves	20
Apricots, fresh..........	2 medium	100
Banana.................	½ small	50
Berries (blackberries, raspberries, and strawberries)..........	1 cup	150
Blueberries.............	⅔ cup	100
Cantaloupe............	½ (6″ diameter)	200
Cherries...............	10 large or 15 small	75
Dates.................	2	15
Figs, dried.............	1 small	15
Figs, fresh.............	2 large	50
Grapefruit.............	½ small	125
Grapefruit.............	½ cup	100
Grapes................	12	75
Grape juice............	½ cup	60
Honeydew melon.......	⅛ (7″ diameter)	150
Mango................	½ small	70
Nectarines.............	1 medium	100
Orange................	1 small	100
Orange juice...........	½ cup	100
Papaya................	⅓ medium	100
Peach.................	1 medium	100
Pear..................	1 small	100
Pineapple..............	½ cup, cubed	80
Pineapple juice..........	⅓ cup	80
Plums.................	2 medium	100
Prunes, dried...........	2 medium	25
Raisins................	2 tbsp level	15
Tangerine..............	1 large	100
Watermelon............	1 cup diced	
	1 slice 3″ × 1½″	175

LIST 4. BREAD EXCHANGES

Carbohydrate 15 Gm, protein 2 Gm, fat negligible.

Food	Approximate measure 1 exchange	Weight, Gm
Bread, baker's..........	1 slice	25
Biscuit, roll............	2″ diameter	35
Muffin................	2″ diameter	35
Cornbread.............	1½″ cube	35
Cereals, cooked........	½ cup, cooked	100
Cereals, dry (flakes, puffed, and shredded varieties)............	¾ cup, scant	20
Rice, macaroni, noodles, spaghetti............	½ cup, cooked	100
Crackers:		
Graham..............	2 (2½ × 2¾″)	20
Oyster...............	20 (½ cup)	20
Saltines..............	5 (2″ square)	20
Soda................	3 (2½ × 2½″)	20
Round, thin varieties...	6–8 (½″ diameter)	20
Vegetables:		
Beans, peas, dried (cooked) Includes limas, navy, kidney beans, black-eyed peas, cowpeas, split peas, etc...........	½ cup, scant	100
Corn.................	⅓ cup or ½ ear	80
Parsnips..............	½ cup	125
Potatoes:		
White, baked........	2″ diameter	100
White, boiled, mashed..........	½ cup	100
Sweet or yam.......	¼ cup	50
Ice cream, vanilla[3]......	⅛ qt	70
Sponge cake, no icing....	1½″ cube	25

[3] Omit 2 fat exchanges.

EXAMPLE. Total calories based on an ideal weight of 180 lb are 1800. Assigned for carbohydrate $180 \times 4 = 720$, for protein $90 \times 4 = 360$ Cal, there remain $(1800 - 720 - 360)$ 720 Cal. These are given as fat, or $720 \div 9 = 80$ Gm fat. The final diet then consists of carbohydrate 180 Gm, protein 90 Gm, and fat 80 Gm. In Tables 86-2 and 86-3 food equivalents are presented in a simplified form as exchange lists. Food can be measured with a standard 8-oz measuring cup, a teaspoon, and a tablespoon.

Oral Hypoglycemic Agents. These have a definite place in the treatment of maturity-onset diabetes, provided it is of the nonketotic type and that dietary treatment alone is unsuccessful in achieving adequate control. Patients falling into this category constitute approximately one-third of all maturity-onset diabetics. It should be emphasized that none of the oral hypoglycemic agents is insulin, nor can they replace it in conditions such as diabetic ketoacidosis. The agents presently in use are of two types: the sulfonylureas and the biguanides.

SULFONYLUREAS. The sulfonylureas available by prescription are tolbutamide (Orinase), acetohexamide (Dymelor), and chlorpropamide (Diabinese). Although there is some evidence that they directly decrease hepatic glucose output, they act primarily by enhancing the secretion of endogenous insulin. Thus, to be effective, at least residual function of the beta cells is necessary. Their use as the only therapeutic agents in growth-onset diabetes is precluded. They are indicated in the maturity-onset diabetic patient in whom diet alone has failed and acetonuria has not been demonstrated. Such a patient can be started on sulfonylureas without the prior use of

Table 86-2. FOOD EXCHANGES (Continued)

LIST 5. MEAT EXCHANGES
Carbohydrate negligible, protein 7 Gm, fat 5 Gm per serving. All items expressed in cooked weight.

Food	Approximate measure 1 exchange	Weight, Gm
Meat: Beef, fowl, lamb, veal (medium fat), liver, pork, ham (lean).......	1 oz	30
Cold cuts: Salami, minced ham, bologna, cervelat, liver sausage, luncheon loaf	1 slice 4½″ diam. × ⅛″	45
Frankfurters (8 to 9 per lb) Fish:	1	50
Cod, haddock, halibut, herring, etc.........	1 oz	30
Salmon, tuna, crab-meat, lobster.......	¼ cup	30
Shrimp, clams, oysters (medium)..........	5	45
Sardines.............	3 medium	30
Cheese:		
Cheddar type........	1 oz	30
Cottage.............	3 tbsp level	45
Peanut butter[4].........	2 tbsp scant	30
Egg.................	1	50

[4] Limit to one serving per day unless adjustment is made to balance carbohydrate content.

LIST 6. FAT EXCHANGES
Carbohydrate and protein negligible, fat 5 Gm per serving. Fat exchanges utilized in cooking should be accounted for.

Food	Approximate measure 1 exchange	Weight, Gm
Avocado...............	⅛ (4″ diam.)	24
Butter or margarine......	1 tsp level	5
Bacon, crisp............	1 slice	10
Cream, light, sweet, or sour—20%...........	2 tbsp level	30
Cream, heavy—40%.....	1 tbsp level	15
Cream cheese.........	1 tbsp level	15
French dressing.........	1 tbsp level	15
Mayonnaise...........	1 tsp level	5
Nuts.................	6 small	10
Oil or cooking fat.......	1 tsp level	5
Olives...............	5 small	50

Table 86-3. EXAMPLE OF AN 1800 CALORIE DIABETIC DIET ORDER
(CARBOHYDRATE 181 GM, PROTEIN 90 GM, FAT 80 GM)

Exchange	Break-fast	Lunch	Snack	Supper	Snack
Milk..........	½	1	—	—	½
Bread.........	2	2	1	2	1
Meat.........	1	2	1	3	1
Fat..........	1	1	—	2	—
Fruit.........	1	1	—	1	—
Vegetable......	—	1	—	1	—
Partition in Gm:					
Carbohydrate...	46	52	15	47	21
Protein.......	15	26	9	27	13
Fat...........	15	25	5	25	10

these agents have a good record, especially with respect to hepatic function. Occasionally, in elderly undernourished patients, severe hypoglycemia may follow their administration. If this occurs, prolonged and intensive treatment with intravenous glucose (200 Gm within 24 hr) and close medical supervision for at least 72 hr is mandatory. Between 20 to 30 per cent of diabetic patients, initially considered to be good candidates for treatment with sulfonylurea, will fail to respond after several months or years. This secondary failure can often be attributed to poor adherence to a prescribed diet, the presence of infection, or the gradual progression of the diabetes to a more insulin-deficient state. Sometimes a secondary failure is due to destruction of the pancreatic islets by carcinoma or hemochromatosis.

TOLBUTAMIDE. This is the most widely used oral hypoglycemic agent. Each tablet contains 500 mg. The biologic half-life is approximately 6 hr. It is administered before breakfast *and* before supper, the total daily dose ranging from 1 to 3 Gm. The excretory product in the urine may give a false positive test for albumin since it is precipitated by acidifying the urine.

ACETOHEXAMIDE. Each tablet also contains 500 mg; however, its half-life is longer, and therefore a *single* dose of 500 to 1,000 mg is occasionally effective.

CHLORPROPAMIDE. Tablets are available containing 100 or 250 mg. The biologic half-life is approximately 36 hr, and daily administration may result in a cumulative effect. The recommended daily dose is 100 to 250 mg before breakfast; it should not exceed 500 mg. Because of its long action, a bedtime snack containing carbohydrate, protein, and fat, e.g., milk with crackers, is advisable. As it has a slightly greater toxic effect on the liver than has tolbutamide or acetohexamide, and since its long half-life may occasionally result in hypoglycemia in the early morning, it is advisable to keep the daily dose as low as possible. A

insulin, or he can be transferred from insulin to sulfonylureas. The chance of therapeutic success with these agents is better when clinical diabetes has been present for a relatively short period of time. A large initial loading dose is now not considered necessary for the sulfonylureas. In general, side effects are rare; and except for chlorpropamide in high doses, trial with chlorpropamide is justified in the patient who fails to respond to tolbutamide.

BIGUANIDES. Of the biguanides, *phenformin*, a phenethyl biguanide (DBI), is commercially available. The mechanism of action differs fundamentally from that of the sulfonylureas in that it can correct hyperglycemia in the pancreatectomized animal and the hypoglycemic effect cannot be produced in nondiabetic subjects. The mechanism of action is still poorly understood, but it appears that phenformin influences the anaerobic pathway of glucose. As phenformin makes a diabetic patient occasionally more sensitive to exogenous insulin, it has been suggested that phenformin inhibits an insulin antagonist. As such an anti-insulin factor would be present only in a patient with diabetes, this could explain the ineffectiveness of this substance in nondiabetics. The use of phenformin as the only antidiabetic agent is limited because the effective dose is frequently associated with gastrointestinal side effects such as anorexia, nausea, vomiting, and diarrhea, probably of central origin. Furthermore, phenformin may produce excess lactic acid; it should not be used in those circumstances in which marked tissue hypoxia might be expected to occur, i.e., myocardial infarction, hypotension, low arterial blood oxygen saturation, etc. Fatalities have been reported in which severe lactic acidosis apparently facilitated by the administration of phenformin, constituted an important contributory effect. Phenformin is available as a 25-mg tablet with a biologic half-life of 3 to 4 hr and as a 50-mg timed-disintegration capsule of longer half-life, provided it is absorbed. The indications for its use are few: (1) in the very rare diabetic patient of maturity onset who is allergic to the sulfonylureas (the daily recommended dose of phenformin ranges from 50 to 200 mg, to be given either as tablets t.i.d. or as capsules b.i.d.); (2) in combination with sulfonylurea in the elderly patient who fails to respond to a maximum dose of a sulfonylurea; (3) in the brittle diabetic on insulin with frequent hypoglycemic reactions, in whom the addition of phenformin might result in reduction of the insulin requirement and thus facilitate control. Unfortunately, the use of phenformin in this type of patient is often disappointing.

Insulin Treatment. The use of insulin is clearly indicated in the youth-onset diabetic and in those patients with maturity-onset diabetes in whom diet and oral hypoglycemic agents have proved inadequate to maintain satisfactory levels of blood glucose in both the fasting and the postprandial state. Furthermore, the use of insulin is mandatory in ketoacidosis, severe infections, and during major surgery.

TYPES OF INSULIN. In the United States the animal sources for insulin are beef and pork. As human insulin has a structure similar to that of pork, the use of pure pork insulin rather than a beef-pork mixture may be preferred; this insulin should produce fewer antibodies in man. Apart from the species difference, seven types of insulin are commercially available. They can be divided into insulins of fast, intermediate, and long action. Their properties are summarized in Table 86-4.

Each of the insulins is available in two different strengths, namely, 40 or 80 units per milliliter. The choice between the two is governed according to the amount of insulin required by the patient. If only a small amount is necessary, for example, 16 units, the use of U 40 will allow a more accurate dosage; if a larger amount is required, U 80 has the advantage of a smaller volume.

CHOICE OF INSULIN. (1) Crystalline insulin is best for emergencies, such as the treatment of diabetic ketoacidosis, or the achievement of fast control in the patient with severe glycosuria; it is also employed for daily use in combination with an intermediate insulin to bring on earlier action. (2) Intermediate insulins in a single dose injected before breakfast will control the majority of diabetics. The dosage will be gauged by the prelunch, midafternoon, and fasting blood sugar values. The midafternoon blood glucose corresponds to the peak of insulin action and will dictate the maximum morning dose. It is advisable that all patients receiving an intermediate insulin be given a midafternoon snack. If the midafternoon blood glucose level is between 80 and 120 mg per 100 ml, and the prelunch value is still unduly elevated, the addition of a small amount of crystalline insulin at breakfast time is indicated. It can be mixed with NPH or Lente in the same syringe. Almost all maturity-onset diabetics

Table 86-4. INSULIN ACTION CURVES

Action	Insulin	Modifier	Duration of action, hr	Maximum effect, hr postinjection
Fast.....................	Crystalline zinc (regular)	None	8	2–3
	Semi-Lente	Zinc	12	3–6
Intermediate.............	Globin	Globin	18	6–8
	NPH	Protamine	24	8–12
	Lente	Zinc	24	8–12
Long....................	Ultra-Lente	Zinc	36	20–30
	Protamine zinc	Protamine	36	20–30

Table 86-5. CASES ILLUSTRATING VARIATIONS IN INSULIN THERAPY

Case	Chemistry	Prebreakfast	Prelunch	Presupper	HS	Insulin therapy
A	Glycosuria[1]	+	+	+	+	Start NPH[2]
	Blood glucose	Elevated	Elevated	Elevated	Elevated	
B	Glycosuria	0	+	0	0	If on NPH, add crystalline
	Blood glucose	Normal	Elevated	Normal	Normal	
C	Glycosuria	+	0	0	0	If on NPH and crystalline, add NPH at HS or before supper
	Blood glucose	Elevated	Normal	Low	Normal	
D	Glycosuria	+	0	0	+	If on NPH and crystalline in A.M., add NPH *and* crystalline before supper
	Blood glucose	Elevated	Normal	Normal	Elevated	

[1] Test for urinary glucose performed on second voided specimen.
[2] Unless indicated otherwise, insulin is given before breakfast.

can be adequately controlled by intermediate insulins alone or in combination with crystalline insulin administered before breakfast.

The patient with youth-onset diabetes often develops nocturnal hyperglycemia and consequently will exhibit a high fasting blood glucose associated with glycosuria. Further increase in the morning dose of intermediate insulin will often lead to hypoglycemia in the midafternoon. To reduce the fasting blood glucose to normal levels a long-acting insulin can be tried, but often a second small dose of the intermediate insulin before supper or at bedtime is preferable. The latter regime is eminently satisfactory in the 24-hr control of the juvenile diabetic, and usually patients do not complain about the second injection as they feel so much better. Very rarely, sugar is spilled at bedtime, but none before supper. Then the addition of a small amount of crystalline insulin to the evening dose of NPH is indicated, and both are given before supper (Table 86-5). As a general rule, it can be stated that whenever insulin is given in the evening in addition to the morning dose, the latter should be reduced. (3) The use of long-acting insulin with the hope of establishing control with a single morning injection has been disappointing.

INITIATION OF INSULIN THERAPY. If the patient has massive glycosuria and elevated blood glucose, insulin therapy is begun immediately with crystalline insulin. The following schedule is recommended: a minimum of 20 units for a 4+, 15 units for a 3+, and 10 units for a 2+ urine test. Once the acute syndrome is under reasonable control or if the metabolic derangement is less dramatic, a longer-acting insulin can be started. It is best to start with 10 or 20 units of NPH or Lente and increase this by 5 units per day, as indicated by urine tests and blood glucose levels.

Complications of Insulin Therapy. INSULIN REACTIONS. These are commonly caused by excess insulin dosage, delayed food intake, or unusual physical activity. Very rarely, an increased sensitivity to insulin is due to early adrenal or pituitary hypofunction and, even more exceptionally, to development of a functioning islet cell tumor. Occasional insulin reactions are almost un-

avoidable, especially in the juvenile insulin-sensitive diabetic, but they are harmless if recognized and treated early. To reduce them to a minimum it is essential that the patient know how to test his urine for glucose and, provided he does not have an elevated renal threshold for glucose, how to reduce his insulin dose when his urine tests indicate absence of glucose for several days. The patient also has to be instructed to eat his meals on time and, when unusual physical activity is anticipated, either to reduce his morning insulin dose or to ingest extra calories to compensate for the blood-sugar-lowering effect of exercise.

The signs and symptoms of an insulin reaction vary with the type of insulin used. Crystalline insulin produces a characteristic reaction of rapid onset consisting of hunger, a peculiar abdominal sensation, sweating, palpitation, tremor, tachycardia, weakness, irritability, and pallor. Patients usually recognize these symptoms early, and they are relieved within minutes by ingestion of carbohydrate—sugar, orange juice, candy, etc. To prevent any awkward situation every diabetic patient on insulin should carry several lumps of sugar with him at all times. As a patient in insulin reaction may act as though he were intoxicated. it is further recommended that all diabetics carry a card identifying them as such. This is especially important in patients with a long history of diabetes. Due to neuropathy, sympathetic nervous system signs may gradually be lost and thus the patient lacks indications of impending reaction and may exhibit only impairment of cerebral functions. The intermediate and long-acting insulins produce a more gradual decline in blood glucose with consequently less release of epinephrine; symptoms are produced by deficient glucose metabolism of the higher nervous centers. They consist of headache, blurred or double vision, fine tremor, uncontrollable yawning, hypothermia, mental confusion, incoordination, and eventually unconsciousness. In elderly persons an insulin reaction may mimic a cerebrovascular accident. Treatment is administration of glucose by mouth or by vein. In severe and prolonged insulin reactions it is advisable to administer a glucocorticoid to produce maximum stimulation of gluconeogenesis. Relatives of diabetic patients prone to severe insulin reactions, and especially parents of diabetic children, should be instructed in the use of glucagon. It can be injected subcutaneously, just as insulin is, and will lead to a transient rise in blood glucose, long enough to wake the patient up and enable him to receive some carbohydrate by mouth.

Recurrent hypoglycemic attacks, with their attendant anxiety, headache, loss of concentration power, etc., constitute a nuisance to the diabetic patient, but only *severe and prolonged* attacks of hypoglycemia will lead to intellectual deterioration as a result of irreversible damage to cortical neurones.

An insulin reaction initiates a counterregulatory mechanism, characterized by release of epinephrine, adrenal corticoids, and growth hormone. This will result in a rebound hyperglycemia, for "hypoglycemia begets hyperglycemia." Knowledge of this physiologic defense mechanism will prevent the physician from administering extra insulin to combat this hyperglycemia. If the insulin reaction is due to excess insulin, the patient will benefit from a reduced insulin dosage.

REACTIONS AT THE SITE OF INSULIN INJECTION. Such reactions are not uncommon at the beginning of treatment. They are characterized by redness, swelling, pain, and nodule formation. As they usually disappear within a few days or weeks, the patient can be reassured and no treatment is indicated. If the local reaction persists, it can be improved by changing to an insulin of the Lente type, which does not contain protamine. Skin infections at the site of injection are extremely rare; but when they occur, they call for prompt treatment.

INSULIN LIPODYSTROPHY. This reaction is characterized by either hypertrophy or atrophy of the subcutaneous adipose tissue at the site of insulin injection. This is frequent and affects children and females more than males. If the patient is bothered by the esthetic aspect of this complication, injection of insulin into other sites is recommended until the lesion improves; then the atrophic area may again be used in the hope of inducing lipogenesis.

INSULIN RESISTANCE. Almost all diabetic patients treated with insulin for several months will develop circulating antibodies to insulin. However, only a few (approximately 1 in 1,000 insulin-treated diabetics) will develop insulin resistance. By definition, insulin resistance is present if the daily insulin requirement in the absence of diabetic ketoacidosis exceeds 200 units. Patients with insulin resistance may require several thousand units daily. When insulin resistance is associated with hemochromatosis, severe infections, Cushing's syndrome, acromegaly, or hyperthyroidism, it is secondary. Occasionally, no obvious cause can be detected. Examination of serum will demonstrate the presence of large quantities of antibodies to insulin and an increased insulin-binding capacity.

TREATMENT. A trial with pure pork insulin is always justified, and very often a sizable reduction in insulin requirement can be achieved. If such a simple measure fails, the use of steroids is indicated, for their anti-insulin effect is outweighed by their antiallergic effect. The natural course of idiopathic insulin resistance is characterized by spontaneous remission within several weeks or months. Frequently, the resistance breaks abruptly and the patient exhibits episodes of severe hypoglycemia as the antibody-bound insulin is released and becomes suddenly available.

DIABETIC ACIDOSIS AND COMA. Lack of insulin is the cause of diabetic ketoacidosis. The patient may be (1) an undiagnosed diabetic, (2) a known diabetic who fails to increase his insulin dose despite poor urine tests, or (3) a known diabetic who suffers from nausea and vomiting and, as he does not eat, reasons that he does not need his daily insulin. Omission of insulin probably constitutes the single largest cause of diabetic acidosis.

DIAGNOSIS. Among clinical signs and symptoms, vomiting is present in approximately two-thirds of patients with acidosis. Abdominal pain and tenderness may be related to nausea and vomiting or sodium depletion and may be so severe as to mimic an abdominal emergency ("pseudoappendicitis" of diabetic acidosis). Air hunger and heavy, labored breathing as described by Kussmaul are expressions of the acidosis and correlate with the reduction in serum CO_2. There is dehydration as evidenced by soft eyeballs, dry skin, poor urinary output, and hypotension. Laboratory findings include the following: the urine usually contains massive amounts of glucose and acetone; frequently there is also transient albuminuria. The diagnosis of diabetic ketoacidosis is made, however, by finding hyperglycemia, ketonemia, and reduction of serum CO_2 content. The acidosis is metabolic and is caused by accumulation of ketone bodies and loss of sodium and potassium. The azotemia is due partly to dehydration and partly to tissue protein breakdown. Serum lipids are generally increased. The rise in hematocrit indicates dehydration; usually there is leukocytosis.

DIFFERENTIAL DIAGNOSIS. On clinical grounds alone it is sometimes difficult to distinguish between diabetic acidosis and an insulin reaction. If any doubt exists, blood should be drawn for laboratory tests and 50 ml 50 per cent glucose injected intravenously. If the coma is due to insulin reaction, the patient will wake up immediately; if he is in diabetic coma, no harm has been done. Other diagnoses to be considered (provided there is acidosis) are salicylate poisoning; lactic acidosis; hyperglycemic, hyperosmolaric, nonketotic coma; or far advanced renal failure—all conditions which can occur in a diabetic patient.

TREATMENT. This will vary greatly from patient to patient; however, the general principles are as follows: (1) through a large needle blood is withdrawn for laboratory tests, and the vein is kept open with an infusion of normal saline. The rationale for this rests on the observation that patients in diabetic coma may decompensate very rapidly, and precious time will be lost in finding a vein and performing a venous cut-down. (2) Crystalline insulin is administered both subcutaneously and intravenously. The average dosage of insulin required for patients in diabetic coma in the first 3 hr is 200 units, 100 units intravenously and 100 units subcutaneously. The dosage, of course, will vary from patient to patient and may have to be larger in an obese diabetic and less in a frail, elderly diabetic. If the patient has been in diabetic coma previously and required 300 units to respond, chances are he may require a similar dose again. Severe acidosis necessitates reevaluation of blood glucose, serum CO_2, and serum acetone levels every 2 hr; if less severe, every 4 hr will suffice. If the blood glucose level remains above 500 mg per 100 ml and serum acetone is positive at 1:4 dilution, another 100 units of insulin should be given. If the patient does not respond at all or if he deteriorates, successive doses are increased rapidly and given at hourly intervals. An occasional patient may require 5,000 or 10,000 units within the first 24 hr of treatment. If, on the other hand, at the fourth hour the level of blood glucose has decreased but remains above 400 mg per 100 ml, administration of another 50 units of insulin is indicated. (3) All patients in diabetic acidosis are severely dehydrated and depleted of sodium chloride and potassium. They will require a large amount of fluid, usually a total of 4 to 8 liters during the first 24 hr. Many electrolyte formulas have been proposed for adequate replacement, and though their value is not doubted, it is important to start fluid therapy *immediately,* which is best done with the universally available normal (0.9 per cent) saline solution. Once treatment is under way and the laboratory has reported values for blood glucose, serum CO_2, and electrolytes, finer adjustments can be made. The addition of bicarbonate is certainly indicated if the acidosis is severe (CO_2-combining capacity less than 10). It may also counteract the inhibitory effect a lowered pH has on insulin activity and therefore restore the patient's sensitivity to insulin. Once the blood glucose approaches 200 mg per 100 ml, feedings with orange juice should be started and the intravenous fluid changed to 5 per cent glucose in saline in order to avoid hypoglycemia. Usually there is also a deficiency of potassium, and this should be replaced, starting at the second or third hour, at a rate not exceeding 20 mEq per hour; rarely more than 80 mEq are needed during the initial 24 hr of treatment. The need for and administration of potassium can be monitored with an electrocardiograph. Signs of hypokalemia are flattening or inversion of T waves and prolongation of the QT intervals. (4) There are useful accessory procedures in treatment of diabetic acidosis. If the patient is unconscious, gastric lavage should be performed to prevent aspiration pneumonia. If the patient is in obvious circulatory collapse, blood, plasma, or a plasma volume expander should be given. Finally, the precipitating cause for the development of diabetic acidosis has to be established, for each patient, before specific treatment can be initiated. (5) The acute phase of diabetic acidosis is considered ended once the patient is completely responsive, the blood glucose is below 200 mg per 100 ml, the undiluted serum shows no evidence for acetone, serum CO_2 is back to normal, and the urine shows minimal glycosuria and not more than 1+ acetone. Now is the time to start the patient on intermediate insulin in a small dose to prevent a relapse into ketosis and, if needed, to give crystalline insulin in amounts dictated by urine sugar levels. A soft diet should be started. It is essential to begin with frequent small feedings. Intravenous fluid administration may be discontinued as soon as the patient is able to retain liquids by mouth. The overall mortality of patients with diabetic acidosis should be lower than 5 per cent.

COMPLICATIONS OF DIABETES

DIABETIC RETINOPATHY. This can be detected in varying degrees in more than 90 per cent of diabetic patients after 20 years of clinical diabetes. Diabetes is the third most frequent cause of blindness in the United States.

The earliest recognizable lesions on fundoscopy are dilatation of veins and "microaneurysms," which actually consist of small punctate hemorrhages. Preferentially they are located near the macula. Unless they occur within the macula, the vision will not be impaired. Other relatively early lesions are waxy exu-

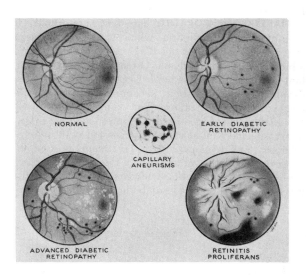

Fig. 86-1. Note the early dilatation of the venules and the punctate hemorrhages in *early diabetic retinopathy* actually representing capillary aneurysms surrounded by hemorrhages, as shown in a microscopic preparation of the retina (*center*). In *advanced diabetic retinopathy,* note in addition the typical hard, waxy exudates. In *retinitis proliferans* is seen the spread of connective tissue, revealed as a white material emanating from the optic disk, together with endovascularization in the form of small irregular vessels. Note the detachment of the retina at the top of the figure, and the larger hemorrhages.

dates, possibly due to lipid leakage from the vessels. This stage of the retinopathy can remain stationary for many years. It is the long-term juvenile diabetic who may progress to a more malignant stage, that of neovascularization and proliferative retinopathy. The new blood vessels usually emanate from the disk and grow toward the vitreous. If a preretinal hemorrhage occurs, organization takes place with formation of fibrous and collagenous tissue. Shrinkage of the scar tissue will produce retinal detachment (Fig. 86-1). Advanced diabetic retinopathy is frequently associated with retinal lesions caused by atherosclerosis, arterial hypertension, and renal insufficiency.

The appearance of retinopathy is fundamentally related to duration of diabetes; one of the reasons for strict chemical control of the metabolic component of diabetes is the possibility of delaying its onset and hopefully making it less severe. If incapacitating retinopathy is present, pituitary ablation should be considered, either by stalk section, total hypophysectomy, or irradiation. Poor vision in one eye and rapidly progressing retinopathy in the other eye constitute the major indication. However, the patient needs to be carefully selected as to emotional stability, long-term willingness to cooperate, and relative freedom from coronary artery disease or nephropathy. As hypoglycemia presents a major hazard after pituitary intervention, the patient should preferably not be living alone. After ablation of the pituitary, preliminary results indicate that two-thirds of patients have stabilized or improved their vision. The factor responsible for improvement has not been identified.

DIABETIC NEPHROPATHY. The first sign usually is asymptomatic albuminuria, which gradually increases over the years, as does the BUN. A decrease in serum albumin will lead to edema. Often there is a concomitant rise in serum cholesterol. Eventually hypertension develops, and the patient succumbs to renal insufficiency, and cardiac failure. The course of the disease is variable and depends on the presence and extent of the specific Kimmelstiel-Wilson lesion with nephrosclerosis and pyelonephritis. Treatment is symptomatic for diabetes, urinary tract infection, hypertension, and the nephrotic syndrome. Abolition of the pituitary has no benefit in diabetic nephropathy. Commonly the terminal stages of nephropathy are associated with *a decrease* in insulin requirement.

DIABETIC NEUROPATHY. This is a common, distressing, and therapeutically unsatisfactory complication of diabetes at any stage. Although it most frequently involves peripheral nerves, it may involve any portion of the nervous system and thus has an almost unlimited range of manifestations (Table 86-6). The peripheral neuropathy is characterized by a *nonsegmental* distribution. An interesting differential diagnosis is presented by the patient with severe headache and ocular palsy. If an intracranial aneurysm can be ruled out by angiogram, diabetic neuropathy may be the underlying cause. The neuropathy may be primarily diabetic, which is potentially reversible, or primarily vascular, which is less amenable to treatment.

Treatment of diabetic neuropathy consists of careful control of the diabetes with supplementary vitamin therapy, especially of the B complex. However, the treatment is not specific, and it may take weeks or months before improvement takes place.

GANGRENE OF THE FEET. This is a serious and frequent complication of diabetes, especially in the older age group. It may be due to vascular lesions ("pulseless" foot) or to neuropathy ("painless" foot), usually with a superimposed infection or injury. Arterial insufficiency is diagnosed by a history of claudication and by finding, on examination, weak or absent pedal pulses, blanching of the foot when raised above a 45° angle, and delayed venous filling when the foot is dependent. An arteriogram is indicated. Amputation is the treatment; hence, prevention, or at least delay of onset, of gangrene is of paramount importance. Simple rules for prevention include: (1) washing the feet with warm but *never* hot water each evening; (2) applying lanolin two or three times weekly if the skin is dry; (3) inserting lamb's wool between overlapping toes; (4) avoiding injuries to feet (the patient should never go barefoot); (5) never cutting toenails if vision is poor; (6) treating corns and calluses by a qualified podiatrist or surgeon.

SURGERY AND DIABETES MELLITUS. Diabetic patients may be affected by any surgical disease, but there are certain conditions, such as gangrene of the foot, cholecystitis, and cholelithiasis, to which they are more prone than the average person. There is also a strong association between diabetes and cancer of the pancreas. In addition, surgical problems may be unrelated to diabetes, such as repair of a hernia. As diabetes is a relatively common condition, from time to time every surgeon and anesthesist will be confronted with a diabetic patient.

The present surgical mortality in diabetics is approximately that of the general population. The surgical risk is increased in diabetics in the presence of poor regulation, obesity, arteriosclerosis, and cardiovascular-renal disease. However, even for the uncomplicated diabetic patient, operation and anesthesia constitute an additional metabolic stress, which will accentuate the predisposition to hyperglycemia and

---

Table 86-6. DIABETIC NEUROPATHIES

1. *Peripheral:*
   Sensory: loss of vibratory sense, paresthesias, pain
   Neuromuscular: weakness, paralysis, absent tendon reflexes, diabetic amyotrophy (thighs)
2. *Autonomic:*
   Eye: extraocular muscle palsies, pupillary changes
   Gastrointestinal: delayed gastric emptying, gallbladder dysfunction, nocturnal diarrhea
   Genitourinary: sexual impotence, atonic urinary bladder
   Vascular: orthostatic hypotension
   Bones and joints: neuropathic foot
   Skin: neurogenic ulcer, absent sweating, dependent edema

ketosis. Nevertheless, diabetes constitutes no contra-indication to surgery; and if the case is an emergency, only a few hours are generally needed to evaluate and prepare such a patient for operation.

Preparation for Surgery of the Diabetic Patient. Minor surgical procedures performed under local anesthesia interfere little with food intake and require no special changes in the administration of insulin or oral hypoglycemic agents. However, major surgery under general anesthesia in patients receiving insulin or oral hypoglycemic agents requires preoperative evaluation and achievement of good control. There should be an adequate carbohydrate intake of 150 to 200 Gm to prevent acetonuria with minimal glycosuria and close to normal premeal blood glucose levels. Patients receiving oral hypoglycemic agents should be given a small dose of insulin the day before surgery, and the oral hypoglycemic agent should be withheld. Dehydration or loss of electrolytes needs to be corrected.

Day of Surgery. Patients on intermediate-acting insulin should receive half the usual dose and, instead of breakfast, an infusion of 5 per cent glucose in water or in saline. From 1,000 to 1,500 ml are infused on the day of surgery and during subsequent days if there is inadequate food intake.

An anesthetic is selected to minimize hypoxia and acidosis and upset the carbohydrate metabolism as little as possible. Local or spinal anesthesia is preferred. Studies on nondiabetic subjects have demonstrated that nitrous oxide, thiopental, trichlorethylene, and cyclopropane have the least effect on blood glucose, whereas chloroform and ether have the most. In general, the anesthetic of choice is the one which will least upset the routine of diabetic treatment and which is familiar to both anesthesiologist and surgeon.

Postoperative Period. For the first hours during and immediately following surgery hypoglycemia need not be feared since any insulin given before surgery should be more than covered by the slow infusion of glucose and the metabolic stress of surgery and anesthesia; also, escape of the diabetic patient into keto-acidosis will be prevented by presence of the exogenous insulin. For treatment after surgery, either of two programs can be followed: one employs NPH or Lente insulin, if needed, in combination with crystalline insulin, and the other employs only crystalline insulin according to urine tests. With the first program, the remainder of the usual morning insulin dose, not given preoperatively, is administered in the recovery room and is covered with infusion of intravenous glucose and oral intake if the postoperative situation permits. If the blood glucose rises above 200 mg per 100 ml or if large amounts of glucose are found in the urine, additional crystalline insulin is administered. The second program does not call for any long-acting insulin postoperatively, but rather the need for extra insulin is gauged by urine tests performed at 4- to 6-hr intervals. A suggested schedule is 20 units for 4+, 15 units for 3+, 10 units for 2+, and none for 1+ or a sugar-free urine specimen. If the patient does not void

spontaneously, it is better to avoid catheterization and obtain a blood glucose level. If the value is above 200 mg per 100 ml, crystalline insulin is given, the dose depending on the individual patient; a rough guideline is 10 units of crystalline insulin for every 100 mg elevation above 200 mg per 100 ml every 6 hr. Regardless of the program employed, the postoperative management must be continued as long as the patient's oral intake is inadequate. Those patients who were well-controlled on diet and an oral hypoglycemic agent before surgery may be reverted to such a regime once the stress of operation and anesthesia has disappeared, which usually takes several days.

Differential Diagnosis. The diagnosis of an acute surgical abdomen may present some difficulty in the diabetic patient for two reasons: diabetic ketoacidosis may simulate an acute appendicitis ("pseudoappendicitis of diabetic coma"), and only lack of improvement after several hours of intensive diabetic therapy will strongly suggest an abdominal surgical emergency; on the other hand, acute appendicitis in the diabetic patient may produce little or no pain in the presence of neuropathy. The response to an infusion of saline may help distinguish "low sodium" muscle spasm from peritoneal irritation.

PREGNANCY AND DIABETES MELLITUS. The problem of management during pregnancy has assumed increasing importance, as young diabetic patients now survive longer and are thus capable of procreation. Infertility in female diabetic patients, common before insulin therapy, is rarely seen with good control of the diabetes. The problems engendered by pregnancy in diabetics concern maternal survival, fetal salvage, and prevention of diabetes in the offspring.

Today pregnancy carries but slightly added risk to the well managed diabetic mother; the maternal survival is 99.7 per cent (White). In contrast, fetal mortality is still high. Stillbirths among diabetics are six times as common as among nondiabetics. Fetal salvage will depend on the duration of the mother's disease and presence or absence of vascular lesions such as nephropathy.

Diagnosis. In patients not previously known as diabetic, pregnancy may induce a temporary state of diabetes. The diagnosis may offer some difficulty since with the lowered renal threshold of pregnancy glycosuria is not uncommon even among nondiabetic pregnant women. If urinary glucose is found during pregnancy and there is, in addition, a history of frequent miscarriages or of babies with a birth weight exceeding 9 lb, plus a family history of diabetes, diabetes should be suspected. The diagnosis can be firmly established only by the presence of abnormal blood glucose levels, whether fasting or postprandial. If they are borderline, performance of a glucose tolerance test is definitely indicated.

Treatment. The best results are obtained by close cooperation between the patient, the internist, and the obstetrician. The treatment of pregnant diabetic patients entails the same general health measures as those recommended for nondiabetic pregnant women. It is desirable to maintain a high intake of protein (i.e., at least 2 Gm per kg body weight per day) with a total caloric intake of 30 Cal per kg body weight and an adequate intake of calcium and iron. To prevent edema and minimize hydramnios, a low-salt diet is indicated, and the liberal use of diuretics is advisable. Diabetes is regulated throughout pregnancy with insulin. Usually the patient requires larger amounts given as a morning and an evening dose of NPH or Lente alone or mixed with crystalline insulin. Because of the lowered renal threshold for glucose one should not attempt to keep the urine sugar-free. It is admittedly often difficult to avoid excessive weight gain, but at least 200 Gm carbohydrate must be utilized to prevent ketosis.

Care of a diabetic patient through the first trimester may be difficult because of nausea and vomiting. If antiemetic drugs fail to control nausea and vomiting and frequent small feedings are not well tolerated, intravenous glucose must be administered. In the last trimester the insulin requirement usually increases concurrently with a rise in adrenal cortical activity, the presence of hormonal anti-insulin factors of placental origin, and placental destruction of insulin. It is of utmost importance to detect preeclamptic toxemia and hydramnios, since treatment will reduce fetal mortality. Timing of delivery is also important. The more advanced the diabetic state of the mother, the earlier the delivery should be attempted. Patients with only chemical diabetes can be delivered at term, patients with vascular complications should be delivered at the thirty-sixth week. The child may be delivered vaginally or by section. Early delivery has the advantage of removing the infant before it becomes too large and before placental circulation is impaired. The latter may be either the cause or the effect of the tendency to toxemia. A sudden decrease of insulin requirement to prepregnancy level usually follows delivery; therefore, it is advisable to omit or at least reduce the insulin dose on the day of delivery and to administer glucose intravenously.

Care of the Newborn. Special attention has to be paid to the predisposition of newborn infants of diabetic mothers to develop the respiratory distress syndrome (hyaline membrane disease) and hypoglycemia. The administration of 5 to 10 mg hydrocortisone intramuscularly during the first few days after delivery may minimize the tendency to hypoglycemia.

The incidence of diabetes later in life in a child delivered of a diabetic mother is 22 per cent and thus not essentially different from that of the general population with either a diabetic mother or a diabetic father.

REFERENCES

Antoniades, H. N., A. M. Huber, B. R. Boshell, C. A. Saravis, and S. N. Gershoff: Studies on the State of Insulin in Blood: Properties of Circulating "Free" and "Bound" Insulin, Endocrinology, 76:709, 1965.

Beaser, S. B.: Oral Treatment of Diabetes Mellitus, J.A.M.A., 187:887, 1964.

Berson, S. A., and R. S. Yalow: Insulin Antagonists, Insulin Antibodies and Insulin Resistance, Am. J. Med., 25:155, 1958.

Cameron, M. P., and M. O'Connor (Eds.): "Aetiology of Diabetes Mellitus and Its Complications," Ciba Foundation Colloquia on Endocrinology, vol. 15, Boston, Little, Brown & Co., 1964.

Cogan, D. G., and T. Kuwabara: Capillary Shunts in the Pathogenesis of Diabetic Retinopathy, Diabetes, 12:293, 1963.

Conn, J. W., and S. S. Fajans: The Prediabetic State: A Concept of Dynamic Resistance to a Genetic Diabetogenic Influence, Diabetes, 11:335, 1962.

Danowski, T. S. (Ed.): "Diabetes Mellitus, Diagnosis and Treatment," American Diabetes Association, New York, 1964.

Field, J. B.: Factors Concerned with Insulin Synthesis and Release, Metabolism, 13:407, 1964.

Freinkel, N., and C. J. Goodner: Insulin Metabolism and Pregnancy, Arch. Int. Med., 109:235, 1962.

Katsoyannis, P. G.: The Synthesis of the Insulin Chains and Their Combination to Biologically Active Material, Diabetes, 13:339, 1964.

Marble, A., and J. Steinke: Physiology and Pharmacology in Diabetes Mellitus: Guiding the Diabetic Patient Through the Surgical Period, Anesthesiology, 24:442, 1963.

Renold, A. E., and G. F. Cahill, Jr.: Diabetes Mellitus, in "The Metabolic Basis of Inherited Disease," J. Stanbury, J. Wyngaarden, and D. Frederickson (Eds.), New York, McGraw-Hill Book Company, Inc., 1966.

Spiro, R. G.: Glycoproteins and Diabetes, Diabetes, 12:223, 1963.

Steinke, J., J. S. Soeldner, R. A. Camerini-Davalos, and A. E. Renold: Studies on Serum Insulin-like Activity in Prediabetes and Early Overt Diabetes, Diabetes, 12:502, 1963.

U.S. Department of Health, Education, and Welfare: "Diabetes Source Book," No. 1168, May, 1964.

Vallance-Owen, J., and P. H. Wright: Assay of Insulin in Blood, Physiol. Rev., 40:219, 1960.

Warren, S., P. M. LeCompte, and M. A. Legg: "The Pathology of Diabetes Mellitus," 4th ed., Philadelphia, Lea & Febiger, 1965.

White, P. (Ed.): "Diabetes," Med. Clin. N. Am., 49, no. 4, 1965.

Wolff, F. W., and W. W. Parmely: Further Observations Concerning the Hyperglycemic Activity of Benzothiadiazines, Diabetes, 13:115, 1964.

Wrenshall, G. A., and B. S. Leibel (Eds.): "On the Nature and Treatment of Diabetes," Proceedings of the 5th Congress of the International Diabetes Federation, Toronto, 1964, Amsterdam, Excerpta Medica Foundation, 1965.

Yalow, R. S., and S. A. Berson: Plasma Insulin Concentrations in Nondiabetic and Early Diabetic Subjects, Diabetes, 9:254, 1960.

87 NONDIABETIC MELITURIA
Alexander Marble

DEFINITION. Nondiabetic melituria includes a variety of conditions in which, in the absence of diabetes mellitus, sugar appears in the urine in amounts large enough to yield positive tests by methods in common use clinically. It is, therefore, not a precisely defined entity. Certain of the conditions appear to be inborn errors of metabolism, and most, though not all, are asymptomatic anomalies with no apparent influence on longevity.

CLASSIFICATION. The nondiabetic meliturias may be classified by whether or not the sugar found in the urine is glucose, as shown in Table 87-1.

GLUCOSURIC MELITURIA

PHYSIOLOGY. Normally, the concentration of glucose in the glomerular filtrate is the same as that in the plasma water. Glucose is reabsorbed in the proximal convoluted tubules, chiefly in their proximal portions. As the concentration of glucose in the plasma increases, the amount of glucose absorbed by the tubules reaches a transfer maximum (Tm_G), which in the normal adult is about 350 mg per minute. When the arterial blood glucose exceeds a certain level (usually about 150 to 180 mg per 100 ml) and the amount of glucose presented to the tubules for reabsorption is greater than the Tm_G, glucose appears in the urine. However, this concentration of blood glucose, often called the *renal threshold,* is not rigidly fixed and is not the sole factor concerned. Changes in the glomerular filtration rate may alter the total quantity of glucose reaching the proximal tubules per unit of time.

RENAL GLUCOSURIA. "True" renal glucosuria with glucose in the urine constantly and persistently even during the fasting state (with blood glucose levels below 100 mg per 100 ml) is a rare condition. Among approximately 50,000 patients with melituria, this type and degree of renal glucosuria was recognized in only 85 cases. However, if the designation of renal glucosuria is made more loosely so as to include situations in which the renal threshold is lower than average but not below 100 mg per 100 ml, the number of cases may be large. Whether or not there is any basic difference in the situations responsible for these varying degrees of lowering of the renal threshold, and whether or not one is justified in considering "true" renal glucosuria an entity, cannot be answered with the information available. Indeed, the cause and nature of the tubular abnormality in renal glycosuria remain obscure.

Renal glucosuria is a condition set apart from diabetes mellitus. Glucosuria is invariably present, and the blood glucose is unquestionably normal both on random sampling and during an oral glucose tolerance test. Measures designed to evaluate carbohydrate utilization yield normal results, and ketosis develops during starvation rather than after dietary excesses. Symptoms characteristic of diabetes are lacking, and without treatment the condition is not progressive.

Renal glucosuria is thought to be inherited as a dominant trait. Although, as stated above, it appears to be unrelated to diabetes mellitus, diabetes seems to occur in the families of persons with renal glucosuria with a frequency greater than expected. There is no evidence that diabetes develops later among persons with renal glucosuria to a greater extent than would be expected in the general population. Care must be taken at the time of original study to exclude those persons in whom glucose tolerance tests yielded borderline results. It is important that persons thought to have renal glucosuria be observed closely, particularly for the first few years, in order to establish with reasonable certainty the diagnosis of a benign condition.

Decreased capacity of the renal tubules to reabsorb glucose may be part of a more extensive disturbance of tubular function, as in the *Fanconi syndrome,* which is characterized also by defective reabsorption of amino acids, phosphate, and bicarbonate (see Chap. 96). Glucosuria may also occur in nephropathies in which there is tubular damage and impaired absorption of glucose. These include certain nephritides and particularly nephrosis resulting from chemical agents such as mercury, uranium salts, and cyanide.

Temporary renal glucosuria occurs frequently in *pregnancy,* particularly during the latter half. The mechanism is poorly understood. The chief responsibility of the physician is to make sure that the condition is benign glucosuria and not diabetes mellitus, which may well have its onset or be recognized first during pregnancy. "Screening" tests should be made by determining the level of blood glucose at 1 hr

Table 87-1. TYPES OF NONDIABETIC MELITURIA

I. Glucosuric melituria
  A. Renal glucosuria
    1. Permanent
      a. "True" renal glucosuria with glucosuria invariably present even during fasting
      b. Associated with other renal tubular defects, as in the Fanconi syndrome
    2. Temporary
      a. Pregnancy
      b. Nephropathy affecting renal tubular absorption
  B. Transient glucosuria in diverse conditions in which there is temporary hyperglycemia considered not to be due to diabetes
II. Nonglucosuric melituria
  A. Pentosuria
  B. Fructosuria
    1. Essential fructosuria
    2. Hereditary fructose intolerance
  C. Lactosuria
  D. Galactosuria
  E. Mannoheptulosuria
  F. Other conditions

after 50 gm glucose, after a meal liberal in carbohydrate, or after the intravenous administration of glucose (see Chap. 86).

Patients with diabetes mellitus may also have a renal threshold lower than normal. When insulin is used in treatment, the dosage must be chosen carefully with special attention to the blood glucose. Parallel studies of blood and urine glucose will furnish a practical guide as to what degree of glucosuria must be allowed to prevent episodes of hypoglycemia.

TRANSIENT GLUCOSURIA IN DIVERSE CONDITIONS. Glucose may appear in the urine transiently and intermittently in a wide variety of conditions, including disorders of the pituitary (acromegaly, pituitary basophilism), adrenals (Cushing's syndrome, pheochromocytoma), and thyroid (hyperthyroidism); stimulation of intracranial nerve centers as with brain tumors, cerebral hemorrhage and injuries of the skull; infections, toxemias, anesthesia, and asphyxia; administration of carbohydrate following starvation ("hunger glucosuria"); following subtotal gastrectomy; acute myocardial infarction; and malignant disease. In most of these conditions hyperglycemia is present temporarily and affords a satisfactory explanation for the glucosuria. However, recent studies and experience suggest that in many of the conditions mentioned, diabetes mellitus is actually present in early or latent form and has been brought to the level of clinical recognition by the stressful situation. Accordingly, patients with temporary hyperglycemia and glucosuria require careful observation and periodic examinations over years of time so that if overt diabetes should develop, it may be recognized early. Such individuals should be encouraged to keep body weight throughout life at a level appropriate for age, height, and body build.

NONGLUCOSURIC MELITURIA

In patients with persistent normoglycemic melituria it is important to ascertain the type of sugar excreted. In most instances the reducing substance will be found to be glucose, but in a number of cases sufficiently great to make special study definitely worthwhile, the sugar is not glucose but pentose, fructose, or some other sugar less commonly encountered. These sugars bear no relation to diabetes mellitus, and their recognition has practical importance as regards eligibility for employment, life insurance, etc., since for the most part these conditions are benign. A systematic study includes the following procedures:

1. Benedict's test, or a modification. This is positive for all sugars found in the urine. The ketoses, particularly fructose, the pentoses, and mannoheptulose, reduce Benedict's solution after a few hours at room temperature (i.e., without heating) and within 10 min at 50 to 60°C.

2. Glucose oxidase test (specific for glucose). Paper strips (Tes-tape and Clinistix) are available for quick testing.

3. Bial (orcinol hydrochloride) reaction. It is positive for pentose.

4. Seliwanoff (resorcinol hydrochloride) reaction. It is positive for fructose.

5. Paper chromatography. This is to confirm the identity of the sugar.

6. Fermentation with baker's yeast. Glucose and fructose are always, galactose usually, lactose occasionally, and pentose and mannoheptulose never fermented.

PENTOSURIA. Essential pentosuria is a benign condition inherited as an autosomal recessive trait. Its rarity is indicated by the fact that among 50,000 patients with melituria, only 11 cases of essential pentosuria have been recognized. It is characterized by the constant presence in the urine of pentose 1-xylulose, in small amounts varying from 1 to 4 Gm daily. With Benedict's method one usually obtains constantly a green test. All reported cases have been in Jews and predominantly in males. Most of the families of pentosurics, at least those in the New York area studied by Lasker, came originally from geographical foci of relatively limited extent, largely Poland and Germany. The condition is harmless, asymptomatic, and unrelated to diabetes. It requires no treatment.

The enzymatic defect concerned in pentosuria appears to be related to the metabolism of glucuronic acid. Normally, uronic acids are converted to a pentose (1-xylulose), then to a sugar alcohol (xylitol), and finally through a series of steps to hexose. In individuals with pentosuria the enzyme responsible for the conversion of 1-xylulose to xylitol apparently is deficient. As a result, 1-xylulose accumulates and is excreted in the urine.

FRUCTOSURIA. Essential Fructosuria. Like pentosuria, this is a benign condition probably inherited as an autosomal recessive trait. All reported cases have been in Jews. Fructosuria appears in males and females with about equal frequency. Fructosuria is rarer than pentosuria. Among 50,000 persons seen with melituria, only 4 cases of fructosuria, 2 in males and 2 in females, were recognized. Two of the patients were brother and sister.

Individuals with fructosuria do not metabolize ingested fructose normally. As a consequence, the concentration of fructose in the blood increases and the sugar is excreted in the urine. During the course of fructose tolerance tests there is a slight to moderate *decrease* in the *blood glucose* concomitant with the rise in blood fructose. This hypoglycemia may be symptomatic.

There is no evidence to suggest a renal defect in fructosuria. Since fructose is primarily metabolized in the liver, the defect responsible for fructosuria has been sought in this organ. Available evidence favors the suggestion of deficient hepatic fructokinase, an enzyme that catalyzes the conversion of fructose to fructose 1-phosphate. However, this idea lacks confirmation by direct enzyme studies in affected persons.

Hereditary Fructose Intolerance. In 1956 Chambers

and Pratt, and in 1957 more extensively Froesch, Prader, et al., described an uncommon and hitherto unrecognized inborn error of metabolism characterized by symptomatic hypoglycemia and vomiting after the ingestion of fructose. In this condition, thought to be inherited as an autosomal recessive trait, the primary defect is a deficiency of fructose 1-phosphate aldolase in the liver. The accumulation of fructose 1-phosphate supposedly inhibits fructose phosphorylation by fructo-kinase and this results in fructosemia and fructosuria. The mechanism for the secondary hypoglycemia is not clear. Indirect evidence favors inhibition of glucose production or release by the liver by fructose 1-phos-phate, although the details of this action have not been clarified.

Treatment consists of elimination of fructose-con-taining foods from the diet. The outlook is excellent if the condition is recognized early in infancy and ap-propriate steps taken. If fructose is not avoided, long-term effects may include mental retardation, liver damage, and renal impairment.

LACTOSURIA. Lactose appears in the urine toward the end of pregnancy and during lactation. It may be considered as a physiologic event and need cause no concern. However, particularly during pregnancy, the finding of sugar in the urine should prompt the determination of the blood glucose at 1 hr after 50 Gm glucose or a meal liberal in carbohydrate in order to detect diabetes if present. Lactose gives a positive test with Benedict's solution. It is best identified by paper chromatography.

GALACTOSURIA. See Chap. 105.

MANNOHEPTULOSURIA. Mannoheptulose appears in the urine of certain persons in small amounts after the eating of avocado. It is of no importance clinically.

OTHER MELITURIAS. Maltosuria has been reported rarely but has not been shown to be of clinical signifi-cance. The finding of sucrose, or cane sugar, in the urine has been reported only rarely, except, of course, following the administration of this sugar intra-venously, in which case it is promptly excreted, since under these conditions there is no provision in the body for hydrolyzing it to simpler sugars. There is room for reasonable doubt whether there is such a condition as spontaneous sucrosuria, although there are a few reports of it in the literature. In reported cases the specific gravity of the urine reached values as high as 1.070. One must be on guard for cases of deception in which patients add cane sugar to urine brought for examination, not realizing that sucrose will not reduce Benedict's solution. An unusually high specific gravity of the urine leads one to think of the possibility of sucrose in the urine.

REFERENCES

Lasker, M.: Mortality of Persons with Xyloketosuria, Hu-man Biol., 27:294, 1955.

Marble, A.: Nondiabetic Melituria, pp. 717–738, in E. P. Joslin, H. F. Root, P. White, and A. Marble: "The Treatment of Diabetes Mellitus," 10th ed., Philadel-phia, Lea & Febiger, 1959.

Stanbury, J. B., J. B. Wyngaarden, and D. S. Frederick-son: "The Metabolic Basis of Inherited Disease," New York, McGraw-Hill Book Company, Inc., 1960; see chapters on Pentosuria, p. 121, Fructosuria, p. 144, and Renal Glycosuria, p. 1246.

Froesch, E. R., H. P. Wolf, H. Baitsch, A. Prader, and A. Labhart: Hereditary Fructose Intolerance. An Inborn Defect of Hepatic Fructose-1-phosphate Splitting Al-dolase, Am. J. Med., 34:151, 1963.

Cornblath, M., I. M. Rosenthal, S. H. Reisner, S. H. Wybregt, and R. K. Crane: Hereditary Fructose In-tolerance, New England J. Med., 269:1271, 1963.

88 HYPERINSULINISM AND HYPOGLYCEMIA

Stefan S. Fajans and George W. Thorn

Introduction

The maintenance of a constant blood glucose level is an essential part of homeostasis. The blood glucose level at any given time reflects the balance of two groups of physiologic processes: (1) those which add glucose to the blood, namely, (*a*) mobilization of glucose from glycogen stores, (*b*) formation of carbo-hydrate from nonglucose sources (gluconeogenesis), and (*c*) absorption of ingested carbohydrate; and (2) those which remove glucose from the blood, namely, utilization of glucose by liver, adipose tissue, muscle, brain, and other tissues.

CLASSIFICATION. Hypoglycemia may be produced by a variety of factors. In some the mechanism is poorly understood. Hence, a complete classification based on pathologic physiology is difficult. Neverthe-less, the common causes of spontaneous hypoglycemia can be grouped as listed in Table 88-1. From the clinical view, patients with hypoglycemia can be di-vided into two groups, according to the usual relation-ship of hypoglycemia to the fasting or postprandial state. Regardless of etiology, the conditions listed in Table 88-1 interfere with the homeostatic mechanism, which regulates the blood glucose level. Such inter-ference may take place at different levels, even if the underlying cause of hypoglycemia is a single one. For example, in patients with functioning islet cell tumors, hypoglycemia is the result not only of increased glu-cose uptake in insulin-sensitive tissues and decreased hepatic glucose output but also of decreased inflow to the liver of substrates needed for gluconeogenesis. For example, the mobilization of amino acids from muscle is reduced.

CLINICAL PICTURE. The clinical symptoms and signs of hypoglycemia are the same regardless of the under-lying cause. The symptoms which occur in any given

Table 88-1. ETIOLOGIC CLASSIFICATION OF
SPONTANEOUS HYPOGLYCEMIA

I. Organic hypoglycemia
   A. Pancreatic islet cell tumor, functioning
   B. Nonpancreatic tumors associated with hypoglycemia
   C. Anterior pituitary hypofunction
   D. Adrenocortical hypofunction
   E. Acquired extensive liver disease
II. Hypoglycemia due to specific hepatic enzyme defect
   A. Glycogen storage diseases
   B. Hereditary fructose intolerance
   C. Galactosemia
   D. Familial fructose and galactose intolerance
III. Functional hypoglycemia
   A. Reactive functional
   B. Reactive secondary to mild diabetes
   C. Alimentary hyperinsulinism
   D. "Idiopathic hypoglycemia" of infancy and childhood
   E. Alcohol and poor nutrition
IV. Exogenous hypoglycemia
   A. Iatrogenic ⎫
   B. Factitious ⎭ insulin or sulfonylurea compounds

patient vary with the degree and the rate of decline of blood glucose levels and with the variable and individual susceptibility of the underlying state of the central and autonomic nervous systems. Symptoms associated with a rapid decline in blood glucose levels are due in part to activation of the autonomic nervous system and the ensuing release of epinephrine. These symptoms are sweating, shakiness, trembling, tachycardia, anxiety, nervousness, weakness, fatigue, hunger, nausea, and vomiting. Other symptoms of hypoglycemia result from decreased uptake of glucose and decreased utilization of oxygen by the brain and usually occur when the decline in blood glucose levels is slow and/or when hypoglycemia is severe or prolonged. These symptoms are headache, visual disturbances, lethargy, yawning, faintness, restlessness, and difficulty with speech and thinking. Other manifestations may be agitation, mental confusion, somnolence, stupor, prolonged sleep, loss of consciousness, and coma. Twitching, convulsions, "epilepsy," and bizarre neurologic signs, motor as well as sensory in nature, may occur. Repeated hypoglycemic episodes may lead to loss of intellectual ability and personality changes characterized by outbursts of temper or queer, bizarre, and psychotic behavior. Extensive and permanent mental or neurologic damage may result from frequent and prolonged episodes of hypoglycemia.

FUNCTIONING ISLET CELL TUMORS

PATHOLOGY. Approximately 90 per cent of functioning islet cell tumors are benign adenomas; approximately 10 per cent are definitely malignant with identified metastases. Hyperplasia of the islet cells has not been proved to occur in adults. Functioning islet cell tumors may be diagnosed at any age, with a majority of cases occurring between thirty and sixty years. Benign islet cell adenomas vary in size from 0.14 to 15 cm in diameter, but the majority are between 0.5 and 3.0 cm. They are usually encapsulated, firmer than the normal pancreas, highly vascular, purplish and occasionally whitish in color, and they present an irregular surface. They are found to be equally distributed throughout the head, body, and tail of the pancreas. Benign adenomas of islet cell tissue rarely occur outside the pancreas. Multiple adenomas are found in approximately 5 to 10 per cent of cases. Multiple adenomas of islet cells may be associated with adenomas of the pituitary, parathyroids, and other endocrine glands and with peptic ulceration. In recent years it has been emphasized that this association frequently has a familial basis. A family history of diabetes has been found also in 25 to 30 per cent of patients with functioning islet cell tumors.

CLINICAL PICTURE. Symptoms of hypoglycemia due to islet cell adenoma may develop insidiously, with periodic hypoglycemic attacks becoming more frequent and more severe. Fasting and exercise precipitate attacks. Attacks usually occur in the early morning hours, during the longest daily fasting period, or they may occur in late afternoon, especially if the noon meal is missed. Symptoms may also occur 2 to 5 hr after meals. Symptoms and signs secondary to decreased cerebral oxygen utilization usually predominate over symptoms secondary to hyperepinephrinemia. The pattern of symptoms is usually repetitive in the same patient, but it may differ from patient to patient. Many patients learn to avert symptoms by taking frequent feedings, including a feeding at 2:00 or 3.00 A.M. Obesity may thereby result. Chronic hypoglycemia may not only produce profound personality changes but may result also in damage to anterior horn cells of the spinal cord, with progressive muscular atrophy.

DIAGNOSIS. A typical symptomatic attack with demonstrated hypoglycemia and relief of symptoms and signs by administration of glucose constitute the diagnostic criteria outlined by Whipple. This *triad of Whipple* is not specific for patients with functioning tumors of the pancreas, as it may occur in patients with other types of hypoglycemia. The level of the overnight fasting blood glucose is usually below normal. Prolonged fasting is the most helpful diagnostic procedure and will cause a fall in blood sugar below 30 to 35 mg per 100 ml (true blood glucose method). In the majority of cases, a typical attack with associated hypoglycemia can be induced within the first 24 hr of fasting. If hypoglycemia and typical symptoms are not induced, fasting should be prolonged for up to 72 hr, at which time the patient should be exercised vigorously. In patients with insulinomas exercise produces a further fall in blood sugar levels, but it produces a rise in blood glucose in patients with functional hyperinsulinism.

The intravenous tolbutamide test is valuable in the

differential diagnosis of spontaneous hypoglycemia. After blood for a fasting blood glucose determination is obtained, 1 Gm sodium tolbutamide dissolved in 20 ml distilled water is injected intravenously over 2 min. Subsequently blood levels of glucose are determined every 15 min for the first hour and every 30 min during the second and third hours of the test. If plasma levels of insulin can be obtained during the test (see below), blood samples for insulin assay should be obtained every 10 min during the first half-hour after administration of tolbutamide. The greatest usefulness of the test is in ruling out the diagnosis of insulinoma. It enables one to rule out insulinoma with confidence in patients suspected of having functional hyperinsulinism but whose history is unusual or in whom fasting blood glucose levels are in the lower range of normal. In such patients a normal 3-hr intravenous tolbutamide test (return of blood glucose to 70 per cent or more of fasting blood sugar level) may obviate hospitalization and determination of blood glucose during prolonged fasting. In patients suspected of harboring insulinoma the test can be used for confirmation, but it should be carefully performed with the patient in the hospital. Tolbutamide-induced hypoglycemia persisted for 3 hr in 50 of 55 patients subsequently proved to have insulinomas. In these 55 patients fasting blood sugar levels were 50 mg per 100 ml or above. The lower the fasting blood sugar, the more frequently will the test have to be terminated early because of severe neurologic symptoms. False positive responses can occur in association with severe liver disease, alcoholic hypoglycemia, idiopathic hypoglycemia of infancy, severe undernutrition, and azotemia. They also may occur in some patients with nonpancreatic tumors and associated hypoglycemia, particularly in those patients in whom blood sugar levels decrease rapidly on fasting. In contrast, no false positive responses have occurred in patients with functional hyperinsulinism, diabetes mellitus with reactive hypoglycemia, or patients without spontaneous hypoglycemia. Obviously the test is of little help if the fasting blood glucose level is very low.

Assays of blood insulin (Chap. 86) in conjunction with the intravenous tolbutamide test may be valuable in diagnosing insulinoma. The finding of excessive increases in plasma insulin levels within the first 30 min after intravenous administration of tolbutamide (1) increases the specificity of this test in patients with insulinoma, (2) increases the usefulness of the test in patients with low fasting blood sugar levels, and (3) may differentiate insulinoma patients from patients with false positive blood glucose responses. However, an increase in plasma levels of insulin in the high normal range after intravenous tolbutamide does not rule out the existence of an insulinoma.

Elevated fasting levels of plasma insulin in peripheral blood are found in only two-thirds of patients with functioning islet cell tumors. Thus, diagnosis of insulinoma is strengthened by an elevated fasting insulin level, but a normal level does not rule out this diagnosis. When fasting insulin levels are measured daily for several days in the same patient, an elevated level can frequently be found in at least one specimen. A plasma insulin level in the normal range associated with a fasting blood sugar level in the hypoglycemic range may also be significant. An elevated fasting level of plasma insulin is not specific for insulinoma, as it has also been reported in one patient with a large fibrosarcoma and in patients with galactosemia and familial fructose and galactose intolerance.

Sensitivity to leucine may be useful diagnostically. In adult patients a large decrease in blood glucose (over 25 mg per 100 ml) and a large increase in plasma insulin after administration of leucine strongly suggest diagnosis of an insulinoma. In childhood, sensitivity to leucine does not differentiate between idiopathic hypoglycemia and insulinoma. Severe leucine hypoglycemia will also be obtained in factitious hypoglycemia due to surreptitious administration of sulfonylureas, since profound sensitivity to leucine hypoglycemia can be produced in normal subjects by pretreatment with such compounds. A negative response to leucine does not rule out the existence of an insulinoma.

The oral glucose tolerance test (Chap. 86) may give a relatively flat curve with rapid return of the blood glucose into the hypoglycemic range due to excessive insulin release from the tumor in response to a rising concentration of blood glucose. Occasionally a high plateau curve may be found due to factors counterregulatory to chronic hypoglycemia, such as excessive secretion of growth hormone and possibly glucagon, and normal or subnormal release of insulin from the tumor in response to a rising blood glucose level. The intravenous glucose tolerance test with calculation of an index of glucose utilization is also of limited usefulness, as variable results are obtained in patients with functioning islet cell tumors.

TREATMENT. When the diagnosis of functioning islet cell tumor is made, relief of hypoglycemia by early surgery is indicated to prevent any further damage to the central nervous system and to prevent obesity, which makes surgical management more difficult. After excision of the adenoma or subtotal pancreatectomy to find the adenoma, the patient is usually cured except in cases of multiple tumors or unlocated tumors in the head of the pancreas.

Glucocorticoids may be useful as an adjunct in the preoperative preparation of patients with insulinomas or in patients with persistent hypoglycemia following unsuccessful surgery. Cortisone, 100 to 200 mg per day, may be required preoperatively, but, of course, continued administration at this level will lead to increased obesity and signs of Cushing's syndrome.

The surgical approach to insulinomas may be complicated by difficulty in identifying the tumor, by difficulty encountered in "shelling out" completely all tumor tissue, and by the fact that multiple tumors are not at all uncommon. In the absence of a definite insulinoma resection of the tail and body of the pancreas is justified, as a significant proportion of tumors are located in these areas. Difficulty in shelling out the complete tumor is undoubtedly a significant factor in tumor recurrence. In approximately 20 per cent of cases diagnosed histologically as carcinoma, follow-up observations have failed to reveal a recurrence of symptoms or tumor for several years.

Patients with nonresectable metastatic islet cell tumors present a management problem, as their hypoglycemia may be so severe as to respond only poorly to oral and even intravenous glucose administration. In these the use of glucocorticoids is valuable. The toxicity of alloxan has prevented its use as a more specific agent. However, recently it has been noted that certain antihypertensives or compounds of the benzothiadiazine type induce hyperglycemia, partly by inhibiting pancreatic insulin release; their use as antihypoglycemic agents is under investigation.

NONPANCREATIC TUMORS ASSOCIATED WITH HYPOGLYCEMIA

Severe hypoglycemia has been reported in more than 85 patients harboring nonpancreatic tumors of mesothelial, epithelial, or endothelial origin. Most of these tumors are mesothelial in type and are classified as fibromas, sarcomas, or fibrosarcomas. They are usually situated in the thorax, the retroperitoneal space, or the pelvis. They may be attached to the diaphragm or found within the liver. Other cases of nonpancreatic tumors associated with severe hypoglycemia include 28 patients with primary hepatic carcinoma, 9 patients with carcinoma of the adrenal cortex, 4 patients with gastrointestinal carcinomas, 2 patients with pseudomyxoma peritonei, and 2 patients with bronchogenic carcinoma. The common clinical characteristics of these tumors, particularly of the fibrosarcomas, are their slow growth and their massive size (up to 9 kg). Hypoglycemia disappears after resection or occasionally after irradiation of the tumor. Many theories have been advanced to explain the mechanism by which these tumors cause hypoglycemia. Twelve reports indicate that extracts of tumors from some of these patients contain an insulinlike substance stimulatory in either isolated rat diaphragm or epididymal fat pad systems. Only rarely have these extracts contained immunologically recognizable insulin. An extremely high level of serum insulin has been reported in one other patient with hypoglycemia due to a large fibrosarcoma. It is likely that these tumors synthesize a polypeptide closely related to insulin but which in the majority of instances is not recognized immunologically as insulin. Other theories proposed to explain the hypoglycemia occurring with these tumors are excessive glucose consumption by tumor tissue and release of a factor from tumor that causes increased sensitivity to pancreatic insulin.

OTHER CAUSES FOR FASTING HYPOGLYCEMIA

Although it is infrequent, fasting hypoglycemia may occur in patients with hypofunction of the anterior pituitary (Chap. 80) or hypofunction of the adrenal cortex (Chap. 84). Usually other stigmas of these disorders enable one to make a diagnosis.

Alcohol ingestion superimposed upon an inadequate dietary intake can precipitate acute hypoglycemia. Blood glucose levels as low as 10 or 20 mg per 100 ml have been observed. Inhibition of gluconeogenesis is primarily responsible for hypoglycemia in conjunction with depletion of liver glycogen stores.

Occasionally diffuse hepatic disease (Chap. 190) may be associated with hypoglycemia. Very seldom fasting hypoglycemia can be traced to a glycogen storage disease (Chap. 104) or to galactosemia (Chap. 105).

In children the most common type of fasting hypoglycemia is that classified as *idiopathic hypoglycemia of infancy and childhood*. This entity is probably heterogeneous. Fasting hypoglycemia may begin in early postnatal life or in the first two or three years of life. The hypoglycemia may be mild and intermittent or more persistent and severe. Usually by seven to nine years of age these children "outgrow" the occurrence of hypoglycemia. Differentiation from functioning islet cell tumor is most difficult, although the occurrence of insulinoma is rare in this age group.

POSTPRANDIAL HYPOGLYCEMIA
REACTIVE FUNCTIONAL HYPOGLYCEMIA

This condition of functional hyperinsulinism occurs almost uniformly in patients with emotional problems and is thought to be due to excessive secretion of insulin in response to a normal rise of blood glucose following meals. The diagnosis is suspected by a history of hypoglycemic symptoms occurring 2 to 4 hr after ingestion of a meal rich in carbohydrates, and it is confirmed by an oral glucose tolerance test extended for 4 or 5 hr, blood samples being obtained at half-hour intervals. It is not unusual in such patients to find blood glucose levels of 30 or 40 mg per 100 ml between the second and fourth hour of the test.

However, the usual symptoms produced by reactive hypoglycemia are transitory and often subside spontaneously in 15 to 30 min. Weakness, hunger, inward trembling, sweating, and tachycardia are the most common symptoms in these patients. Loss of consciousness or convulsions do not occur, and the severity of symptoms is not progressive. In patients with functional hyperinsulinism attacks are more frequent when emotional stress and anxiety are greater. A 72-hr fast is well tolerated, and the concentration of blood glucose rarely drops below 45 mg per 100 ml. The intravenous tolbutamide test is normal. A family history for diabetes mellitus is usually absent.

In some patients with advanced cerebrovascular disease, reactive functional hypoglycemia may be the trigger which initiates a cerebral ischemic episode and its subsequent potential chain of events. Similarly, in patients with a hypersensitive carotid sinus or with postural hypotension, the same procedures that do not induce the vascular response at other times may do so during an episode of reactive hypoglycemia. Likewise, there are a number of patients with ectopic tachycardias of various types in which an episode of reactive hypoglycemia is either the sole "trigger" initiating the attacks, which is quite rare, or one of several "triggers," which is quite common. Episodes of reactive hypoglycemia may precipitate attacks of angina as well as bouts of acute pulmonary edema in predisposed cardiac patients. For this small but important group of patients serious cerebral and cardiovascular complications may be minimized by *recognizing* the possible role that reactive functional hypoglycemia may play as an initiating factor.

TREATMENT. The distressing symptoms experienced by patients with functional hypoglycemia may be prevented by a diet low in carbohydrate and high in protein, with adequate fat to maintain caloric requirements. The diet is divided into three to six feedings, with protein and carbohydrate proportions divided equally among the meals. In patients with a history suggestive of reactive hypoglycemia but in whom the diagnosis cannot be substantiated by a glucose tolerance test, diet therapy may be tried. An important approach is to improve the psychologic and emotional status of the patient with functional hyperinsulinism. In this regard the use of sedatives such as Phenobarbital, 30 mg at 10:00 A.M., 3:00 P.M., and bedtime, as well as tranquilizers such as Meprobamate, 200 mg two to three times daily, may prove useful. The prognosis is good, as usually it is a self-limiting disease within a few months or years.

REACTIVE HYPOGLYCEMIA SECONDARY TO MILD DIABETES

This condition has to be distinguished from reactive functional hypoglycemia, for both the underlying mechanism and the prognosis are different. Whereas in patients with reactive functional hypoglycemia the pancreatic insulin release is thought to be excessive but well-timed in response to the rising postprandial blood glucose, in patients with mild diabetes the insulin release is delayed. It is not until the blood glucose rises to frank diabetic levels that insulin is secreted in excess. Measurements of serum insulin during glucose tolerance tests in such patients have demonstrated that relatively large amounts of insulin are released, albeit late; the blood glucose then decreases from diabetic to normal levels and further to hypoglycemic levels. This type of hypoglycemic response is most likely to occur between the third and the fifth hours. It is apparent that these patients have only mild diabetes, as endogenous insulin is available and

their fasting blood glucose is within normal limits. Their carbohydrate intolerance can only be detected by a postprandial blood glucose determination or an oral glucose tolerance test. Frequently there is a family history of diabetes mellitus.

Treatment consists of a diabetic diet with frequent feedings. Weight reduction in the obese patient may normalize glucose tolerance, with disappearance of reactive hypoglycemia. Contrary to the relatively benign prognosis of reactive functional hypoglycemia, the disorder is not self-limiting and such patients may eventually progress to a more advanced state of insulin deficiency and the clinical syndrome of diabetes mellitus (Chap. 86).

ALIMENTARY HYPOGLYCEMIA

In patients with gastroenterostomy or subtotal gastrectomy, hypoglycemia is due to excessive insulin release in response to excessive postprandial hyperglycemia (alimentary hyperinsulinism). The diagnosis is made by history of abdominal surgery, an *abnormal oral glucose tolerance test* with elevation of the peak blood glucose level, but a *normal intravenous glucose tolerance test.*

OTHER CAUSES OF POSTPRANDIAL HYPOGLYCEMIA

Leucine sensitivity in the adult is extremely rare. Approximately 70 per cent of patients with functioning islet cell tumors and 30 per cent of patients with idiopathic hypoglycemia of infancy and childhood may be sensitive to leucine. Recently, hypoglycemia following the ingestion of fructose has also been described, due to an inborn error of metabolism in which there is a deficiency of the enzyme hepatic fructose 1-phosphate aldolase. It is very infrequent.

EXOGENOUS HYPOGLYCEMIA

The possibility of factitious hyperinsulinism as a result of surreptitious administration of insulin or sulfonylureas should always be considered, particularly in nurses, other medical personnel, and relatives of diabetic patients. If self-administration of insulin is suspected, presence of *insulin antibody in serum* from such patients may point to the proper diagnosis, provided there is no history of previous insulin administration.

REFERENCES

Conn, J. W., and H. S. Seltzer: Spontaneous Hypoglycemia, Am. J. Med., 19:460, 1955.

Crain, E. L., Jr., and G. W. Thorn: Functioning Pancreatic Islet Cell Adenomas: A Review of the Literature and Presentation of Two New Differential Tests, Medicine, 28:427, 1949.

DiGeorge, A. M., and V. H. Auerbach: Leucine-induced Hypoglycemia: A Review and Speculations, Am. J. Med. Sci., 240:792, 1960.

Dormandy, T. L., and R. J. Porter: Familial Fructose and Galactose Intolerance, Lancet, 1:1189, 1961.

Fajans, S. S., J. M. Schneider, D. E. Schteingart, and J. W. Conn: The Diagnostic Value of Sodium Tolbutamide in Hypoglycemic States, J. Clin. Endocrinol. & Metab., 21:371, 1961.

Fajans, S. S., R. F. Knopf, J. C. Floyd, Jr., L. Power, and J. W. Conn: The Experimental Induction in Man of Sensitivity to Leucine Hypoglycemia, J. Clin. Invest., 42:216, 1963.

Field, J. B., H. Keen, P. Johnson, and B. Herring: Insulin-like Activity of Nonpancreatic Tumors Associated with Hypoglycemia, J. Clin. Endocrinol. & Metab. 23:1229, 1963.

Floyd, J. C., Jr., S. S. Fajans, R. F. Knopf, and J. W. Conn: Plasma Insulin in Organic Hyperinsulinism: Comparative Effects of Tolbutamide, Leucine and Glucose, J. Clin. Endocrinol. & Metab., 24:747, 1964.

Frantz, V. K.: Tumors of the Pancreas, sec. 7, fasc. 27 and 28, pp. F 27-142–F 27-149, in "Atlas of Tumor Pathology," Washington, D.C., Armed Forces Institute of Pathology, 1959.

Freinkel, N., D. L. Singer, R. A. Arky, S. J. Bleicher, J. B. Anderson, and C. K. Silbert: Alcohol Hypoglycemia: I. Carbohydrate Metabolism of Patients with Clinical Alcohol Hypoglycemia and the Experimental Reproduction of the Syndrome with Pure Ethanol, J. Clin. Invest., 42:1112, 1963.

Froesch, E. R., H. P. Wolf, H. Baitsch, A. Prader, and A. Labhart: Hereditary Fructose Intolerance: An Inborn Defect of Hepatic Fructose-1-Phosphate Splitting Aldolase, Am. J. Med., 34:151, 1963.

Samols, E., and V. Marks: Insulin Assay in Insulinomas, Brit. Med. J., 1:507, 1963.

Steinke, J., J. S. Soeldner, and A. E. Renold: Measurement of Small Quantities of Insulin-like Activity in Rat Adipose Tissue. IV. Serum Insulin-like Activity and Tumor Insulin Content in Patients with Functioning Islet Cell Tumors, J. Clin. Invest., 42:1322, 1963.

89   DISEASES OF THE TESTES

George W. Thorn and John F. Crigler

History

Androgen deficiency resulting from loss of testicular tissue was undoubtedly recognized by prehistoric man, as was the associated sterility; indeed, testicular tissue was recommended for impotence over 30 centuries ago. This dual function of the testes, as both the site of spermatogenesis and the primary site of male hormone production, was clearly defined in the middle of the nineteenth century when Berthold returned to the capon the characteristics, both physical and behavioral, of the cockerel by testicular grafts and when his contemporaries, the anatomists von Kolliker, Leydig, Sertoli, and Schweigger-Seidel, defined the morphology of the gland. They recognized the spermatogonia, spermatids, the Sertoli (or sustentacular) cells, and cells located interstitially between the tubules (the Leydig or interstitial cells).

The tropic role played by the anterior pituitary gland in the development and maintenance of testicular function was demonstrated by Smith and Engle in 1927, and several years later Butenandt isolated androsterone from male urine. By 1935, testosterone had been both chemically synthesized from cholesterol and isolated in crystalline form from bull testes. In addition, it was conclusively shown to be the most significant natural androgenic material.

DEVELOPMENT

EMBRYOGENIC. In the fourth to sixth week of fetal development, the primitive genital ridge differentiates into cortical and medullary components. If the sperm bears a Y chromosome, the embryo is a genotypic male (XY) and its destiny is to be a phenotypic male. Normally, in the presence of this genotypic pattern, the primitive interstitial cells direct somatic development along masculine lines, the cortical component of the gonad atrophies, and the medullary component develops into fetal seminiferous tubules. Assuming normal production of fetal masculinizing hormone(s), the male infant develops a normal infantile male soma with persistence of the Wolffian system, atrophy of the Mullerian system, and complete closure of the urogenital sulcus except for the urinary meatus at the end of the phallus. If the sperm bears an X chromosome, the embryo is genotypically female (XX), the medullary component of the gonad atrophies, and the cortical component persists as the future ovary. More important, in the absence of the masculinizing factors of the primitive interstitial cells, presumably evoked by the presence of a Y chromosome, normal female somatic development takes place with the formation of the upper part of the vagina, uterus, and fallopian tubes from the Mullerian ducts, regression of the Wolffian system, and persistence of a small genital tubercle and unfused labroscrotal folds.

POSTNATAL. Shortly after birth, the testes are approximately 1 cm in length and weigh but 0.5 Gm each. The interstitial cells, active during uterine life as a result of chorionic gonadotropin, undergo dedifferentiation and remain quiescent or semiquiescent until puberty, when further alterations occur. In childhood, however, the testes may change in location at any time, from the abdominal cavity into the scrotum. The age at which this descent takes place is highly variable, occurring most often in utero but occasionally as late as 15 or 16 years after birth. During adolescence, each testis increases 4 to 5 cm in length and 15 to 20 Gm in weight as a result chiefly of changes in the size of the seminiferous tubules under stimulation of pituitary follicle-stimulating hormone (FSH). Subsequently, luteinizing hormone (LH) induces interstitial cell differentiation with the production of male sex hormones, genital enlargement, and the development of secondary sexual characteristics. Mature male genitalia vary considerably in size. Normal function, including demonstrated fertility, has been noted when testes were less than half the mean size.

ABERRATIONS IN EMBRYONIC DEVELOPMENT. When the interstitial cells in the genotypic male (XY) fail to develop or function, the genital ducts and external genitalia then differentiate according to the female pattern. If gonadal tissue is absent (gonadal dysgenesis, often genotypic XO), both internal and external genitalia may be entirely female. A similar total lack of masculinization of the external genitalia can occur in genotypic males (XY) who have histologically normal-appearing testes (syndrome of testicular feminization). The latter appears to represent a functional defect in either the metabolism (production or degradation) of fetal masculinizing hormone(s) or in the response of tissues to them. Indeed, the feminization in these patients may be so complete that the abnormality is only discovered later in life because of primary amenorrhea, the absence of sexual hair (reported as an associated anomaly in approximately one-third of the patients), or the presence of inguinal masses in an otherwise apparent female. Surgical exploration of these patients usually reveals absence of uterus and fallopian tubes and presence of testes showing clumps of Leydig cells but small undeveloped seminiferous tubules.

Partial failure in the elaboration of fetal masculinizing hormone results in ambiguous external genitalia and variations in internal genitalia depending upon the nature and degree of the gonadal defect and the developmental stage at which it occurred. This type of gonadal defect can produce defects in genital development ranging from the complete feminization just described above through failure of fusion of the labioscrotal folds with some enlargement of the genital tubercle to encompass males with mild degrees of hypospadius. In addition, animal experiments have demonstrated that many of the effects of fetal masculinizing hormone occur locally in the gland, probably by direct diffusion of hormone into the tissues. Thus, unilateral damage or developmental abnormalities of the fetal gonad (including the formation of an ovotestis) may produce feminization on one side and masculinization on the other resulting in the findings described in patients with true hermaphroditism. In an analogous fashion and to complete the picture, since development proceeds along female lines unless directed by the masculinizing hormone, administration of androgenic or potentially androgenic agents to a pregnant female may induce in a genotypic female fetus various degrees of irreversible masculinization. Fortunately, the defects so induced seem limited to the external genitalia (clitoral hypertrophy and labioscrotal fusion) so that if the condition is recognized, an appropriate sex assignment can be made and the genital abnormality corrected by surgery.

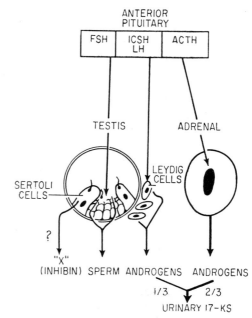

Fig. 89-1. Scheme showing anterior pituitary–testis relationship.

Physiology

The role of fetal testicular function on genital development has been described above. The precise interrelationships of hypothalamic-pituitary and testicular functions (Fig. 89-1) at adolescence and in adult life are not completely defined. The hormone elaborated by the anterior pituitary gland that appears to induce development and then functional maintenance of the testicular interstitial (Leydig) cells has been appropriately labeled interstitial cell–stimulating hormone (ICSH) and reportedly is identical to LH in the female. Pituitary FSH stimulates development of the seminiferous tubules. It is generally accepted that the Leydig cell is the principal site of steroid hormonal (testosterone plus others) synthesis. The role of the Leydig cell and possibly that of LH in hormonal production in human beings has been suggested by observations on so-called "fertile eunuchs," patients who show spermatogenesis but lack masculine secondary sexual changes and in whom testicular biopsies show an absence of Leydig cells. Production of estrogens by the testes has been demonstrated, and it has been suggested that they may arise from Sertoli cells and serve to inhibit pituitary production of gonadotropins.

Production of androgenic hormones by the testes at puberty effects the numerous somatic changes noted in the adolescent male. These include enlargement and increased pigmentation of the external genitalia, hypertrophy of the larynx with lowering of the voice, a generalized increase in hirsutism with growth of a beard and a typical masculine pelvic escutcheon and forehead hair line, enlargement of the prostate and seminal vesicles, and an overall increase in muscular development. Metabolic balance studies demonstrate

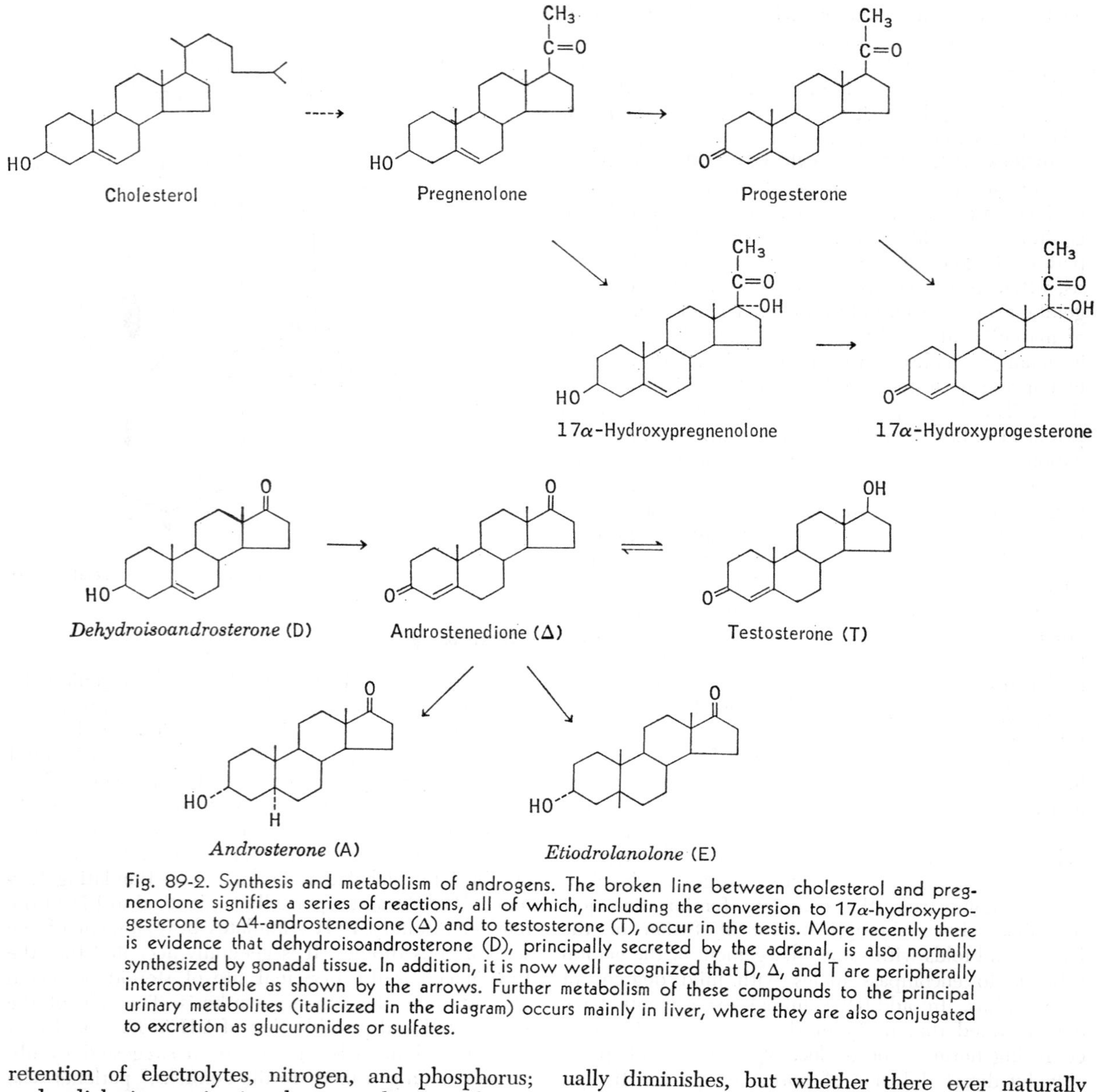

Fig. 89-2. Synthesis and metabolism of androgens. The broken line between cholesterol and pregnenolone signifies a series of reactions, all of which, including the conversion to 17α-hydroxyprogesterone to Δ4-androstenedione (Δ) and to testosterone (T), occur in the testis. More recently there is evidence that dehydroisoandrosterone (D), principally secreted by the adrenal, is also normally synthesized by gonadal tissue. In addition, it is now well recognized that D, Δ, and T are peripherally interconvertible as shown by the arrows. Further metabolism of these compounds to the principal urinary metabolites (italicized in the diagram) occurs mainly in liver, where they are also conjugated to excretion as glucuronides or sulfates.

retention of electrolytes, nitrogen, and phosphorus; and radiologic examination shows acceleration of osseous development with subsequent epiphyseal fusion.

The testes in the normal male elaborate between 6 and 10 mg testosterone daily. Approximately half this amount appears in the urine as measurable 17-keto-steroids, primarily androsterone and etiocholanolone (Fig. 89-2). The total 17-ketosteroid daily excretion for males, which includes the steroid derivatives from the testes and adrenal cortex, amounts to approximately 13 to 20 mg, of which approximately 5 mg is derived from the testes and the remainder from the adrenals. Mean plasma testosterone concentrations in young adult males are approximately 0.8 μg per 100 ml, whereas normal females of similar age show a concentration of 0.05 μg per 100 ml. With increasing age, 17-ketosteroid secretion in the normal man gradually diminishes, but whether there ever naturally occurs a sudden cessation in gonadal function analogous to the female menopause is dubious.

HYPOGONADISM

The clinical term *hypogonadism* refers to failure in interstitial cell function, resulting in decreased or absent production of androgenic hormones. Interstitial cell function may be decreased either by a primary defect in their number or activity or secondarily by a lack of pituitary tropic hormone (LH).

PREPUBERAL HYPOGONADISM. The clinical picture of hypogonadism is directly related to the time of development of androgen deficiency. Prepuberal deficiency results in varying degrees of failure to develop the expected secondary sexual characteristics associated with maturity. Total lack of androgen production by the testes is associated with persistent infantile morphology, a high voice, partial or total lack of facial, axillary, and pubic hair, infantile genitalia, and a barely palpable prostate. Because of lack of osseous maturation, epiphyseal closure is delayed, resulting in a tall "eunuchoid" habitus with long graceful arms and legs and wide hips. Gynecomastia and girdle obesity may also be present. The skin is pale and delicate and may show early wrinkling. Acne is absent.

Prepuberal hypogonadism remains obviously inapparent (unless there are gross physical anomalies of the testes, which may signal pathologic changes at an earlier age) until the expected time of puberty. A total absence of any of the usual changes of adolescence at approximately age fourteen or fifteen suggests that interstitial cell function may be abnormal. However, as in other developmental states, there is a wide range of normal variation so that puberal changes may not be noticeable in some normal boys until the sixteenth year, when voice, genital, and hirsutic changes may begin to be apparent. This delay in adolescent development causes much concern to patient, family, and physician and not infrequently some form of hormonal therapy is given, followed by somatic changes that undoubtedly would have occurred without treatment.

POSTPUBERAL HYPOGONADISM. Postpuberal hypogonadal changes decrease or are minimized when the hypogonadal state develops late in adult life; thus castration of elderly men may cause none of the alterations seen in younger individuals. In the latter, there is usually diminished beard growth and thinning axillary and other body hair. The skin becomes smoother, the prostate atrophies to the point of being barely palpable, and sexual desire and performance wane. The genitalia lose pigmentation and may decrease somewhat in size. The voice does not change, but gynecomastia may appear. In older men none of these changes may be noted; beard and body hair growth usually persist, and there may be no noticeable change in libido or sexual function.

PRIMARY HYPOGONADISM. Primary hypogonadism (not secondary to failure of elaboration of pituitary tropic hormone) may result from numerous causes. It may be present at birth as either a genetic or an embryologic defect, or it may occur at any time later in life as a result of either testicular infections such as mumps, tuberculosis, brucellosis, leprosy, syphilis or following trauma, irradiation, neoplasm, or castration, either surgical or accidental. In this group, besides the obvious physical characteristics of hypogonadism, the patient may excrete excessive quantities of pituitary gonadotropins in the urine. The immature mouse uterine weight assay, which measures both FSH and LH, is used most frequently. In addition, because of lack of testosterone synthesis, there will be a slightly lower excretion of total urinary 17-ketosteroids due to a significant decrease in urinary androsterone and etiocholanolone. This decrease in the

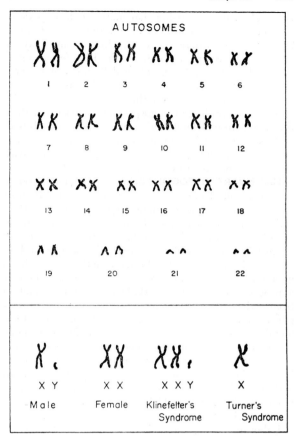

Fig. 89-3. Schematic drawing of 22 pairs of autosomes and aberrations in the number of sex chromosomes as seen in patients with Klinefelter's or Turner's syndrome.

urinary excretion of androgens and their metabolites is often more apparent when the total biologic activity is bioassayed (growth of cockerel's comb, etc.). It should be stated here with emphasis, however, that the patient's own tissues clinically observed frequently provide the most significant assay of androgen production. The following syndrome is an example of primary hypogonadism.

KLINEFELTER'S SYNDROME (SEMINIFEROUS TUBULE DYSGENESIS). Klinefelter, Reifenstein, and Albright described in 1942 a clinical syndrome of hypogonadism that includes gynecomastia, eunuchoidism, elevated urinary gonadotropins, and decreased testicular size associated with hyalinization of the tubules. Barr demonstrated that many of these patients were *chromatin-positive*, exhibiting nuclei similar to those seen in females (see Chap. 55). Culture of marrow cells and leukocytes in vitro in the presence of colchicine has permitted direct chromosomal counting and classification (see Fig. 89-3); and indeed, many patients with the triad described by Klinefelter et al. have been shown to possess an extra sex chromosome, resulting in a karyotypic classification of 22 autosomes plus 2 X chromosomes and 1 Y chromosome (see Chap. 55). Thus, they have 47 instead of 46 chromosomes, and it is therefore not surprising that many of these patients also have various degrees of mental deficiency (similar to mongolism, where the extra chromosome may be autosomal). Some patients with Klinefelter's syndrome, however, lack the clinical findings of gynecomastia, hypoplastic testes, and eunuchoidism and may be discovered only when they appear in a fertility clinic with a finding of oligospermia or aspermia; thus, the spectrum of Klinefelter's syndrome is quite broad, including obviously feminized males on one end and on the other end grossly normal, virilized men with only abnormal microscopic testicular anatomy.

SECONDARY HYPOGONADISM. Secondary hypogonadism results from failure of pituitary elaboration of the necessary tropic hormones, specifically interstitial cell–stimulating hormone. In most cases there is an associated loss of other pituitary tropic hormones resulting in growth failure before adolescence and in decreased thyroid and adrenal function as well as gonadal function at all ages. However, when there is a progressive loss of hypothalamic-pituitary function from either a granulomatous process (sarcoid), neoplasm (chromophobe, astrocytoma, hamartoma, teratoma), or cyst (craniopharyngioma), the first deficiency observed is often in the secretion of gonadotropic hormones, and the patient may therefore appear in the clinic as a case of isolated hypogonadism. In addition, idiopathic deficiency of gonadotropic hormones without demonstrable loss of other hormones occurs not infrequently.

Laboratory tests may demonstrate an absence of pituitary gonadotropins and skull x-ray may reveal enlargement of the sella turcica or erosion of the clinoids. Thyroid and adrenal studies may also reveal clinically unsuspected hypofunction, and visual field examination may show an early involvement of the optic nerves. The following syndromes are examples of secondary hypogonadal states.

FROELICH'S SYNDROME AND THE LAURENCE–MOON–BIEDL SYNDROME. In 1901, Froelich described an obese, hypogonadal boy with signs of a tumor in the hypothalamic area. Since then, Froelich's name has been inappropriately applied to a large group of overweight boys with slightly retarded maturation but without any demonstrated hypothalamic lesion and,

therefore, without any real clinical significance. On the other hand, the Laurence-Moon-Biedl syndrome encompasses a group of congenital malformations (the trait being inherited as a recessive characteristic) including hypogonadism, dwarfism, mental retardation, polydactyly, syndactyly, obesity, retinitis pigmentosa, and diabetes insipidus.

ANDROGEN–ESTROGEN IMBALANCE. This ill-defined group of diseases includes hepatic decompensation with supposed failure in the removal of circulating estrogens, as exemplified by Laennec's cirrhosis, various feminizing tumors of the testes and adrenals with excessive production of estrogens, and, lastly, intentional or unintentional intake of exogenous estrogen. All of these may be associated with decreased sexual function and desire, decreased testicular size, gynecomastia, and loss of hair. The changes, however, are highly variable, depending on the duration and intensity of female hormone exposure and the age and individual characteristics of the patient.

TREATMENT OF HYPOGONADISM. Preparations of testosterone, representing replacement therapy, are administered to hypogonadal males when treatment is indicated. Most commonly used are the long-acting depot injections listed in Table 89-1. The usual method of therapy is to start with a relatively small dose, such as 150 mg, of a depot preparation of testosterone, given intramuscularly every 3 to 4 weeks. The dosage then may be gradually increased to 250 or 300 mg monthly. Excessive acne formation, edema from retention of sodium, and undesirable personality changes all indicate overtreatment, and the dosage should be diminished appropriately.

In patients with hypogonadism in the puberal or prepuberal age group, testosterone administration has been reported to cause pathologic changes in the seminiferous tubules, resulting in azoospermia and sterility. Hence, it must be used cautiously with this group. If hypogonadism is secondary to failure of gonadotropin secretion by the pituitary, a trial on chorionic or pituitary gonadotropins may be indicated, starting with injections of 500 to 1,000 units two or three times weekly, increasing the dosage over a period of several weeks. In most patients this form of therapy will ultimately fail, possibly due to the development of antibodies to the nonhuman origin of commercial gonadotropins. In contrast, a similar schedule of gonadotropin therapy has been suggested for the treatment of undescended testes in the adolescent. In these patients, therapy may prove effective since the course is a self-limited one. A discussion of impotence and libido may be found in Chap. 22 and of sterility in Chap. 91.

Table 89-1. TESTOSTERONE PREPARATIONS COMMONLY USED

Short acting	Dosage
Testosterone proprionate in oil..................	10–25 mg intramuscularly 3 to 5 times per week
Methyltestosterone tablets	10–100 mg by mouth

Long acting	
Testosterone cyclopentyl-proprionate in oil.......	100–300 mg intramuscularly every 3 to 4 weeks
Testosterone enanthate in oil..................	100–300 mg intramuscularly every 3 to 4 weeks
Testosterone phenylacetate, aqueous suspension.....	100–300 mg intramuscularly every 3 to 4 weeks

HYPERGONADISM

The production of excessive quantities of androgenic hormone in the adult male results in little, if any, morphologic or functional change. However, in the child, the somatic changes associated with puberty may be induced at an early age and therefore become clinically apparent (precocious puberty).

Hypergonadism may be due to excessive androgen production from a functioning testicular tumor, the Leydig or interstitial cell carcinoma. Children with these tumors show all the changes associated with puberty, such as increased hair growth and phallic enlargement, and usually have a palpable testicular tumor. However, the presence of the tumor may be difficult to determine if the testes are undescended or if the tumor is extremely active in producing hormone but still very small in size. The urine may contain excessive quantities of biologically active androgen. Because of the marked potency of testosterone, the total 17-ketosteroids may be normal or only slightly increased in the presence of marked androgenicity. Urinary pituitary gonadotropins are absent.

Hypergonadism may also result from an early onset of puberty due to altered hypothalamic-pituitary function. The sequence of development is similar to that observed in adolescence, with enlargement of genitalia, appearance of pubic and axillary hair, deepening of the voice, and appearance of acne and seborrhea occurring in that order and beginning at two to three years of age or earlier. The testes are large for the patient's chronologic age but are in accord with the size expected for the degree of maturity exhibited by the remainder of his somatic development. Gonadotropins may be present in the urine but are not invariably measurable by routine assay procedures. In the early stages, 17-ketosteroids may not be significantly elevated for the patient's chronologic age (in contrast to virilism produced by adrenal abnormalities), but subsequently they increase to levels appropriate for his developmental age. Isosexual precocity of this type in males, although uncommon, is often familial in contrast to the more frequently occurring true precocity in females, from whom a family history of early puberty is seldom obtained. When true precocity occurs in males without a family history, it is almost always associated with space-occupying lesions in the region of the third ventricle (pinealoma, astrocytoma, hamartoma, teratoma, and rarely a craniopharyngioma) (Table 89-2). The continued production of

Table 89-2. CAUSES OF MALE SEX PRECOCITY

Type of precocity	Cause	%
Complete genital precocity, true precocious puberty	Idiopathic	55
	Pineal neoplasm	12
	Cerebral (hypothalamic disease)	13
Incomplete genital precocity, precocious pseudopuberty, dissociated virilization (failure of testes to mature)	Adrenal cortical lesion	16
	Interstitial cell tumor of testis	4

SOURCE: Seckel, and Dorfman and Shipley.

androgens excessive for their age in these patients results in accelerated growth during childhood, followed by early closure of the epiphyses, ending in an adult who frequently is smaller than his contemporaries.

Isosexual precocity in the male may also result from excessive quantities of adrenal androgens. The pattern of accelerated growth and development is similar to that produced by testicular hormones. The testes remain, however, infantile and atrophic; and gonadotropins are invariably absent. The diagnosis is made on the basis of markedly elevated urinary 17-ketosteroids. For further discussion, see Chap. 84.

NEOPLASMS OF THE TESTES

Neoplasms of the testes are relatively uncommon. It is generally believed that they occur more commonly in the cryptorchid testis (1 in 2,000) than in the normal testis (1 in 100,000). They may be classified as follows, in their relative order of frequency:

1. Seminoma (germinoma)
2. Teratocarcinoma
3. Embryonal carcinoma
   a. Chorioepithelioma
4. Teratoma
5. Interstitial cell tumor
6. Fibroma, lipoma, adrenoma, myxoma
7. Unclassified varieties

The incidence of teratocarcinoma is roughly constant throughout life, whereas the incidence of seminoma tends to rise with age. One-year survival is rare for embryonal carcinomas and chorioepitheliomas, not uncommon for teratocarcinomas and teratomas, and the rule for seminomas.

Endocrine changes such as gynecomastia and increased secretion of gonadotropins giving a positive Aschheim-Zondek test result are occasionally seen in chorioepitheliomas as well as in embryonal carcinomas and teratocarcinomas. The endocrine effects of interstitial cell tumors have been discussed.

DIAGNOSIS. The diagnosis is made by palpating a mass, usually firm, smooth, and painless. Neoplasms must be distinguished from the changes induced by tuberculosis or gonorrheal epididymitis from syphilis (usually accompanied by a positive serologic test and a response to specific therapy), and from the various fluid-containing cysts (hydrocele, spermatocele), which may be transilluminated. The diagnosis may be aided also by increased urinary excretion of 17-ketosteroids, estrogens, or gonadotropins; the latter give a positive Aschheim-Zondek test. Rarely, tumor cells may be identified in the semen.

TREATMENT. Surgical removal is always indicated in any tumor of the testes and will usually effect a cure in the benign varieties. If the tumor is malignant, a radical operation followed by irradiation should be employed. X-ray therapy has been shown to effect a cure in the majority of cases of seminoma. Results of therapy may be followed by repeated determinations of the 17-ketosteroids or estrogens or by the Aschheim-Zondek test, if originally positive. Certain testicular tumors, particularly the chorioepitheliomas, have been shown to be exquisitely sensitive to certain antimetabolic agents such as 4-amino-N^{10}-methylpteroylglutamic acid (Methotrexate).

DISEASES OF THE PROSTATE

BENIGN PROSTATIC HYPERTROPHY. This pathophysiologic disorder, which affects a high proportion of elderly men, is a significant cause of dysuria and incontinence (see Chap. 18) and urinary tract obstruction (see Chap. 155). It has also been considered a potentially precancerous lesion. Hormonally, the prostate is significant as a clinical indicator of androgen secretion, since appreciable reduction in prostatic size accompanies either primary or secondary hypogonadism as well as those disorders of liver function characterized by excessive estrogen activity.

CARCINOMA OF THE PROSTATE. Adenocarcinoma of the prostate is one of the most common tumors of men. It is rare before the age of forty, and the incidence rises rapidly with advancing age, occurring microscopically in 10 to 15 per cent of men in the fifth decade and as high as 40 per cent in those in the eighth decade. However, only one-fourth may become clinically apparent before death. Three-fourths of these tumors arise in the posterior lobe. The majority are easily palpable; hence, routine frequent rectal examinations are indicated to demonstrate early and operable tumors. Although the whole gland need not be enlarged, the presence of stony, hard, indurated nodules or masses strongly suggests the presence of an adenocarcinoma. Frequently, there may be an elevation in the "prostatic" fraction of serum acid phosphatase while the tumor is still located within the prostatic capsule, and elevation of this enzyme may serve to differentiate a benign hypertrophic nodule from a malignancy. Once the tumor has spread locally from the gland, and particularly after it has metastasized, total serum acid and alkaline phosphatase may be greatly elevated.

Therapy consists of radical prostatectomy; irradiation by x-ray, radium, or radioactive isotopes (colloidal gold); and estrogen hormonal treatment (especially when metastatic disease develops). Androgens are decreased by orchidectomy and by adrenalectomy or adrenal cortical suppression following cortisone administration (50 to 100 mg cortisone given orally in divided doses); estrogen levels are increased by administering diethylstilbestrol, 10 to 15 mg daily, or the equivalent dosage of other estrogenic products.

REFERENCES

Albert, A., L. O. Underdahl, L. F. Greene, and N. Lorenz: Male Hypogonadism: I, II, III, IV, V, VI, VII, Proc. Staff Meet. Mayo Clinic, 28:409, 557, 698, 1953; 29:131, 317, 368, 1954; 30:31, 1955.

Dorfman, R. I., and R. A. Shipley: "Androgens–Biochemistry, Physiology and Clinical Significance," New York, John Wiley & Sons, Inc., 1956.

Ferguson-Smith, M. A., and A. W. Johnston: Chromosome Abnormalities in Certain Diseases of Man, Ann. Intern. Med., 53:359, 1960.

Howard, R. P., R. C. Sniffen, F. A. Simmons, and F. Albright: Testicular Deficiency: A Clinical and Pathological Study, J. Clin. Endocrinol., 10:121, 1950.

Kleinfelter, H., E. Reifenstein, Jr., and F. Albright: Kleinfelter Syndrome Characterized by Gynecomastia, Aspermatogenesis without A-Leydigism, and Increased Excretion of Follicle-stimulating Hormone, J. Clin. Endocrinol., 2:615, 1942.

Leadbetter, W. F.: Treatment of Testis Tumors Based on Their Pathological Behavior, J.A.M.A., 151:275, 1953.

McCullagh, E. P., J. C. Beck, and C. A. Schaffenburg: A Syndrome of Eunuchoidism with Spermatogenesis: Normal Urinary FSH and Low or Normal ICSH ("Fertile Eunuchs"), J. Clin. Endocrinol. & Metab., 13:489, 1953.

Seckel, H. P. G.: Precocious Sexual Development in Children, Med. Clin. North America, 30:183, 1946.

90 DISEASES OF THE OVARY AND UTERUS

Kendall Emerson, Jr. and John C. Laidlaw

History

The ovulatory function of the ovaries was first described by a Dutch physician, Reinier de Graaf, in 1673. He recognized small fluid blisters, now known as *graafian follicles*, which had succeeded in reaching the surface of the ovaries before ovulation. The hormonal function of the ovaries was first demonstrated in 1896, by the German biologist, Knauer, who showed that ovarian grafts in the dog would prevent the uterine atrophy that follows castration. It was next observed by Marshall and Jolly, that the ovarian secretion which produced estrus differed from that which was formed by the corpus luteum. The presence of estrogens in the follicles was proved by R. T. Frank, and their occurrence in urine was established by Allen and Doisy, who demonstrated the effectiveness of potent urinary extracts in producing estrus in the vaginal mucosa of rodents. This relatively simple biologic assay method became of incomparable help in the isolation and synthesis of estrogenic compounds. In 1929, Butenandt and Doisy and associates isolated estrone in a crystalline form from the urine of pregnant women. In 1930, estriol was identified by Browne in human placentas, and in 1936, MacCorquodale obtained estradiol, the most potent natural estrogen, from ovarian follicular fluid. The progestational activity of the corpus luteum hormone was first demonstrated by Corner and Allen in 1929. Five years later progesterone was isolated and identified simultaneously and independently by Butenandt, Allen, Slotta, and Hartmann.

Embryogenesis

A brief description of the embryologic development of the ovary is of great importance in understanding some of the disorders that may occur in later life.

The mature ovary, like the testis, is basically composed of three primitive cell types: the primordial germ cells and the somatic cortical and medullary cells. The germ cells are found in the genital ridge of the five-week embryo and possess bisexual potential. If the somatic cells contain the female XX chromosomal configuration and lack the male Y chromosome, the somatic cells of the cortex become the dominant cell type, growing in from the adjacent median edge of the mesonephric body to surround the germ cells, determine their future development as oocytes, and become the female-hormone-producing theca and granulosa cells of the future ovary.

The medulla of the ovary shares a common origin with the adrenal cortex in the medial mesonephros, but in the absence of the Y chromosome it is dominated and invaded by the cortex and ultimately concentrated toward the hilus of the ovary. It provides the bulk of the interstitial cells of the prepuberal ovary and probably of the stroma of the adult organ. Recent in-vitro evidence by Savard indicates that under the stimulation of gonadotropic hormones these cells can synthesize androgens in far greater quantities than any other cellular constituents of the ovary and may be the source of the testosterone produced in small amounts by the normal ovary, chiefly at the time of ovulation, and in larger amounts in certain pathologic conditions, to be described later. In the course of the invasion and confinement of the medulla by the cortex, nests of embryonic medullary cells may be sequestered, with the potential to become androgen-producing tumors. With the dominance of the cortex and relative suppression of the medulla, the Mullerian duct system prevails over the Wolffian and the further development of the urogenital system is female.

Physiology

The human ovaries possess three closely related functions: (1) the secretion of estrogenic hormones, primarily growth-promoting agents acting on the uterus, genitalia, breasts, and skeletal bone and essential for the development and maintenance of secondary sex characteristics; (2) the storage of oocytes and their periodic release as ova during ovulation; (3) the formation of the corpus luteum following ovulation, from the theca and granulosa cells of the ovulating follicle. The corpus luteum secretes progesterone, the second ovarian hormone, which stimulates the secretory activity of the uterine endometrium, already primed by estrogen, and suppresses the growth effect of the latter. The net effect of these two hormones is to prepare the uterus for the implantation and nourishment of the fertilized ovum. All three functions of the ovary depend upon a delicately maintained balance between the hypothalamus, the gonadotropins of the anterior pituitary, and the circulating levels of the ovarian hormones themselves.

The manifestations of ovarian estrogen secretion first make their appearance about the age of ten with the development of budding of the nipples and breasts and growth of the bony pelvis. There follows in gradual fashion the growth of pubic hair, thickening and cornification of the vaginal epithelium, and growth of the external and internal genitalia. Pigmentation of the nipples and axillary hair growth appear next, and finally, about the age of thirteen, menstruation begins. The menstrual flow consists of endometrial cells, secretions, and blood. It lasts 3 to 7 days, occurs approximately every 4 weeks, and brings to a conclusion a regularly occurring series of changes in the uterine mucosa. These changes reflect cyclic fluctuations in ovarian estrogen and progesterone secretion. At first the menstrual periods are irregular and anovulatory, but by the middle teens, when full sexual maturation has taken place, ovulation and menstruation occur at regular intervals. All these signs of sexual maturation are maintained through the reproductive period into the forties, when estrogen production diminishes, ovulation and progesterone production cease, and menstruation, after a period of irregularity, gradually disappears. This is the menopause. Thereafter, regressive changes in the breasts and genitalia slowly evolve.

Of the large number of follicles present at puberty, the vast majority degenerate either as primitive follicles or at various stages of development (atretic follicles). With each menstrual cycle many follicles begin to mature, but only one "favored follicle" reaches full maturity, penetrates the surface of the ovary, and discharges its ovum into the peritoneal cavity. This phenomenon, *ovulation*, occurs approximately 2 weeks before onset of menstrual flow. The ovum then finds its way into the fallopian tube and thence is carried to the uterine cavity. There, within a few days, it disintegrates unless it has been fertilized in transit, in which case it implants itself within the uterine mucosa. Following ovulation, the ruptured follicle is transformed into the corpus luteum, a richly vascularized body composed of progesterone- and estrogen-secreting cells. This body reaches maturity about 1 week before the next menstrual period and then, over the course of weeks to months, gradually involutes to a tiny scar (the corpus albicans). If the previously discharged ovum has been fertilized and pregnancy has occurred, the corpus luteum does not regress but becomes larger. This "corpus luteum of pregnancy" continues to secrete progesterone and estrogen until the second half of gestation, when involution occurs in the usual way. The syncytial trophoblasts of the placenta then assume the major responsibility for estrogen and progesterone synthesis.

The maturation of the graafian follicle depends upon

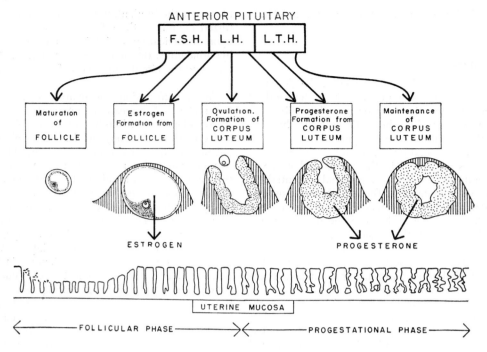

Fig. 90-1. Semidiagrammatic representation of the relation of anterior pituitary gonadotropic hormones to ovarian and uterine changes during the menstrual cycle in normal women.

the anterior pituitary follicle-stimulating hormone (FSH) (Fig. 90-1). This hormone stimulates the growth of the granulosa cells and the production of follicular fluid, which surrounds the ovum. Along with the luteinizing hormone (LH or ICSH), FSH induces the cells of the theca interna to secrete estrogens. Estrogen secretion increases rapidly during the week before ovulation, maintains a plateau over the ensuing 2 weeks, and diminishes rapidly just before menstruation. The increased estrogen secretion is responsible for the proliferative changes that occur in the endometrium during the first half of the menstrual cycle. If fertilization occurs and pregnancy ensues, luteotropin continues to maintain the corpus luteum through the first few months of the gestation period. In this action LTH is aided by the placental secretion of chorionic gonadotropin.

Like all the tropic hormones of the pituitary, the primary initiating stimulus for the release of gonadotropins arises from the neurosecretory neurones of the hypothalamus. The so-called LH and probably FSH "releasing factors" are found in the median eminence and perhaps elsewhere in the hypothalamus and form the connection between the pituitary and the external environment. In many animal species these hypothalamic centers can be activated to induce estrus by sexual stimulation or a variety of other environmental stimuli. What it is that sets the human biologic alarm clock to the spontaneous estrus cycle of 28 days remains one of nature's mysteries.

OVARIAN HORMONES

Ovarian hormones are steroids. The estrogens are characterized chemically by the presence of a benzene ring and a phenolic hydroxyl group, which makes them soluble in alkali, a property used to separate them chemically from the adrenal cortical steroids. Estradiol is the principal and most potent estrogen secreted by the human ovary. Wherever estradiol appears, it is in a reversible equilibrium with its less potent ketone derivative, estrone, and both these steroids are converted irreversibly to the least potent, water-soluble, trihydroxide estriol, by the liver and probably other tissues. Estradiol and estrone circulate in the blood and are selectively concentrated to a high degree in the target organs, the uterus, vagina, and breast, as the free hormone. All three steroids are ultimately conjugated with glucuronic and sulfuric acids by the liver and excreted in the bile and urine. Because of its water solubility estriol is excreted almost entirely in the urine. Only a small portion of the estradiol produced by the ovary has been accounted for by these three metabolites, however. Some 11 different metabolites of estradiol have now been isolated from human urine, mostly in small quantities. When urine is hydrolyzed with acid in the presence of zinc during the proliferative phase of the menstrual cycle, a much greater quantity of biologically active estrogens is obtained than can be accounted for by chemical analysis. This extra biologic activity disappears during the secretory phase of the cycle and is thought to be due to as yet unidentified oxidative products of estrogen metabolism, which may play an important role in stimulating the release of pituitary FSH.

It has recently been shown that estradiol in molecular quantities is capable of speeding up the tricarboxylic acid cycle by catalytic activation of a DPN-linked isocitric dehydrogenase. This activity may be of fundamental importance in its growth-promoting properties. In addition, small doses of estrogens will stimulate pituitary gonadotropins and cause sodium, calcium, phosphorus, nitrogen, and water retention. Undesirable side effects of estrogen administration include painful breasts, uterine bleeding, nausea, and vomiting. The salt and water retention observed with large doses of estrogens may precipitate or aggravate cardiac failure. The specific growth-stimulating properties of these substances for the breast and uterus requires that one be alert to the possibility of malignant changes occurring in these organs during long-term estrogen therapy in women with a genetic predisposition to cancer.

Progesterone bears a striking chemical resemblance to the adrenal cortical steroids. It is largely degraded in the liver, and a small fraction appears in the urine as the inactive pregnanediol glucuronide (Fig. 90-2). The major metabolites of progesterone are unknown. In addition to its effect on the endometrium, progesterone decreases uterine motility and activates the secretory tissue of the breast. No undesirable side effects accompany progesterone administration. Such is not the case, however, for the synthetic progestational compounds 17-α-ethinyl-19-nortestosterone (Norlutin) and its $\Delta^{5(10)}$ isomer, norethynodrel. The administration of these substances during early pregnancy may result in masculinization of the female fetus.

Biosynthesis of Ovarian Hormones

In-vitro studies employing radioactive precursors have recently shown that the ovary contains enzymes capable of synthesizing its steroid hormones from simple acetate fractions by a pathway involving cholesterol → pregnenolone → progesterone → testosterone → estradiol ⇄ estrone (Fig. 90-2). During the proliferative phase of the menstrual cycle, estradiol, formed by the cells of the theca interna, and its metabolites estrone and estriol, are the principal ovarian hormones found in the urine. Very little progesterone appears until after ovulation when the corpus luteum synthesizes all the hormones depicted in Fig. 90-2, and progesterone is produced in the largest quantities. It has been suggested that in the cells of the theca interna estrogen synthesis goes by way of pregnenolone, bypassing progesterone, whereas in the granulosa cells of the corpus luteum estrogen synthesis switches to the progesterone pathway (see Fig. 90-2). Reduced nicotinamide adenine dinucleotide phosphate (TPNH)

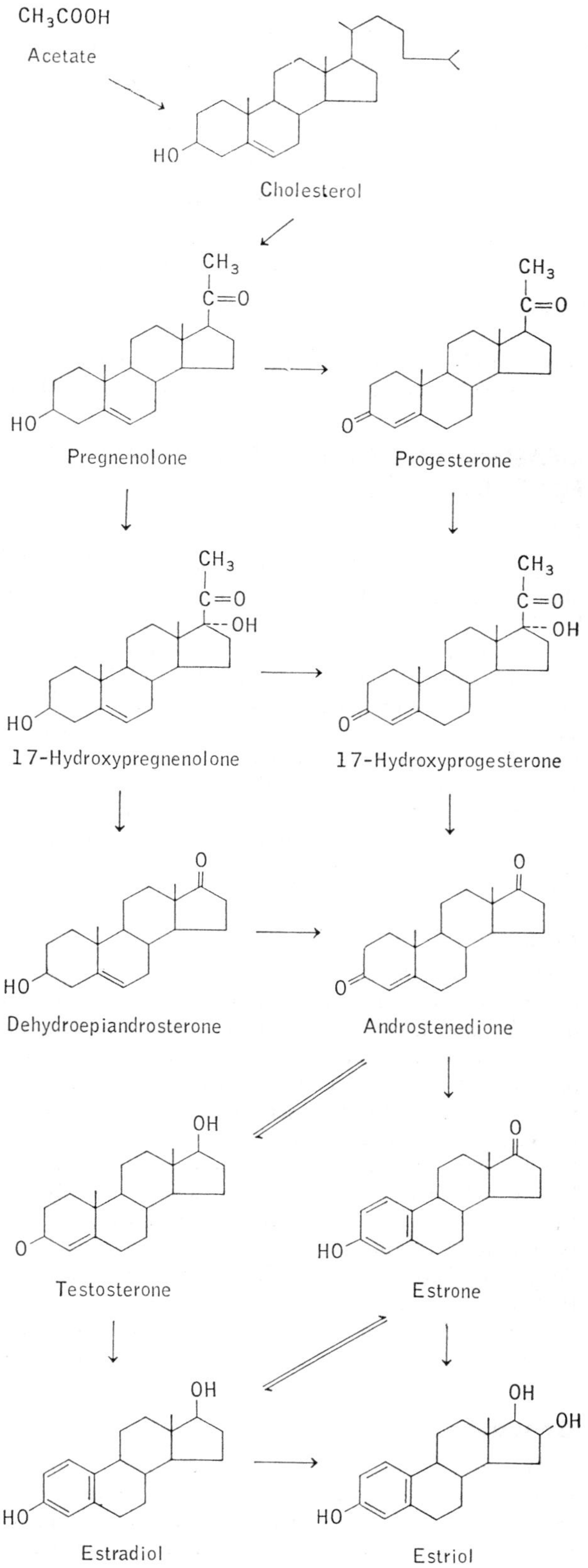

Fig. 90-2. Biosynthesis of ovarian steroids.

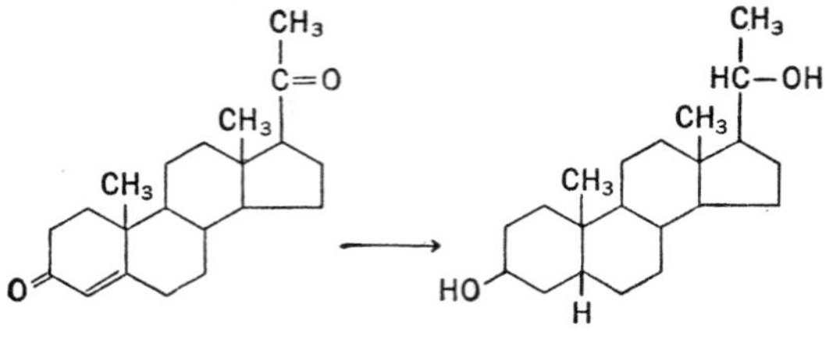

Fig. 90-3. Progesterone and its principal urinary metabolite.

appears to be an essential cofactor for LH activity, but not a specific mediator as it is thought to be for ACTH.

MEASUREMENT OF PITUITARY–OVARIAN FUNCTION

Estrogens

The chemical and biologic methods presently available for the assay of urinary estrogens are hampered by the relatively small quantities present in the urine of the nonpregnant female. A gross and indirect estimate of estrogen secretion may be obtained from examination of an endometrial biopsy or vaginal smear. The absence of cornification in the latter specimen indicates marked diminution of estrogen production. When estrogen is present and progesterone absent or diminished, a drop of cervical mucus allowed to dry on a glass slide will crystallize out in a characteristic fernlike pattern, the *ferning phenomenon*.

Progesterone

Once progesterone secretion has been detected by any procedure, it may be assumed that ovulation has occurred and a corpus luteum has formed. Adequate progesterone production is indicated by the presence of 3 to 10 mg pregnanediol glucuronide in a 24-hr urine collection during the second half of the menstrual cycle. A further indication of progesterone activity is the finding of secretory changes in an endometrial biopsy, which is preferably taken a few days before the expected onset of menstruation or soon after the beginning of uterine bleeding. A daily record of basal body temperature, taken each morning before arising, that reveals an abrupt rise of approximately 1° in the middle of the menstrual cycle and persisting until its end suggests a functioning corpus luteum.

Gonadotropins

An estimate of combined FSH and LH activity in urine can be determined by the ability of urine extracts to produce uterine growth in mice. Normal values in women during the reproductive period range from 10 to 15 mouse units. High levels are found in primary ovarian deficiency, but little or none can be measured if the deficiency is secondary to pituitary or hypo-

thalamic disease. Until recently the separation of LH and FSH in urine has been extremely difficult. This has been accomplished both by immunologic techniques and by bioassay methods involving ovarian ascorbic acid or cholesterol depletion in pseudopregnant rats as a specific measure of LH activity.

A rapid and simple immunologic test for urinary chorionic gonadotropin is now available and may well supplant the Aschheim-Zondek, Friedman, and male frog tests of pregnancy.

OVARIAN PREPARATIONS FOR CLINICAL USE

Four types of estrogenic substances are available: (1) The naturally occurring estrogens related to estradiol. These include estrone, estradiol, and its long-acting esters, estradiol benzoate and dipropionate. These substances are less active by mouth than by injection. They may be given intramuscularly as solutions in oil. Estrone sulfate isolated from pregnant mare's urine may be given orally and does not induce gastric irritation. This preparation is administered in doses ranging from 0.625 to 5 mg per day. (2) The synthetic ethynyl derivative of estradiol may be given by mouth. It may occasionally produce nausea. The dose of this compound is 0.05 to 0.2 mg per day. (3) Synthetic estrogens made up of two aromatic rings joined by a short aliphatic chain are also available. The most commonly used preparation is diethylstilbestrol. This is potent by mouth, but occasionally it causes nausea. The dose ranges from 0.5 to 2.0 mg per day. (4) A synthetic compound having a prolonged action, tri-para-anisylchloro-ethylene (TACE), may be given by mouth in daily doses of 12 to 24 mg.

Progesterone may be given by intramuscular injection in oil in doses ranging from 5 to 50 mg per day. An oral preparation, anhydrohydroxyprogesterone, is administered in doses of 20 to 100 mg per day. Two synthetic progestational compounds, 17-α-ethinyl-19-nortestosterone (Norlutin) and its $\Delta^{5(10)}$ isomer, norethynodrel (Enovid), which also contains ethinyl estradiol, may be given orally in doses of 5 to 20 mg per day. As previously noted, some of the synthetic progestational compounds, if given during pregnancy, may bring about masculinization of the female fetus.

DISEASES OF THE OVARY

The diseases discussed in this section are associated with disturbances in the secretion of ovarian hormones. These disturbances may occur as the result of disease in the ovaries themselves or may be due to hypothalamic or pituitary disorders that alter gonadotropin secretion. Such hypothalamic or pituitary conditions lead to changes in ovarian hormone secretion because both ovaries are secondarily involved. In contrast, not all forms of primary ovarian disease are accompanied by an endocrine disturbance. A number of congenital, inflammatory, cystic, degenerative, and neoplastic diseases of the ovary may cause no endocrine disorder when the lesion is confined to one ovary and the uninvolved gonad can maintain adequate hormone secretion. In certain instances, however, unilateral ovarian disease does lead to endocrine disturbances, as in the case of the hormone-producing tumors. These disorders are characterized by increased rather than decreased hormone production.

Conditions that disturb ovarian hormone secretion may be conveniently divided into those which result in diminished secretion (ovarian hypofunction) and those which lead to excessive secretion (ovarian hyperfunction).

Ovarian Hypofunction

The manifestations of this state differ according to whether it is present before or after puberty. In prepuberal ovarian hypofunction sexual maturation fails to occur. The uterus does not enlarge, and the infantile cervicouterine ratio is preserved. Menstruation does not begin (primary amenorrhea), and sterility is invariably present. The breasts do not develop, and the growth of pubic and axillary hair is sparse. The pelvis fails to enlarge. Osteoporosis may be present. The patient may grow excessively tall because of failure of epiphyseal union. In addition, there may be a disproportion between the extremities and the trunk such that the arm span exceeds the height. This type of skeletal development is referred to as *eunuchoidism*.

It is well to remember that there are marked individual variations in the time of onset of puberty and the rapidity with which it develops. Menstruation in normal girls may begin at any time between the ages of nine and sixteen years. In the absence of menstruation and sexual development in a sixteen-year-old girl, it is often difficult to distinguish between a physiologic delay in maturation and a pathologic ovarian insufficiency. A family history of delayed adolescence and the presence of some breast development are favorable indications that sexual maturation will eventually occur.

Primary Ovarian Insufficiency

This condition results from congenital hypoplasia or absence of ovaries, from castration due to surgery, x-ray irradiation, or infection such as tuberculosis, brucellosis, or mumps or from the spontaneous cessation of ovulation occurring when all available follicles have discharged their ova at the time of the menopause. In all instances when the patients are beyond the age of puberty there will be a high level of gonadotropins in the urine.

Gonadal Dysgenesis (Turner's Syndrome)

This is a special form of congenital ovarian hypoplasia in which the "ovaries" consist of a fibrotic streak or cord in each broad ligament. Examination of nuclei in skin biopsies, smears of buccal mucosa, and leukocytes has shown that approximately 80 per cent of patients have chromatin-negative (male pattern) nuclear sex. Furthermore, such cases have an XO sex chromosome constitution, with no Y chromosome and a diploid number of 45. Patients with gonadal dysgenesis show signs of estrogen deficiency: infantile female genitalia, primary amenorrhea, lack of breast development, and osteoporosis. Axillary and pubic hair usually develop normally, though their appearance may be somewhat delayed. Rarely androgenic manifestations such as hirsutism and clitoral enlargement may be present; these findings have been attributed to the presence of androgen-secreting hilus cells in the ovarian anlagen. The condition of gonadal dysgenesis is usually associated with shortness of stature and multiple congenital abnormalities. The commonest of these are short metacarpals, cubitus valgus, eye disorders, webbing of the neck, shieldlike chest, coarctation of the aorta, and lymphedema of the extremities. The appearance of the patient is often sufficient to suggest the diagnosis.

These patients should receive continuous estrogen replacement therapy from the chronologic age of puberty. Estrogen may be given as diethylstilbestrol in doses of 0.5 to 2 mg daily. The therapy should be administered cyclically, with 3 weeks of treatment followed by 1 week of rest, whether or not withdrawal bleeding occurs. On this therapy sexual maturation is achieved, but sterility, of course, remains.

Adrenogenital Syndrome

The most common adrenal disease of childhood is congenital adrenal cortical hyperplasia with increased androgen secretion. In females this condition leads to pseudohermaphroditism and failure of sexual maturation. The ovarian insufficiency is believed to be due to the inhibitory effect of the adrenal androgens on gonadotropin secretion (Chap. 84).

Female Climacteric or Menopause

This state has its onset, in the majority of instances, between the ages of forty-five and fifty-five years. Commonly there is a progressive irregularity in the frequency, duration, and amount of menstrual flow until finally amenorrhea ensues. Persistent metrorrhagia, or a recurrence of bleeding after a period of amenorrhea, in a woman of menopausal age requires careful investigation and must be considered due to uterine or ovarian neoplasm until proved otherwise. Along with the disappearance of menstruation at the climacteric a more gradual regressive change in the uterus, vagina, and breasts occurs. Pubic and axillary hair tend to become sparse, and, after some time, osteoporosis may become evident. Mild hirsutism, usually confined to the face, is not infrequent. In keeping with the view that the menopausal state is a type of primary ovarian insufficiency, one finds a high urinary gonadotropin excretion.

Certain vasomotor and nervous symptoms may accompany the menopausal changes just described. These include periodic feelings of warmth in the face, neck, and upper thorax ("hot flushes"). Less frequently, sudden surges of heat involve the whole body and are accompanied by drenching sweats ("hot flashes"). There may be nervousness, irritability, fatigability, and lassitude. These symptoms appear in many women at the climacteric, but in only a small proportion are they of a marked degree or more than a few months in duration. Most patients with climacteric symptoms respond well to simple psychotherapy and the administration of mild sedatives. These measures should always be employed first before hormonal substitution therapy is considered. Estrogen treatment is reserved for a relatively small group of patients whose distress is not relieved by the simple measures described. Diethylstilbestrol, in an initial dose of 0.5 mg per day, or equivalent doses of other estrogen preparations may be given cyclically, with 3 weeks of treatment followed by 1 week of rest. Once benefit is achieved, the hormone dose may be lowered to the level that maintains relief. Estrogen should not be used indefinitely, however, in these patients. It is suggested that after a period of 3 to 6 months the hormone be gradually withdrawn. The treatment of postmenopausal osteoporosis is discussed in Chap. 227.

Premature Climacteric

The spontaneous onset of the climacteric before the age of forty is regarded as premature. Treatment is as described for the normal climacteric, except that estrogens are more frequently required and in somewhat larger doses (initial dose of diethylstilbestrol, 1 to 2 mg per day). The estrogen therapy is usually maintained until the early forties, when it is gradually withdrawn. It is important to continue cyclic estrogen therapy up to the normal menopausal age in order to prevent premature onset of degenerative disease.

SECONDARY OVARIAN INSUFFICIENCY

This condition arises from diseases that directly or indirectly affect the hypothalamus or anterior pituitary in a manner that interferes with gonadotropin secretion. Urinary excretion of gonadotropins will consequently be low or absent.

Hypothalamic Infantilism

Ovarian insufficiency occurring in association with destructive lesions of the hypothalamus and with congenital conditions such as the Laurence-Moon-Biedl syndrome has been described previously (see Chap. 80).

Psychogenic Amenorrhea

Emotional disturbances are one of the most common causes of amenorrhea and sterility. Other signs of ovarian insufficiency, however, are usually absent. It is believed that emotional disorders induce amenorrhea through their influence on hypothalamic centers that control gonadotropin secretion. In these patients successful psychotherapy is usually followed by restoration of normal menstrual function.

General Metabolic Disturbances Associated with Ovarian Insufficiency

A number of metabolic disturbances may be accompanied by failure of sexual maturity in the prepuberal child or amenorrhea and sterility after puberty has been attained. Such disorders include obesity, chronic malnutrition, of which anorexia nervosa is a classic example, uncontrolled diabetes mellitus, hyperthyroidism, and chronic renal disease. It is believed that hypogonadism is due to a failure of normal synthesis of hypothalamic or pituitary hormones. Successful treatment of the primary condition usually results in the resumption of normal ovarian development and function.

Hypopituitarism

In the prepuberal period hypopituitarism most commonly results from damage to the pituitary by an expanding craniopharyngioma, more rarely from trauma or inflammatory disease. After puberty, the commonest cause during the childbearing period is pituitary necrosis associated with postpartum hemorrhage (Sheehan's syndrome). Pressure atrophy due to tumors of the pituitary (chromophobe or eosinophil adenoma) or surrounding structures (meningiomas), metastatic tumors (especially from breast), or granulomatous diseases (sarcoid, Hand-Schüller-Christian syndrome) may occur at any age. Under these conditions gonadotropin secretion is usually the first and may be the only pituitary function to be compromised, or the full picture of panhypopituitarism with thyroid, adrenal, and ovarian hypofunction may develop (see Chap. 80).

FSH replacement therapy, utilizing extracts of human pituitaries or, a more practical source, extracts of human postmenopausal urine, when supplemented with LH provided by human placental chorionic gonadotropin, has proved effective in permitting conception and successful parturition to take place in women with pituitary gonadotropin deficiency. These extracts are so remarkably potent that they may cause the simultaneous maturation of several follicles, resulting in a high incidence of multiple pregnancies, unless the dosage is carefully regulated.

Virilizing Syndromes

Congenital adrenal cortical hyperplasia with increased androgen production, *the adrenogenital syndrome,* leads to pseudohermaphroditism and failure of sexual maturation in prepuberal females. A milder form of this condition may not become apparent until after puberty but may then lead to amenorrhea, sterility, and varying degrees of masculinization. The ovarian insufficiency is believed to result from the inhibition of gonadotropin secretion by adrenal androgens, and suppression therapy with cortisone usually allows normal sexual maturation in the child and restores menses with fertility in the adult (see Chap. 84). Ovarian insufficiency may be caused in a similar manner by androgen-producing tumors of the adrenal or of the ovary, such as the arrhenoblastoma and hilus cell tumor, but such lesions will not be affected by cortisone therapy and must be removed surgically.

Stein-Leventhal Syndrome

One of the commonest causes of amenorrhea and sterility in the young postpuberal female is the *polycystic ovary syndrome,* described by Stein and Leventhal. The etiology of this syndrome remains obscure and is probably multiple. It usually appears within the first 5 to 10 years after the menarche and is characterized clinically by absent or irregular anovulatory menses, infertility, and varying degrees of hirsutism and obesity. Pathologically there is enlargement of the ovaries (except in early cases) with a thick tunica albuginea, increased stroma, many follicular cysts and hyperplasia, and, not infrequently, luteinization of the theca interna. Urinary 17-ketosteroid excretion may be normal or elevated, and urinary LH has been found to be elevated by some investigators. The failure of the follicles to reach full maturation and rupture is thought to result in a persistence of estrogen production, which inhibits the normal cyclic FSH release. In-vitro studies of the biosynthesis of ovarian hormones by these polycystic ovaries, however, have revealed a decrease in the conversion of testosterone to estradiol, resulting in an accumulation of the androgenic precursor. Recent evidence suggests that this may be due to excessive activity of the ovarian stroma, which produces primarily testosterone, as noted above under Embryogenesis. The refinement of chemical methods sufficiently sensitive to measure blood levels of testosterone has now made it possible to demonstrate that the amount of testosterone circulating in the blood of patients with the Stein-Leventhal syndrome, as well as those with hirsutism from other causes, known or unknown, is significantly increased above those of the normal female. Bilateral wedge resection of the polycystic ovaries with removal of a generous quantity of ovarian stroma and cortex frequently restores normal menstrual function, but the hirsutism is rarely ameliorated by this procedure.

Some patients with amenorrhea and Stein-Leventhal ovaries also have bilateral adrenal hyperplasia and increased 17-ketosteroid excretion. In this group of patients the menses may be restored and conception may occur following suppression of the adrenals with small doses of a glucocorticoid such as Prednisone, 2.5 mg three times a day.

An analog of the nonsteroidal estrogen TACE (see under Ovarian Preparations), Clomiphene citrate (1-[p-(β-diethylaminoethoxy) phenyl]-1,2-diphenyl-2-chloroethylene), which is by itself a weak estrogen and in intact animals a potent estrogen antagonist, has recently been shown to cause ovulation, corpus luteum formation, and fertility in a significant number of patients with polycystic ovaries. It is given in oral doses of 100 mg daily for 5 days, and during this time there occurs a marked increase in the urinary excretion of estrone and to a lesser extent of estradiol but not of estriol. If treatment is successful, ovulation will take place 4 to 7 days after cessation of therapy and a normal luteal phase will ensue. Excessive dosage may produce large, painful follicular cysts, whereas continuous therapy with smaller doses will prolong the survival of the corpus luteum and ultimately cause endometrial hypoplasia due to the anti-estrogenic effect of the drug.

This compound is also of value in the treatment of amenorrhea resulting from partial FSH deficiency and in postpuberal ovarian hyperfunction with abnormal functional bleeding (metropathia hemorrhagica, see below). Its mode of action is as yet not clear. Very recent evidence suggests that it inhibits cytochrome oxidase. As a result the rate of oxidation of TPNH by cytochrome C is reduced and more TPNH is present to catalyze the aromatization of testosterone to estrone in the ovary.

OVARIAN HYPERFUNCTION

As with hypofunction, a state of hyperfunction in the ovary may be due to primary gonadal changes or may be secondary to alterations in hypothalamic or pituitary function. Ovarian hyperfunction may be said to be present when there is a premature appearance of ovarian hormone secretion (prepuberal hyperfunction) or when there is an excessive hormone secretion in adult life (postpuberal hyperfunction).

Prepuberal Hyperfunction

The early onset of normal (adult) ovarian hormone secretion leads to precocious puberty. This syndrome includes premature appearance of pubic and axillary hair, enlargement of the genitalia and breasts, periodic uterine bleeding, and rapid skeletal growth but also premature closure of the epiphyses. Ovulation is present, and conception is possible. Precocious puberty is usually associated with hypothalamic disorders that prematurely initiate gonadotropin secretion.

The appearance of an abnormal quantity of ovarian hormone secretion in the prepuberal period leads to the syndrome of precocious pseudopuberty. In this syndrome, which is produced by granulosa cell tumors of the ovary, ovulation does not occur and only the signs of estrogen hypersecretion are present.

Precocious puberty may be (1) constitutional, i.e., occurring before the age of nine and without demonstrable disease, or (2) due to hypothalamic irritation from tumors, cysts, degenerative lesions following meningitis or encephalitis, or from the fibrous dysplasia of the floor of the skull seen in Albright's disease (see Chap. 231). Precocious pseudopuberty is very rare and may result from the premature secretion of gonadotropin or ovarian hormones by embryonic placental syncytium contained in a teratoma of the ovary (choriocarcinoma or chorionepithelioma) or of estrogens and progesterone secreted by a functioning granulosa cell tumor in the prepuberal ovary.

Postpuberal Hyperfunction: Abnormal Uterine Bleeding

The prime manifestation of postpuberal ovarian hyperfunction is abnormal uterine bleeding. No overt changes in the external genitalia or secondary sexual characteristics occur. The abnormal uterine bleeding may be a reappearance of bleeding after a normal menopause or changes in the menstrual cycle during the childbearing period. In the latter instance there may be metrorrhagia (excessive intermenstrual bleeding), menorrhagia (excessive menstrual bleeding), or both. There may be periods of amenorrhea irregularly interrupted by periods of uterine hemorrhage (metropathia hemorrhagica).

It is important to emphasize that abnormal uterine bleeding may be caused by a multitude of conditions, only a few of which are associated with ovarian hyperfunction (see Table 90-1). It is evident that abnormal menstrual flow during the active reproductive period or the reappearance of uterine bleeding following the menopause requires extremely thorough investigation. The causes of abnormal uterine bleeding

Table 90-1. CAUSES OF ABNORMAL
UTERINE BLEEDING

General

Abnormalities in blood coagulation
Hypothyroidism
Estrogen therapy

Local

Pregnancy states: abortion, ectopic pregnancy
Tumors of cervix and body of uterus
Feminizing ovarian tumors
Infections of uterus and adnexa
Endometriosis
Functional uterine bleeding

associated with ovarian hyperfunction include the feminizing ovarian tumors, choriocarcinoma (chorionepithelioma) of the uterus, and "functional uterine bleeding." The feminizing ovarian tumors will be discussed below. Choriocarcinoma of the uterus may produce bleeding partly through its local effect, partly by virtue of its secretion of estrogen and progesterone, and also because of its elaboration of chorionic gonadotropin, which stimulates ovarian estrogen secretion. The urinary excretion of this tropic hormone will give rise to a positive pregnancy test.

Three common gynecologic conditions with an endocrine background must be considered in the differential diagnosis of abnormal uterine bleeding: midcycle bleeding, endometriosis, and leiomyoma of the uterus. Midcycle bleeding may occur at the time of ovulation. It is painful at times (*mittelschmerz*) and associated with light staining. No treatment is necessary. Leiomyomas of the uterus ("fibroids") develop during the childbearing period. Their growth is stimulated by estrogen. Further growth of these tumors ceases at the menopause. Bleeding associated with leiomyomas occurs when the tumor involves the endometrium. Treatment is by myomectomy or hysterectomy, depending on the age of the patient.

Endometriosis is a disease of young women in which uterine mucosa may be found around the large bowel, the adnexa, and, most commonly, the ovaries. The ectopic or metastatic endometrium frequently participates in the cyclic changes induced by ovarian hormones. Chocolate cysts are the characteristic lesions. Local irritation, intraabdominal hemorrhages, and adhesions may occur. In many patients there are no symptoms. When present, they include abdominal pain, dysmenorrhea, irregular menses, and infertility. Treatment is aimed at suppressing the cyclic changes in the mucosal implants or removal of the ectopic endometrium. The former may be achieved with gradually increasing doses of norethynodrel and ethinyl estradiol (Enovid) to a limit of 50 mg per day over a period of 6 months. Such treatment suppresses ovarian function and leads to degeneration of the ectopic endometrial tissue. On withdrawal of therapy, prolonged palliation frequently results. Surgical treatment of endometriosis involves removal of implants, presacral neurectomy for relief of pain, and uterine suspension if retroversion is present. Sterilization by ovariectomy should be reserved for the most intractable cases.

FUNCTIONAL UTERINE BLEEDING. This condition is common but often transitory during the active reproductive period. It is physiologic at the extremes of this period, that is, for a short time following the menarche and just before the cessation of menstruation. Its exact etiology is not known. Whatever the cause may be, an anovulatory state frequently exists and there is a deficiency of progesterone in the presence of normal or elevated estrogen production. The abnormal pattern of hormone secretion may lead to menorrhagia, metrorrhagia, or metropathia hemorrhagica. The diagnosis of functional uterine bleeding should be made only after the other causes of abnormal uterine bleeding have been carefully eliminated (see Table 90-1). There are two aims in the treatment of functional uterine bleeding. Of first importance is to control excessive blood loss. Secondly, it is hoped, particularly in the young adult female, to restore normal menstrual function and fertility. Functional uterine bleeding that is mild in degree and of short duration requires no therapy; the condition is frequently temporary, and normal menstrual periods may soon be resumed. When bleeding is more severe or prolonged, the curettage, which is carried out to exclude other causes of uterine bleeding, is not infrequently followed by normal menstrual function. When this procedure fails, medical therapy should first be tried. Progestational agents alone may be administered as progesterone in oil, 50 mg in a single intramuscular injection, or as Norlutin or Enovid, 10 mg by mouth daily for 7 days. The course of progesterone is repeated every 4 weeks for a period of 3 to 4 months. Occasionally following such a regimen, normal menstrual periods are resumed. When progesterone alone is unsuccessful in controlling the excessive bleeding, the patient may be given cyclic estrogen and progesterone therapy. The estrogen may be administered as diethylstilbestrol, 0.5 to 1 mg by mouth per day for a 3-week period, followed by a course of progesterone as described above. At the end of the period of withdrawal bleeding, the course of treatment is resumed and repeated cyclically over a period of 3 to 4 months. Prolonged functional uterine bleeding results in iron deficiency, not always demonstrable by hematocrit or red cell count alone, and may be cured in some cases by restoration of normal body stores of iron. Only when medical treatment has failed to control prolonged and excessive blood loss should surgical treatment be considered. The surgical procedure of choice is hysterectomy without removal of the ovaries. This operation is preferable to simple sterilization by ovariectomy since the chief focus of symptoms may be removed without the loss of secondary sexual characteristics or the appearance of menopausal symptoms.

FUNCTIONAL NEOPLASMS OF THE OVARY

Table 90-2 lists ovarian tumors that may be considered in the differential diagnosis of ovarian masses. Relatively few of these tumors secrete hormones. They may produce androgens or estrogens, occasionally progesterone, and very rarely chorionic gonadotropin. The uncommon struma ovarii may secrete thyroid hormone.

FEMINIZING TUMORS. Feminizing ovarian tumors, when they occur in the prepuberal period, give rise to the syndrome of precocious pseudopuberty. In the adult female little change in secondary sexual characteristics results. When the tumors develop before

Table 90-2. NEOPLASMS OF THE OVARY

Tumors arising from celomic epithelium (vaginal, endocervical, endometrial, endosalpingial)

Cystadenoma (endometrioma, endosalpingioma, adenoma, fibroadenoma)
Papillary cystadenoma
Malignant papillary cystadenoma
Solid carcinoma

Tumors arising from primitive mesenchyme

Arrhenoblastoma*
Granulosa cell, theca cell*
Hilus cell*
Luteoma*
Dysgerminoma
Fibroma
Sarcoma

Tumors arising because of continuity

Adrenal cell*
　Kidney cell (hypernephroma)
　Mesonephroma
　Brenner (renal pelvis, ureter, or urethra)

Tumors arising from ova

Teratoma, chorionepithelioma,* struma*
Dermoid cyst

Metastatic tumors

From uterus (endometrial)
From stomach (Krukenberg)
From intestine (small or large), eye, rectum, breast, bile duct, etc.

* Only these seven are endocrinologically active.
SOURCE: Modified from J. V. Meigs: New Engl. and J. Med., 228:53, 1943.

the menopause, there is commonly excessive uterine bleeding, though occasionally amenorrhea is observed. Sterility is present. In the postmenopausal female, feminizing ovarian tumors are associated with a reappearance of uterine bleeding. When these tumors are removed surgically, the signs of feminization disappear.

GRANULOSA CELL TUMOR. These are the most common hormone-producing tumors, comprising about 10 per cent of all solid ovarian neoplasms. They are usually unilateral, often cystic, and not infrequently malignant. The uninvolved ovary is atrophied, presumably because of pituitary inhibition, by the high level of circulating estrogen arising from this type of tumor. The incidence of uterine leiomyoma and adenocarcinoma is increased. While pure granulosa cell tumors have been occasionally encountered, commonly a mixture of granulosa and theca cells is found. These cells may rarely secrete progesterone as well as estrogen. The majority of the tumors are found after the menopause, but they may appear during the reproductive period and before puberty. The clinical picture has been described above. Biopsy of the uterine mucosa usually reveals a proliferative endometrium, though occasionally secretory changes are observed. Urinary assays show increased estrogen but decreased gonadotropin excretion. Surgical therapy is the treatment of choice. In premenopausal patients with a well-encapsulated unilateral tumor, the affected ovary is removed, but the uterus and opposite ovary may be left intact. If there is evidence of malignancy, a radical pelvic dissection is performed. The latter procedure is recommended for the postmenopausal patient because of the higher incidence of recurrence and of associated uterine cancer. Postoperative radiotherapy should be used when the tumor is malignant.

THECA CELL TUMOR (THECOMA). Pure theca cell tumors are rare. They are almost always unilateral, usually solid, and seldom malignant. The average age incidence is similar to that of granulosa cell tumors. Theca cell tumors, however, are uncommon during the reproductive period and extremely rare in infancy. The clinical picture, laboratory findings, and therapy are as described for granulosa cell tumors.

LUTEOMA. When all or the greater portion of an ovarian tumor is transformed into luteal tissue, the tumor is known as a luteoma. Luteomas accompanied by a syndrome of feminization are believed to represent luteinization in a granulosa cell or theca cell tumor. Treatment, therefore, is as described for these tumors.

CHORIOCARCINOMA (CHORIONEPITHELIOMA) OF THE OVARY. This extremely rare tumor, a type of teratoma, may be found in the ovaries of prepuberal females. It is highly malignant. Its ability to secrete chorionic gonadotropin, estrogen, and progesterone leads to the syndrome of precocious pseudopuberty. An ovarian mass in conjunction with a positive pregnancy test in a prepuberal female may suggest the diagnosis. Treatment consists of radical pelvic surgery followed by chemotherapy, methotrexate or vincoleucoblastin. It should be noted that in the adult female choriocarcinoma of the uterus frequently metastasizes to the ovaries.

MASCULINIZING TUMORS. The manifestations of masculinizing ovarian tumors may vary from a mild increase of facial hair to a full picture of virilization with generalized hirsutism, loss of scalp hair, acne, muscularity, deepening of the voice, atrophy of breasts and uterus, amenorrhea, and sterility. The urinary 17-ketosteroid excretion is often normal and only rarely very high. Hence, the finding of normal urinary 17-ketosteroids in a patient with masculinization does not exclude the presence of an ovarian tumor. Surgical removal of such tumors is followed by the disappearance of most of the clinical manifestations. Not infrequently, however, the hirsutism is unaffected or only slightly diminished. It is important to emphasize that virilization in the adult female is only rarely due to a functioning ovarian tumor. The differential diagnosis and management of the syndrome of masculinization have been discussed previously (see Chap. 84).

ARRHENOBLASTOMA. This uncommon tumor is believed to arise from male-directed embryonic rests in the ovary. It is usually unilateral and only rarely malignant. The tumor is commonly solid, though occasionally cystic degeneration may be observed. The uninvolved ovary is often atrophied, presumably because of inhibition by high circulating androgen levels of pituitary gonadotropin secretion. Microscopically there are strands of primitive cells arranged in adenomatous formation, in cords, or in tubules.

Interstitial cells resembling testicular Leydig cells can often be identified. The arrhenoblastoma is found predominantly during the reproductive period. It occasionally occurs beyond the menopause. No patient under sixteen years of age has been known to develop this tumor. Signs of masculinization are found in association with a pelvic mass and a normal or slightly elevated urinary 17-ketosteroid excretion. In younger patients simple removal of the ovary and tube on the affected side is sufficient. In older women, particularly if they are past the menopause, hysterectomy and removal of the adnexa on both sides are advised because of the greater incidence of malignancy at this later age.

HILUS CELL (LEYDIG CELL) HYPERPLASIA OR ADENOMA. Characteristic cells, indistinguishable from testicular Leydig cells, have been found in the hilus of the normal ovary. On very rare occasions these cells may show hyperplasia or adenomatous formation and give rise to a syndrome of virilization. The hyperplastic tissue may be bilateral and large in size, but the tumors are usually small and confined to one ovary. The urinary 17-ketosteroid excretion may be normal or slightly increased. Treatment is surgical removal.

MISCELLANEOUS MASCULINIZING TUMORS. Rare tumors, variously described as adrenal-like tumors, luteomas, masculinovoblastomas, and virilizing lipoid cell tumors have been described in association with a syndrome of virilization. The confusion regarding the cellular origin of these tumors arises from difficulty in distinguishing between proliferating adrenocortical and luteal cells. These tumors may be highly malignant. Urinary 17-ketosteroid levels are usually increased. Treatment consists of surgical removal.

STRUMA OVARII. Struma ovarii is an extremely rare type of ovarian teratoma in which the predominant tissue is thyroid. These tumors are unilateral and usually benign. Hyperthyroidism may be present as a result of excessive production of thyroid hormone. Treatment is surgical removal.

THE PLACENTA

Anatomy

Within 7 to 8 days after conception the fertilized ovum has developed into the blastocyst, which consists of an inner cell mass, the site of the growing fetus, surrounded by a layer of cells, the primordial trophoblasts, from which the placenta and fetal membranes are derived. The trophoblasts soon separate into two layers, the outer syncytiotrophoblasts and the inner cytotrophoblasts. The syncytiotrophoblasts are created by division of the cytotrophoblasts but are not themselves capable of further division. It has been postulated that they are haploid, that is, have only a single set of 23 chromosomes, presumably all maternal. Thus they form a protective barrier around the embryo that is genetically identical to the maternal cells and prevents the development of antibodies by the mother to the foreign protein introduced into the fetus with the sperm. As long as this layer of syncytiotrophoblasts remains intact, growth and differentiation of the fetus can take place even when it is transplanted to other sites in the maternal organism such as the kidney. Whenever it is disrupted, a foreign body rejection phenomenon is initiated. The syncytiotrophoblasts have the capacity to lyse and invade the decidual cells of the uterine endometrium, carrying with them the cytotrophoblasts from which the placental villi with their connective tissue and blood vessels are formed in close approximation to the intrauterine vessels of the maternal circulation.

Physiology

First and foremost, the placenta acts as the fetal lung, transporting oxygen to the fetus and removing carbon dioxide from it. This process is carried out by simple diffusion aided and abetted by the greater affinity of fetal hemoglobin for oxygen and the wise provision of nature whereby the maternal and placental blood flows are in opposite directions. Thus maternal arterial blood first comes into approximation with fetal venous blood and oxygen diffusion is greatly facilitated by the high maternal fetal gradient.

In addition to the passive transport of gases, the placenta carries on a wide variety of exceedingly active metabolic functions and acts in lieu of the fetal liver until that organ has developed sufficiently to assume its own role. A long list of enzymatic activities has been demonstrated in placental tissue. These include all those enzymes necessary for the metabolism of glycogen and glucose through the carboxylic acid cycle and for the normal synthesis of cellular proteins and lipids, those required to furnish energy for the active transport of nutrients across cell membranes, and a large number with activities specific for the synthesis of protein and steroid hormones. A clinically important function of the placenta is its ability to sequester and enzymatically inactivate insulin in relatively large amounts. Notably lacking in the placenta are the enzymes required to carry out the urea cycle, to conjugate bilirubin with glucuronic acid, and to convert acetate to estrogens.

Placental Hormone Synthesis

The inability of the placenta to form estrogen either from acetate or progesterone has always puzzled investigators seeking the source of the abundant placental estrogen production. The elegant studies of Dicfaluzy and others appear to have solved this puzzle. These investigators, starting with the knowledge that the placenta is rich in hydrolytic and aromatizing enzymes, have shown that dehydroepiandrosterone (DHA) sulfate, derived from both the fetal and maternal adrenals, is rapidly hydrolyzed, converted to androstenedione and testosterone, and aromatized by the placenta almost quantitatively to estrone and

estradiol-17B. Chorionic gonadotropin is thought to stimulate this process by facilitating the hydroxylation of C19 just before the aromatization step. These estrogens are then converted to estriol by maternal hepatic enzymes in the same proportion as in the nonpregnant state. The disproportionately large quantities of estriol found in human pregnancy urine appear to be derived directly from conversion of DHA, or 16 α-hydroxylated intermediates arising from the fetus, to estriol by the placenta. The importance of the contribution of precursors derived from the fetal adrenal cortex to estriol synthesis in pregnancy is suggested by the characteristic hypertrophy of these glands and confirmed by the fact that in women bearing anencephalic monsters, where absence of fetal ACTH prevents development of the fetal adrenal cortex, and in patients with chorioepitheliomas (where no fetus exists), there is no increase in estriol excretion out of proportion to that in estrone and estradiol-17B.

Although the placenta can convert small quantities of cholesterol to progesterone, it exhibits an exceedingly great capacity to convert pregnenolone and 17 α-hydroxypregnenolone almost quantitatively to progesterone and it seems likely that the large quantities of progesterone produced in pregnancy are derived from these precursors. Evidence suggests that the bulk of the precursor arises from the maternal endocrine system, ovaries and adrenals, rather than the fetal, as in the case of estrogen precursors. In summary, then, the placenta appears to be poorly equipped to synthesize steroid hormones de novo but to have an extraordinary capacity to produce compounds with potent specific biologic activities from relatively inactive steroid precursors provided from other endocrine sources. Although other adrenal cortical hormones have been detected in small amounts in placental extracts, it seems probable that they were produced elsewhere and merely trapped in the placenta.

The principal protein hormone produced by the placenta, so-called "chorionic gonadotropin," appears very early after implantation, rises to a peak in the second or third month, and then reaches a plateau at a lower level for the remainder of pregnancy. Immunologic studies suggest that, whereas chorionic gonadotropin as extracted from urine has properties of both FSH and LH, when it is obtained directly from the placenta, it exhibits the immunologic specificity of pure LH only, indicating that the FSH fraction must be derived from the maternal pituitary. Chorionic gonadotropin appears to be either inactivated by, or used up in, the synthesis of placental steroids, because whenever premature failure of placental function occurs, as in diabetes, renal insufficiency, or for reasons unknown, the urinary titer of gonadotropins will rise as that of estriol and pregnanediol fall.

A second quantitatively important protein hormone, isolated in relatively large amounts from human placentas by Josimovich and MacLaren and also found in human pregnancy serum, has been shown to be biologically similar to prolactin (LTH) and at the same time to enhance markedly the biologic activity of growth hormone. It is immunologically similar to but not identical with growth hormone and has very weak growth-promoting properties in itself. This hormone, currently known as human placental lactogen (Josimovich) or chorionic "growth hormone-prolactin" (Grumbach), is found in relatively large and increasing amounts during pregnancy in maternal blood but is absent from cord blood. Increase in growth hormone production, on the other hand, is confined to the fetus. Human placental lactogen may be of fundamental importance in the maternal adaptation to the metabolic demands of pregnancy.

REFERENCES

Ferguson-Smith, M. A.: Cytogenetics in Man, A.M.A. Arch. Int. Med., 105:159, 1960.

Grumbach, M. M., and M. L. Barr: Cytological Tests of Chromosomal Sex in Relation to Sexual Abnormalities in Man, Recent Progr. Hormone Res., 14:255, 1958.

Katzman, P.: Metabolism of Steroids, Ann. Rev. Biochem., 28:257, 1959.

Morris, J. Mc., and R. E. Scully: "Endocrine Pathology of the Ovary," St. Louis, The C. V. Mosby Company, 1958.

Pincus, G.: The Physiology of Ovarian and Testis Hormones, vol. III in "Hormones: Physiology, Chemistry and Applications," G. Pincus and K. V. Thimann (Eds.), New York, Academic Press, Inc., 1955.

Sohval, A. R.: Physiology of the Ovary, in "Diseases of the Endocrine Glands," 2d ed., L. J. Soffer (Ed.), Philadelphia, Lea & Febiger, 1956.

Villee, C. A. (Ed.): "The Placenta and Fetal Membranes," Baltimore, The Williams & Wilkins Company, 1960.

——: Physiology Symposium: Physiology of the Placenta, Fed. Proc., 23:773–798, July–August, 1964.

Wilkins, L.: "The Diagnosis and Treatment of Endocrine Disorders in Childhood and Adolescence," 2d ed., Springfield, Ill., Charles C Thomas, Publisher, 1957.

91 INFERTILITY

Melvin L. Taymor

DEFINITION. Infertility may be defined as the inability to conceive during the course of normal sexual activity. It is generally held that a marriage should not be considered infertile until a year of unprotected coitus has been allowed to pass. However, each couple's problems should be judged individually, and diagnosis and treatment instituted at an earlier or later date as indicated.

ETIOLOGY. The two fundamental concepts to be kept in mind are (1) the multiplicity of etiologic factors and (2) the equal responsibility of male and female partners. To delineate these possible factors working either singly or in concert, one need only review the pathways of conception in male and female and the disorders of these pathways that may ensue.

Deficiency of sperm production in quantity and quality accounts for the majority of the *male's* contribution to the problem of infertility. Sperm production may be adversely affected by congenital influences such as germinal aplasia or cryptorchidism, by hormonal deficiencies of the pituitary or thyroid glands, by infection such as mumps orchitis, and by environmental factors such as nutritional deficiencies, noxious chemicals and drugs, radiation, excess local heat, and altitude. Often the cause is not ascertainable by diagnostic methods available at present. Sperm transport is affected by congenital malformations, surgical trauma, and infections. Impotency, an important factor in many cases, is commonly on a psychologic basis, although local infection or general systemic disorders may play a contributory role.

Defects in the *female* are related to production of ova and interference with their union with spermatozoa. Vaginal causes are organic or functional.

TREATMENT. The treatment of any defects, minor or major, in both the husband or the wife should be carried out concomitantly so that the total fertility potential of the couple will be raised to an optimum level.

In the *male* with azoospermia, in whom spermatogenesis is normal as shown by testicular biopsy, and in whom a block has been demonstrated, epididymovasostomy can result in return of fertility in 10 to 20 per cent of cases. When hormonal studies reveal a deficiency of pituitary gonadotropin, treatment with human chorionic gonadotropin (5,000 units APL intramuscularly twice weekly for 2 to 6 months) is indicated. However, sperm deficiencies not associated with specific pituitary defects will not respond to pituitary or pituitarylike extract. Azoospermia or severe oligospermia will not respond in any significant degree to the administration of hormones, vitamins, thyroid preparations, or diet unless a specific deficiency can be demonstrated. In the present state of knowledge, little can be offered in the vast majority of cases of azoospermia or severe oligospermia.

This degree of pessimism should not be carried over to the infertile male with moderate degree of oligospermia (10 to 30 million per ml) or to the male partner of an infertile couple with only a moderately lowered sperm count (30 to 60 million per ml), particularly if one considers the "couple as a unit" concept of infertility. A modest improvement in the sperm count or motility combined with attention to the factors in the female partner may raise the fertility of the couple above a critical level. Avoidance of excess alcohol and tobacco, sufficient sleep and exercise, an optimum diet, adjustment of local excesses of heat, administration of thyroid preparations in minor degrees of hypofunction—all these singly or together may prove of definite benefit.

In the *female* specific attention should be directed to the cervical factor by correction of unfavorable coital habits, correction of retroversion of the uterus by

Table 91-1. TESTS FOR INFERTILITY

I. In the male.
   A. Routine.
      1. Semen analysis. The semen is delivered into a clean glass container by withdrawal or masturbation. The following characteristics are considered normal:
         a. Volume—3 to 5 ml.
         b. Sperm count—above 60 million per ml is unquestionably normal, below 30 million per ml unquestionably indicates reduced fertility. The significance of counts between 30 million and 60 million depends upon the quality of motility and the degree of fertility in the female partner. A highly fertile female would be more susceptible to a count of borderline fertility.
         c. Motility—40 per cent or more still actively motile 4 to 5 hr after collection.
         d. Morphology—at least 60 per cent of the spermatozoa should be of normal size and shape.
      2. Examination of prostatic smear—excess leukocytes indicate that infection may play a contributory role.
   B. Special tests—for the male with reduced fertility as indicated by semen analysis.
      1. Evaluation of thyroid function by basal metabolic rate, protein-bound iodine, or radioactive iodine uptake.
      2. Testicular biopsy—in most cases this will result in a definitive diagnosis. In only a few cases, however, will it demonstrate a remediable defect.
      3. Urinary gonadotropins—these may be low in pituitary deficiency. Excretion is high in primary gonadal failure.
      4. Sex chromatin determination.
II. In the female.
   A. Routine.
      1. Postcoital test—examination of the cervical mucus for its preovulatory qualities of clarity, spinnbarkeit (ability of the mucus to form a thread 5 to 10 cm in length when stretched between slide and cover slip), ferning (ability of the mucus to form fernlike pattern when dried and examined under low power of microscope), and for the number of viable spermatozoa 8 to 12 hr after coitus.
         a. Good test—more than 20 active spermatozoa per high-power field.
         b. Fair test—5 to 20 spermatozoa per high-power field.
         c. Poor test—less than 5 spermatozoa per high-power field. A poor postcoital test in the presence of good preovulatory mucus suggests a semen deficiency, a deficiency of the coital method, or malposition of the cervix. A poor postcoital test combined with poor mucus in the preovulatory phase and a normal semen analysis indicates a hostile cervix either on an inflammatory or an endocrine basis.
      2. The evaluation of tubal patency—initially by insufflation with carbon dioxide (Rubin test) and followed at a later date by hysterosalpingography in those cases which show failure of carbon dioxide to pass or who fail to conceive after an interval of time despite a normal Rubin test.

Table 91-1. TESTS FOR INFERTILITY (*Continued*)

      3. Evaluation of ovulation and hormonal factors by:
         a. Measurement of basal body temperature, which characteristically shows a sustained rise after ovulation. Studies have shown that actual ovulation may occur as long as 2 days before or 2 days after the beginning of the temperature rise. The value of the temperature chart as an exact indicator of ovulation timing for purposes of timing coitus or insemination treatments can be overestimated.
         b. Endometrial biopsy with the demonstration of secretory changes in the endometrium is valid evidence that ovulation has occurred. The presence of endometrium out of phase with the time of biopsy is evidence of a progestational deficiency.
   B. Special tests should be carried out when indicated.
      1. Evaluation of thyroid function.
      2. Endocrine assays, such as urinary gonadotropin and 17-ketosteroid determination, in cases of anovulation or inadequate luteal function.
      3. Further studies of ovulation timing utilizing vaginal or urinary smears and studies of cervical mucus.
      4. Culdoscopy to detect early endometriosis, pelvic adhesions interfering with tube-ovarian function, or polycystic ovaries.

a pessary, improvement in quality and quantity of preovulatory mucus by the daily administration of small dosages of estrogen (0.1 mg diethylstilbestrol daily for three or four cycles), by the use of a plastic cervical cap, and by the correction of cervicitis by systemic and local antibiotics or by cervical cauterization. Cauterization must be conservative lest more harm than good be produced by cervical stenosis or obliteration of mucus-secreting glands. When cervical stenosis is found, dilatation under anesthesia is of definite value.

Attempts to overcome tubal occlusion by repeated insufflations, diathermy, and high dosage of estrogen occasionally meet with success. Plastic repair of tubes or cornual implantation is followed by success in only 10 to 20 per cent of cases. Surgery for tube-ovarian blockade, due to ovaries fixed by endometriosis or peritubal or periovarian adhesions, but associated with essentially normal tubes, results in a higher percentage of success. Infrequent ovulation accompanied by gross irregularity will respond to thyroid preparations when specifically indicated and to the correction of a specific dietary or vitamin deficiency. Ovulation accompanied by an inadequate luteal phase should be treated with progesterone preparations (17-ethinyl-19-nortestosterone, 2.5 mg daily for 10 days) or injections of human chorionic gonadotropin (HCG, 1,000 units intramuscularly every other day for five doses). Treatment should begin on the fifth or sixth day after the midcycle rise in the basal body temperature.

When anovulation is caused by a specific defect in thyroid function, nutrition, adrenal activity, or the psyche, correction of these defects will improve the condition. Wedge resection of polycystic ovaries, if bilaterally enlarged, is accompanied by 60 to 80 per cent resumption of ovulatory cycles.

Recently two approaches to the medical induction of ovulation, although still experimental and as yet commercially unavailable, show promise for future clinical application. The first is an extract of gonadotropins, high in FSH activity, prepared from the urine of postmenopausal females (Pergonal). The usual dosage is 150 to 200 FSH units administered intramuscularly daily for 7 to 12 days. When there is evidence of follicular activity, as indicated by increased cornification of the vaginal smear or increasing fern formation in cervical mucus, HCG is administered, 2,000 to 4,000 units daily for 4 days. Each patient responds differently. Overstimulation can result in enlarged cystic ovaries, so each patient should be followed carefully. Polycystic ovaries are most susceptible to massive enlargement and possible rupture.

Clomiphene, a chemical closely related to stilbestrol, also can stimulate ovulation. It, too, is only available experimentally at the present time. The mode of action is not completely clarified, but after a 3- to 5-day course of the medication, 100 mg daily, a burst of gonadotropins 3 to 10 days later often results in ovulation. It, too, should be used with caution in patients suspected of having polycystic ovaries.

Psychotherapy is of value in improving the coital habits of the couple, in reducing tubal spasm, and in correcting some deficiencies of hormonal nature. Finally, the manner and attitude of the physician plays a role in the outcome by preventing undue feelings of guilt and depression from gaining the upper hand, and by instilling sufficient hope and fortitude to allow the couple to carry through with the tedious and sometimes painful diagnostic testing and therapeutic maneuvers.

REFERENCES

Buxton, C. L., and A. L. Southam: "Human Infertility," New York, Paul B. Hoeber, Inc., Medical Department of Harper & Brothers, 1958.

Gemzell, C. A.: Induction of Ovulation with Human Pituitary Gonadotropins, Fertil. & Steril., 13:153, 1962.

MacLeod, J., R. Z. Gold, and C. M. McLane: Correlation of Male and Female Factors in Human Infertility, Fertil. & Steril., 6:112, 1955.

Meeker, S. R.: "Human Sterility, Causation, Diagnosis and Treatment: A Practical Manual of Clinical Procedures," Baltimore, The Williams & Wilkins Company, 1933.

Nelson, W. O.: The Klinefelter Syndrome, Fertil. & Steril., 8:527, 1957.

Rosenberg, E.: Clinical Effects of Human Urinary Menopausal Gonadotrophin, J. Clin. Endocrinol. & Metab., 23:181, 1963.

Stone, A., and M. E. Ward: Factors Responsible for Pregnancy in 500 Infertility Cases, Fertil. & Steril., 7:1, 1956.

92 DISEASES OF THE BREAST
Kendall Emerson, Jr.

HISTORY. The earliest description of cancer of the breast, and probably of cancer in any form, is credited to the Egyptian physician Imhotep in 3000 B.C. and is recorded in the Edwin Smith Surgical Papyrus under Case number 39, "Bulging Tumor of the Breast." The gross anatomy of the lactating breast must have been familiar to the author of the Song of Solomon in the year 1014 B.C., who likened it to "a cluster of grapes." Aside from its obvious function of lactation, however, little was known about the mammary gland, and interest in it throughout the ages has been more esthetic and symbolic than scientific until the studies of Sir Astley Cooper in 1845 provided us with an adequate morphologic description of this organ and the first suggestion of its possible relationship to menstrual dysfunction. In the latter half of the nineteenth century the German investigators discovered that normal breast development in animals depended upon intact ovarian function, and in 1896 Sir George Beatson first demonstrated the inhibition of the growth of mammary cancer by oophorectomy in human beings. The role of the corpus luteum and pituitary in the development of the breasts has been brought to light during the present century by the works of L. Loeb, Gardner, Riddle, Corner, Turner, and many others.

CONGENITAL ANOMALIES

The occurrence of aberrant breast tissue (polymastia) and supernumerary nipples (polythelia) situated along the so-called "milk line" extending from the midclavicle to the inguinal ligament has been noted in art and legend since recorded time. One wonders if these anomalies may not have been more common when man was closer in evolution to his multiparous animal forebears, since the number of breasts allotted to each member of the animal kingdom is in proportion to the average size of its litter. Absence of one or both breasts (amastia) occurs very rarely but was recorded long ago by the aforementioned author of the Song of Solomon.

ENDOCRINE RELATIONSHIPS

The most comprehensive recent studies of the endocrine factors determining the growth and function of the mammary glands in rats are those of Lyons, which are very briefly summarized here because they seem to support most of the observations in human beings. The development of the normal nonlactating breast is directly dependent upon the synergistic action of three major hormones: estrogens, pituitary growth hormone, and adrenal cortical steroids. Growth hormone alone will cause some growth of mammary ducts, whereas estrogens and adrenal hormones have no effect by themselves. Prolactin (luteotropic hormone, LTH) and progesterone are essential for the functional development of the alveolar lobules and the secretion of milk, whereas in the adult gland estrogens inhibit lactation by suppressing LTH activity. Prolactin with adrenal steroids can induce lactation in the absence of progesterone. The hormones of greatest clinical importance in relation to the breast in man are the estrogens. Painful engorgement of the breasts may be seen as a transient phenomenon in newborn infants due to the high level of circulating estrogens of placental origin. The normal development of the female breast at puberty, which is sometimes accompanied by intermittent tenderness and edema, results from the rising level of circulating estrogens secreted by the maturing ovarian follicles just prior to the menarche. Precocious breast development may occur as a result of inherited or constitutional factors, of abnormal pituitary, ovarian, or adrenal activity associated with functional tumors or hyperplasia of these organs, or of locally irritating lesions such as tumors of the pineal or fourth ventricle, fibrous dysplasia of the bones of the base of the skull, as occurs in Albright's disease (polyostotic fibrous dysplasia), or rarely following viral encephalitis.

Gynecomastia occurs physiologically in normal males at puberty and may persist through adolescence. (In some animals such as the bat, the function of lactation is retained by the male who may assist his partner in suckling their young.) This breast enlargement usually subsides spontaneously, but if it presents a sufficiently serious psychologic problem simple mastectomy with preservation of the nipples is justified since any hormonal treatment is ineffective. Gynecomastia should always raise the suspicion of seminiferous tubule dysgenesis with fibrosis, a variant of Klinefelter's syndrome, in which there is usually an elevated urinary excretion of follicle-stimulating hormone and a female pattern of sex chromatin (see Chap. 89).

Marked degrees of breast development in adolescent males or the onset of gynecomastia in later life may indicate the presence of an estrogen-secreting tumor of the adrenal. These tumors are usually associated with an elevation of the urinary 17-ketosteroids, the excretion of which is not further stimulated by ACTH or suppressed by adrenal steroids. Every effort should be made to locate such tumors by radiographic means and to remove them surgically because, though rare, a high percentage, if not all, are malignant.

Choriogenic tumors, and more rarely interstitial cell and granulosa cell tumors of the testes, may produce gynecomastia. This condition is also seen in males with cirrhosis of the liver and in states of severe malnutrition, presumably in both instances due to failure of inactivation of circulating estrogens. It regularly follows iatrogenic administration of estrogenic compounds in the treatment of carcinoma of the prostate and even occasionally occurs during testosterone therapy in eunuchoidism. Transient gynecomastia occurs as a normal physiologic phenomenon in elderly men.

INFECTIOUS DISEASES

Acute pyogenic infections of the breast are largely confined to the first 2 months of lactation and usually involve the staphylococcus, less often a beta streptococcus. They should be prevented by proper hygiene and treated with appropriate antibiotics. Very rarely an acute mastitis may occur during the course of paratyphoid or typhoid fever, brucellosis, or mumps, unassociated with lactation.

Chronic tuberculous mastitis is a rarity today. It usually results from the extension of tuberculosis of the underlying bone into the breast tissue and should be suspected from the presence of multiple sinus tracts and the finding of active tuberculosis elsewhere.

INFLAMMATORY LESIONS

Mammary duct ectasia (Haagensen) is a benign condition usually seen in elderly women with atrophic breasts wherein the mammary ducts in or just beneath the nipple become dilated and filled with cellular debris and lipid-containing material. Intermittent pain and local inflammatory changes may be present, and because a discharge, at times bloody, and retraction of the nipple may occur, this condition must be differentiated from carcinoma. Excision of the nipple is usually indicated.

Fat necrosis is a common occurrence following trauma, which may be so slight as not to have been noticed. It presents as a painful lump usually associated with some ecchymosis and may be followed by local atrophy and dimpling of the skin, at which stage biopsy must be performed to distinguish it from carcinoma.

Thrombosis of the thoracoepigastric veins and sclerosing subcutaneous phlebitis (Mondor's disease) occur after trauma or for no apparent reason and are manifest by the appearance of long cordlike structures, initially tender, in the outer half of the breast, frequently extending up into the axilla or down toward the epigastrium. They may persist up to a year, but no treatment is indicated.

Sarcoid may very rarely involve the skin of the chest. Eosinophilic granuloma may occur in the submammary folds.

It must not be forgotten that carcinoma of the breast may rarely present as a subacute red, warm, indurated mass, resembling a bacterial cellulitis, the so-called "inflammatory carcinoma." This lesion may be suspected when the skin over it presents the characteristic *peau d'orange* appearance.

FIBROCYSTIC DISEASE

With each menstrual cycle there is a recurring biphasic stimulation first of proliferation of breast tissue by estrogens, then of alveolar secretory activity by progesterone, followed by a period of involution. In most women these changes are of such slight degree as to cause few if any clinical symptoms. Not infrequently, however, well-marked inflammatory changes may occur preceding each menses, with tenderness, engorgement, and increasing nodularity of the breasts. This is more often seen in nulliparous women and may subside after childbearing and lactation. Methyl testosterone, 5 mg daily for 7 to 10 days before each menstrual period, will often provide relief.

In the later years of reproductive life the continued recurrent stimulation and involution of the breasts in the course of each menstrual cycle may result in diffuse and nodular fibrosis and the formation of cysts of varying sizes, so-called "chronic cystic mastitis." This condition can simulate carcinoma but is usually distinguishable by the fact that it is intermittently painful and may subside to some extent following menstruation. Nevertheless carcinoma may coexist and be masked by the diffuse nodularity of the cystic disease. Moreover, the incidence of mammary carcinoma is greater in patients with fibrocystic disease of the breasts, and it is unwise to delay biopsy of suspicious areas in the hope that they may subside by the end of the next menstrual cycle. In severe cases simple mastectomy is fully justified.

TUMORS OF THE BREAST

Benign fibroadenomas of the breast may occur at any age but are more common in women under the age of thirty. They may be distinguished from carcinomas by their mobility and well-defined margins, but biopsy is nonetheless imperative.

Benign intraductal papillomas may occur and cause a bloody discharge from the nipple. They are usually small and difficult to feel but may be located by noting that area of the breast on which pressure causes the bleeding. Excision is always advisable.

Sarcomas of all types make up less than 3 per cent of all breast tumors. Fibrosarcomas are the most frequent; lymphosarcomas occasionally originate in the breast. Liposarcomas and hemangiosarcomas have been reported rarely. Cystosarcoma phyllodes is a curious, very large, relatively rapidly appearing tumor arising usually from a preexisting fibroadenoma. It presents as a tender, warm, cystic mass often replacing the whole breast. The skin over it is thinned, and the superficial veins are dilated. The tumor consists of fibrous cords covered with epithelium arising from the duct system. The cords are separated by cystic areas which become filled with leaflike (phyllodes) projections of epithelial tissue. Although these tumors are usually benign, blood-borne metastases have been reported and surgical removal of the tumor is always indicated.

CARCINOMA. Carcinoma of the breast is the most frequent malignant tumor to which the human female is subject and accounts for a greater number of deaths than any other single form of cancer in women. It occurs with increasing frequency from the age of twenty-five or thirty up to the menopause, when its incidence levels off until a second rise in frequency occurs after the age of sixty-five.

Etiology. In common with most forms of malignant disease, the etiology of breast cancer is not known. A few factors affecting its incidence are, however, reasonably well established. The very strong hereditary influence seen in mice can be carried over, though in a much smaller degree, to human beings. A two- to sevenfold increase in the familial incidence of the disease is reported. There is good evidence that the frequency of mammary cancer is inversely related to the number of children nursed, a fact which many modern pediatricians fail to realize. The role of the estrogenic hormones in the genesis of breast cancer in human beings has not yet been settled. The view most widely accepted at the present time is that estrogens do not initiate the cancer but may, nevertheless, hasten its development in genetically susceptible individuals. The prolonged use of these hormones, especially at or beyond the menopause or in patients with a family history of cancer, should be discouraged.

Pathology. The primary site is usually in the ducts, less often in the alveoli. Multicentric origins are a frequent occurrence, and all gradations of differentiation may be observed. It is common to see a marked proliferation of dense connective tissue surrounding groups of malignant cells, whether primary or metastatic, the so-called "scirrhous carcinoma." Unfortunately all degrees of differentiation may be found in different portions of the same tumor, and little prognostic value can be attached to the histologic appearance of any one area of such a malignancy.

Mammary carcinoma is prone to metastasize relatively early to the regional lymph nodes—axillary and supraclavicular if the primary site is in the outer half of the breast, the internal mammary chain if the disease arises in the inner quadrants of breast tissue. From thence spread occurs primarily to bone, lungs, liver, skin, and subcutaneous tissues generally, less frequently to the brain. Blood-borne metastases may occur even before lymphatic spread is clinically evident. It is interesting that there is a predilection for metastases to occur in the ovaries, adrenals, and pituitary—areas rich in the hormones stimulating the growth of this type of epithelial cell.

Diagnosis. The diagnosis of breast cancer is facilitated by the fact that it is possible to palpate directly this type of neoplasm, a procedure which should be done gently because of the possibility of spreading the disease. Unfortunately, the diffuse nodularity of the adult female breast makes it difficult to detect early lesions. As a rule the physician must depend on such evidence as hardness, fixation to underlying structures, or dimpling of the overlying skin to distinguish a malignant mass from a benign nodule of breast tissue, and by the time these distinguishing signs have become apparent the cancer has all too often metastasized. The majority of patients with breast cancer suggest the diagnosis themselves because of their ready detection of abnormal lumps or masses during self-examination. Although the procedure of periodic self-examination of the breasts may be decried as tending to encourage neuroticism and cancerphobia, it is the only practical way by which we can succeed in reducing the death rate from cancer of the breast until a final cure for cancer has been found.

Treatment. Total surgical excision provides the only permanent cure for carcinoma of the breast and x-ray therapy the best palliation for localized disease. The technical details of the surgical and radiologic treatment of breast cancer are beyond the scope of this chapter, as is the controversy over radical versus simple mastectomy and extensive local irradiation, as advocated by McWhirter and others. Because of the susceptibility of breast cancer to changes in its endocrine environment, however, every physician should be cognizant of the remarkable palliative effect which can be achieved in inoperable mammary cancer by intelligent hormonal manipulations.

In considering appropriate therapy for metastatic breast cancer, it is convenient to divide the patients into four age groups which may be termed premenopausal, intramenopausal, postmenopausal, and senescent. The primary growth stimulant for the malignant mammary cell in the premenopausal and the majority of intramenopausal patients is the estrogens; it follows, therefore, that in these patients every effort should be made to remove all sources of these hormones. Oophorectomy or adequate x-ray castration will induce subjective and/or objective remissions in approximately 40 per cent of such patients, lasting from 4 months to more than 2 years. The addition of small doses of adrenal cortical hormones, such as prednisone, 5 mg twice daily, has been advocated in order to prolong this remission by suppressing the compensatory synthesis of adrenal estrogens that follows ovarian ablation. There is increasing evidence, but not universal agreement, that prophylactic castration and prednisone suppression at the time of mastectomy may significantly prolong the survival of those patients with metastases ostensibly confined to axillary lymph nodes.

When the regression following oophorectomy has ended, or if it fails to occur, prednisone in doses of 15 to 20 mg per day, or the equivalent amounts of other synthetic adrenal cortical steroids, may induce a very satisfactory remission in a significant number of cases. At this point bilateral adrenalectomy, as advocated by Huggins, or hypophysectomy, as first carried out by Olivacrona, should be seriously considered whenever adequate facilities are available. These procedures provide objective remissions in 40 to 50 per cent of patients in the early postmenopausal period and are more likely to be successful in patients who have previously responded favorably to oophorectomy or adrenal cortical hormones. Similarly successful results have been reported following hypophyseal stalk section or the transnasal implantation of yttrium 91 and other radioactive substances, as well as by proton beam bombardment of the pituitary. The usefulness of these procedures is obviously limited by the requirement of a cooperative team of skilled surgeons to carry out the procedures and conscientious internists to handle the subsequent hormone replacement problems of adrenal or pituitary insufficiency. When these facilities are not available, further benefit may be obtained from the use of androgens or pharmacologic doses of estrogens, as will be described below.

As ovarian activity wanes during the course of the menopause, the estrogens come to play a lesser role and other factors, some at least of pituitary origin, a more important one in stimulating the growth of breast cancer. There appears to be a small group of patients in this age group who may actually be adversely affected by oophorectomy, perhaps because the secretion and stimulating activity of growth hormone or other pituitary factors on the cancer cell is enhanced by removal of estrogen inhibition. There is no way of predicting such a result in the present state of our knowledge, but fortunately it is a rare occurrence. Such patients may well be the ideal candidates for hypophyseal ablation or sex hormone administration.

In the postmenopausal group, treatment must be individualized. Some patients may show continued ovarian activity even up to the age of seventy; a very high incidence of ovarian stromal hyperplasia, which is considered to be evidence of persistence of estrogen synthesis beyond the period of ovulation, has been observed among postmenopausal patients with mammary cancer. Such estrogen activity may be most easily detected by demonstrating the presence of more than 10 per cent of cornified cells in the vaginal smear stained by the Papanicolaou method. When this activity is present, oophorectomy is indicated and may produce dramatic remissions even in patients over the age of seventy years.

Bulbrook and associates have recently presented statistical evidence to indicate that in women under the age of sixty-five who excrete a low ratio of androgens (11-deoxy-17-ketosteroids) to 17-hydroxy corticosteroids (17-OH-CS) in their urine, breast cancer has a poorer prognosis, in terms of recurrence rate, 3-year survival, and response to adrenalectomy, than in women of similar age with a higher androgen excretion rate. The following discriminant function was derived from their data to separate these two groups: 80-80(17-OH-CS, mg/24 hr) + etiocholanolone, mcg/24 hr. When the value of this function was over 1, a good response to adrenalectomy occurred in 50 per cent of cases, whereas when it was less than 1, only 10 per cent showed a definitely favorable response. This finding, if confirmed, may be an important step in helping to solve the difficult problem of selecting those patients who are most likely to benefit from endocrine ablative therapy.

In the older postmenopausal patients and the senescent group, 15 years or more past the menopause, large doses of estrogens may provide remarkable palliation and this is the treatment of choice. This paradoxic effect of estrogens, first clearly described by Nathanson, has never been fully explained.

The place of androgens and estrogens in the treatment of metastatic breast cancer has been well defined by the recent report of the American Medical Association's Council on Drugs, based on a 10-year nationwide cooperative study. In summary, androgens produced objective remissions in approximately 20 per cent of patients both before and after the menopause. Estrogens, which should not be used before the menopause, will induce remissions in about 36 per cent of patients during the first 8 postmenopausal years and in more than 38 per cent in later years. Estrogens have a greater relative effect on soft tissue and visceral metastases than on bone but equal or exceed the effect of androgens on all types of tissue. It should be emphasized that estrogens must be employed in large doses to achieve these results, such as stilbestrol, 15 mg, or ethinyl estradiol, 3 mg daily. Smaller amounts may adversely affect the tumor. Nausea and vomiting may occur at the onset of treatment but can be controlled by antiemetic agents and will disappear in time. Uterine bleeding may be troublesome but can usually be controlled by the cyclic administration of progesterone or methyl testosterone.

The optimum dose of androgens has been found to be equivalent to 100 mg of testosterone propionate given intramuscularly three times weekly. Recent experience indicates that the newer anabolic androgens such as fluoxymestrone in oral doses of 20 mg daily may be equally effective with much less tendency to produce the undesirable masculinizing side effects of testosterone.

All patients, but especially those within the first 8 postmenopausal years, should be observed carefully during the first few days and weeks of treatment because both androgens and estrogens may cause an exacerbation of their disease, estrogens by a direct stimulating effect and androgens presumably by being converted in small but effective amounts to estrogens. One of the most serious complications produced by administration of these hormones in patients who exhibit extensive skeletal metastases is calcium intoxication. This is presumed to result from the sudden stimulation of growth of the bony metastases by the hormone, with correspondingly rapid destruction of bone and flooding of the circulation with calcium. There is a marked increase in urine calcium excretion, and the serum calcium level may rise to as high as 15 to 20 mg per 100 ml, and drowsiness, coma, convulsions, and death from renal failure may ensue. It is important to distinguish this condition from cerebral or liver metastases or the terminal effects of widespread cancer because it can be reversed by forcing fluids, withdrawal of the offending hormone, and administration of large amounts of hydrocortisone, 200

mg daily by slow intravenous drip or in divided oral doses daily, until symptoms subside.

Currently, extensive studies are being made of the value of carcinolytic chemical agents as adjuncts to other forms of therapy for mammary cancer. To date, definite and repeated regression of cutaneous and subcutaneous metastases have been observed following the use of thio-triethylene phosphoramid and 5-fluorouracil. Unfortunately, these effects are transient and the value of these agents is limited at present by their bone marrow toxicity.

Carcinoma occurs in the male breast at least 100 times less frequently than in the female. Otherwise it behaves in exactly the same manner. The treatment is the same except that orchiectomy replaces oophorectomy. Prednisone and hypophysectomy have both been shown to induce remissions when the primary disease has metastasized, and progestational compounds may be of value.

REFERENCES

Bulbrook, R. D., J. L. Hayward, and B. S. Thomas: "The Relation Between the Urinary 17-Hydroxy Corticosteroids and 11-Deoxy-17-Oxysteroids and the Fate of Patients After Mastectomy," Lancet, 1:947, 1964.

Haagensen, C. D.: "Diseases of the Breast," Philadelphia, W. B. Saunders Company, 1956.

Lyons, W. R., C. H. Li, and R. E. Johnson: "Hormonal Control of Mammary Growth and Lactation," Recent Prog. Hormone Res., 14:219, 1958.

Pincus, Gregory (Ed.): "Recent Progress in Hormone Research," New York, Academic Press, Inc., 1958.

Pincus, G., and E. P. Vollmer (Eds.): "Biological Activities of Steroids in Relation to Cancer," New York, Academic Press, Inc., 1960.

Segaloff, Albert (Ed.): "Breast Cancer," The Second Biennial Louisiana Cancer Conference, St. Louis, The C. V. Mosby Company, 1958.

93 DISEASES OF THE PINEAL GLAND
Julian I. Kitay

INTRODUCTION. Histochemical studies of the pineal gland in monkeys, rats, and other animals have shown the presence of ribonucleoprotein, deoxyribonucleoprotein, glycogen, acid and alkaline phosphatase, and succinic dehydrogenase in the parenchymal cells. Radioisotope experiments in rats have demonstrated that the uptake of P^{32} per 100 mg fresh tissue is greater in the pineal gland than in any other organ studied. Hypophysectomy in rats results in an even greater pineal uptake of P^{32}, whereas corticotropin administration decreases the uptake to prehypophysectomy levels. Pinealectomy in chicks, mice, rabbits, or rats is associated with gonadal hypertrophy and acceleration of vaginal opening in immature animals and with prolongation of estrus and shortening of diestrus in mature animals. On the other hand, pineal extract administered to these animals consistently reversed the changes.

More recently, the mammalian pineal gland has been demonstrated to contain a number of amines, including serotonin, norepinephrine, and histamine, and enzymes concerned with their synthesis and metabolism. In 1959, Lerner et al. isolated 5-methoxy N-acetyl tryptamine (melatonin) in bovine pineal glands. This compound has since been synthesized in vitro by N-acetylation of serotonin followed by O-methylation. The enzyme hydroxyindole-O-methyl transferase, associated with the latter step, has been shown to be located uniquely in the pineal gland of man and a variety of animal species. Its activity has been correlated with light stimulation. Melatonin is extremely potent in lightening frog skin both in vivo and in vitro. An interesting paradox has resulted from the observation that melatonin is not demonstrable in amphibian pineal glands despite the striking changes it produces in skin pigmentation of the frog. On the other hand, the compound exerts no effect on human skin, although it is abundant in the human pineal and is stored in human peripheral nerve. Melatonin has been shown to inhibit ovarian function in the rat, consistent with older reports of studies with crude gland extracts. Other experiments have associated the pineal gland with regulation of aldosterone secretion. These studies and many others suggest that the pineal is a functioning endocrine organ. Confirmation and further research is indicated, however, before its function can be defined.

ANATOMY AND PATHOLOGY. The human pineal gland is a small, gray, conical organ, that lies deep in the brain along the quadrigeminate groove between the superior colliculi. It is attached anteriorly to the posterior wall of the third ventricle by the pineal stalk, which is continuous with the superior habenular and posterior commissures. It is considered to contain two types of cells, pineal parenchymal cells and neuroglia, and pineal weight does not decrease at puberty or in senescence. The normal human pineal gland weighs between 140 and 200 mg.

Calcification in the pineal gland is seen in about 50 per cent of routine skull roentgenograms. The incidence of such calcification is negligible in the first decade of life; it approximates 25 per cent in the second decade; and it increases gradually from the third to the eighth decades. The visible calcium deposits in the gland are frequently used as an anatomic landmark in roentgenographic localization of brain tumors. It should be noted that similar deposits occurring in the habenular region may be confused with pineal calcification.

Many pineal lesions have been described, including tumors, fibrosis, infarction, atrophy, agenesis, and a variety of histopathologic changes that occur in association with diseases elsewhere in the body. With the exception of tumors, none of these lesions has demonstrable clinical significance.

PINEAL TUMORS. Neoplasms are the most common pineal lesions; however, their incidence is low in most series of intracranial tumors. Over 50 per cent of the total cases have been reported in patients twenty years of age or younger. The incidence is three times as frequent in men as in women. Histopathologic descriptions are varied and confusing, and more than 25 types of tumor have been described. All these types may be generally classified as either tumors of parenchymal origin (e.g., pinealomas) or tumors of nonparenchymal origin (e.g., teratomas, gliomas, and cysts). However, such classification may be difficult because pinealomatous and teratomatous tissues have frequently been noted to coexist in the same lesion. Ectopic pinealomas have also been described with no pathologic changes in the pineal gland itself.

Clinical Features. The neurologic signs most frequently associated with pineal tumors include headache, hydrocephalus, papilledema, cerebellar dysfunction, and paralysis of upward gaze (Parinaud's syndrome) with weakened convergence and decreased pupillary reaction to light (Chap. 206). Diabetes insipidus is occasionally present, usually in association with tumors of parenchymal origin. The course is generally one of local expansion with involvement of neighboring areas. Occasionally, distant metastases may occur to various parts of the central nervous system.

Precocious puberty (Pellizzi's syndrome) has been observed in 30 per cent of boys with pineal tumors. The lack of a corresponding syndrome in girls has not been explained. A contributory factor may be the relatively low incidence of pineal lesions in prepuberal females. The current explanation of the mechanism whereby a pineal tumor causes precocious puberty is that the expanding lesion indirectly stimulates the pituitary gland by compressing or destroying hypothalamic areas that regulate anterior pituitary function. This trauma presumably increases the secretion of gonadotropins, with consequent development of precocity. Proponents of this theory believe that the histologic composition of the tumor is not important and that only its location is significant. It should be noted, however, that this hypothesis was formulated because sexual precocity occurs in connection with both pineal and other intracranial lesions, and some workers wished to explain all sexual precocity due to intracranial disease on the basis of a single mechanism.

Although the above-mentioned theory has been widely held, reexamination of the available data has called attention to certain findings that tend to controvert it. Pineal tumors of parenchymal origin and those of nonparenchymal origin are equally distributed in children one to sixteen years of age. However, sexual precocity is associated with nonparenchymal tumors four times as often as with parenchymal tumors—a statistically significant disproportion.

Moreover, hypogenitalism also has been reported in association with pineal tumors, and in these cases parenchymal tumors predominate by a ratio of 2.5:1. The "pressure" hypothesis outlined above is incompatible with these findings. A better explanation must await more definitive experimental studies.

Treatment. Conservative therapy consists of decompression by ventriculostomy or shunting (Torkildsen procedure) followed by irradiation. Such treatment has yielded a 10-year survival rate of greater than 60 per cent. Direct attempts at surgical resection have generally resulted in a prohibitively high mortality.

REFERENCES

Kitay, J. I., and M. D. Altschule: "The Pineal Gland: A Review of the Physiologic Literature," Cambridge, Mass., Harvard University Press, 1954.

Lerner, A. B., J. D. Case, and R. V. Heinzelman: The structure of melatonin, J. Am. Chem. Soc., 81:6084, 1959.

Smith, R. A.: Pineal Tumors, Michigan Univ. Med. Bull., 27:33, 1961.

Wurtman, R. J., J. Axelrod, and E. W. Chu: Melatonin, a pineal substance: effect on rat ovary, Science, 141: 277, 1963.

Section 3

Errors of Metabolism

INTRODUCTION

W. Eugene Knox

The errors of metabolism constitute a very large group of individually rare hereditary conditions, each distinguished by some striking biochemical departure from the usual. Far from being curiosities of no general importance, these conditions provided the conceptual schemes that linked the sciences of genetics and biochemistry to each other and to the science of medicine. The central idea emerged in 1902, in a paper by Sir Archibald Garrod entitled "The Incidence of Alkaptonuria, A Study in Chemical Individuality." To alkaptonuria he later added cystinuria, albinism, and pentosuria, calling them "inborn errors of metabolism." He realized that these conditions, biochemical peculiarities "which advertised their presence in some conspicuous way," were only prototypes of a potentially large number of differences between individuals of greater or less significance:

If it be, indeed, the case that in alkaptonuria and the other conditions mentioned, we are dealing with individuality in metabolism and not with the results of morbid processes, the thought naturally presents itself that these are merely extreme examples of variations of chemical behavior which are probably everywhere present in minor degrees and that just as no two individuals of a species are ever absolutely identical in bodily structure neither are their chemical processes carried out on exactly the same lines. Such chemical differences will be obviously far more subtle than those of form, for whereas the latter are evident to any careful observer the former will only be revealed by elaborate chemical methods.

Since then, many further examples of the same kind of thing have been discovered, adding detail to Garrod's concept without altering his general principles.

The central idea of Garrod's concept was the relationship between gene, enzyme, and disease. At a time when mendelian inheritance was not known in man, Garrod saw that the aggregation of cases of an inborn error of metabolism in particular families followed the law of recessive inheritance. At a time when the mysteries of metabolism were still unexplored, Garrod hypothesized that metabolism occurred in a series of chemical steps, each catalyzed by a specific enzyme and with each enzyme produced by a specific genetic factor. The gene-determined inactivity of a single enzyme blocked that step in metabolism. Accumulation of the intermediate before the block, or deficiency of the intermediate coming after the block, produced the signs and symptoms of the associated disease. At a time when morbidity was being ascribed with great success to extraneous agents such as bacteria or poisons, Garrod perceived that morbid processes could also be inborn.

The idea of the relationship of gene, enzyme, and disease has flowered with time. The excretion of homogentisic acid in alkaptonuria and of L-xylulose in pentosuria and the signs and symptoms of these conditions can now be traced back to the gene-determined inactivity of the specific enzymes that normally metabolize these compounds. The same relationship in the form of the *one gene, one enzyme hypothesis* became the key for the study of intermediary metabolism in the lower forms of life by experimental genetics. The purview of Garrod's idea has also extended beyond the inborn abnormalities of intermediary metabolism. The cystine excretion of cystinuria results not from a block in metabolism but from failure of a specific renal tubular reabsorption mechanism. Therefore genes play a role in the formation not only of the enzymes of metabolism but also of the specific enzymelike transport systems. Still more recently it has been learned that genes determine the detailed structure of functional proteins such as the hemoglobins. There are still other subtle chemical differences among individuals, such as the blood group antigens, that are genetically determined. The present development of Garrod's concept envisages the primary equipment of the cell as a cadre of molecules, for the most part functional proteins, whose molecular structures and therefore functions are determined by the arrays of nucleotides of deoxyribonucleic acid in the genes. These molecules fashion the cell from its environment. The inborn structural variations of these molecules account for the inborn diversities in the biochemical makeup of human beings. When the physiologic consequences of a particular molecular alteration are sufficiently grave, the condition may appropriately be considered a hereditary molecular disease. The term *molecular disease*, first introduced by Pauling to describe sickle-cell anemia, indicates both the modern chemical definition of the "error" first conceived by Garrod and our modern knowledge of the detailed pathologic consequences to the individual from such a molecular alteration.

The enduring fruitfulness of Garrod's concept results from the happy combination of its esthetic attractiveness and its wide applicability to biologic problems. The discrete alteration in a single type of functional molecule represents an experiment of nature whose subtlety has long captivated biologists. Through such errors we have gained insight about pathways and functions whose existence was unsuspected so long as they operated smoothly. The discovery of new examples of such errors has continued unabated since Garrod's time, and no decrease is to be expected. The possible number of such diseases is commensurate with the number of genes. All variant genes should produce variant molecules. Therefore, the molecular abnormalities are not restricted to the recessively inherited types that were first singled out. Individuals with one or two abnormal genes and even the heterozygous carriers of a recessive disease have a portion of abnormal molecules produced by their abnormal gene. Because heterozygous carriers of a gene for a rare recessive disease are so enormously more frequent than patients with the disease, it turns out that most individuals must possess some abnormal genes and therefore some abnormal molecules.

The specifically medical interest in the inborn errors centers on the pathogenetic pathways by which a chemical abnormality of a molecule produces the signs and symptoms of disease. The pathologic consequences of the precise chemical disturbances in these conditions contributes fundamental information about disease mechanisms in general. Such information is equally applicable to the mechanisms of nonheritable diseases, which share similar final common pathways. The inborn errors studied so far have inexorably produced certain pathologic consequences with little influence by ordinary environmental conditions. Now examples are being recognized in which the molecular

abnormality does not lead inevitably to disease: environmental influences must interact in some essential way for a pathologic result. Such a hereditary abnormality that is a necessary but not sufficient cause for disease is the deficiency of glucose 6-phosphate dehydrogenase in red cells. In this condition hemolytic anemia results only when there is exposure to certain substances like the fava bean. The participation of environmental influences in the pathogenesis of a disease promises to clarify the hereditary basis of many common diseases whose familial occurrence is too highly variable to be proved hereditary by simple mendelian expectations.

It is not to be anticipated that environmental influence can alter the primary defect either in a gene or in the functional molecule made by the gene. But the consequences of gene action are being continuously altered by environmental influences. Given knowledge of how a disease results from the fundamental chemical disturbance, the play of environment can often be altered by design to minimize or prevent the disease consequences that would otherwise result from an inborn error of metabolism.

REFERENCES

Garrod, A. E.: Inborn Errors of Metabolism, Lancet, II:1, 73, 142, 214, 1908.

Harris, H.: "Garrod's Inborn Errors of Metabolism," London, Oxford University Press, 1963.

Knox, W. E.: Sir Archibald Garrod's "Inborn Errors of Metabolism," Am. J. Human Genetics, 10:3, 95, 249, 385, 1958.

Stanbury, J. B., J. B. Wyngaarden, and D. S. Fredrickson (Eds.): "The Metabolic Basis of Inherited Disease," 2d ed., New York, McGraw-Hill Book Company, Inc., 1964.

94   PHENYLKETONURIA (Phenylpyruvic Oligophrenia)

W. Eugene Knox

DEFINITION. Phenylketonuria is a recessively inherited failure to oxidize phenylalanine to tyrosine, characterized by the excretion of phenylpyruvic acid, mental deficiency, epileptic seizures, and mild pigmentation.

HISTORY. Følling in 1934 described 10 mentally deficient patients whose urine contained phenylpyruvic acid, identified by the blue-green color produced with $FeCl_3$. Surveys in the Western world based on this urine test revealed that about 0.7 per cent of the inmates in institutions for the mentally defective were so affected. Jervis proved that phenylketonuria was recessively inherited through a single autosomal gene. He also located the metabolic error by demonstrating a very large accumulation of phenylalanine in the body fluids and the absence of the normal rise in plasma tyrosine following a dose of phenylalanine. In 1953, Jervis demonstrated the inactivity of phenylalanine hydroxylase of the liver in these patients, thus completing for the first time a proof of the relationships between gene, enzyme, and disease postulated for the inborn errors of metabolism by Garrod.

ETIOLOGY. The parents of a phenylketonuric child each have one defective gene for phenylalanine hydroxylase, manifesting itself in a slightly reduced capacity to oxidize phenylalanine but without any mental or clinical abnormalities. On the average, one in four children of such a union receives two defective genes and so has no active phenylalanine hydroxylase. This enzyme is restricted to liver, where it appears during the first few weeks after birth. The failure of active enzyme to appear in the phenylketonuric infant results in the gradual accumulation of phenylalanine from the diet to as much as thirty times the normal blood level after several weeks. It then overflows via transamination into the rapidly excreted phenylpyruvate. Several other related metabolites are also excreted in abnormal amounts. Among these phenylalanine and o-hydroxyphenylacetic acid may have diagnostic usefulness.

The high levels of phenylalanine in body fluids inhibit transport of amino acids into cells. A pronounced deficit of cerebral cerebrosides occurs. The mental disease results from these changes.

By six months of age, mental development is retarded, and seizures and other neurologic abnormalities suggesting extrapyramidal disease appear. Since the mental defect is stationary and not progressive in older children or adults, the brain injury appears to be limited to a particularly sensitive stage in brain development. Delayed myelination has been found at autopsy in the youngest children, but there are no other neuropathologic findings to account for the mental disease.

The mild pigmentation of hair, eyes, and skin results from the competitive inhibition by phenylalanine of the melanin formation by tyrosinase. Eczema has been commonly described, but it is not a specific sign.

DIAGNOSIS. Chemical diagnosis is essential for successful treatment, since the neurologic abnormalities, once established, are largely irreversible. The $FeCl_3$ urine test is remarkably effective after one month of age: several drops of 5 per cent $FeCl_3$ in 5 ml fresh urine produces first some precipitation of phosphates, then with several more drops a blue- or olive-green color slowly appears within 2 min and fades after 1 or 2 hr. Paper strips for the test are available. Confirmation is obtained by formation of a yellow precipitate on addition to the urine of a few drops of saturated 2,4-dinitrophenylhydrazine in 2 N HCl. Diagnosis before one month of age must depend upon the grossly elevated level of plasma phenylalanine, as should the final corroboration of the diagnosis before treatment is started.

TREATMENT. The biochemical abnormalities can be corrected by preventing the accumulation of phenylalanine. This is done by a special diet in which protein is replaced by an amino acid mixture low in phenylalanine (Ketonil, Lofenolac). Supplementary foods are given to supply only the amount of L-phenylalanine needed for body growth. An infant requires at least three times as much per kg body weight as an older child. Normal weight gain and near normal plasma phenylalanine levels should be maintained. Treatment should continue at least until four years of age. Normal development has been obtained in some patients treated from early infancy. Little permanent improvement can be achieved by treatment begun after the age of three years.

REFERENCES

Harris, H.: "Garrod's Inborn Errors of Metabolism," London, Oxford University Press, 1963.

95 ALKAPTONURIA AND OCHRONOSIS

W. Eugene Knox

DEFINITION. Alkaptonuria is the lifelong excretion in the urine of the strongly reducing compound homogentisic acid (2,5-dihydroxyphenylacetic acid). Old or alkaline *urine turns dark,* and after middle life the darkened mesenchymal tissues (*ochronosis*) appear blue through the skin and *degenerative joint changes* occur.

HISTORY. The condition was named by Bödeker in 1859. He found in the urine of a patient with lumbar arthritis a substance which, when alkalinized, darkened the urine from the surface down and caused the urine to take up more than its own volume of oxygen: "I call it for this reason 'Alkapton' (admittedly a somewhat barbarous combination from the Greek participle of καπτεἰν, to suck up greedily, and the Arabic, *alkali*), after its outstanding behaviour toward oxygen in alkaline solution." Virchow in 1866 reported as a pathologic curiosity a patient with "arthritis deformans," the coal blackness of whose cartilages and tendons he called ochronosis. Albrecht in 1902 demonstrated the connection between ochronosis and alkaptonuria at the section of a patient with gray-blue ears "like dilated veins" and with residual bladder urine which darkened on standing. Sir William Osler (1904) was the first to diagnose ochronosis during life on the basis of the darkened scleras, ears, and nose of two alkaptonurics. He failed to connect the disabling arthritis in one of his patients with the alkaptonuria. This was done in 1913 by Umber on the basis of a family with five alkaptonurics, all five with arthritis.

Alkaptonuria was the prototype of the inborn errors of metabolism. It was the first of these diseases that Garrod studied, and the one to which he fitted the definition of the group.

ETIOLOGY. Alkaptonuria is inherited as a very rare autosomal recessive characteristic. The sexes are equally affected, but parents and offspring of a patient are usually unaffected. An average of one in four siblings is affected, and the parents are often related. The incidence is about 1 in 200,000 persons. The molecular basis is the complete hereditary inactivity of homogentisate oxidase, which normally catalyzes a step in tyrosine metabolism. Approximately 4 Gm per day of homogentisic acid accumulates at this metabolic block to be rapidly excreted by the kidneys. The amount excreted can be decreased by a low-protein diet (short of negative nitrogen balance) and increased by administration of extra protein or the amino acids, phenylalanine and tyrosine. At neutral pH or above, homogentisic acid is rapidly oxidized to the brown or black polymer, which accounts for the darkening of the urine on standing and the staining of wetted linen. A slower accumulation in the body of a similar polymer bound to cartilages and related tissues produces the ochronosis and the degeneration of the stained structures seen by middle life.

CLINICAL PICTURE. Most patients have been found by an atypical positive test for reducing substances in the urine, raising the question of diabetes. More males than females are found because more males have urine tests. Less commonly the darkening of the urine leads to the diagnosis. Wet diapers turn black in hours. It is remarkable how often this phenomenon will go unnoticed throughout the life of an affected individual. The condition is completely benign until thirty or forty years of age, when the degenerative joint changes begin in at least half the cases. The large joints and spine are affected with pain and stiffness, sometimes there are acute inflammatory episodes, and the process progresses in time to ankylosis. Degeneration of the intervertebral disks with subsequent calcification and vertebral osteophyte formation makes the spine appear radiologically like the ties and rails of a railroad track. The ochronosis can be seen in the transmitted blueness of cartilages of the ear, nose, costochondral junctions, and the superficial tendons, and brown areas in the scleras at the rectus insertions on both sides of the irides. The affected tissues, when exposed, present an arresting sight of coal blackness. Staining also occurs in the arterial intima, sclerotic plaques, and other elements of the cardiovascular system. Older patients often exhibit degenerative cardiovascular disease. The association may be one of chance.

DIAGNOSIS. Chemical identification of homogentisic acid should be required even in the presence of the triad of arthritis, ochronosis, and darkening urine. Undarkened urine plus sodium hydroxide turns red brown and then blackens as it absorbs oxygen. The urine strongly reduces alkaline copper solutions, but since it turns black in the process the erroneous diagnosis of glucosuria can be avoided. It does not give a positive test with glucose oxidase test papers, nor does it reduce bismuth reagents for sugar (Nylander's test). Undeveloped photographic film exposed to the light will be immediately blackened by the urine just as it will be by the chemically similar hydroquinone developer. This is the clinical test of choice.

In carbolochronosis from the long-continued absorption of large amounts of phenol or its derivatives, the tissues are stained as in alkaptonuria, and the urine may be dark from hydroquinone formed metabolically. Acute phenol poisoning and rarely melanomas will also produce dark urines.

TREATMENT. A low but adequate protein diet for life should be instituted at an early age to avoid excessive homogentisate formation and possibly to delay the degenerative changes. "Wishful" treatments should be avoided, including insulin, liver extracts and cortisone, and ascorbic acid, which merely keep homogentisate in the urine bleached.

REFERENCES

Garrod, A. E.: The Incidence of Alkaptonuria, A Study in Chemical Individuality, Lancet, II:1616, 1902.

96 CYSTINURIA, CYSTINOSIS, AND THE FANCONI SYNDROME

W. Eugene Knox

CYSTINURIA

DEFINITION. Cystinuria is the inborn and lifelong excretion in the urine of large amounts of the dibasic amino acids, cystine (about 1 Gm per day), lysine, arginine, and ornithine. It results from a hereditary defect in a specific reabsorptive process of the renal tubule. Recurrent cystine urinary calculi and their sequelae are the sole clinical manifestations.

HISTORY. The first amino acid available in relatively pure form was the cystine in the stones from cystinurics. The condition has been recognized by the stones or by the microscopic crystalluria since the early nineteenth century, but its critical definition dates from the medical thesis of Niemann in 1876. On the basis of 53 cases then known, he defined the disease, excluded age and environmental factors as causes, noted its familial occurrence, and suggested an arrest of cystine metabolism as the cause. Garrod's contribution, coming after the rediscovery of Mendel's laws of inheritance, was to recognize that most of the familial cases followed the pattern of recessive inheritance. The erroneous belief that intermediary cystine metabolism was defective persisted in the face of evidence to the contrary until recently. Then three other amino acids, previously unnoticed because of their high solubility in urine, were found to be excreted by cystinurics along with cystine. Dent and Harris thereupon promptly and completely explained the renal physiology and genetics of cystinuria.

ETIOLOGY. In two-thirds of the families so far studied, cystinuria was inherited as a recessive condition, with the parents of affected individuals having no abnormality of amino acid excretion. In the remaining third of the families the condition was incompletely recessive, with the heterozygous carriers of one abnormal gene showing raised excretions of cystine and lysine. The amount of cystine excreted is almost always less than 250 mg per Gm creatinine. Above this amount stone formation may occur. These heterozygotes account for the high incidence (1 in 250) of chemically detectable cystinuria without stones found in the population. Matings between the two types are needed to determine if the two kinds of genes are allelic.

The four amino acids excreted in cystinuria have two basic groups separated by four or five carbon atoms. Possibly this is the structural basis for their reaction with a single transport system that has an enzymelike specificity. Because of the inactivity of this specific transport system in a cystinuric, the renal clearances of these amino acids closely approach the glomerular filtration rate. In the normal or heterozygous person an administered load of one of these amino acids will competitively inhibit the reabsorption of the others. The blood levels of the four amino acids are low in cystinuria rather than elevated as would be expected from a blocked metabolism with an overflow type of excretion.

The same four amino acids are also poorly absorbed by the gut, indicating that the same genetic system acts in this organ and in the kidney. Chronic lysine deficiency results in decreased growth.

The amount of cystine excreted depends directly upon its blood level. Methionine, and not cystine itself, is the component of dietary protein that elevates the blood cystine level and so increases cystine excretion. The amount excreted is usually 0.4 to 1.2 Gm per day or 0.3 to 0.8 mg per min, and this amount is primarily determined by body size and diet. The solubility of cystine in urine at body temperature is less than 0.4 mg per ml through the readily attainable range of urine pH. A urine flow above 2 ml per min (3 liters per day) may therefore be needed throughout the 24 hr to carry in solution the cystine that will be excreted. The decreased urine flow in the early morning hours is often responsible for the supersaturation of cystine, its crystallization, and the accretion into calculi unless washed away by the daytime diuresis. First stones appear randomly at all ages among cystinurics when this precarious equilibrium fails, as it eventually does in nearly all untreated cystinurics. Recurrent calculi and progressive renal damage then usually occur.

DIAGNOSIS. The only clinical manifestations are those referable to recurrent urinary calculi of the kidney, ureters, bladder, or urethra, or to the passing of gravel. These are not clinically distinguishable from other urologic conditions of this type. With infection, the urine may develop a particularly foul odor from the decomposition of ornithine and lysine to putrescine and cadavarine. Because of the high atomic number of sulfur, the cystine stones are radiologically dense, more so than urate and comparable to the density of calcium oxalate. Because effective treatment is possible, every effort should be made to identify the 1 per cent of urinary calculi that are cystine and, when

possible, to diagnose the condition before calculi appear.

The microscopic appearance of cystine crystals in the sediment of the first morning urine is a sufficiently sensitive test to detect cystinuria, especially if combined with a urine concentration test and if the urine plus glacial acetic acid to pH 4.5 is chilled for a few hours before centrifuging. The crystals are hexagonal plates resembling the formula of a benzene ring. Crystalluria is nearly restricted to those cystinurics excreting more than 250 mg cystine per day. These are the ones who may develop stones. Their incidence is perhaps 1 in 50,000 persons.

The nitroprusside tests for cystine in urine will detect the cystinurics and also the very much more frequent heterozygotes of the incompletely recessive form (1 in 250 persons). It will also detect some rarer conditions in which cystine excretion is part of a general aminoaciduria. Urinary cystine must first be reduced to cysteine with sodium cyanide to give this test.

The specific aminoaciduria consisting of the excretion of cystine, lysine, arginine, and ornithine in comparable amounts is diagnostic. The specific pattern can be demonstrated with paper chromatography. It distinguishes cystinuria from all other diseases, including cystinosis.

TREATMENT. Medical treatment can prevent formation and growth of stones. Over a long period it can sometimes also bring about stone dissolution, but usually the accepted urologic procedures for dealing with calculi should be followed. The progressive renal insufficiency that follows recurrent episodes of calculi complicates the medical treatment even while it produces a more dilute urine that diminishes the cystine precipitation.

The basis of the medical treatment is the quantitative estimation of the 24-hr cystine excretion. From this and the known solubility of cystine in urine, an adequate urine flow to carry the excreted cystine in soluble form can be calculated. The flow must be maintained throughout the 24 hr by nocturnal fluids. The total amount of cystine excreted can be minimized by a diet low in methionine, obtained by replacing animal protein with vegetable protein. The diet must be chosen for its long-term adequacy for the patient. The efficiency of the regimen is monitored by periodic checks to determine that cystine saturation is not exceeded in either the day or night urines. Occasionally it may be necessary to use in addition the small increase in cystine solubility obtainable by alkalinizing the urine.

Penicillamine is excreted as a mixed disulfide with cysteine, which is more soluble than cystine. This offers an additional means of therapy.

CYSTINOSIS AND THE FANCONI SYNDROME

DEFINITION. Two groups of cases will be distinguished from the tubular nephropathies that share some or all of the features of generalized amino-aciduria, renal glucosuria, hypophosphatemia, chronic acidosis, and defective mineralization of bone matrix (resistant rickets or osteomalacia). These are the features of the *adult Fanconi syndrome*. Cystinosis is seen in infants and children. They have, in addition, cystine crystals deposited throughout most tissues.

HISTORY. In 1903, Abderhalden described the finding at autopsy of crystalline cystine deposits in the tissues of a twenty-one-month-old infant dead of "inanition." He called the disease *familial cystine diathesis* since two siblings died in a similar way, and moderate excretion of cystine occurred in adult members of the family. The next child, described in 1924 by Lignac-Leider, was unique in also having cystine urinary calculi. Nevertheless, there is no justification for confusing the condition with the quite different disease of cystinuria. Later cases in adults and children were described from different points of view under a variety of eponyms such as the Fanconi-Lignac-Debré-de Toni syndrome to refer to various combinations of signs. Central to all these is the renal tubular disorder.

ETIOLOGY. Cystinosis and adult Fanconi syndrome appear to be genetically distinct entities transmitted as recessive characters. In families with one of these conditions, it would be unusual to find the other (or cystinuria).

In both conditions there is a shortened and narrowed "swan neck" deformity of the proximal renal tubule. This has been demonstrated by microdissection. It is probable that the morphologic and functional defects are related, since most of the findings can be attributed to failure of many reabsorptive and other functions of the (proximal) renal tubule. There is absence of alkaline phosphatase in the proximal tubule, probably a secondary effect of the disease.

Glucose reabsorption is certainly a proximal tubule function, and possibly so are the reabsorptions of amino acids, phosphate, bicarbonate, and potassium. Glucosuria, scant and intermittent or profuse and constant, occurs with a normal blood sugar level. The carbohydrate wastage is extreme enough to produce ketosis in about one-fourth of the patients. This may contribute to the acidosis. The generalized aminoaciduria occurs without an increased blood level of α-amino nitrogen. The pattern of amino acids excreted resembles that of plasma. The aminoaciduria is innocuous, amounting perhaps to a loss of as much as one-tenth of the dietary protein in the urine. This loss may contribute to the dwarfism and body wastage and may participate in calcium excretion by chelation. The phosphaturia produces hypophosphatemia and, together with the acidosis, results in osteomalacia. The loss of phosphate from bone counteracts acidosis because dissolution of bone converts PO_4^{3-} to $HPO_4^=$ and so buffers one hydrogen ion. Low bicarbonate resorption results in bicarbonate excretion at a lower urine pH than normal and in depletion of body alkali stores. It also contributes to the defect in urinary acidification. Thus bicarbonate loss also contributes to the acidosis and to the hyperchloremia. The potassium wastage results in hypokalemia and sometimes causes profound muscular weakness or paralysis. Potassium depletion may in turn produce renal tubular damage by positive feedback, resulting in polyuria and inability to concentrate urine and inability to excrete urine more acid than pH 6 to 7 despite the severe acidosis. Potassium depletion can by itself cause the vacuolation of proximal tubule cells seen in this condition and can predispose to the development of renal infection. Thus the proximal tubular anomaly can be considered to initiate a self-maintained renal injury with widespread metabolic consequences. The condition often produces glomerular damage with hyalinization, often pyelonephritis, and eventual death with hypertension and uremia.

CLINICAL PICTURE. In addition to the distinction between young and adult cases, each individual patient differs considerably from others in the particular combination and severity of his pathologic changes. In the adult Fanconi cases, at least, renal tubular dysfunction precedes the development of the usual presenting complaints caused by osteomalacia. The typical urinary abnormalities have been found in relatives without bone disease who were then followed until bone changes did develop. Such individuals also have hypophosphatemia and mild acidosis. Over a period of years, rheumatic-type pains develop, which restrict movement until the patient is bedridden. Severe osteomalacia is seen radiologically with its characteristic pseudofractures. These are bilateral, symmetric lines of decalcification whose location can be predicted since they occur adjacent to the course of blood vessels curving round the bones.

The condition seen in children is more fulminating. Failure to thrive and severe resistant rickets with dwarfing develop in the first few months of life. In children death usually occurs by ten years of age, although treated cases have survived as long as 35 years. The intracellular deposition of considerable amounts of cystine (about 0.5 Gm per Gm tissue nitrogen) in most tissues (not only in the reticuloendothelial system) is a unique and puzzling feature in the young cases. An altered active transport of cystine and possibly of other amino acids into cells might be suggested, but such a mechanism cannot now be related to the renal abnormality that determines the main clinical features. The presence of these crystalline rods or plates in the cornea and conjunctivas, demonstrable by a slit lamp, is of diagnostic importance.

Usually there is no difficulty in assigning a patient to this general group, but classification within the group is seldom satisfactory because of the variations between patients and in the same patient at different stages of the disease. A closely related group of patients with renal tubular acidosis shares many of the defects of the Fanconi syndrome, including low reabsorption of bicarbonate. However, formation of renal calculi, nephrocalcinosis, and absence of aminoaciduria distinguish renal tubular acidosis from the Fanconi syndrome. The differential diagnosis may consider diabetes or even diabetic acidosis on the basis of the urine findings, but the normal blood glucose level should warn against this error.

TREATMENT. Because patients vary widely in the severity of the several defects making up this syndrome, they will also vary in their response to the several therapeutic procedures available. These are merely replacement therapies and are not curative: alkali therapy with Shohl's solution (98 Gm sodium citrate and 140 Gm citric acid per liter) to correct acidosis when present; 50,000 to 400,000 units of vitamin D daily to improve the calcium balance by decreasing the fecal loss without expectation of reducing the urinary loss; supplementary neutral phosphate to improve the phosphate balance despite a continued or even increased urinary loss; correction of hypokalemia, especially before any glucose tolerance tests, which may precipitate a "dextrose shock" by further reduction of the serum potassium to a critical value. Potassium and calcium supplements should be given only when indicated by plasma measurements; otherwise the basic regimen should be continued indefinitely. Great symptomatic improvement is possible, but the treatment does not prevent the slow progression of renal impairment with ultimate glomerular failure and uremia. Because of this and the increased susceptibility of potassium-deficient subjects to renal infection, urinary tract infections should be carefully sought and specifically treated.

REFERENCES

Schwartz, W. B.: Case 44341 (Fanconi Syndrome), New England J. Med., 259:392, 1958.

97 OTHER DISORDERS OF AMINO ACID METABOLISM

W. Eugene Knox

TYROSINOSIS

The excretion of large amounts of *p*-hydroxyphenylpyruvate, the α-keto acid of tyrosine, was reported in a single adult about 1935 but has been seen in a number of children. These show hepatomegaly, hypophosphatemic rickets, and elevated tyrosine in blood and urine. Treatment of one case with a low phenylalanine and tyrosine diet similar to that used in phenylketonuria reversed the biochemical abnormalities and improved renal function.

ALBINISM

The virtual absence of melanin pigment from skin, hair, and eyes is recessively inherited. The sole consequence is sensitivity to light: the skin sunburns easily, and the pink-appearing eyes are affected with photophobia and nystagmus. The melanocytes, which are normally recognized by their pigment in mitochondrialike organelles, have unpigmented organelles in human albino tissues. They are present as "clear" cells in the skin of certain albino mice. The known occurrence of (amelanotic) melanomas in two human albinos suggests that melanocytes are functional and that the albino defect is subcellular, probably a missing enzyme. The tyrosinase system, which oxidizes tyrosine through dopa to melanin, can normally be detected histochemically by the dopa oxidase reaction, but it is inactive in human albino skin. A sex-linked form of ocular albinism is also known in which the pigment defect is limited to the eye structures. Other localized absences of pigment occur commonly, often dominantly inherited as "white streaks," or as part of more serious congenital anomalies.

ARGININOSUCCINIC ACIDURIA

This ninhydrin-positive amino acid intermediate of the urea cycle was excreted in large amounts (1 to 2 Gm per day) by two siblings who were both seriously mentally retarded. Other siblings and the parents were normal. Presumably the condition represents a new inborn error of metabolism. Systemic urea formation was not abnormal, as would be expected if the "splitting enzyme" normally acting on argininosuccinate was lacking in the liver. Some particular defect in the central nervous system is suggested by the fact that two to three times as much argininosuccinic acid has been noted in the cerebrospinal fluid as in the blood.

HARTNUP DISEASE

This condition, also called *H disease*, was first detected in four of eight children from a first-cousin marriage. At least 13 cases are now known. It is characterized by intermittent attacks of a red, scaly, pellagralike rash appearing after exposure to sunlight, attacks of cerebellar ataxia, and occasionally psychiatric changes ranging from emotional instability to delirium. There is massive aminoaciduria, renal in origin, with at least 12 amino acids excreted in a characteristic pattern. For example, the four amino acids excreted in cystinuria and the proline excreted in generalized aminoacidurias such as the Fanconi syndrome are not abnormally excreted in Hartnup disease. There is also excretion of large amounts of indican and other indole derivatives formed from tryptophan by bacteria in the gut. A specific active transport system for the monocarboxylic amino acids is defective. In consequence, renal reabsorption fails and produces the aminoaciduria. Slowed intestinal absorption occurs and permits the bacterial action on tryptophan, and diversion of tryptophan from its normal route of degradation to nicotinic acid results in niacin deficiency. Oral doses of nicotinamide have markedly improved the pellagralike dermatitis and the neurologic signs. A high-protein diet is also recommended to offset the urinary amino acid loss.

MAPLE SYRUP URINE DISEASE

Several familial cases of a disease uniformly fatal in the first years of life have been observed, characterized by the onset of central nervous system symptoms soon after birth (muscular hypertonicity, poor feeding, vomiting, and mental retardation) and intermittently by the odor of maple syrup to the urine. The disease is analogous to phenylketonuria: there is an accumulation of ten times the normal plasma levels of methionine and the branched amino acids leucine, isoleucine, and valine; an overflow type of excretion of these amino acids in the urine; and the urinary excretion of α-keto acids, mainly those derived from isoleucine and leucine. Identification of the latter compounds by precipitation with a solution of 2,4-dinitrophenylhydrazine in 2 N HCl added to urine is diagnostically more reliable than the urine odor. The metabolic defect leading to accumulation of these amino acids is unknown. One patient has been successfully treated by restricted intake of the accumulated amino acids.

PRIMARY HYPEROXALURIA AND OXALOSIS [1]

This is a rare recessive condition beginning in childhood, with continuous high urinary oxalate excretion, progressive bilateral calcium oxalate urolithiasis and nephrocalcinosis, and extrarenal crystalline calcium oxalate deposits of "oxalosis." It results in death from renal failure by early adult life. Oxalate is normally not further metabolized. The 0.02 mg oxalate per mg creatinine (<50 mg per day) normally excreted comes from the small proportion of that in the diet which is absorbed plus that formed endogenously. In hyperoxaluria the excretion of oxalate is consistently several times the maximum normal value. The extra oxalate is formed endogenously. Some ingested ascorbic acid is converted to oxalate, but the amount cannot account for the extra oxalate formed in hyperoxaluria. The other major route of oxalate formation involves the conversion of glycine (and serine through glycolic acid) to glyoxylic acid. Normally and in hyperoxaluria about half the oxalate excreted comes from glycine, representing a normal conversion of about 0.5 per cent of the daily glycine turnover. The metabolic defect in hyperoxaluria therefore probably consists of a failure to metabolize glyoxylic acid by some other route, leaving more to be oxidized to oxalate. The possible routes of glyoxylic acid metabolism that may be defective include its transamination to glycine, oxidation to formic acid, and reduction to glycolic acid. Administration of pyridoxine, necessary as a coenzyme of transamination, will decrease the normal excretion of oxalate. Attempts to decrease oxalate excretion in hyperoxaluria by a restricted protein diet or by administration of sodium benzoate to trap glycine produced only small or temporary changes. All three measures warrant further trial, in conjunction with avoidance of oxalate-rich foods.

REFERENCES

Halvorsen, S., and L. R. Gjessing: Studies on Tyrosinosis: 1. Effect of Low-tyrosine and Low-phenylalanine Diet, Brit. Med. J., 2:1171, 1964.

Stauffer, M.: Oxalosis: Report of a Case, with a Review of the Literature and Discussion of the Pathogenesis, New England J. Med., 263:386, 1960.

98 SEROTONIN AND THE CARCINOID SYNDROME

Seymour J. Gray

Although the presence of a vasopressor substance in clotted blood has been known since 1868, the responsible factor has been isolated only recently and identified as 5-hydroxytryptamine, a powerful smooth-muscle stimulant and vasoconstrictor known as *serotonin*. This compound is formed predominantly in the argentaffin cells of the gastrointestinal tract. It is transported in the blood by the platelets and is present in the brain and other tissues.

Serotonin was discovered in considerable quantities in carcinoid tumors (argentaffinomas) by Lembeck in 1953. One year later Thorson, Biorck, Bjorkman, and Waldenstrom described the clinical picture of the "carcinoid syndrome" in patients with metastatic (malignant) carcinoids. The syndrome is characterized by episodic flushing of the skin, patchy cyanosis, telangiectasia, diarrhea, asthma, and valvular heart disease.

The excess secretion of serotonin by the endocrine tumors and a disturbance in tryptophan metabolism appear to be responsible for the various manifestations. The profound and dramatic effects of serotonin upon various organ systems have stimulated considerable investigation of the physiologic and pharmacologic properties of this hormone and related hydroxyindoles.

SEROTONIN METABOLISM

The metabolic pathway involved in the formation and breakdown of serotonin (5-HTA) is presented in Fig. 98-1. The amino acid, tryptophan, a constituent of many dietary proteins, is hydroxylated to form 5-hydroxytryptophan (5-HTP), or serotonin precursor. 5-HTP then undergoes rapid decarboxylation to form 5-hydroxytryptamine (5-HTA), or serotonin. The enzyme monoamine oxidase converts serotonin by oxidative deamination to 5-hydroxyindoleacetic acid (5-HIAA), which is excreted in the urine.

HYDROXYLATION OF TRYPTOPHAN TO 5-HYDROXYTRYPTOPHAN. Approximately 1 per cent of dietary tryptophan is normally metabolized by the 5-hydroxy-

[1] See also Chap. 155.

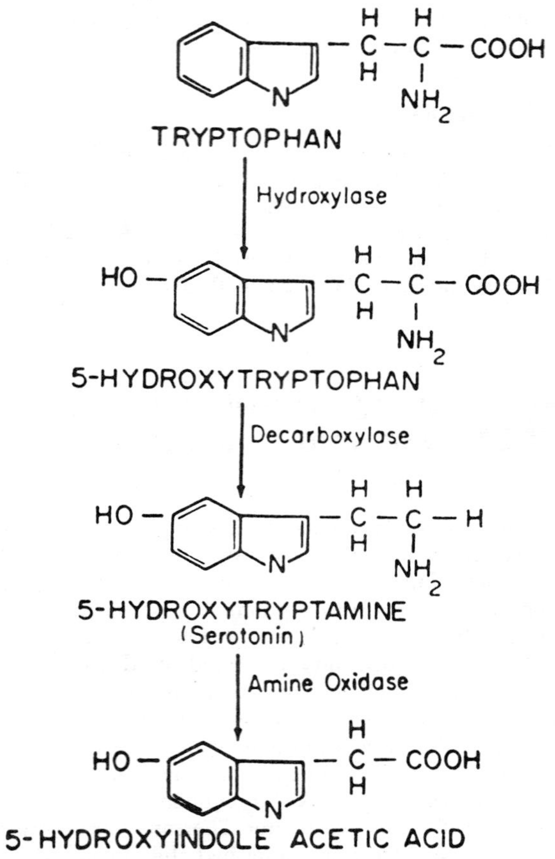

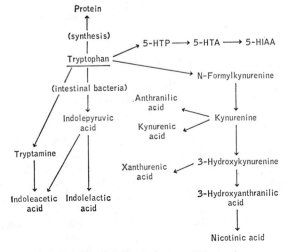

Fig. 98-1. Metabolic pathway of serotonin.

indole pathway. Its relationship to the major catabolic pathway of tryptophan to kynurenine and nicotinic acid is depicted in Fig. 98-2. Patients with carcinoidosis can convert as much as 60 per cent of dietary tryptophan to 5-hydroxyindole compounds. The excessive diversion of tryptophan in this direction may decrease the amount available for protein and nico-

tinic acid, resulting in a pellagralike picture (Fig. 98-2).

Although the site of tryptophan hydroxylation is unknown, it may take place in the argentaffin cell. 5-HTP has been identified chromatographically in the urine of certain patients with malignant carcinoidosis, and C[14]-labeled tryptophan has been shown in the human being to be converted to C[14]-labeled 5-HTP, lending considerable support to the concept that 5-HTP is an intermediate in the biosynthesis of serotonin.

DECARBOXYLATION OF 5-HYDROXYTRYPTOPHAN TO 5-HYDROXYTRYPTAMINE. The enzymatic decarboxylation of 5-HTP to 5-HTA takes place in the liver, kidney, gastrointestinal mucosa, brain, lung, and carcinoid tumor. Only the L-form of 5-HTP is normally decarboxylated to serotonin. In the cental nervous system the localization of the enzyme 5-hydroxytryptophan decarboxylase in the hypothalamus and upper brain stem parallels the distribution of serotonin. The presence of a metal as well as pyridoxal phosphate (vitamin B_6) is required for its activity. Diminished formation of serotonin from 5-HTP has been demonstrated in pyridoxine-deficient animals.

SEROTONIN. Serotonin is the biologically active compound resulting from tryptophan hydroxylation. The major depot in the body is the gastrointestinal tract. Serotonin is also found in blood platelets, brain, spleen, lungs, and other tissues. Post-mortem examination of the human brain for 5-HTA content has revealed highest quantities in the mesencephalic and diencephalic structures. In nature serotonin may be found in bananas, tomatoes, pineapples, certain mushrooms, insect venoms, and crustacea.

Serotonin is active only in the free form. Biologic activity is apparently lost when it is bound to tissues or platelets. The mechanism of binding and release remains uncertain, although ATP may play a role. When 5-HTA is released from tissue stores into the blood, it is rapidly taken up by the platelets. There is no evidence that platelets synthesize or metabolize serotonin or that serotonin plays a role in platelet function or hemostasis. Normal human whole blood contains only 0.1 to 0.3 μg serotonin per milliliter, virtually all of which is bound to the platelets and released into the plasma when the platelets disintegrate.

5-HYDROXYINDOLEACETIC ACID. In the presence of monoamine oxidase, free serotonin rapidly undergoes oxidative deamination to form 5-HIAA, the final major metabolic derivative of the 5-hydroxyindole pathway. Monoamine oxidase activity has been demonstrated in gastrointestinal mucosa, lung, kidney, brain, and liver. Very small amounts of serotonin may be degraded by mechanisms other than oxidative deamination.

Physiology and Pharmacology

GASTROINTESTINAL TRACT. Approximately 90 per cent of the total body serotonin is found in the

Fig. 98-2. Metabolic pathways of tryptophan.

argentaffin cells of the gastrointestinal tract. Serotonin is present in the stomach, small intestine, appendix, and colon. The human small intestine contains the largest quantities. Small doses of serotonin or serotonin precursor administered intravenously to man produce marked intestinal contractions, increased intestinal tone, abdominal cramps, nausea, and vomiting. Although the intestinal response has been attributed to stimulation of postganglionic cholinergic fibers, animal experiments indicate that serotonin acts directly on autonomic ganglions at sites different from those of acetylcholine. In vitro studies suggest that serotonin may sensitize the mucosal stretch receptors for initiation of the peristaltic reflex, indicating an important function for 5-HTA in the regulation of normal gastrointestinal motility.

Pathologic Physiology. Serotonin has little effect upon gastric secretion in animals but may enhance the gastric acid response to histamine stimulation. An increase in gastric blood flow has been observed. The gastric secretory response to serotonin in human beings is variable. Achlorhydria is present in some patients with carcinoidosis, but there is no consistent abnormality of gastric acid secretion. An increased incidence of gastric and duodenal ulcerations has been noted in patients with metastatic carcinoid and in animals after the administration of 5-HTP or serotonin. The exact mechanism of ulcer production is unknown. Smooth-muscle spasm, vasoconstriction, or histamine release may be implicated.

An increase in urinary 5-HIAA is observed in some patients with nontropical sprue, with a return to normal following the elimination of gluten or gliadan from the diet, suggesting a possible abnormality in serotonin metabolism. Similar increases in blood and platelet serotonin levels have been reported.

A release of serotonin from the small intestine has been observed to follow the instillation of hypertonic glucose into the jejunum of animals or intestinal perfusion with physiologic solutions of hydrochloric acid. It has been postulated that the serotonin released into the circulation may initiate the vasomotor and other symptoms of the postgastrectomy "dumping" syndrome.

CENTRAL NERVOUS SYSTEM. A physiologic role for serotonin in brain function as a chemical mediator of parasympathetic impulses has been proposed by Brodie and Shore. Serotonin, 5-hydroxytryptophan decarboxylase, and monamine oxidase are present in the brain, particularly in the hypothalamus and those areas where autonomic integration occurs. Although serotonin itself does not enter the brain from peripheral tissues, it can be synthesized within the brain from its precursor 5-HTP, which can pass the blood-brain barrier.

The concept that 5-HTA may be of physiologic importance in cerebral function is based on the following: (1) the finding of serotonin in brain tissue; (2) the hallucinogenic effects of certain antagonists and analogs of serotonin; (3) the depressant effects of reserpine, which liberates serotonin (and epi-nephrine) from the brain; (4) the stimulatory effects of the amine oxidase inhibitor, iproniazide, which blocks serotonin degradation; (5) the pronounced central nervous system effects of exogenously administered 5-HTP. Further studies are necessary, however, to establish the importance of serotonin in brain function. There is no proof that serotonin metabolism is disturbed in mental disease. Evidence that 5-hydroxyindole metabolism may be altered in schizophrenia has not been confirmed, and abnormal mental function or striking emotional disorders are observed only rarely in patients with carcinoidosis. A significant increase in the total 5-hydroxyindoles of the cerebrospinal fluid in hydrocephalus and an increased serotonin level in tuberculous meningitis have been reported.

ANAPHYLAXIS. In animals, both histamine and serotonin are released by anaphylaxis. Although mast cells of rats and mice contain serotonin as well as histamine, serotonin is not demonstrable in the mast cells of man. There is no conclusive evidence, furthermore, linking serotonin to allergic manifestations in man. Serotonin antimetabolites neither suppress anaphylactic reactions nor influence asthma in patients with malignant carcinoidosis.

SMOOTH MUSCLE. Serotonin is an extremely powerful smooth-muscle constrictor, and the bioassay of serotonin utilizes the constrictor effects upon the guinea pig ileum, pulmonary artery of dogs, rat uterus, and clam heart. The actions of serotonin on smooth muscle may be responsible in part for the cutaneous vascular changes, the bronchoconstriction, and the abnormal intestinal motility observed in patients with malignant carcinoidosis. Aerosolized serotonin may induce bronchial constriction in some asthmatic patients.

CARDIOVASCULAR–RENAL EFFECTS. Serotonin constricts arteries and veins and dilates capillaries. Infusion of the amine decreases blood flow, increases vascular volume, and produces flushing and cyanosis of the skin. It induces intense spasm of the infused vein. Serotonin has been reported to increase cardiac output in human beings and may elevate the pulmonary artery pressure in human beings and animals. Its effect on the systemic blood pressure is variable and inconsistent. Serotonin may act as a regulator of glomerular filtration by constricting the afferent renal arterioles. It can exert an antidiuretic effect in animals and human beings and may cause ischemic cortical necrosis of the kidneys in rats.

THE CARCINOID SYNDROME (Carcinoidosis)

The clinical aspects of the carcinoid syndrome reflect the effects of excess serotonin upon the cardiovascular and respiratory systems and the gastrointestinal tract. Abnormal tryptophan metabolism, malnutrition, and diarrhea may predispose the patient to protein deficiency or a pellagralike state. The generalized signs and symptoms of the syndrome do not usually appear until the carcinoid metastasizes to the liver and high levels of blood serotonin are attained.

Carcinoids occur from adolescence to extreme old age. Metastasizing carcinoids are commoner in the older age group and are seen equally among the sexes. The symptoms may extend over many years in spite of metastases because of the slow growth of the tumor.

Clinical Features

VASOMOTOR. The most distinctive and often the earliest symptom of the carcinoid syndrome is the acute, reddish, cutaneous flush, which starts in the face and neck and may extend to the chest, arms, and legs. Colors range from bright red to violaceous. The flush usually lasts only a few minutes but may persist longer and recur many times during the day, precipitated at times by emotional disturbances, physical exertion, manipulation of the tumor, food, or alcohol intake. Periorbital edema, hypotension, tachycardia, abdominal pain, diarrhea, and wheezing often accompany the flushing. The flush tends to be more frequent and severe as the disease progresses. Facial vascular congestion may become permanent, and some patients develop localized telangiectasia in the affected area or chronic cyanosis resembling polycythemia.

Ballistocardiograms demonstrate involvement of the entire circulatory system during the flushing episode. Observation of the peritoneum during abdominal laparotomy reveals peritoneal flushing as well. Cardiac catheterization performed during flushing demonstrates an elevated pressure in the pulmonary vasculature—a well-described serotonin effect in animals.

The flushing reaction has been attributed to the release of serotonin into the general circulation. There is some doubt, however, that serotonin is the sole cause. An increase of free serotonin in the hepatic vein has not been demonstrated regularly during flushing, nor do the plasma serotonin or urinary 5-HIAA levels rise consistently during spontaneous or induced flushes. Moreover, it is difficult to induce the characteristic facial flush with intravenous serotonin, although its infusion into the brachial artery produces a deep flush in the injected arm. Other factors that appear to be implicated in the flushing are epinephrine, histamine, and a recently discovered flush mediator, bradykinin, which is found in hepatic vein blood and in the circulation during flushing. The intravenous administration of epinephrine, norepinephrine, or a variety of sympathomimetic amines provokes the typical flush in patients with malignant carcinoid. Recent evidence indicates that the catecholamines induce flushing through the release of serotonin or by the liberation into the blood of the vasoactive peptide, bradykinin. The peptide-forming enzyme (kallikrein) responsible for bradykinin has been found in the metastatic hepatic carcinoids and is apparently released from the tumors into the blood, thereby initiating the flushing reaction.

Increased histamine excretion has also been demonstrated during the flush in some patients with the carcinoid syndrome. Since carcinoid tumors do not contain excess histamine, it has been postulated that serotonin may release histamine from normal tissue stores, producing a peculiar bright red, patchy flush. Tumors secreting both 5-HTP and serotonin may be more potent in histamine release.

GASTROINTESTINAL. Recurrent or chronic diarrhea is one of the most frequent manifestations of the disease and may be accompanied by borborygmi, colicky abdominal pain, and other signs of hyperperistalsis. Diarrhea is often the first symptom noted. An enlarged liver usually signifies metastatic involvement, although metastases may be present without hepatomegaly. An increased incidence of peptic ulcer has been reported.

Carcinoids of the appendix may obstruct the lumen, presenting the picture of acute appendicitis; in the small bowel they may cause symptoms of intestinal obstruction. Rarely tumors obstructing the biliary system may produce jaundice or steatorrhea.

CARDIAC INVOLVEMENT. Right-sided cardiac involvement, primarily pulmonary stenosis, appears late in the disease and occurs in about 50 per cent of advanced cases. Although the tricuspid and pulmonic valves are most commonly involved, either alone or in combination, all four valves may become sclerotic. Characteristically, the pulmonic and tricuspid valves present a pearly-gray fibrosis with sclerosis, thickening, and retraction of the chordae tendinae. Rigidity, thickening, and contractures may explain the physical findings of stenosis and regurgitation. Right-sided heart failure may develop. In some instances, the mural endocardium becomes markedly thickened. The cause of endocardial fibrosis is unknown. It has been attributed to chemical irritation from the high levels of blood serotonin. Hepatic metastases are invariably present when cardiac involvement appears.

The serotonin in the blood passing from the right to the left side of the heart may be rapidly oxidized by the monamine oxidase in the lungs, which explains the predominance of right-sided cardiac lesions. This concept is supported by the finding of valvular heart lesions involving both sides of the heart in a patient with carcinoidosis and a patent foramen ovale. However, the serotonin content of pulmonary artery blood is not consistently greater than that of the pulmonary vein. There is no significant change in systemic blood pressure.

RESPIRATORY. Asthmatic wheezing attacks and dyspnea are noted in some patients, particularly during flushing episodes, and are presumably related to bronchiolar constriction produced by serotonin.

OTHER SYMPTOMS. Other symptoms include abnormal pigmentation of the skin with pellagralike lesions and hyperkeratosis in severe cases, arthritis with swelling and stiffness of the joints, sudden localized edema of the hands or face, dependent edema, and weight loss. Rarely a malabsorption syndrome or scleroderma may accompany the carcinoid syndrome.

The Carcinoid Tumor

The term *carcinoid* was first proposed by Oberndorfer in 1907, to emphasize the malignant appearance but benign course of the tumor. Carcinoid tumors of the intestine arise from the argentaffin cells (Kultschitzky cells) of the intestinal mucosa near the bases of the crypts of Lieberkuhn, and they often contain cytoplasmic granules with an affinity for silver or chromium compounds. The fresh tumors are firm and yellow and consist of clumps or strands of epithelial cells with a tendency to tubular or acinar formation. In contrast to the intestinal argentaffin tumors, which secrete serotonin, bronchial carcinoids and carcinoids of the stomach and pancreas rarely give an argentaffin staining reaction and secrete the serotonin precursor 5-HTP predominantly.

SITE. Serotonin-producing tumors may be found anywhere from the stomach to the rectum, although 80 to 95 per cent are located in the region of the ileocecal valve, principally in the appendix and the terminal ileum. Carcinoids may also be present in the gallbladder, bile ducts, pancreatic ducts, ampulla of Vater, stomach, or in a Meckel's diverticulum. They are multiple in 15 to 25 per cent of cases. Occasionally a carcinoid may arise from an ovarian or testicular teratoma. Bronchial adenomas of the carcinoid type and carcinoids of the stomach and pancreas may give rise to the syndrome.

METASTASIS. Appendiceal carcinoids metastasize rarely, if at all. Carcinoid tumors involving the ileum, cecum, colon, or stomach metastasize more frequently, usually to the liver and regional lymph nodes and occasionally to the ovaries, lungs, and bones. Bronchial carcinoids are usually benign but metastasize occasionally. Carcinoids of the bronchus, stomach, and pancreas tend to metastasize to liver, bone, and skin. Metastatic lesions may appear late, grow slowly, and assume massive proportions.

Relationship of Liver Metastases to the Clinical Syndrome. The clinical features of the carcinoid syndrome in most instances signify malignant carcinoidosis of the liver and a high blood level of serotonin. The serotonin formed by metastatic tumors in the liver escapes destruction and enters the hepatic vein and the general circulation. In the absence of liver metastases, serotonin secreted by the intestinal carcinoid is inactivated in the liver by monamine oxidase, resulting in an increased excretion of 5-HIAA in the urine without clinical manifestation of the carcinoid syndrome. Serotonin secreted by extraportal carcinoids, such as ovarian tumors, enters the systemic circulation directly through the vena cava and may produce the syndrome without metastasis to the liver. The role of the hepatic metastases in the flushing reaction has been described previously.

Diagnosis and Management of the Carcinoid Syndrome

LABORATORY ASPECTS AND DIAGNOSIS. The diagnosis can be established by demonstrating a high level of 5-HIAA in the urine. Urinary levels of 50 to 1,000 mg per day are found in patients with the carcinoid syndrome, compared to normal values of 2 to 10 mg. A simple screening test for 5-HIAA, consisting of a purple color when a nitrosonaphthol solution is added to urine, becomes positive when the daily excretion of 5-HIAA exceeds 40 mg. Marked increases do not occur except in carcinoidosis, although a slight elevation may be observed in some patients with nontropical sprue and transiently after the administration of reserpine. The ingestion of bananas, which contain significant amounts of serotonin (4 mg per banana), or pineapples can also increase the urinary excretion of 5-HIAA. Decreased excretion has been noted in renal insufficiency and in some instances of phenylketonuria. Medications containing mephenesin carbamate and phenothiazines interfere with the determination.

The malignant carcinoid usually contains 1.0 to 3.0 mg 5-HTA per Gm tumor. The level of 5-HIAA in the urine is a measure of the extent of the functioning tumor mass and may be helpful in following the clinical course of the patient after surgery or other therapy. It returns to normal when the carcinoid is completely removed if no metastases are present.

The serotonin pool in the body of a carcinoid patient approximates 2,800 mg. The blood serotonin levels vary from 0.5 to 3.0 μg per ml (normal, 0.1 to 0.3 μg per ml). Normally serotonin in the urine is barely detectable, compared to 0.5 to 12 mg daily in the carcinoid patient. Hypoalbuminemia and hypoproteinemia are seen in some instances.

In a variant of the syndrome in which the carcinoid tumors secrete 5-HTP predominantly (carcinoids of the bronchus, stomach, and biliary or pancreatic ducts), the urine contains large amounts of 5-HTP, 5-HTA, and 5-HIAA. In some patients with 5-HTP–secreting tumors, notably of gastric origin, large amounts of histamine may be excreted as well.

PROGNOSIS. Since carcinoids often grow very slowly, patients may live as long as 10 to 20 years after the symptoms have developed. The immediate prognosis is not necessarily poor with inoperable carcinoids or those which have already metastasized. Death is caused by heart failure, metastatic liver disease, malnutrition, or intercurrent infection.

MANAGEMENT. Surgery is indicated in spite of metastases, because of the remarkably slow progression of the carcinoid tumors. Surgical removal of the primary lesion and metastases, when feasible, may decrease, delay, or ameliorate symptoms by reducing serotonin production. Removal of the primary tumor is advisable to prevent local complications such as obstruction. Vitamin supplements, particularly nicotinic acid, are recommended.

There is no single treatment of choice for the carcinoid syndrome. A number of serotonin antagonists and antimetabolites, including lysergic acid diethylamide (LSD), brominated LSD, and the benzyl analog of serotonin (BAS), have proved ineffective therapeutically. Phenylacetic acid diminishes 5-HIAA excretion in some patients, probably by its action on renal clearance, but it does not ameliorate the symptoms. Reserpine, which releases serotonin from tissue stores, is also of little value. X-ray therapy, radioactive gold, 5-fluorouracil, and nitrogen mustard have been tried without success.

The decarboxylase inhibitor, α-methyl-dopa (α-methyl-3,4-dihydroxyphenylalanine), which blocks serotonin formation by inhibiting decarboxylase activity, may alleviate flushing in patients with tumors secreting large quantities of 5-HTP, such as that noted in the variant of the carcinoid syndrome (gastric carcinoid). Presumably this agent inhibits the conversion of 5-HTP to serotonin in the skin and other target organs, resulting in a decrease in urinary serotonin and 5-HIAA and an increase in the urinary excretion of 5-HTP. The drug is ineffective in patients with carcinoid tumors secreting chiefly serotonin, and the side effects may be severe.

Chlorpromazine, 25 mg every 6 hr, may diminish the diarrhea and the severity of the flush in some instances. Cyproheptadine, a serotonin antagonist, may also alleviate symptoms, particularly diarrhea. Another potent serotonin antagonist, 1-methyl-D-lysergic acid butanolamide tartrate (Deseril), 2 mg three times daily, appears to be effective against diarrhea but has little influence upon the flushing. These drugs do not decrease the urinary excretion of 5-HIAA. They apparently block the action of serotonin rather than inhibit its metabolic pathway.

Two adrenolytic drugs, phentolamine methane sulfonate (Regitine), 50 mg every 4 hr, and dibenzyline, 10 mg daily, may relieve the flushing in some patients. Prednisone and 6-methyl prednisolone have also been noted to alleviate the flushing.

REFERENCES

Thorson, A. H.: Studies on carcinoid disease, Acta med. Scandinav., 161:1, 1958 (Supp. 334).

Page, I. H.: Serotonin (5-hydroxytryptamine); The last four years, Physiol. Rev., 38:277, 1958.

Resnick, R. H., and Gray, S. J.: Serotonin metabolism and the carcinoid syndrome, Med. Clinics N. America, 44:1323, 1960.

Sjoerdsma, A., H. Weissbach, and S. Udenfriend: Clinical, physiologic and biochemical study of patients with malignant carcinoid (argentaffinoma), Am. J. Med., 20:520, 1956.

Robertson, J. I. S., W. S. Peart, and T. M. Andrews: The mechanism of facial flushes in the carcinoid syndrome, Quart. J. Med., 31:103, 1962.

99 GOUT AND OTHER DISORDERS OF URIC ACID METABOLISM

Warren E. C. Wacker
and George W. Thorn

HISTORY. Gout is an inherited disturbance of uric acid metabolism characterized by acute arthritic episodes and the eventual deposition of sodium urate crystals in various tissues. It has been recognized since ancient times and is mentioned in the writings of Hippocrates. The name is derived from the Latin *gutta*, a drop, signifying the presence of noxious drops (of sodium urate) in the joints. Uric acid was first associated with gout by Scheele in 1776, through the demonstration of its presence in urine; Wollaston shortly thereafter identified it in a renal calculus obtained from a gouty patient. The hyperuricemia of gout was discovered by Garrod in 1848. Emil Fischer derived the structural formula of uric acid, and Folin developed the first adequate method for its measurement.

INCIDENCE. Gout is not rare; in the United States almost half a million persons are estimated to be afflicted. In careful genealogic studies the familial incidence is found to be as high as 75 per cent. In addition to clinical gout, however, the incidence of asymptomatic hyperuricemia is even higher in the families of gouty patients. The defect in uric acid metabolism is probably due to a single autosomal dominant gene, and clinical gout occurs in a small percentage of heterozygotes. Clinical gout occurs chiefly in men; only about 5 per cent of patients are women. The incidence of asymptomatic hyperuricemia is much more nearly the same in both sexes. In women clinical gout is rare before the menopause, whereas the most frequent age of onset for men is in the third and fourth decades. The infrequent occurrence in women probably represents an altered expression of the defect rather than a sex-linked genetic process. The common perception that gout is due primarily to overindulgence in food and wine is without basis in fact.

ETIOLOGY. Gout represents the accumulation of large amounts of uric acid, identified by an increased concentration in serum, by an increased total body uric acid pool, and in advanced gout by the precipitation of urates in various tissues.

In man uric acid is the end product of purine metabolism. The two purines, adenine and guanine, are present in the body chiefly as components of the nucleic acids, ribonucleic acid (RNA) and deoxyribonucleic acid (DNA). Normally two purine sources are responsible for uric acid production, purines obtained by the hydrolysis of ingested nucleic acids and those obtained by the hydrolysis of endogenous nucleic acids. Uric acid, 2-6-8 trioxypurine, is formed by the stepwise enzymatic oxidation of adenine and guanine. The further degradation of uric acid to allantoin appears not to occur in man, though it does in most other mammalian species; however, there is evidence that limited uricolysis may occur in man, although the biochemical mechanism is currently unknown.

Uric acid may accumulate in patients with gout (Fig. 99-1) through several possible mechanisms. Simple overingestion of dietary nucleic acid has been excluded; a constantly increased degradation of endogenous nucleic acids, although it occurs in patients with gout secondary to diseases associated with excessive cell destruction sufficient to provide this amount of nucleic acid, such as polycythemia vera, leukemia, or lymphoma, has been ruled out as a cause of primary gout. Direct overproduction of uric acid from simple purine precursors or impedance of the normal excretory process are the remaining possibilities.

The biochemical pathways of uric acid synthesis have been elucidated in detail; it is formed from several simple precursors, glycine, aspartic acid, CO_2, and glutamine. Uric acid is normally derived from the degradation of purines previously incorporated into nucleic acids; however, in some patients with primary gout, there exists an alternate pathway for the direct synthesis of uric acid, which does not involve prior incorporation into nucleic acid. The rate and extent of incorporation of isotopically labeled glycine into urinary uric acid has been employed to demonstrate this abnormal mechanism. Some patients with gout given isotopically labeled glycine excrete an amount greater than normal in urinary uric acid; the rapid appearance of the isotope precludes the possibility that the labeled uric acid is derived from the normal degradation of nucleic acid purines. The accumulation of uric acid in these patients may thus be explained on the basis of an abnormally *increased synthesis*. The enzymatic defect(s) responsible for the shunt mechanism are not known; however, an abnormality in purine biosynthesis in patients with gout is revealed by an altered excretory pattern of several purine compounds, 8-hydroxy-7-methylguanine and 6-succinoaminopurine.

Abnormal synthesis of uric acid, however, does not occur in all patients with primary gout; it appears to be limited to those who excrete an excessive amount of uric acid in the urine. In many patients, despite an elevated serum uric acid content, urinary uric acid excretion does not exceed the normal range of 300 to 600 mg per 24 hr. In these patients it is not possible to demonstrate increased synthesis as measured by the incorporation of N^{15}-labeled glycine into uric acid; this suggests an impairment of the excretory mechanism. The major mechanism of uric acid excretion is the renal pathway. It appears that uric acid is excreted largely by tubular secretion; most, if not all, of that filtered by the glomerulus is reabsorbed. The ability of chlorothiazide and pyrizinamide to cause hyperuricemia by altering the renal excretory process strongly supports the concept of tubular secretion. In a converse fashion, so does the occurrence of hypouricemia in Wilson's disease and the deToni-Fanconi syndrome, diseases characterized by other known renal tubular defects. Therefore, in those patients with primary gout in whom it is impossible to demonstrate increased synthesis, and the concomitant hyperexcretion of uric acid, an abnormality of the tubular secretory mechanism may be the primary pathologic defect. This hypothesis is supported by the observation that the renal clearance of uric acid in these gouty patients is much lower than that achieved by normal persons in whom the plasma uric acid concentration has been raised

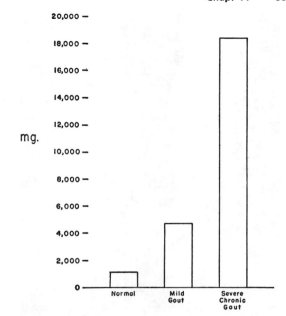

Fig. 99-1. Uric acid pool in normal and gouty persons.

artificially by the administration of urate precursors.

Thus, at least two biochemical defects can cause primary gout: a defect in purine biosynthesis, leading to a direct overproduction of uric acid, and an abnormal renal tubular secretory mechanism for uric acid. They may operate independently or jointly.

There is a simple relationship between the clinical manifestations of chronic tophaceous gout and the biochemical alterations leading to an increase in plasma uric acid and the total body uric acid pool. Sodium urate is quite insoluble and therefore precipitates to form tophi in the joints, bones, cartilage, kidneys, and other soft tissues. In the pathogenesis of acute gouty arthritis only recently has there been demonstrated a direct relationship between the accumulation of uric acid and the symptoms and signs of acute attacks. Microcrystals of sodium urate are always present in the synovial fluid of the joints affected with acute gouty arthritis. Moreover, while injection of amorphous sodium urate does not produce a syndrome similar to acute gouty arthritis, injection of microcrystals of sodium urate does indeed produce an inflammatory reaction that has all the characteristics of acute gouty arthritis. Thus, gout in all its forms can be related to an excess of uric acid, which exceeds the limit of solubility, precipitates in inappropriate areas, and thus gives rise to the pathologic and clinical manifestations of the disease. In support of this view of the pathogenesis of gout, it should be pointed out that clinical gout appears to occur simply as a result of hyperuricemia in patients with polycythemia or leukemia. In these diseases there is no disturbance in purine metabolism that would be expected to give some evanescent product able to produce the symptomatology of acute gout.

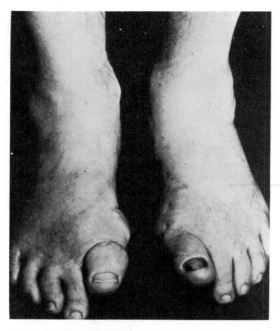

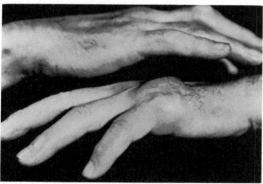

Fig. 99-2. *Upper,* appearance of feet in chronic gout. Note swelling of the great toes as well as subcutaneous deposits of uric acid opposite the first metatarsal joint. *Lower,* appearance of hands in chronic gout. Note joint enlargement due to deposits of uric acid.

PATHOLOGY. The pathognomonic lesion of gout is the deposit of sodium urate crystals, resulting in inflammatory and eventual degenerative changes. The lesions occur chiefly in joints, bones, bursae, and cartilaginous structures. The marked insolubility of urates at the acid pH characteristic of these tissues may account for the preferential precipitation at these sites. Any joint may be affected; however, those of the lower extremities, and chiefly those of the great toe, are favored. Urate deposits occur in the articular cartilage and periarticular structures, causing bone destruction, joint narrowing, degeneration of the synovium, bony ankylosis, and exostoses. The precipitates

in nonarticular tissues are called *tophi,* meaning "chalkstones." The cartilage of the ears, the tendons, the tarsal plates of the eyes, and the olecranon and patellar bursae are the most common locations. Urates also precipitate in the collecting tubules of the kidney, leading to obstruction and pyelonephritis. Glomerular fibrosis and arteriolar and arterial nephrosclerosis are invariably present to some extent in the kidneys of patients with gouty nephropathy. Arteriosclerosis, with its attendant hypertension and cardiac hypertrophy, occurs more frequently in patients with gout than in others of comparable age.

CLINICAL PICTURE. Gout is often unrecognized in early stages before the obvious destructive changes of chronic tophaceous gout have appeared. Its onset is characterized by acute attacks of joint pain with intervals of complete well-being. Later, the intervals become progressively shorter until the final state of persistent deforming arthritis is reached.

Acute Gout. Acute arthritis usually heralds the disease, although occasionally renal colic, from urate stones, may be the initial manifestation. The metatarsophalangeal joint of the great toe is the primary site of attack in 60 per cent of cases, according to Scudamore (Fig. 99-2); frequently the arthritis is bilateral. Other common sites, in the order of their frequency, include the instep, ankle, heel, knee, and hand. Acute attacks are often preceded by a stressful or traumatic episode, i.e., mild physical trauma to the joint, acute infection, surgery, cold exposure, and injection of foreign protein or drugs such as mercurials, epinephrine, ergotamine, or liver extract. The onset of acute joint pain following surgery in a male patient should immediately suggest an acute episode of gout. Attacks may also be associated with sudden changes in atmospheric pressure. The attack often occurs at night and awakens the patient from sleep. Some patients are able to recognize that an attack is imminent by a mild sensation of burning, tingling, numbness, or warmth in the affected joint. Often, however, the attack begins suddenly, the joint becoming swollen, tender, violaceous, and excruciatingly painful. Lymphangitis and true cellulitis are rare complications. The involvement may be monarticular or of a migratory polyarticular type. General malaise, headache, tachycardia, and fever associated with an elevated leukocyte count and erythrocyte sedimentation rate and an elevated serum uric acid concentration complete the clinical picture. The duration of the attack is a function of the time before the initiation of therapy and of its effectiveness. Untreated, an acute episode may last 2 weeks.

Interval Gout. Early in the course of the disease symptom-free periods between acute attacks may vary from months to years. As the disease progresses, however, the asymptomatic periods become shorter and shorter, until finally persistent deforming arthritis supervenes.

Chronic Gout. This stage of the disease occurs after a variable period of time; it is characterized by irreversible, deforming changes in the joint spaces, capsules, tendons, and bursae. Tophi in the cartilaginous structures and subcutaneous tissues are usually present. Ankylosis, multiple draining sinus tracts, and complete crippling inactivation are the hallmarks of the final stages of untreated gout.

Complications. Renal disease, secondary to the deposition of urates in the kidney parenchyma, is the major, direct, serious complication of gout. Although autopsy studies indicate that renal damage is present to some degree in most patients with the disease, severe renal failure does not occur in more than 10 per cent of patients. Clinically the earliest manifestation of gouty renal disease is albuminuria, which may persist for several decades before nitrogen retention ensues. The terminal stage of gouty renal disease is the uremic syndrome, with its attendant hypertension and anemia. Secondary pyelonephritis, causing additional renal impairment, is a frequent occurrence in gout.

About 20 per cent of patients with gout have a history of renal colic. Most frequently the stones are composed entirely of urate salts; however, they may have a mixed composition consisting of calcium phosphate or oxalate as well as urate. The passage of urate stones may be the first indication of the disease. The complete combustion of a urate stone in a flame allows its differentiation from a calcium stone, which imparts a brick-red color to the flame.

Hypertension and atherosclerosis occurring at an earlier age than in the normal population are quite common in patients with gout and are reflected in a high incidence of myocardial infarction in young men with the disease.

DIAGNOSIS. Acute gouty arthritis is easily recognized by its explosive onset. The severe pain and exquisite tenderness of the affected joint, the elevated serum uric acid concentration (greater than 7 mg per 100 ml in men), and the rapid response to treatment with colchicine confirm the diagnosis. The disease, however, is frequently overlooked in the interval phases. Specific interrogation of all patients who complain of arthritic symptoms will prevent misdiagnosis in most instances. Since gout is the only variety of chronic arthritis for which an effective form of therapy is known, it is important to recognize it as early as possible. The most valuable clues are a family history of gout (or rheumatism), delayed onset of acute joint symptoms following mild trauma, or the passage of renal stones.

Chronic gout may be diagnosed by the presence of deposited urates, either as tophi in soft tissues or in the joints and bursae. Removal of the chalky contents of a tophus and chemical identification of the material as sodium urate provide an absolute diagnosis. Roentgenologic changes in affected joints are often lacking in the early stages of gout. The typical roentgenologic finding is a punched-out, destructive lesion representing a urate deposit (Fig. 99-3). Narrowing and destruction of the joint spaces also occur. The extent

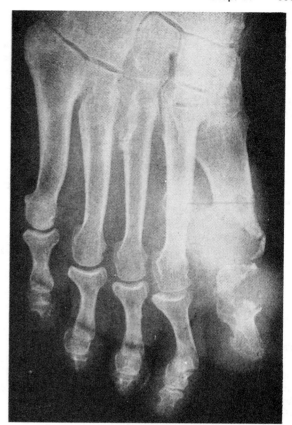

Fig. 99-3. X-ray of a foot in a case of chronic gout. Note marked destruction of the first and second metatarsal joints and adjacent punched-out areas of diminished density.

of these processes depends, of course, on the stage of the disease.

Although an elevated serum uric acid concentration (7.0 mg per 100 ml in men; 5.0 mg per 100 ml in women) is a necessary accompaniment of gout, it is not pathognomonic. Hyperuricemia also occurs secondary to renal disease; for this reason, the blood urea nitrogen should be determined simultaneously with the serum uric acid. In patients with renal disease hyperuricemia will correlate with the increased blood urea nitrogen (Table 99-1).

Hyperuricemia not due to gout also occurs under other circumstances. Individuals who have fasted for as short a time as 24 hr develop hyperuricemia due to reduced renal excretion of uric acid. It may well be

Table 99-1. SERUM URIC ACID AND BLOOD UREA NITROGEN LEVELS IN PATIENTS WITH GOUT AND NEPHRITIS

	Normal	Gout	Nephritis
Serum uric acid (mg per 100 ml)	2–5	8	6
Blood urea nitrogen (mg per 100 ml)	8–15	15	45

that the frequently reported elevations of serum uric acid in patients with acute myocardial infarction may be the result of the fasting that attends the onset of this acute disease. Similar elevations of serum uric acid also occur in patients with diabetic acidosis and in acute alcoholism (see also Chap. 104). Also, several drugs are known to increase serum uric acid, for example, small doses of aspirin as well as continued administration of chlorothiazide.

Differential Diagnosis. Acute gout must be differentiated from acute rheumatic fever, rheumatoid arthritis, infectious arthritis, osteoarthritis, cellulitis, bursitis, tendonitis, and thrombophlebitis. Palindromic arthritis in women, manifested by episodes of acute arthritis with periods of complete remission, is unusually similar to gout. The presence of incipient and persistent hyperuricemia without azotemia and the response to colchicine strongly point to gout as the diagnosis.

Secondary Gout. The accumulation of uric acid by a direct increase of nucleic acid catabolism occurs in patients with hematologic disorders, chiefly polycythemia, leukemia, and lymphoma. In these diseases an episode of acute gout may represent the first clinical manifestation of the underlying disorder.

TREATMENT. The knowledge that the metabolic abnormalities of gout result in an accumulation of uric acid provides the basis for the long-term therapy of this disease, i.e., the potentiation of uric acid excretion. Therapy, however, may be separated conveniently into the treatment of the acute attack, of chronic gout, of interval gout, and of the azotemia secondary to progressive renal involvement.

Acute Gouty Arthritis. Colchicine remains the most effective drug for the treatment of acute gout. To be maximally effective, treatment should be started as early in the course of an attack as possible. The drug should be administered according to the following schedule: 0.5 to 0.6 mg every hour until the arthritis abates or gastrointestinal side effects (nausea, vomiting, or diarrhea) appear. The maximum tolerable dosage is 4 to 10 mg; since it varies from person to person, it must be established empirically for each individual. The distressing diarrhea, if it occurs, may be controlled with tincture of opium.

Phenylbutazone is also effective in treating acute gout. Following an initial dose of 0.4 Gm, 0.1 Gm should be given four times a day for 2 to 3 days. The serious toxicity of phenylbutazone is reduced when it is given for this short period of time.

Chronic tophaceous gout may also be treated with 4-hydroxypyrazole-(3,4-*d*) pyrimidine, a potent inhibitor of xanthine oxidase. This drug prevents the conversion of hypoxanthine and xanthine to uric acid thereby permitting these uric acid precursors to be excreted. Clinical trials indicate that 4-hydroxypyrazole-(3,4-*d*) pyrimidine, in doses of 300 to 600 mg/day is effective in lowering serum uric acid and reducing tophi. Since it decreases uric acid excretion it is par-

ticularly useful in patients who have a propensity to develop uric acid renal calculi. The drug has minimal side effects, the most troublesome being attacks of acute gout and occasional diarrhea.

Adrenocorticotropic hormone (ACTH) is a potent uricosuric agent and also effective in the treatment of acute gout; 100 units ACTH gel should be administered daily until symptoms subside. The dose should then be decreased gradually over the next several days to prevent exacerbation due to sudden withdrawal of adrenal stimulation. Cortisone, 100 to 200 mg daily, or its analog may also be employed. It is probably wise to terminate the steroid therapy with ACTH (20 to 40 units per day for 2 to 3 days). ACTH and cortisone in smaller doses may also be used to minimize undue gastrointestinal sensitivity to colchicine.

Supportive therapy consists of bed rest and immobilization of the affected joint. In contrast, however, to other forms of acute arthritis, mobilization may be allowed as soon as the joint is no longer painful. Codeine may be used if pain is severe.

Chronic Gout. Since the precipitation of urate crystals is responsible for the deforming arthritis of chronic gout, the major therapeutic goal must be the mobilization and excretion of excess urate. The discovery of the potent uricosuric agent, probenecid, has provided the means to achieve this goal. This drug promotes the excretion of uric acid by a direct effect on the kidney, preventing the reabsorption of uric acid from the glomerular filtrate.

Probenecid has been used extensively and is known to have a very low order of serious toxicity. It should be given in amounts varying between 1.0 and 2.0 Gm per day in divided doses. Initially a dose of 0.5 to 1 Gm per day is employed to minimize the precipitation of uric acid crystals in the renal tubules. For the same reason all patients, throughout the initial course of therapy, should maintain a high fluid intake (2.5 to 3 liters per day). Patients with a history of urate stones may be treated with sodium citrate or bicarbonate to alkalinize the urine and render uric acid more soluble.

Probenecid medication prevents the extension of the disease and reduces the size of tophi and the deposits of urate in the joints. Salicylates antagonize the uricosuric action of these agents; therefore the two drugs should not be given concomitantly.

Strict dietary limitations have not been beneficial in the management of gout; only those few foods containing a large amount of purine, such as sweetbreads, liver, kidneys, etc., should be prohibited.

Although uricosuric therapy ultimately diminishes the attack rate of acute gout, initially it is unaltered; therefore, therapy to prevent acute attacks is indicated. Colchicine, 0.5 to 2 mg per day, is optimal therapy to prevent acute gout. The necessary dose should be established for each patient such that, while it is therapeutically adequate, it does not cause gastrointestinal side effects. Continuous combined therapy with a potent uricosuric agent and colchicine provides a simple, effective program to prevent the disabling consequences of gout.

Surgical treatment may occasionally be employed to remove large, painful subcutaneous tophi or discharging sinuses associated with a tophaceous deposit.

Prophylaxis. Hyperuricemia occurs frequently in relatives of patients with gout; however, only a relatively small number of these individuals will develop symptomatic gout. It is accepted that those who develop clinical gout should be treated. There is, however, no universal agreement concerning the management of patients with asymptomatic hyperuricemia. The facts concerning the prophylactic treatment of affected relatives are as follows:

1. The incapacitating and potentially lethal effects of gout are *certainly* caused by the deposition of uric acid.

2. The accumulation of uric acid, reflected by *hyperuricemia,* can be prevented by a safe and simple program of drug therapy.

Therefore, to prevent the disease, relatives of gout patients who show significantly elevated concentrations of uric acid in serum (above 8 mg per 100 ml) should be treated with a uricosuric drug. To be successful, such a program of preventive medicine *requires* the full understanding and cooperation of the patient and the recognition by the physician of the absolute necessity for frequent, detailed, and continued close observation.

REFERENCES

Buchanan, J. M.: The Enzymatic Synthesis of the Purine Nucleotides, Harvey Lecture Series, 14:104, 1960.

Nugent, C. A., and F. H. Tyler: The Renal Excretion of Uric Acid in Patients with Gout and Non-gouty Subjects, J. Clin. Invest., 38:1890, 1959.

Seegmiller, J. E., and A. I. Grayzel: Use of the New Uricosuric Agents in the Management of Gout, J.A.M.A., 73:106, 1960.

——, L. Laster, and R. R. Howell: Biochemistry of Uric Acid and Its Relation to Gout, N. England J. Med., 268:712, 1963.

Stetten, D., Jr.: Recent Contributions to the Understanding of the Metabolic Defect in Gout, Geriatrics, 9:163, 1964.

Talbott, J. H.: "Gout," New York, Grune & Stratton, Inc., 1964.

——, and K. L. Terplan: The Kidney in Gout, Medicine, 39:405, 1960.

Weissmann, B., and A. B. Gutman: The Identification of 6-Succinoaminopurine and 8-Hydroxy-7-methylguanine as Normal Urinary Constituents, J. Biol. Chem., 229:239, 1958.

Yu, T. F., and A. B. Gutman: Effect of Allopurinol (4-Hydroxypyrazole-(3,4-*d*) pyrimidine) on Serum and Urinary Uric Acid in Primary and Secondary Gout, Am. J. Med., 37:885, 1964.

Yu, T. F., B. Weissmann, L. Sharney, S. Kupfer, and A. B. Gutman: On the Biosynthesis of Uric Acid from Glycine N[15] in Primary and Secondary Polycythemia, Am. J. Med., 21:901, 1956.

100 HEMOCHROMATOSIS
George E. Cartwright

DEFINITION. Idiopathic hemochromatosis (bronze diabetes, pigment cirrhosis) is characterized pathologically by excessive deposits of iron in the body and clinically by hepatomegaly with eventual liver insufficiency, pigmentation of the skin, diabetes mellitus, and frequently cardiac failure.

HISTORY. The first clinical description of the disease was given by Trousseau in 1865. In 1889 von Recklinghausen named the disease *hemochromatosis* and described the iron-containing pigment, hemosiderin. Sheldon, in a now classic monograph, reviewed the world's literature in 1935. Finch and Finch in 1955 reviewed the literature since 1935 and added 80 cases of their own.

INCIDENCE. Hemochromatosis is a rare disease, recognized once in approximately 20,000 hospital admissions, and once in 7,000 hospital deaths. It is observed ten times as frequently in males as in females. Nearly 70 per cent of all patients with this disease develop their first symptoms between the ages of forty and sixty years. Hemochromatosis is rarely recognized below the age of twenty years.

PATHOGENESIS. One of the earliest measurable alterations in iron metabolism in hemochromatosis is the elevation of the plasma iron and saturation of the plasma iron-binding protein, transferrin. As the disease progresses, the amount of storage iron increases. In advanced disease, the tissues contain over 20 Gm of iron; total body iron in normal persons is in the range of 3 to 5 Gm. The excess iron is deposited primarily in parenchymal cells in the form of ferritin and hemosiderin. Increased amounts of iron are found in almost all body tissues, especially those in which there is organ dysfunction. Iron in the liver and pancreas is increased fifty to one hundred times; in the heart, ten to fifteen times; in the spleen, kidney, and skin, about five times.

Since iron is not excreted from the body in appreciable amounts even in normal persons, the conclusion that iron absorption is increased in idiopathic hemochromatosis is inescapable. There are two quite differing explanations as to why this occurs. The classical concept is that idiopathic hemochromatosis is due to an inherited inborn error in metabolism in which the basic abnormality is the increased absorption of iron. According to this view the excessive deposition of iron is the cause of the tissue damage. The other point of view is that hemochromatosis is a variant of portal cirrhosis of the liver. A high incidence (30 to 85 per cent) of alcoholism has been observed in patients with idiopathic hemochromatosis, and it has been noted that the iron content of alcoholic beverages, particularly various wines, is high.

Hemochromatosis has been observed (1) as a familial occurrence without apparent cause other than an inherited inborn error of metabolism; (2) in alcoholic subjects with a high dietary intake of iron; (3) in malnourished Bantu subjects in South Africa secondary to long-term iron overload ("Bantu siderosis"); (4) in isolated instances of parenchymal iron overload following intake of medicinal doses of iron over many years; (5) in association with various types of refractory anemia; and (6) in a few patients given 100 or more transfusions of blood. Therefore, it would seem that hemochromatosis is a syndrome with several possible causes. The common denominator in all cases is the presence of excessive iron in parenchymal tissues.

PATHOLOGY. At autopsy the enlarged, nodular liver and pancreas present a striking ochre color. Histologically, hemosiderin is deposited in many organs, particularly the liver and pancreas. The liver shows considerable fibrosis. Testicular atrophy is frequently present, both grossly and histologically. There are hemosiderin deposits in the myocardium, and they may be associated with myocardial edema, fibrosis, and necrosis. The epidermis of the skin is thin, and melanin pigment is found in the cells of the basal layer. Hemosiderin is deposited almost entirely in the corium.

CLINICAL MANIFESTATIONS. The symptoms and signs of hemochromatosis are related to the skin pigmentation, diabetes, liver impairment, and cardiac disease. Of these the cirrhosis of the liver is the most constant abnormality.

The initial symptoms most frequently encountered are related to the onset of diabetes. Weakness, lassitude, weight loss, change in skin color, abdominal pain, dyspnea, edema, ascites, loss of libido, and peripheral neuritis are also frequent initial symptoms. Hepatomegaly, pigmentation, spider angiomas, splenomegaly, ascites, evidences of congestive failure or cardiac arrhythmias, loss of body hair, testicular atrophy, jaundice, and hypertension are the most prominent physical signs, given in decreasing order of frequency.

The liver is the first tissue known to be damaged, and hepatomegaly is present in about 93 per cent of symptomatic cases. Hepatic enlargement may exist in the absence of symptoms or in the presence of normal liver function test results. Indeed, over half the patients with symptomatic hemochromatosis have little or no laboratory evidence of functional impairment of the liver in spite of hepatomegaly and proved fibrosis. Loss of body hair, palmar erythema, testicular atrophy, gynecomastia, spider angioma, and, particularly, loss of libido are often seen and are related to the severity of the liver damage. Manifestations of portal hypertension and esophageal varices may occur but are less commonly observed than in Laennec's cirrhosis. A nontender, slightly enlarged spleen is present in approximately half the cases. Primary carcinoma of the liver develops in about 14 per cent. The incidence of this last complication increases greatly with age.

Excessive skin pigmentation is present in about 90 per cent of the patients at the time the diagnosis is established. Pigmentation may be due to deposition of melanin or iron or both. In general, melanin deposition gives rise to bronzing, iron deposition to a metallic gray hue. Pigmentation usually is diffuse and generalized, but frequently it is deeper on the face, neck, extensor aspects of the lower forearms, dorsae of the hands, lower legs, genital regions, and in scars. In only 10 to 15 per cent of cases is there demonstrable pigmentation of the oral mucosa.

About 82 per cent of all patients develop diabetes mellitus and symptoms therefrom. The diabetes may appear rapidly, and insulin requirements may increase rapidly. About 72 per cent of the patients require insulin for the control of the diabetes. In some instances severe insulin resistance develops, in others there may be sensitivity to insulin. In most instances, the diabetes is controlled with little difficulty. Since the diabetes is usually present for less than a decade, the late degenerative sequelae of this complication are not prominent.

Approximately one-third of patients with idiopathic hemochromatosis die of cardiac failure. The heart disease is extremely common in young adults, and symptoms may develop suddenly, with rapid progression to death. The most important manifestations of heart disease are congestive failure and cardiac arrhythmias, particularly ventricular extrasystoles and paroxysmal atrial tachycardia. Other arrhythmias may occur as well.

DIAGNOSIS. The classical triad of skin pigmentation, diabetes mellitus, and hepatomegaly, especially in the presence of heart disease and evidence of hypogonadism, should always suggest the diagnosis. Confirmation of the presence of liver, pancreatic, heart, and gonadal disease should then be obtained by customary tests of the functions of these organs. It then remains to demonstrate that there is excessive storage iron.

The diagnosis is enhanced considerably if the plasma iron level is found to be elevated (above 150 μg per 100 ml) and the iron-binding protein of the plasma is 75 to 100 per cent saturated. However, the only definitive test is liver biopsy. Other procedures which indicate an excess of body iron stores are bone marrow aspiration for hemosiderin, examination of the urine sediment for hemosiderin, skin biopsy, and gastric mucosal biopsy.

Finch and Finch state that there are no unique features in idiopathic hemochromatosis by which it may be distinguished pathologically from the terminal stage of other iron-storage diseases, such as dietary or transfusion hemochromatosis. They define *hemosiderosis* as a focal increase in tissue iron or a general increase in iron stores without associated tissue damage, and *hemochromatosis* as a general increase in body iron stores with resultant tissue damage. From these definitions, the differentiation of hemosiderosis from hemochromatosis can be easily made by the presence or absence of organ dysfunction. Dietary and transfusion hemochromatosis can be differentiated from idiopathic hemochromatosis on the basis of a history of excessive iron intake by mouth, by injection, or intravenously in the form of blood. In evaluating dietary iron exposure, the dietary iron content, type of diet, type of cooking utensils, intake of medicinal iron, and iron content of the drinking water or other beverages must be considered.

PROGNOSIS. The life expectancy of patients after signs of clinical hemochromatosis have become manifest averages 4.4 years, but several instances have been recorded of patients living up to 20 or 30 years after manifestation of signs. The average duration of life after diabetes has developed is 3 years. The principal causes of death are cardiac failure (30 per cent), hepatic coma (15 per cent), hematemesis (14 per cent), hepatoma (14 per cent), and pneumonia (12 per cent). The most recent advance in the therapy of this disease, the introduction of methods for removal of iron, is expected to increase life expectancy further.

TREATMENT. The therapy of idiopathic hemochromatosis involves removal of the excess body iron by phlebotomy and supportive treatment of damaged organs. The management of the hepatic failure, cardiac failure, and diabetes differs little from the conventional management of these conditions. Loss of libido and change in secondary sex characteristics are relieved by testosterone therapy. Iron is best removed from the body by a weekly phlebotomy of 500 ml. Since the average amount of iron in a patient with hemochromatosis is approximately 25 Gm, about 2 years of weekly bleeding will be required to deplete the iron stores. Desferrioxamine, an iron-chelating agent, is of value in the treatment of hemochromatosis secondary to aplastic and other refractory anemias and may be used in conjunction with weekly phlebotomy in patients with primary hemochromatosis.

REFERENCES

Bothwell, T. H., and C. A. Finch: "Iron Metabolism," Boston, Little Brown and Company, 1962.

Finch, S. C., and C. A. Finch: Idiopathic Hemochromatosis, an Iron Storage Disease, Medicine, 34:381, 1955.

MacDonald, R. A.: Idiopathic Hemochromatosis: Genetic or Acquired? A.M.A. Arch. Internal Med., 112:184, 1963.

Sheldon, J. H.: "Hemochromatosis," Fairlawn, N.J., Oxford University Press, 1935.

101 DISORDERS OF PORPHYRIN METABOLISM

George E. Cartwright

DEFINITIONS. *Porphyrins* are pigments that possess a basic structure of four pyrrole rings linked by methene($=CH-$) bridges (Fig. 101-1). The individual

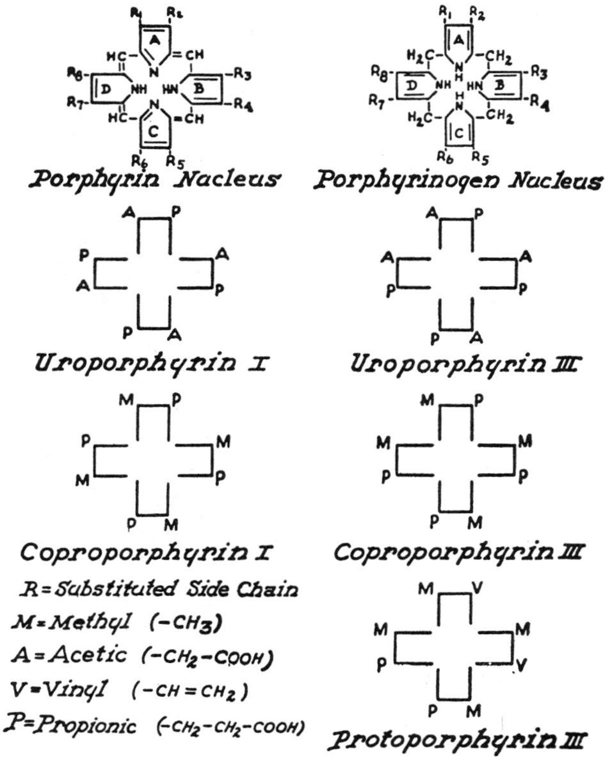

Fig. 101-1. The structural formulas of the porphyrin and porphyrinogen nuclei and diagrammatic formulas of the important naturally occurring porphyrins.

porphyrins differ from each other according to the nature of the eight possible side chains. Each porphyrin has a number of stereoisomers. *Porphyrinogens* are colorless compounds (reduced porphyrins) with a basic structure of four pyrrole rings linked by methane (—CH$_2$—) bridges.

Porphyrin pigments are widely distributed throughout the plant and animal worlds in chlorophyll, hemoglobin, catalase, and a number of cytochrome and peroxidase enzymes.

The term *porphyrinuria* refers to excessive excretion of porphyrins in the urine. *Coproporphyrinuria*, the excretion of increased amounts of coproporphyrin, is not uncommon and occurs in a variety of conditions. The term *porphyria* embraces a group of diseases, each with unusual and characteristic manifestations, which have in common the excessive excretion of one or more of the porphyrins, porphyrinogens, and/or porphyrin precursors (Δ-aminolevulinic acid and porphobilinogen) in the urine and/or feces.

HISTORY. Congenital porphyria was first described by Günther in 1911. Much of the knowledge of the chemistry of the porphyrins came from Hans Fischer and his school in Munich. In 1915, these workers described, named, and isolated in crystalline form the uroporphyrins and coproporphyrins from the urine of the patient in their famous case of congenital porphy-

ria (Petry). Shemin and Granick and their groups in New York have made substantial contributions to knowledge of the biosynthesis of the porphyrins. Contributions to the understanding of the types and manifestations of porphyria have come from Waldenström in Sweden, Rimington in England, Barnes and Dean in South Africa, and Watson, Schwartz, and Schmid in the United States.

BIOSYNTHESIS. The rather complex porphyrin molecule is synthesized in the body from two simple precursors, acetate and glycine (Fig. 101-2). Acetate enters the Krebs tricarboxylic acid cycle (Chap. 62, p. 336) and is converted into succinate. Succinyl CoA (active succinate) is then formed in the presence of Mg^{++} ion, adenosine triphosphate (ATP), and coenzyme A (CoA). The activated form of succinate condenses with a pyridoxal phosphate-glycine enzyme (glycine-PE) to form the 5-carbon compound, Δ-aminolevulinic acid (Δ-ALA), and carbon dioxide by the decarboxylation of glycine. This step is enzymatically controlled (ALA synthetase) and several intermediate compounds have been suggested. Two molecules of Δ-aminolevulinic acid, in the presence of glutathione (GSH) and an enzyme, Δ-aminolevulinic acid dehydrase (Δ-ALA DH), condense to form a substituted monopyrrole, porphobilinogen, which contains acetic acid (A) and propionic acid (P) side

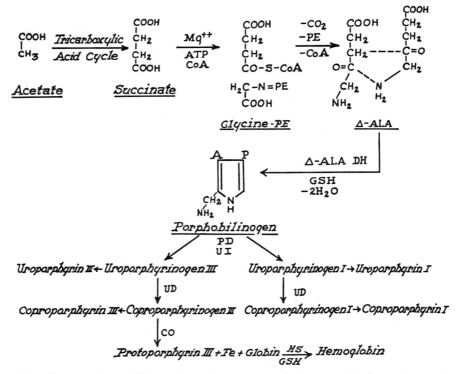

Fig. 101-2. The biosynthesis of the porphyrins from acetate and glycine and the biosynthetic pathway of hemoglobin. CoA, coenzyme A; ATP, adenosine triphosphate; PE, pyridoxal phosphate enzyme (ALA synthetase); Δ-ALA, delta-aminolevulinic acid; Δ-ALA DH, delta-aminolevulinic acid dehydrase; GSH, glutathione; PD, porphobilinogen deaminase; UI, uroporphyrinogen isomerase; UD, uroporphyrinogen decarboxylase; CO, coproporphyrinogen oxidase; HS, heme synthetase; A, acetic; P, propionic.

chains. In the next step in heme synthesis, four molecules of porphobilinogen condense to form the reduced tetrapyrrolic structure, uroporphyrinogen. This step is catalyzed by at least two enzymes, porphobilinogen deaminase (PD) and uroporphyrinogen isomerase (UI). Details of the action of these enzymes and the sequence of reactions leading from porphobilinogen to uroporphyrinogen types I and III are not known. Uroporphyrin III is not in the direct pathway of heme synthesis, as was formerly assumed, but is a by-product. Uroporphyrinogen III (reduced uroporphyrin) is converted to coproporphyrinogen by the enzyme, uroporphyrinogen decarboxylase (UD). Coproporphyrinogen III is then converted to protoporphyrin III in the presence of the enzyme coproporphyrinogen oxidase. Coproporphyrin III is a by-product, whereas the available evidence suggests that protoporphyrin III is in the direct pathway of heme synthesis. Protoporphyrin III is converted to hemoglobin in the presence of iron, glutathione, globin, and the enzyme heme synthetase (HS). The intermediate steps between protoporphyrin and hemoglobin have not been identified. It is not known whether heme or a porphyrin-globin compound is an intermediate in this reaction, although the former possibility seems more likely.

METABOLISM. The most important of the naturally occurring porphyrins are uroporphyrin (isomer types I and III), coproporphyrin (types I and III), and protoporphyrin (type III).

Protoporphyrin III is present in hemoglobin and is, therefore, the most important of the porphyrins from the physiologic standpoint. It is normally absent from urine. The concentration of fecal protoporphyrin is related to the amount of blood in the gastrointestinal tract and the rate of liberation of protoporphyrin from hemoglobin by fecal bacteria.

Coproporphyrin is the predominant porphyrin in urine and feces under normal circumstances. Coproporphyrinuria occurs in a variety of clinical conditions, such as lead poisoning, poliomyelitis, liver disease, acute alcoholism, hemolytic anemia, and Hodgkin's disease. In all these disorders the increased coproporphyrinuria accompanies the underlying disease, and it is unlikely that the abnormality in porphyrin metabolism contributes significantly to the clinical picture. Coproporphyrinuria is also found in patients with porphyria. Abnormally high fecal coproporphyrin values are found in patients with hemolytic anemia, and low values occur in patients with liver disease.

Uroporphyrin is normally excreted in urine in only trace amounts. The urinary excretion of this porphyrin is moderately increased in lead poisoning and is greatly increased in patients with porphyria.

PORPHYRIA

Porphyria may be divided into two general groups (Table 101-1). In porphyria erythropoietica, excessive quantities of porphyrins are synthesized in the bone marrow. The predominant porphyrin synthesized in erythropoietic uroporphyria (congenital porphyria) is uroporphyrin. The predominant porphyrin synthesized in erythropoietic protoporphyria is protoporphyrin. In porphyria hepatica, excessive porphyrin production occurs in the liver. Hepatic porphyria may be subdivided further into at least three different types: acute intermittent porphyria, porphyria cutanea tarda hereditaria, and porphyria cutanea tarda symptomatica. Not all patients with hepatic porphyria can be so classified; there is some degree of overlapping, and it is entirely possible that more than a single entity is included in each subtype of hepatic porphyria.

Table 101-1. DISTINGUISHING FEATURES OF THE SEVERAL TYPES OF PORPHYRIA

Characteristics	Erythropoietic		Hepatic				
	Uroporphyria	Proto-porphyria	Acute intermittent		Cutanea tarda hereditaria		Cutanea tarda symptomatica
Inheritance...............	Recessive	Dominant	Dominant		Dominant		Acquired
Sex......................	Both	Both	Both		Both		Both
Age of onset..............	0–5 yr	0–5 yr	15–40 yr		10–30 yr		Any age
Phase of disease...........	....	....	Latent	Acute	Latent	Acute	
Cutaneous lesions.........	++++*	++	0	0	0	+ or 0	++
Abdominal colic, psychoses, and/or neurologic disease	0	0	0	+	0	+	0
Urine Δ-ALA†.............	N	N	+	++	N	++	N
Urine PBG†	N	N	++	++++	N	++	N
Uroporphyrinuria..........	++++	N	++	++	N	+++	++++
Coproporphyrinuria........	++	N	++	++	N	+++	++
Fecal porphyrins..........	++	N to ++	N	+	++++	+++	+

* 0, absent; N, normal; +, increased; ++++, greatly increased.
† Δ-ALA, Δ-aminolevulinic acid; PBG, porphobilinogen.

Porphyria Erythropoietica

ERYTHROPOIETIC UROPORPHYRIA (CONGENITAL PORPHYRIA)

This is a very rare disorder, inherited probably as a recessive mendelian characteristic. The clinical manifestations occur very early in life, sometimes even a few days after birth, but often they are not observed until after an interval of a year or two. The disease is characterized by the excessive deposition of porphyrin in the tissues, leading to pronounced photosensitization. The early lesions of photodynamic origin are the blisters of hydroa estivale (hydroa vacciniforme) on skin surfaces exposed to light, especially of the face and hands. In time, scarring and mutilation occur. After years of continued photosensitivity, the mutilation becomes extensive, with loss of fingers, portions of the nose, ears, scarring of the cheeks and about the mouth, ectropion, or symblepharon. Skin not exposed to light remains unaffected. Hemolytic anemia and splenomegaly are an integral part of the disease. Erythrodontia may be observed in those cases in which sufficient porphyrin has been deposited in the teeth to make them grossly red or reddish brown. Teeth which do not show erythrodontia in ordinary light may exhibit red fluorescence in Wood's light. Red fluorescence may be seen in the phalangeal bones if a strong source of ultraviolet light is allowed to shine through the fingers. There is no marked disturbance of the nervous system, nor is there abdominal colic.

Because of the demonstration of large quantities of uroporphyrin and coproporphyrin in the normoblasts in the bone marrow, it has been suggested that in this type of porphyria the excessive quantities of porphyrin are formed in the marrow. It is for this reason that the disease has been called *erythropoietic porphyria* rather than congenital porphyria.

The color of the urine varies from pink to red. Uroporphyrin I and coproporphyrin I are the predominant porphyrins excreted. If the concentration of uroporphyrin is sufficiently great, the urine, on the addition of hydrochloric acid, exhibits an intense band at about 552 mμ and a weaker band at 596 mμ when viewed in a hand spectroscope. The excretion of porphyrin precursors, Δ-aminolevulinic acid and porphobilinogen, is not increased.

The disease is slowly progressive, and death is usually due to an intercurrent infection or severe hemolytic anemia. At autopsy there is extensive deposition of porphyrins in the skeleton and tissues. This may be so pronounced as to color the bones red. Erythroid hyperplasia of the bone marrow and splenomegaly are additional pathologic features.

TREATMENT. Exposure to sunlight should be avoided. The harmful and disfiguring effects of light may be ameliorated by the use of quinine cream. Splenectomy is indicated if there is evidence of increased erythrocyte destruction. Splenectomy may be associated not only with amelioration of the hemolytic anemia but also with a reduction in photosensitivity and porphyrin excretion.

ERYTHROPOIETIC PROTOPORPHYRIA CONGENITA

This is a rare disorder, which appears in childhood and is probably transmitted as a mendelian dominant characteristic. The disorder is characterized clinically by the sudden onset of itching, erythema, and edema following exposure to ultraviolet light. Vesicles, bullae, scars, and pigmentation do not occur. Biochemically the disorder is characterized by an increase in the protoporphyrin and coproporphyrin content of the normoblasts and erythrocytes. The urinary excretion of Δ-ALA, porphobilinogen, coproporphyrin, and uroporphyrin is not increased. The fecal excretion of protoporphyrin and coproporphyrin is usually but not always increased. The fecal excretion of uroporphyrin is normal.

Porphyria Hepatica

ACUTE INTERMITTENT PORPHYRIA

This is an uncommon but not a rare disease which affects both sexes, with a slight predilection for the female. Young adults or the middle-aged are most frequently affected. Acute porphyria is extremely rare below the age of fifteen and after the age of sixty. The familial occurrence of the disease is marked. It is probably transmitted as a mendelian dominant characteristic. The disease is characterized clinically by (1) periodic attacks of intense abdominal colic, usually accompanied by nausea and vomiting; (2) obstinate constipation; (3) neurotic or even psychotic behavior; and (4) neuromuscular disturbances. The mortality rate is high.

Abdominal pain is frequently the presenting complaint. The pain is usually colicky in nature and may be extremely severe and associated with spasm without localizing signs but with fever, tachycardia, and leukocytosis. The abdominal signs may be, and frequently are, mistaken for manifestations of renal colic, acute appendicitis, cholelithiasis, or pancreatitis. It is not uncommon for patients with porphyria to have multiple surgical scars on the abdomen. The neurologic manifestations are quite varied and may include neuritic pain in the extremities, areas of hypoesthesia and paraesthesia, and foot and wrist drop. Paraplegia or a complete flaccid quadriplegia may ensue and may be followed by bulbar paralysis and death. Except for pain in the extremities, sensory changes are usually not prominent and signs of upper motor neurone changes are usually absent. The neurologic manifestations may simulate a wide variety of conditions, including poliomyelitis, encephalitis, and arsenic or lead poisoning. A true ascending paralysis of the Landry type is not observed.

The patients frequently have many vague "neurotic" complaints, even when in remission from an attack.

With an attack they may become confused or even psychotic. Hypertension may accompany an attack, there may be temporary loss of vision, and convulsions have been described.

The course of the disease is extraordinarily variable. Recurrent abdominal crises may be present for years, or the patient may die in the first attack. It is not at all uncommon to find in one parent or in several siblings of a patient with porphyria that porphobilinogen, the diagnostic feature of porphyria, is present in the urine, even though they have never had active symptoms of the disease. This condition is called *latent porphyria*. In general, the neuromuscular and psychotic symptoms are late manifestations, and with their appearance the prognosis becomes more grave. Between attacks there may be no symptoms. The mechanism by which the latent disease is converted to manifest disease, i.e., an attack of acute porphyria, is unknown, but it is known quite definitely that attacks may be provoked by the administration of certain drugs, particularly barbiturates. Menstruation, pregnancy, infection, alcohol, or lead may be the precipitating factor in a few patients.

The freshly voided urine is frequently normal in color and on standing in the sunlight turns to a Burgundy wine color or even black. This color change can be hastened by adding a small amount of acid to the urine and boiling for 30 min. The explanation for these color changes is that porphobilinogen (colorless) and not uroporphyrin (red) is excreted in the urine. Heating of porphobilinogen in an acid medium results in the nonenzymatic formation of uroporphyrin, together with a dark-brown or reddish-brown nonporphyrin pigment.

In acute intermittent porphyria during relapse the presence of porphobilinogen is a constant feature. During remission the porphobilinogen reaction is usually positive, but a negative test does not exclude the diagnosis of this type of porphyria. The qualitative determination of porphobilinogen by the Watson-Schwartz modification of the Ehrlich reaction is, therefore, a simple and valuable screening procedure. In this test 5 ml freshly voided urine is mixed with 5 ml Ehrlich's reagent (0.7 Gm paradimethylaminobenzaldehyde, 150 ml concentrated hydrochloric acid, and 100 ml water). After mixing, 10 ml aqueous saturated sodium acetate is added. The solution is then extracted successively with 10 ml chloroform and 10 ml *n*-butanol. A positive test for porphobilinogen gives an intense red color remaining in the aqueous layer. This test is quite specific for acute intermittent porphyria. The test is negative in erythropoietic porphyria and in porphyria cutanea tarda symptomatica. It is positive in patients with porphyria cutanea tarda hereditaria during acute attacks but is negative in the interval between such episodes.

In addition to porphobilinogen, patients with acute intermittent porphyria excrete excessive quantities of uroporphyrin (types I and III), coproporphyrin (types I and III), and other as yet unidentified porphyrins. As mentioned previously, the porphyrins are formed in the renal tubules by the nonenzymatic transformation of porphobilinogen into uroporphyrin at an acid pH. Examination of the tissues of such patients, in contrast to the findings in erythropoietic porphyria, has revealed that the porphyrin content of the bone marrow is normal. The liver, on the contrary, regularly exhibits increased quantities of porphyrin, especially porphyrin precursors. For this reason, acute intermittent porphyria is classified among the hepatic porphyrias.

TREATMENT. The use of barbiturates should be avoided completely at all times because of their known action in precipitating acute attacks. Chloral hydrate and paraldehyde may be used for sedation. Opiates, Demerol, or ganglioplegics such as tetraethylammonium may be used for relief of pain. Chloropromazine, in doses of 50 to 100 mg, is reported to effect rapid relief of acute symptoms but without change in the underlying disease process. The rauwolfia derivatives may have supplementary value as maintenance therapy. ACTH, corticosteroids, and chelating agents such as BAL (2,3-dimercaptopropanol) and EDTA (disodium ethylenediaminetetraacetate) have been reported to be effective in alleviating acute attacks. However, evaluation of drugs is made difficult by the intermittent nature of the disease.

PORPHYRIA CUTANEA TARDA HEREDITARIA

Porphyria cutanea tarda hereditaria is characterized clinically by cutaneous lesions or acute attacks of abdominal colic and not infrequently by both. The disease is inherited as a non-sex-linked mendelian dominant. The onset of symptoms is usually between the ages of ten and thirty years. The outstanding biochemical feature of the disorder is the increased excretion of coproporphyrin and protoporphyrin in the feces *at all times* in the course of the disease.

During the latent phase of the disease the patients are entirely asymptomatic. Porphyrinuria is usually absent and the porphyrin precursors, Δ-aminolevulinic acid and porphobilinogen, are not excreted in increased amounts. The disease can be diagnosed only during the latent phase by examination of the stools for porphyrins. A simple screening test can be done by obtaining a small specimen of stool on a glove. The specimen is extracted with about 2 ml of solvent containing equal parts of glacial acetic acid, amyl alcohol, and ether. The supernatant solution is then decanted and viewed in a Wood's lamp. Negative specimens show a green or gray fluorescence, a positive specimen a brilliant pink. Excess chlorophyll may give rise to a false positive test.

In a number of patients, particularly males, the skin is unusually sensitive to light and blisters and abrades easily. Healed depigmented scars may be present over the exposed surfaces, particularly the hands. Hyperpigmentation of the skin may occur, and hirsutism has been observed in females. The photosensitivity and cutaneous deformities are not so great as in erythropoietic porphyria.

Acute attacks of jaundice and abdominal colic accompanied in some cases by psychotic manifestations and motor paralysis may intervene in the course of the disease. Indeed, any or all of the manifestations of acute intermittent porphyria may make their appearance. As in acute intermittent porphyria, death or recovery may occur. During the acute attacks the excretion of porphyrins in the feces frequently decreases and the excretion of coproporphyrin and uroporphyrin in the urine increases. Both Δ-aminolevulinic acid and porphobilinogen are usually excreted in increased amounts in the urine during acute attacks. It has been suggested that the disease remains asymptomatic as long as the liver is capable of excreting the porphyrins in the bile (latent phase); when this capacity is impaired bilirubinemia, porphyrinemia, porphyrinuria, and cutaneous lesions appear (cutaneous phase); and finally when porphyrin metabolism is greatly disturbed, Δ-aminolevulinic acid and porphobilinogen appear in the urine and all the manifestations of acute intermittent porphyria may develop (acute phase). Porphyria cutanea tarda hereditaria is not an entirely suitable name for this disorder since not all patients develop cutaneous lesions. It is for this reason that the designation *porphyria variegata* has been suggested.

PORPHYRIA CUTANEA TARDA SYMPTOMATICA

This type of porphyria is characterized clinically by cutaneous lesions, hyperpigmentation of the skin, evidences of liver disease, and hypertrichosis; and chemically by the excretion of large amounts of uroporphyrin and lesser amounts of coproporphyrin in the urine. Abdominal pain and neurologic complications are conspicuously absent. The urine does not contain increased quantities of Δ-aminolevulinic acid or porphobilinogen. The excretion of protoporphyrin in the feces is normal; the excretion of coproporphyrin in the feces is usually increased.

The skin lesions are indistinguishable from those observed in porphyria cutanea tarda hereditaria. The skin is unusually sensitive both to light and to mechanical trauma. Blisters appear on the exposed skin areas, frequently ulcerate, and finally lead to scar formation. The photosensitivity is similar to that in erythropoietic porphyria but not as marked.

This disorder has been described (1) in male subjects, forty to seventy years of age, with alcoholic cirrhosis of the liver; (2) in Bantu subjects in South Africa with nutritional cirrhosis of the liver; (3) in children and adults in Turkey who have ingested the fungicide hexachlorobenzene; (4) in three elderly subjects with a tumor of the liver; and (5) in an occasional young adult without a history of alcoholism or drug exposure. Porphyria cutanea tarda symptomatica is probably acquired, but constitutional factors may be involved in some cases.

EXPERIMENTAL PORPHYRIA

A condition resembling in many respects porphyria erythropoietica in human beings has been produced experimentally in rats, rabbits, and chickens by the administration of lead, phenylhydrazine, or the dye rose bengal, as well as by excessive exposure to sunlight. A bovine form of porphyria erythropoietica, inherited as a recessive trait, has been recognized and studied in some detail.

A condition resembling porphyria hepatica of the acute intermittent type has been produced in animals and in chick embryos by the administration of the sedative Sedormid (allyl-isopropyl-acetylcarbamide).

REFERENCES

Goldberg, A., and C. Rimington: "Diseases of Porphyrin Metabolism," Springfield, Ill., Charles C Thomas, Publisher, 1962.

Mauzerall, D.: Normal Porphyrin Metabolism, J. Pediat., 64:5, 1964.

Waldenström, J., and B. Haeger-Aronsen: Different Patterns of Human Porphyria, Brit. Med. J., 2:272, 1963.

Watson, C. J.: The Problem of Porphyria—Some Facts and Questions, New England J. Med., 263:1205, 1960.

Watson, C. J., I. Bossenmaier, and R. Cardinal: Acute Intermittent Porphyria: Urinary Porphobilinogen and Other Ehrlich Reactors in Diagnosis, J.A.M.A., 175:1087, 1961.

102 DISORDERS OF MELANIN METABOLISM

Thomas B. Fitzpatrick

Definition

Melanin is the basis of the coloration of human skin, hair, and eyes. In man it functions primarily as a screen that shields the dermis from the deleterious effects of solar radiation. Since the amount and distribution of melanin in skin and hair is changed in a number of diseases, a detailed study of irregularities of pigmentation may provide important diagnostic clues.

The term *melanin* is derived from the Greek word *melas,* black, and is the name given to a biochrome of high molecular weight formed by enzymatic oxidation of the phenol tyrosine. The biochrome is therefore often referred to as *tyrosine-melanin.* Tyrosine-melanin is the product of unique unicellular glands, *melanocytes,* that secrete this substance into epidermal cells. The exact chemical nature of melanin has not been determined, because tyrosine-melanin (both natural and synthetic) is so extremely insoluble that all attempts to degrade it into identifiable fragments have failed.

Biosynthesis

Melanocytes are situated at the dermoepidermal interface, in the hair bulb, the uveal tract and retinal pigment epithelium, and the leptomeninges. These scattered groups of cells are known as the *melanocyte system.* They may be considered to constitute a unit, because the melanocytes in all these locations are derived from the neural crest and can hydroxylate tyrosine to dihydroxyphenylalanine and ultimately to the pigment tyrosine-melanin. The melanocyte system is analogous, but not known to be related, to the chromaffin system. Like melanocytes, the cells of the chromaffin system are derived from the neural crest and possess biochemical mechanisms for the hydroxylation of tyrosine to dihydroxyphenylalanine; unlike melanocytes, however, they convert this substance to adrenochrome and not to tyrosine-melanin. Benign and malignant neoplasms arise in all parts of the melanocyte system except the retinal pigment epithelium and the hair bulbs.

The melanocytes present at the dermoepidermal interface form a horizontal network that is closely connected to the epidermal cells by means of numerous cytoplasmic processes, or dendrites. That this intimate relationship permits cytocrine transference of melanin particles (melanosomes, melanin granules) from melanocytes to malpighian cells has been clearly demonstrated by electronmicroscopy in a study of the fine structure of cortical cells and hair melanocytes and more recently by tissue culture studies of human epidermis.

It has been possible to demonstrate by electronmicroscopy that melanocytes contain specialized organelles with a distinctive internal structure. These organelles, known as *melanosomes,* contain tyrosinase, the melanin-synthesizing enzyme. Under normal conditions, melanin is progressively formed and deposited on the surface of melanosomes until they are transformed into *melanin granules,* i.e., into particles of amorphous melanin that contain no tyrosinase activity (Fig. 102-1). Melanosomes are believed to originate in the Golgi area, appearing first as unmelanized vesicles that gradually increase in size and become dark in color and increasingly dense.

Tyrosinase is one of a large group of copper-containing aerobic oxidases that catalyze the oxidation of both monohydric and dihydric phenols to orthoquinones. In man and other mammals, this oxidase catalyzes the hydroxylation of the melanin precursor, tyrosine, to dihydroxyphenylalanine (dopa) and dopaquinone (Fig. 102-2). Tyrosinase is required only for the first step in the biosynthesis of tyrosine-melanin, i.e., the orthohydroxylation of tyrosine. It is noteworthy that zinc ions catalyze the conversion of dopachrome to 5,6-dihydroxyindole and that melanosomes have recently been shown to contain zinc in high concentration.

In the hair and skin of man, characteristic coloration is determined not by variations in the number of melanocytes present but by variations in the number and type of melanin granules produced by existing melanocytes. The amount of pigment present in individual

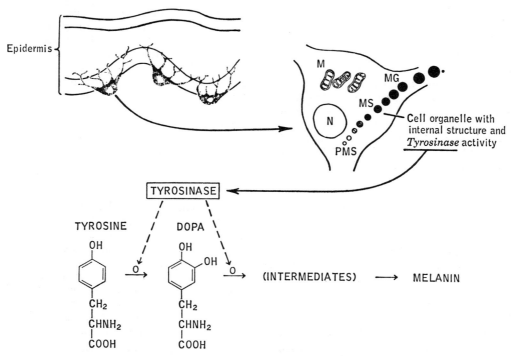

Fig. 102-1. Melanogenesis in human skin, as seen in the light microscope and the electron microscope and at the molecular level. PMS = premelanosome; MS = melanosome; MG = melanin granule; M = mitochondria. (*Modified from The New England Journal of Medicine, 265:330, 1961.*)

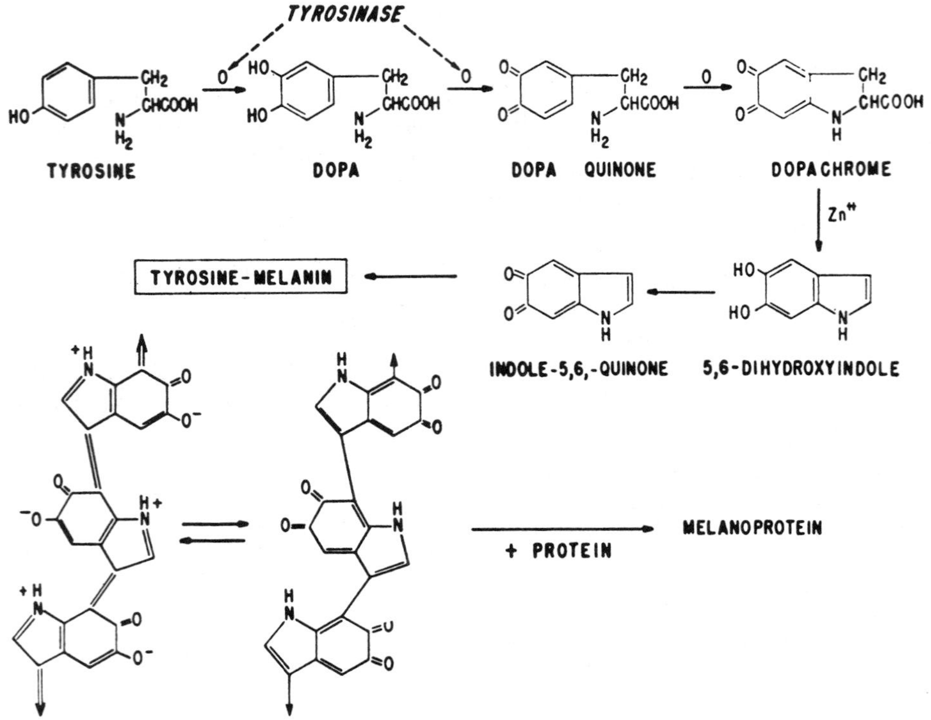

Fig. 102-2. Biosynthesis of tyrosine melanin. (*By permission from The New England Journal of Medicine, 265:330, 1961.*)

melanosomes is related to their tyrosinase content; for example, melanosomes that lack tyrosinase remain unpigmented, as in albinism.

PATHOGENESIS OF PIGMENTARY DISORDERS

To explain the pathogenesis of a disturbance of melanin pigmentation, it is necessary to evaluate the rate at which tyrosinase is synthesized on the ribosomes; to determine the rate at which premelanosomes progress through successive stages to melanin granules; to understand the role played by factors that regulate the biosynthesis of melanin; and to examine the transference of melanin granules to epidermal cells.

Availability of free tyrosine is essential for the biosynthesis of melanin. Tyrosine that is bound in a peptide linkage cannot act as a substrate if the amino group is blocked.

Aggregation and dispersion of melanin granules probably play no part in the pigmentary anomalies of man. Such movement of pigment has thus far been observed only in the specialized effector cells, *melanophores,* present in vertebrates below mammals in the phylogenetic scale.

CLINICAL DISORDERS OF MELANIN PIGMENTATION (MELANOSES)

CLASSIFICATION. Disorders of melanin pigmentation that involve the melanocyte system may be classed as *hypomelanoses* and *hypermelanoses.* On a morphologic basis, they can be divided into three main categories: (1) hypomelanosis, in which paucity of pigment renders the skin white or lighter than normal; (2) hypermelanosis (brown), in which excess pigment produces a brown-black color; and (3) hypermelanosis (blue), in which excess pigment produces a blue, slate, or gray hue. Pigmentary disorders with similar etiology may also be grouped together. Table 102-1 incorporates these various methods of classification. Hypomelanosis (decreased pigmentation) may result from loss of melanocytes, as in thermal burns, or from absence or paucity of melanin. In the disorders listed in Table 102-1 under the heading of Brown Hypermelanosis, the brown pigmentation results from an increase in the *activity* of epidermal melanocytes and not from an increase in the number of these cells. Gray, slate, or blue hypermelanosis results from the presence of melanin within dermal phagocytes or ectopic dermal melanocytes. The blue, slate, or gray hue is related to the Tyndall light-scattering phenomenon.

DIAGNOSIS. Recognition of hypomelanosis and gray, slate, or blue hypermelanosis is usually not difficult. When the degree of hypomelanosis is very slight, diagnosis may be facilitated by the use of black light.[1] Differentiation between abnormal diffuse brown hyperpigmentation and normal pigmentation frequently poses a problem because there is such a wide range of coloration in different individuals. It is usually possible, however, to determine whether the patient has

[1] Melanin pigment appears darker in black light than in normal light. Black light, which emits 3,660 Å, primarily emphasizes the contrast between hypopigmented and normal skin.

Table 102-1. DISTURBANCES OF HUMAN MELANIN PIGMENTATION*

Cause	Hypomelanosis (decreased melanin pigmentation)	Hypermelanosis (increased melanin pigmentation)	
	White *(or lighter than normal)*	*Brown*	*Gray, slate, or blue†*
Genetic or nevoid....	*Albinism, oculocutaneous‡* Albinism, cutaneous (white forelock, piebaldism, Waardenburg's syndrome, etc.) Phenylketonuria (hair and iris) Vitiligo (may be universal)‡	Neurofibromatosis (*café au lait*) Polyostotic fibrous dysplasia (Albright's syndrome) Acanthosis nigricans (juvenile type) *Gaucher's disease‡*	
Metabolic..........		*Hemochromatosis‡* *Hepatolenticular disease‡* (Wilson's disease) Porphyria‡ (congenital and cutanea tarda)	Hemochromatosis‡
Nutritional.........	Chronic protein deficiency or loss, as in kwashiorkor, nephrosis, ulcerative colitis, malabsorption syndrome (hair gray or reddish)	Kwashiorkor Pellagra (may be diffuse) Sprue (may be diffuse)	Chronic nutritional insufficiency
Endocrine..........	*Hypopituitarism‡* Addison's disease (vitiliginous) Hyperthyroidism (vitiliginous)	*ACTH- and MSH-producing* pituitary tumors‡ *ACTH therapy‡* Pregnancy (may be diffuse) *Addison's disease‡* Estrogen therapy (nipple)	
Chemical...........	Chloroquine and hydroxychloroquine (hair) Mephenesin carbamate (hair) Arsenical intoxication	*Arsenical intoxication‡* Busulfan‡ Photochemical (drugs, tar)	Quinacrine toxicity Chlorpromazine
Physical............	Burns: thermal, ultraviolet, ionizing radiation (loss of melanocytes) Trauma (loss of melanocytes)	Ultraviolet light Heat Alpha-, beta-, and gamma-radiation Trauma (e.g., chronic pruritus)	
Inflammatory and infectious.........	Syphilis Leprosy§	Postinflammatory (dermatitis, exanthems, drug eruptions)	
Neoplasmic..........	In sites of melanoma after disappearance (therapeutic or spontaneous) of tumor	Urticaria pigmentosa Adenocarcinoma with acanthosis nigricans	*Malignant melanoma‡* advanced (generalized dermal pigmentation syndrome, with melanuria)
Miscellaneous........	Vogt-Koyanagi syndrome Scleroderma§ (circumscribed or systemic) Horner's syndrome, congenital and acquired (iris)	*Scleroderma, systemic‡* *Chronic hepatic insufficiency‡* *Whipple's syndrome‡* Melasma (chloasma)	

* This classification includes disorders of interest to physicians in general; many pigmentary disorders not listed are of special interest to the dermatologist.

† Gray, slate, or blue color results from the presence of *dermal* melanocytes or phagocytized melanin in the dermis.

‡ Pigment change is generalized and diffuse, not spotty; no identifiable borders.

§ Loss of pigmentation usually partial. Viewed with Wood's light, the lesions are not chalk-white as in vitiligo.

observed an unusual or progressive change in coloration that has had no obvious cause. A summer tan may not have faded, or the patient's associates may have detected a gradual deepening of his skin color. The degree of brown hypermelanosis that develops appears to be related to the basic skin color of the patient. For example, a patient of Mediterranean extraction (Italian, French, Spanish) may become intensely pigmented with the onset of primary adrenocortical insufficiency, while a light-skinned patient will have only a minimal degree of hypermelanosis that may or may not be detectable. Localized pigmentation that develops newly in the mucous membranes and in certain areas such as the axillas and palmar creases is usually

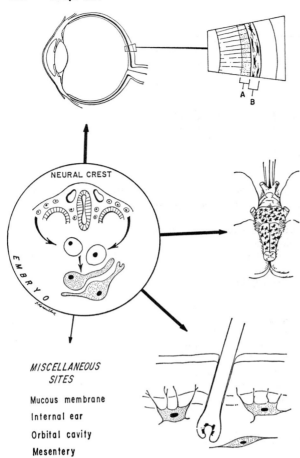

MISCELLANEOUS
SITES

Mucous membrane

Internal ear

Orbital cavity

Mesentery

Fig. 102-3. Diagram showing the embryonic origin, dispersal, and developmental fate of melanocytes in man. *A* = retinal pigment epithelium; *B* = choroidal melanocytes. (*By permission from The Metabolic Basis of Inherited Disease, 2d ed., 1965.*)

easier than generalized hyperpigmentation[2] to identify as a pathologic change.

GENETIC OR NEVOID

ALBINISM. Albinism is characterized by paucity or absence of melanin in affected areas of the body. In this disorder whatever tyrosinase may be synthesized by the melanocytes is functionally defective and unable to catalyze the oxidation of tyrosine to melanin. The formation of melanin granules is interrupted in the premelanosome stage; few or no mature melanosomes are present in albinotic skin or hair (Fig. 102-3). Albinism is diagnosed and classified on the basis of ocular and cutaneous findings. The same ocular abnormalities, e.g., hypopigmentation of the fundus oculi, translucency of the irides, and nystagmus, are found in both the oculocutaneous and the ocular types of the dis-

[2] Pigmentation of the gums, tongue, and buccal mucosa is a normal finding in the Asiatic, American Indian, and Negroid races and often in the East Indian.

order. In *oculocutaneous* albinism these ocular changes are associated with cutaneous manifestations of universal, unpatterned hypopigmentation; in *ocular* albinism, pigmentation of the skin is normal. *Cutaneous albinism* involves the skin and hair only; it has been known as white forelock, piebaldism, and Waardenburg's syndrome. In cutaneous albinism, melanin is lacking in patterned areas on the extremities and ventral thorax, and there is commonly a white forelock; the melanin content of the eyes, however, remains normal. The deficiency of melanin in oculocutaneous albinism has two disturbing consequences for man: decreased visual acuity and an abnormal degree of intolerance to sunlight. The sensitivity of human albinos to ultraviolet light leads to the development of carcinoma in exposed areas of the skin, especially in albinos living in the tropics.

PHENYLKETONURIA. In phenylketonuria there is a single metabolic block in the conversion of phenylalanine to tyrosine. The condition is associated with subnormal pigmentation of the hair and the iris. The hair of patients with phenylketonuria ranges in color from light blond to dark brown, and it is only by comparison with the hair of siblings that the characteristic dilution of color becomes evident. The diminution of melanin formation results from the fact that the large amounts of phenylalanine and its metabolites present in serum and extracellular fluid act as competitive inhibitors of tyrosinase activity, thus blocking melanin synthesis (Chap. 94).

VITILIGO. Vitiliginous macules are sometimes associated with *Addison's disease*, hyperthyroidism, and pernicious anemia but are usually idiopathic.

Idiopathic vitiligo is an inherited disorder, probably an irregular dominant trait. It is caused by a defect of melanocytes that leads to failure of melanin formation. The lesions may be localized, generalized, or universal, but the pigment of the eye is never involved in the process of pigment loss.

NEUROFIBROMATOSIS (VON RECKLINGHAUSEN'S DISEASE). This condition is inherited as a dominant trait. It is characterized by the presence, primarily on the trunk but also on the extremities, of numerous pale yellow-brown macules, so-called *café au lait* spots, that vary in diameter from less than 1 to more than 15 cm. Spotty generalized pigmentation may also be present, especially in the axillas. Often, but not always, a few or myriads of soft, rounded, cone-shaped or pendulous cutaneous tumors covered by normal skin are seen. Nerve-sheath tumors may occur.

The presence of six or more *café au lait* spots with a diameter greater than 1.5 cm is diagnostic of neurofibromatosis even when there is no familial history of the condition. In *polyostotic fibrous dysplasia* there are rarely more than three or four macules, unilaterally distributed usually on the buttocks or cervical area (Chap. 231). It may be difficult to differentiate the single, large, isolated *café au lait* spot of neurofibromatosis from the pigmented macule of *polyostotic fibrous dysplasia* (*Albright's disease*). Recently, however, it has been possible to detect peculiar, large, extracellular globules of melanin in whole mounts of epidermis prepared from the *café au lait* macules of neurofibromatosis; these extracellular melanin globules are not present in polyostotic fibrous dysplasia.

METABOLIC

Generalized brown hypermelanosis of the skin is a characteristic manifestation of *hemochromatosis* and *cutaneous porphyria (porphyria cutanea tarda)* (Chap. 101). The hyperpigmentation observed in hemochromatosis (Chap. 100) may have a grayish-brown hue or be indistinguishable from that of Addison's disease (Chap. 84). The diagnosis of hemochromatosis is established by the presence of hemosiderin in the sweat glands of the skin. Porphyria may be recognized by the abnormally large amounts of *uroporphyrin* in the urine, stools, and plasma and by other characteristic clinical features, such as the presence of bullae, atrophic scars, and milia on the exposed surfaces of the face and hands.

NUTRITIONAL

Chronic protein deficiency, as, for example, in kwashiorkor, chronic nephrosis, ulcerative colitis, and malabsorption syndrome, is sometimes associated with diminished hair color, appearing first as a reddish-brown and eventually as gray. In chronic nutritional insufficiency, splotches of dirty-brown hyperpigmentation appear, especially on the trunk. In *sprue* brown hypermelanosis may be generalized. In *pellagra* hypermelanosis is limited to areas of skin that have been exposed to light.

ENDOCRINE

Diffuse brown hypermelanosis is a striking feature of primary adrenocortical insufficiency (Chap. 84). Although this hypermelanosis is diffuse, there is marked accentuation of pigmentation in certain areas, namely, in the pressure points (vertebras, knuckles, elbows, knees), the body folds, the palmar creases, and the gingival mucous membrane. An identical type of diffuse hyperpigmentation has also been reported to follow adrenalectomy in patients with Cushing's syndrome due to adrenal hyperplasia. In these patients there are usually signs and symptoms of pituitary tumors; all the tumors recorded have been chromophobe adenomas. A third example of the Addisonian type of melanosis described above has recently been reported in patients with tumors of organs other than the adrenal or pituitary glands. The generalized brown hypermelanosis found in all these conditions results from overproduction of two hormones: alpha-melanocyte-stimulating hormone (MSH) and ACTH. Both peptides, MSH and ACTH, share common peptide sequences, and it is not yet known which one plays the dominant role in the pigmentation that oc-

curs in adrenocortical insufficiency; both MSH and ACTH are increased as a result of the decreased output of hydrocortisone by the adrenals. Hypermelanosis of the Addisonian type can be produced in adrenalectomized human subjects by administering large amounts of homogeneous ACTH and alpha-MSH.

CHEMICAL

Chemicals can induce both hypo- and hypermelanosis. Hydroquinone and its derivatives block the conversion of tyrosine to dopa and thereby prevent the formation of melanin. Striking generalized Addisonian hypermelanosis of the skin follows Busulfan therapy; the mechanism of action of this drug is not known. Inorganic trivalent arsenicals produce both generalized Addisonian hypermelanosis and scattered macular hypomelanosis, as well as punctate keratoses of the palms and soles.

PHYSICAL

Mechanical trauma as well as burns caused by either heat, ultraviolet light, or alpha-, beta-, and gamma-radiation can lead to hypo- or hypermelanosis. The effect of these physical agents on pigmentation is determined by the intensity and duration of exposure and is limited to the site of injury. The hypomelanosis results from destruction of melanocytes.

Chronic pruritus, such as that associated with chronic biliary tract disease and lymphoma, may lead to generalized brown hypermelanosis.

INFLAMMATORY AND INFECTIOUS

Circumscribed hypomelanosis is a characteristic feature of *tuberculoid leprosy.* It occurs in areas of anesthesia and the degree of pigment loss is only partial; the lesions are lighter in color than areas of surrounding skin but are not chalk-white as in vitiligo. Generalized, spotty hyperpigmentation not uncommonly follows *exanthems* and *eruptions due to drugs;* it usually disappears spontaneously within 2 or 3 months.

NEOPLASTIC

Hypomelanosis is seen in rare instances at the site of a *malignant melanoma* that has undergone remission spontaneously or as the result of therapy. During the terminal stages of malignant melanoma, striking generalized blue hypermelanosis sometimes develops and large amounts of a conjugated derivative of 5,6-dihydroxyindole are excreted in the urine (so-called "melanuria"). This intermediate in the metabolic pathway from tyrosine to melanin can be oxidized to melanin in the absence of tyrosinase, and therefore melanin can be synthesized at almost any site in which oxidation can take place. Consequently, diffuse black pigmentation may develop in the peritoneum, liver, heart muscle, and dermis of patients during the late stages of malignant melanoma. The brown melanin present in the dermal phagocytes appears as a blue skin color because of the Tyndall light-scattering effect.

The multiple, irregular, round or oval, yellow-brown to red-brown macules and papules characteristic of *urticaria pigmentosa* are related to the presence in the dermis of clusters of mast cells. Urticarial wheals develop when the individual lesions are stroked vigorously. In rare instances (*systemic mastocytosis*), mast cells infiltrate diffusely into the liver, spleen, gastrointestinal system, and bones, as well as into the skin.

MISCELLANEOUS

Generalized brown hypermelanosis of the type seen in Addison's disease is not infrequently associated with *systemic scleroderma* and may appear very early in the course of the disorder. Generalized hyperpigmentation occasionally develops in patients with *chronic hepatic insufficiency*, especially that due to portal cirrhosis. The pathogenesis of the pigmentation in both these conditions is unknown.

Melasma (chloasma) is seen most commonly in pregnant women, but it also occurs in men and in nonpregnant women. The lesions consist of large macules with irregular borders on the exposed areas of the face and vary in color from yellow-brown to red-brown and very dark brown. Recently, melasma has been observed in women receiving oral progestational agents.

REFERENCES

Fitzpatrick, T. B., and W. C. Quevedo, Jr.: Albinism, in "The Metabolic Basis of Inherited Disease," rev. ed., J. B. Stanbury, J. B. Wyngaarden, and D. S. Fredrickson (Eds.), New York, McGraw-Hill Book Company, Inc., 1965.

——, M. Seiji, and A. D. McGugan: Melanin Pigmentation, New England J. Med., 265:328, 374, 430, 1961.

Lerner, A. B.: Melanin Pigmentation, Am. J. Med., 19: 902, 1955.

——, and J. S. McGuire: Melanocyte-stimulating Hormone and Adrenocorticotrophic Hormone; Their Relation to Pigmentation, New England J. Med., 270: 539, 1964.

Riley, V., and J. G. Fortner (Eds.): The Pigment Cell: Molecular, Biological and Clinical Aspects, Ann. New York Acad. Sci., 100, parts I and II, February, 1963.

103 HEPATOLENTICULAR DEGENERATION (Wilson's Disease)

George E. Cartwright

DEFINITION. Hepatolenticular degeneration (progressive lenticular degeneration, Wilson's disease, pseudosclerosis of Westphal and Strümpell, tetanoid chorea of Gowers) is an uncommon, familial, progressive, fatal disease which becomes manifest usually in the first three decades of life and is characterized by the triad of basal ganglion degeneration, cirrhosis of the liver, and a ring of brown pigment at the corneal margins known as the Kayser-Fleischer ring.

HISTORY. Kinnier Wilson, in 1912, in his classic monograph, "Progressive Lenticular Degeneration," first clearly defined the disease entity to which his name is now affixed. A similar condition had previously been described in 1883 by Westphal and later by Strümpell. The symptoms resembled those of multiple sclerosis, but no demyelinative plaques were observed. For that reason it was called *pseudosclerosis*. The cirrhosis of the liver was overlooked until Spielmeyer reexamined the cases many years later. His studies and the clinical observations of Hall left little doubt that hepatolenticular degeneration and pseudosclerosis were the same disease. The corneal ring was described in 1902 by Kayser in a case diagnosed as "multiple sclerosis," but to Fleischer is due the credit for appreciating its significance in relation to the disease as it is now known.

A marked increase in the copper content of both the brain and the liver was demonstrated by Haurowitz in 1930 and was later confirmed by Glazebrook and Cummings. Mandelbrote and his associates in 1948 observed by chance that the urinary output of copper was high and that this output is increased by the administration of BAL (British antilewisite). In the same year Uzman and Denny-Brown found that a persistent aminoaciduria is associated with the disease.

INHERITANCE. The condition is inherited as an autosomal recessive trait, the affected individuals inheriting the gene from both parents who, while phenotypically normal, are heterozygous for the abnormal allele. Since the frequency of the abnormal gene is low in the general population, affected individuals may be expected to be, most often, the products of consanguineous marriages. This has proved to be the case.

PATHOGENESIS. Two different types of metabolic disturbance have been described, namely (1) abnormalities in the metabolism of copper and (2) impairment in renal tubular reabsorption.

A number of alterations in the metabolism of copper has been described (Table 103-1). The amount of copper in the tissues, particularly in the liver and brain, is increased about tenfold above the normal. The golden-brown pigment of the Kayser-Fleischer ring contains copper. The amount of copper excreted in the urine is increased. The specific copper protein of plasma, ceruloplasmin, is almost invariably decreased. On the other hand, the "direct-reacting" fraction of plasma copper, the copper which is probably loosely bound to albumin, is increased. Since there is a greater reduction in ceruloplasmin copper than there is increase in direct-reacting copper, the net effect on the total plasma copper is such that there is usually hypocupremia. In an occasional patient the total plasma copper concentration may be as high as 116 μg per 100 ml. Patients with this disease retain more than the normal amount of copper in the body. This is apparently because of an increased rate of absorption of copper from the gastrointestinal tract. Whether or not copper is excreted by the liver into the bile at the normal rate has not yet been determined with certainty. There may be a normal copper content in the bile, but this is not normal when the total copper content of the liver is considered.

Renal dysfunction which is present in many, but not all, patients includes abnormalities in tubular reabsorption manifested by aminoaciduria, peptiduria, proteinuria, glucosuria, uricosuria, or phosphaturia. The aminoaciduria involves most of the amino acids found in normal urine and, in addition, proline and citrulline. Taurine, aspartic acid, isoleucine, methyl histidine, and arginine are excreted in amounts close to the normal range. The urinary amino acid pattern and the severity of the aminoaciduria depend in part on the amount and type of protein ingested and vary considerably from patient to patient without relation to the type, duration, or stage of disease. The aminoaciduria is not accompanied by any significant elevation in the blood α-amino nitrogen level. The uricosuria may be associated with a diminished level of uric acid in the serum. The phosphaturia may result in hypophosphatemia and eventually in osseous changes.

The pathogenesis of the metabolic and pathologic changes is not fully understood. Because of the excessive deposition of copper in the tissues of patients with Wilson's disease, it has been suggested that the lesions in the liver and in the lenticular nuclei are the consequence of the excessive deposition of copper in these tissues and that the accumulation of copper in the kidney causes a functional impairment in the reabsorption of amino acids, peptides, and other substances. In support of this concept is the observation that excessive deposition of copper in the liver precedes the development of significant parenchymal damage. In at least some patients with the disease, the mobilization of copper from the body is apparently associated with dramatic improvement in the clinical state of the patient.

Copper absorbed from the gastrointestinal tract enters first into the direct-reacting fraction of plasma copper. Therefore, the increase in this fraction reflects the increased turnover of copper between the gastrointestinal tract, the tissues, and the excretory routes. The copper in this fraction is easily dissociable from the albumin, and the increase in the direct-reacting fraction probably accounts for the increased excretion of copper by the kidneys.

The most widely held concept of the disease is that the inherited defect is an inability to synthesize ceruloplasmin. However, some individuals heterozygous for the gene may have as low a ceruloplasmin concentration as some patients with the disease. Furthermore, there is a poor correlation between the ceruloplasmin

Table 103-1. BIOCHEMICAL ALTERATIONS IN WILSON'S DISEASE

Determination	Normal subjects*	Wilson's disease
Total plasma copper, μg/100 ml	114 (81–147)	60 (19–103)
Direct-reacting plasma copper, μg/100 ml	7 (0–20)	26 (12–40)
Ceruloplasmin, mg/100 ml......	33 (25–43)	9 (0–19)
Urine copper, μg/24 hr........	15 (5–25)	522 (95–1,300) †
Liver copper, μg/Gm wet tissue	5 (3–10)	79 (53–100) †
Urine α-amino nitrogen, mg/day	164 (118–204)	337 (90–519)

* The figures in parentheses refer to ±2 standard deviations.

† Determined range.

level and the severity or duration of the disease. An additional difficulty with this theory is that a mechanism whereby a deficiency of ceruloplasmin can lead to excessive tissue deposits of copper is not known.

Another theory which has been proposed is that the genetically determined abnormality in protein metabolism results in the formation of abnormal tissue proteins which have a high avidity for copper. The difficulty with this theory is that it does not explain the low concentrations of the plasma copper protein, ceruloplasmin.

PATHOLOGY. The characteristic pathologic findings are in the liver and the brain. The liver is usually small, firm, and coarsely nodular. It may or may not be bile-stained. Nodules of regenerating liver cells are separated by trabeculae of fibrous connective tissue. The picture is that of healed subacute yellow atrophy or the nonalcoholic variety of Laennec's cirrhosis. The most striking gross finding in the brain is cavitation of the putamen on each side and rarely of cerebral cortex and white matter. In many cases, probably more than half, the putamen and caudate nuclei are atrophic and of light, grayish-brown color, and there is no evidence of cavitation. Microscopic examination almost invariably reveals a remarkable hyperplasia of protoplasmic astrocytes in the cerebral cortex, lenticular and caudate nuclei, subthalamic nuclei of Luys, substantia nigra, dentate and red nuclei. Nerve cell loss is widespread but is most pronounced in the lenticular and dentate nuclei and cerebral cortex. The protoplasmic astrocytosis does not differ from that observed in hepatic coma. Splenomegaly is a common finding.

CLINICAL MANIFESTATIONS. The disease usually begins in adolescence, but it may appear as early as the age of four or as late as age forty. The mode of onset is somewhat variable. In a few cases the first manifestation is related to liver insufficiency, i.e., jaundice, ascites, or splenomegaly. More often the initial symptom is related to the neurologic system: tremor, dysarthria, ataxia, incoordination, or personality change. The disease may run an acute course of several months' duration associated with fever, rapid emaciation, and mental deterioration, or an extremely chronic afebrile course of 30 or 40 years' duration. The usual course is 5 to 10 years.

The clinical picture of a well-developed case is quite characteristic. *Tremor* of one or both of the upper extremities is an outstanding as well as an early manifestation. The tremor consists of regular, rhythmic, alternating contractions and may occur in the earliest stages only on movement of the extremity. Later it is also present when the arm is maintained in an attitude of repose. It is accentuated by excitement or by attention being drawn to it. One of the most certain ways of demonstrating the tremor is by having the patient extend the arms in front of the body. In this position "flapping" or "wingbeating" may be noted. The tremor may also increase during fine volitional movements, taking a form that resembles intention tremor. Indeed, in some cases cerebellar ataxia and tremor are the principal neurologic manifestations. In severe cases a tremor of the mandible or even of the entire head is present. *Abnormal movements* of choreic or choreoathetoid type are present in some patients but are not frequent. *Rigidity* of the skeletal muscles, often reaching an extreme degree, is another characteristic. The rigidity may be intermittent or constant, and the resulting clinical state may vary from transient spasms in the acute cases to permanent *contractures* and *deformities* in the chronic. In the late stages of the disease the facial muscles become set in a stiff, vacuous smile, the neck and trunk become rigid, the upper extremities are held rigidly in flexion at the elbow, wrist, and metacarpal joints, and the lower extremities are held in a position of extension. *Dysarthria* or even anarthria in advanced cases is an almost constant finding. *Cachexia* and muscular wasting may be extreme. Some form of *mental disturbance* is common, and in severely affected patients changes in character and personality and terminally marked mental deterioration may be present. The sensory system is intact, and the reflexes are essentially normal. Pyramidal signs are usually absent.

The clinical course of the liver disease is extremely variable. In many patients signs of liver insufficiency are completely lacking, even though the liver function tests are abnormal and cirrhosis can be demonstrated by needle biopsy. In other patients the signs of liver insufficiency, such as splenomegaly, ascites, jaundice, hepatomegaly, hematemesis, and spider angiomas, dominate the clinical picture. When liver function is markedly impaired, anemia, leukopenia, and thrombocytopenia may be found to accompany the splenomegaly.

The most remarkable, unique, and consistent feature of the disease is the Kayser-Fleischer ring (see Chap. 109), a golden-brown or greenish-brown ring of pigment located at the periphery of the cornea in Descemet's membrane. The pigment usually goes completely around the cornea; occasionally there may be only a crescent-shaped distribution. Although the rings are frequently visible in ordinary light, in the early stages of the disease or in patients in whom the color of the iris is brown, it may be necessary to use a slit lamp to visualize the rings. Under slit-lamp examination, the ring is seen to be composed of a multitude of granular specks. When present the rings are pathognomonic of the disease. Since the metabolic changes in Wilson's disease have been recognized, not a single patient has been reported with the disease without Kayser-Fleischer rings. The presence of the rings is a more reliable and consistent feature of the disease than any single one of the biochemical alterations.

Skeletal abnormality, manifested by roentgenographic evidences of osteomalacia, cartilage injury, or bone fragmentation, is a frequent finding in the disease. Azure lunulas, bluish crescent areas at the nail bases, have been observed in several patients.

DIAGNOSIS. The triad of Kayser-Fleischer rings, cirrhosis of the liver, and signs of basal ganglion disease is pathognomonic of this condition.

The various clinical findings combine to form several different clinical pictures, the most frequent of which is Parkinson's syndrome. Occasionally cerebellar ataxia, chorea, choreoathetosis, or dystonia predominates. If signs of liver insufficiency are not evident from physical examination, liver function studies or needle biopsy of the liver will demonstrate the presence of liver disease. Rubeanic acid stain may be used to demonstrate the excessive deposition of copper. In young patients in whom neurologic disease is not manifest and the signs of liver disease are marked, the condition has been confused with "juvenile" or "familial" cirrhosis.

The presence of hypocupremia, hypoceruloplasminemia, hypercupruria, and hyperaminoaciduria confirms the diagnosis, although it is rarely necessary to perform the difficult laboratory examinations in order to establish the diagnosis. In a rare patient with the disease, hypocupremia and hypoceruloplasminemia may not be present. Hypocupremia and hypoceruloplasminemia may be present in some normal individuals who are heterozygous for the gene. These two biochemical alterations are also present in all normal newborn infants and in at least some patients with kwashiorkor, sprue, celiac disease, and the nephrotic syndrome. Hypercupruria may be present only in the last condition mentioned. Hypercupruria may be present in patients with alcoholic cirrhosis of the liver, but the copper excreted rarely exceeds 200 μg per day; in this condition the concentration of copper and ceruloplasmin in the plasma is either normal or increased.

PROGNOSIS. The disease is progressive and invariably fatal if untreated. It is still too early to know for certain if death can be prevented or delayed by the early continuous and energetic therapy outlined below. Death results from intercurrent infection or hepatic failure.

TREATMENT. The therapy of Wilson's disease is directed toward (1) the prevention of the continued accumulation of copper in the body and (2) the removal of copper already deposited. Potassium sulfide (potash sulfurated technical, 20 mg three times daily with meals) prevents the absorption of copper by the formation of insoluble, unabsorbable copper sulfide in the gut. No undesirable side effects have been observed when such therapy has been given continuously for periods up to 5 years. The administration of copper-chelating agents such as BAL (2,3-dimercapto-propanol), amino acids, Versenate (calcium disodium salt of ethylenediaminetetraacetic acid), or penicillamine (β,β-dimethyl cysteine), results in the mobilization of copper from the tissues and an increase in its excretion in the urine. Of the chelating agents, penicillamine is the most effective. D-Penicillamine, 1 to 4 Gm daily in four divided doses, on an empty stomach, should be given continuously for the lifetime of the patient. Fever, skin rashes, leukopenia, and thrombocytopenia may result from penicillamine therapy but are rarely sufficiently severe to require more than temporary cessation of therapy and gradual desensitization by the administration of increasing amounts of the agent. A diet high in protein promotes the urinary excretion of copper and may be of value in the treatment of the liver disease.

Therapy as outlined above has resulted in some degree of improvement in the clinical manifestations in about 1 month in some but not all patients. If mental changes are present they may revert toward normal, while the tremors and rigidity become less pronounced, sometimes to a remarkable degree. Improvement in liver function or in plasma copper aberrations is not observed with therapy. The partial remissions may last for months to years.

REFERENCES

Scheinberg, I. H., and I. Sternlieb: The Pathogenesis and Clinical Significance of the Liver Disease in Hepatolenticular Degeneration (Wilson's Disease), Med. Clin. N. Am., 44:665, 1960.

Walshe, J. M., and J. N. Cumings: "Wilson's Disease: Some Current Concepts," Oxford, Blackwell Scientific Publications, Ltd., 1961.

Wilson, S. A. K.: Progressive Lenticular Degeneration: A Familial Nervous Disease Associated with Cirrhosis of the Liver, Brain, 34:395, 1912.

104 DISORDERS OF GLYCOGEN SYNTHESIS AND MOBILIZATION

Richard A. Field

The glycogen deposition diseases occupy a noteworthy place in the evolution of the conceptual approaches to the modern methods of study of disease. In 1952, Dr. Gerty T. Cori demonstrated by specific enzymatic studies of tissue from patients that von Gierke's disease is due to the loss of activity of a single tissue enzyme, and thus she provided a prototype for the study of genetically determined metabolic aberrations. Since the points of enzymatic abnormality of most of the syndromes to be discussed in this chapter concern the steps of synthesis and degradation between glucose 6-phosphate and glycogen, a working schema of these pathways is presented in Fig. 104-1. The Cori Classification of glycogen deposition diseases is shown in Table 104-1.

GLUCOSE 6–PHOSPHATASE DEFICIENCY HEPATORENAL GLYCOGENOSIS

First described pathologically by von Gierke in 1929, this condition, characterized by enlargement of liver and kidneys and bouts of severe hypoglycemia, is probably the most frequent form of glycogenosis. Symptoms and recognizable clinical signs usually appear in the first year of life, and hepatomegaly may be detectable at birth. The disorder is transmitted as an autosomal, mendelian recessive characteristic.

PATHOLOGIC PHYSIOLOGY. Under normal conditions hepatic glycogen serves as the main reservoir compound in the overall economy of blood glucose homeostasis. During and after ingestion of carbohydrate foods, a major portion of the glucose arriving in the liver via the portal system is phosphorylated and, by several intermediary steps, is stored as the regularly branched polysaccharide, glycogen (Chap. 62). During the postcibal period, peripheral utilization of glucose depletes circulating glucose, with the result that liver glycogen is depolymerized and free glucose is released into the hepatic vein (Chap. 62). The overall intracellular reactions in this process are called glycogenolysis, and the final enzymatic step is the hydrolytic dephosphorylation by the specific enzyme, hepatic glucose 6-phosphatase (Fig. 104-1). Absence or marked reduction of this enzyme activity can be demonstrated by direct tissue assay in hepatorenal glycogenosis and accounts for most, if not all, of the metabolic disturbances noted in patients with this condition. The central feature of this limitation of hepatic glucose release is hypoglycemia, and it follows that little or no elevation of blood glucose concentration occurs following the injection of glucagon or epinephrine. Likewise, the normal expected rise in blood glucose level is not observed in patients with this hepatic enzyme deficiency following the intravenous administration of fructose or galactose. For all intents and purposes, these hexoses are metabolized solely by the liver and ultimately are converted intracellularly to glucose 6-phosphate, which, like the molecules of the same compound derived from glycogen depolymerization, cannot be dephosphorylated in the absence of glucose 6-phosphatase so as to appear in the blood stream as free glucose. Apparently large quantities of glucose

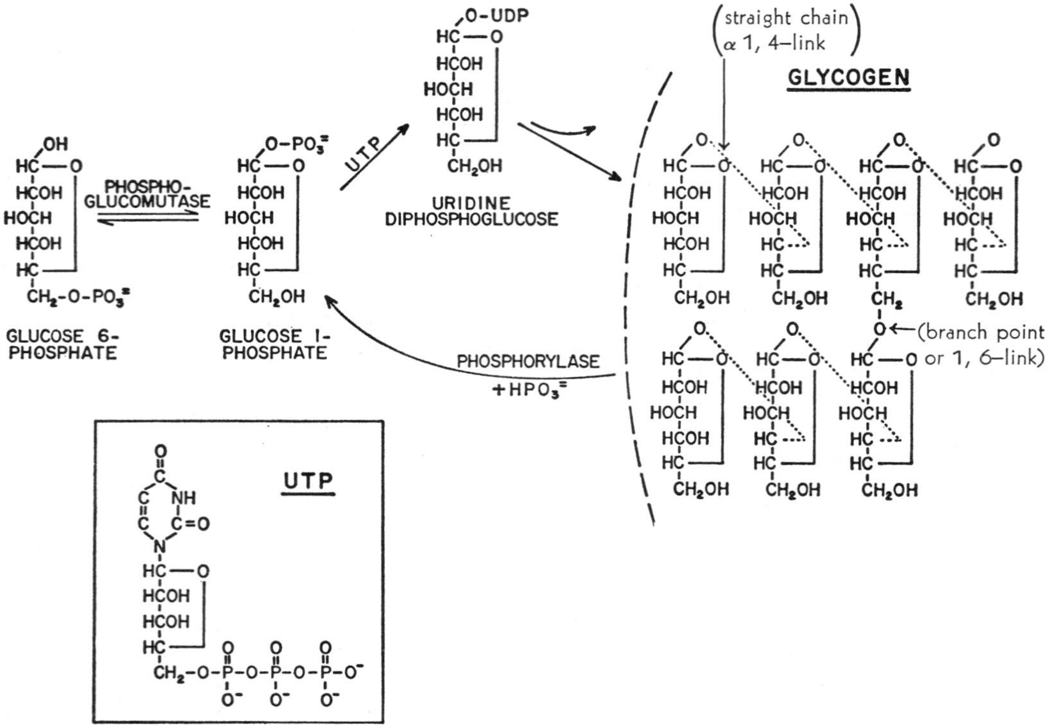

Fig. 104-1. Pathways of glycogen synthesis and breakdown.

6-phosphate are disposed of by increasing the amounts carried through the steps of anaerobic glycolysis resulting in an increased production and release of lactic and pyruvic acids; thus, hyperlacticacidemia is a characteristic finding in the syndrome and can be strikingly augmented by the administration of glucagon or other stimuli of hepatic glycogenolysis. Although ketonemia, lipemia, and ketonuria are frequently observed, because of the relative unavailability of glycogen stores and the resultant hypoglycemia which triggers mobilization of fat to meet energy requirements, marked and dangerous lacticacidosis is also frequent and may supervene precipitously. It is believed that the chronic hyperlacticacidemia is responsible for disturbance in renal clearance of water and accounts for the hyperuricemia seen in this condition. Chronic acidosis on a cellular level may play a role in the generally retarded growth, mild normochromic unresponsive anemia, hypophosphatemia, and generalized decreased bone density with mushrooming of the metaphyses and frequent fractures observed in these patients. Glycosuria and nonspecific aminoaciduria without aminoacidemia also occur and may be striking. It has been suggested that these findings correlate with the severity of glycogen infiltration and the hypothetically intracellular accumulation of phosphorylated hexoses in the renal tubular cells; but other impairments of renal function are not prominent.

PATHOLOGY. The liver is markedly enlarged, smooth, firm, and brownish in color. Microscopic study shows the liver cells to be enlarged up to three times

the normal size and to be filled with glycogen and at times excessive amounts of fat. In the kidneys, which are usually at least double normal size, intracellular excess of glycogen is found in the cells of the proximal tubules. That the excess of glycogen persists in these organs long after death is not surprising when the nature of the biochemical defect is recalled.

CLINICAL PICTURE. The child is pale and undersized, with a fat face and neck and a markedly distended abdomen containing a huge, easily palpable liver without associated ascites or splenomegaly. Xanthomas with prominent lipemia may be a feature. Occasionally, epileptiform seizures and vomiting occur; however, more often the gravity and prevalence of the low blood sugar level are not appreciated until serious central nervous system deterioration has resulted.

LABORATORY EXAMINATIONS. These examinations reveal fasting hypoglycemia, hyperlipidemia, hyperlacticacidemia, anemia, and, at times, ketonemia and ketonuria. After glucose ingestion or infusion, the fall of blood levels may be delayed, yielding a pseudo-diabetic curve. This may be explained as impaired capacity to increase the already superabundant stores of liver glycogen, rather than as a failure to utilize glucose at a normal rate in peripheral tissues. There is hypersensitivity to insulin, and severe prolonged hypoglycemia may follow its administration. Suspicion of this disorder is warranted when typical clinical characteristics are present and consonant results with glucagon or epinephrine challenge tests and of galactose or fructose infusion have been obtained. Final

Table 104-1. DISORDERS OF GLYCOGEN DEPOSITION AND MOBILIZATION

Cori type	Enzyme defect	Organ	Glycogen structure	Eponymic name	Suggested clinical name
1	Glucose 6-phosphatase	Liver, kidney, intestine (?)	Normal	von Gierke's disease	Glucose 6-phosphatase deficiency hepatorenal glycogenosis
2	α-Glucosidase (maltase)	Generalized	Normal	Pompe's disease	α-Glucosidase deficiency generalized glycogenosis
3	Amylo-1,6-glucosidase (debrancher)	Liver, heart, muscle, leukocytes	Abnormal; missing or very short outer chains	Forbes's disease	Debrancher deficiency limit dextrinosis
4	Amylo-(1,4:1,6) transglucosidase (brancher)	Liver, probably other organs	Abnormal; very long inner and outer unbranched chains	Andersen's disease	Brancher deficiency amylopectinosis
5	Muscle phosphorylase	Skeletal and cardiac muscle	Normal	McArdle-Schmid-Pearson disease	Myophosphorylase deficiency glycogenosis
6	Liver phosphorylase	Liver	Normal	Hers's disease	Hepatophosphorylase deficiency glycogenosis

diagnosis, as with all glycogenoses, rests on biochemical assay of enzyme activity in biopsy material, in this instance, liver. In typical cases, liver glucose 6-phosphatase activity is found to be absent or reduced to less than 10 per cent of normal. There is no ready explanation for the three cases reported in which glucose 6-phosphatase activity was either normal or only moderately reduced despite the careful characterization of the cases as clinically and pathophysiologically entirely consistent with the diagnosis.

DIFFERENTIAL DIAGNOSIS. The sporadic reports of cases of liver glycogenosis in which multiple enzymatic abnormalities in the glycogen pathways can be demonstrated and other cases in which members of the same kinship have distinctly different enzymatic lesions have given rise to both diagnostic and conceptual confusion. At present, it is not clear whether such cases result from secondarily induced adaptations, a close relationship of chromosomal genetic loci for determining and controlling the formation of the different enzymes, or from the influences of environmental factors. Until further investigations clarify these situations or augment the details of pathways of glycogen metabolism, the nonrestrictive labeling of such cases as do not fit, either biochemically or functionally, into the classical groupings as simply "liver glycogen disease" seems wise.

TREATMENT. Although no means of increasing tissue activity levels of glucose 6-phosphatase in typical cases is available, earlier diagnosis, combined with recognition of hypoglycemia, acidosis, and intercurrent infection as the causes of morbidity and mortality, has markedly improved the life expectancy in this disease. The observation that the disturbances in metabolism and function in patients who survive beyond the fifth year tend to ameliorate provokes inquiry into the biochemical mechanisms by which such could occur and points to the necessity for assiduous care of the afflicted infant. It appears that in cases with prolonged survival the hyperuricemia and urate deposition which result, especially in the kidneys, become the major causes of difficulties. For this the daily administration of 0.5 to 2.0 Gm probenecid (Benemid) may be employed (Chap. 99).

α-GLUCOSIDASE DEFICIENCY GENERALIZED GLYCOGENOSIS

This disorder, the most devastating form of glycogenosis, causes death within the first 2 years of life. It is marked by a generalized deposition of glycogen and by striking cardiomegaly. Symptoms and signs appear within 1 or 2 months after birth and quickly produce an infant with marked muscular hypotonia, enlarged tongue, cretinoid appearance, cardiomegaly, and neurologic deficits. Increased susceptibility to recurrent respiratory infections is based on poor ventilative and tussive efforts.

The structure of isolated glycogen is normal, and hyperglycemia promptly follows glucagon or epinephrine administration or the infusion of galactose or fructose. Glycogen accumulation in vacuoles located in the cytoplasm of almost all body cells occurs to a variable degree and is a process in which the leukocytes participate. The principal mechanisms of death are cardiac failure and aspiration pneumonitis. The disease is familial in occurrence, and the mode of inheritance appears to be through a single recessive autosomal gene.

Hers has demonstrated in the tissues of five affected infants the absence of a normally ubiquitous α-$(1 \rightarrow 4)$ glucosidase which has optimum activity in the acid range. The enzyme characteristically hydrolyzes maltose and glycogen to glucose and can catalyze the transglucosylation from maltose to glycogen. Present hypotheses regarding glycogen metabolism do not provide a locus of influence at which this enzyme could effect glycogen deposition. Furthermore, spontaneous glycogenolysis occurs in excised tissues. Hers emphasizes the possible lysosomal nature of the enzyme and suggests that the polysaccharide accumulation is the result of a failure of physiologic digestion of areas of cytoplasm by the defective lysosomes. This interpretation is in agreement with the clinical observations of an absence of hypoglycemia, ketosis, and hyperlipidemia and the concept that the manifestations are the result of disruption of muscle fibers by the progressive glycogen accumulation. Although the clinical picture is highly characteristic, diagnosis depends on the demonstration of the absence of the acid α-$(1 \rightarrow 4)$ glucosidase in biopsy material.

Treatment is unavailing, although chemotherapy of intercurrent bacterial respiratory infections appears to prolong life.

DEBRANCHER ENZYME DEFICIENCY (LIMIT DEXTRINOSIS) AND BRANCHER ENZYME DEFICIENCY (AMYLOPECTINOSIS)

These two conditions are the result of defects of the enzymes concerned with the formation and the disengagement of the branch points of the typically arborized glycogen molecule (3 and 4 in Table 104-1). In the first instance, there is a deficiency of the specific enzyme required for cleavage of the branch point bond, and therefore glycogenolysis is interrupted as the first branch point is reached and a glycogen of abnormal structure with excessively frequent branch points and shortened inner and outer chains results. When the branching enzyme is deficient, an unusually structured glycogen which possesses excessively lengthened inner and outer chains and a paucity of branch points is produced. Apparently, this structure formation, which resembles that of plant starch, gives the polysaccharide the physical characteristics which lead to its sequestration within the cells, where it acts as an irritative nidus, producing a characteristic increase in periportal connective tissue.

Limit dextrinosis is a relatively frequent type of glycogenosis; amylopectinosis is exceedingly rare, only

two cases having been recognized. Since the clinical picture of the debrancher deficiency disturbance (limit dextrinosis) so closely resembles a mild form of the glucose 6-phosphatase deficiency, many cases of the former were mistakenly diagnosed as the latter before precise enzymatic assay techniques were available. The confusion need no longer arise even on clinical grounds or on the basis of functional tests, for in limit dextrinosis infusions of galactose lead to prompt intrahepatic conversion to glucose, with prompt hyperglycemia, there being no impediment to dephosphorylation and release. In the differential diagnosis in cases with equivocal hyperglycemic responses to glucagon or epinephrine and in which hepatomegaly, growth retardation, and a tendency to hypoglycemia and ketonuria contribute uncertainty, a liver biopsy need not be done, since it has been demonstrated that the debrancher enzyme is also absent in leukocytes, muscle, and erythrocytes. Furthermore, fasting levels of lactate and pyruvate are likely to be normal, in contrast to the situation with the Type I case (glucose 6-phosphatase deficiency), where they are distinctly elevated. In the Type III case, erythrocyte glycogen content is elevated, but again this is not so in the Type I individual.

Prognosis for the Type III defect appears to be relatively good, and at least two patients with this condition have reached the fifth decade of life. Logical treatment consists of a high protein, relatively low fat diet, with frequent feedings, prompt treatment of intercurrent infections, and prohibition of strenuous exercise, cardiodepressant drugs, and anesthetics, since the myocardium is involved.

GLYCOGEN DEPOSITION SYNDROMES DUE TO DEFICIENCIES OF GLYCOGEN PHOSPHORYLASES

Glycogen phosphorylase (5, Table 104-1) catalyzes glycogen depolymerization by phosphorylytic cleavage to yield glucose 1-phosphate and thus mediates the major initiating step in making the glucose moieties available for metabolism. In the liver the bulk of the glucose derived from the action of this enzyme ultimately defends the level of blood sugar and maintains an adequate supply for the peripheral tissues, while in the muscle the phosphorylase-produced hexose phosphate provides an immediate fuel source for the energy demanded by quick, sharp increases in contractile activity. Muscle and liver phosphorylase are distinctly different proteins immunologically, structurally, and functionally, and it appears that each has its own genetic determinant. Both enzyme activities are enhanced by epinephrine, while only liver phosphorylase responds in vivo to injections of glucagon.

MYOPHOSPHORYLASE DEFICIENCY GLYCOGENOSIS (McArdle)

A group of patients consisting of members of several unrelated families have been shown to be lacking in muscle phosphorylase activity. None has any growth retardation, disturbance in carbohydrate economy, or abnormality of response to glucagon or epinephrine administration. However, they have in common an incapacity to perform prolonged or strenuous muscle work and are excessively sensitive to ischemic conditions in this regard because of the occurrence of weakness, pain, and spasm of the exercised muscle. The demonstration of the isolated absence of muscle phosphorylase adequately explains the clinical phenomena when the importance of brisk glycogenolysis in supplying substrate for anaerobic glycolysis during ischemic muscle work is recalled. The impediment limiting the acceleration and augmentation of anaerobic glycolysis thus curtails increased lactate production. The failure to detect a significant rise in lactate concentration in the venous return from a muscle working under imposed ischemic conditions is a useful diagnostic test. A modest excess of glycogen in the muscles has been described, and in some cases prolonged exercise may cause breakdown of muscle cells and myoglobinuria. Although it has been shown that cardiac muscle shares the defect, no cardiac disturbance on this account has been described.

Since liver phosphorylase is normal in amount and activity, patients do quite well provided they accept limitations in exertion, protect themselves from tight garments that produce muscle ischemia, and fortify themselves with exogenous carbohydrates before attempting unusual physical tasks.

HEPATOPHOSPHORYLASE DEFICIENCY GLYCOGENOSIS (Hers)

Isolated development of hepatomegaly in infancy or childhood with a tendency to fasting hypoglycemia due to excessive accumulation of hepatic glycogen of normal structure characterizes this condition. Little in the way of other metabolic or developmental disturbance accrues as a consequence of the sluggish glycogenolysis which results from the absent or markedly reduced hepatophosphorylase activity. The deficiency of the enzyme can be demonstrated biochemically in hepatic tissue or in leukocytes. A possibly contingent deficiency of glucose 6-phosphate dehydrogenase has been described in some cases. No therapy beyond avoidance of prolonged fasting and the administration of a high protein diet with frequent feedings appears to be necessary. The mechanism of failure of hyperglycemic response to glucagon or epinephrine is obvious, and the normal response to galactose infusion as well as the normal serum lactate level and lack of hyperlipemia allow easy differentiation of this disease from the more devastating glucose 6-phosphatase deficiency. Transmission appears to be by means of an autosomal recessive gene.

REFERENCES

Cori, G. T.: Glycogen Structure and Enzyme Deficiencies in Glycogen Storage Disease, Harvey Lectures, 48: 145, 1952–1953.

——— "Glycogen Metabolism," Ciba Symposium, Boston, Little, Brown and Company, 1964.

Hers, H. G.: Glycogen Storage Disease, in "Advances in Metabolic Disorders," Vol. 1, Academic Press Inc., New York, 1964.

Stanbury, J. B., J. B. Wyngaarden, and D. S. Fredrickson: "The Metabolic Basis of Inherited Disease," p. 156, New York, McGraw-Hill Book Company, 1960.

Van Creveld, S.: Glycogen Disease, Arch. Disease Childhood, 34:298, 1959.

105 GALACTOSEMIA
Kurt J. Isselbacher

Galactosemia is an inborn error of metabolism associated with an impairment in the conversion of galactose to glucose and its derivatives. The disease is due to a congenital absence of a specific enzyme, galactose 1-phosphate uridyl transferase.

CLINICAL FEATURES. The disease manifests itself shortly after birth when the afflicted infant is exposed to galactose (in the form of lactose) in cow's milk or breast milk. Vomiting and diarrhea occur, and as a result there is an impairment in nutrition or failure to thrive. Jaundice may then become evident, together with enlargement of the liver and spleen. The clinical picture at this point may readily be confused with that of hepatitis. If the dietary ingestion of milk or galactose continues, cataracts are likely to form followed by the development of mental retardation. Cataracts may be evident at three or four weeks of age; several months may elapse before mental retardation is recognized. When blood galactose levels are very high, episodes of hypoglucosemia may occur and may be associated with convulsions.

If the infant is examined shortly after the ingestion of milk, galactose will be found in the blood as well as in the urine. The urine will also show an increase in amino acids (predominantly of the neutral type), and occasionally albuminuria is observed. It must be remembered that if, because of vomiting, no milk has been ingested, galactosuria will probably not be found.

All the clinical features except for mental retardation may regress completely when galactose is removed from the diet. The jaundice will readily subside, together with a diminution of the hepatosplenomegaly. Although cirrhosis of the liver may occur in the untreated galactosemic patient, only a residual fibrosis may remain in later years in patients who have been treated. Cataracts may improve greatly and, in fact, have been known to disappear completely on a galactose-free diet. Unfortunately, mental retardation is a lifelong feature, and once it has developed it is not reversible.

PATHOLOGIC PHYSIOLOGY. Both breast milk and cow's milk have as their sole content of carbohydrate the disaccharide lactose. This sugar is split within the intestinal epithelial cell into its component monosaccharides, namely, galactose and glucose. The infant with galactosemia has difficulty in converting galactose which is liberated to glucose and its derivatives. The main enzymes and the reactions involved in galactose utilization by the mammalian organism are as follows:

1. *Galactokinase:*

$$\text{Galactose} + \text{ATP} \rightarrow \text{galactose 1-phosphate} + \text{ADP}$$

2. *Galactose 1-phosphate uridyl transferase:*

$$\text{Galactose 1-phosphate} + \text{UDP-glucose}$$
$$\rightleftharpoons \text{UDP-galactose} + \text{glucose 1-phosphate}$$

3. *UDP-galactose-4-epimerase:*

$$\overset{\text{DPN}}{\text{UDP-galactose} \rightleftharpoons \text{UDP-glucose}}$$

4. *UDP galactose-pyrophosphorylase:*

$$\text{UTP} + \text{galactose 1-phosphate} \rightleftharpoons \text{UDP-galactose}$$
$$+ \text{pyrophosphate}$$

It is seen from these reactions that the first step in galactose utilization consists in its conversion to galactose 1-phosphate by the enzyme galactokinase. The galactose 1-phosphate must then be converted to glucose 1-phosphate; this is accomplished by the second reaction, catalyzed by the enzyme galactose 1-phosphate uridyl transferase. It is this enzyme and this reaction which are deficient in galactosemia. As a consequence, galactose 1-phosphate accumulates in the tissues. The epimerase serves to interconvert UDP-galactose and UDP-glucose and is a mechanism whereby normally in a galactosemic individual, galactose-containing substances, especially those found in brain lipids, may be synthesized from glucose even in the absence of dietary galactose. The fourth enzyme occurs mostly in liver, and it will be observed that it allows for some conversion of galactose 1-phosphate to UDP-galactose by a mechanism other than the transferase reaction. It is believed that the presence of this enzyme may serve as an accessory or alternate pathway in patients with galactosemia and may account for the improvement of galactose tolerance which occurs in some of these patients with increasing age.

The present evidence indicates that a number of the toxic symptoms found in galactosemia may be related to the accumulation of galactose 1-phosphate in the tissues. This sugar accumulates in lens, liver, and red cells and has been shown to inhibit the enzyme phosphoglucomutase. However the mechanism whereby this accumulation and subsequent enzyme inhibition lead to changes such as hepatic fibrosis and central nervous system damage has not yet been determined. One recent observation suggests that cataract formation may be related to the accumulation of a non-phosphorylated derivative of galactose (dulcitol) in the lens. The reduction in blood glucose levels in association with elevated galactose levels in the blood appears to be due to a decreased hepatic output of glucose. The basis for the aminoaciduria is not completely understood, but in animal studies (with intestine and kidney slices) it has been observed that sugars such as galactose tend to inhibit the transport of certain groups of amino acids.

DIAGNOSIS. The usual clue to the diagnosis consists of the clinical picture described above, together with the finding of a reducing sugar in the urine. Such a urine will give a positive reaction to Benedict's test (copper reduction) but a negative glucose oxidase test. If the urine is chromatographed, it shows predominantly galactose rather than glucose. If these initial screening tests suggest the diagnosis of galactosemia, then more specific tests are necessary.

In the past galactose tolerance tests have been performed which typically show a delayed clearance of galactose from the blood stream when the sugar was given by mouth or intravenously. However because of the toxicity of this sugar in the patient with galactosemia and because of the availability of more specific tests, this procedure is no longer recommended. The specific diagnostic test for this disease consists in the demonstration of the absence of galactose 1-phosphate uridyl transferase in the patient's red blood cells. In this test, the cells are incubated together with the two substrates, galactose 1-phosphate and UDP-glucose. After a period of incubation, the amount of uridine diphosphate glucose remaining is determined. In the normal individual the UDP-glucose disappears, because of the presence of the transferase in the red cells, but in galactosemia no utilization of UDP-glucose occurs when it is incubated in the presence of galactose 1-phosphate.

It is also possible to measure the transferase deficiency indirectly by a number of other procedures. For example, one may incubate red cells with galactose and demonstrate either enzymatically or chromatographically that galactose 1-phosphate accumulates. One may also incubate red cells or whole blood with radioactive galactose. Normal cells will oxidize the galactose, and, thus, radioactive carbon dioxide (CO_2) will be produced, but in the galactosemic cells, very little if any radioactive CO_2 will be liberated because of the defect in the oxidation of galactose.

DIFFERENTIAL DIAGNOSIS. The most important condition from which galactosemia needs to be differentiated in the neonatal period is primary liver disease, either acute or chronic. It must be recalled that in the presence of decreased liver function, galactose removal from the blood stream is impaired, and as a consequence, both elevated blood galactose levels and galactosuria may be found. However in liver disease (either hepatitis or cirrhosis) normal levels of red cell transferase are found and galactose utilization and oxidation by red cells or whole blood is completely normal.

Since these patients are often seen when nausea, vomiting, and diarrhea have developed and therefore dietary intake of galactose may be minimal, it must be emphasized that neither elevated blood nor urine galactose levels will be found in the absence of recent dietary intake of this sugar. Hence, an analysis of the blood and urine at these times may be misleading.

TREATMENT. The treatment of this disease consists in the exclusion of galactose and galactose-containing foods from the diet. In early infancy this involves the elimination of lactose as well as galactose. The milk substitutes which have been used effectively are Dextrimaltose and Nutramigen. Soy bean preparations have been used in the past, but they possess galactose-containing polysaccharides and should be avoided. As indicated above, fairly dramatic improvement will occur when the infant is placed on a galactose free-diet, and all symptoms except for the mental retardation may improve completely. These patients must remain on very restricted galactose diets until they have reached adequate physical and neurologic development.

GENETICS. Abundant evidence has been obtained to indicate that this is a disorder transmitted by an autosomal recessive gene. Specific enzyme studies have demonstrated both parents to be heterozygous with respect to galactose 1-phosphate uridyl transferase activities in their red cells. The exact incidence of this disease has not been determined, but the most recent data indicate that cases may be as frequent as 1 in 18,000 births. The occurrence of the carrier state is believed to be 1 out of 130 individuals.

REFERENCES

Bretthauer, R. K., R. G. Hansen, G. Donnell, and W. R. Bergren: Procedure for Detecting Carriers of Galactosemia, Proc. Nat. Acad. Sci. U.S., 45:328, 1959.

Hansen, R. G., R. K. Bretthauer, J. Mayes, and J. H. Nordin: Estimation of Frequency of Occurrence of Galactosemia in the Population, Proc. Soc. Exptl. Biol. Med., 115:560, 1964.

Isselbacher, K. J.: Galactosemia, pp. 208–225, in "The Metabolic Basis of Inherited Disease," J. B. Stanbury, J. B. Wyngaarden, and D. S. Fredrickson (Eds.), New York, McGraw-Hill Book Company, 1960.

Kalckar, H. M., E. P. Anderson, and K. J. Isselbacher: Galactosemia, Congenital Defect in a Nucleotide Transferase, Biochim. Biophys. Acta, 20:262, 1956.

106 LIPIDOSIS AND XANTHOMATOSIS

Donald S. Fredrickson

Lipidosis is a general term applied to disorders characterized by abnormal concentrations of lipids in tissues or in extracellular fluid. Sometimes it is restricted to only those abnormalities of lipid metabolism that are inheritable. *Xanthomatosis*, earlier employed in a broader sense, has now become a morphologic term referring to lipid accumulation in tissues in association with large "foam cells." The list of lipidoses and xanthomatoses in Table 106-1 encompasses most of the *primary* disturbances in lipid metabolism and includes some disorders in which secondary lipid stor-

Table 106-1. LIPIDOSES AND XANTHOMATOSES

I. Abnormal plasma lipoprotein concentrations (dyslipoproteinemias)
  A. Hyperlipoproteinemia
    1. Hyperbetalipoproteinemia (familial hypercholesterolemia)
      a. Definition and history
      b. Etiology
      c. Clinical picture
      d. Diagnosis
      e. Treatment
    2. Hyperprebetalipoproteinemia (endogenous hyperlipemia)
      a. Definition
      b. Clinical picture
      c. Etiology and diagnosis
      d. Treatment
    3. Hyperchylomicronemia (exogenous hyperlipemia)
      a. Definition and history
      b. Etiology
      c. Clinical picture
      d. Diagnosis
      e. Treatment
    4. Mixed types of hyperlipoproteinemia
  B. Hypolipoproteinemia
    1. Familial low-density lipoprotein deficiency (Abetalipoproteinemia)
    2. Familial high-density lipoprotein deficiency (Tangier disease)
II. Tissue lipid storage diseases
  A. Familial sphingolipidoses
    1. Glucocerebroside lipidosis (Gaucher's disease)
    2. Sphingomyelin-sterol lipidosis (Niemann-Pick disease)
    3. Cerebroside sulfatide lipidosis (metachromatic leukodystrophy)
    4. Ceramide-trihexoside lipidosis (Fabry's disease)
    5. Ganglioside lipidosis (amaurotic family idiocy; Tay-Sachs disease)
  B. Other rare storage diseases
    1. Phytanic acid (3,7,11,15-tetramethyl hexanoic acid) storage (Refsum's disease)
    2. Cholesterol storage with adrenal calcification (Wolman's disease)
    3. Cephalin storage
    4. Ceroid storage
III. Granulomatous diseases with lipid storage
  A. Histiocytosis X (xanthoma disseminatum, eosinophilic granuloma, Hand-Schüller-Christian disease, Letterer-Siwe disease)
  B. Lipoid proteinosis (Urbach-Wiethe disease)
  C. Lipoid dermatoarthritis
  D. Disseminated lipogranulomatosis (Farber's disease)
IV. Xanthomas
  A. Simple (xanthelasma, juvenile xanthoma)
  B. Associated with trauma and chronic infections
V. Adipose tissue disorders
  A. Relapsing panniculitis (Weber-Christian disease)
  B. Lipodystrophy
    1. Lipomas
    2. Adiposis dolorosa (Dercum's disease)
    3 Insulin lipodystrophy

Table 106-1. (Continued)

C. Lipoatrophy
   1. Partial (progressive lipodystrophy)
   2. Total (lipoatrophic diabetes mellitus)

age is prominent and some of the disorders of adipose tissue.

PLASMA LIPOPROTEIN ABNORMALITIES

The commonest of the lipidoses are those associated with primary alterations in concentrations of the plasma lipids. These can be better understood when considered in terms of lipoproteins, the form in which all lipids, except for free fatty acids, are present in plasma. Both selective increases or severe deficiency and absence of some of the groups or classes of lipoproteins can occur.

Hyperlipoproteinemia

Increased concentrations of plasma lipids and lipoproteins not explained by other primary disease represent metabolic problems that are difficult both to classify and to treat. Diagnosis requires (1) a careful history with special effort to gather evidence of familial involvement, (2) particular examination of skin and tendons for xanthomas, and (3) measurement of plasma cholesterol and triglyceride concentrations *plus* at least qualitative estimation of lipoprotein classes. For clinical purposes the simple technique of paper electrophoresis so adapted as to provide at least four major groups of lipoproteins (Table 106-2) is of great value. Helpful ancillary information can also be gained by estimates of glucose tolerance, response of lipoproteins to controlled diets, and measurements of plasma postheparin lipolytic activity.

The classification of blood lipid excess simply as either *essential hypercholesterolemia* or *hyperlipemia*

is inadequate. These traditional designations are included here to avoid confusion; but their evolution to more specific terms is encouraged, particularly since it is now possible to differentiate certain syndromes of hyperlipidemia which at least partially respond to quite different forms of therapy. The lipoprotein abnormalities offer a key to such differentiation.

Three syndromes in which the concentration of a single group of lipoproteins is elevated can now be distinguished:
1. Hyperbetalipoproteinemia (familial hypercholesterolemia)
2. Hyperprebetalipoproteinemia (endogenous hyperlipemia)
3. Hyperchylomicronemia (exogenous hyperlipemia)

In other kindreds several of these lipoprotein abnormalities may be combined, adding several more poorly differentiated syndromes to this list. High-density (α_1) lipoproteins are often decreased in association with hyperlipoproteinemia; pathologic increases have been recognized only with obstructive hepatic disease.

HYPERBETALIPOPROTEINEMIA
(Familial hypercholesterolemia)

DEFINITION AND HISTORY. This syndrome was first described in terms of its xanthomatous manifestations by Addison and Gull in 1851. Associated atheromatous involvement of the heart and arteries was soon recognized and observed to be familial. Hypercholesterolemia was only later discovered to be the common denominator. Now the disease is widely accepted as an elevation of plasma low-density lipoprotein, which secondarily leads to lipid accumulation in skin, tendons, and vascular tissues, with a high incidence of complications from premature atherosclerosis. A single abnormal gene for the disease may be associated with the lipoprotein abnormality and all its complications. A double dose of the abnormal gene will usually result in severer abnormalities occurring earlier in life.

Table 106-2

Lipoproteins*	Synonyms	Component Lipids†		
		Cholesterol	Phospholipids	Triglyceride
Chylomicrons..............	Primary and secondary particles; exogenous glyceride	+	+	++++
β-Lipoprotein..............	Low-density lipoproteins of S_f 0–20; density 1.006–1.063	++++	+++	+
Pre-β-lipoprotein...........	Low-density lipoproteins of $S_f > 20$; density < 1.006; α_2-lipoprotein; "hyperlipemic" particles; endogenous glyceride	++	++	+++
α₁-Lipoprotein..............	High-density lipoproteins; density 1.063–1.21	+++	++++	+

* As defined by paper electrophoresis according to technique of Lees and Hatch (J. Lab. & Clin. Med., 61:518, 1963).
† Indicating the relative degree to which the concentrations of plasma lipids will be altered by an increase in the species of lipoproteins.

ETIOLOGY. The biochemical abnormality responsible for this syndrome remains unknown. It has long been considered that cholesterol metabolism is the locus of abnormality; but this has not been demonstrated so far by measurements of hepatic cholesterol synthesis or in removal of cholesterol by the two major pathways, excretion into the gut or conversion to bile acids. Since not only plasma concentrations of cholesterol but also of phospholipids and the specific beta-polypeptide found in low-density lipoproteins are increased, abnormalities in the metabolism of these constituents or of the lipoprotein as a whole remain to be excluded. A number of factors, genetic and environmental, may affect the penetrance or expressivity of the abnormal gene since manifestations range over a broad spectrum.

CLINICAL PICTURE. An increase in plasma cholesterol, phospholipids, and beta-lipoprotein may be the only manifestation. In the heterozygote excessive lipoprotein concentrations are usually detectable by the first decade but may not be expressed until later. Xanthelasma and corneal arcus occur in about 50 per cent of patients. Somewhat less commonly this is associated with xanthomatous deposits in the Achilles tendons, extensor tendons of the hands, and sometimes elbows, tibial tuberosities, and other sites. These are usually painless and rarely, if ever, interfere with joint function. Deposition of carotene and lipid in the creases of the hands and feet (plane xanthomas) may be seen in some patients but also occur in hyperlipoproteinemia associated with obstructive liver disease. Coronary artery disease and peripheral claudication are quite common. Clinically detectable involvement of renal or cerebral vessels is much less common. The homozygous abnormal subject may have cholesterol concentrations exceeding 500 mg per 100 ml and xanthomas in early childhood with sufficient involvement of coronary vessels and endocardium to be fatal in the first decade. Either sex is equally affected. Hyperuricemia is common. Abnormal glucose tolerance is not a distinguishing feature of this syndrome.

DIAGNOSIS. The abnormality in plasma is usually the same—an increase in cholesterol and lesser elevation in phospholipids. Beta-lipoprotein (Table 106-2) is discretely elevated; and increased amounts of carotene, carried in this lipoprotein, are easily visible. Plasma glycerides are characteristically normal and the plasma clear. Modest increases in glyceride and pre-beta-lipoprotein may be seen, particularly in all affected members of a family; and it is likely that these represent different mutations, discussed below under Endogenous Hyperlipemia. An upper limit of normal for plasma cholesterol concentration has not been defined. Below the age of twenty to twenty-five years a concentration greater than 250 mg per 100 ml, in the absence of other primary disease, is abnormal and most likely due to this familial syndrome. The mean cholesterol and low-density lipoprotein concentrations rise slowly in the general population during the third to fifth decades. Beyond age twenty-five values above 250 to 350 mg per 100 ml are suspicious and over 350

are most certainly abnormal. All hyperbetalipoproteinemia is doubtless not ascribable to this familial syndrome, and there is no biochemical test for ascertainment. The presence of tendon xanthomas makes the diagnosis very likely, but in every case it should be confirmed by demonstration of similar abnormalities in parents and other relatives.

TREATMENT. There is no universally effective therapy. The use of hypocholesterolemic agents such as sitosterol, nicotinic acid, d-thyroxin, or ethyl α-p-chlorophenoxyisobutyrate is generally unsuccessful. Promising experimental results have been obtained with long-term oral administration of cholestyramine, a resin that binds bile acids in the gut, preventing their recirculation and thus increasing catabolism of cholesterol, the precursor of bile acids. Dietary modifications usually do not bring the lipoprotein concentrations to normal but can produce some reduction. Generally accepted recommendations include (1) maintenance of ideal weight, (2) reduced intake of foods high in cholesterol and saturated fats, including substitution of skim for whole milk products and of fish and chicken for meats of higher saturated fat content, and (3) liberal use of unsaturated oils for salads, cooking, and baking. Very low fat, high carbohydrate diets are to be avoided.

HYPERPREBETALIPOPROTEINEMIA
(Endogenous hyperlipemia)

DEFINITION. Many different diseases may be associated with hyperprebetalipoproteinemia. These include poorly controlled diabetes mellitus, glycogen storage disease, and possibly starvation. Here the mechanism is suspected to be excessive free fatty acid mobilization in response to inadequate utilization of glucose. The cause must yet be delineated in other conditions such as severe lipoatrophy, chronic pancreatitis, nephrotic syndrome, multiple myeloma or macroglobulinemia, myxedema, idiopathic hypercalcemia, and acute alcoholism. When these diseases have been excluded, there remain a significant number of patients with unexplained elevated concentrations of this lipoprotein class, or *endogenous hyperlipemia*.

CLINICAL PICTURE. Patients with unexplained hyperprebetalipoproteinemia have a number of features in common. Practically all have abnormal glucose tolerance or tolbutamide tests, and many have mild maturity-onset diabetes and evidence of premature arteriosclerosis. Family history of diabetes and of coronary artery disease is common. Features common to severe hyperlipemia due to any cause may be present. These include lipemia retinalis, hepatosplenomegaly, and presence of foam cells in bone marrow. Eruptive, tuberous, planar, and tendon xanthomas may be present. Occasional patients may have hyperuricemia and even gout. Genetic data are inadequate, but more than one familial syndrome is represented. One syndrome resembles familial hypercholesterolemia, but is characterized by hyperlipemia and beta-migrating lipoproteins of abnormally low density (< 1.006). In other families, there is no associated increase in beta-lipoprotein concentrations and the cholesterol concentration may be normal despite significant hyperglyceridemia.

ETIOLOGY AND DIAGNOSIS. Several undifferentiated diseases are doubtless included under this generic term. One of the most significant features, possibly a common denominator in all, is *carbohydrate induction*. A diet low in fat and containing 70 per cent or more of calories as carbohydrate frequently exacerbates the hyperlipemia, whereas a diet containing 70 per cent fat and 15 per cent carbohydrate greatly diminishes it. The diets must be isocaloric, and each, ideally, should be maintained for 3- to 4-week periods to be certain of the response. Carbohydrate induction can be followed in a briefer period, however, by changes in pre-beta-lipoprotein observable on paper electrophoresis. The aberrant mechanisms accounting for diversion of carbohydrate to glyceride or its possible retention in plasma are not yet known. Patients with *exogenous* hyperlipemia and normal subjects are also "carbohydrate-inducible," and it is premature to ascribe all instances of endogenous elevation in glycerides to this single phenomenon. Demonstration of sensitivity of plasma glycerides to the carbohydrate content of the diet, however, is very useful in prescribing dietary therapy.

TREATMENT. The association of chronically elevated levels of pre-beta-lipoproteins with coronary artery disease is now well established, and endogenous hyperlipemia should not be ignored. Most patients show improvement in hyperlipemia and glucose tolerance, if it is present, with hospitalization alone. This is frequently dramatic and may occur even if the prehospital diet is duplicated, suggesting that their usual activities or environment may contribute unknown factors exacerbating the disease. Adjustment of occupation or environment to eliminate apparently stressful factors may be beneficial. Reduction to ideal weight often improves considerably both hyperlipemia and glucose tolerance. The demonstration of carbohydrate induction of hyperlipemia justifies recommendation of an isocaloric diet containing not more than 25 per cent of calories as carbohydrate. Fats, preferably unsaturated and low in cholesterol content, may constitute at least 50 per cent of calories. Abnormal concentrations of these low-density lipoproteins can sometimes be dramatically lowered by 2 to 3 Gm daily of nicotinic acid or 1.5 to 2.5 Gm per day of ethyl-α-*p*-chlorophenoxyisobutyrate. Serious side effects of these drugs have not so far been recognized. They may prove useful in long-term therapy but should still be employed with caution.

HYPERCHYLOMICRONEMIA (Exogenous hyperlipemia)

DEFINITION AND HISTORY. Hyperlipemia dependent upon dietary fat intake was first reported in a child by Bürger and Grütz in 1932, and familial incidence was recorded by Holt, Aylward, and Timbres shortly thereafter. Reports of about 40 similar cases have appeared

subsequently. The disease is now defined by the presence in postabsorptive plasma of chylomicrons, which disappear only when the diet contains less than 5 to 10 Gm fat per day.

ETIOLOGY. This exogenous, or *fat-induced, hyperlipemia* is due to an inherited defect in removal of chylomicrons from plasma. The enzyme lipoprotein lipase probably plays an important role in this process in adipose tissue and at the endothelial wall in perhaps other tissues. The enzyme is "released" into plasma by heparin, and most patients have uniquely low postheparin lipolytic activity. There are exceptions, which perhaps can be explained by measurement of nonspecific lipolytic activity or the remoteness of the plasma assay from the important tissue sites. The metabolic defect in the disease, however, must still be demonstrated precisely.

CLINICAL PICTURE. The disease is usually detected within the first decade, although sometimes not until early adulthood, usually when marked hyperlipemia is discovered during work-up for either sudden appearance of eruptive xanthomas, moderate hepatosplenomegaly, or bouts of severe abdominal pain. These abnormalities are only suggestive and not diagnostic for this type of hyperlipemia. The episodic abdominal pain usually follows a period of high fat intake. It is usually epigastric or midabdominal, rarely radiates to the back, and can be associated with signs of peritoneal irritation and fever, mimicking a number of "acute abdominal emergencies." Sometimes the pain is localized to the left upper quadrant, associated with a tender spleen and probably due to splenic infarction. Pancreatitis may develop, although, when associated with chronic pancreatitis, hyperlipemia may often be the result rather than the cause. There is no evidence that familial hyperchylomicronemia is associated with accelerated vascular disease, and the major hazard appears to be accumulation of fat in reticuloendothelial tissues and the precipitation of abdominal crises. Glucose tolerance is usually normal.

DIAGNOSIS. Hyperlipemia due to chylomicron accumulation can be suspected when plasma glycerides exceed 3,000 mg per 100 ml with relatively normal cholesterol concentrations. When glycerides rise, as they may, to 10,000 to 15,000 mg per 100 ml, cholesterol and phospholipid concentrations also rise since these lipids make up about 10 per cent of chylomicron lipid. On a regular diet chylomicrons are easily demonstrable on paper electrophoresis. The concentrations of all other lipoproteins are usually decreased. An isocaloric diet containing 5 to 10 Gm fat per day will result in disappearance of chylomicrons within a week. Mere *reduction* of hyperlipemia, which occurs in many patients on low-fat diets, is not diagnostic of this particular syndrome. If this diet is continued, pre-beta-lipoprotein will appear since these patients are also especially susceptible to carbohydrate induction of hyperlipemia, presumably because even a normal output of these lipoproteins cannot be cleared from plasma because of the same defect that interferes with removal of chylomicrons. Postheparin lipolytic activity is almost always markedly subnormal and a useful diagnostic test. Hyperlipemia and low lipolytic activity may or may not be found in other family members, but the pedigree should be thoroughly screened. The full-blown disease appears in either sex.

TREATMENT. To avoid the crippling attacks of abdominal pain, pancreatitis and foam cell accumulation in liver, spleen, and bone marrow seen in most cases, it is recommended that the daily intake of fat not represent more than 25 per cent of calories, or 50 Gm fat per day. Commercial preparations of glycerides containing short-chain fatty acids (less than 12 carbons) offer means of occasionally satisfying craving for fat without inducing chylomicronemia since these glycerides go directly to the liver in the portal vein. They may reappear in plasma as pre-beta-lipoprotein, however. Since excessive plasma concentrations of the latter are frequently associated with premature atherosclerosis, neither excessive amounts of these glycerides nor diets extremely high in carbohydrates can be considered wise therapy in this disease.

MIXED TYPES OF PRIMARY HYPERLIPOPROTEINEMIA

There are patients, sometimes with familial involvement, who have certain features of both fat-induced and carbohydrate-induced hyperlipemia to a degree that prevents their ready classification. Usually the patients have poor glucose tolerance, and nearly all have plasma postheparin lipolytic activity that is normal or only slightly subnormal. Diet therapy must be judiciously determined from observation of response to test diets. Present experience suggests that moderate excesses of chylomicrons are associated with less serious long-term disability than hyperprebetalipoproteinemia, and the diet should be adjusted accordingly. In addition, it is usually desirable to (1) reduce body weight to the ideal value; (2) cut back excessive alcohol intake; and (3) consider possible ways to reduce the environmental stresses on the patient. In some patients these maneuvers will decrease hyperlipoproteinemia.

LIPOPROTEIN DEFICIENCIES

LOW–DENSITY LIPOPROTEIN DEFICIENCY
(Abetalipoproteinemia)

Abetalipoproteinemia is a rare familial disease, uniquely characterized by severe deficiency, usually complete absence, of the polypeptide typical of beta-lipoproteins. The plasma contains low-density lipoproteins of abnormal composition, and no chylomicrons are formed when fat is ingested. The syndrome follows a fairly uniform course, beginning before the age of one year, with *malnutrition* and growth retardation, lordosis, abdominal distension, and steatorrhea. *Ataxia*, nystagmus, weakness and areflexia, and other signs of progressive neurologic dysfunction, particularly involving the posterolateral columns and spinocerebellar tracts, then appear. *Pigmentary retinal degeneration*

develops during adolescence. The erythrocytes have a crenated appearance (*acanthocytosis*). The esterified lipids of these cells and of the plasma are deficient in both lecithin and linoleic acid. Dietary fat is assimilated but is held up in the intestinal mucosal cells, creating a pathognomonic picture detectable by peroral biopsy. Some fat is absorbed, possibly by direct passage through the portal system into the liver.

The disease may occur in siblings and is likely due to a double dose of a mutant autosomal gene, since the consanguinity rate in affected families is high. Most relatives have normal concentrations of plasma lipoproteins. Whether the primary defect is related to formation of beta-polypeptide or some other aspect of fat absorption is not known, and the prognosis is uncertain.

DIAGNOSIS. The diagnosis is suspected when a plasma cholesterol concentration less than 100 mg per 100 ml is associated with the above clinical picture. It must be confirmed by immunochemical evidence of the absence of plasma beta-lipoprotein.

TREATMENT. There is no definitive therapy. Medium-chain triglycerides may help provide some fat intake in the absence of chylomicron formation, and low vitamin A levels have been increased with supplements.

HIGH–DENSITY LIPOPROTEIN DEFICIENCY
(Tangier disease)

Familial high-density lipoprotein deficiency is also called *Tangier disease*, after the island home of the first cases. The disease has been detected in other children and adults and must be suspected when hypocholesterolemia is associated with orange or yellowish-gray discoloration of the tonsils and pharyngeal or rectal mucosa or *enlargement of spleen, liver, or lymph nodes*. Reticuloendothelial tissues are infiltrated with *foam cells* containing large amounts of cholesterol esters. In adults *corneal infiltration*, hypersplenism, papular skin lesions containing foam cells, and possibly premature coronary artery disease have been seen as complications. There are no abnormalities in absorption, in neurologic function, or in erythrocytes.

Parents and other relatives of patients with Tangier disease have lower than normal amounts of plasma high-density (alpha$_1$) lipoprotein. The propositi are probably *homozygous* for a mutant gene that normally governs the synthesis of this lipoprotein.

Diagnosis is established by immunochemical evidence that the alpha-polypeptide characteristic of plasma high-density lipoprotein is present in only trace amounts. Splenectomy may be required for hypersplenism. There is no definitive therapy.

THE SPHINGOLIPIDOSES

There are other storage diseases characterized by tissue rather than plasma lipid abnormalities. The sphingolipidoses represent one group of these disorders and are so-called because they have in common the accumulation of a different derivative (—R) of acyl-sphingosine (ceramide).

$$CH_3(CH_2)_{12}CH=CH-\underset{\underset{\text{CH}_3-(CH_2)_n-CO-NH}{|}}{\overset{\overset{\text{H}}{\overset{\text{O}}{|}}}{C}}-C-C-O-R$$

Ceramide

These are all inheritable disorders; the defect has not been proved to involve specifically the metabolism of the stored lipid. Each disease may involve the nervous system. Most occur in several clinical forms or syndromes, probably reflecting mutations at different genetic loci.

GAUCHER'S DISEASE (See Chap. 125)

First described by Gaucher in 1882, this is a rare disease in which glucocerebrosides (ceramide-glucose) accumulate in reticuloendothelial cells, producing marked splenomegaly, hepatomegaly, and bone lesions. In adults, there is often associated skin pigmentation and characteristic pingueculae of the scleras. In infants progressive neurologic disturbances also may occur, and they are usually associated with a rapidly fatal course.

NIEMANN–PICK DISEASE (See Chap. 125)

This is a rare familial disorder, first described in 1914, in which sphingomyelin (ceramide-phosphoryl-choline) and cholesterol accumulate in reticuloendo-thelial cells throughout the body. There is associated destruction of ganglion cells in both central and autonomic nervous systems. Hepatosplenomegaly and retarded nervous and physical development are usually observed within the first 6 months of life, and death from inanition or intercurrent infection usually occurs within 3 years. The disease may progress slowly, and the typical tissue changes have been unsuspectingly found at autopsy in adults.

METACHROMATIC LEUKODYSTROPHY (See Chap. 209)

This is a disorder of children in which abnormal amounts of cerebroside-sulfatide (ceramide-galactose-SO₃H) accumulate in the brain and kidney. The material is also excreted in bile, causing fibrosis of the gall-bladder, and in urine, where it may be detected as an aid to diagnosis.

FABRY'S DISEASE (See Chap. 122)

In this sex-linked disorder, the manifestations are usually only seen in males and are due mainly to deposition of glycolipid, mainly a trihexoside (ceramide-glucose-galactose-galactose), in blood vessels and nerves. The disease is also known by its unusual skin manifestations, *angiokeratoma corporis diffusum*.

AMAUROTIC FAMILY IDIOCY (See Chap. 211)

This is a general term for several closely related familial neurologic disorders characterized by varying degrees of blindness and dementia. Other terms, such as *cerebromacular* or *retinocerebral degeneration*, are sometimes employed to describe this group which includes Tay-Sachs, Bielschowsky, Spielmeyer-Vogt, Kufs, and Hallevorden types. They are considered as a lipidosis because, at least in the infantile or Tay-Sachs form within the group, the characteristic lesions in the nervous system have been shown to be associated with an increase in abnormal gangliosides and other aminoglycolipids, having the general molecular structure of ceramide-glucose-(galactose, galactosamine, N-acetylneuraminic acid).

OTHER RARE TISSUE LIPID STORAGE DISEASES

In addition to the sphingolipidoses, there are several other rare disorders in which lipids pile up in tissues apparently because of enzymatic defects not yet understood. In *Refsum's disease* there is accumulation of phytanic acid (3,7,11,15-tetramethyl hexadecanoic acid) in the esterified lipids present in both tissues and plasma. This familial disease is characterized by ataxic neuropathy and retinitis pigmentosa and is commonest in children or young adults of Scandinavian ancestry. Parents may have high levels of phytanic acid in plasma without other abnormalities, and the basis of the disease is not understood.

Familial xanthomatosis with adrenal calcification (Wolman's disease) resembles Niemann-Pick disease in the presence of hepatosplenomegaly, foam cell deposition in tissues, and death in early childhood. The stored lipids are mainly triglycerides and cholesterol, much of it esterified. The etiology and effective treatment are unknown.

Cephalin lipidosis is a very rare syndrome clinically identical to Niemann-Pick disease but with accumulation of a lipid reported to be an inositol-containing phospholipid rather than a sphingolipid.

Ceroid storage disease, or the accumulation of ceroid, a pigmented lipid of unknown chemical composition, may also include sufficient organ involvement to produce a clinical picture similar to severe Niemann-Pick disease. It may also be associated with cirrhosis of the liver and intestinal malabsorption. Ceroid may be identified histochemically by the combination of red periodic acid-Schiff stain, acid-fastness, and fluorescence. Deposition of this material has also been seen in aorta, liver, intestinal musculature, and other tissues in a variety of conditions, including tocopherol deficiency. The biochemical basis for ceroid formation and storage is not known.

GRANULOMATOUS DISEASES WITH LIPID STORAGE

Frequently considered among the lipid storage diseases are certain tissue proliferative disorders sometimes accompanied by lipid deposition. *Histiocytosis X* (see Chap. 125) is the generic term for a group of disorders that affect the reticuloendothelial system and which may be either different stages or forms of the same disease. *Letterer-Siwe disease* and *xanthoma disseminatum* may be the two extremes of such abnormalities, with *eosinophilic granuloma* and *Hand-Schüller-Christian disease* representing intermediate and special forms. The usual order of progression of the pathologic lesions is reticuloendothelial cell proliferation and hyperplasia, granulomatous changes featuring eosinophils and giant cells, conversion of reticulum cells and histiocytes to foam cells or xanthomas, and, finally, fibrosis.

Several other uncommon diseases are associated with proliferation of histiocytes and deposition of material considered to represent both lipid and carbohydrate because it stains by both the Sudan and periodic acid-Schiff techniques. The chemical composition of the lesions has not been characterized. It is likely that any faulty metabolism of lipid is secondary to some other processes, perhaps involving mucopolysaccharide metabolism.

In *lipoid proteinosis* (cutaneous-mucosal hyalinosis; Urbach-Wiethe disease) the lesions share enough histologic features of *histiocytosis X* to suggest an etiologic relationship. The skin and mucous membranes of the pharynx and larynx are infiltrated by extracellular deposits of hyaline material. Clinical manifestations include hoarseness or aphonia, widely distributed skin papules, dental anomalies, and symmetric calcifications in the region of the sella turcica as seen by x-ray. The disease is not incompatible with long life.

In *lipoid dermatoarthritis* polyarthritis is associated with multiple nodular or papular skin lesions. In both skin and synovial tissues there is an infiltration of histiocytes, eosinophils, lymphocytes, red blood cells, and multinucleated giant cells. The joint changes may be extremely destructive, producing *arthritis mutilans,* or the "opera-glass hand." Serologic reactions for rheumatoid arthritis are negative.

Disseminated lipogranulomatosis (*Farber's disease*) is an extremely rare disease, appearing in infancy as generalized nodular periarticular swelling and dysphonia. There is progressive systemic involvement with widespread proliferation of histiocytes and neuronal abnormalities. Storage cells appear containing both mucopolysaccharide and lipids. The basic disorder probably involves the metabolism of certain acid mucopolysaccharides similar to those in Hurler's disease (Chap. 246).

Many chronic infections, particularly accompanied by exudates, and other proliferative processes, such as osteitis fibrosa cystica or traumatic lesions, may be associated with collections of foam cells (*xanthomas*) and sometimes crystals of cholesterol. Most skin xanthomas are secondary to hyperlipoproteinemia, but *juvenile xanthomas* (nevoxanthoepithelioma) are benign skin lesions that can appear without abnormal plasma lipids. *Xanthelasmas* need not always be associated with hyperlipoproteinemia.

ADIPOSE TISSUE DISORDERS

Adipose tissue can be a site of expression of many disorders including those of connective tissue, lipid, and carbohydrate metabolism. There is therefore no simple classification of the adipose tissue diseases.

Relapsing panniculitis (*Weber-Christian disease*) may represent several diseases that share similar but rather nonspecific histologic changes (see Chap. 241).

Although the term *lipodystrophy* is sometimes used to describe *lipoatrophy,* it also has a generic meaning that allows it to encompass several disorders in which adipose tissue is abnormal but not necessarily absent. Several abnormalities may properly be considered forms of lipodystrophy.

Lipomas are benign mesenchymal tumors consisting of circumscribed masses of adipose tissue. There is usually a capsule, but the cells are histologically indistinguishable from ordinary fat. They may occur nearly anywhere in the body, singly or as multiple fatty growths (lipomatosis), most commonly in subcutaneous tissues. They also arise in retroperitoneal or peritoneal areas, in breast, mesentery, and mediastinum, and in other body cavities and organs. Lipomas have caused intestinal obstruction, or dyspnea by superior mediastinal obstruction and may embarrass the function of other vital tissues. Rarely they may calcify; and it has been presumed that they may on occasion give rise to liposarcomas or other malignant tumors, but there is no general agreement on this. Multiple lipomas may be symmetrically placed and may run in families. The therapy is surgical excision; occasionally they will recur in the same site.

Adiposis dolorosa (*Dercum's disease*) refers to a poorly defined disorder in which painful subcutaneous lipomas, often widely and symmetrically situated, are sometimes associated with asthenia, decreased cutaneous sensation, motor weakness, or other evidence of peripheral neuropathy. Some patients have also had adenomas in the pituitary, thyroid, or adrenal glands. They may or may not be accompanying generalized obesity. Siblings may be similarly involved. The interstitial neuritis observed in the original adipose tissue nodules by Dercum has not been seen in many subsequent cases. There is no specific therapy.

Insulin lipodystrophy refers to changes in subcutaneous fat at the site of insulin injection (see Chap. 86) and may involve either localized hypertrophy or atrophy of adipose tissue.

Lipoatrophy may be partial or complete. *Partial lipoatrophy* (also called *progressive lipodystrophy*) is characterized by the absence of subcutaneous fat over wide, symmetric areas of the body. The remaining parts of the body have normal or sometimes increased subcutaneous fat deposits. It occurs predominantly in females and often begins in childhood. The onset is usually insidious and may begin with loss of subcutaneous fat in the face and subsequently involve that of the upper extremities and upper trunk. In other instances the disorder may begin at the level of the iliac crest and extend downward. There are no subjective symptoms. The cause is unknown, although experiments that resulted in disappearance of normal fat when grafted into areas of lipoatrophy suggest that the disorder is due to disturbed autonomic trophic regulation. There is no known therapy.

Total lipoatrophy (lipoatrophic diabetes mellitus) is a rare disorder in which generalized atrophy of body fat occurs gradually. In addition to subcutaneous fat deposits, all other body fat, sometimes excepting that in the breasts, may disappear. This is usually but not always associated with diabetes, which may precede or follow the onset of lipoatrophy. There is also hyperlipemia, hepatomegaly, and sometimes acanthosis nigricans; serious nephropathy, including both nephritic and nephrotic manifestations, may occur whether the patient has diabetes or not. Some patients may also have hypermetabolism, others have features suggestive of "leprechaunism," and the syndrome undoubtedly results from several different causes. The diabetes is associated with high plasma insulin levels and may be very difficult to control. The course of the disease may be either indolent or rapidly progressive. No therapy is known.

REFERENCES

Abul-Haj, S. K., D. G. Martz, W. F. Douglas, and L. J. Geppert: Farber's Disease, J. Pediat., 61:221, 1962.

Bortz, A. I., and M. Vincent: Lipoid Dermato-arthritis and Arthritis Mutilans, Am. J. Med., 30:951, 1961.

Hartroft, W. S., and E. A. Porta: Pathology and Bacteriology—Ceroid, Am. J. Med. Sci., 250:324, 1965.

McCusker, J. J., and R. M. Caplan: Lipoid Proteinosis (Lipoglycoproteinosis), Am. J. Pathol., 40:599, 1962.

Oppenheimer, E. H., and E. C. Andrews, Jr.: Ceroid Storage Disease in Childhood, Pediatrics, 23:1091, 1959.

Richterich, R. W. Kahlke, P. Van Mechelen, and E. Rossi: Refsum's Syndrome, Heredopathia Atactica Polyneuritiformis, Klin. Wschr., 41:800, 1963.

Schwartz, R., I. A. Schafer, and A. E. Renold: Generalized Lipoatrophy, Hepatic Cirrhosis, Disturbed Carbohydrate Metabolism and Accelerated Growth (Lipoatrophic Diabetes), Am. J. Med., 28:973, 1960.

Senior, B., and S. S. Gellis: The Syndromes of Total Lipodystrophy and of Partial Lipodystrophy, Pediatrics, 33:593, 1964.

Stanbury, J. B., J. B. Wyngaarden, and D. S. Fredrickson (Eds.): "The Metabolic Basis of Inherited Disease," 2d ed., chaps. 22–29, New York, McGraw-Hill Book Company, Inc., 1966.

Tedeschi, C. G., and W. H. Lyon: Fat Tissue Growths, J. Mt. Sinai Hosp., 24:1272, 1957.

Thannhauser, S. J.: "Lipidoses," New York, Grune & Stratton, Inc., 1958.

Wolman, M., V. V. Sterk, S. Gatt, and M. Frenkel: Primary Familial Xanthomatosis with Involvement and Calcification of the Adrenals, Pediatrics, 28:742, 1961.

107 AMYLOIDOSIS
Evan Calkins

Although amyloidosis is infrequent in occurrence and as yet uncertain in its pathogenesis, it has attracted increasing attention in recent years. In part this reflects an increased awareness of its diverse clinical forms, which may mimic a number of other clinical entities. In part this interest is due to a growing conviction that further knowledge of the nature and pathogenesis of amyloidosis may lead to a better understanding of the numerically more important diseases with which it is frequently associated.

DEFINITION AND CHARACTERISTICS. The term *amyloid* was originally proposed to designate the hyaline material, accumulating in the kidney, liver, and spleen of patients with prolonged inflammatory disease, by virtue of staining properties which suggested a possible relationship to starch. It is now realized that amyloid represents a complex of substances, predominately protein in nature, but also containing carbohydrate. Although its distribution varies with the clinical syndrome, the material usually accumulates in the walls of the blood vessels, chiefly small arterioles, as well as in the kidneys, especially glomeruli, liver, and spleen. Frequently observed adjacent to basement membranes, it appears on electron microscopy to be distinct from the membrane. Amyloid usually exhibits characteristic staining reactions (eosinophilic with hematoxylin and eosin, metachromatic with crystal violet, positive staining with Congo red, and birefringent when viewed with polarized light, especially after Congo red staining). Weakly autofluorescent, it is strikingly fluorescent after staining with Congo red. When viewed in the electron microscope, amyloid is seen to contain numerous fibrils, which do not resemble either collagen or elastin.

CLASSIFICATION. The classification of amyloidosis is still in a process of evolution. Most investigators agree, however, that there are at least three general categories. Secondary amyloidosis is that which may accompany prolonged inflammatory or infectious diseases. Histologic evidence of amyloidosis is seen in approximately 25 per cent of all patients with rheumatoid arthritis, dying of any cause. It becomes clinically manifest in only a small percentage of these cases however. Secondary amyloidosis is a common cause of death in paraplegics who have developed decubitus ulcers and urinary tract infections. It is seen in approximately one-third of patients with leprosy at the U.S. Public Health Service Hospital in Carville, La., and is one of the chief causes of death at this hospital. Secondary amyloidosis is clinically manifested chiefly by nephrosis and subsequent azotemia; hepatomegaly and splenomegaly may also be seen. At autopsy the predominant sites of involvement are the kidney, spleen, liver, and adrenal glands. Microscopic traces of amyloid may be widely distributed, especially in blood vessel walls.

A second category of amyloidosis is that which accompanies multiple myeloma. Between 10 and 20 per cent of patients with multiple myeloma are known to develop this complication. Clinical involvement may resemble that seen in "secondary" amyloidosis. More widespread manifestations, such as neuropathy of the carpal tunnel syndrome may also be seen.

In the third and probably most common category of amyloidosis seen today the disease develops without any known predisposing disease. Recent studies have provided increasing evidence that this so-called "primary" form of amyloidosis is, in turn, comprised of a number of relatively discrete syndromes, each with characteristic clinical expression and pattern of occurrence.

In several of these entities the involvement resembles that seen in the secondary form. One example is the amyloidosis which often occurs in association with familial Mediterranean fever (FMF), primarily in members of the Sephardic and Iraqui Jewish races. The two disorders appear to be inherited as independent recessive traits; amyloidosis may be seen in members of a family who do not have FMF and vice versa.

Other varieties of "primary" amyloidosis are manifested by more widespread evidences of the disease. One example is the primary familial amyloidosis described by Andrade. In this entity, which occurs predominately in individuals of Portuguese ancestry, one encounters severe impairment of the sensory function of the peripheral nerves, as well as less severe impairment of motor function. This is often accompanied by involvement of the sympathetic ganglions, with postural hypotension, impotence, absence of sweating, and intestinal hypermotility and malabsorption. Adie's pupil is apt to be present. The patients usually succumb to severe malnutrition and inanition. Another example of primary amyloidosis occurring in families is that described by Rukavina et al. in a family of Swiss ancestry. Although some members of the family resembled the patients described by Andrade; others exhibited a variety of different clinical manifestations. Other family constellations, yielding a variety of syndromes, have also been described.

Despite the increasing awareness of the familial incidence of amyloidosis, many patients who develop the disease, without known predisposing cause, do not appear to have any genetic or familial predisposition. In some of these cases the distribution of the amyloid resembles that seen in the secondary form of the disease; others exhibit diffuse involvement, especially of the skin or the heart. In many patients the accumulation may be localized to a single area, such as the respiratory passages, without evidence of widespread involvement.

NATURE OF AMYLOID. What is amyloid, and why does it occur? Unfortunately definitive answers to these questions are not yet available. For example we do not know if *all* amyloid is the same, or if amyloid as seen in one clinical syndrome may differ in significant respects from that seen in other syndromes. Increasing evidence favors the latter alternative. Similarly we do not know if amyloid is deposited from the blood or arises *in situ*. It seems probable, however, that both mechanisms apply. In some instances, such as secondary amyloidosis involving the spleen, the substance may arise *in situ*. In other instances, such as diffuse vascular involvement in patients with multiple myeloma or macroglobulinemia, it is hard to avoid the impression that the amyloid is deposited from the blood.

A number of different theses have been developed concerning the nature of amyloid. One of the most persistent of these has been the suggestion that this substance is composed of γ-globulin or material related to γ-globulin. This hypothesis holds that these globulins may have been precipitated in the tissue either as an antigen-antibody complex or as a metabolically altered protein. Alternatively it has been suggested that amyloid may represent an accumulation of imperfectly synthesized globulins or globulin fragments.

Unfortunately, serologic, immunochemical, and immunohistologic studies have shown that while γ-globulin can almost always be detected in or in association with amyloid, the quantity is highly variable. It appears increasingly unlikely that the γ-globulin is the sole or most important ingredient.

Recent attention has been focused on the fibrillar component, which is present in all forms of amyloid studied so far. The nature of this material and the reason for its accumulation are still uncertain.

CLINICAL MANIFESTATIONS. The clinical manifestations of amyloidosis depend on the organ or system involved. Since the symptoms may resemble those of a variety of other disorders, amyloidosis must frequently be considered in differential diagnosis.

Amyloidosis of the skin is most typically characterized by hyaline plaques, occurring chiefly in or near the folds of the skin, as in the inguinal regions. Occasionally, the disease results in widespread purpura.

Although in most cases this purpura is thought to be due to involvement of the walls of small blood vessels, other mechanisms may be involved. These may include thrombocytopenia, deficiencies of several different clotting factors, and increased plasmin activity. As a result of the defects in hemostasis, prolonged bleeding may follow such minor surgical procedures as a gingival biopsy. Parameters of coagulation are usually within normal limits. The bleeding time may be prolonged, presumably because of increased rigidity of small blood vessels.

Ocular involvement may be of different sorts. Diffuse infiltrates in the posterior chamber have been described in some types of primary amyloidosis. Discrete deposits of amyloid may be seen beneath the bulbar conjunctiva. An Adie pupil is frequently noted in primary systemic amyloidosis of Andrade.

Amyloid infiltration of the heart classically results in enlargement, which is due to an increased thickness of the myocardial wall, without change in intracardiac volume. The resultant syndrome, due to a stiffened myocardium, may yield results on cardiac catheterization which closely resemble those seen in constrictive pericarditis. In other cases, the clinical picture may more nearly resemble that seen in diffuse arteriosclerotic heart disease, with an enlarged and insufficient myocardium. Electrocardiogram often reveals low voltage in the QRS complex. Arteriovenous block and arrhythmias may also be seen. In summary, therefore, amyloidosis is one of a group of conditions which may cause cardiac failure, without detectable murmurs. Unfortunately, it is very seldom correctly diagnosed ante mortem.

Amyloid involvement of the liver is characterized primarily by hepatomegaly. Clinical evidences of hepatic dysfunction and jaundice are rarely observed. Liver function tests characteristically show minimal abnormalities, which are usually suggestive of biliary obstruction. Although liver biopsy has been recommended and often yields diagnostic information, it has been followed in a few instances by intractable bleeding and/or rupture of the liver. It is our belief that liver biopsy should be avoided when amyloidosis is suspected.

Renal amyloidosis is manifested predominantly by the nephrotic syndrome. The appearance of progressively severe proteinuria in patients with chronic inflammatory diseases such as rheumatoid arthritis should always lead to a suspicion of amyloidosis. In attempting to differentiate renal amyloidosis from chronic pyelonephritis, the size of the kidneys, as seen on x-ray, may be helpful. In pyelonephritis the kidneys are usually reduced in size; amyloid-laden kidneys are likely to be normal in size or may be enlarged. Hypertension is not commonly observed in amyloidosis. Azotemia is a very late manifestation. Kidney biopsy is a satisfactory method of confirming the diagnosis of renal amyloidosis in cases in which the clinical syndrome, plus rectal or gingival biopsy, has not already led to a definite diagnosis.

Amyloidosis may result in a variety of neurologic lesions. Diffuse motor and sensory neuropathy, together with interference with function of the sympathetic nervous system, is characteristic of the primary familial amyloidosis of Andrade. Sensory involvement may also be seen in amyloidosis secondary to multiple myeloma, because of diffuse involvement of the sheaths of the peripheral nerves.

Accumulations of amyloid in the trachea or bronchi may result in serious obstruction to the respiratory passages. Local excision, often with epithelial grafting, is the preferred form of treatment. Recurrences are frequent but by no means invariable.

Amyloid may infiltrate any portion of the gastrointestinal tract, resulting in a variety of syndromes, ranging from esophageal obstruction to malabsorption syndrome. Infiltration of the endocrine organs may also ensue. This rarely results in insufficiency of function of the involved gland, however.

DIAGNOSIS, COURSE, AND TREATMENT. Correct diagnosis of amyloidosis involves, first of all, an awareness of this possibility when one encounters any of the widespread syndromes alluded to above. Although certain clinical clues may heighten one's suspicion, confirmation of this diagnosis is best obtained by biopsy. The gingival biopsy has been helpful, permitting confirmation of the diagnosis in between one-half to two-thirds of the cases. In the experience of Sohar and his associates, the rectal biopsy has proved even more sensitive.

Both metachromasia, with the crystal violet stain, and birefringence, under polarized light, following staining with Congo red, have proved useful guides to the presence of amyloid in biopsy specimens. Since the material characteristically appears in trace amounts, the biopsy specimens should be interpreted by someone experienced in the technique. Renal biopsy may be performed, when it seems advisable, but liver biopsy is, in the opinion of the author, to be avoided. The Congo red test has also proved helpful in corroborating the diagnosis of amyloidosis. In performing this test, aliquots of blood are obtained at 4 min and 60 min following the intravenous administration of 10 ml of 1 per cent *recrystallized* Congo red in water. Serum retention of 20 per cent or less of the dye, seen in comparison of 4-min and 60-min blood values, provides strong evidence for the presence of amyloidosis. This test is positive in approximately 60 per cent of patients with secondary amyloidosis and in approximately one-third of patients with primary amyloidosis. Injection of the dye has been followed by serious and even fatal reactions unless the dye is recrystallized and suspended in distilled water and has been screened for absence of precipitate. Because of the need for these special precautions this technique does not lend itself to widespread use.

The course of amyloidosis is usually progressive and downhill, especially if the organs involved include the kidneys, heart, or gastrointestinal tract. Of the fifty-odd cases studied by the author, none has exhibited a remission, except for those cases of localized amyloidosis in which surgical extirpation has been possible. The course may be prolonged, however, lasting for periods of many years. Treatment with large doses of ascorbic acid (1,000 mg per day) or of lightly seared liver (¼ lb per day) has been attempted, chiefly on empirical grounds, but there is no sound clinical evidence, to date, to support this program. If amyloidosis accompanies other inflammatory conditions, vigorous efforts to treat the underlying condition should be initiated. If these efforts are successful, remission of the amyloidosis may ensue. This outcome is rarely seen, however, chiefly because potentially treatable chronic inflammatory conditions usually receive treatment prior to the onset of amyloidosis.

REFERENCES

Andrade, C.: A Peculiar Form of Peripheral Neuropathy; Familial Atypical Generalized Amyloidosis with Special Involvement of the Peripheral Nerves, Brain, 75: 408, 1952.

Cohen, A. S., and E. Calkins: A Study of the Fine Structure of the Kidney in Casein-induced Amyloidosis in Rabbits, J. Exptl. Med., 112:479, 1960.

Gafni, J., and E. Sohar: Rectal Biopsy for the Diagnosis of Amyloidosis, Am. J. Med. Sci., 240:332, 1960.

Giles, R. B., Jr., and E. Calkins: Studies of the Composition of Secondary Amyloid, J. Clin. Invest., 34:1476, 1955.

Heller, H., E. Sohar, J. Gafni, and J. Heller: Amyloidosis in Familial Mediterranean Fever: An Independent Genetically Determined Character, A.M.A. Arch. Internal Med., 107:539, 1961.

Osserman, E. F., K. Takatsuki, and N. Talal: The Pathogenesis of "Amyloidosis." Studies on the Role of Abnormal Gamma Globulin and Gamma Globulin Fragments of the Bence Jones (L-polypeptide) Type in the Pathogenesis of "Primary" and "Secondary Amyloidosis," and the "Amyloidosis" Associated with Plasma Cell Myeloma, in "Seminars in Hematology," New York, Grune & Stratton, Inc., 1964.

Rukavina, J. G., W. D. Block, C. E. Jackson, H. F. Falls, J. H. Carey, and A. C. Curtis: Primary Systemic Amyloidosis: A Review and an Experimental, Genetic, and Clinical Study of 29 Cases with Particular Emphasis on the Familial Form, Medicine, 35:239, 1956.

Schultz, R. T., E. Calkins, F. Milgrom, and E. Witebsky: Association of Gamma Globulin with Amyloid, Am. J. Path., in press.

Index